HISTOLOGY
A Text and Atlas

THIRD   EDITION

HISTOLOGY
A Text and Atlas
THIRD EDITION

Michael H. Ross, Ph.D.

Professor and Chairman
Department of Anatomy and Cell Biology
University of Florida School of Medicine
Gainesville, Florida

Lynn J. Romrell, Ph.D.

Professor
Department of Anatomy and Cell Biology
University of Florida School of Medicine
Gainesville, Florida

Gordon I. Kaye, Ph.D.

Alden March Professor of Anatomy, Cell Biology and Neurobiology
and
Professor of Pathology
Albany Medical College
Albany, New York

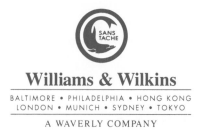

Williams & Wilkins

BALTIMORE • PHILADELPHIA • HONG KONG
LONDON • MUNICH • SYDNEY • TOKYO

A WAVERLY COMPANY

Editor: Patricia A. Coryell
Copy Editor: Bill Cady
Designer: Norman W. Och
Illustration Planner: Wayne Hubbel
Production Coordinator: Charles E. Zeller
Cover Designer: Bob Och

Cover credit
_____

The triple-exposure micrograph appearing on the cover was provided courtesy of Kevin J. McCarthy, Department of Cell Biology, University of Alabama, Birmingham.

Printed in the United States of America

First Edition 1985
Second Edition 1989

Library of Congress Cataloging-in-Publication Data

Ross, Michael H.
    Histology : a text and atlas / Michael H. Ross, Lynn J. Romrell, Gordon I. Kaye.
    —3rd ed.
      p.   cm.
    Includes index.
    ISBN 0-683-07369-9
    1. Histology.   2. Histology—Atlases.   I. Romrell, Lynn J.   II. Kaye, Gordon
    I.   III. Title.
    [DNLM: 1. Histology—atlases.   QS 517 R825h 1995]
    QM551.R67   1995
    611′.018—dc20
    DNLM/DLC   94-9400
    for Library of Congress   CIP

                                                94 95 96 97 98
                              1   2   3   4   5   6   7   8   9   10

Preface

This third edition of *Histology: A Text and Atlas* appears at a time of continued change both in the knowledge base underlying the subject and in the nature of the medical and the premedical curriculum. To incorporate a large body of new information that has been developed since the second edition, a substantial revision of the text was indicated. At the same time, we felt that a change in format could facilitate better management of information and respond to the different forms of curriculum that are developing today. Both objectives call for a greater degree of independent learning on the part of the student. To accomplish this, several new features have been incorporated.

A new style of sentence headings has been utilized that provides a focus on the text material. This style also lends itself to review by allowing the student to read the headings more rapidly and to mentally ascertain one's recollection and understanding of the underlying text information.

The introduction of lists highlighted by bullets further emphasizes important facts and relationships. In addition, the use of boxed material for clinical and certain physiologically relevant information and the highlighting of key words have been expanded. This is largely due to response from both our own students and those who have written to us with suggestions for improving the text.

Another improvement is to the legends in the Atlas section. They have been restyled and laid out to correspond to the position of the figures on the facing page. This allows easier correlation of the figures with the explanatory text, requiring less time to find pertinent information.

Lastly, many black-and-white figures have been replaced with new full-color figures, and new text illustrations have been developed to explain the material more fully.

As in the first edition, all of the current changes were undertaken with student needs in mind, namely, to be able to understand the subject matter and to apply it as a base in the understanding of body function, normal as well as abnormal.

Michael H. Ross
Lynn J. Romrell
Gordon I. Kaye

Acknowledgments

This third edition of *Histology: A Text and Atlas* reflects considerable change from the previous editions. A major impetus for this change has come from our students, those at our own institutions as well as those students from other schools, who have taken the time and effort to tell us what they liked about the book and, more importantly, have provided suggestions for change to help them better understand the subject material. Their comments and suggestions have been extremely helpful in preparing this new edition.

Many of our colleagues who teach histology and cell biology courses, likewise, were most helpful in producing this new edition. Some of them suggested increasing the clinical relevance. We responded to this as best we could within the page limitation. Others were most helpful in providing new micrographs and suggestions for redrawing existing diagrams. Finally, there are many of our colleagues who suggested adding specific new information and, in some cases, deleting older material. Our special thanks go to a number of these colleagues including Drs. Johannes Rhodin, George Pappas, Albert Pawlina, Tom Hollinger, Craig Tisher, Alvin Telser, John Aris, Carl Feldherr, Kelly Selman, and Kevin McCarthy. Our appreciation goes out again to Dr. Albert Pawlina for helping to reor-ganize the chapter on the female reproductive system. We are particularly grateful to Dr. Nancy Kaye for her many comments and suggestions as well as her critical reading of final chapter revisions. We are also indebted to a number of people who were involved in the technical aspects of producing this book. Todd Barnash provided invaluable assistance in preparing the text as well as a number of the computer-rendered diagrams. Denny Player provided superb technical expertise in producing new color photographs and electron micrographs. We also express our appreciation to Pauletta Sanders for the special histologic preparations that she was able to produce.

Lastly, we wish to acknowledge the outstanding support and cooperation of many of the people at Williams & Wilkins. Particular thanks go to Nancy Evans, who helped us develop the new style of the text; to Tim Satterfield and Pat Coryell, our editors, who constantly provided us with encouragement and assistance; to Chuck Zeller, Bob Och, Wayne Hubbel, and Bill Cady in their specific roles during the preparation and production of this edition; and to Paula Huber for her expertise and management during production.

Contents

Methods

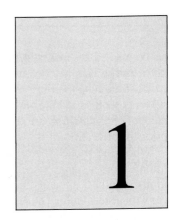

The Objective of a Histology Course Is to Lead a Student to Understand the Microanatomy of Cells, Tissues, and Organs and to Correlate Structure With Function

The methods employed by histologists are extremely diverse. Much of the histology course content can be framed in terms of light microscopy, which the students will use in the laboratory exercises. More detailed interpretation of microanatomy rests with the electron microscope (EM), both the transmission electron microscope (TEM) and the scanning electron microscope (SEM), because of its greater useful magnification and the many auxiliary techniques of cell and molecular biology for which use of the EM is the last step in data acquisition. These auxiliary techniques include

- Histochemistry and cytochemistry
- Autoradiography
- Organ and tissue culture
- Cell and organelle separation by differential centrifugation
- Specialized microscopic techniques and microscopes

The student might feel removed from such techniques and experimental procedures because direct experience with them is usually not available in current curricula. Nevertheless, it is important to know something about specialized procedures and the data they yield. *This chapter provides a survey of methods and offers an explanation of how the data provided by these methods can help the student acquire a sound appreciation of histology.*

One of the problems faced by the student in histology is understanding the nature of the two-dimensional image of a histologic slide or an electron micrograph and how it relates to the three-dimensional structure from which it came. To bridge this conceptual gap, we must first present a brief description of the methods by which slides and electron microscopic specimens are produced.

TISSUE PREPARATION

Hematoxylin and Eosin Staining With Formalin Fixation

The Routinely Prepared Hematoxylin and Eosin-Stained Section Is the Specimen Most Commonly Studied

The slide set given each student to study with the light microscope consists mostly of formalin-fixed, paraffin-embedded, hematoxylin and eosin (H&E)-stained specimens. The light micrographs in the Atlas section of this book are from slides of actual student sets. Also, most photomicrographs used to illustrate tissues and organs in histology lectures and conferences are taken from such slides. Other techniques are sometimes used to demonstrate specific cell and tissue components; several of these are described below.

The First Step in Preparation of a Tissue or Organ Sample Is *Fixation* to Preserve Structure

Fixation, usually by a chemical or mixture of chemicals, stops cell metabolism and preserves the tissue structure for subsequent treatments. *Formalin,* a 37% aqueous solution of formaldehyde, at various dilutions and in combination with other chemicals and buffers, is the most commonly used fixative. Formaldehyde preserves the general structure of the cell and extracellular components by reacting with the amino groups of proteins; formaldehyde does not react with lipids and, therefore, is a poor fixative of membranes.

In the Second Step, the Specimen Is Prepared for *Embedding* in Paraffin to Permit *Sectioning*

To allow the specimen to be examined, it must be infiltrated with an embedding medium that allows it to be thinly sliced, 5–15 μm [1 micrometer (μm) equals 1/1000th of a millimeter (mm); see Table 1.4, page 11)]. This is accomplished by *washing* the specimen after fixation and *dehydrating* it in a series of alcohol solutions of ascending concentration up to 100% alcohol to remove water. Organic solvents such as xylol or toluol, which are miscible in both alcohol and *paraffin,* are then used to remove the alcohol prior to infiltration of the specimen with melted paraffin.

When the melted paraffin is cool and hardened, it is trimmed into an appropriately sized block. It is then mounted in a specially designed slicing machine, a *microtome,* and cut with a steel knife. The resulting sections are then mounted on glass slides with albumin used as an adhesive.

In the Third Step, the Specimen Is Stained to Permit Examination

Because the paraffin sections are colorless, the specimen is not yet suitable for light microscopic examination. To color or stain the tissue sections, the paraffin must be dissolved out, again using xylol or toluol, and the slide must then be rehydrated through a descending series of alcohol solutions to water. The tissue on the slides is then stained with *hematoxylin* in water. Because the counterstain, *eosin,* is more soluble in alcohol than in water, the specimen is again dehydrated through an ascending series of alcohol solutions to 100% alcohol and stained with eosin in alcohol. It is then passed through xylol or toluol to a nonaqueous mounting medium and covered with a coverslip to obtain a permanent preparation such as those used in teaching and diagnostic laboratories. A summary of H&E staining reactions of various cell and tissue components is presented in Table 1.1.

Other Fixatives

Formalin Does Not Preserve All Cell and Tissue Components

Although H&E-stained sections of formalin-fixed specimens are convenient to use because they display general structural features adequately, the stains are nonspecific in terms of the chemical composition of cell components. Also, many components are lost in the preparation of the specimen. To retain certain components and structures known to be lost in formalin fixation, other fixation methods must be employed. These are generally based on a clear understanding of the chemistry involved. For instance, the use of the alcohols and organic solvents in routine preparations removes neutral lipids.

To retain neutral lipids, such as that in adipose cells, frozen sections of formalin-fixed tissue and dyes that dissolve in the fat must be used; to retain membrane structures, special fixatives containing heavy metals, such as permanganate and osmium, that bind to the phospholipids must be used. The routine use of osmium tetroxide as a fixative for electron microscopy is the primary reason for

TABLE 1.1. Summary of Hematoxylin and Eosin (H&E) Staining

CELL AND EXTRACELLULAR COMPONENT	STAIN REACTION
Nucleus	
Heterochromatin	Blue
Euchromatin	Negative
Nucleolus	Blue
Cytoplasm	
Ergastoplasm	Blue
General cytoplasm	Pink
Cytoplasmic filaments	Pink
Extracellular material	
Collagen fibers	Pink
Elastic fibers[A]	Pink, but not usually distinguishable from collagen fibers
Reticular fibers[B]	Pink, but not usually distinguishable from collagen fibers
Ground substance	Blue, but only if present in large amounts, as in cartilage matrix
Bone matrix (decalcified)	Pink
Basement membrane[B]	Pink

[A]Special staining procedure used for their demonstration, such as one containing resorcin-fuchsin or orcein.
[B]Special staining procedure used for their demonstration, such as silver impregnation or periodic acid-Schiff (PAS) stain.

the excellent preservation of membranes in electron micrographs.

Other Staining Procedures

Hematoxylin and Eosin Are Used in Histology Because They Display Structural Features; They Provide No Information on Chemical Characteristics

Despite the merits of H&E staining, the procedure does not adequately reveal certain structural components of histologic sections, including elastic material, reticular fibers, basement membranes, and lipids. When it is desirable to display these components, other staining procedures, most of them selective, can be used. These procedures include the use of orcein and resorcin-fuchsin for elastic material and the use of silver impregnation for reticular fibers and basement membrane material. Although the chemical bases of many staining methods are not always understood, they work. Knowing what a procedure reveals is often more important than knowing precisely how the procedure works.

HISTOCHEMISTRY AND CYTOCHEMISTRY

Specific Chemical Procedures Can Provide Detailed Information on the Function of the Cells and Extracellular Components of the Tissues

Histochemical and cytochemical procedures may be based either on *specific binding* of a dye or a *fluorescent dye-labeled antibody* to a particular cell component or on the *inherent enzymatic activity* of a cell component. In addition, incorporation by cells and tissues prior to fixation of radioactively tagged precursors of many of the large molecules normally found in cells can be used to localize the large molecules by *autoradiography*. Many of these procedures can be used with both light microscopic and electron microscopic preparations.

Before we discuss the chemistry of routine staining and of some of the histochemical and cytochemical methods, it will be useful to examine briefly what is contained in a routinely fixed and embedded section of a specimen.

Chemical Composition of Histologic Samples

The Chemical Composition of a Tissue Ready for Routine Staining Differs Greatly From Tissue in the Living State

The components that remain after fixation consist mostly of large molecules that are not readily dissolved, especially after treatment with the fixative. Such large molecules, particularly those that have reacted with other large molecules to form macromolecular complexes, are most consistently preserved in a tissue section. Examples of such large macromolecular complexes are

- *Nucleoproteins,* formed from nucleic acids bound to protein
- *Intracellular cytoskeletal proteins* complexed with other proteins
- *Extracellular proteins* in large, insoluble aggregates bound to similar molecules due to cross-linking of neighboring molecules, as in collagen fiber formation
- *Membrane phospholipid-protein (or carbohydrate) complexes*

For the most part, these molecules constitute the structure of cells and tissues, in that they make up the formed elements of the tissue. They are the basis for the organization that is seen in tissue with the microscope.

In many cases a structural element is at the same time a functional unit. For example, in the case of proteins that make up the contractile filaments of muscle cells, the filaments are the visible structural components and the actual participants in the contractile process. The RNA of the cytoplasm is visualized as part of a structural component (ergastoplasm of gland cells, Nissl bodies of nerve cells) while being the actual participant in the synthesis of protein.

Many Tissue Components Are Lost During the Preparation of the Hematoxylin and Eosin-Stained Section

Despite the fact that nucleic acids, proteins, and phospholipids are mostly retained in tissue sections, many are also lost. Small proteins and small nucleic acids, such as transfer RNAs, are generally lost during the preparation of the tissue. Large molecules also may be lost, for example, by being hydrolyzed due to an unfavorable pH of the fixative solutions. Examples of large molecules lost during routine fixation in aqueous fixatives are

- *Glycogen* (an intracellular storage carbohydrate common in liver and muscle cells)
- *Proteoglycans* and *glycosaminoglycans* (extracellular complex carbohydrates found in connective tissue; see page 105)

Such molecules can be preserved, however, by the use of nonaqueous fixative for glycogen or by the addition to the fixative solution of specific binding agents that preserve extracellular carbohydrate-containing molecules. Also, as described above, neutral lipids are usually lost during routine tissue preparation because of dissolution in organic solvents.

Soluble Components, Ions, and Small Molecules Are Also Lost From the Tissue Samples During the Preparation of Paraffin Sections

Intermediary metabolites, glucose, sodium, chloride, and similar substances are no longer present in the specimen. Although these small substances are lost during the preparation of routine H&E paraffin sections, many of these substances can be studied in special preparations, sometimes with considerable loss of structural integrity. These small soluble ions and molecules do not make up the formed elements of a tissue; they constitute substances being processed or participating in cellular reactions. When they can be preserved and demonstrated by specific methods, they can provide invaluable information on cell metabolism, active transport, and other vital cellular processes. Water, a highly versatile molecule, participates in these reactions and processes and contributes to the stabilization of macromolecular structure through hydrogen bonding.

TABLE 1.2. Some Basic and Acid Dyes

	COLOR
Basic dyes	
Methyl green	Green
Methylene blue	Blue
Pyronin G	Red
Toluidine blue	Blue
Acid dyes	
Acid fuchsin	Red
Aniline blue	Blue
Eosin	Red
Orange G	Orange

Chemical Basis of Staining

Hematoxylin and Eosin Are the Most Commonly Used Dyes in Histology

An *acid dye,* such as eosin, carries a *net negative charge* on its colored portion and is described by the general formula Na^+dye^-.

A *basic dye* carries a *net positive charge* on its colored portion and is described by the general formula dye^+Cl^-.

Hematoxylin is not strictly a basic dye but has properties that closely resemble those of a basic dye. The color of a dye is not related to whether it is basic or acid, as can be noted by the list of some basic and acid dyes in Table 1.2.

Basic Dyes React with Anionic Components of Cells and Tissue (Components That Carry a Net Negative Charge)

Basic Dyes. Anionic components include the phosphate groups of nucleic acids, the sulfate groups of glycosaminoglycans, and the carboxyl groups of proteins. The ability of such anionic groups to react with a basic dye is called *basophilia.* Tissue components that stain with hematoxylin are also said to exhibit basophilia.

The reaction of the anionic groups varies with pH. Thus,

- At a *high pH* (about 10), all three groups are ionized and available for reaction by electrostatic linkages with the basic dye.
- At a *slightly acid to neutral pH* (5–7), sulfate and phosphate groups are ionized and available for reaction with the basic dye by electrostatic linkages.
- At *low pH* (below 4), only sulfate groups remain ionized and react with basic dyes.

Therefore, staining with basic dyes at controlled pH can be used to focus on specific anionic groups and, because the specific anionic groups are found predominantly on certain macromolecules, the staining serves as an indicator of these macromolecules.

An additional procedure used in conjunction with staining at controlled pH is the use of enzymes for selectively removing substrates from the tissue section prior to staining (Fig. 1.1).

As already mentioned, hematoxylin is, strictly speaking, not a basic dye. It is used with a mordant, i.e., an intermediate link between the tissue component and the dye. It is the mordant that causes the staining to resemble a basic dye. The linkage in the tissue-mordant-hematoxylin complex is not a simple electrostatic linkage, and when sections are placed in water, hematoxylin does not dissociate from the tissue. Because of this, hematoxylin lends itself to those staining sequences in which it is followed by aqueous solutions of acid dyes. True basic dyes, as distinguished from hematoxylin, are not generally used in sequences wherein the basic dye is followed by an acid dye. The basic dye then tends to dissociate from the tissue during the washes in aqueous solutions between the two dye solutions.

Acid Dyes React With Cationic Groups in Cells and Tissues, Particularly the Ionized Amino Groups of Proteins

Acid Dyes. The reaction of such cationic groups with an acid dye is called *acidophilia.* Reactions of cell and tissue components with acid dyes are neither as specific nor as precise as reactions with basic dyes.

Although the electrostatic linkage is the major factor in the primary binding of an acid dye to the tissue, it is not the only one; because of this, acid dyes are sometimes used in combinations to color different tissue constituents selectively. For example, three acid dyes are used in the *Mallory staining technique:* aniline blue, acid fuchsin, and orange G. These dyes selectively stain collagen, ordinary cytoplasm, and red blood cells, respectively. The acid fuchsin also stains the nuclei.

In other multiple acid dye techniques, hematoxylin is used to stain nuclei first, then the acid dyes are used to stain cytoplasm and extracellular fibers selectively. The selective staining of tissue components by acid dyes is not due to specific properties of the dye or tissue but rather to relative factors. They include such factors as size and degree of aggregation on the part of the dye and permeability and degree of "compactness" on the part of the tissue.

Basic dyes can also be employed in combinations or sequentially (e.g., methyl green and pyronin to study protein synthesis and secretion), but those combinations are not as widely used as acid dye combinations.

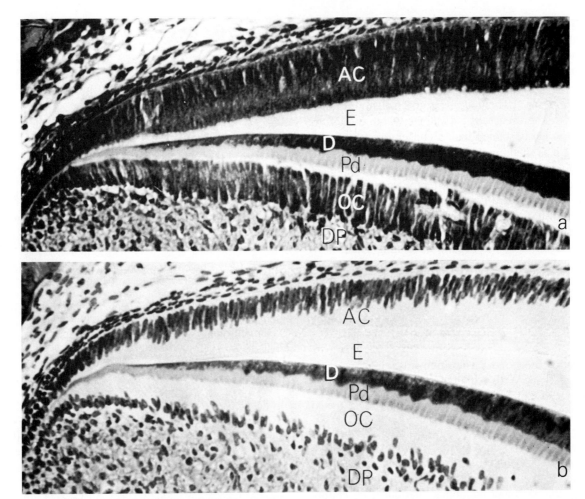

Figure 1.1. **a.** Developing tooth germ stained with toluidine blue at pH 6.5. Note the staining of ameloblast cytoplasm (AC), dentin (D), predentin (Pd), odontoblast cytoplasm (OC), and components of the dental papilla (DP). The developing enamel (E) is unstained. The toluidine blue stains anionic groups, e.g., COO^-, PO_4^{3-}, and SO_4^{2-}; consequently, little specificity is displayed by the dye. **b.** This specimen (a serial section to the specimen shown in **a**) was treated with the enzyme RNAse to remove RNA from the tissue prior to staining with toluidine blue, again at pH 6.5. Note that the ameloblast cytoplasm (AC) and the odontoblast cytoplasm (OC) have lost their intense staining due to digestion of the RNA. As the nuclei contain chiefly DNA, which is unaffected by the RNAse, they retain their intense staining and resemble the same structures seen in **a**. In like manner, the matrix of dentin (D), predentin (Pd), and dental papilla (DP) retain their staining, probably due to presence of sulfated compounds within the matrix. In this example, the enzyme RNAse was employed as a reagent prior to staining in order to aid in the identification of RNA when used in combination, as in **a** and **b**. A variety of other enzymes, e.g., DNAse and enzymes used to focus on the presence of polysaccharides, can be employed according to the same principles.

Tissue Components That React With Basic Dyes or With Hematoxylin Are Called *Basophilic*

Basophilia and Acidophilia. A limited number of substances within cells and the extracellular matrix display basophilia (Gr. for base-loving), i.e., react with basic dyes. These include

- *Heterochromatin* and *nucleoli* of the nucleus (both due chiefly to ionized phosphate groups in nucleic acids)
- *Cytoplasmic components* such as the ergastoplasm (also due to ionized phosphate groups in RNA)
- *Extracellular materials* such as the complex carbohydrates of the matrix of cartilage (due to ionized sulfate groups)

Tissue Components That Stain With Acid Dyes Are Called *Acidophilic*

Staining with acid dyes is less specific, but more substances within cells and the extracellular matrix exhibit acidophilia. These include

- Most *cytoplasmic filaments,* especially those of muscle cells
- Most *intracellular membranous components* and much of the otherwise unspecialized cytoplasm
- Most *extracellular fibers* (primarily due to ionized amino groups)

Certain Basic Dyes React With Tissue Components Such That Their Normal Color Shifts From Blue to Red or Purple; This Absorbance Change Is Called *Metachromasia*

Metachromasia. The underlying mechanism for metachromasia is the presence of polyanions within the tissue. When such tissue is stained with a concentrated basic dye solution, such as toluidine blue, the dye molecules are sufficiently close to form dimeric and polymeric aggregates whose absorption properties are different from those of the individual nonaggregated dye molecules.

Cell and tissue structures that have high concentrations of ionized sulfate and phosphate groups, such as the ground substance of cartilage, the heparin-containing granules of the mast cell, and the rough endoplasmic reticulum of plasma cells, will exhibit metachromasia. Therefore, toluidine blue will appear purple to red when it stains these components.

Aldehyde Groups and the Schiff Reagent

The Ability of Bleached Basic Fuchsin (Schiff Reagent) to React With Aldehyde Groups to Give a Distinctive Red Color Is the Basis of the *Periodic Acid-Schiff* **and** *Feulgen Reactions*

The *periodic acid-Schiff (PAS) reaction* stains carbohydrates and carbohydrate-rich macromolecules. It is used to demonstrate glycogen in cells, mucus in various cells and tissues, the basement membrane that underlies epithelia, and reticular fibers in connective tissue. The *Feulgen reaction,* employing a mild hydrochloric acid hydrolysis, is used to stain DNA.

The PAS reaction is based on the following facts:

- Hexose rings of carbohydrates contain adjacent carbons, each of which bears a hydroxyl (—OH) group.
- Hexosamines of glycosaminoglycans contain adjacent carbons, one of which bears an —OH group, while the other bears an amino (—NH$_2$) group.
- Periodic acid cleaves the bond between these adjacent carbon atoms and forms aldehyde groups.
- These aldehyde groups react with the Schiff reagent to give a distinctive magenta color.

The PAS staining of basement membrane (Fig. 1.2) and reticular fibers is based on the content or association of proteoglycans (complex carbohydrates associated with a protein core). PAS staining is an alternative to silver impregnation methods, which are also based on reaction with the sugar molecules in the proteoglycans.

The Feulgen reaction is based on the fact that the mild acid hydrolysis cleaves the purines from the deoxyribose of DNA; the sugar ring then opens with the formation of aldehyde groups. Again, it is the newly formed aldehyde

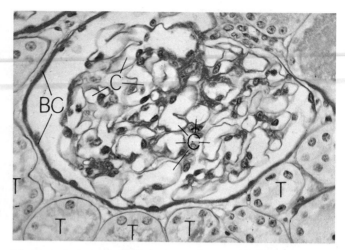

Figure 1.2. Photomicrograph of kidney tissue stained by the PAS method to demonstrate and localize histochemically carbohydrate. The basement membranes are PAS positive, as evidenced by the deep pink staining of these sites. The kidney tubules *(T)* are sharply delineated by the stained surrounding basement membrane. The glomerular capillaries *(C)* and the epithelium of Bowman's capsule *(BC)* also show PAS-positive basement membranes.

groups that react with the Schiff reagent to give the distinctive magenta color. The reaction of the Schiff reagent with DNA is *stoichiometric* and can be used, therefore, in spectrophotometric methods to quantitate the amount of DNA in the nucleus of a cell. RNA does not stain with the Schiff reagent because it lacks the deoxy sugar.

FEULGEN MICROSPECTROPHOTOMETRY

Feulgen microspectrophotometry is a technique that was developed to study DNA increases in developing cells and to analyze *ploidy,* i.e., the number of times the normal DNA content of a cell is multiplied (a normal, nondividing cell is said to be *diploid,* a sperm or egg cell is *haploid;* see page 51). Recently, it has become a valuable tool for surgical pathologists in evaluating the metastatic potential of a malignant tumor and in making prognostic and treatment decisions. The technique of *static cytometry* of Feulgen-stained sections of tumors (contrasted with *flow cytometry,* which can only be used on isolated individual cells) uses microspectrophotometry coupled with a digitizing imaging system to measure the absorption of light at 560 nm by cells and cell clusters in Feulgen-stained sections. This allows the pathologist to describe ploidy patterns in specific *adenocarcinomas* (epithelial cancers). This method has been particularly useful in studies of breast cancer, kidney cancer, colon and other gastrointestinal cancers, endometrial cancer (uterine epithelium), and ovarian cancer. Adenocarcinomas that have a largely diploid pattern are said to be well differentiated and have a better prognosis than the same cancers with *aneuploidy* (nonintegral multiples of the haploid amount of DNA) and *tetraploidy.*

Enzyme Digestion

Enzyme Digestion of a Section Serial to One Stained for a Specific Component, Such as Glycogen, DNA, or RNA, Can Be Used to Confirm the Identity of the Stained Material

Intracellular material that stains with the PAS reaction may be identified as glycogen by pretreatment of sections with diastase or amylase. Abolition of the staining after these treatments positively identifies the stained material as glycogen.

Similarly, the predigestion of tissue sections with deoxyribonuclease (DNAse) will abolish the Feulgen staining in those sections, and digestion of sections of protein secretory epithelia with ribonuclease (RNAse) will abolish the staining of the ergastoplasm with basic dyes (see Fig. 1.1).

Enzyme Histochemistry

Histochemical Methods Are Also Used to Identify and *Localize Enzymes* in Cells and Tissues

To localize enzymes in tissue sections, special care must be taken in fixation so as to preserve the enzyme activity. Usually, mild aldehyde fixation is the preferred method.

In these procedures the reaction product of the enzyme activity, rather than the enzyme itself, is visualized. In general, a *capture reagent,* either a dye or a heavy metal, is used to trap or bind the reaction product of the enzyme activity by precipitation at the site of reaction. In a typical reaction to display a hydrolytic enzyme, the tissue section is placed in a solution containing a substrate *(AB)* and a trapping agent *(T)* that will precipitate one of the products as follows:

$$AB + T \xrightarrow{\text{enzyme}} AT \downarrow + B,$$

where AT is the trapped end product and B is the hydrolyzed substrate.

Using such methods, the lysosome (see page 35), first identified in differential centrifugation studies of cells, was equated with a vacuolar component seen in electron micrographs. In lightly fixed tissues, the acid hydrolases and acid esterases contained in lysosomes are reacted with an appropriate substrate. The reaction mixture also contains lead ions to precipitate, for instance, lead phosphate derived from the action of acid phosphatase. The precipitated reaction product can then be observed with both light and electron microscopy.

Similar light and electron histochemical procedures have been developed to demonstrate alkaline phosphatase, adenosinetriphosphatases (ATPases) of many varieties including the Na^+-K^+-activated ATPase that is the enzymatic basis of the sodium pump in cells and tissues, various esterases, and many respiratory enzymes (Fig. 1.3).

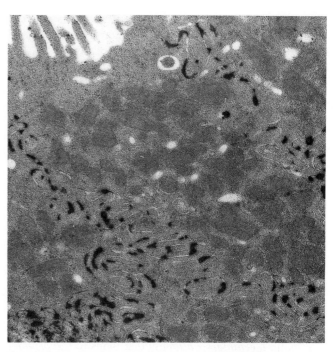

Figure 1.3. Electron micrograph demonstrating the localization of ATPase along the complex lateral plications in the apical region of rabbit gallbladder epithelial cells. This histochemical localization corresponds with the location of the sodium transport system in these very active transporting cells. ×26,000.

Immunocytochemistry

A Foreign Protein or Other *Antigen* Injected into an Animal Results in Production of *Antibodies*

An antibody is a protein produced by certain blood cells that binds to and usually precipitates the foreign substance that stimulated its production. In the laboratory, antibodies can be purified and conjugated (i.e., chemically bound) to a fluorescent dye such as fluorescein. This reagent can then be applied to sections of lightly fixed or frozen tissue on glass slides in order to localize the antigen in cells and tissues. The reaction can then be examined and photographed with a fluorescence microscope.

The Specificity of the Reaction Between Antigen and Antibody Is the Underlying Basis of Immunocytochemistry

In a typical procedure, a specific protein, such as actin, would be isolated from the muscle cells of one species, such as rat, and injected into the circulation of another species, such as rabbit. The actin would stimulate the formation of antiactin antibodies that would circulate in the blood of the rabbit. The antibodies would then be removed from the blood of the rabbit, conjugated with a fluorescent dye, and used to stain tissues or cells suspected of containing actin, such as fibroblasts in connective tissue. If actin were present, the antibodies would bind to it, and the reaction could be visualized by virtue of the fluorescent dye bound to the antibodies (Fig. 1.4). A fluorescence microscope is used to display the fluorescein now attached indirectly to the antigen. It is also possible to conjugate substances such as gold or ferritin (an iron-containing molecule) to the antibody molecule. These markers can be visualized directly with the EM.

Enzyme Histochemical Methods Are Combined With Traditional Immunocytochemical Methods to Give Greater Amplification of the Localization Reaction Than Is Possible With Fluorescein

In these methods, horseradish peroxidase enzyme is conjugated with the *primary antibody,* and after the antigen-antibody reaction has occurred, the histochemical procedure for demonstrating peroxidase activity is run to reveal the location of the complex (direct reaction). A further refinement of this method attaches the peroxidase to an anti-γ-globulin *(secondary antibody)* that binds to the *primary antibody,* further amplifying the reaction (indirect reaction). Because the end product of the peroxidase reaction

is also visible in the EM, this method is easily adapted to EM immunocytochemistry. Monoclonal antibodies conjugated with ferritin or gold particles may be used as primary antibody stains to achieve even more precise localization of antigens in tissue sections examined in the TEM than is possible with traditional polyclonal antibodies.

An additional advantage of the indirect labeling method is that a single secondary antibody can be used to localize the intracellular or tissue-specific binding of several different primary antibodies. For light microscopic studies, the secondary antibody can be conjugated with different fluorescent dyes so that multiple labels can be shown in the same tissue section (see page 570).

Autoradiography

Autoradiography Makes Use of a Photographic Emulsion Placed Over a Tissue Section to Localize Radioactive Material Within the Tissue

Many small molecular precursors of larger molecules, such as the amino acids that are incorporated into proteins and the nucleotides that are incorporated into nucleic acids,

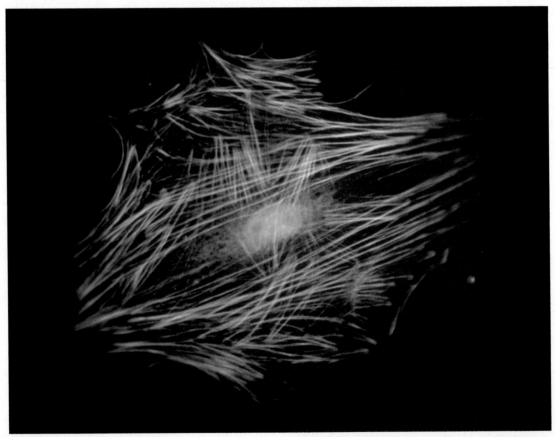

Figure 1.4. Human skin fibroblast in culture, photographed in the fluorescence microscope. The cell was stained with an actin-specific antibody conjugated with the dye fluorescein. The antigen-antibody reaction, performed directly in the culture, re-sults in localization of the actin. The actin filaments, organized in linear bundles, fluoresce and thus show their distribution in this nonmigrating cell. (Courtesy of Dr. E. S. Lazarides.)

may be tagged by substitution of a radioactive atom or atoms in their molecular structure and the consequent radioactivity used to localize the larger molecules in cells and tissues. The procedure has been used effectively by injecting the labeled precursor molecules into animals or by introducing the labeled precursors into cell or organ cultures. In this way, synthesis of DNA and subsequent cell division, synthesis and secretion of proteins by cells, and localization of synthetic products within cells and in the extracellular matrix have been studied.

In this technique, sections of specimens that have incorporated the radioactive material are mounted on slides. In the dark, the slide is usually dipped in a melted photographic emulsion, thus producing a thin photographic film on the surface of the slide. After appropriate exposure in a light-tight box, usually days to weeks, the exposed emulsion on the slide is developed by standard photographic techniques and permanently mounted with a coverslip. The slides may be stained either before or after the exposure and development. The silver grains in the emulsion over the radioactively labeled molecules will be exposed and developed by this procedure and will appear as dark grains overlying portions of the tissue when examined with the light microscope (Fig. 1.5a).

The silver grains in the developed emulsion may be used simply to indicate where a substance is localized, or the silver grains may be counted to provide semiquantitative information on the amount of a given substance in a specific location. For instance, after injection of an animal with tritiated thymidine, cells that have incorporated this nucleotide into DNA prior to dividing but that have not yet divided will have approximately twice as many silver grains overlying their nuclei as will cells that have divided after incorporating the labeled nucleotide.

Autoradiography can also be carried out by using thin plastic sections for examination with the EM. Essentially the same procedures are used, but as with all TEM preparation techniques, the processes are much more delicate and more difficult; however, they also yield results of much greater resolution and localization (Fig. 1.5b).

Historadiography

Historadiography Is the Production of an X-ray Photograph (Microradiograph) of a Specimen on a Slide

A historadiograph displays mass just as a regular x-ray does. Although x-rays can be used to examine soft tissues, their greatest utility is in the examination of ground sections of bone or other mineralized tissue. In practice, the ground section of bone is placed in contact with a photographic emulsion on a glass slide and exposed to a beam of x-rays. The photographic emulsion is then developed and viewed with a microscope (Fig. 1.6). Standards of known mass can be added to the slide or to a companion slide treated in the

same manner in order to provide semiquantitative information on the amount of bone mineral in different parts of the ground section.

MICROSCOPY

Light Microscopy

A microscope, whether simple (one lens) or compound (multiple lenses), is an instrument that magnifies an image and allows visualization of greater detail than is possible with the unaided eye. The simplest microscope is a magnifying glass or a pair of reading glasses.

The resolving power of the human eye, i.e., the distance by which two objects must be separated to be seen as two objects (0.2 mm) is determined by the spacing of the photoreceptor cells in the retina. The role of a microscope is to magnify an image to a level at which the retina can resolve the information that would otherwise be below its limit of resolution. Table 1.3 compares the resolution of the eye to various instruments.

Resolving Power Is the Ability of a Microscope Lens or Optical System to Produce Separate Images of Closely Positioned Objects

The resolution depends not only on the optical system but also on the wavelength of the light source and on other factors, such as specimen thickness, quality of fixation, and staining intensity. With light whose wavelength is 540 nm (Table 1.4), a green-filtered light to which the eye is extremely sensitive, and with appropriate objective and condenser lenses, the greatest attainable resolving power of a bright-field microscope would be about 0.2 μm (see page 17 for method of calculation). This is the theoretical resolution and, as already mentioned, depends on all conditions being optimal. *The ocular lens magnifies the image produced by the objective, but it cannot increase resolution.*

Various light microscopes are available for general and specialized use in modern biologic research and study. Their differences are based largely on such factors as the wavelength of specimen illumination, physical alteration of the light coming to or leaving the specimen, and specific analytic processes that can be applied to the final image. These instruments and their applications are described briefly in this section.

The Microscope Used by Both Students and Researchers Is Referred to as the *Bright-field Microscope*

Bright-field Microscope. The bright-field microscope is the direct descendant of the microscopes that became widely available in the 1800s and opened the first major

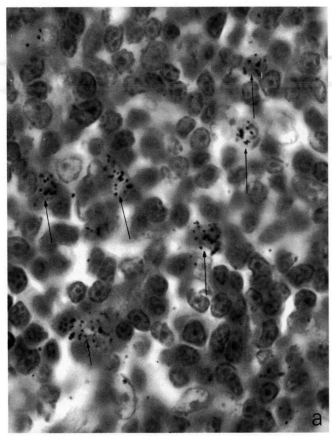

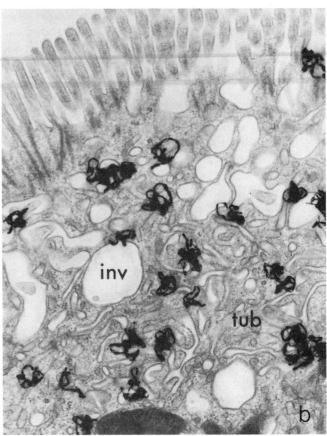

Figure 1.5. **a.** Photomicrograph of a lymph node section from an animal treated with tritiated thymidine. Some of the cells exhibit aggregates of metallic silver grains, which appear as small black particles *(arrows)*. These cells are preparing for division and have incorporated the thymidine into their nuclei. The low-energy radioactive particles emitted from the tritiated thymidine, on striking silver halide crystals in a photographic emulsion covering the specimen over a period of time (exposure), create a latent image (much like light striking photographic film in a camera). On photographic development of the slide with its covering emulsion, the latent image, actually the activated silver halide in the emulsion, is reduced to the metallic silver, which then appears as the black grains in the microscope. (Original slide specimen courtesy of E. Kallenbach.) **b.** Electron microscopic autoradiograph of the apical region of an intestinal absorptive cell. In this specimen, ^{125}I bound to nerve growth factor (NGF) was injected into the animal, and the tissue was removed 1 hour later. The specimen was prepared in a manner similar to that for light microscopy, as in **a**. Because of the greater resolution and cytologic detail and the relatively small size of the silver grains, however, the localization of the ^{125}I-NGF is extremely precise. Note that the silver grains are concentrated over apical invaginations *(inv)* and endocytic tubules *(tub)*. (Micrograph courtesy of Marian R. Neutra.)

era of research in histology. The bright-field microscope (Fig. 1.7) essentially consists of

- **Light source** for illumination of the specimen, e.g., a substage lamp
- **Condenser lens** to focus the beam of light at the level of the specimen
- **Stage** on which the slide or other specimen is placed
- **Objective lens** to gather the light that has passed through the specimen
- **Ocular lens** (or a pair of ocular lenses in the more commonly used binocular microscopes) through which the image formed by the objective lens may be examined directly

A specimen to be examined with the bright-field microscope must be sufficiently thin for light to pass through it. Although some light is absorbed while passing through the specimen, the optical system of the bright-field microscope does not produce a useful level of contrast in the unstained specimen. For this reason, the various staining methods discussed earlier are employed. Other optical systems, described below, may be used to enhance the contrast without staining.

The Phase Contrast Microscope Enables the Examination of Unstained Cells and Tissues and Is Especially Useful for Living Cells

Phase Contrast Microscope. The phase contrast microscope takes advantage of the fact that there are small differences in the index of refraction in different parts of a

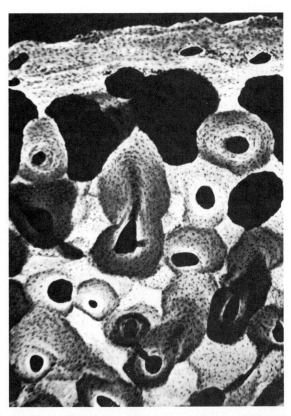

Figure 1.6. Microradiograph of a 200-μm-thick section of bone. *Black areas* are sites of soft tissue; *white areas* contain high concentrations of calcium salts; and *light gray to dark gray areas* reflect decreasing amounts of calcium salts. (Courtesy of Dr. J. Jowsey.)

cell and in different parts of a tissue sample. Light passing through areas of relatively high refractive index (denser areas) is deflected and becomes out of phase with the rest of the beam of light that has passed through the specimen. By adding other induced-out-of-phase wavelengths by the use of a series of optical rings in the condenser and objective lenses, the phase contrast microscope essentially abolishes the amplitude of the initially deflected portion of the beam and produces a useful amount of contrast in the image. Dark portions of the image correspond to dense portions of the

TABLE 1.3. Eye versus Instrument Resolution

	DISTANCE BETWEEN RESOLVABLE POINTS
Human eye	0.2 mm
Bright-field microscope	0.2 μm
SEM	2.5 nm
TEM	
Theoretical	0.05 nm
Tissue section	1.0 nm

TABLE 1.4. Linear Equivalents[A]

1 Angstrom (Å)	=	0.1 nanometer (nm)
10 Angstroms	=	1.0 nanometer [formerly millimicron (mμ)]
1000 nanometers	=	1.0 micrometer (μm) [formerly micron (μ)]
1000 micrometers	=	1.0 millimeter (mm)

specimen; light portions of the image correspond to less dense portions of the specimen. The phase contrast microscope is, therefore, used to examine living cells and tissues, such as cells in tissue culture, and is used extensively to examine unstained semithin (approximately 0.5-μm) sections of plastic embedded tissue.

Two modifications of the phase contrast microscope are the *interference microscope,* which also allows for quantitation of tissue mass, and the *differential interference microscope* (using Nomarski optics), which is especially useful for assessing surface properties of cells and other biologic objects.

In Dark-field Microscopy, No Direct Light From the Light Source Is Gathered by the Objective Lens

Dark-field Microscope. In dark-field microscopy, only light that has been scattered or diffracted by structures in the specimen reaches the objective. To achieve this, the dark-field microscope is equipped with a special condenser that illuminates the specimen with strong, oblique light. Thus, the field of view appears as a dark background on which small particles in the specimen that reflect some light into the objective appear bright.

The effect is similar to dust particles that are seen in the light beam emanating from a slide projector in a darkened room. The reflected light from the dust particles reaches the retina of the eye, thus making the particles visible.

The resolution of the dark-field microscope cannot be better than that of the bright-field microscope, using, as it does, the same wavelength source. Smaller individual particles can be detected in dark-field images, however, because of the enhanced contrast that is created.

The dark-field microscope is useful in examining autoradiographs, in which the developed silver grains appear white in a dark background. Clinically, it is useful in examining urine for crystals, such as those of uric acid and oxalate, and in demonstrating spirochetes, particularly *Treponema pallidum,* the organism that causes syphilis, a sexually transmitted disease.

The Fluorescence Microscope Utilizes the Fact That Certain Molecules Fluoresce Under Ultraviolet Light

Fluorescence Microscope. A molecule that fluoresces emits light of wavelengths in the visible range when ex-

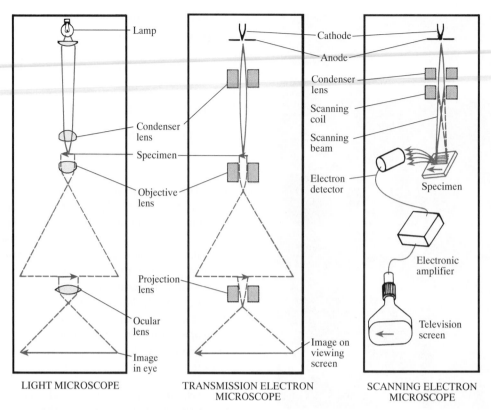

Figure 1.7. Diagram comparing the optical paths of the light microscope *(left)*, shown as if it were turned upside down, the TEM *(middle)*, and the SEM *(right)*. The specimen and the projected magnified image are depicted by the *arrows*.

posed to an ultraviolet (UV) source. The fluorescence microscope is used to display naturally occurring fluorescent (autofluorescent) molecules, such as vitamin A and some neurotransmitters. Because autofluorescent molecules are not numerous, however, its most widespread application is the display of introduced fluorescence, as in the detection of antigens or antibodies in immunocytochemical staining procedures (see Fig. 1.4). Specific fluorescent molecules can also be injected into an animal or directly into cells and used as tracers. Such methods have been useful in studying intercellular (gap) junctions, in tracing the pathway of nerve fibers in neurobiology, and in detecting fluorescent growth markers of mineralized tissues.

Various filters are inserted between the UV light source and the specimen to produce monochromatic or near-monochromatic (single wavelength or narrow band of wavelength) light. A second set of filters inserted between the specimen and the objective allows only the narrow band of wavelength of the fluorescence to reach the eye or to reach a photographic emulsion or other analytic processor.

The Confocal Scanning Microscope Combines Components of a Light Optical Microscope With a Scanning System to Optically Dissect a Specimen

Confocal Scanning Microscope. The confocal scanning microscope is a relatively new microscope system used to study the structure of biologic materials. The illuminating laser light system that it employs is very strongly convergent and, therefore, produces a very shallow scanning spot. The light emerging from the spot is directed to a photomultiplier tube, where it is analyzed. A mirror system is used to move the laser beam across the specimen, illuminating a single spot at a time (Fig. 1.8). The data from each point of the specimen scanned by this moving spot is recorded and stored in a computer. The information can then be displayed on a high-resolution video monitor to create a visual image. The major advantage of this system is its ability to image the specimen in very thin optical sections (approximately 1 μm thick). The out-of-focus regions are subtracted from the image by the computer program, thus creating extreme sharpness of the image. In these aspects, confocal microscopy resembles the imaging process in computed axial tomography (x-ray) scanning (CAT scans). Ordinary or nonconfocal light imaging contains superimposed in-focus and out-of-focus specimen parts, thereby reducing image quality.

Furthermore, by utilizing only the narrow depth of the in-focus image, it is possible to create multiple images at varying depths within the specimen. Thus, one can literally dissect layer by layer through the thickness of the specimen. It is also possible to use the computer to make three-dimensional reconstructions of a series of these images. Be-

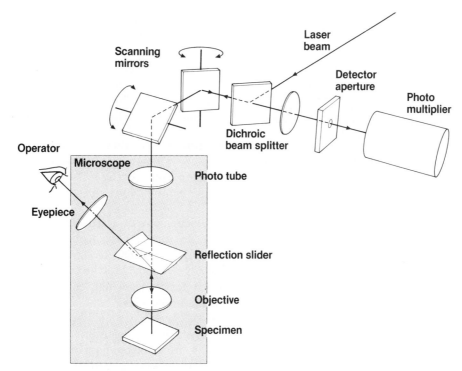

Figure 1.8. Diagram of the beam path in the confocal microscope. (Courtesy of Sarastro, Inc., USA.)

cause each individual image located at a specific depth within the specimen is extremely sharp, the resulting assembled three-dimensional image is equally sharp. Moreover, once the computer has assembled each of the sectioned images, one can rotate the reconstructed three-dimensional image and view it from any orientation desired.

The Ultraviolet Microscope Uses Quartz Lenses With an Ultraviolet Light Source

Ultraviolet Microscope. The image in the UV microscope is dependent on the absorption of UV light by molecules in the specimen. The UV source has a wavelength of approximately 200 nm. Thus, it may achieve a resolution of 0.1 μm. In principle, UV microscopy is not unlike the workings of a spectrophotometer; the results are usually recorded photographically. The specimen cannot be inspected directly through an ocular because the UV light is not visible and is injurious to the eye.

The method is useful in detecting nucleic acids, specifically the purine and pyrimidine bases of the nucleotide. It is also useful for detecting proteins that contain certain amino acids. Using specific illuminating wavelengths, UV spectrophotometric measurements are commonly made through the UV microscope to determine quantitatively the amount of DNA and RNA in individual cells. As described on page 6, it is used clinically to evaluate the degree of ploidy (multiples of normal DNA quantity) in sections of tumors.

The Polarizing Microscope Utilizes the Fact That Highly Ordered Molecules or Arrays of Molecules Can Rotate the Angle of the Plane of Polarized Light

Polarizing Microscope. The polarizing microscope is a simple modification of the light microscope in which a polarizing filter, called the *polarizer,* is located between the light source and the specimen and a second polarizer, called the *analyzer,* is located between the objective lens and the viewer.

Both the polarizer and the analyzer can be rotated; the difference between their angles of rotation is used to determine the degree by which a structure affects the beam of polarized light. The ability of a crystal or paracrystalline array to rotate the plane of polarized light is called ***birefringence*** (double refraction). Striated muscle and the crystalloid inclusions in the testicular interstitial cells (Leydig cells), among other common structures, exhibit birefringence.

Electron Microscopy

Two kinds of EMs can provide morphologic and analytic data on cells and tissues: the ***transmission electron microscope (TEM)*** and the ***scanning electron microscope (SEM).*** The primary improvement in the EM versus the light microscope is that the wavelength of the EM beam is approximately 1/2000th that of the light microscope beam, thereby increasing resolution by a factor of 10^3.

The *Transmission Electron Microscope* Uses the Interaction of a Beam of Electrons With a Specimen to Produce an Image

Transmission Electron Microscope. The "optics" of the TEM are, in principle, very similar to those of the light microscope (see Fig. 1.7), except that the TEM uses a beam of electrons rather than a beam of light. The principle of the microscope is as follows:

- There is a *source,* a heated tungsten filament that emits electrons *(cathode).*
- There is an *anode* toward which the electrons are attracted.
- A potential difference between the cathode cover and the anode imparts an accelerating voltage of between 20,000 and 200,000 volts to the electrons, creating the beam.
- The beam then passes through a series of *electromagnetic lenses* that serve the same functions as do the glass lenses of a light microscope.

The *condenser lens* shapes the beam and changes the diameter of the beam that reaches the specimen plane. The beam that has passed through the specimen is then focused and magnified by an *objective lens* and further magnified by one or more *projector lenses*. The final image is viewed on a phosphor-coated *screen*. Portions of the specimen through which electrons have passed appear bright; portions of the specimen that have absorbed or scattered electrons because of their inherent density or because of heavy metals added during specimen preparation, appear dark. A photographic plate or video detector can be placed above or below the viewing screen in order to record permanently the image on the screen.

Specimen Preparation for Transmission Electron Microscopy Is Similar to That for Light Microscopy Except That It Requires Finer Methods

The principles in the preparation of sections for viewing with the TEM are essentially the same as those for light microscopy, with the added constraint that at every step one must work with specimens 3–4 orders of magnitude smaller or thinner than those used for light microscopy. The TEM, with a wavelength in the electron beam of approximately 0.1 nm, has a theoretical resolution of 0.05 nm.

Because of the great resolution of the TEM, the quality of fixation, i.e., the degree of preservation of subcellular structure, must be the best achievable.

Routine Preparation of Specimens for Transmission Electron Microscopy Begins With Glutaraldehyde Fixation Followed by a Buffer Rinse and Fixation With Osmium Tetroxide

Glutaraldehyde, a dialdehyde, preserves protein constituents by cross-linking them; the osmium tetroxide reacts with lipids, particularly phospholipids. The osmium also imparts electron density to cell and tissue structures because it is a heavy metal, thus enhancing subsequent image formation in the TEM.

Ideally, tissues should be perfused with buffered glutaraldehyde before excision from the animal. More commonly, tissue pieces no more than 1 mm³ are fixed for the TEM (as compared with light microscope specimens that may be measured in centimeters). The dehydration process is identical with that used in light microscopy, and the tissue is infiltrated with a monomeric resin, usually an epoxy resin, that is subsequently polymerized.

The Plastic-Embedded Tissue Is Sectioned on Specially Designed Microtomes Using *Diamond Knives*

Because of the limited penetrating power of electrons, sections for routine transmission electron microscopy range from 50 nm to no more than 150 nm. These sections are much too thin to handle; they are floated away from the knife edge on the surface of a fluid-filled trough and picked up from the surface onto plastic-coated copper mesh grids. The grids have 50–400 holes/inch or special slots for viewing serial sections.

For viewing in the TEM, the plastic need not be removed from the specimen; rather, it is essential to have it remain to impart structural stability to the extremely thin sections. The beam passes through the holes in the copper grid, then through the specimen, and the image is then focused on the viewing screen or photographic film.

Routine Staining of Transmission Electron Microscopy Sections Is Necessary to Increase the Inherent Contrast So That the Details of Cell Structure Are Readily Visible and Photographable

In general, staining of transmission electron microscopy sections is done by adding materials of great density, such as ions of heavy metals, to the specimen. Heavy-metal ions may be bound to the tissues during fixation or dehydration or by soaking the sections in solutions of such ions after sectioning. The osmium tetroxide routinely used in the fixative binds to the phospholipid components of membranes, imparting additional density to the membranes.

Uranyl nitrate is often added to the alcohol solutions used in dehydration in order to add density to components of cell junctions and other sites. Sequential soaking in solutions of uranyl acetate and lead citrate is routinely used to stain sections before viewing in the TEM. Although the chemistry of these reactions is still imperfectly understood, the empirically derived procedures allow the production of high-resolution, high-contrast electron micrographs.

SPECIAL STAINING OF TRANSMISSION ELECTRON MICROSCOPY SECTIONS

Many of the histochemical methods that are used in light microscopy have been adapted for electron microscopy. The use of the low-molecular-weight dialdehydes, particularly glutaraldehyde, as primary fixatives has allowed the application of many of the standard enzyme histochemical methods to tissue for TEM examination, often requiring only minor modifications of buffers and capture reagents. The phosphatase and esterase procedures have been very well adapted for the TEM. The reactions are usually run on 50-μm tissue slices that are subsequently fixed in osmium tetroxide and embedded for TEM sectioning (see Fig. 1.3).

Substitution of a heavy metal-containing compound for the fluorescent dye usually conjugated with an antibody has allowed adaptation of immunocytochemical methods to transmission electron microscopy, as has the adaptation of the diaminobenzidine-based peroxidase reaction. These have been particularly useful in elucidating the cellular sources and intracellular pathways of certain secretory products, the location on the cell surface of specific receptors, and the intracellular location of ingested drugs and substrates. Similarly, refinement of techniques has also allowed development of routine EM autoradiography as an investigative method (see Fig. 1.5b).

Freeze Fracture Is a Special Method of Sample Preparation for Transmission Electron Microscopy Especially Important in the Study of Membranes

The tissue to be examined may be fixed or unfixed; if it has been fixed, the fixative is washed out of the tissue before proceeding. A cryoprotectant, such as glycerol, is allowed to infiltrate the tissue, and the tissue is then rapidly frozen to about −160°C. Ice crystal formation is prevented by the use of cryoprotectants, rapid freezing, and extremely small tissue samples. Following this, the frozen tissue is then placed in vacuum in the freeze fracture apparatus and struck with a knife edge or razor blade.

The Fracture Plane Passes Preferentially Through the Hydrophobic Portion of the Plasma Membrane, Exposing the Interior of the Plasma Membrane

The resulting fracture of the plasma membrane produces two new surfaces. The surface of the membrane that is backed by extracellular space is called the **E-face;** the face that is backed by the protoplasm (cytoplasm) is called the **P-face.** The fractured tissue may be allowed to remain in the apparatus for a variable, but short period of time during which frozen water evaporates (sublimes), causing certain structural details of the inside of the plasma membrane to stand out in greater relief. The specimen is then coated, typically with evaporated platinum, to create a replica of the fracture surface. The tissue is then dissolved, and the surface replica, not the tissue itself, is picked up on grids to be examined with the TEM. Such a replica displays details at the macromolecular level (Fig. 2.6, page 24).

In Scanning Electron Microscopy, the Electron Beam Does Not Pass Through the Specimen but Is *Scanned* Across Its Surface

Scanning Electron Microscope. The SEM in many ways resembles more closely than the TEM the television tubes from which electron microscopy derived. For the examination of most tissues, the sample is fixed, dehydrated by critical point drying, coated with an evaporated gold-carbon film, mounted on an aluminum stub, and placed in the specimen chamber of the SEM. For mineralized tissues, it is possible to remove all the soft tissues with a bleach and then examine the structural features of the mineral.

The scanning is accomplished by the same type of raster that scans the electron beam across the face of a television tube. Electrons reflected from the surface (**backscattered electrons**) and electrons forced out of the surface (**secondary electrons**) are collected by one or more detectors and reprocessed to form a three-dimensional image on a high-resolution CRT (television tube).

Photographs may then be taken of the CRT to record data or the image may be recorded on videotape. Other detectors can be used to measure x-rays emitted from the surface, cathodoluminescence of molecules in the tissue below the surface, and Auger electrons emitted at the surface.

Many Microscopes Combine the Features of a Transmission Electron Microscope and Scanning Electron Microscope to Give a *Scanning-Transmission Electron Microscope* and Allow Electron Probe X-ray Microanalysis

The SEM configuration can be used to produce a transmission image by inserting a grid holder at the specimen level, collecting the transmitted electrons with a detector, and reconstructing the image on a CRT. This latter configuration of an SEM or scanning-transmission electron microscope (STEM) facilitates the use of the instrument for *electron probe x-ray microanalysis.*

Detectors can be fitted to the microscope to collect the x-rays emitted as the beam bombards the section, and with appropriate analyzers, a map can be constructed showing the distribution in the sections of elements having an atomic number greater than 12 and a concentration sufficient to produce enough x-rays to analyze. Semiquantitative data can also be derived for elements in sufficient concentration. Thus, both the TEM and the SEM can be converted into sophisticated analytical tools in addition to their uses as ''optical'' instruments.

High-Voltage Electron Microscopes Have Been Constructed That Have Accelerating Voltages Ranging From 500,000 to 1.2 Million Volts

High-voltage EMs (HVEMs) have been particularly useful in the examination of sections in the range of 0.25–0.5 μm, i.e., 3–5 times as thick as those used in the conventional TEM. Using stereo pairs of photographs, it has been possible to develop a better understanding of the three-dimensional structure of organelles and cell surfaces and to examine the relationships among the various cytoplasmic organelles.

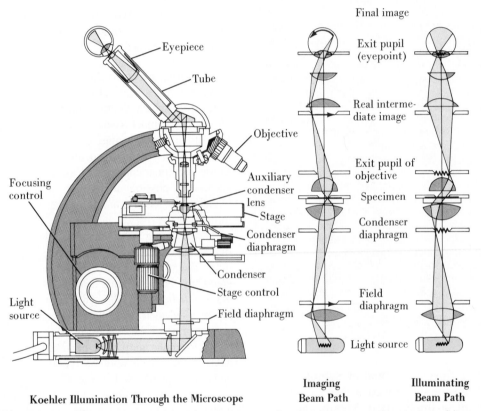

Figure 1.9.   Diagram of a modern light microscope showing a cross-sectional view of its operating components and light path. (Courtesy of Carl Zeiss, Inc., Thornwood, NY.)

PROPER USE OF THE LIGHT MICROSCOPE

This brief introduction to the proper use of the light microscope is directed to those students who will be using the microscope for the routine examination of tissues. If the following comments appear elementary, it is only because most users of the microscope fail to use it to its fullest advantage. Despite the availability of today's fine equipment, there is relatively little formal instruction on the correct use of the light microscope.

Expensive and highly corrected optics can perform optimally only when the illumination and observation beam paths are centered and properly adjusted. The use of proper settings and proper alignment of the optic pathway will contribute substantially to the recognition of minute details in the specimen and to the faithful display of color for the visual image and for photomicrography.

Köhler illumination is one key to good microscopy and is incorporated in the design of practically all modern laboratory and research microscopes. Figure 1.9 shows the two light paths and all the controls for alignment on a modern laboratory microscope and should be referred to in following the instructions given below to provide appropriate illumination in your microscope.

The alignment steps necessary to achieve good Köhler illumination are few and simple. They are

- Focus the specimen.
- Close the field diaphragm.
- Focus the condenser by moving it up or down until the outline of its field diaphragm appears in sharp focus.
- Center the field diaphragm with the centering controls on the (condenser) substage. Then, open the field diaphragm until it covers the full field observed.
- Remove the eyepiece (or use a centering telescope or a phase telescope accessory if available) and observe the exit pupil of the objective. You will see an illuminated circular field, the radius of which is directly proportional to the numerical aperture of the objective. As you close the condenser diaphragm, its outline will appear in this circular field. For most stained materials, set the condenser diaphragm to cover approximately two-thirds of the objective aperture. This setting results in the best compromise between resolution and contrast.

By using only these five simple steps, the image obtained will be as good as the optics allow. Now let us find out why.

Principles of Bright-field Microscopy

First, why do we adjust the field diaphragm to cover only the field observed? Illuminating a larger field than the optics can "see" only leads to internal reflections or stray light, resulting in more "noise" or a decrease in image contrast.

Second, why is there emphasis on the setting of the condenser diaphragm or, in other words, the illuminating aperture? This diaphragm greatly influences the resolution and the contrast with which specimen detail can be observed.

For most practical applications the resolution is determined by the equation

$$d = \frac{\lambda}{NA_{objective} + NA_{condenser}}$$

where

d = point-to-point distance of resolved detail (in nm)
λ = wavelength of light used (green = 540 nm)
NA = numerical aperture or sine of half angle picked up by the objective or condenser of a central specimen point multiplied by the refractive index of the medium between objective or condenser and specimen

How do wavelength and numerical aperture directly influence resolution? Specimen structures diffract light. The diffraction angle is directly proportional to the wavelength and inversely proportional to the spacing of the structures. According to Ernst Abbé, a given structural spacing can be resolved only when the observing optical system (objective) can see some of the diffracted light produced by the spacing. The larger the objective's aperture, the more diffracted light participates in the image formation, resulting in resolution of smaller detail and sharper images.

Our simple formula, however, shows that the condenser aperture is just as important as the objective aperture. This is only logical when you consider the diffraction angle for an oblique beam or one of higher aperture. This angle remains essentially constant but is presented to the objective in such a fashion that it can be picked up easily.

How does the aperture setting affect the contrast (contrast simply being the intensity difference between dark and light areas in the specimen)? The closest to the real contrast transfer from object to image theoretically would be obtained by the interaction (interference) between nondiffracted and all the diffracted wavefronts.

For the transfer of contrast between full transmission and complete absorption in a specimen, the intensity relationship between diffracted and nondiffracted light would have to be 1:1 in order to get full destructive interference (black) or full constructive interference (bright). When the condenser aperture matches the objective aperture, the nondiffracted light enters the objective with full intensity, but only part of the diffracted light can enter, resulting in decreased contrast. In other words, closing the aperture of the condenser to two-thirds of the objective aperture brings the intensity relationship between diffracted and nondiffracted light close to 1:1 and thereby optimizes the contrast. Closing the condenser aperture (or lowering the condenser) beyond this equilibrium will produce interference phenomena or image artifacts such as diffraction rings or lines around specimen structures. Most microscope techniques used for the enhancement of contrast, such as dark-field, oblique illumination, phase contrast, or modulation contrast, are based on the same principle; i.e., they suppress or reduce the intensity of the nondiffracted light to improve an inherently low specimen contrast.

By observing the steps outlined above and maintaining clean lenses, the quality and fidelity of visual images will vary only with the performance capability of the optical system.

The Cell

2

Cells Are the Basic Structural and Functional Units of All Multicellular Organisms

The processes we normally associate with the daily activities of organisms, such as protection, ingestion, digestion, absorption of metabolites, elimination of wastes, movement, reproduction, and even death, are all reflections of similar processes occurring within each of the billions of cells that constitute the human body. To a very large extent, similar mechanisms are used by cells of different types to synthesize protein, to transform energy, and to move essential substances into the cell; they utilize the same kinds of molecules to engage in contraction, and they duplicate their genetic material in the same manner.

Specific Functions Are Identified With Specific Structural Components and Domains Within the Cell

Some cells develop one or more of these functions to such a degree of specialization that they are identified by the function and the cell structures associated with it. For example, although all cells contain contractile filamentous proteins, some cells, such as *muscle cells,* contain large amounts of these proteins in specific arrays. This allows them to carry out their specialized function of contraction at both the cell and tissue level.

Most Cells Are Specialized (Differentiated) to Perform One or More Specific Activities With Great Efficiency

The specialized activity or function of a cell may be reflected not only by the presence of a larger amount of the specific structural component performing the activity but also by the shape of the cell, by its organization with respect to other similar cells, and by its products (Fig. 2.1).

The Purpose of This Chapter Is to Examine Those Structural Components Common to Virtually All Cells

Cells can be divided into two major compartments, the *cytoplasm* and the *nucleus.* The term *protoplasm* applies to both compartments. The cytoplasm and the nucleus not only manifest distinct functional roles but also work in concert to maintain the cell's viability as well as to contribute to the viability of the organism as a whole.

CYTOPLASM

The Cytoplasm Contains Organelles and Inclusions in a Cytoplasmic Matrix

The *organelles* or "little organs" include the membrane systems of the cell and the membrane-limited compartments that are responsible for the metabolic, synthetic, energy-requiring, and energy-generating functions of the cell, as well as nonmembranous structural components.

The *inclusions* are materials in the cytoplasm that may or may not be surrounded by a membrane. They comprise such diverse materials as secretory granules, pigment, neutral fat, glycogen, and stored waste products.

The cytoplasmic ground substance was called *cytosol* in older texts because it was believed to be an amorphous fluid. It is now termed *cytoplasmic matrix* to emphasize that it has an organized structure.

Intracellular Membranes Increase Surface Area and Delimit Compartments

Many of the organelles and inclusions are membrane-limited structures; i.e., they are surrounded by a membrane. The membranes form vesicular, tubular, and other structural patterns that may be convoluted (as in the case of the smooth-surfaced endoplasmic reticulum) or plicated (as in the case of the inner mitochondrial membrane). These convoluted and plicated membrane configurations provide an immense augmentation of surface within the cell. This is important because many essential physiologic and biochemical reactions occur on membranes.

Moreover, the spaces enclosed by membranes constitute intracellular microcompartments in which substrates, prod-

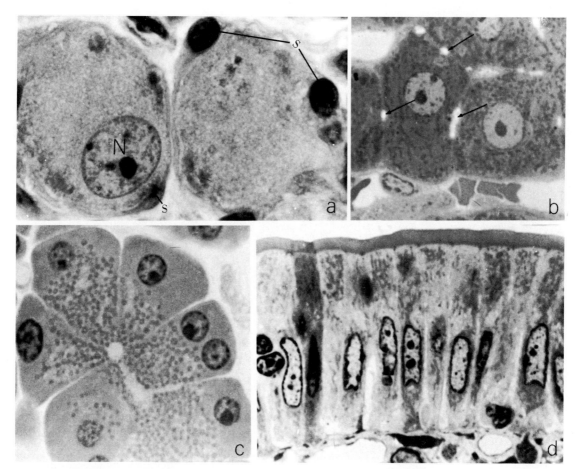

Figure 2.1. Photomicrographs of different cell types, each of which displays certain specific characteristics, such as size, shape, orientation, and cytoplasmic contents, that can be related to its specialized activity or function. All figures are from plastic-embedded specimens and are of the same magnification. **a.** Two ganglion cells. Note the large size of these cells and the large nucleus *(N),* compared with the surrounding satellite cells *(S)* and the cells seen in the other figures. The size of the ganglion cell reflects the extensive synthetic activity required in providing for the exceedingly long processes (axons) that these cells possess. **b.** Several liver cells. They are generally cuboidal in shape and exhibit small spaces or canaliculi *(arrows)* between neighboring cells into which they secrete bile. The small and very numerous dark bodies within the cell are mitochondria, a reflection of the liver cells' high metabolic activity. **c.** Acinus or secretory unit composed of pancreatic cells. Note how the cells here tend to have a pyramidal shape. The narrow apical end of the cell faces a lumen, created by the organization of the cells, into which enzyme precursors, the small granules within the cell, are emptied. The basal part of the cell (the part away from the lumen) is highly basophilic, reflecting the abundant RNA that is localized in this region of the cytoplasm. **d.** Tall (columnar) epithelial cells of the small intestine. The apical surface of these cells has minute cytoplasmic processes known as microvilli that when seen at the light microscope level appear as a dark band across the top of the cells. The processes greatly expand the apical surface area of the cell to facilitate absorption. (Fig. 2.2 provides a TEM of the apical part of one of these cells and shows to advantage the microvilli.)

ucts, or other substances can be segregated or concentrated. For example, the enzymes of lysosomes are separated by a membrane from the cytoplasmic matrix because their hydrolytic activity would be detrimental to the cell.

Organelles Are Described as Membranous (Membrane-Limited) and Nonmembranous

The membranous organelles include

- *Plasma* (cell) *membrane*
- *Rough-surfaced endoplasmic reticulum (rER)*
- *Smooth-surfaced endoplasmic reticulum (sER)*
- *Golgi apparatus*
- *Mitochondria*
- *Lysosomes* (and their derivatives)
- *Endosomes*
- *Peroxisomes*

The nonmembranous organelles include

- *Microtubules*
- *Filaments* (of various varieties)
- *Centrioles* (and their derivatives)
- *Ribosomes* (both those attached to membranes of the rER and those free in the cytoplasm)

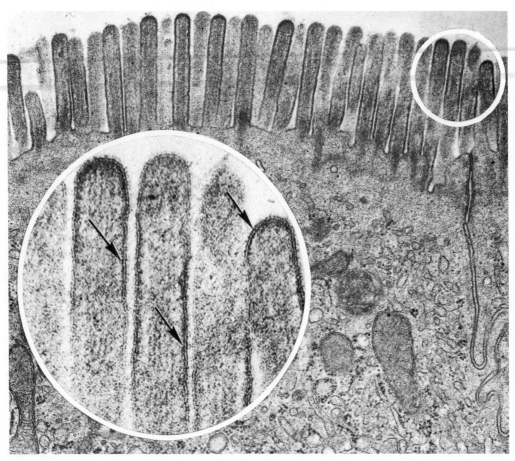

Figure 2.2. Electron micrograph of the apical portion of an absorptive cell of the small intestine. The **inset** is a higher magnification (×95,000) of the area within the *circle.* Note that at this magnification the plasma membrane appears as a trilaminar structure *(arrows);* i.e., there are two electron-dense lines separated by a clear or electron-lucent intermediate layer.

Microtubules and filaments form elements of the *cytoskeleton,* a semipermanent structural scaffolding in the cytoplasmic matrix.

Plasma Membrane

The plasma membrane (cell membrane) is not visible with the light microscope. Even when the light microscope was the only optical tool of the cytologist, however, it was known that some boundary structure enclosed the cell and that the integrity of this boundary structure was essential to the integrity of the cell. It is now clear that the plasma membrane actively participates in many physiologic and biochemical activities essential to cell function and survival.

The Plasma Membrane Has a Trilaminar Appearance in Transmission Electron Microscopy

Although the plasma membrane is usually drawn in diagrams as a single line, when it is properly fixed, sectioned, stained, and viewed on edge with the transmission electron microscope (TEM), the plasma membrane displays a characteristic trilaminar appearance that has been designated as the *unit membrane.* The components referred to by the designation trilaminar are

- An outer electron-dense layer
- An inner electron-dense layer
- An intermediate, electron-lucent or nonstaining layer (Fig. 2.2)

The total thickness of the plasma membrane is about 8–10 nm. On its outer surface, the plasma membrane has a coat consisting of high-density carbohydrates that are covalently linked[1] to proteins and lipids in the membrane.

The Plasma Membrane Is a Fluid and Dynamic System, Not a Static Structure

The current interpretation of how the plasma membrane is organized at the molecular level, referred to as the *mod-*

---

[1]Covalent bonds, i.e., bonds in which electrons are shared by adjacent atoms in a molecule, are the strongest bonds in biologic systems. Such bonds are used to make large, complex molecules from simpler precursor molecules. For example, the covalent bonding of a complex carbohydrate to a protein or a lipid creates a glycoprotein or glycolipid, respectively. Enzymatic activity is usually needed to disrupt these bonds. Weaker bonds that occur in biologic systems include electrostatic bonds, as in salts (Na^+Cl^-), and hydrogen bonds, which play an essential role in establishing the final three-dimensional molecular structure of proteins.

ified fluid-mosaic model, is shown in Figure 2.3. The membrane consists primarily of *phospholipid, cholesterol,* and *protein* molecules. The lipid molecules form a bilayer with their fatty acid chains facing each other, thereby making the inner portion of the membrane hydrophobic (i.e., having no affinity for water). The surfaces of the membrane are formed by the polar head groups of the lipid molecules, thereby making the surfaces hydrophilic (i.e., having an affinity for water).

Hydrophobic regions of proteins extend through or partially through the lipid bilayer as *integral proteins* of the membrane. On the extracellular surface of the plasma membrane, carbohydrate is attached to protein, thereby forming a glycoprotein, or to lipids of the bilayer, thereby forming a glycolipid. These surface molecules constitute a layer at the surface of the cell, referred to as the *cell coat* or *glycocalyx* (Fig. 2.4). They contribute to the establishment of extracellular microenvironments at the membrane surface that have specific functions in metabolism, cell recognition, and cell association and as receptor sites for hormones.

Integral Membrane Proteins Are Made Visible With the Special Tissue Preparation Technique of Freeze Fracture

Confirmation of the existence of protein within the substance of the plasma membrane, i.e., integral proteins, came from freeze fracture studies. When tissue is prepared for electron microscopy by the freeze fracture process (Fig. 2.5*a*), membranes typically split or cleave along the hydrophobic plane, i.e., between the two lipid layers, to expose two interior faces of the membrane, an E-face and a P-face (Fig. 2.5*b*).

The *E-face* is backed by *e*xtracellular space, whereas the *P-face* is backed by *p*rotoplasm. The numerous particles seen on the E- and P-faces with the TEM represent the integral protein of the membrane. Usually, the P-face displays more particles, thus more protein, than the E-face (Fig. 2.6).

Integral Membrane Proteins Have Important Functions in Cell Metabolism, Regulation, and Integration

Six broad categories of membrane proteins have been defined in terms of their function. These are pumps, channels, receptors, enzymes, transducers, and structural proteins. The categories are not mutually exclusive; e.g., a structural membrane protein might simultaneously serve as a receptor, an enzyme, a pump, or any combination of these functions.

- *Pumps* serve to transport certain ions, such as Na$^+$ actively across membranes. Pumps also transport metabolic precursors of macromolecules such as amino acids

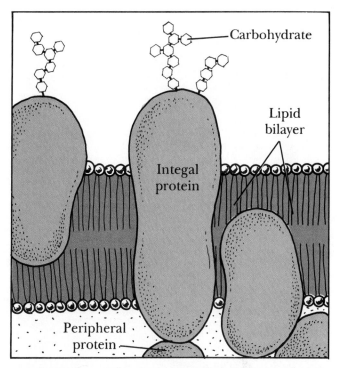

Figure 2.3. Diagram of a plasma membrane showing lipid molecules forming a bilayer. The fatty acid chains in each layer face each other. The polar heads of the lipid molecules form the outer and inner surfaces of the membrane. The integral proteins are inserted in the membrane. Some extend entirely through the membrane, whereas others are restricted to the internal or external domain of the membrane. Most integral proteins that extend through the outer domain of the membrane have carbohydrate molecules attached.

and sugars across membranes either by themselves or linked to the Na$^+$ pump.

- *Channels* allow for the passage of small ions and molecules across the plasma membrane in either direction, i.e., passive diffusion. Gap junctions (described below) are formed by aligned channels in the membranes of adjacent cells that permit passage of ions and small molecules from the cytoplasm of one cell to the cytoplasm of the other cell.

- *Receptor proteins* allow for the recognition and localized binding of substances to the outer surface of the plasma membrane in such processes as hormonal stimulation, coated vesicle endocytosis, and antibody reactions.

- *Transducers* are involved in the coupling of membrane receptors to cytoplasmic enzymes following the binding of a *ligand,* such as a hormone, to the receptor. (The term *ligand* refers to any molecule that binds to a receptor on the surface of a cell; some ligands, such as hormones, serve as messenger molecules.) Through the action of a transducer, an enzyme may activate the formation of a second messenger, such as cyclic adenosine monophosphate (cAMP), in the cytoplasm.

- *Enzymes,* particularly adenosine triphosphatases

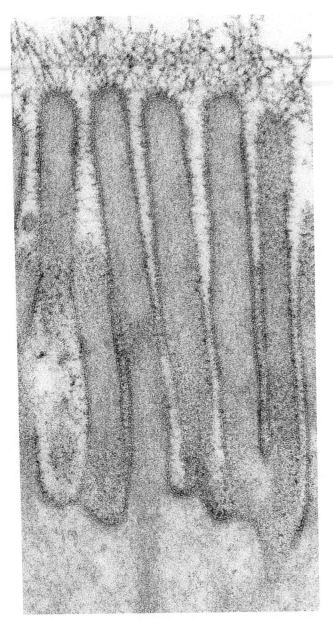

Figure 2.4. Electron micrograph of microvilli on the apical surface of an absorptive cell in the rat colon. The glycoproteins of the glycocalyx can be seen extending from the tips of the microvilli into the lumen. At this magnification, the relationship between the outer plasma membrane leaflet and the glycocalyx is particularly well demonstrated. Glycoproteins of the glycocalyx include terminal digestive enzymes such as dipeptidases and disaccharidases. ×100,000. (Courtesy of Dr. Ray C. Henrikson.)

(ATPases), that have specific roles in ion pumping and digestive enzymes such as disaccharidases and dipeptidases are integral membrane proteins.

- *Structural proteins* have been visualized specifically by the freeze fracture method, especially where they form junctions with neighboring cells. Often, certain proteins and lipids are concentrated in localized regions of the plasma membrane to carry out specific functions. Ex-

amples of such regions can be recognized in polarized cells such as those of epithelia.

Integral Membrane Proteins Move Within the Lipid Bilayer of the Membrane

The fluidity of the plasma membrane is not revealed in static electron micrographs of cells. Experiments, however, reveal that the membrane behaves as though it were a two-dimensional lipid fluid. Proteins with their hydrophobic regions localized in the interior of the lipid bilayer are free to diffuse laterally.

Particles bound to the membrane can be shown to move on the surface of a cell; even integral membrane proteins, such as enzymes, may be shown to move from one surface of a cell to another, e.g., from apical to lateral, when barriers to flow, such as cell junctions (see page 59), are disrupted. The fluidity of the membrane is a function of the types of phospholipids in the membrane and of variations in the local concentration of those phospholipids.

Movement of integral membrane proteins may occur in order for these protein molecules to mediate a hormone response (as receptors are coupled with transducers) or for them to sort (or move) to a different region of the plasma membrane. It is important to recognize that the lateral diffusion of proteins is often limited by physical connections between membrane proteins and intracellular or extracellular structures. Such connections may exist

- Between proteins associated with cytoskeletal filaments of the cell and the portions of the membrane proteins that extend into the adjacent cytoplasm
- Between the cytoplasmic domains of membrane proteins
- Between proteins associated with the extracellular matrix and the portions of the membrane proteins that extend from the surface of the cell, i.e., the extracellular domain

By these mechanisms, proteins can be localized or restricted to specific "specialized" regions of the plasma membrane or act as transmembrane linkers between intracellular and extracellular filaments (see below).

Any Substance That Enters or Leaves the Cell Must Pass the Barrier of the Plasma Membrane

Some substances cross the plasma membrane by *diffusion* down their concentration gradient; others, by *active transport* against their concentration gradient. Some substances enter and leave cells by processes that involve configurational changes in the plasma membrane at localized sites, namely, *vesicular transport*. This activity involves the formation of vesicles from the membrane or the fusion of vesicles with the membrane (Fig. 2.7). Vesicular transport, in its various modes, may be defined in more specific terms:

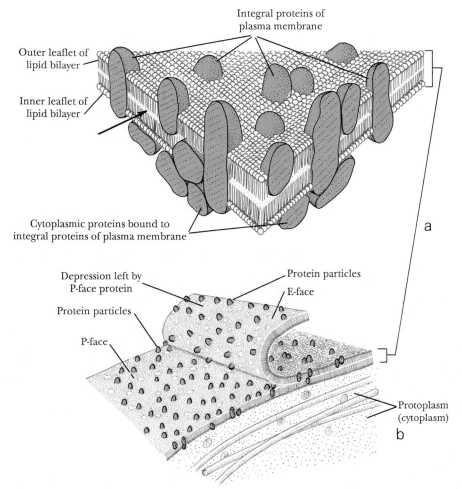

Integral proteins of
plasma membrane

Outer leaflet of
lipid bilayer

Inner leaflet of
lipid bilayer

Cytoplasmic proteins bound to
integral proteins of plasma membrane

a

Depression left by
P-face protein

Protein particles

P-face

Protein particles

E-face

Protoplasm
(cytoplasm)

b

Figure 2.5. Diagram showing where cleavage occurs in *freeze fracture* of a plasma membrane. **a.** View of plasma membrane seen on edge with *arrow* indicating preferential split of lipid bilayer along the hydrophobic plane of the membrane. Some proteins are carried with the outer leaflet; most proteins are retained within the inner leaflet. **b.** View of plasma membrane with the leaflets separating along the cleavage plane. Before examination with the TEM, the surfaces are coated, forming replicas; the replicas are separated from the tissue and examined in the electron microscope. Proteins appear as bumps. The replica of the inner leaflet is called the P-face; it is backed by protoplasm. A view of the outer leaflet is called the E-face; it is backed by extracellular space.

- *Endocytosis* is the name given to the process of vesicular transport when it involves substances entering the cell.
- *Exocytosis* is the name given to the process of vesicular transport when it involves substances leaving the cell.

Both processes can be visualized with the electron microscope.

Two forms of endocytosis are recognized:

- *Phagocytosis* (Gr. for cell eating) is the ingestion of particulate matter, including bacteria and other cells.
- *Pinocytosis* (Gr. for cell drinking) is the ingestion of substances initially in molecular dispersion and the ingestion of bulk fluid stimulated by ionic changes. Two forms of pinocytosis are recognized with the TEM. In one form, smooth *pinocytotic vesicles* are produced; in the other form, *coated vesicles* are produced.

Pinocytotic Vesicles Form by Invagination of the Plasma Membrane

The plasma membrane invaginates to form small pits or *caveolae* that project into the cell. The opening of the pit constricts into a narrow neck, and further constriction results in the separation of a vesicle from the membrane. These smooth pinocytotic vesicles are especially numerous in the endothelium of blood vessels (see Figs. 12.5 and 12.9, pages 308 and 313) and under the plasma membrane of smooth muscle cells but are present in nearly every cell type.

The formation of coated vesicles is similar except that the plasma membrane acquires a localized concentration of short bristle-like projections on its inner surface where the vesicle is to form. In the formation of vesicles by this method, the coated membrane first forms a depression, then a small pit; finally, the coated pit pinches off to become a *coated vesicle.*

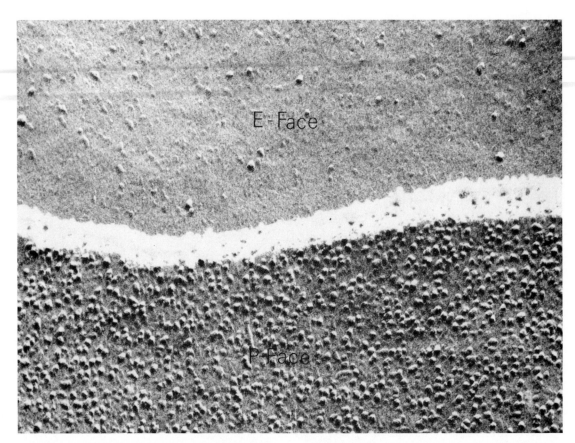

Figure 2.6. Electron micrograph of a freeze-fracture replica showing the E-face of the membrane of one epithelial cell and the P-face of the membrane of the adjoining cell. The cleavage plane has jumped from the membrane of one cell to the membrane of the other cell as indicated by the clear space (intercellular space) across the middle of the figure. Note the paucity of particles in the E-face compared with the P-face from which the majority of the globular proteins project. (Courtesy of Dr. G. Raviola.)

Coated Vesicles Participate in a Selective Process of Absorption Referred to as *Receptor-Mediated Endocytosis*

In receptor-mediated endocytosis, certain molecules within the plasma membrane recognize and bind specific substances that come in contact with the plasma membrane. Smooth pinocytotic vesicles, by contrast, are relatively nonselective. Modification of the environment of the membrane, such as ionic changes, and nonspecific binding of charged particles to the glycocalyx, however, can stimulate pinocytosis.

Exocytosis Is the Process by Which a Vesicle Moves From the Cytoplasm to the Plasma Membrane Where It Discharges Its Contents to the Extracellular Space

There are two general pathways of exocytosis:

- Constitutive pathway
- Regulated secretory pathway

The *constitutive pathway* identifies a process that is continuous. Proteins that leave the cell by this process are secreted immediately after their synthesis and exit from the Golgi apparatus, as seen in the secretion of immunoglobulins by plasma cells and of tropocollagen by fibroblasts (pages 114 and 101). Proteins that are concentrated and transiently stored in secretory granules pass along the *regulated secretory pathway*. In this case, a regulatory event must be activated for secretion to occur, as in the release of zymogen granules by chief cells of the gastric mucosa and by acinar cells of the pancreas (pages 449 and 514).

The membrane that is added to the plasma membrane by exocytosis is recovered into the cytoplasmic compartment by an endocytic process.

Modified Portions of the Plasma Membrane Allow Adjacent Cells to Interact

Cell Junctions. The junctions that bind cells to one another to form tissues are described in Chapter 4, Epithelial Tissue. Junctions that allow the cytoplasmic compartments of adjacent cells to communicate are special adaptations of *membrane channels* and are called *gap junctions*.

Organized Concentrations of Integral Membrane Proteins Form the Gap Junctions

Gap Junctions. Membrane channels are particularly important in nerve cells and in cells engaged in fluid and

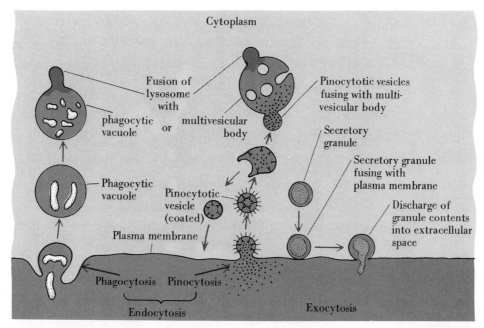

Figure 2.7. Endocytosis (phagocytosis and pinocytosis) and exocytosis. Both phagocytosis and pinocytosis are mechanisms whereby substances are brought into the cell. Phagocytosis involves the ingestion of particulate substances. The particles make contact with the outer surface of the membrane. The plasma membrane may partially enclose or envelop the particles; then the membrane and particles are internalized by the cell. Finally, the invaginated membrane becomes pinched off from the plasma membrane; it is then a phagocytic vacuole. Pinocytosis involves the ingestion of non-particulate substances (e.g., molecules in solution). Again, contact is made with the outer surface of the plasma membrane; it becomes indented, and finally, the invaginated portion of the membrane pinches off from the membrane to become a pinocytotic vesicle within the cell. Exocytosis is the discharge of a substance from the cell. The illustration shows a secretory granule surrounded by a membrane. This membrane makes contact and fuses with the inner surface of the plasma membrane. The fused region then opens, allowing the contents of the secretory granule to escape from the cell.

electrolyte transport. The **gap junction** is a concentration of such channels in an organized array that allows communication between adjacent cells; it bridges the space or gap between the cells.

Various experiments have been used to study gap junctions, including the injection of dyes, radiolabeled compounds, or electric current into cells and the measurement of these probes in adjacent cells. In the dye studies, a fluorescent dye is injected with a micropipette into one cell of an epithelial sheet. The readily visualized dye can be seen to pass to the immediately adjacent cells. Experiments of this sort have led to the conclusion that adjacent cells share communicating channels that allow small molecules and ions to pass directly between cells without entering the extracellular space.

Gap Junctions Reduce Resistance to Passage of Electric Current Between Adjacent Cells

Electrical conductance studies of gap junctions involve the introduction of microelectrodes into neighboring cells and the establishment of a voltage difference between the electrodes. Current flow between the cells is then measured. If there are no gap junctions between the neighboring cells, the current flow is low, primarily due to the high electrical resistance of the plasma membranes. In contrast, if neighboring cells are joined together by gap junctions,

there is little electrical resistance between them, and current flow is high. The low resistance is a reflection of the direct cytoplasmic continuity between the two cells due to the presence of the gap junctions, which are, therefore, also called **low-resistance junctions.** Such junctions are present in a wide variety of tissues to allow coordinated activity in neighboring cells. Examples are readily found in epithelia, smooth and cardiac muscle, and certain connective tissues, as well as nerve.

Gap Junctions Can Be Visualized in Transmission Electron Microscope Sections and Freeze Fracture Preparations

When viewed with the TEM, the gap junction appears as an area of contact between the plasma membranes of adjacent cells (Fig. 2.8a). With the application of uranyl acetate as a "stain" before embedding of the tissue **(en bloc staining),** a gap junction appears as two parallel, closely apposed plasma membranes separated by a gap of 2 nm.

Freeze fracture images of the plasma membrane in the region of the gap junction show groups of 2-nm channels formed by the apposition of identical structures in the facing membranes, specifically a set of six circularly arranged integral membrane proteins with a central 2-nm opening. This structure is a **connexon.** Each channel is composed of two connexons, with one belonging to each cell. Many such

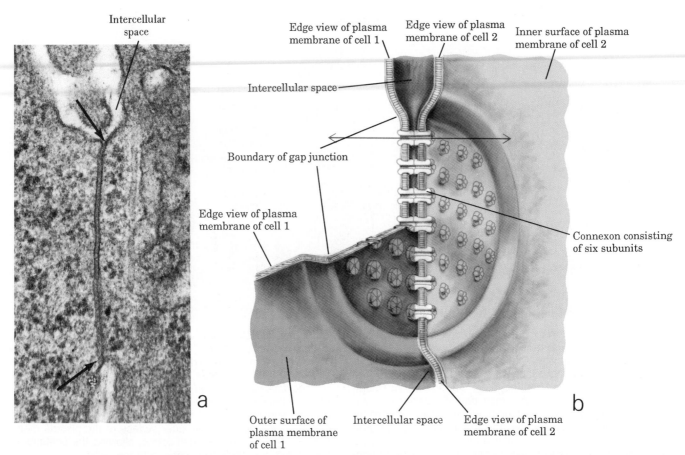

Figure 2.8.   a. Electron micrograph showing the plasma membranes of two adjoining cells forming a gap junction. The unit membranes *(arrows)* approach one another (note *top* and *bottom* of micrograph) narrowing the intercellular space to produce a 2-nm-wide gap. **b.** Model of a gap junction showing the membranes of adjoining cells creating the 2-nm gap and the structural components of the membrane that form channels or passageways between the two cells *(double-headed arrow).* Each passageway is formed by a circular array of six subunits, dumbbell-shaped particles that span the membrane of each cell. These complexes, called connexons, have a central opening of about 2 nm in diameter. The channels formed by the registering of the adjacent complementary pairs of connexons permit the flow of small molecules through the channels but not into the intercellular space. Conversely, substances in the intercellular space can permeate the area of a gap junction by flowing around the connexon complexes but cannot enter into the channels. (Redrawn from Staehelin LA, Hull BE: Junctions between living cells. *Scientific American,* 238:41, 1978.)

channels are closely packed at the site of the gap junction (Fig. 2.8*b*).

The Plasma Membrane Is Both a Dynamic Structure and a Boundary Structure

The plasma membrane participates in the functional and metabolic activities of the cell. It serves as both a selective and a nonselective barrier between the inside and the outside of the cell, allowing the cell to maintain an internal environment distinctly different from the external environment. Portions of the plasma membrane continuously turn over; membrane leaves the cell surface as the membranes of endocytic vesicles. Membrane is added to the cell surface by fusion of exocytic vesicles with the plasma membrane. Finally, as is discussed in detail in Chapter 4, the plasma membrane participates in the formation of several other types of intercellular junctions, namely, adhering junctions and tight junctions.

Rough-Surfaced Endoplasmic Reticulum

The Protein Synthetic System of the Cell Consists of Rough-Surfaced Endoplasmic Reticulum and Ribosomes

The cytoplasm of a variety of cells engaged chiefly in protein synthesis stains intensely with basic dyes. The basophilic staining is due to the presence of RNA. That portion of the cytoplasm that stains with the basic dye is called **ergastoplasm.** The ergastoplasm in secretory cells, e.g., pancreatic acinar cells, is the light microscopic image of the organelle called the **rough-surfaced endoplasmic reticulum** or **rER.**

In the TEM, the rER appears as a series of interconnected, membrane-limited flattened sacs called **cisternae,** with particles studding the exterior surface of the membrane (Fig. 2.9). The particles, called **ribosomes,** measure

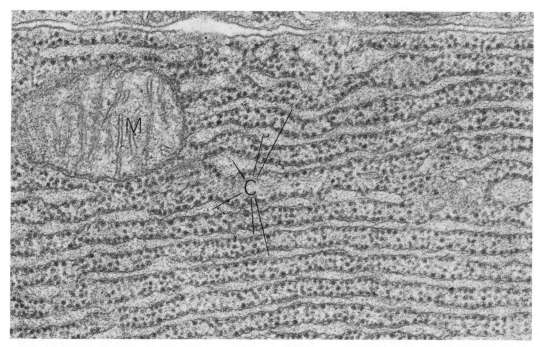

Figure 2.9. Electron micrograph showing the rER in a chief cell of the stomach. Note the cisternae *(C)* are closely packed in parallel arrays. Each is bounded by a ribosome-studded membrane. *M,* mitochondrion. ×50,000.

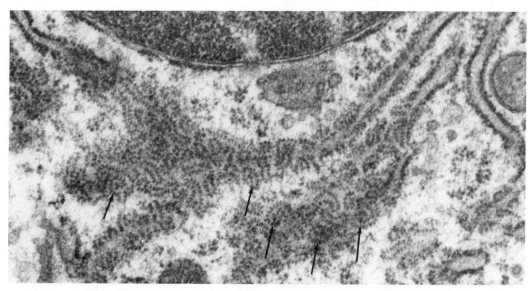

Figure 2.10. Fortuitous section showing the rER in two planes. The reticulum has turned within the section. Thus, in the upper right and left of the electron micrograph, the membranes of the reticulum have been cut at a right angle to their surface. In the center, the reticulum has twisted and is seen as though one were looking down on the surface of the membrane. Viewed in this aspect, it becomes evident that most of the ribosomes are arranged in a spiral configuration on the membrane *(arrows).* ×38,000.

15–20 nm in diameter and contain RNA and protein. In many instances, the rER is continuous with the outer membrane of the nuclear envelope (see below). Groups of ribosomes form short spiral arrays called *polyribosomes* or *polysomes* (Fig. 2.10), in which many ribosomes are attached to a thread of *messenger RNA (mRNA).*

Copying the Genetic Message from DNA to Messenger RNA Is Called *Transcription;* Reading the Message in Messenger RNA to Synthesize Polypeptides Is Called *Translation*

mRNA is synthesized (transcribed) in the *nucleolus* (see page 48) and travels from the nucleus to the cytoplasm through *nuclear pores*. The mRNA attaches to the polysomes that then translate the genetic message carried in the mRNA into a sequence of amino acids that are linked to form a polypeptide, the basic building block of proteins. All mRNA initially attaches to free ribosomes in the cytoplasm to form polysomes.

If the protein to be synthesized is one that will be exported or will become part of the plasma membrane, the first group of amino acids that are linked to one another form a *signal peptide* (signal sequence) that will bind to a receptor on the membrane of the rER (Fig. 2.11). When the ribosome (polysome) binds to the rER membrane, the signal peptide or a subsequent sequence instructs the newly formed peptide to pass through the membrane into the lumen of the rER cistern. For simple secretory proteins, the polypeptide continues to be inserted into the lumen as it is synthesized (Fig. 2.11). For integral membrane proteins, sequences along the polypeptide may instruct the forming protein to pass back and forth through the membrane, creating the functional domains that the protein will exhibit at its final membrane site.

Polysomes of the Rough-Surfaced Endoplasmic Reticulum Synthesize Proteins for Export From the Cell and Integral Proteins of the Plasma Membrane

As polypeptide chains are synthesized by the membrane-bound polysomes, the protein is injected into the lumen of the cistern, where it may be further modified, concentrated, or carried to another part of the cell in the continuous channels of the rER. The rER is particularly well developed in those cells that are making protein destined to leave the cell as well as in cells with very large amounts of plasma membrane, such as nerve cells. The secretory cells include glandular cells, fibroblasts, plasma cells, odontoblasts, ameloblasts, and osteoblasts. The rER is not limited, however, to secretory cells and neurons. Virtually every cell of the body contains profiles of rER, but they may be few in number, a reflection of the degree of protein secretion, and dispersed so that with the light microscope they are not evident as areas of basophilia.

In agreement with the observation that the rER is most highly developed in active secretory cells, secretory proteins are exclusively synthesized by the ribosomes of the rER. In all cells, however, proteins that are to become permanent components of the lysosome, Golgi apparatus, rER, or nuclear envelope (these structures are discussed below) or integral components of the plasma membrane are also synthesized on the ribosomes of the rER.

Secretory Proteins Pass Through the Membrane of the Rough-Surfaced Endoplasmic Reticulum to Its Lumen, Where They May Be Modified and Stored

Proteins destined for secretion are unique in that they have a hydrophobic signal domain or region of the molecule at their initial forming end (Fig. 2.11). The signal domain of the forming protein induces its receptor-mediated attachment to the membrane of the rER and then the insertion of the protein into and through the membrane as it is being synthesized. This is referred to as *contranslational insertion* of protein into the rER cisternae. If the forming protein is not to be threaded in its entirety through the membrane, a new hydrophobic domain will stop the threading process and cause the protein to be anchored permanently in the membrane at this site.

On completion of protein synthesis, the ribosome detaches from the rER membrane and is again free in the cytoplasm. The region of the newly formed protein that extends into the lumen of the rER is exposed to modification by enzymes present there. For example, most proteins receive an oligosaccharide transferred from a lipid donor to the amide N of certain asparagine residues (thus referred to as N-linked oligosaccharide). The initial hydrophobic domain is usually cleaved by a protease. Disulfide bonds and internal hydrogen bonds are established to achieve the correct three-dimensional conformation of the molecule.

Except for those few proteins that remain permanent residents of the rER membranes and those proteins secreted by the constitutive pathway, the newly synthesized proteins are normally delivered to the Golgi apparatus within minutes. In some cells in which the constitutive pathway is dominant, namely, plasma cells and developing fibroblasts, newly synthesized protein may accumulate in the rER cisternae, causing their engorgement and distension.

"Free" Ribosomes Synthesize Proteins That Will Remain in the Cell as Cytoplasmic Structural or Functional Elements

Cytoplasmic basophilia is also associated with cells that are producing large amounts of protein that will remain in the cell. Such cells and their products include developing red blood cells (hemoglobin), developing muscle cells (the contractile proteins actin and myosin), nerve cells (neurofilaments), and keratinocytes of the skin (keratin). In addition, most enzymes of the mitochondrion are synthesized by free polysomes and transferred into that organelle.

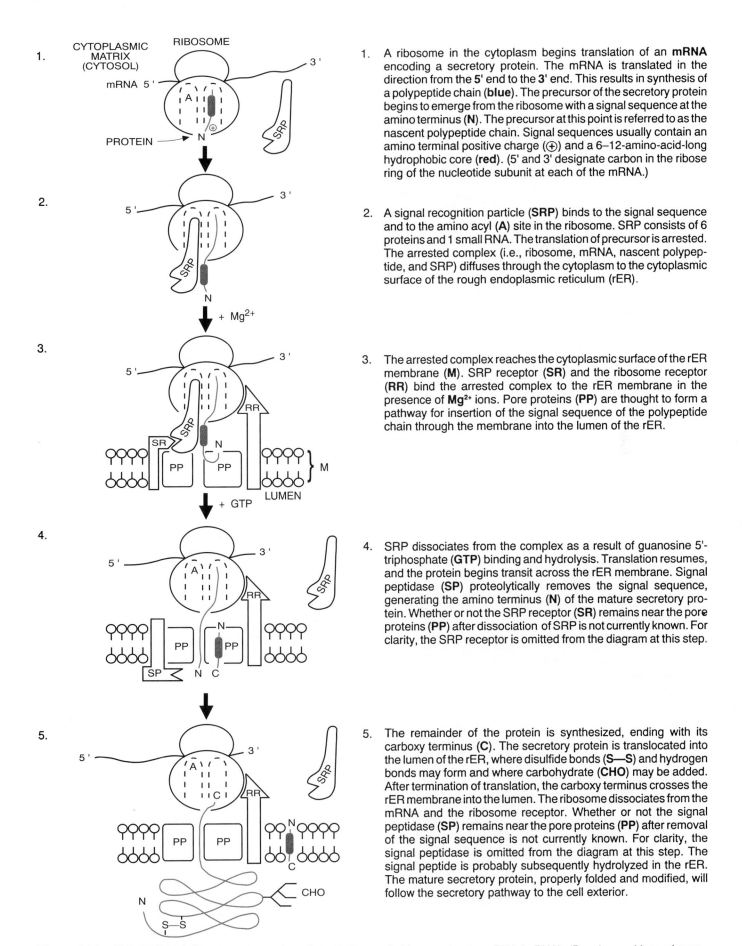

1. A ribosome in the cytoplasm begins translation of an **mRNA** encoding a secretory protein. The mRNA is translated in the direction from the **5'** end to the **3'** end. This results in synthesis of a polypeptide chain (**blue**). The precursor of the secretory protein begins to emerge from the ribosome with a signal sequence at the amino terminus (**N**). The precursor at this point is referred to as the nascent polypeptide chain. Signal sequences usually contain an amino terminal positive charge (⊕) and a 6–12-amino-acid-long hydrophobic core (**red**). (5' and 3' designate carbon in the ribose ring of the nucleotide subunit at each of the mRNA.)

2. A signal recognition particle (**SRP**) binds to the signal sequence and to the amino acyl (**A**) site in the ribosome. SRP consists of 6 proteins and 1 small RNA. The translation of precursor is arrested. The arrested complex (i.e., ribosome, mRNA, nascent polypeptide, and SRP) diffuses through the cytoplasm to the cytoplasmic surface of the rough endoplasmic reticulum (rER).

3. The arrested complex reaches the cytoplasmic surface of the rER membrane (**M**). SRP receptor (**SR**) and the ribosome receptor (**RR**) bind the arrested complex to the rER membrane in the presence of **Mg²⁺** ions. Pore proteins (**PP**) are thought to form a pathway for insertion of the signal sequence of the polypeptide chain through the membrane into the lumen of the rER.

4. SRP dissociates from the complex as a result of guanosine 5'-triphosphate (**GTP**) binding and hydrolysis. Translation resumes, and the protein begins transit across the rER membrane. Signal peptidase (**SP**) proteolytically removes the signal sequence, generating the amino terminus (**N**) of the mature secretory protein. Whether or not the SRP receptor (**SR**) remains near the pore proteins (**PP**) after dissociation of SRP is not currently known. For clarity, the SRP receptor is omitted from the diagram at this step.

5. The remainder of the protein is synthesized, ending with its carboxy terminus (**C**). The secretory protein is translocated into the lumen of the rER, where disulfide bonds (**S—S**) and hydrogen bonds may form and where carbohydrate (**CHO**) may be added. After termination of translation, the carboxy terminus crosses the rER membrane into the lumen. The ribosome dissociates from the mRNA and the ribosome receptor. Whether or not the signal peptidase (**SP**) remains near the pore proteins (**PP**) after removal of the signal sequence is not currently known. For clarity, the signal peptidase is omitted from the diagram at this step. The signal peptide is probably subsequently hydrolyzed in the rER. The mature secretory protein, properly folded and modified, will follow the secretory pathway to the cell exterior.

Figure 2.11. This series of diagrams summarizes the events that occur during the translation of the genetic information carried by a messenger RNA (mRNA). (Drawing and legend courtesy of Dr. John P. Aris.)

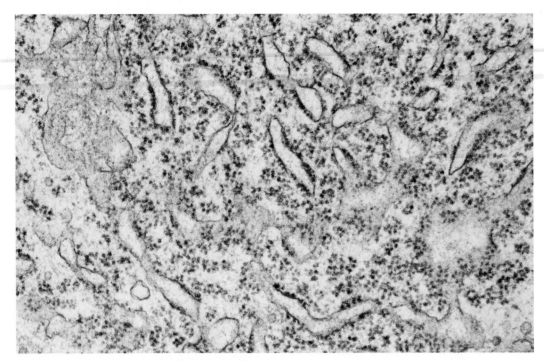

Figure 2.12. Electron micrograph of a nerve cell body showing profiles of endoplasmic reticulum with attached ribosomes. The cytoplasm between the reticulum contains numerous free ribosomes. Collectively, the free ribosomes and membrane-attached ribosomes are responsible for the cytoplasmic basophilia observed with the light microscope. ×45,000.

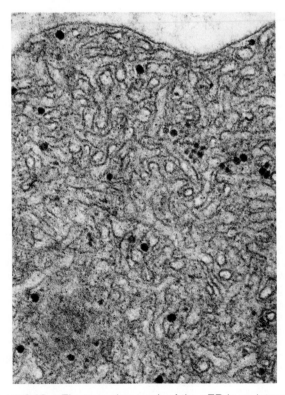

Figure 2.13. Electron micrograph of the sER in an interstitial cell of the testis. The reticulum seen here is a complex system of anastomosing tubules. The small dense objects are glycogen particles. ×60,000.

Basophilia in these cells was also called ergastoplasm and is due to the presence of large amounts of RNA. In this case, the ribosomes and polysomes are "free" in the cytoplasm; i.e., they are not attached to membranes of the endoplasmic reticulum. The large basophilic bodies of nerve cells, called Nissl bodies, consist of both rER and large numbers of free ribosomes (Fig. 2.12). All ribosomes contain RNA; it is the phosphate groups of the RNA of the ribosomes, not the membranous component of the endoplasmic reticulum, that accounts for basophilic staining of the cytoplasm.

Smooth-Surfaced Endoplasmic Reticulum

Smooth-Surfaced Endoplasmic Reticulum Consists of Short Anastomosing Tubules That Are Not Associated With Ribosomes

Cells with large amounts of sER may exhibit distinct cytoplasmic acidophilia (eosinophilia) or may appear empty when viewed with the light microscope. The sER is well developed in cells that synthesize and secrete steroids, such as adrenal cortical cells and testicular interstitial cells (Fig. 2.13). In skeletal and cardiac muscle, where it is also called sarcoplasmic reticulum, the sER segregates calcium ions that are essential in the contractile process and is closely apposed to the plasma membrane invaginations that conduct the contractile impulse to the interior of the cell.

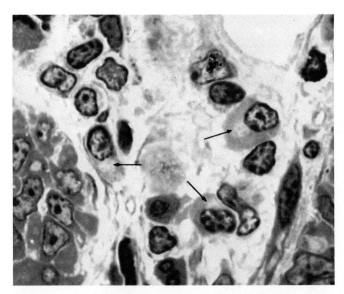

Figure 2.14. Light micrograph of a plastic-embedded specimen from the intestine, stained with toluidine blue. The plasma cells, where appropriately oriented, exhibit a clear area in the cytoplasm (i.e., are negatively stained) that represents the Golgi area. The surrounding cytoplasm is deeply stained due to the presence of the ribosomes associated with the extensive rER. ×1200.

Smooth-Surfaced Endoplasmic Reticulum Is the Principal Organelle Involved in Detoxification of Drugs and Conjugation of Other Noxious Substances

The sER is particularly well developed in the liver. The degree to which the liver may be involved in detoxification at any given time may be estimated by the amount of sER present in liver cells. The sER is also involved in

- *Lipid absorption and metabolism*
- *Glycogen metabolism*
- *Membrane formation and recycling*

Because of these widely disparate functions, numerous enzymes, including hydrolases, methylases, glucose-6-phosphatase, Ca^{2+}-ATPase, and lipid oxidases are associated with the sER.

Golgi Apparatus

The Golgi Apparatus Functions in the Posttranslational Modification, Packaging, and Sorting of Proteins Secreted by the Cell

The Golgi apparatus was described more than 100 years ago by Camillo Golgi. In studies of osmium-impregnated nerve cells, he discovered an organelle that formed networks around the nucleus. It was also described as well developed in secretory cells. Changes in the shape and location of the Golgi complex relative to secretory state were described even before it was viewed with the electron microscope and its functional relationship to the rER was es-

tablished. It is very active both in cells that secrete protein by exocytosis and in cells, such as nerve cells, that synthesize large amounts of plasma membrane and membrane-associated proteins.

The Golgi Apparatus Does Not Stain With Hematoxylin or Eosin

In the light microscope, secretory cells that have a large Golgi apparatus, e.g., plasma cells, osteoblasts, or cells of the epididymis, typically exhibit a clear area partially surrounded by ergastoplasm (Fig. 2.14). In electron micrographs, the Golgi appears as stacks of flattened membrane-limited sacs or cisternae that are closely associated with vesicles (Fig. 2.15).

The Golgi Apparatus Has a Convex Outer Face Closest to the Rough-Surfaced Endoplasmic Reticulum and a Concave Inner Face Closest to the Plasma Membrane

The Golgi apparatus is polarized both morphologically and functionally. The outer face is also called the *forming face* or *cis-Golgi,* and the inner face is called the *maturing face* or *trans-Golgi.* Small vesicles called *transport vesicles* carry newly synthesized protein from the rER to the forming face of the Golgi. It is unclear precisely how this material then moves through the Golgi stacks, but its progress is related to changes in the oligosaccharides associated with the newly synthesized protein. The secretory product subsequently appears at the maturing face where *condensing vacuoles* pinch off from the ends of the concave stacks. The condensing vacuoles are further modified to form mature secretory vacuoles of protein-secreting cells (Fig. 2.16). These vacuoles eventually fuse with the plasma membrane to release the secretory product by exocytosis.

The Golgi is often described as the packing and shipping department of the protein-secretory factory. However, many other vital functions occur there. It is in the Golgi (as well as in the rER) that oligosaccharides are added to proteins in the synthesis of most glycoproteins and that sulfate groups are added to proteoglycans. The Golgi has a major role in membrane synthesis and in membrane recycling, particularly membrane retrieved from the apical plasma membrane of protein-secreting cells.

There is also evidence that the Golgi complex may have a dehydrating function relative to the packaging of secretory material. A proton pump has been identified in the Golgi of some cells and is believed to be involved in the concentration (dehydration) of secretory granules.

The Golgi Apparatus Also Modifies, Sorts, Packages, and Delivers Enzymes to *Lysosomes*

The production of *lysosomes* (see below) involves the interaction of the rER and the Golgi apparatus but in a manner different from that for secretory proteins. Although the

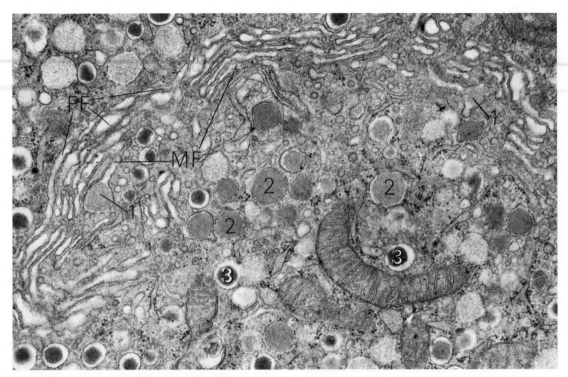

Figure 2.15. Electron micrograph of the Golgi apparatus in an islet cell of the pancreas. The flattened membrane sacs of the Golgi are arranged in layers. The forming face (FF) of the Golgi is represented by the flattened vesicles on the outer convex surface, whereas the flattened vesicles of the inner convex region constitute the maturing face (MF) of the Golgi. Budding off the maturing face are several condensing vacuoles (1). These are released (2) and eventually become the mature secretory granules (3).

lysosomes contain hydrolytic enzymes, which are proteins synthesized in the rER, the route these enzymes take from the rER to the Golgi is different from that taken by proteins destined for export. In lysosome production, there is evidence that there is a direct link between some rER cisternae and those of the inner face of the Golgi complex, providing a direct route for lysosomal enzymes between these two membrane-limited compartments. There is also evidence that posttranslational modifications of newly synthesized lysosomal enzymes make them subject to receptor-mediated sorting in the maturing face of the Golgi apparatus. This ensures that they are segregated from secretory proteins entering condensing vacuoles at the same level of the Golgi apparatus. The maturing face of the Golgi apparatus and the associated tubulovesicular array, referred to as the ***trans-Golgi network,*** thus serves as the sorting station for shuttling vesicles that deliver protein to various locations, such as to the basolateral membrane of an epithelial cell, to the luminal surface, or to the lysosomes.

The Golgi Apparatus Handles the Distribution of Newly Synthesized Membranes and Membrane-Associated Proteins

The Golgi apparatus also processes proteins that are to remain membrane-associated throughout their lifetime. The principles involved in modifying and sorting these proteins is similar to those described for proteins that pass through the Golgi lumen. Membrane-associated protein is subject to an additional set of modifications that involves the addition or alteration of fatty acids or glycolipids that may influence the subsequent association of these proteins with the membrane.

Mitochondria

Mitochondria Occur in Large Numbers in Cells That Generate and Expend Large Amounts of Energy

Mitochondria were also known to early cytologists who could observe them in cells vitally stained with Janus green B. They described movement, branched and other pleomorphic states, and division of mitochondria in living cells. It is now evident that mitochondria increase in number by division.

The early suggestion that mitochondria evolved from a prokaryote that lived symbiotically in primitive eukaryotic cells has received support with the demonstration that mitochondria possess DNA and RNA and that they divide as well as synthesize some of their structural (constituent) proteins. The remaining mitochondrial proteins, particularly the many enzymes they contain, are dependent on DNA and free ribosomes of the cell for synthesis.

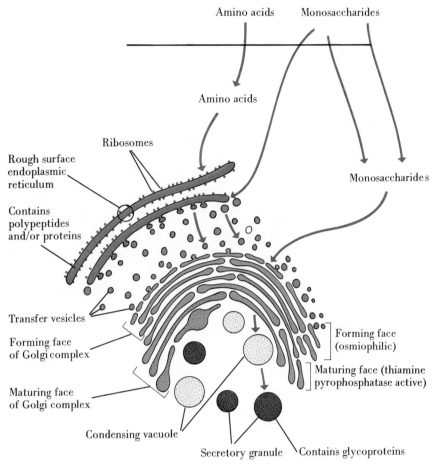

Figure 2.16. Diagram of the relationship between rER, Golgi apparatus, and secretory granules. The rER synthesizes polypeptides and protein from amino acids; these are conveyed to the Golgi apparatus by transfer vesicles; and then carbohydrates are added to the protein both in the rER and in the Golgi to form glycoproteins. The product is condensed in vacuoles to form secretory granules, which are discharged from the cell by exocytosis. (Based on Bloom W, Fawcett DW: *A Textbook of Histology,* 10th ed. Philadelphia, WB Saunders, 1975, p 56.)

Mitochondria Are Present in All Cells Except Red Blood Cells and Terminal Keratinocytes

The number, shape, and internal structure of mitochondria are often characteristic for specific cell types. When present in large numbers, mitochondria contribute to the acidophilia of the cytoplasm because of the large amount of membrane they contain. Mitochondria may be stained specifically by histochemical procedures that demonstrate some of their constituent enzymes, such as those involved in ATP metabolism (ATPase and phosphorylases) and in oxidation.

Mitochondria Contain the Enzyme System That Generates ATP by Means of the Krebs Cycle and Oxidative Phosphorylation

Because they can generate ATP, mitochondria are more numerous in cells that use large amounts of energy, such as striated muscle cells and cells engaged in fluid and electrolyte transport. Mitochondria also localize at sites in the cell where the energy is needed, as in the middle piece of the sperm, the interfibrillar space in striated muscle cells, and adjacent to the basolateral plasma membrane infoldings in the cells of the proximal convoluted tubule of the kidney. Mitochondria contain dense *matrix granules* that are storage sites for divalent cations. These granules increase in number and size when the concentration of divalent (and polyvalent) cations increases in the cytoplasm. Mitochondria can accumulate cations against a concentration gradient. Thus, in addition to ATP production, mitochondria also function to regulate the concentration of certain ions of the cytoplasmic matrix, a role they share with the sER.

Mitochondria Use an Inner Membrane to Create Functional Compartments

Mitochondria are membrane-limited organelles possessing a smooth, 6–7-nm outer membrane and a somewhat thinner, plicated inner membrane (Fig. 2.17). The space between the two membranes is the outer compartment (Fig. 2.18). The folds of the inner membrane, called *cristae,*

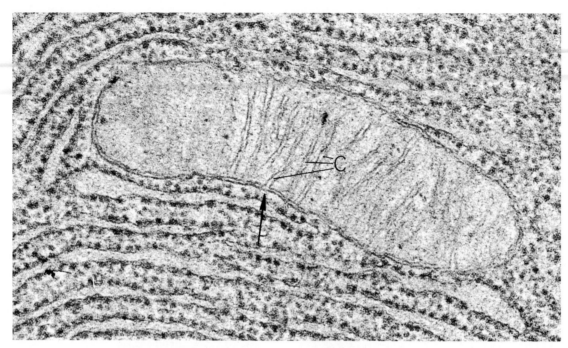

Figure 2.17. Electron micrograph of a mitochondrion in a pancreatic acinar cell. Note the inner mitochondrial membrane forms the cristae *(C)* through a series of infoldings. This is evident in the region of the *arrow.* The outer membrane is a smooth continuous envelope that is separate and distinct from the inner membrane.

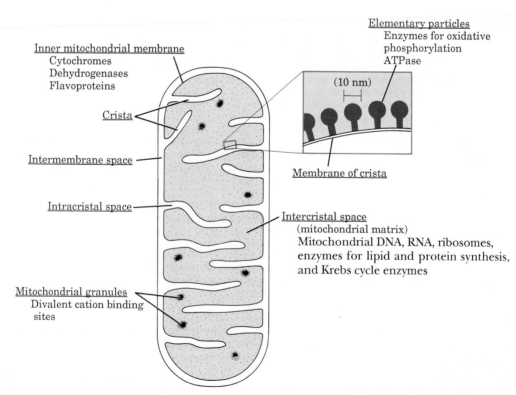

Figure 2.18. Schematic diagram of a mitochondrion and some activities of mitochondrial components. Note that the intercristal space is synonymous with the *inner* compartment. The intracristal space and the intermembrane space are synonymous with the *outer* compartment. (Based on Bloom W, Fawcett DW: *A Textbook of Histology,* 10th ed. Philadelphia, WB Saunders, 1975, p 47.)

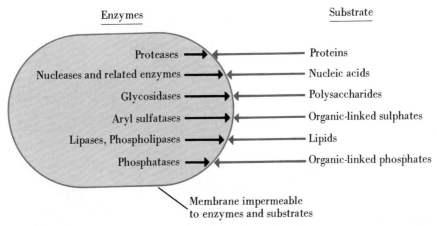

Figure 2.19. Schematically depicted lysosome with a list of some lysosomal enzymes. The respective substrates are listed outside of the lysosome. In order to act, the lysosome typically discharges the enzyme into the cellular microcompartment containing the substrate. More than 40 lysosomal enzymes have been identified. (From Novikoff AB, Holtzman E: *Cells and Organelles,* 2nd ed. New York, Holt, Rinehart & Winston, 1976, p 138, copyright 1976 by Holt, Rinehart & Winston. Reprinted by permission of CBS College Publishing.)

project into the *matrix* that constitutes the inner compartment of the organelle. In some cells involved in steroid metabolism, the inner membrane may form tubular or vesicular projections into the matrix.

Elementary particles that appear as tennis racquet-shaped structures are attached to the inner membrane and project their heads into the matrix (Fig. 2.18, *rectangle*). The heads measure about 10 nm in diameter and contain the enzymes of the electron transport system and an ATPase.

Mitochondrial DNA, RNA, and ribosomes, as well as the enzymes for mitochondrial protein and lipid synthesis, the Krebs cycle enzymes, and the divalent cation-containing granules, are located in the matrix.

Mitochondria Undergo Morphologic Changes Related to Their Functional State

Mitochondria may appear in two distinct configurations in the TEM. In the *orthodox configuration,* the cristae are prominent, and the matrix compartment occupies a large part of the total mitochondrial volume. This configuration has been shown to correspond to a *low level* of oxidative phosphorylation. In the *condensed configuration,* cristae are not easily recognized, the matrix is concentrated and reduced in volume, and the intermembrane (outer) compartment increases in volume to as much as 50% of the total. This configuration has been shown to correspond to a *high level* of oxidative phosphorylation.

Lysosomes

Lysosomes May Be Recognized Only After Using Histochemical Procedures to Demonstrate Lysosomal Enzymes

Lysosomes were not recognized as a distinct family of membrane-limited organelles until the simultaneous devel-opment of the techniques of differential cell fractionation and transmission electron microscopy of sectioned tissues, nearly 45 years ago. Nearly 100 different hydrolytic enzymes had been demonstrated in membrane-limited vesicles isolated from cells by centrifugation. In electron micrographs, a population of vesicles could be recognized either by their content of partially digested material or by specific histochemical demonstration of one of their contained hydrolytic enzymes. The demonstration that these two populations were identical earned Dr. Christian deDuve a share of the Nobel Prize in Medicine in 1974.

Lysosomes Are the Digestive Organelles of the Cell

Newly formed lysosomes, those that have pinched off from the ends of the Golgi cisternae, are called *primary lysosomes* and contain all the enzymes that are used in digestion in the cell (Fig. 2.19). These digestive enzymes are adapted to function in the low-pH environment created within the lysosome by proton pumps located in the lysosomal membrane. They participate in digestion of extracellular substances (and organisms) brought into the cell by endocytosis and in digestion of other cellular components that are isolated from the cytoplasmic matrix by newly formed membrane (autophagy).

Primary lysosomes fuse with the membrane of the structure that contains the material to be digested and release their enzymes, thus forming a *secondary lysosome.* Secondary lysosomes may also be called *phagosomes, digestive vacuoles,* or *autophagic vacuoles,* depending on the origin (intracellular or extracellular) of the material to be digested (Fig. 2.20).

Some cells, e.g., osteoclasts involved in bone resorption and neutrophils involved in acute inflammation, may release lysosomal enzymes directly into the extracellular space to digest components of the extracellular matrix.

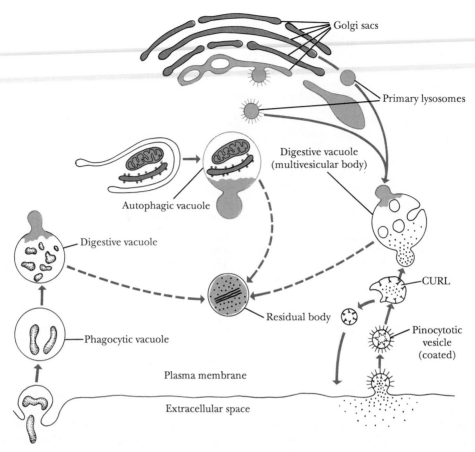

Figure 2.20. Schematic diagram of origins of primary lyso-somes from the Golgi and trans-Golgi network. Primary lyso-somes fuse with and discharge hydrolytic enzymes into auto-phagic, pinocytotic (or endosome), and phagocytic vacuoles to form secondary lysosomes (digestive vacuoles). Residual bod-ies contain undigested residue. Endosomes fuse to form a compartment where uncoupling of the ligands and surface re-ceptors occurs (CURL, see text for explanation). The com-partment containing the free ligands subsequently fuses with the lysosome; the receptors remain bound to the membrane of vesicles, which is partitioned off from the CURL and recy-cled to the plasma membrane. (Modified from Novikoff AB, Holtzman E: *Cells and Organelles,* 2nd ed. New York, Holt, Rinehart & Winston, 1976, p 139, copyright 1976 by Holt, Rinehart & Winston. Reprinted by permission of CBS College Publishing.)

Lysosomes in Some Cells Are Recognizable With the Light Microscope Because of Their Number, Size, or Contents

The numerous azurophilic granules of the *neutrophil (polymorphonuclear neutrophilic leukocyte or PMN)* are lysosomes and are recognized in aggregate by their specific staining; secondary lysosomes that contain phagocytized bacteria and fragments of damaged cells are often recog-nized in macrophages.

Hydrolytic breakdown of the contents of secondary lyso-somes often produces a debris-filled vacuole that is called a *tertiary lysosome* or *residual body.* Residual bodies may remain in cells for the life of the cell, as in nerve cells, in which they have been called ''age pigment'' or *lipofuscin granules.* Residual bodies are a normal feature of cell ag-ing.

LYSOSOMAL STORAGE DISEASES

Absence of certain lysosomal enzymes can lead to the pathologic accumulation of undigested substrate in resid-ual bodies. This can lead to several disorders collectively termed *lysosomal storage diseases.* In *Tay-Sachs dis-ease,* for example, the absence of a lysosomal galacto-sidase in nerve cells produces concentric lameliated structures in residual bodies that accumulate in the nerve cell and interfere with normal functions. Lysoso-mal storage diseases must be distinguished from other metabolic storage diseases such as glycogen storage dis-ease and the numerous mucopolysaccharidoses (Hurler's syndrome, Hunter's syndrome, etc.) in which incompletely synthesized or incompletely digested products accumulate in the cell because of the absence of specific enzymes in the rER, Golgi apparatus, sER, or cytoplasmic matrix.

Endosomes

Endosome-Associated Vesicles. As previously explained, vesicles formed as the result of phagocytosis, i.e., large endosomes, typically fuse with lysosomes, leading to the degradation of the phagocytosed material.

The Pathway That *Endosomes* Follow Within the Cell Depends on Their Contents

One of the following pathways is usually traced by an endosome once it is in the cell:

- The endosome may fuse with another domain or region of the plasma membrane to release its product from the cell; this process is referred to as *transcytosis.* It allows substances to be altered as they are transported across the cells of an epithelium; this occurs during the secretion of immunoglobulins into saliva, milk, and the intestinal lumen.
- The endosome may fuse with a lysosome, forming a *phagosome.* As explained above, this pathway allows substances taken into the cell to be digested or hydrolyzed.
- The endosome may fuse with another vesicular structure, sometimes referred to as the *compartment for uncoupling of receptor and ligand (CURL)* (Fig. 2.20). This pathway allows a *ligand,* a general name for any molecule that is recognized by a receptor, to be segregated from its receptor.[2] This pathway is important because it allows surface receptors to be recycled. Surface receptors allow the cell to bring substances into the cell selectively through the process of endocytosis. Tracer ligands such as charged molecules or plant carbohydrates can be used as markers that are taken up by the cell to identify the vesicles of the three pathways described above.

Peroxisomes (Microbodies)

Peroxisomes Contain *Oxidative* Enzymes

Peroxisomes (microbodies) are small (0.5-μm-diameter), membrane-limited spherical bodies that contain oxidative enzymes, particularly catalase and other peroxidases that break down hydrogen peroxide (H_2O_2). They are numerous in liver and kidney cells but are found in most cells.

---

[2]In the CURL pathway, the phase of the process involving the dissociation of the ligand and receptor is usually mediated by the acidic pH of this compartment. After dissociation, the ligand leaves the CURL en route to the lysosome by way of the vesicle-mediated pathway; the receptor typically returns to the plasma membrane along another vesicle-mediated pathway. Ligand-receptor dissociation does not always accompany receptor recycling. For example, the low pH of the endosome and CURL dissociates iron from the iron-carrier protein transferrin, but transferrin remains associated with its receptor. Once the transferrin-receptor pair returns to the cell surface, however, transferrin is released. This occurs because at the neutral extracellular pH, transferrin requires bound iron to be recognized by its receptor.

The number of peroxisomes present in a cell increases in response to diet, drugs, and hormonal stimulation.

In most animals, but not humans, peroxisomes also contain urate oxidase (uricase), which often appears as a characteristic crystalloid inclusion *(nucleoid).* In addition to peroxidases, peroxisomes contain D-amino acid oxidase, β-oxidation enzymes, and nearly 20 other enzymes. Virtually all of these produce hydrogen peroxide as a product of the oxidation reaction. Hydrogen peroxide is a toxic substance. The catalase universally present in peroxisomes carefully regulates the hydrogen peroxide content in cells, thus protecting the cell.

The β oxidation of fatty acids is also a major function of peroxisomes. In some cells, peroxisomal fatty acid oxidation may equal that in mitochondria. The proteins contained in the peroxisome lumen and membrane are synthesized on cytoplasmic ribosomes and appear to gain entry into the peroxisome by a receptor-mediated mechanism.

NONMEMBRANOUS ORGANELLES

Microtubules

Microtubules Are Ubiquitous Elements of the Cytoskeleton and of Specialized Structures Involved in Subcellular Movements

Microtubules are found in the

- *Axoneme* of *cilia* and *flagella*
- *Basal bodies* of cilia
- *Mitotic spindle* "fibers"
- *Centrioles* from which the spindle fibers radiate
- Elongating cell processes, such as growing axons
- Cytoplasm, generally

Microtubules may be seen with the light microscope by using special stains, polarization, or phase contrast optics. They have often, erroneously, been called fibers, such as the "fibers" of the mitotic spindle. Microtubules may be distinguished from filamentous and fibrillar cytoplasmic components at the light microscopic level by using antibodies to tubulin, the primary protein component of microtubules, conjugated with fluorescent dyes. Microtubules are the principal components of centrioles and basal bodies, cytoplasmic organelles easily recognized in sections viewed with the light microscope.

Microtubules are involved in numerous essential cellular activities that relate to cytoskeletal functions. These activities include

- Cell elongation and movement (migration)
- Intracellular transport of secretory granules
- Movement of chromosomes during mitosis and meiosis
- Maintenance of cell shape, particularly asymmetric shape
- Beating of cilia and flagella

In the activities listed above that involve movement of cells or their organelles, microtubules serve as guides for

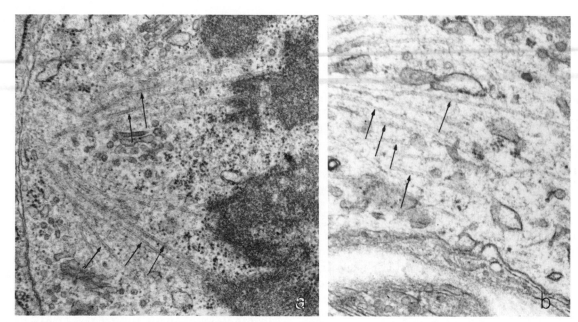

Figure 2.21. Electron micrographs of cytoplasmic microtubules. In **a** the microtubules *(arrows)* are associated with the chromosomes in a dividing (metaphase) cell. In **b** the microtubules *(arrows)* are in the axon of a nerve cell. In both examples the microtubules are seen in longitudinal profile. ×30,000.

molecular motors, molecules that are attached to the moving structures and that ratchet along a tubular or filamentous track. The energy required for these motors is derived from ATP hydrolysis.

Microtubules Are Elongated Polymeric Structures Made Up of Equal Parts of α-Tubulin and β-Tubulin

Microtubules are nonbranching, hollow cylinders that measure 20–25 nm in diameter (Fig. 2.21). The wall of the microtubule is about 5 nm thick and consists of 13 circularly arrayed globular protein subunits called ***protofilaments.*** Axial periodicity seen along the 5-nm-diameter protofilaments corresponds to the length of the ***dimeric tubulin molecules.*** These are the basic subunits of the protofilaments (Fig. 2.22). The tubulin dimer has a molecular weight of 110,000 and is formed from an α- and a β-tubulin molecule, with each having a molecular weight of 55,000. The

dimers polymerize in an end-to-end fashion, head to tail, with the α molecule of one dimer bound to the β molecule of the next dimer in a repeating pattern, to form protofilaments.

A Pool of Tubulin Dimers Exists in the Cytoplasm and Is in Equilibrium With the Polymerized Tubulin in the Microtubules

This equilibrium can be shifted in the direction of the unpolymerized dimer by exposure of cells or isolated microtubules to low temperature or high pressure. Repeated exposure to alternating low and high temperature is the basis of the purification technique for tubulin and microtubules. Alkaloids, such as colchicine, vincristine, and vinblastine, bind to tubulin and prevent polymerization into protofilaments and microtubules. This effect is the basis of the experimental inhibition of mitosis by colchicine and for

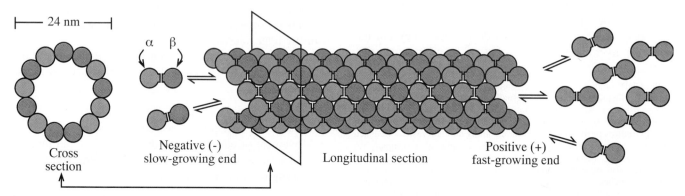

Figure 2.22. Diagram of microtubule in cross section and in longitudinal profile, depicting the reversible process of polymerization and depolymerization between tubulin dimers and microtubules.

the use of vincristine and vinblastine as chemotherapeutic agents in cancer treatment. Calcium also inhibits assembly of microtubules from tubulin. The particular structure and the function of microtubules in mitosis and in cilia and flagella are discussed further later in this chapter and in Chapter 4.

Filaments

Two Basic Types of Filaments—*Microfilaments and Intermediate Filaments*—Occur Within Cells

Microfilaments. Some cells, such as muscle cells, are characterized by the size, amount, and nature of the filaments they contain. There are two types of microfilaments *(myofilaments)* present in muscle cells: 6–8-nm microfilaments (called thin filaments) of *actin* and 15-nm microfilaments (called thick filaments) of *myosin.* The specific structural and functional relationships among actin, myosin, and *tropomyosin* in muscle contraction are discussed in Chapter 10 (Muscle Tissue).

Actin Microfilaments Are Present in Virtually All Cell Types

Actin may constitute up to 10% of the total protein of some nonmuscle cells. Actin microfilaments are often grouped as bundles close to the plasma membrane. These membrane-associated microfilaments function in the

- Anchorage and movement of membrane proteins
- Movement of the plasma membrane (as in endocytosis, exocytosis, and cytokinesis)
- Formation of the structural core of microvilli on absorptive cells
- Extension of cell processes
- Locomotion of cells

Microfilaments are distributed in three-dimensional networks throughout the cell (Fig. 2.23a; see also Fig. 1.4). Contraction of these microfilaments is essential in cytoplasmic streaming, i.e., the stream-like movement of cytoplasm that can be observed within cells in culture.

Microfilaments may also function in maintaining a ''flat'' apical cell surface in epithelial cells; e.g., the apical terminal web of actin filaments serves as tensioning cables under the cell surface. Other cross-linked microfilament networks are also thought to be an important component of the cytoskeleton, the underlying three-dimensional organization of the cytoplasmic matrix (see below).

Contraction in All Cells Involves Interactions of Actin and Myosin

In nonmuscle cells, contractile molecules other than actin are not organized into well-defined filaments. Small, wispy myosin filaments can, however, usually be identified by immunocytochemical techniques.

It is now apparent that some movements relative to microfilaments are also due to ''molecular motors'' as described above for microtubules. Myosin that is not organized in filaments may function in this manner. Other possible mechanisms of movement involving microfilaments include the force exerted by polymerization at the growing end of the filaments and syneresis (the contraction of a gel, such as a blood clot, by squeezing out some of the dispersion medium).

MICROFILAMENTS AND WOUND HEALING

Unlike most organelles, microfilaments and microtubules are transient structures that, unless organized into specialized arrays (as in myofilaments of muscle cells or microtubules of cilia), persist for periods of time ranging from only minutes to hours. Thus, cells can regulate the activity of microfilaments and microtubules by their selective placement during polymerization. This placement is achieved, in part, by local fluctuations in the concentration of divalent calcium ions, the concentration of specific actin-binding proteins (both monomer-binding and filament-end-binding proteins), and the pH. It is because of the dynamic nature of microtubules and microfilament networks that antipolymerization agents (such as colchicine for microtubules and cytochalasin for actin) can result in their disappearance from the cytoplasm. The transient nature of microfilament organization may have many significant functions. In one important instance, actin filaments in structural arrays that resemble those present in smooth muscle (see page 107) may be seen in developing fibroblasts in healing skin wounds. These arrays are so well developed that the wound fibroblasts have been called *myofibroblasts.* The myofibroblasts serve to pull together the edges of a skin wound with loss of substance (wound contraction).

Intermediate Filaments. Intermediate filaments have a supporting or general structural role. Nearly all of them consist of subunits with a molecular weight of about 50,000. There is some evidence that many of the stable structural proteins in intermediate filaments have been derived in evolution by minor genetic modification of highly conserved enzymes.

Intermediate Filaments Are a Heterogeneous Group of 8–10-nm Cytoskeletal Elements Found in Various Cell Types

Intermediate filaments (Fig. 2.23b) have been separated into five major classes on the basis of protein composition and cellular distribution:

- *Cytokeratin (or prekeratin)*
- *Vimentin*

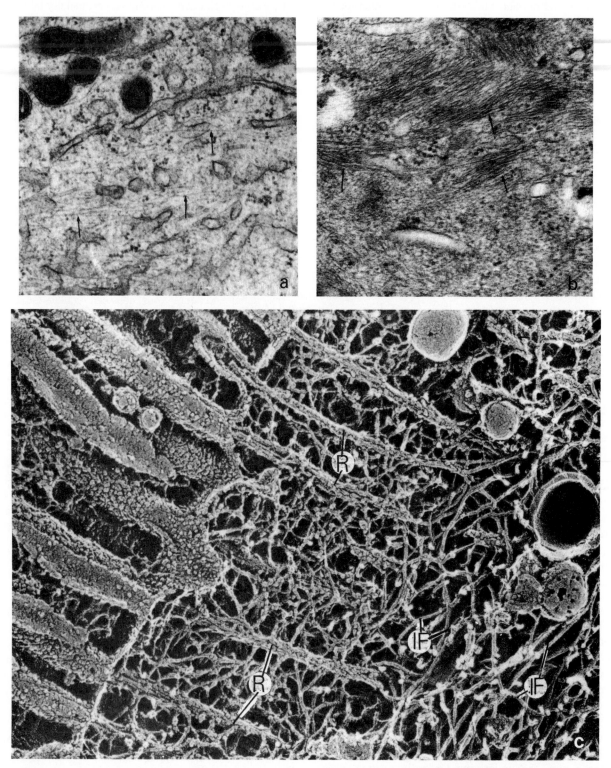

Figure 2.23.   a. Electron micrograph showing the very thin microfilaments *(arrows)* within a Sertoli cell in human testis. ×45,000. **b.** Electron micrograph showing aggregates of intermediate filaments *(arrows)* in the cytoplasm of a urinary bladder epithelial cell. The filament bundles are passing through the thickness of the section at oblique angles. Thus, their length within the cell cannot be appreciated. ×45,000. **c.** Electron micrograph showing terminal web portion of an epithelial cell and underlying intermediate filaments. The epithelial cells were treated with glycerin after incubation in a medium containing no ATP. The long straight rootlets extending from the bases of the microvilli are cross-linked by a dense and complicated network of cross-linkers. Intermediate filaments can be seen at the base of the rootlets forming a foundation for these processes. *IF,* intermediate filaments; and *R,* rootlets. (From Hirokawa et al: *The Journal of Cell Biology* 96:1325, 1983, by copyright permission of The Rockefeller University Press.)

TABLE 2.1. Distribution of the Primary Types of Intermediate Filaments

TYPE OF FILAMENT (MW)[A]	CELL(S) WHERE FOUND
Cytokeratin (prekeratin) (40,000–65,000)	Epithelial cells
Vimentin (55,000)	Cells of mesenchymal origin, including endothelial cells and some smooth muscle cells and myofibroblasts; and some cells of neuroectoderm origin
Desmin (51,000)	Muscle cells
Neurofilament (70,000, 140,000, and 210,000)	Neuronal cells
Glial fibrillary acidic protein (50,000)	Neuroglial cells, including oligodendroglia, astrocytes, microglia, Schwann cells, and ependymal cells and pituicytes

[A]The approximate molecular weight values of the polypeptide subunits are listed in the table. The neurofilament consists of three different filament polypeptides, which are sometimes referred to as a neurofilament triplet. Cytokeratin is a family of polypeptides that has a range of molecular weights.

- *Desmin*
- *Neurofilaments*
- *Glial fibrillary acidic protein (GFAP)*

Spectrin found in red blood cells (see page 190) and the nuclear lamins associated with the nuclear envelope (see page 49) are also intermediate filaments but do not belong to any of the five major classes.

Although the various classes of intermediate filaments differ in amino acid sequence and show some variation in molecular weight, they all share a homologous region that is important in filament self-assembly. In addition, they all contain a region of variable length that allows them to make molecular contact with other intracellular structures and, thus, to participate in many functions within the cell and between cells.

Some of the intermediate filaments of muscle and epidermis connect internal structures or organelles to transmembrane proteins that are bound to similar transmembrane proteins of neighboring cells or to extracellular matrix filaments (see pages 227 and 72). Intermediate filaments also do not typically disappear and re-form in the continuous manner characteristic of most microtubules and microfilaments. It is for these reasons that intermediate filaments are believed to play a primarily structural role within the cell and to comprise the cytoplasmic link of a tissue-wide continuum of cytoplasmic, nuclear, and extracellular filaments (Fig. 2.23c).

INTERMEDIATE FILAMENTS AND TUMOR DIAGNOSIS

Immunolabeling techniques have been used to determine the distribution of these five types of intermediate filaments (Table 2.1). The use of antibodies that are specific to the various filament types has also been useful in clinical medicine to aid in the diagnosis of tumors. For example, in the diagnosis of gliomas, a pathologist can utilize immunolabeling techniques and look for cells that are reactive with anti-GFAP antibody. Similarly, anti-keratin antibodies are used to identify tonofilaments in epithelial (particularly skin) tumors, and antivimentin antibodies are used to identify tumor cells of mesenchymal origin.

Centrioles

Centrioles Are Paired, Short, Rod-Like Cytoplasmic Bodies Visible With the Light Microscope

Early cytologists recognized centrioles as forming the ends of the mitotic spindle (see page 37). In nondividing cells, the centrioles are usually found close to the nucleus, often partially surrounded by the Golgi apparatus. This part of the cell was called the *cell center, centrosome,* or *centrosphere.*

The TEM reveals that each rod-shaped centriole is about 0.2 μm long and consists of nine triplets of microtubules that are oriented parallel to the long axis of the organelle (Fig. 2.24). The three microtubules are fused to one another, with adjacent microtubules sharing a common wall. The innermost or *A* microtubule is a complete ring of 13 protofilaments; the middle and outer microtubules, *B* and *C,* respectively, appear C-shaped because of the protofilaments they share with each other and with the *A* microtubule.

The Paired Centrioles in a Resting Cell Are Arranged at Right Angles to Each Other but Are Not Connected

Prior to cell division, when DNA is being replicated, during the S phase of the cell cycle (see page 50), the centrioles also duplicate themselves. A small mass of granular and fibrillar material, the *procentriole,* appears at the side of each centriole and gradually enlarges to form a right-angle appendage to the parent. Microtubules develop in the mass as it grows, appearing first as single tubules, then as doublets, and finally as triplets. After duplication, the parent-daughter pairs separate and, in doing so, define the poles between which the mitotic spindle develops.

Centrioles and Adjacent Dense Material (Centriolar Satellites) Constitute a General Microtubule Organizing Center in Both Interphase and Mitosis

Centrioles are equally important in organizing the new microtubule system that forms in daughter cells from the

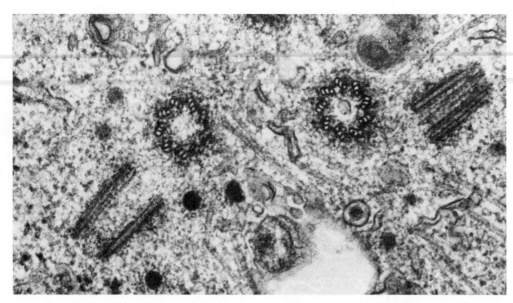

Figure 2.24. Electron micrograph showing both parent and daughter centrioles in a fibroblast. Note that the transverse-sectioned centriole in each of the pairs reveals the triplet configuration of microtubules. The lower left centriole represents a midlongitudinal section, whereas the upper right centriole has also been longitudinally sectioned, but along the plane of its wall. ×90,000. (Courtesy of M. McGill, D. P. Highfield, T. M. Monahan, and B. Brinkley.)

tubulin dimers resulting from dismantling of the mitotic spindle. The presence of a single microtubule organizing center (MTOC) in interphase cells, together with the inherent polarity of tubulin dimer assembly, provides a radial coordinate system by which the cell can distinguish center from periphery for the localization of its organelles and enzymes. At the time of division, the centriolar satellites appear to be the actual points of polar attachment of the microtubules of the mitotic spindle.

Basal Bodies

Development of Cilia on the Cell Surface Requires the Presence of Basal Bodies, Structures Derived From Centrioles

Each cilium must have a basal body. Basal bodies are produced by the repeated replication of centrioles and the migration of the newly formed organelles to the apical surface of a cell. Each centriole-derived basal body serves as the organizer for the assembly of the microtubules of a cilium. The core structure (axoneme) of a cilium is a complexly organized set of microtubules consisting of two central microtubules surrounded by nine microtubule doublets (see Fig. 4.22, page 76). The organizing role of the basal body is different from that of the MTOC; in this case, the axonemal microtubule doublets are continuous with the A and B microtubules of the basal body from which they develop by addition of tubulin dimers at the growing end.

Inclusions

Inclusions Are "Nonliving" Components of the Cell; They Include *Secretory Granules, Pigment Granules, Neutral Fat* and *Other Lipid Droplets,* and *Glycogen*

Secretory granules and pigment granules are surrounded by a membrane; lipid droplets and glycogen are not. Secretory granules and neutral fat may often fill most of the cytoplasmic volume, compressing the other formed organelles into a thin rim at the margin of the cell. This is the typical structure of the intestinal goblet cell (see Fig. 16.15, page 456) and the adipose cell of the connective tissue (see Fig. 6.2, page 128), respectively.

The density of secretory granules in secretory cells is sensitive to the presence or absence of signaling agents or "secretagogues" that trigger granule exocytosis by a receptor-activated second messenger cascade. Some highly active secretory cells lack secretory granules altogether because they exocytose their secretory proteins continuously, i.e., by constitutive exocytosis (page 24), rather than in a secretagogue-dependent regulated manner, i.e., regulated exocytosis (page 24).

Glycogen may be seen with the light microscope only after special fixation and staining procedures. It is usually lost during the routine processing of tissue for light microscopy. Liver and striated muscle cells, which usually contain large amounts of glycogen, may display empty regions where the glycogen was localized. *Glycogen* appears in electron micrographs as granules of 25–30-nm diameter and as clusters of such granules that often occupy significant portions of the cytoplasm (Fig. 2.25).

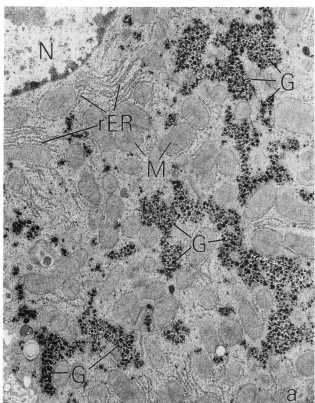

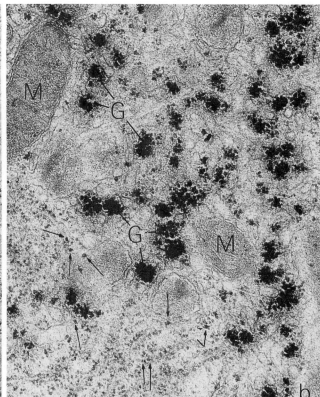

Figure 2.25. a. Low-magnification electron micrograph showing a portion of a liver cell with part of the nucleus (*N*) in the upper left. The glycogen (*G*) appears as irregular electron-dense masses. Profiles of rough endoplasmic reticulum (*rER*) and mitochondria (*M*) are also evident. ×10,000. **b.** The higher magnification electron micrograph reveals the glycogen (*G*) as aggregates of small particles. Even the smallest aggregates (*arrows*) appear to be composed of several smaller glycogen particles. The density of the glycogen is considerably greater than that of the ribosomes (lower left region of the micrograph). ×52,000.

Lipid inclusions (fat droplets) are also usually extracted by the organic solvents used to prepare tissues for both light and electron microscopy. What is seen as a "fat droplet" in light or electron microscopy is actually a hole in the cytoplasm, showing the site from which the lipid was extracted.

Certain cells contain crystalline inclusions that are recognized with the light microscope. In the human, such inclusions are found in the sustentacular (Sertoli) and interstitial (Leydig) cells of the testis. With the electron microscope, crystalline inclusions have been found in many cell types and in virtually all parts of the cell, including the nucleus and most cytoplasmic organelles. Although some of these inclusions are storage material, the significance of others is not clear.

Cytoplasmic Matrix

The Cytoplasm Has a Complex Three-Dimensional Architecture That Provides a Substratum for Cytoplasmic Functions

The cytoplasmic matrix (ground substance or cytosol) shows little specific structure by light microscopy or conventional transmission electron microscopy and has traditionally been described as a solution containing electrolytes, metabolites, RNA, and synthesized proteins. Studies with high-voltage electron microscopy (HVEM) of 0.25–0.5-μm sections, however, reveal a very complex three-dimensional structural network of thin ***microtrabeculae.***

This ***microtrabecular lattice*** or ***cytoskeleton*** is composed, in part, of the filaments and tubules described above and appears to anchor most of the other cytoplasmic organelles. It provides a structural substratum on which cytoplasmic reactions occur, such as those involving free ribosomes, and along which regulated and directed cytoplasmic transport may occur.

NUCLEUS

The Nucleus Is a Membrane-Limited Compartment That Contains the *Genome* (Genetic Information) in Eukaryotic Cells

The nucleus of a nondividing cell, also called an ***interphase cell,*** consists of the following components:

- *Chromatin,* organized as euchromatin and heterochromatin
- *Nucleolus* (or nucleoli)
- Membranous *nuclear envelope*
- *Nuclear skeleton*
- *Nucleoplasm*

Chromatin

Chromatin, a Complex of DNA and Proteins, Is Responsible for the Characteristic Basophilia of the Nucleus

In most cells, the chromatin does not have a homogeneous appearance; rather, clumps of densely staining chromatin are embedded in a more lightly staining background. The densely staining material is highly condensed chromatin called *heterochromatin,* and the lightly staining material is a dispersed form called *euchromatin.* It is the phosphate groups of the DNA of the chromatin that gives the characteristic basophilia of chromatin (page 5). The proteins of chromatin include five basic proteins called *histones* and others called *nonhistone proteins.*

Heterochromatin is disposed in three locations (Fig. 2.26):

- *Marginal chromatin* is found at the perimeter of the nucleus (the structure light microscopists formerly referred to as the *nuclear membrane* actually consists largely of marginal chromatin).
- *Karyosomes* are discrete bodies of irregular size and shape found throughout the nucleus.
- *Nucleolar associated chromatin* is chromatin found in association with the nucleolus.

Heterochromatin stains with basic dyes and hematoxylin; it is also readily displayed with the Feulgen procedure (a specific histochemical reaction for the deoxyribose of DNA, page 6) and fluorescent vital dyes such as Hoechst dyes and propidium iodide. It is the heterochromatin that accounts for the conspicuous staining of the nucleus in hematoxylin and eosin preparations.

Euchromatin is indicative of active chromatin, i.e., chromatin that is stretched out so that the genetic information in the DNA can be read and transcribed. It is prominent in metabolically active cells such as neurons and liver cells. Heterochromatin predominates in metabolically inactive cells such as small circulating lymphocytes and sperm or in cells that are making only one major product, such as plasma cells.

Euchromatin is not evident with the light microscope. It is present within the nucleoplasm in the "clear" areas between the heterochromatin. In routine electron micrographs, there is no sharp delineation between euchromatin and heterochromatin; both have a granular-filamentous appearance, but the euchromatin is less tightly packed.

The Smallest Units of Chromatin Structure Are Macromolecular Complexes of DNA and Histones Called *Nucleosomes*

Nucleosomes. Nucleosomes are found in both euchromatin and heterochromatin and in chromosomes (see below). A nucleosome is a particle of about 10-nm diameter, consisting of a core of eight histone molecules with approximately two loops of DNA wrapped around the octamer. The DNA extends between each particle as a 1.5-nm filament that joins adjacent nucleosomes. This structure gives rise to the description of the nucleosomal substructure of chromatin as *"beads on a string."*

A long strand of nucleosomes is coiled to produce a unit chromatin fibril that is about 25–30 nm in diameter. Six nucleosomes form one turn in the coil of the chromatin fibril. Both interphase chromatin and chromosomes are formed from the 25–30-nm unit fibril. In heterochromatin, the unit chromatin fibrils are tightly packed and folded on each other; in euchromatin, the unit fibrils are more loosely arranged. This allows the DNA polymerases to have access to the DNA in euchromatin.

In Dividing Somatic *(Mitotic)* Cells, Chromatin Is Condensed and Organized Into Discrete Bodies Called *Chromosomes*

Chromosomes. Chromosomes (literally, colored bodies) are formed in the process of mitosis by condensation of the euchromatin and combination with heterochromatin. Each chromosome is formed by two *chromatids* that are joined together at a point called the *centromere.* The double nature of the chromosome is produced in the preceding synthetic (S) phase of the cell cycle (see below) during which DNA is replicated in anticipation of the next mitotic division.

With the exception of the mature gametes, the egg and sperm, human cells contain *46 chromosomes* organized as *23 homologous pairs.* Twenty-two of the pairs have identical chromosomes and are called *autosomes.* There is one pair of *sex chromosomes,* designated X and Y. The female contains two X chromosomes; the male contains one X and one Y chromosome. The chromosomal number, 46, is found in most of the somatic cells of the body and is called the diploid $(2n)$ number. Diploid chromosomes will have the $2n$ amount of DNA immediately after cell division but will have twice that amount, i.e., the $4n$ amount of DNA, after the S phase.

The mature sex cell, egg or sperm, as a result of *meiosis* (see below) has only 23 chromosomes, the haploid $(1n)$ number, as well as the haploid $(1n)$ amount of DNA. The somatic chromosome number and the diploid $(2n)$ amount of DNA are reestablished at the time of *fertilization* by the fusion of the sperm nucleus with the egg nucleus.

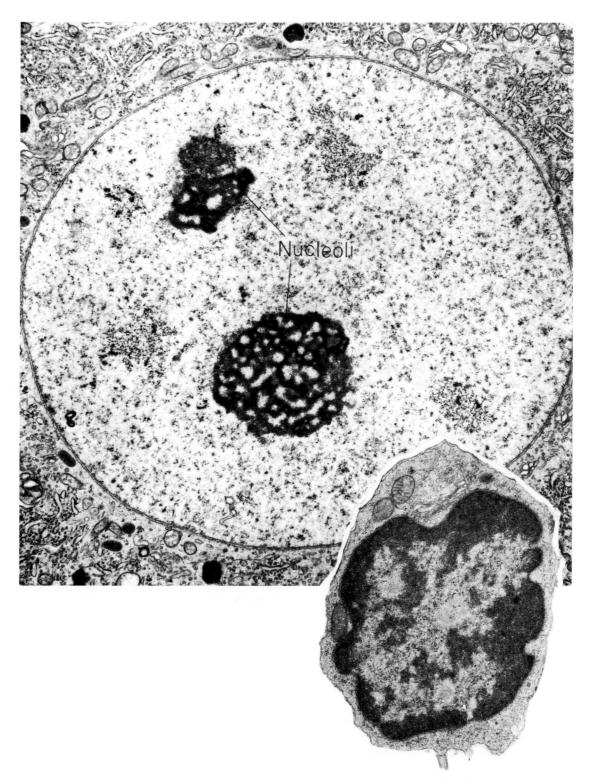

Nucleoli

Figure 2.26. Electron micrographs of nuclei from two different cell types. The large micrograph shows the nucleus of a nerve cell. Two nucleoli are included in the plane of section. The nucleus of this very active cell, exclusive of the nucleoli, is comprised almost entirely of extended chromatin or euchromatin. The smaller nucleus **(inset)** belongs to a small circulating lymphocyte (the entire cell is shown in the micrograph). It is a relatively inactive cell. Note the paucity of cytoplasm and cytoplasmic organelles. The chromatin in the nucleus is largely condensed or heterochromatin. The *lighter areas* represent euchromatin. Nerve cell, ×10,000; lymphocyte, ×13,000.

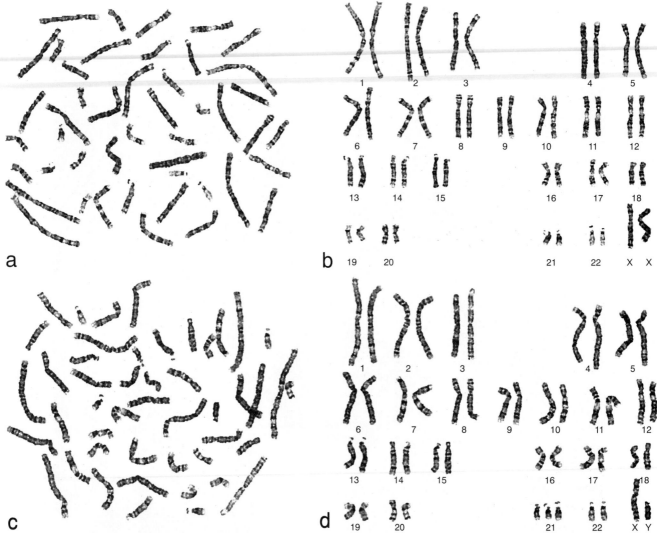

Figure 2.27. Metaphase spread **(a)** and karyotype **(b)** of a normal female and metaphase spread **(c)** and karyotype **(d)** of a male with Down's syndrome. The paired chromosomes are numbered in each of the karyotypes, and the sex chromosomes are indicated by *x* and *y*. The identification of the chromosomes as well as alterations is facilitated by standard G-banding techniques. Note that the sex difference between the male and female is seen in the karyotypes of the sex chromosomes. Females have two X chromosomes **(b)**, and males have one X chromosome and one Y chromosome **(d)**. Down's syndrome is reflected in the trisomy chromosome 21. Note that there are three number 21 chromosomes present in **d** as opposed to the normal paired compliment of chromosome 21 present in **b**. (Courtesy of the University of Florida Cytogenetics Laboratory.)

Karyotypes Are Chromosome Pairs Sorted According to Their Morphology

Karyotype. A preparation of chromosomes derived from mechanically ruptured, dividing cells that are then fixed, plated on a microscope slide, and stained with Giemsa stain is called a metaphase spread (Fig. 2.27, *a* and *c*). Such spreads are then photographed. The chromosome pairs are cut from the photograph and sorted according to their morphology to form what is called a *karyotype* (Fig. 2.27, *b* and *d*). Karyotypes are used to analyze for chromosome abnormalities such as deletions, nondisjunctions, and additions, for determination of sex in fetuses, and for prenatal diagnosis of certain endocrine disorders. Special stains (banding techniques) allow the study of localized regions of specific chromosomes to determine duplications or deletions of specific gene sites (loci).

The Barr Body Can Be Used to Identify the Sex of a Fetus

Some chromosomes are *repressed* in the interphase nucleus and exist only in the tightly packed heterochromatic form. One X chromosome of the female is an example of such a chromosome. This fact can be used to identify the sex of a fetus. This chromosome was discovered in 1949 by Barr and Bartram in nerve cells of female cats, where it appears as a well-stained round body, now called the *Barr body,* adjacent to the nucleolus.

Sex chromatin

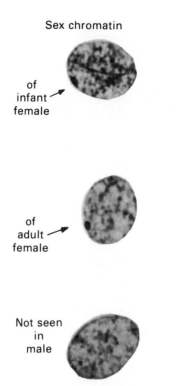

of infant female →

of adult female →

Not seen in male

Figure 2.28. Photomicrographs of nuclei of oral mucosal cells showing Barr bodies only in the female *(arrows).* (Courtesy of K. I. Moore and M. L. Barr, 1955).

Although it was originally found in sectioned tissue, it was subsequently shown that any relatively large number of cells prepared as a smear (e.g., scrapings of the oral mucous membrane from the inside of the cheeks) might be used to search for the Barr body. In cells of the oral mucous membrane, the Barr body is located adjacent to the nuclear envelope (Fig. 2.28). In both sections and smears, many cells must be examined to find those whose orientation is suitable for the display of the Barr body.

Nucleolus

The Nucleolus Is the Site of Ribosomal RNA Synthesis and Initial Ribosomal Assembly

The nucleolus is a nonmembranous, intranuclear structure formed by filamentous and granular material (Fig. 2.29). It varies in size, being particularly well developed in cells active in protein synthesis. In some cells, there may be more than one nucleolus. The nucleolus consists largely of RNA and protein and is the site of synthesis of subunits of ribosomal RNA that leave the nucleus, presumably via nuclear pores (see below), to be assembled into functional ribosomes in the cytoplasm.

The Nucleolus Stains Intensely With Hematoxylin and Basic Dyes and Metachromatically With Thionine Dyes

That the basophilia and metachromasia are due to the phosphate groups of the nucleolar RNA is confirmed by

predigestion of specimens with RNAse, which abolishes the staining. There is DNA in the nucleolus but in such small amounts that it appears Feulgen negative when examined with the light microscope. However, Feulgen-positive material, nucleolus-associated chromatin, often rims the nucleolus.

Both the granular, **pars granulosa,** and fibrillar, **pars fibrosa,** material of the nucleolus consist of RNA, with the first organized as granules and the second as extremely fine filaments packed very tightly together. The pars fibrosa is the most densely staining compartment of the nucleolus and the densest component seen in transmission electron microscopy. The network formed by the pars granulosa and the pars fibrosa is called the **nucleonema.** The DNA that is responsible for the synthesis of the ribosomal subunits is localized in the interstices of that network.

Nucleoplasm

Nucleoplasm Is the Material Enclosed by the Nuclear Envelope Exclusive of the Chromatin and the Nucleolus

Although crystalline, viral, and other inclusions are sometimes described in the nucleoplasm, until recently morphologic techniques showed it to be amorphous. It must

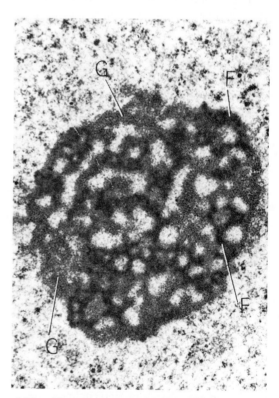

Figure 2.29. Electron micrograph of the nucleolus from a nerve cell showing the DNA-containing interstices *(light areas),* the pars granulosa *(G)*-containing accumulated ribonucleoprotein particles, and the pars fibrosa *(F),* which has a more electron-dense appearance.

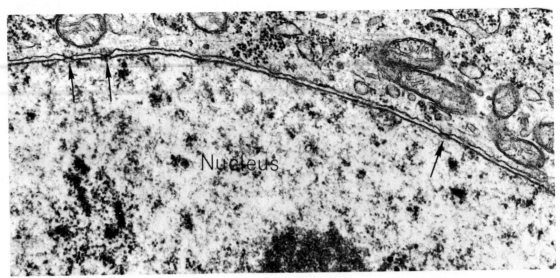

Figure 2.30. Electron micrograph of the nuclear envelope showing the nuclear pores *(arrows)* and the two membranes that constitute the "envelope." At the periphery of each pore the outer and inner membranes of the nuclear envelope are continuous. A diaphragm-like structure appears to cross the pore structure. ×30,000.

be assumed, however, that many proteins and other metabolites must be resident in or must pass through the nucleus in relation to the synthetic and metabolic activity of the chromatin and nucleolus. It is likely that improved procedures for transmission electron microscopy preparation, HVEM, and immunocytochemical methods will elucidate further the nature of the nucleoplasm as they have done for the cytoplasm.

Nuclear Envelope

The Nuclear Envelope, Formed by Two Unit Membranes With a Perinuclear Cisternal Space Between Them, Serves as a Membranous Boundary Between the Nucleoplasm and the Cytoplasm of the Interphase Cell

In the interphase cell, the perinuclear cisternal space is continuous with the cisternal space of the rER; the outer membrane of the nuclear envelope is continuous with the membranous component of the rER. Polyribosomes are often present on the cytoplasmic side of the nuclear envelope. During cell division, the components of the nuclear envelope dissociate. At the end of mitosis (and meiosis), the nuclear envelope re-forms from elements of the rER.

Fibrous (Nuclear) Lamina

The Nuclear Lamina Lies Adjacent to the Inner Surface of the Nuclear Envelope, Between the Membrane and the Marginal Heterochromatin

The *fibrous (nuclear) lamina,* a thin, electron-dense protein layer, has a supporting or "nucleoskeletal" function. If the membranous component of the nuclear envelope is disrupted by exposure to detergent, the fibrous lamina remains, and the nucleus retains its shape.

The major components of the lamina, as determined by biochemical isolation, are the *nuclear lamins,* a specialized type of intermediate filament (see page 39). The lamins appear to serve as a scaffolding for chromatin, chromatin-associated proteins, nuclear pores, and the membranes of the nuclear envelope.

The Nuclear Envelope Possesses an Array of Perforations Called Nuclear Pores

Nuclear Pores. At numerous sites on the surface of the nucleus there are small 70–80-nm "openings" in the nuclear envelope. The openings or *nuclear pores,* as they are designated, are a result of the union of the inner and outer membranes of the nuclear envelope. With an ordinary TEM the pores appear to have a diaphragm-like structure crossing the pore opening (Fig. 2.30). Often, but not always, a small dense body is observed in the center of the opening. Such profiles are now thought to represent ribosomes and other particulate material caught during their passage through the pore.

With special techniques, such as negative staining and high-resolution transmission electron microscopy, the nuclear pore exhibits additional structural detail. Each pore possesses eight protein subunits arranged in an octagonal array at the periphery of the pore to form what is known as the *nuclear pore complex.* Although a number of different nuclear pore complex proteins have been identified, they are collectively referred to as *nucleoporins.*

The Nuclear Pore Complex Mediates Bidirectional Nucleocytoplasmic Transport

On the basis of various experiments it has been shown that the nuclear pore complex regulates the passage of pro-

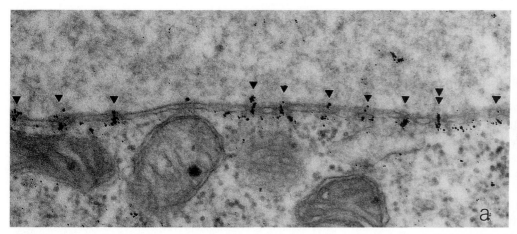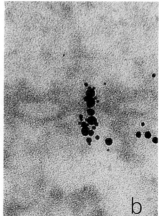

Figure 2.31. Electron micrographs showing the nuclear envelope and protein-coated gold particles that had been injected into the cytoplasm of an oocyte. In **a**, 15 minutes after injection, the coated gold particles are seen largely concentrated in the region of the pore complexes of the nuclear envelope (*arrowheads*). ×60,000. **b**. A higher magnification of the area marked by the *double arrowhead* in **a**, shows an elongate cluster of gold particles at the site of the nuclear pore complex. The particles are in a linear array and appear to be in transit through the nuclear pore complex from the cytoplasm to the nucleoplasm. This illustrates the pathway taken by proteins synthesized in the cytoplasm that must be transported into the nucleus. ×200,000. (Courtesy Carl M. Feldherr.)

teins between the nucleus and the cytoplasm (Fig. 2.31). The significance of the nuclear pore complex can be readily appreciated, as the nucleus does not carry out protein synthesis. The ribosomal proteins that are incorporated into ribosomes in the nucleolus, as well as the nuclear proteins, such as histones and lamins, are produced in the cytoplasm. Thus, the nuclear pore serves in the transport of these substances into the nucleus. Similarly, mRNAs and ribosomes must exit the nucleus to reach the cytoplasm and do so by the same route. The passage of large molecules is dependent on the presence of specific receptor-binding sites on the pore complex. They are then actively transported through the pore by an ATP energy-dependent mechanism. Ions and smaller molecules may cross the nuclear pores by diffusion. It has been shown that the effective size of the pore is ≈9 nm for substances that diffuse, rather than the 70–80-nm measurement of the pore boundary. Thus, any globular and nonnuclear proteins less than 9 nm can traverse the pore. Even the smaller nuclear proteins that are capable of diffusion are selectively transported, however, presumably because the rate is faster than by simple diffusion.

RENEWAL

Somatic Cells in the Adult Organism May Be Classified According to Their Mitotic Activity

The level of mitotic activity can be judged by the number of mitotic metaphases visible in a single high-magnification light microscopic field or by autoradiographic studies of the incorporation of tritiated thymidine, indicative of DNA syntheses prior to mitosis. By use of these methods,

cell populations may be classified as either static, stable, or renewing:

- *Static cell populations* consist of cells that no longer divide (postmitotic cells), such as cells of the central nervous system, or of cells that divide only rarely, such as skeletal and cardiac muscle cells.
- *Stable cell populations* consist of cells that divide episodically and at slow rates to maintain normal tissue or organ structure and that may be stimulated by injury to become more mitotically active. Periosteal and perichondrial cells, smooth muscle cells and endothelial cells of blood vessels, and fibroblasts of the loose connective tissue may be included in this category.
- *Renewing cell populations* may be slowly renewing or rapidly renewing but display *regular mitotic activity*. The division of such cells usually results in one daughter cell that differentiates both morphologically and functionally and one cell that remains as a stem cell. Daughter cells may divide one or more times before their mature state is reached. The differentiated cell may, ultimately, be lost from the body.

Slowly renewing populations include smooth muscle cells of most hollow organs, fibroblasts of the uterine wall, and epithelial cells of the lens of the eye. Slowly renewing populations may actually slowly increase in size during life, as do the smooth muscle cells of the gastrointestinal tract and the lens of the eye.

Rapidly renewing populations include blood cells, epithelial cells and dermal fibroblasts of the skin, and the epithelial cells and subepithelial fibroblasts of the mucosal lining of the alimentary tract.

CELL CYCLE

Somatic Cell Division Is a Cyclic Process Divided Into Two Phases, Mitosis and Interphase

For renewing cell populations and growing cell populations, including embryonic cells, cells in tissue culture, and even tumor cells, a *cell cycle* may be described that has two principal phases, *mitosis* (M phase) and *interphase,* and three other phases, G_1, *S,* and G_2, that further subdivide interphase (Fig. 2.32).

Mitosis, which nearly always includes both karyokinesis (division of the nucleus into two daughter nuclei) and cytokinesis (division of the cell into two daughter cells), lasts about 1 hour. It is usually followed by the G_1 or gap 1 phase, a period in which no DNA synthesis occurs. The G_1 *phase* is usually a period of *cell growth* and may last only a few hours in a rapidly dividing cell or may last a lifetime in a nondividing cell. A cell that leaves the cycle in G_1 to begin "terminal" differentiation is considered to begin the G_O *phase,* "O" for "outside" the cycle.

The *S* or *DNA synthesis phase* follows the G_1 phase and usually lasts for about 7 hours. The DNA of the cell is doubled during the S phase, and new chromatids are formed that will become obvious at the prophase or metaphase (Figs. 2.32 and 2.33) of the next M phase. It is the brevity of the S phase that allows the use of tritiated thymidine to label only those cells engaged in DNA synthesis at the time the radioactively labeled nucleotide is present.

The S phase is also followed by a period in which no DNA synthesis occurs, a second gap or G_2 *phase.* The G_2 phase may be as short as 1 hour in rapidly dividing cells or of indefinite duration in some polyploid cells and in cells, such as the primary oocyte, that may leave the cell cycle for extended periods from the G_2 phase.

Cells identified as *reserve stem cells* may be thought of as G_O cells that may be induced to reenter the cell cycle in response to injury of the cell populations within the tissues of the body. Such activation of the reserve stem cells may occur in normal wound healing and in the repopulation of the seminiferous epithelium after intense acute exposure of the testis to x-irradiation or during regeneration of an organ, such as the liver, after removal of a major portion. If the damage to the tissues is too severe, even the reserve stem cells die, and there is no potential for regeneration.

Cell Division—Mitosis and Meiosis

In both developing and growing individuals and in adult individuals, it is necessary for cells to divide in order to increase in numbers, to permit renewal of cell populations, and to allow wound repair.

Mitosis Is a Cell Division Process That Produces Two Daughter Cells With the Same Chromosome Number (n) and DNA Content as the Original Cell

At fertilization in the human, fusion of the haploid nuclei from the egg and a spermatozoon results in the formation of the zygote with 23 pairs of chromosomes (22 pairs of autosomes plus XX in females and 22 pairs of autosomes plus XY in males). Each chromosome pair contains one member of maternal origin and one of paternal origin. The chromosome number is called *diploid (2n),* and the DNA content is called *2n.* Subsequent growth of the multicellular organism, except for gametogenesis, occurs through the process of mitotic cell division.

The process of cell division usually includes division of both the nucleus *(karyokinesis)* and the cytoplasm *(cytokinesis).* In strict sense, the terms mitosis and meiosis are used to describe the duplication and distribution of the chromosomes. If cytokinesis does not follow karyokinesis, a binucleate cell is formed.

Cells that are not in the process of dividing are called

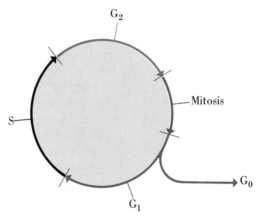

Figure 2.32. Scheme of cell cycle of rapidly dividing cells in relation to DNA synthesis. After *mitosis,* the cell is in interphase. G_1 represents the period in which there is a lull or gap in DNA synthesis. S represents the period during which DNA synthesis occurs. This is the period during which (tritiated) thymidine is incorporated into the DNA to serve as an experimental tracer. G_2 represents a second lull or gap in DNA synthesis. G_O represents the path of a cell that no longer stays in the compartment of rapidly dividing cells. Such a cell is said to be outside of the cycle.

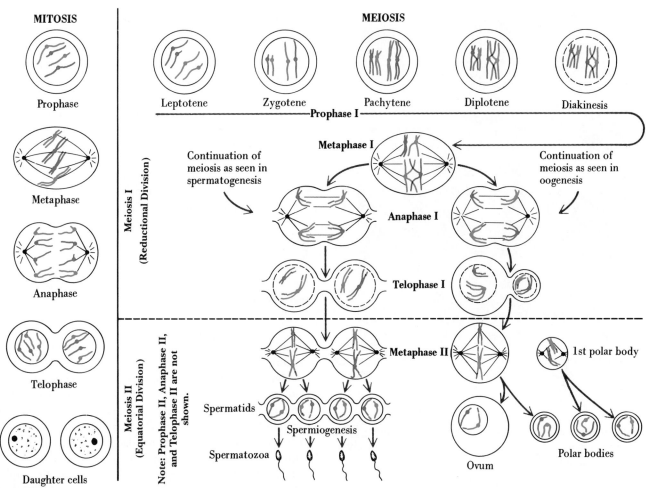

Figure 2.33. Comparison of mitosis and meiosis in an idealized cell having two pairs of chromosomes (2*n*). The chromosomes of maternal and paternal origin are depicted in red and blue, respectively. The mitotic division produces daughter cells that are genetically identical to the parental cell (2*n*). The meiotic division, which has two components, a reductional division and an equational division, produces a cell, which un-like the parental cell has only two chromosomes (*n*). In addition, during the chromosome pairing in prophase I of meiosis there is exchange of chromosome segments leading to further genetic diversity. It should be noted that in the human the first polar body does not divide. Division of the first polar body does occur in some species.

resting or interphase cells. Prior to entering mitosis or entering the first meiotic division (but not the second meiotic division), cells duplicate their DNA. This phase of the cell cycle is called the *S* or *synthesis phase.* At the beginning of this phase, the chromosome number is 2*n*, and the DNA content is 2*n*; at the end, the chromosome number is 4*n*, and the DNA content is 4*n*.

Mitosis Follows the S Phase and Is Defined in Four Phases

Mitosis consists of four phases:

• *Prophase* (Fig. 2.33) begins as the chromosomes become visible. As the chromosomes continue to condense, each can be seen to consist of two strands called *chromatids.* They are held together by the *centromere* or *kinetochore.* Other changes include disappearance of the nucleolus, replication of the centrioles, and disintegration of the nuclear envelope.

• *Metaphase* begins as the mitotic spindle, consisting of microtubules, becomes organized around the centrioles located at opposite poles of the cell and directs the movements of the chromosomes to the plane in the middle of the cell, the *equatorial* or *metaphase plate.*

• *Anaphase* begins as the chromatids separate and are pulled to opposite poles of the cell by the microtubules of the spindle that are attached to the *centromeres.*

• *Telophase* is marked by the reconstitution of a nuclear envelope around the chromosomes at each pole. The chromosomes uncoil and become indistinct except at regions that remain condensed in the interphase nucleus. The nucleoli reappear, and the cytoplasm divides to form two daughter cells. Because the chromosomes in the daughter cells contain identical copies of the duplicated DNA, the daughter cells are genetically identical and

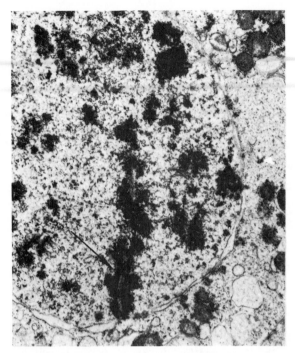

Figure 2.34. Electron micrograph of synaptonemal complex (*arrow*) in the nucleus of a pachytene primary spermatocyte. ×10,000.

contain the same kind and number of chromosomes. The daughter cells are 2*n* in DNA content and 2*n* in chromosome number.

Meiosis Is a Process Consisting of Two Sequential Cell Divisions That Produces Gametes Containing Half the Number of Chromosomes and Half the DNA Found in Somatic Cells

The zygote and all the somatic cells derived from it are described as *diploid (2n)* in chromosome number; the *gametes,* having only one member of each chromosome pair, are described as *haploid (1n).* During gametogenesis, reduction in chromosome number to the haploid state (23 chromosomes in the human) occurs through the two meiotic divisions. This reduction is necessary to maintain a constant number of chromosomes in the species. Reduction in chromosome number also produces reduction in DNA content to the haploid (1*n*) amount.

During meiosis, the chromosomes pair and may exchange chromosome segments, thus altering the genetic composition of the chromosomes. This genetic exchange, called *crossing-over,* and the random assortment of each member of the chromosome pairs into haploid gametes give rise to infinite genetic diversity.

The nuclear events of meiosis are the same in the male and female, but the cytoplasmic events are markedly different. Figure 2.33 illustrates the key nuclear and cytoplasmic events of meiosis as they occur in spermatogenesis and oogenesis. The events of meiosis through metaphase I are the same in both sexes. Therefore, the figure illustrates

the differences in the process as they diverge after metaphase I.

The Cytoplasmic Events Associated with Meiosis Differ in the Male and Female

In the male, the two meiotic divisions of a primary spermatocyte result in the formation of four structurally identical, although genetically unique haploid spermatids. Each spermatid has the capacity to differentiate into a spermatozoon. In contrast, in the female, the meiotic divisions of a primary oocyte result in the formation of one haploid ovum and three haploid polar bodies. The ovum receives the majority of the cytoplasm and becomes the functional gamete. The polar bodies receive very little cytoplasm and undergo degeneration.

The Nuclear Events of Meiosis Are Similar in Males and Females

During the *S phase* that precedes meiosis, the chromosomes are replicated. The DNA content becomes *4n,* and the chromosome number becomes *4n.* The cells then undergo a *reductional division (meiosis I)* and an *equatorial division (meiosis II).* During meiosis I, the maternal and paternal chromosomes pair and exchange segments. They then separate from one another. This results in one member of each pair of chromosomes in the daughter cells and the DNA being reduced to the *2n* amount. In meiosis II, the chromatids separate from one another, establishing the haploid number *(n)* of chromosomes and reducing the DNA to the haploid amount *(n).*

Phases in the Process of Meiosis Are Similar to the Phases of Mitosis

Prophase. The prophase of meiosis I is an extended phase that is subdivided into five stages (see Fig. 2.33):

1. *Leptotene.* The chromosome becomes visible as thin strands.
2. *Zygotene.* Homologous chromosomes of maternal and paternal origin pair. This pairing involves the formation of a *synaptonemal complex,* a tripartite structure that brings the chromosomes into physical association so that crossing-over may occur (see Fig. 2.34).
3. *Pachytene.* As the chromosomes condense, the individual chromatids become visible. Crossing-over occurs early in this phase.
4. *Diplotene.* The chromosomes condense further, and *chiasmata* or contacts between the chromatids appear. The chiasmata indicate crossing-over may have occurred.
5. *Diakinesis.* The chromosomes reach their maximum thickness, the nucleolus disappears, and the nuclear envelope disintegrates.

Metaphase I. Metaphase I is similar to the metaphase

of mitosis except that the paired chromosomes are aligned at the equatorial plate with one member on either side. *Anaphase I* and *telophase I* are similar to the same phases in mitosis except that the centromeres do not split and the paired chromatids, held by the centromere, remain together. A maternal or paternal member of each homologous pair, now containing exchanged segments, moves to each pole. *Segregation* or *random assortment* occurs because the maternal and paternal chromosomes of each pair are randomly aligned on one side or the other of the metaphase plate. This is an important contributor to genetic diversity. At the completion of meiosis I or the reductional division, the cytoplasm divides. Each resulting daughter cell (a secondary *spermatocyte* or *oocyte*) is haploid in chromosome number ($1n$), containing one member of each chromosome pair, but is still diploid in DNA content ($2n$).

Meiosis II. The cells quickly enter meiosis II or the equatorial division, which is more like mitosis because the centromeres divide. The chromatids then separate at *anaphase II* and pass to opposite poles of the cell. During meiosis II the cells pass through prophase II, metaphase II, anaphase II, and telophase II. These stages are essentially the same as those described in mitosis except that they involve a haploid set of chromosomes and produce daughter cells that have only the haploid DNA content ($1n$). *Unlike the cells produced by mitosis that are genetically identical with the parent cell, the cells produced by meiosis are genetically unique.*

Tissues: Concept and Classification

3

Tissues May Be Defined as Aggregates or Groups of Cells Organized to Perform One or More Functions

In examining the structure of the body at the light microscope level, it soon becomes apparent that the cells and extracellular components comprising the various organs of the body exhibit certain recognizable and often very distinctive patterns of organization. This organized arrangement is a reflection of the cooperative effort that like cells perform in carrying out a particular function. Thus, when we speak of an organized aggregation of cells that function in a collective manner, we are, by definition, referring to a tissue.

Although it is frequently said that the cell is the basic functional unit of the body, it is really the tissues, through the collaborative efforts of their individual cells, that are responsible for maintaining body functions. Furthermore, it is now well known that cells within certain tissues can communicate through specialized intercellular junctions (gap junctions, page 24), thus facilitating collaborative effort and allowing the cells to operate as a functional unit. Other mechanisms also exist that permit cells of a given tissue to function in a unified manner. This includes the presence of specific membrane receptors, neural innervation, and noncommunicating junctions between cells.

Despite Disparate Structure and Physiologic Properties, All Organs Are Made Up of Four Basic Tissue Types

The concept of tissues provides a basis for understanding and recognizing the many cell types within the body and how they interrelate. Despite variations in general appearance, structural organization, and physiologic properties of the various body organs, the cell aggregations that make them up are reduced to and classified under four tissue types. These *basic* or *fundamental tissues* are

- *Epithelial tissue* (epithelium), which covers body surfaces, lines body cavities, and forms glands

- *Connective tissue,* which underlies or surrounds and supports the other three basic tissues, both structurally and functionally
- *Muscular tissue,* which is made up of contractile cells and is responsible for movement of the body and its parts
- *Nervous tissue,* which gathers, transmits, and integrates information from outside and inside the body to control the activities of the body and its parts

Each of these basic tissues is defined by a set of general morphologic characteristics or by functional properties. Each type may be further subdivided on the basis of more specific characteristics of the various cell populations as well as on the basis of intercellular substances in those cases where they present special characteristics.

In considering the basic tissues, recognize that two different definitional parameters are employed. The basis for definition of epithelium and connective tissue is primarily morphologic, whereas the basis for the definition of muscular and nervous tissue is functional. Moreover, the same variations in parameters exist in designating the tissue subclasses. For example, while muscle tissue itself is defined by its function, it is subclassified into smooth and striated categories, a purely morphologic distinction, not a functional one. Another kind of contractile tissue, though functionally muscle, is typically designated as an epithelium (myoepithelium) because of its location.

For these reasons, the student must rely more on remembering the features or characteristics used in categorizing the many different cell aggregations that define the basic tissues and their subclasses rather than in relying on those that a simple formula, i.e., definition, might provide.

EPITHELIUM

Epithelium Is Characterized by the Close Apposition of Its Constituent Cells and Its Presence at a Free Surface

Epithelial cells, whether arranged in a single layer or in multiple layers, are always contiguous with one another. In

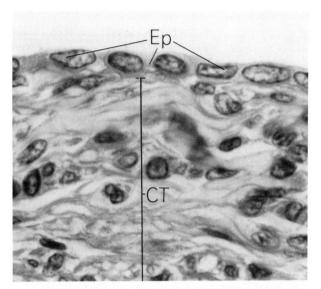

Figure 3.1. Comparison of an epithelium *(Ep)* and connective tissue *(CT)*. Note that the epithelial cells possess one surface that is not adherent to other cells. This is the free surface. Furthermore, the epithelial cells have established themselves in a single layer to form a continuous surface cover. Their nuclei have a uniform appearance and orientation. The cells of the connective tissue are of several types and appear randomly disposed. The nuclei exhibit varied sizes and shapes. The cytoplasm is difficult to discern and tends to blend with the connective tissue fibers.

addition, they are usually joined by specialized junctions, thus creating a barrier between the free surface and the adjacent tissue. The intercellular space between epithelial cells is very limited and is devoid of any structure except where junctional attachments are present.

The free surface of an epithelium is defined as that surface to which no cellular or extracellular formed elements adhere. Such surfaces are characteristic of the exterior of the body, the outer surface of many internal organs, and the lining of the body cavities, tubes, and ducts, both those that ultimately communicate with the exterior of the body and those that are enclosed, such as the lining endothelium of the vascular system.

Subclassifications of epithelium are usually based on the shape of the cells and the number of cell layers. However, they may also be based on the functions of the epithelium.

CONNECTIVE TISSUE

Connective Tissue Is Characterized on the Basis of the Extracellular Material That Is Present

Unlike epithelium, connective tissue cells are conspicuously separated from one another. The intervening spaces are occupied by material produced by the connective tissue cells. The nature of the cells and the intercellular material vary according to the function of the tissue and, thus, its type. The subclassification of connective tissue takes into

consideration not only the cells but also the composition and organization of the intercellular material.

Figure 3.1 demonstrates the essential difference between a typical epithelium and its subjacent connective tissue. Note that the epithelial cells are organized in a single uniform layer. In contrast, the underlying connective tissue displays cells whose nuclei are of variable appearance, thus representing nuclei of different cell types. Moreover, there is no distinct pattern of organization of the nuclei of connective tissue compared with those of the epithelium. The extracellular material, consisting largely of fibers, occupies the greater volume of the tissue. The subclassification of the connective tissue shown here is designated *loose connective tissue.* It is typically found in association with epithelia and contains both cells that originate and reside there permanently and cells that migrate into it from other sites.

Other types of connective tissue are subclassified mainly on the basis of the nature of the extracellular material. In some cases, the connective tissue, for purposes of strength, contain numerous closely packed fibers with fewer cells present. This type of connective tissue would be described as *dense connective tissue.* Bone and cartilage, for example, are two other types of connective tissue. Again, in both of these instances, it is the nature of the extracellular material that is present that characterizes the tissue, not the cellular component.

NERVOUS TISSUE

Nervous Tissue Consists of Nerve Cells (Neurons) and Associated Supporting Cells of Several Types

Although all cells exhibit electrical properties, *neurons* are highly specialized to transmit electrical impulses from one site in the body to another; they are also specialized to integrate those impulses. Neurons are characterized by having processes, an *axon* and *dendrites,* through which they interact with other nerve cells and with cells of epithelia and muscle. The axon is a long process (sometimes longer than a meter) that carries impulses away from the part of the cell that contains the nucleus (cell body); dendrites receive impulses and carry them toward the cell body.

Nerve cells receive and process information from the external and internal environment; they may develop specific sensory receptors and sensory organs to accomplish this.

In the central nervous system (CNS), i.e., the brain and spinal cord, the supporting cells are called neuroglial cells. In the peripheral nervous system (PNS), i.e., the nerves in all other parts of the body, the supporting cells are called Schwann (neurilemmal) cells and satellite cells.

In an ordinary hematoxylin and eosin (H&E)-stained section, nervous tissue may be observed in the form of a nerve, consisting of varying numbers of neuronal processes along with their supporting cells (Fig. 3.2). Nerves are most commonly seen, in longitudinal or cross section, in loose

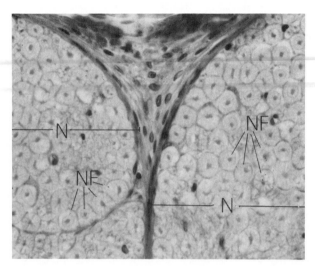

Figure 3.2. A section through a nerve showing part of two smaller nerve bundles *(N)*. The bulk of the nerve is comprised of long thread-like nerve fibers *(NF)*. The fibers are tightly packed together, and because they have been cut in cross section, they give a circular profile pattern. The dot-like units represent the thin cytoplasmic processes or axons of the nerve fibers. The surrounding material is myelin, which forms a highly specialized insulating cover.

connective tissue. Nerve cell bodies in the PNS, including the autonomic nervous system (ANS), are seen in aggregations called ganglia, where they are surrounded by satellite cells (Fig. 3.3).

Nerve cells and all of their associated cells are derived from the cells of the neuroectoderm (page 82) that constituted the neural tube in the embryo. Neuroectoderm originates by invagination of an epithelial layer, the dorsal ectoderm of the embryo. Some cells of the nervous system, such as the ependymal cells and the cells of the choroid plexus in the CNS, retain the absorptive and secretory functions characteristic of epithelial cells.

MUSCLE TISSUE

Muscle Tissue Is Categorized on the Basis of a Functional Property, the Ability of Its Cells to Contract

Muscle cells are characterized by the large amounts of the contractile proteins actin and myosin (pages 39 and 214) in their cytoplasm and by the particular cellular relationships in the tissue.

To function efficiently to effect movement, the muscle cells are most often aggregated into distinct bundles that are easily recognized as different from surrounding tissue. The cells are usually oriented with their long axes in the

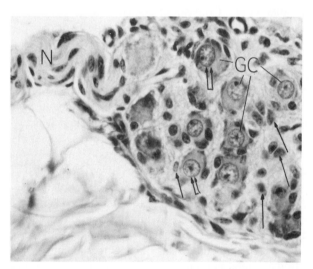

Figure 3.3. A section through a small ganglion. Here, the principal feature is the relatively large ganglion cells *(GC)* or nerve cell bodies that possess large nuclei *(double arrows)*. Many other smaller cells are present, as evidenced by the small nuclei *(arrows)*. Most of these are supporting or satellite cells, which are intimately associated with the nerve cell bodies. A longitudinal section of a nerve *(N)* leaving (or entering) the ganglion is also evident. The nerve fibers are longitudinally disposed in this section. Furthermore, they are unmyelinated, and without a myelin cover, the small nerve process is difficult to define.

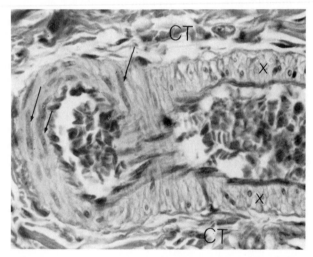

Figure 3.4. A section of a small artery with surrounding connective tissue *(CT)* making a right-angle turn within the section. The right portion of the micrograph shows the vessel longitudinally cut, whereas the left shows the vessel in cross section. The wall of the vessel is composed largely of smooth muscle cells, which have an elongate shape. They are packed together, parallel to one another, and tend to circumscribe the lumen of the vessel. Thus, where the vessel is longitudinally sectioned, the smooth muscle cells are seen in cross section *(X)*, and the elongate nuclei appear as small circular profiles. Where the vessel has turned and is cross-sectioned, the nuclei of the smooth muscle cells are seen as elongate profiles *(arrows)*. The pattern of the nuclei is distinctive in both instances.

same direction. This is evident in Figures 3.4 and 3.5, which show examples of smooth and striated muscle, respectively. The arrangement of nuclei seen in these figures confirms the parallel orientation of the cells.

Although the shape and arrangement of cells in particular muscle types, e.g., smooth muscle, skeletal muscle, and cardiac muscle, may be quite different (Figs. 3.4 and 3.5), all muscle types share the common characteristic that the bulk of the cytoplasmic volume consists of the contractile protein fibrils actin and myosin. Although these same proteins are ubiquitous in cells, it is only in muscle cells that they are present in such large amounts that their contractile activity can affect an entire organ or organism.

IDENTIFYING TISSUES

Recognition of Tissues Is Based on the Presence of Specific Structures Within Cells and on Specific Cellular Relationships

By keeping in mind these few basic facts and concepts concerning the fundamental tissues, the task of examining and interpreting histologic slide material can be greatly facilitated. The first goal is that of recognizing aggregates of cells as tissues and determining what special characteristics they present. Are the cells present at a surface? Are they in contact with their neighbors, or are they separated by a definable intervening material? Do they belong to a group having special properties, such as muscle or nerve?

The elements that characterize each of the fundamental tissues and relate to its functional aspects are examined in subsequent chapters. It is important to realize that in focusing on a single specific tissue we are, in a sense, artificially separating the constituent tissues of organs just as we previously concentrated on the specific characteristics of cells, divorced from tissues. However, only after having dealt with each of the basic tissues and their subtypes in this way is it possible to understand and appreciate the histology of the various organs of the body and the means by which they operate as functional units and integrated systems.

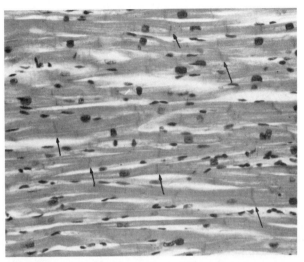

Figure 3.5. A section of cardiac muscle that consists of elongate cells larger in size than the smooth muscle cells just examined. As in the case of smooth muscle, the muscle cells seen here are arranged in parallel arrays, and when longitudinally sectioned, a linear pattern is readily discernible. The cells are attached end to end, forming a fiber structure. The muscle fibers anastomose with one another, as evidenced by branching of the fibers. The faint vertical lines *(arrows)* seen at this magnification are specialized sites that maintain adhesion between adjoining cells.

Detailed Knowledge of the Structure of Normal Cells and Tissues Helps Us Understand Abnormal Tissues

When tissues undergo abnormal change, as in tumors and teratomas, the nature of the tissue may not be recognizable by routine histologic examination. However, as we develop our understanding of the nature of tissue-specific components of cells, such as the various types of intermediate filaments described briefly on pages 30 and 41, we can begin to apply that detailed knowledge and sophisticated specific antibody staining procedures (see page 41) to identifying the origins of such abnormal tissues. For example, antibodies to tissue-specific intermediate filaments are used to determine whether certain poorly differentiated tumors are of epithelial or connective tissue origin. This allows diagnostic and therapeutic decisions to be made with greater confidence.

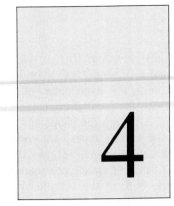

Epithelial Tissue

4

Epithelium Covers Body Surfaces, Lines Body Cavities, and Constitutes Glands

Epithelium is an avascular tissue comprised of cells that cover the exterior surfaces of the body and line both the internal closed cavities of the body and those body tubes that communicate with the exterior (the alimentary, respiratory, and genitourinary tracts). Epithelium also forms the secretory portion (parenchyma) of glands and their ducts and the receptors of certain sensory organs.

The cells that make up an epithelium have three principal characteristics:

- They are closely apposed and adhere to one another by means of special *junctions.*
- They exhibit functionally distinct surface domains, namely, a *free* or *apical surface,* a lateral surface, and a basal surface. (The properties of each are determined by the presence of specific membrane proteins.)
- Their basal surface is attached to an underlying *basement membrane,* a noncellular, protein–polysaccharide-rich layer demonstrable at the light microscopic level by histochemical methods (see Fig. 1.2, page 6).

Special Situations Occur Where Epithelial Cells Lack a Free Surface (Epithelioid Tissues)

In some locations, cells are found aggregated in close apposition to one another but lack a free surface. Although the close apposition of these cells and the presence of a basement membrane would lead to their classification as an epithelium, the absence of a free surface is sufficient to justify terming such cell aggregates as *epithelioid tissues.* Examples of epithelioid tissues include the interstitial cells of Leydig in the testis, the luteal cells of the ovary, the parenchyma of the adrenal gland, and the epithelioreticular cells of the thymus. Epithelioid patterns are also found in pathologic responses to injury and in many tumors.

Epithelium Creates a Selective Barrier Between the External Environment and the Underlying Connective Tissue

Covering and lining epithelia form a continuous, sheet-like cellular investment that separates the underlying or ad-

jacent connective tissue from the external environment and from the environment of internal cavities, both closed cavities and those that lead to the exterior of the body. This epithelial investment serves, among other roles, as a selective barrier capable of facilitating or inhibiting the passage of specific substances between the exterior (as well as the body cavities) and the underlying connective tissue compartment. In the study of the various organs it will be seen that any substance that enters the body as a metabolite or is discharged from the body as a waste product must literally pass through the epithelial cells, not between them (Fig. 4.1).

Furthermore, a given epithelium may serve one or more other functions, depending on the activity of the cell types present:

- It can be an almost impervious *barrier,* as in the epidermis or urinary bladder.
- It can be *secretory,* as in the stomach.

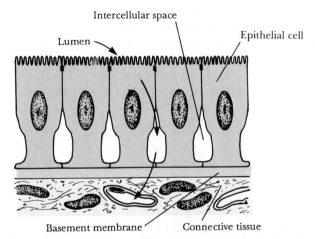

Figure 4.1. Diagram of absorptive epithelial cells, such as those of the intestine. The pathway of fluid movement, indicated by the *arrows,* is from the intestinal lumen into the cell, then across the lateral membrane into the intercellular space, and, finally, across the basement membrane to the connective tissue.

TABLE 4.1. Types of Epithelium

	CLASSIFICATION	SOME TYPICAL LOCATIONS	MAJOR FUNCTION
	Simple squamous	Lining of vascular system (endothelium) Lining of body cavities (mesothelium) Bowman's capsule (kidney) Lining of respiratory spaces in lung	Exchange, barrier in central nervous system Exchange and lubrication Barrier Exchange
	Simple cuboidal	Small ducts of exocrine glands Surface of ovary (germinal epithelium) Kidney tubules	Absorption, conduit Barrier Absorption
	Simple columnar	Lining of small intestine and colon Stomach lining and gastric glands Lining of gallbladder	Absorption and secretion Secretion Absorption
	Pseudo-stratified	Lining of trachea and bronchi Lining of deferens Efferent ductules of epididymis	Secretion, conduit Secretion, conduit Absorption, conduit
	Stratified squamous	Epidermis Lining of oral cavity and esophagus Lining of vagina	Barrier, protection Barrier, protection Barrier, protection
	Stratified cuboidal	Sweat gland, ducts Larger ducts of exocrine glands Anorectal junction	Barrier, conduit Barrier, conduit Barrier, conduit
	Stratified columnar	Largest ducts of exocrine glands Anorectal junction	Barrier, conduit Barrier, conduit
	Transitional	Renal calyces Ureters Bladder Urethra	Barrier, distensible property Barrier, distensible property Barrier, distensible property Barrier, distensible property

- It can be both *secretory* and *absorptive,* as in the intestines.
- It can provide a *transport* system through motile cilia on its surface to move particulates and mucus, as in the trachea and bronchi.
- It can serve to receive *sensory* stimuli, as in the taste buds of the tongue or the retina of the eye.

CLASSIFICATION OF EPITHELIUM

Epithelium Is Classified by Cell Arrangement and Cell Shape, Not by Function

Classification of epithelium is descriptive and based on the combination of the number of cell layers and the shape of the surface cells. The terminology is related only to structure, notto function. Thus, epithelium is described as

- *Simple,* when it is one cell layer thick
- *Stratified,* when it is two or more cell layers

The individual cells that compose an epithelium are described as

- *Squamous,* where the width of the cell is greater than its height
- *Cuboidal,* where the width, depth, and height are approximately the same
- *Columnar,* where the height of the cell appreciably exceeds the width (the term *low columnar* is often used where a cell's height only slightly exceeds its other dimensions)

The cells in a number of exocrine glands have a more or less pyramidal shape, with their apices directed toward a lumen. These cells are classified as either cuboidal or columnar, depending on their height rather than on their width at the base of the cell.

In a stratified epithelium, the shape and height of the cells usually vary from layer to layer, but *only the shape of the cells forming the surface layer is utilized in classifying the epithelium.* Thus, in designating an epithelium as stratified squamous, we are stating that it consists of more than one layer of cells and that the surface layer consists of flat or squamous cells. By describing the number of cell layers, i.e., simple or stratified, and the surface cell shape, the various configurations of epithelia are easily classified.

Pseudostratified Epithelium and Transitional Epithelium Are Special Classifications of Epithelium

Two special categories of epithelium are pseudostratified and transitional. *Pseudostratified epithelium* has the appearance of being stratified. Some of the cells do not reach the free surface; however, all rest on the basement membrane. Thus, it is actually a simple epithelium. Because pseudostratified epithelium has a rather limited distribution in the body and because it is often difficult to discern that all of the cells contact the basement membrane, its identification usually depends on the knowledge of where it exists.

Transitional epithelium is a name applied to the epithelium lining the pelvis of the kidney, the ureters, the urinary bladder, and part of the urethra. It is a stratified epithelium that has rather specific morphologic characteristics and functionally accommodates well to distension. This epithelium is dealt with in more detail in the chapter on the urinary system (Chapter 19).

The cellular configurations of the various types of epithelia and their appropriate nomenclature are illustrated in Table 4.1.

Endothelium and Mesothelium Are Specific Names Given to Simple Squamous Epithelium Lining the Vascular System and Body Cavities

Specific names are applied to epithelium in certain locations:

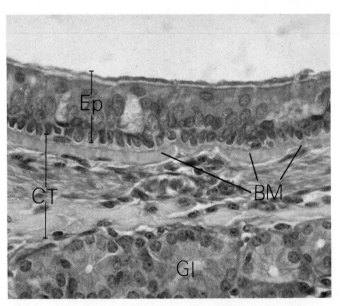

Figure 4.2. Photomicrograph of an H&E-stained section of the basement membrane *(BM)* of the trachea. It appears as a thick homogeneous structure lying immediately below the epithelium *(Ep).* It is actually a part of the connective tissue *(CT)* and is composed largely of densely packed connective tissue fibrils (collagen). Note that the epithelium forming the glands *(Gl)* in the tracheal wall does not exhibit similar structures. To demonstrate the basement membrane associated with the epithelium of the glands, as is the case with most other epithelia, special staining techniques, such as the periodic acid-Schiff (PAS) technique, are required. ×450.

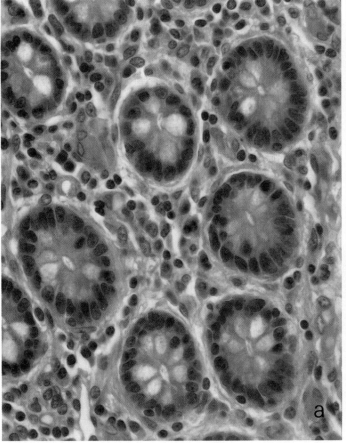
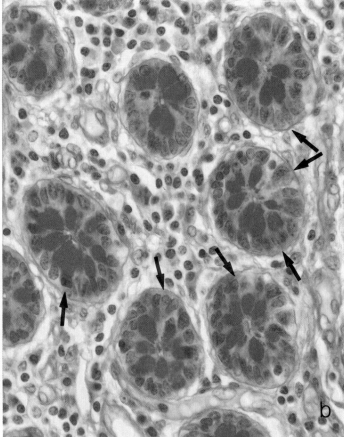

Figure 4.3. Photomicrographs showing serial sections of the intestinal glands of the colon. The glands have been cross-sectioned. **a.** This specimen was stained with H&E. Note that neither the basement membrane nor the mucin in the cells is stained. **b.** This section was stained with the PAS reaction. It reveals the basement membrane as a thin pink band between the base of the epithelial cells of the glands and the adjacent connective tissue *(arrows)*. The mucin within the secretory cells is also PAS positive.

- *Endothelium* is the name given to the epithelial lining of the vascular system.
- *Mesothelium* is the epithelium that lines the walls and covers the contents of the closed cavities of the body, i.e., the thoracic, pericardial, and abdominal cavities.

Both endothelium and mesothelium are almost always classified as simple squamous epithelia. Exceptions are found in postcapillary venules of certain lymphatic tissues where the endothelial cells are cuboidal and in the venous sinuses of the spleen where the endothelial cells are rod shaped and arranged much like the staves of a barrel.

The Morphology of an Epithelium Often Correlates With Its Function

Epithelia involved in secretion or absorption are typically simple or, in a few cases, pseudostratified. The height of the cells often reflects the level of secretory or absorptive activity. Simple squamous epithelia are compatible with a high rate of transepithelial transport if no intracellular pro-

cessing of the transported substance occurs. Stratification of the epithelium usually correlates with transepithelial impermeability. Finally, the pseudostratified arrangement of some epithelia reflects the role of stem cells in maintaining a stable population of cells to balance cell turnover. The basal cells in epithelia of this type usually belong to a renewing cell population that gives rise to mature functional cells of the epithelium.

BASEMENT MEMBRANE

Epithelium Is Attached to Its Underlying Connective Tissue by Basement Membrane

Basement membrane is the term originally given to a layer of variable thickness at the basal surfaces of epithelia. Although a prominent structure referred to as basement membrane is observed with hematoxylin and eosin (H&E) stain in a few locations, such as the trachea (Fig. 4.2) and, sometimes, urinary bladder and ureters, basement mem-

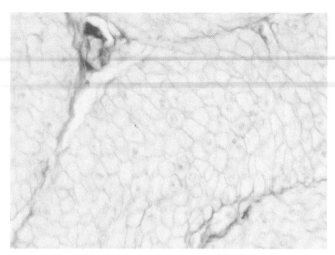

Figure 4.4. Photomicrograph of smooth muscle stained by the PAS method and counterstained with hematoxylin (pale nuclei). The muscle cells have been cut in cross section and appear as polygonal profiles due to the presence of PAS-reactive material surrounding each cell. As the plane of section, passes through each smooth muscle cell, it may or may not pass through the portion of the cell that includes the nucleus. Therefore, in some of the polygonal profiles, pale-staining nuclei can be seen; in other profiles, no nuclei are seen. The cytoplasm is not stained. ×850.

brane requires special staining for its demonstration in the light microscope. In part, this is due to its thinness and its staining with eosin, which makes it indistinguishable from the immediately adjacent connective tissue. In the case of the trachea, the element that is often described as basement membrane is actually a dense layer of closely spaced and aligned collagen fibrils that belong to the connective tissue.

In contrast to H&E (Fig. 4.3*a*), the periodic acid-Schiff (PAS) staining technique (Fig. 4.3*b*) results in a positive reaction at the site of the basement membrane. It appears as a thin, well-defined pink layer between the epithelium and the connective tissue. The stain, which reacts with the sugar moieties of proteoglycans, accumulates in sufficient amounts and density to make the basement membrane visible in the light microscope. A technique involving the reduction of silver salts by the sugars, thus blackening the basement membrane, can also be utilized to demonstrate this structure. Although basement membrane is classically described as being exclusively associated with epithelia, similar PAS-positive and silver-reactive sites can be demonstrated in relation to nerve-supporting cells, adipocytes, and muscle cells (Fig. 4.4); this delineates them from the surrounding connecting tissue. Connective tissue cells, other than adipocytes, do not show a similar PAS-positive or silver reaction. That most connective tissue cells are not surrounded by basement membrane material is consistent with the fact that they are not adherent to the connective tissue fibers and, in fact, require the ability to migrate within the tissue under appropriate stimuli in order to function.

Basal Lamina Is the Structural Attachment Site

Examination of the site of epithelial basement membranes with the electron microscope reveals a discrete layer of electron-dense matrix material, 50–100 nm thick (Fig. 4.5), between the epithelium and the adjacent connective

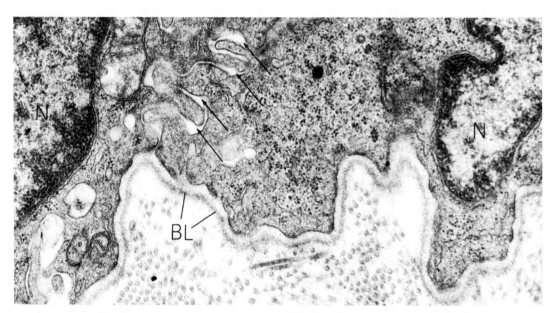

Figure 4.5. Electron micrograph showing only the very basal portion of two adjoining epithelial cells and parts of their nuclei *(N)*. The intercellular space is partially obscured by lateral interdigitations between the two cells *(arrows)*. The basal lamina *(BL)* appears as a thin band that follows the contours of the basal aspect of the overlying cell. Below the basal lamina are numerous cross-sectioned connective tissue fibrils (collagen). ×30,000.

tissue. This layer, referred to as **basal lamina** or sometimes *lamina densa,* reveals a network of fine 3–4-nm filaments when observed at high resolution. Between the basal lamina and the cell is a relatively clear or electron-lucent area, the *lamina lucida.* It contains fine filaments that join the plasma membrane to the basal lamina.

On the opposite side of the basal lamina, the connective tissue side, **anchoring fibrils** (*type IX collagen,* see Table 5.2, page 100) or **microfibrils,** typically one or the other in any given tissue, extend from the basal lamina matrix and appear to attach to reticular fibrils of the connective tissue (Fig. 4.6). The basal lamina thus serves as the structural attachment site for the overlying cells and the underlying connective tissue.

Muscle cells and nerve-supporting cells exhibit a peripheral extracellular electron-dense material having the same appearance as the basal lamina of epithelium. This, too, corresponds to a PAS-positive staining reaction, as described above (see Fig. 4.4). Although the term basement membrane is not ordinarily applied to the extracellular stainable material of these nonepithelial cells in light microscopy, the term basal lamina or *external lamina* is typically used at the electron microscope level.

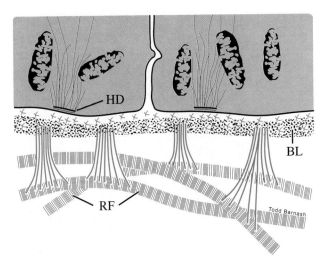

Figure 4.6. Diagram showing some of the components that provide attachment between epithelial cells and the underlying connective tissue. On the connective tissue side of the basal lamina *(BL),* anchoring fibrils (blue) extend from the basal lamina to the reticular fibrils *(RF)* of the connective tissue, providing structural attachment at this site. On the epithelial side, laminin (red) is present in the lamina rara and lamina densa and provides adhesion between the basal lamina and the epithelial cells. The laminin in the lamina rara is shown concentrated at the sites of the hemidesmosomes *(HD),* where the attachment is strongest.

> **BASEMENT MEMBRANE AND BASAL LAMINA: TERMINOLOGY**
>
> There is confusion in the usage of the terms **basement membrane** and **basal lamina.** Some authors use basement membrane interchangeably in both light and electron microscopy. Others dispense with the term basement membrane and use basal lamina in both light and electron microscopy. Because the term basement membrane originated with light microscopy, it is used in this book only in the context of light microscopic descriptions and only in relation to epithelia. The electron microscopic term basal lamina is reserved for the ultrastructural level to denote the layer present at the interface of connective tissue with epithelial cells. The term **external lamina** is often utilized to identify this same layer when it forms a peripheral cellular investment, as in the case of muscle and of nerve-supporting cells.

Basal Laminae Have Multiple Functions

Various functions are now attributed to the basal lamina. These include the following:

- *Structural attachment:* As already noted, the basal lamina serves as an intermediary structure in the attachment of cells to the adjacent connective tissue.
- *Compartmentalization:* Structurally, the basal lamina separates or isolates the connective tissue from epithelia, nerve, and muscle tissues. One can view connective tissue, including all of its specialized tissues, such as bone and cartilage (with the exception of adipose tissue, in that its cells possess a basal lamina), as a continuous single compartment. Epithelia,

muscle, and nerve, in contrast, are separated from adjacent connective tissue by intervening basal lamina. For anything to move from one tissue to another, i.e., from one compartment to another, it must cross a basal lamina.

- *Filtration:* The movement of substances to and from the connective tissue is, in part, regulated by the basal lamina largely through ionic charges and integral spaces. Filtration is well characterized in the kidney, where plasma filtrate must cross the compound basal laminae of capillaries and adjacent epithelial cells to reach the urinary space within a renal corpuscle.
- *Polarity induction:* Epithelial cells exhibit functionally different membrane properties as a result of surface exposure. Specific properties attributable to the basal membrane surface, as opposed to the apical and lateral membrane surfaces, are induced by the presence of the basal lamina. For example, epithelial cells grown in ordinary tissue culture become very flat as they proliferate and grow in the culture. The same cells, when grown on the surface of an artificial basal lamina in the culture medium, display their characteristic in vivo shape with evidence of normal polarity and function.
- *Tissue scaffolding:* The basal lamina serves as a guide or scaffold during regeneration. Newly formed cells or growing processes of a cell utilize basal lamina that remains after cell loss, thus helping to maintain the orig-

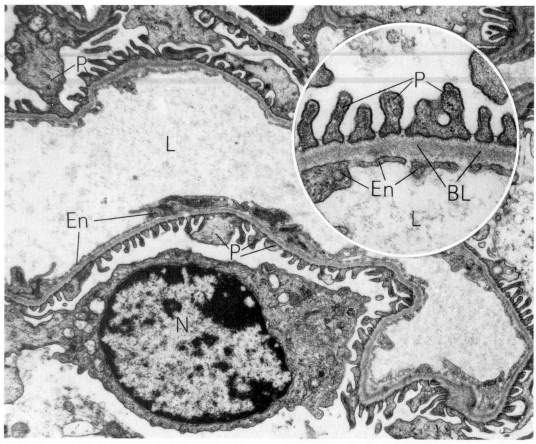

Figure 4.7. Electron micrograph of a kidney glomerular capillary. A basal lamina *(BL)* is seen interposed between the endothelial cell *(En)* of the capillary and the cytoplasmic processes *(P)* of the podocytes, which are located on the outer (abluminal) surface of the endothelial cell. The **inset** shows the relationship at higher magnification. Note that the two epithelial cells are separated by the basal lamina and no collagen fibrils are present. *N*, nucleus of podocyte; and *L*, lumen of capillary. ×12,000; **inset,** ×40,000.

inal tissue architecture. For example, in the case of nerve damage, new neuromuscular junctions from a growing axon will be established only if the basal lamina remains intact after injury.

Composition of Basal Laminae Includes at Least Five Substances

Analyses of basal laminae derived from epithelia in many locations (kidney glomeruli, lung, cornea, lens of the eye) indicate that it consists of at least five substances, namely, collagens, proteoglycans, laminin, and two glycoproteins, entactin and fibronectin.

- *Type IV collagen:* The major collagen, designated *type IV collagen,* represents 1 of approximately 16 types of collagen currently characterized in the body (see Table 5.2, page 100). Type IV collagen does not form fibrils, as do many of the other collagens. It consists of short filaments that are thought to provide structural integrity to the basal lamina. Moreover, it has a much higher content of hydroxyproline, hydroxylysine, and carbohydrate side chains than do other collagens.

- *Proteoglycans:* Much of the bulk volume of the basal lamina is probably due to the *proteoglycans* (heparan sulfate and chondroitin sulfate proteoglycans), molecules that, owing to their highly anionic character, are extensively hydrated (see page 105). Because of their high negative charge density, sulfated proteoglycans are believed to play an important role in the regulation of the passage of ions across the basal lamina.

- *Laminin:* A cross-shaped glycoprotein molecule, *laminin,* bridges the lamina lucida to link the basal lamina to the basal plasma membrane surface of the overlying epithelial cells (Fig. 4.6). Unlike the other collagens that are a product of fibroblasts and related connective tissue cells, type IV collagen is a product of the epithelial cells and other cell types that possess a basal lamina. Laminin and the heparan sulfate and chondroitin sulfate proteoglycans are also products of these cells; when secreted along with the type IV collagen, they self-assemble into basal lamina sheets.

- *Entactin and fibronectin:* The remaining two substances are less well characterized. *Entactin* is a small sulfated glycoprotein whose specific location within the

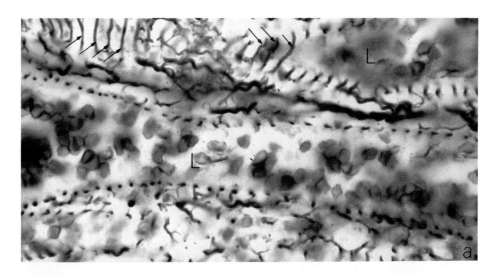

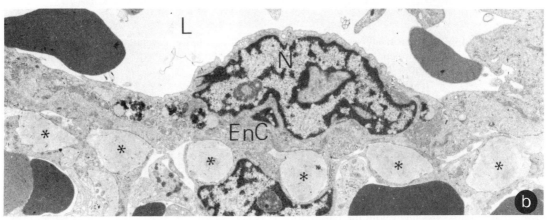

Figure 4.8. **a.** Photomicrograph of a silver preparation revealing two longitudinally sectioned venous sinuses of the spleen. These blood vessels are surrounded by a modified basement membrane, which takes the form of a ring-like structure, much like the hoops of a barrel, rather than a continuous layer or lamina. The rings are blackened by the silver and appear as bands where the walls of the vessel have been tangentially sectioned *(upper left arrows)*. To the right, the cut has penetrated deeper into the vessel, showing the lumen *(L)*, and the cut edges of the rings are seen on both sides of the vessel. In the lower vessel, the cut rings have been sectioned in a virtually perpendicular plane, and the ring appears as a series of dots. ×400. **b.** Electron micrograph of the wall of a venous sinus of the spleen, showing a longitudinally sectioned endothelial cell *(EnC)*. The nucleus *(N)* of the cell is protruding into the lumen. The basal lamina material *(asterisks)* has the same homogeneous appearance seen in other sites except that it is aggregated into ring-like structures rather than into a flat layer or lamina. Moreover, its location and plane of section, as seen here, correspond to the silver-reactive, dot-like material in **a.** ×25,000.

basal lamina and its function are not yet elucidated. Similarly, *fibronectin,* another glycoprotein, acts as an adhesive substance, binding to the plasma membrane and to heparan sulfate proteoglycan. Its specific location and role within basal laminae are still unclear.

• *Anchoring filaments:* Collagen fibrils of still another type, type VII, may form *anchoring filaments* that link the basal lamina to the underlying connective tissue or *reticular lamina* (described below). These molecular associations are reinforced by additional glycoproteins, still incompletely characterized, that interconnect or cross-link the molecules to achieve even greater stability in the interactions between the basal lamina and the structures that interface with it.

A Layer of Reticular Fibers Underlies the Basal Lamina

There is still lack of agreement as to the extent to which the basal lamina seen in the electron microscope corresponds to the structure described as the basement membrane in the light microscope. Some investigators contend that the basement membrane includes not only the basal lamina but also a secondary layer of small unit fibrils of type III collagen (the reticular fibers of light microscopy) that forms the reticular lamina. The reticular lamina, as such, belongs to the connective tissue and is not a product of the epithelium. The reticular lamina was once regarded as the component that reacted with silver, whereas the polysac-

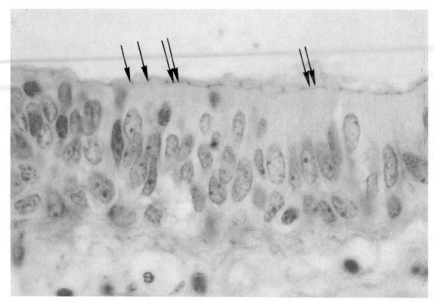

Figure 4.9. Photomicrograph showing the terminal bar in a pseudostratified epithelium. The bar appears as a dot *(single arrows)* when it is seen on its cut edge. When the bar is cours- ing parallel to the cut surface and lying within the thickness of the section, it is seen as a linear or bar-like profile *(double arrows)*.

charides of the basal lamina and the ground substance associated with the reticular fibers were thought to be the component staining with the PAS reaction. However, convincing arguments can be made for the basal lamina being responsible for both the PAS and silver reactions in several sites. In normal kidney glomeruli, for example, there are no collagen (reticular) fibers associated with the basal lamina of the epithelial cells (Fig. 4.7), although a positive reaction occurs with both PAS staining and silver impregnation. Also, in the spleen, where the basal lamina of the venous sinuses forms a unique pattern of ring-like bands rather than a thin, sheath-like layer around the vessel, exactly corresponding images are seen with the PAS and silver techniques as well as with the electron microscope (Fig. 4.8).

Attachment to a Basement Membrane Is Essential for Epithelial Development and Function

The multiple roles of the basal lamina and basement membrane are not yet fully elucidated. It is generally accepted that they facilitate attachment of epithelia to underlying connective tissue and that they influence the differentiation and proliferation of the epithelial cells that contact them.

Other roles for these layers that are currently the subject of intense investigation include their function as selective and regulatory filtration barriers to substances moving between the epithelium and the connective tissue and between the connective tissue and the epithelium and their function in providing a scaffold for the growth and migration of epithelial cells during embryogenesis, regener-

ation, normal tissue cell renewal and migration, and wound healing.

EPITHELIAL CELL ADHESION AND INTERCELLULAR CONTACTS

Epithelial cells are not only characteristically in close apposition but are also, with few exceptions, extremely adherent to one another. Prior to the advent of electron microscopy it was thought that this property of adhesion was due to the presence of a viscous adhesive substance referred to as ''intercellular cement.'' It was also noted that this cement substance stained deeply at the apical-lateral margin of the cells of most cuboidal and columnar types of epithelium. When viewed in a plane perpendicular to the epithelial surface, the stainable material gives the appearance of a dot-like structure. When the plane of section passes parallel to and includes the epithelial surface, however, the dot-like component is seen as a dense bar or line between the apposing cells (Fig. 4.9). The bars, in fact, form a polygonal structure (or band) at the periphery of each cell.

Terminal Bars Represent Epithelial Cell Attachment Sites

Because of its location in the terminal or apical portion of the cell and its bar-like configuration, the stainable material was designated ***terminal bar.*** It is now evident that intercellular cement, as such, does not exist.

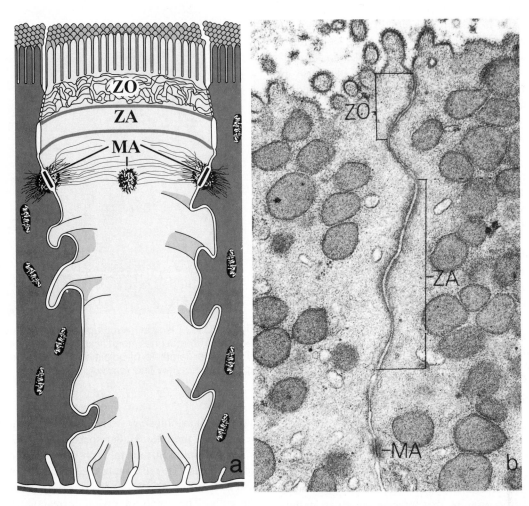

Figure 4.10. **a.** Diagram showing the components of the junctional complex and their relationship in a columnar epithelial cell. (Modified from Kristic RV: *Illustrated Encyclopedia of Human Histology.* Berlin, Springer, 1984, p 213.) **b.** Electron micrograph of the apical portion of two adjoining epithelial cells of the gastric mucosa, showing the junctional complex. *MA,* macula adherens; *ZA,* zonula adherens; and *ZO,* zonula occludens. ×30,000.

BASEMENT MEMBRANE CHANGES IN DISEASE STATES

Under certain pathologic conditions, basement membrane undergoes marked change. In diabetes, a disease that exacts a heavy toll on the vascular system, there is a striking thickening of the basement membrane of the small blood vessels. The capillaries of diabetics are more leaky to plasma proteins than are those of normal patients, despite the increased thickness of the basement membrane. Increased production of type IV collagen and laminin appears to be responsible for the thickening of the basement membrane. Diabetics demonstrate a decreased sulfation of heparan sulfate proteoglycan, however, which may contribute to the increased permeability of the capillaries. In addition, chondroitin sulfate proteoglycan is abnormally present in the vascular basement membranes of animals with induced diabetes. It has also been suggested that thickening may be caused, in part, by enhanced or abnormal binding of proteins to the basement membrane. In membrane glomerulonephritis, as well as in certain other nephritic syndromes, there is a thickening of the basal lamina of the kidney glomerular capillaries. The significance of these changes and their specific effect on tissue function are unclear.

The terminal bar, however, does represent a significant structure. Electron microscopy has shown it to be the site of specialized attachment of adjoining epithelial cells (Fig. 4.10). It is also the site of a barrier to the passage (diffusion) of substances across the epithelium. The specific structural components that make up the barrier and the attachment device are readily identified in the electron microscope and are collectively referred to as a *junctional complex* (Table 4.2). The structures revealed in the electron microscope that constitute the junctional complex are

- *Zonula occludens,* also called a *tight junction,* the diffusion barrier. It is located at the most apical point between adjoining epithelial cells and forms a ring or circumferential band (thus, zonula) around the cell.
- *Zonula adherens,* a continuous band-like adhesion. This device surrounds the cell and joins it to its neighbors.
- *Macula adherens,* also known as a *desmosome,* which is included by many authors as a third component of the junctional complex. It is a localized spot adhesion, as opposed to a zonular adhesion, located at multiple sites on the upper lateral surfaces of adjoining cells.

The Zonula Occludens Is Created by Localized Sealing of the Outer Leaflets of Adjacent Plasma Membranes

Examination of the zonula occludens in the electron microscope reveals a narrow region in which the outer leaflets of the plasma membrane of adjoining cells come in contact to seal off the intercellular space (Fig. 4.11). The seal is created by specific proteins that traverse the outer leaflets of the interacting cells and join in the intercellular space. The arrangement of the protein in forming the seal is best visualized by the freeze fracture technique (Fig. 4.12). When the plasma membrane is fractured at the site of the zonula occludens, the junctional proteins are observed on the P-face of the membrane, where they give the appearance of a ridge-like structure. The opposing surface of the fractured membrane, the E-face, reveals a complementary groove as a consequence of detachment of the protein particles from its surface. The ridges and grooves are arranged as a net-

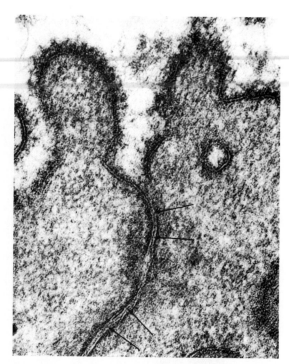

Figure 4.11. Electron micrograph of the zonula occludens from Figure 4.10*b* at higher magnification. Note the intimate contact of the outer lamellae of adjoining plasma membranes, which appear as a single line *(arrows).* ×100,000.

work of anastomosing strands, thus creating a functional seal within the intercellular space (Fig. 4.12).

High-resolution transmission electron microscopy similarly reveals that the zonula occludens is not a continuous seal but, rather, appears as a series of focal fusions between the cells. The points of fusion correspond to the location of the protein particles observed in freeze fracture preparation. Also, observations based on different kinds of epithelia reveal that the complexity and number of strands forming the zonulae occludentes (pl.) varies. In those epithelia where anastomosing strands or fusion sites are sparse, such as certain kidney tubules, the intercellular pathway is partially permeable to water and solutes. In contrast, in those epithelia where the strands are numerous and extensively intertwined, e.g., intestinal and urinary bladder epithelia, the intercellular region is highly impermeable.

TABLE 4.2.   Terminology of Intercellular Contacts

LIGHT MICROSCOPY	ELECTRON MICROSCOPY
Terminal bar = Junctional complex =	{ Zonula occludens = tight junction Zonula adherens Macula adherens
Desmosome = Macula adherens	

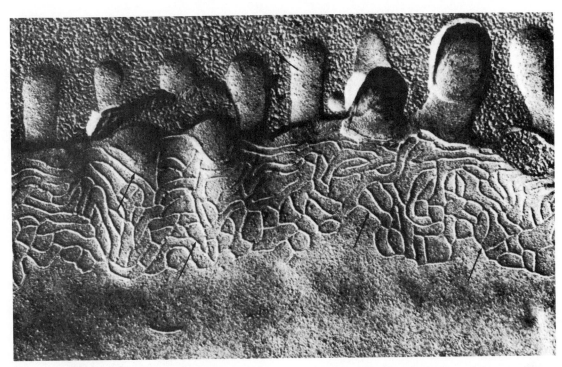

Figure 4.12. Freeze fracture preparation of intestinal epithelium. The zonula occludens appears as an anastomosing network of ridges *(arrows)* seen here on the P-face of the membrane. (The E-face of the fractured membrane would show a complementary pattern of grooves.) The strands or ridges are interpreted as linear arrays of integral protein particles within the membrane. The membrane of the opposing cell contains a similar network, which is in register and is firmly bonded to the first cell. The actual sites of fusion between the cells are thus along the anastomosing network. ×100,000. (From Hull B, Staehelin LA: *The Journal of Cell Biology* 68(3):693, 1976.)

The Zonula Occludens Separates Luminal Space From Intercellular Space and Connective Tissue Compartment

It is now evident that the zonula occludens plays an essential role in maintaining selective passage of substances from one side of an epithelium to the other (see Fig. 4.1). To the degree that water and solutes are restricted from diffusing between cells by the zonula occludens, transport must occur by active means. This requires specialized membrane transport proteins that move selected substances across the apical plasma membrane into the cytoplasm and then across the basolateral membrane below the level of the junction.

The Zonula Occludens Establishes Functional Domains in the Plasma Membrane

As a junction, the zonula occludens restricts not only the passage of water, electrolytes, and other small molecules across the epithelial layer but also the diffusion of molecules within the thickness of the plasma membrane itself. Thus, the cell is able to segregate certain enzymes on the apical (free) surface and restrict others to the lateral or basallateral surfaces. In the intestine, for instance, the enzymes for terminal digestion of peptides and saccharides (dipeptidases and disaccharidases) are localized in the membrane of the microvilli of the apical surface. The Na^+-K^+-activated ATPase (adenosinetriphosphatase) that drives salt and water transport, as well as amino acid and sugar transport, is restricted to the lateral plasma membrane below the zonula occludens.

The Zonula Adherens Provides Lateral Adhesion Between Epithelial Cells

The integrity of epithelial surfaces is, in large part, dependent on the lateral adhesion of the cells with one another and their ability to resist separation. Although the zonula occludens involves a fusion of adjoining cell membranes, resistance to mechanical stress is limited. Reinforcement of this region is dependent on a strong bonding site below the zonula occludens. Like the zonula occludens, the required lateral adhesion device occurs in a band or belt-like configuration around the cell; thus, the adhering junction is referred to as a zonula adherens. The morphologic and functional integrity of the zonula adherens are calcium dependent. Removal of Ca^{2+} from solutions bathing epithelia leads to disruption of this junction.

When examined in the electron microscope, the site of the zonula adherens is characterized by a uniform 15–20-nm space between the opposing cell membranes (Fig. 4.13). The intercellular space is of low electron density, almost appearing clear, but is evidently occupied by a material through which the two membranes maintain their adherence to one another. In the confines of the zonula adherens, a moderately electron dense material is found along the cy-

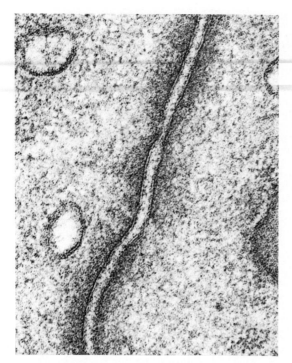

Figure 4.13. Electron micrograph of the zonula adherens from Figure 4.10*b* at higher magnification. The plasma membranes are separated here by a relatively uniform space. The intercellular space appears clear, showing only a sparse amount of diffuse punctate substance. The cytoplasmic side of the plasma membrane exhibits a moderately electron dense material. ×100,000.

toplasmic side of the membrane of each cell. It is believed that this material, largely by virtue of its location, represents the stainable substance in light microscopy, the terminal bar (in contrast, the principal element that constitutes the zonula occludens, namely, the membrane particles, lacks both size and quantity to be resolved in the light microscope as a component of the terminal bar). Associated with the electron-dense material is an array of 6-nm microfilaments (comprised of actin) that stretch across the apical cytoplasm and appear to anchor in the electron-dense material of the junction. These filaments are thought to give structural rigidity to the apical region of the cell.

The Fascia Adherens Is a Sheet-Like Junction That Stabilizes Nonepithelial Tissues

Physical attachments that occur between cells in tissues other than epithelia are usually not prominent, but there are a few notable exceptions. In cardiac muscle, the cells are arranged end to end, forming thread-like contractile units. The attachment is by a combination of typical desmosomes or maculae adherentes and broad adhesion plates morphologically like the zonula adherens of epithelial cells. Because the attachment is not a ring-like configuration but, rather, has a broad face, these attachments are designated *fascia adherens* (Fig. 4.14).

The Macula Adherens (Desmosome) Provides Localized Spot-Like Adhesion Between Epithelial Cells

The macula adherens, the second type of adhesion device, provides a particularly strong attachment structure, as shown by microdissection studies. These junctions are localized on the lateral sides of the cell, much like a series of spot welds (see Fig. 4.10). Originally described in epidermal cells and designated as a ***desmosome*** (fr. Gr. *desmo,* bond; *soma,* body), the name is still retained and often used interchangeably with macula adherens (fr. L. *macula,* spot). In epidermal cells, the desmosome is the only attachment device present. In other epithelia, particularly those with

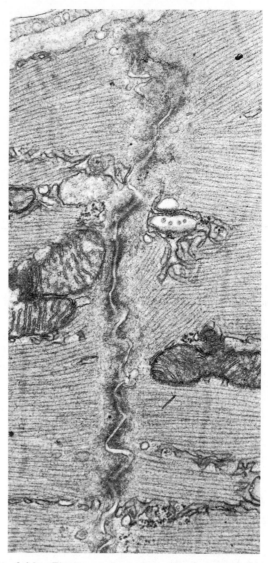

Figure 4.14. Electron micrograph showing the end-to-end apposition of two cardiac muscle cells. The intercellular space appears as a clear undulating area. On the cytoplasmic side of the plasma membrane of each cell there is a dense material similar to that seen in a zonula adherens. Because the attachment site here involves a portion of the end face of the two cells, it is called a fascia adherens. ×38,000.

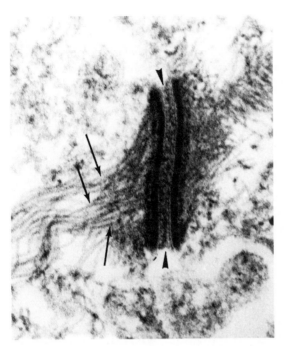

Figure 4.15. Electron micrograph of a macula adherens. The tonofilaments *(arrows)* attach into a dense material or plaque located on the cytoplasmic side of the plasma membrane. The intercellular space is also occupied by a dense material *(arrowheads)*, presumably the adhesion substance. The intercellular space above and below the macula adherens is not well defined due to extraction of the plasma membrane in order to define the integral components of the macula adherens. ×40,000. (Courtesy of Dr. E. Kallenbach.)

cuboidal or columnar cells, the macula adherens or desmosome is found in conjunction with a zonula adherens. The macula adherens occupies small, localized sites on the cell surface, however; it is not a continuous structure around the cell, as is the zonula adherens. Thus, a section perpendicular to the surface of a cell, though it will cut through the entire lateral surface, will often not include a macula adherens. The section will, however, always include the zonula adherens.

When observed in the electron microscope, the macula adherens exhibits a complex structure. On the cytoplasmic side of the plasma membrane of each of the adjoining cells is a very dense material in the shape of a disc; this is referred to as an *attachment plaque* to which intermediate filaments are anchored (Fig. 4.15). The filaments appear to loop through the attachment plaques and extend back out into the cytoplasm. They are thought to play a role in dissipating physical forces throughout the cell from the attachment site. The intercellular space of the macula adherens is conspicuously wider than that of the zonula adherens and is occupied by a dense medial band, the *intermediate line.* Between the intermediate line and the plasma membrane on either side is a fibrillar material that appears to provide attachment of the two cells through interaction of extracellular linker filaments. The intermediate line repre-

sents a condensation of the outer part of the glycocalyx from each cell.

Hemidesmosomes Occur Where Epithelia Require Strong Adhesion to the Connective Tissue

A variant of the desmosome is found in certain epithelia where abrasion and mechanical shearing forces would tend to separate the epithelium from the underlying connective tissue. Typically, it occurs in cornea, skin, and mucosae of the oral cavity, esophagus, and vagina. In these locations, only half the desmosome is present, hence the name **hemidesmosome.** Hemidesmosomes are found on the basal cell surface, where they provide increased adhesion to the basal lamina (Fig. 4.16). Their extracellular linker filaments, instead of interacting with those of a neighboring cell as in the desmosome, enter the basal lamina and give it a more dense appearance at that site.

In some instances, the contact between cells may be at a molecular level, involving individual membrane glycoproteins, which are not visualized with conventional microscopic techniques. These glycoproteins project out into the cell coat and link with individual specific glycoproteins expressed on neighboring cells. The type of glycoprotein varies from cell type to cell type and is believed to help confer a "social identity" onto cells. These molecular-scale contacts have the potential to be reversible and, thus, are found in embryonic as well as adult tissue. Such interactions of cells occur, during embryonic development, to direct the migration and association of cells as organ systems

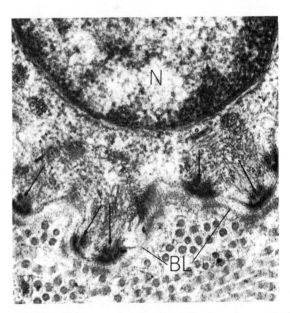

Figure 4.16. Electron micrograph of the basal aspect of a gingival epithelial cell. Below the nucleus *(N)*, tonofilaments are seen converging on the dense attachment plaques *(arrows)* of the hemidesmosome. Below the plasma membrane are the basal lamina *(BL)* and collagen fibrils (most of which are cut in cross section) of the connective tissue. ×40,000.

develop or, in the adult, to direct the function of the cells of the immune system.

In summary, there is a requirement for attachments within certain populations of cells. In epithelium, the junctional complex is particularly significant because it serves to create a long-term barrier, allowing the cells to compartmentalize and restrict the free passage of substances across the epithelium. Although it is the zonula occludens of the junctional complex that principally effects this function, it is the adhesive properties of the zonulae and maculae adherentes that guard against physical disruption of the barrier. Also important is the requirement for very strong attachment sometimes required in other sites. For example, in the stratified epithelial cells of the epidermis, it is the macula adherens that maintains cell adhesion. In cardiac muscle, where there is a similar need for strong adhesion, a combination of the macula adherens and fascia adherens provides this feature.

CELL SURFACE MODIFICATIONS

Epithelial cells exhibit modifications of their cell surfaces that relate to specialized functions. Those surface modifications that are dealt with in relation to epithelia are

- *Microvilli,* cytoplasmic processes that extend from the cell surface
- *Stereocilia,* microvilli of unusual length
- *Cilia,* motile cytoplasmic processes
- *Lateral and basal cell surface folds and processes,* invaginations and evaginations of the cell surface that create interdigitating and interleaving tongue-and-groove margins for neighboring cells

Microvilli Are Finger-Like Cytoplasmic Projections on the Apical Surface of Most Epithelial Cells

As observed in the electron microscope, microvilli are seen to vary in appearance from small, irregular, short bleb-like projections in some cell types to tall, closely packed, uniform projections that provide an enormous increase in the free surface area of other cell types. In general, the number and the shape of the microvilli of a given cell type correlate with its absorptive capacity. Thus, cells whose principal function is the transport of fluid and absorption of metabolites exhibit many closely packed, tall microvilli. Cells in which transport across the epithelium is less active exhibit smaller, more irregular microvilli.

Among the fluid-transporting epithelia, e.g., those of the intestine and kidney tubule, a distinctive border of vertical striations at the apical surface of the cell is readily detectable with the light microscope. This surface structure was originally given the name *striated border* for the intestinal absorptive cell and the name *brush border* for the kidney tubule cell. Where there is no apparent surface modification

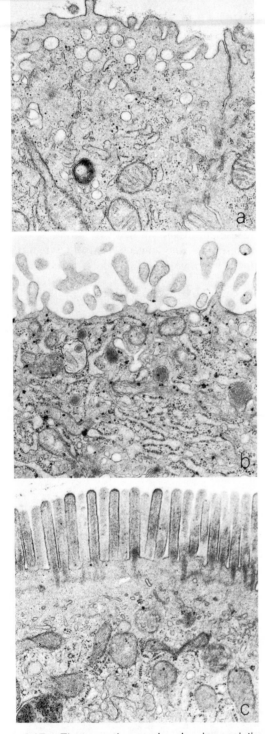

Figure 4.17. Electron micrographs showing variation in microvilli of different cell types. **a.** Cell of uterine gland; very small projections. **b.** Placenta; irregular, branching microvilli. **c.** Intestinal absorptive cell with very uniform and regularly arranged microvilli. All figures, ×20,000.

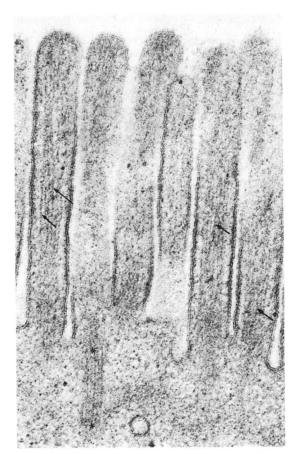

Figure 4.18. Higher-magnification view of the microvilli seen in Figure 4.17c. Note the presence of the microfilaments in the microvilli *(arrows),* which extend into the apical cytoplasm *(asterisks).* ×80,000.

based on light microscope observations, microvilli, if present, are usually short and not numerous; thus, they may escape detection with the light microscope.

The degree to which microvilli may vary among different types of epithelia is illustrated in Figure 4.17. The microvilli of the intestinal epithelium (striated border) are the most highly ordered, being even more uniform in appearance than those that constitute the brush border of kidney cells. They also contain a conspicuous core of microfilaments (actin) that are anchored to the plasma membrane at the tip and sides of the microvillus and extend down into the apical cytoplasm. Here, they interact with a horizontal network of filaments, the **terminal web,** that lies just below the base of the microvilli (Fig. 4.18). The actin filaments primarily provide support and give rigidity to microvilli to help maintain their parallel array. It has been proposed that some of the microfilaments of the zonula adherens and the terminal web have a contractile ability, which could have the effect of decreasing the diameter of the apex of the cell, causing the microvilli, whose stiff actin cores are anchored into the terminal web, to spread apart at their tips and increase the intermicrovillous space. Actin filaments are also

present in the microvilli of other cell types, but they are usually much less well developed and are often so sparse in number that they are difficult to detect.

Stereocilia Are Unusually Long Microvilli

Stereocilia are included in this section not because of their wide distribution among epithelia but because of the traditional treatment of this unusual surface modification as a separate structural entity. They are, in fact, limited to the epididymis of the male reproductive system and to the sensory (hair) cells of the ear.

Stereocilia of the ductus epididymis are extremely long processes that extend from the apical surface of the cell. Electron microscopic examination reveals them to be unusually long microvilli (Fig. 4.19). They lack notable internal structural features. When seen with the light microscope, these processes frequently give the superficial

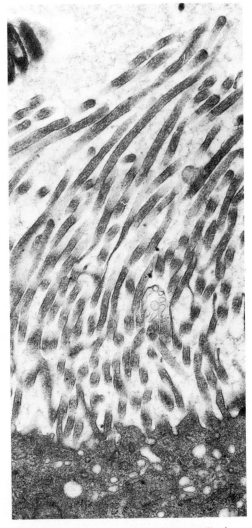

Figure 4.19. Electron micrograph of stereocilia from the epididymis. The cytoplasmic projections are similar to microvilli, but they are extremely long. ×20,000.

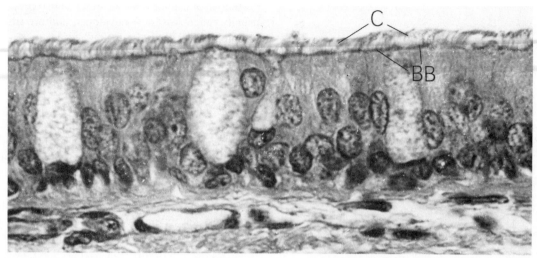

Figure 4.20. Photomicrograph of the pseudostratified, ciliated epithelium of the trachea. The cilia *(C)* appear as hairlike processes extending from the apical surface of the cells. The dark line immediately below the ciliary processes is produced by the basal bodies *(BB)*. ×750.

appearance of the hairs of a coloring brush due to the way the processes often aggregate into pointed bundles.

Stereocilia of the sensory epithelium of the ear are uniform in diameter and possess an internal filamentous structure. They serve as a receptor device rather than an absorptive structure (see page 775).

Cilia Are Motile Cytoplasmic Structures Capable of Moving Fluid and Particles Along Epithelial Surfaces

In contrast to stereocilia, true cilia possess an internal structure that provides for movement of the cilia. In most ciliated epithelia, as in the trachea, bronchi, or oviducts, there may be as many as several hundred cilia to a cell, all arranged in orderly rows. In the tracheobronchial tree, the cilia play a cleansing role by sweeping mucus and trapped particulate material toward the oropharynx where it is swallowed along with saliva and, thus, eliminated. In the oviduct, cilia help sweep ova and fluid along the tract toward the uterus.

In some epithelia, only a single cilium per cell may be present, e.g., the epithelial cells of the rete testis in the male reproductive tract and the vestibular hair cells of the ear. In these instances, the single cilium is regarded as having a sensory role.

Cilia Give a "Crew-Cut" Appearance to the Epithelial Surface

In the light microscope, cilia appear as short, fine, hairlike structures emanating from the free surface of the cell (Fig. 4.20). A thin, dark-staining band is usually seen extending across the cell at the base of the cilia. This darkstaining band is due to structures, known as *basal bodies,* that take up stain and, when viewed with the light micro-

scope, collectively appear as a continuous band. However, each cilium is associated with a single basal body that is separate and distinct from those of adjacent cilia.

Cilia Contain an Organized Core of Microtubules, the 9 + 2 Arrangement

Each cilium, when examined by electron microscopy and viewed in longitudinal profile, reveals an internal content of microtubules (Fig. 4.21). When the cilium is viewed in cross-sectional profile, the microtubules are observed to have a specific arrangement, namely, nine doublets or pairs of circularly arranged microtubules surrounding two central microtubules (Fig. 4.22).

The microtubules comprising each doublet are constructed so that the wall of one microtubule, designated the *B microtubule,* is actually incomplete; it shares a portion of the wall of the other microtubule of the doublet, the *A microtubule.* The two central microtubules are separate from one another; each is a single structure. This 9 + 2 microtubule array courses from the tip of the cilium to its base, where the outer paired microtubules join the basal body. The basal body is a modified centriole consisting of nine short microtubule triplets arranged in a ring. Each of the paired microtubules of the cilium is continuous with two of the triplet microtubules of the basal body. The central two microtubules of the cilium end at the level of the top of the basal body. Therefore, a cross section of the basal body would reveal nine circularly arranged microtubule triplets but not the two central single microtubules of the cilium.

Cilia Develop From Procentrioles

The process of *ciliary formation* in differentiating cells involves the replication of the centriole to give rise

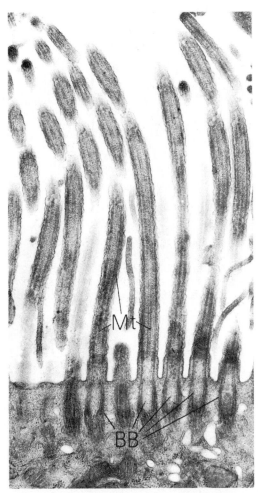

Figure 4.21. Electron micrograph of longitudinally cut cilia from the oviduct. The internal structures within the ciliary process are the microtubules *(Mt)*. The basal bodies *(BB)* appear empty due to the absence of the central pair of microtubules in this portion of the cilium. The other two basal bodies have been sectioned peripherally through the outer microtubule doublets. ×20,000.

ment, the ***recovery stroke.*** The plane of movement of a cilium is perpendicular to a line joining the central pair of microtubules. Through sequential timing, the cilia in successive rows start their beat so that each row is slightly more advanced in its cycle than the following row, thus creating a wave that sweeps across the epithelium. This ***metachronal rhythm*** is responsible for moving mucus over epithelial surfaces or facilitating the flow of fluid and other substances through tubular organs and ducts.

Ciliary activity is based on the movement of the doublet microtubules in relation to one another. Each doublet, when seen in cross section at high resolution, exhibits a pair of ''arms'' that contain ***dynein,*** an ATPase (see Fig. 4.22, *diagram*). The dynein arms extend from the A microtubule to form temporary cross-bridges with the B microtubule of the adjacent doublet. Addition of ATP produces a sliding movement of the bridge along the B microtubule, and as a result, the cilium bends.

KARTAGENER'S SYNDROME

A structural abnormality involving absence of dynein arms has been found in some individuals with Kartagener's syndrome, a hereditary disease associated with chronic respiratory difficulty (including bronchitis and sinusitis) and visceral asymmetry. Ciliary motility is severely impaired or absent in afflicted individuals, and as a consequence, there is reduced or no ciliary transport of mucus in the ***tracheobronchial system.*** As indicated above, individuals afflicted with the disease often demonstrate complete ***situs inversus,*** transposition of the viscera, or some degree of visceral asymmetry. Inversion of the viscera may be related to the lack of ciliary activity during the developmental process. Another possibility is that microtubules that designate a form of polarity within cells may also indirectly influence the polarity of organ systems. Inversion of the viscera may occur as a result of abnormal microtubular structure. Males with Kartagener's syndrome are sterile. The flagellum of the sperm, which is similar in structure to the cilium, is immotile. In contrast, some females afflicted with the syndrome may be fertile. In such individuals, the ciliary movement may be sufficient, though impaired, to permit transport of the ovum through the oviduct.

---

to multiple ***procentrioles,*** one for each cilium that is destined to form. The procentrioles grow and migrate to the apical surface of the cell, where each becomes a basal body. From each of the nine triplets that make up the basal body, a microtubule doublet grows upward, creating a projection containing the nine doublets found in the mature cilium. Simultaneously, the two single central microtubules form de novo within the ring of doublet microtubules, thus yielding the characteristic 9 + 2 arrangement.

Cilia Beat in a Synchronous Pattern

Cilia undergo a regular and synchronous undulating movement. In the living state, each cilium exhibits a rapid forward movement in a rigid state, the ***effective stroke,*** but becomes flexible and bends on the slower return move-

Lateral and Basal Cell Surface Folds Create Interdigitating Cytoplasmic Processes of Adjoining Cells

The lateral surface of certain epithelial cells may show a tortuous boundary due to infoldings or interdigitations of each cell with its neighbor (Fig. 4.23). These infoldings increase the lateral surface of the cell and are particularly prominent in cells that transport fluid rapidly, as in the intestinal epithelium. Water that is in the intestine enters the epithelial cells at their apical surface. It then leaves the cell at the lateral surface by osmotically following sodium ions that are actively transported across the lateral plasma mem-

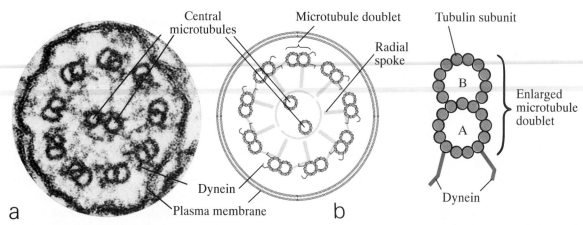

Figure 4.22. Electron micrograph **(a)** and corresponding diagram **(b)** of a cross section of a cilium showing the two central microtubules and the nine surrounding microtubule doublets. The dynein arms extend from the microtubule and make temporary bridges with the B microtubule of the adjacent doublet. The substructure of a microtubule doublet is shown in the adjacent diagram on the right. Note that the A microtubule of the doublet is composed of 13 tubulin dimers arranged in a side-by-side configuration, whereas the B microtubule is composed of 10 tubulin dimers and shares the remaining units with those of the A microtubule. (The length of the microtubules is dependent on the end-to-end addition of the tubulin dimer units. See Figure 2.22.) **a,** ×180,000. (**a** is provided courtesy of Dr. K. Selman.)

brane. The intercellular space becomes distended (see Plate 4, page 91) by the accumulation of fluid as it moves across the epithelium. The hydrostatic pressure gradient established within the intercellular space provides a driving force to move the fluid from the space into the adjoining connective tissue. Because the cells possess an occluding junction at the luminal or free surface, the fluid can move only in the direction of the connective tissue.

Other cells known to transport fluid show infoldings at the basal cell surface. These basal surface modifications are prominent in proximal and distal tubules of the kidney (Fig. 4.24) and in certain ducts of the salivary glands. Mitochondria are typically concentrated at this basal site to provide the energy requirements for active transport. The mitochondria are usually oriented within the folds. The orientation of the mitochondria, combined with the basal membrane infoldings, results in a striated appearance along the basal aspect of the cell when observed with the light microscope. Because of this phenomenon, the salivary gland ducts that possess these cells are referred to as *striated ducts.*

GLANDS

Glands Are Composed of Epithelial Cells Specialized to Synthesize and Secrete a Specific Product

Typically, glands are classified into two major groups reflecting how their products are distributed:

- *Exocrine glands* secrete their products onto a surface through ducts or tubes. The ducts, also composed of epithelial cells, may convey the secreted material in an unaltered form or may modify the secretion by concentrating it or by adding a constituent substance.
- *Endocrine glands* lack a duct system. They secrete their products into the connective tissue from which they enter the bloodstream in order to reach their target cells. The products of endocrine glands are called *hormones.*

In some epithelia, individual cells secrete a substance that does not reach the bloodstream but, rather, has an effect on other cells within the same epithelium. Such secretory activity is referred to as a *paracrine* secretion. The secretory material reaches the target cells by diffusion through the extracellular space.

Exocrine Glands Are Classified as Either Unicellular or Multicellular

Unicellular glands are the simplest in structure. In this instance, the secretory component consists of single cells distributed among other cells that are not secretory. A typical example is the goblet cell, a mucus-secreting cell positioned among other columnar cells (Fig. 4.25). Goblet cells are located in the surface lining and glands of the intestines and in certain passages of the respiratory tract.

Multicellular glands are composed of more than one cell and exhibit varying degrees of complexity. Their structural organization allows for subclassification according to the arrangement of the secretory cells (parenchyma) and the presence or absence of branching of the duct elements.

The simplest arrangement of a multicellular gland is a cellular sheet in which each surface cell is a secretory cell. For example, the entire lining of the stomach and its gastric pits is a sheet of mucus-secreting cells (Fig. 4.26).

Other multicellular glands typically form tubular invag-

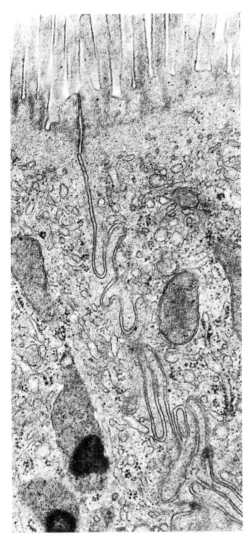

Figure 4.23. Electron micrograph showing infoldings or interdigitations at the lateral surfaces of two adjoining intestinal absorptive cells.

- *Simple branched acinar,* as in the cardiac glands of the stomach (Plate 73, Fig. 4, page 477)
- *Compound acinar,* as in the pancreas (see Fig. 4.29)
- *Compound tubuloacinar,* as in the submandibular gland (Plate 66, Fig. 1, page 431)

Mucous and Serous Glands Are So Named Because of the Type of Secretion Produced

The secretory cells of exocrine glands associated with the various body tubes, i.e., the alimentary canal, respiratory passages, and urogenital system, are often described as being *mucous, serous,* or both.

Mucous secretions are viscous and slimy, whereas serous secretions are watery. Goblet cells, secretory cells of the sublingual salivary glands, and surface cells of the stomach are examples of mucus-secreting cells. The mucous nature of the secretion is the result of extensive gly-

inations from the surface. The end pieces of the gland contain the secretory cells; the portion of the gland connecting the secretory cells to the surface serves as a duct. If the duct is unbranched, the gland is called *simple;* if the duct is branched, it is called *compound.* If the secretory portion is shaped like a tube, the gland is *tubular;* if it is shaped like a flask, the gland is *alveolar* or *acinar;* if the tube ends in a sac-like dilation, the gland is *tubuloalveolar.* Tubular secretory portions may be straight, branched, or coiled; alveolar portions may be single or branched. Various combinations of duct and secretory portion shapes are found in the body (Fig. 4.27). Thus, exocrine glands may be described as

- *Simple tubular,* as in the intestinal glands of the colon (Plate 80, Fig. 2, page 491)
- *Simple coiled tubular,* as in the eccrine sweat glands (Plate 61, Fig. 1, page 399)
- *Simple branched tubular,* as in the submucosal glands of Brunner in the duodenum (Plate 77, Fig. 1, page 485)

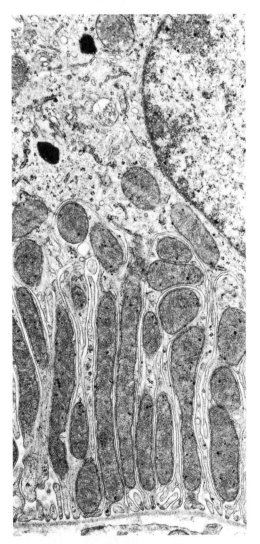

Figure 4.24. Electron micrograph of the basal portion of a kidney tubule cell showing the infolding of the plasma membrane. Note the mitochondria contained within the cytoplasmic folds.

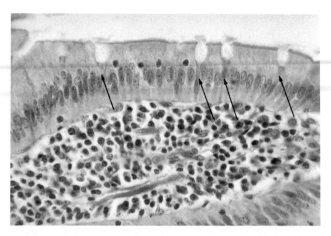

Figure 4.25. Photomicrograph of intestinal epithelium showing single goblet cells *(arrows)* dispersed among absorptive cells.

cosylation of the constituent proteins with anionic oligosaccharides. The mucinogen granules, the secretory product within the cell, are therefore PAS positive (see Fig. 4.3*a*). However, they are water soluble and lost during routine tissue preparation. For this reason the cytoplasm of mucous cells appears to be empty in H&E-stained paraffin sections. Another characteristic feature of a mucous cell is that its nucleus is usually flattened against the base of the cell (Fig. 4.28).

Serous cells, in contrast to mucus-secreting cells, produce poorly glycosylated or nonglycosylated protein secretions. The nucleus typically appears rounded or oval (Fig. 4.29). The apical cytoplasm is often intensely stained with eosin if its secretory granules are well preserved. The perinuclear cytoplasm often appears basophilic due to an extensive rough endoplasmic reticulum, a characteristic of protein-synthesizing cells.

Acini containing serous cells are found in the parotid gland and in the pancreas. Acini of some glands, such as the submandibular gland, contain both mucous and serous cells. In these cases, the serous cells are more removed from the lumen of the acinus and are shaped as crescents or *demilunes* (''half-moons'') at the periphery of the mucous acinus. Their secretions reach the duct of the gland by means of small intercellular channels or *canaliculi* between the mucous cells (Fig. 4.30).

HISTOGENESIS OF EPITHELIUM

Each of the Germ Layers—Ectoderm, Mesoderm, and Endoderm—Has Specific Epithelial Derivatives

The three germ layers in the developing embryo contribute to the formation of the various epithelia.

Ectodermal Derivatives

The derivatives of the *ectoderm* may be divided into two major classes: surface ectoderm and neuroectoderm. *Surface ectoderm* gives rise to

- *Epidermis* and its derivatives (hair, nails, sweat glands, sebaceous glands, and the parenchyma and ducts of the mammary glands)
- *Cornea* and *lens epithelia* of the eye
- *Enamel organ* and *enamel* of the teeth
- *Components of the inner ear*

Neuroectoderm gives rise to the

- *Neural tube* and its derivatives (the central nervous system, including ependyma, pineal body, and neurohy-

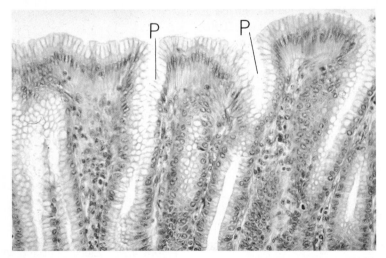

Figure 4.26. Photomicrograph of stomach surface. The epithelial cells lining the surface are all mucus-secreting cells, as are the cells lining the gastric pits *(P)*.

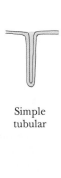

Simple tubular   Simple coiled tubular   Simple branched tubular   Simple branched acinar

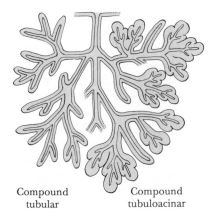
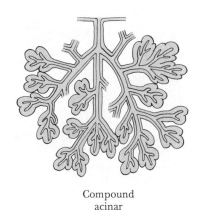

Compound tubular   Compound tubuloacinar

Compound acinar

Figure 4.27. Schematic diagram of various types of glands, showing configuration of the duct and secretory cells. (Based on Weiss L, Greep RO: *Histology,* 4th ed. New York, McGraw-Hill, 1977, fig. 3.28.)

pophysis; and the sensory epithelium of the eye, ear, and nose)

- *Neural crest* and its derivatives (components of the peripheral nervous system, including ganglia, nerves and glial cells, medullary cells of the adrenal gland, the *amine precursor uptake and decarboxylation (APUD)* cells of the diffuse neuroendocrine system (see page 453), melanoblasts, the precursors of melanocytes, and the mesenchyme of the head and its epithelial derivatives, such as corneal endothelium and vascular endothelium)

Mesodermal Derivatives

Mesoderm gives rise to

- *Epithelium* of the kidney and the gonads
- *Mesothelium,* the epithelium lining the pericardial, pleural, and peritoneal cavities
- *Endothelium,* the epithelium lining the cardiovascular and lymphatic vessels
- *Adrenal cortex*

Many of the more atypical epithelia, such as the adrenal cortex, arise from mesoderm. For example, the adrenal cortical cells, the Leydig cells of the testis, and the lutein cells of the ovary, all of which are endocrine components, lack

a free surface, a feature not characteristic of most epithelia. These secretory cells, which are derived from progenitor mesenchymal cells (nondifferentiated cells of embryonic origin found in connective tissue), are referred to as epithelioid. Although the differentiation process may involve a transient exposure of progenitor mesenchymal cells at a free surface, the differentiated cells lack a surface location. Endothelium and mesothelium differ from epithelia derived from the other two germ layers, in that they have no continuity or communication with the exterior of the body.

Endodermal Derivatives

Endoderm (or entoderm) gives rise to

- Respiratory system epithelium
- Alimentary canal epithelium (excluding the epithelium of the oral cavity and anal region, which are of ectodermal origin)
- Extramural digestive gland epithelium, i.e., the liver, pancreas, and gallbladder
- Thyroid, parathyroid, and thymus gland epithelial components
- Lining epithelium of the tympanic cavity and auditory (Eustachian) tubes
- Adenohypophysis (anterior lobe of pituitary gland)

Thyroid and parathyroid glands develop as epithelial

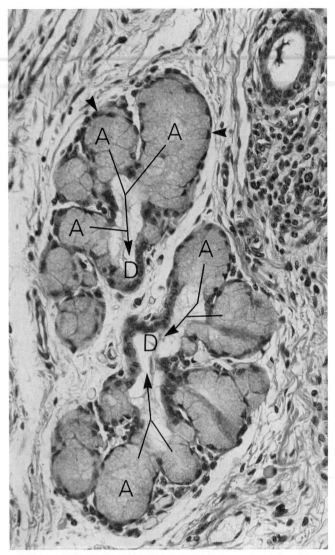

Figure 4.28. Photomicrograph showing two small lobes of a mucus-secreting gland associated with the larynx. Each displays the beginning of a duct *(D)* into which the mucin is secreted *(arrows)*. The individual secretory cells that form the acinus *(A)* are difficult to define. Their nuclei *(arrowheads)* are flattened and located in the very basal portion of the cell, a feature typical of mucus-secreting glands. The cytoplasm is filled with mucin that is very lightly stained.

outgrowths from the floor of the pharynx and then lose their attachments from their sites of original outgrowth. The thymus also originates as an epithelial outgrowth of the floor of the pharyngeal wall; it grows into the mediastinum and also loses its original connection. Similarly, the adenohypophysis develops as an outgrowth of the roof of the pharynx; it joins the neurohypophysis that grows down from the third ventricle of the developing brain to form the pituitary gland. Figure 4.31 summarizes the derivatives of the three germ layers.

Neural Crest Cells Give Rise to Ectomesenchyme

A special class of cells called *ectomesenchyme,* derived from neural crest cells, develops into most of the mesodermal tissues in the head. At about the time that the neural folds in the embryo close to form a tube, some of the neuroectodermal cells at the lateral edges of the neural plate separate and are not incorporated into the tube. These cells migrate and form the **neural crest** over the neural tube. They migrate extensively in the developing embryo and give rise to components of the peripheral nervous system, including Schwann cells, all sensory cells, sympathetic and parasympathetic autonomic ganglia and neurons, as well as the medullary cells of the adrenal gland, APUD cells, and melanoblasts. Neural crest cells in the cranial region also form connective tissue, bone, cartilage, some muscle of the face, and components of the tooth, but not the enamel.

EPITHELIAL CELL RENEWAL

Most Epithelial Cells Have a Finite Life Span Less Than That of the Whole Organism

Surface epithelia and epithelia of many simple glands belong to the category of continuously renewing cell populations as described on page 48. The rate of cell turnover, i.e., the replacement rate, is characteristic of a specific epithelium. For example, the cells lining the small intestine are renewed every 4–6 days in humans. The replacement cells are produced by mitotic activity in the lower portion of the intestinal glands (crypts) (Fig. 4.32). They then migrate to the surface of the intestinal lumen on the villi. The migration of these new cells continues until they reach the tips of the villi, where they die and slough off into the lumen.

Similarly, the stratified squamous epithelium of skin is replaced in most sites over a period of approximately 28 days. In this instance, cells in the basal layer of the epidermis, appropriately named the stratum germinativum, undergo mitotic activity to provide for cell renewal. As these cells differentiate, they are pushed toward the surface by later renewing cells in the basal layer. Ultimately, the cells become keratinized and slough off. In both of the above examples, a steady state relative to the number of cells within the epithelium is maintained, with new cells normally replacing depleted cells at the same rate.

In other epithelia, particularly in the more complex glands, the individual cells may be very long lived, and cell division is rare after the adult state has been reached. The epithelial cells in this instance are characteristic of stable cell populations where relatively little mitotic activity occurs. The liver is a good example of this. However, loss of significant amounts of liver tissue through physical trauma or acute toxic destruction is accommodated by active hepatocyte proliferation. The liver is essentially restored by the mitotic activity of healthy liver tissue.

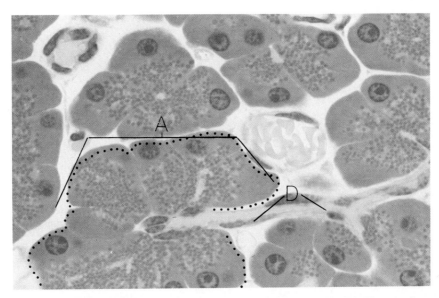

Figure 4.29. Photomicrograph of pancreatic acinus *(A)* with its duct *(D)*. The small round objects within the acinar cells represent the stored secretory precursor material.

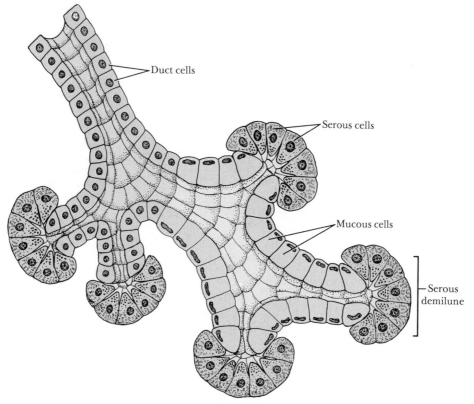

Figure 4.30. Diagram illustrating a tubuloacinar gland. Both tubular and acinar regions are composed of mucus-secreting cells (note the flattened nuclei that are characteristic of these cells). Typically, a number of serous cells form the demilune. The thin, watery serous secretion of the demilune cells makes its way into the alveolar lumen via a narrow canaliculus or channel between mucous cells. (Based on Weiss L, Greep RO: *Histology,* 4th ed. New York, McGraw-Hill, 1977, fig. 3.27.)

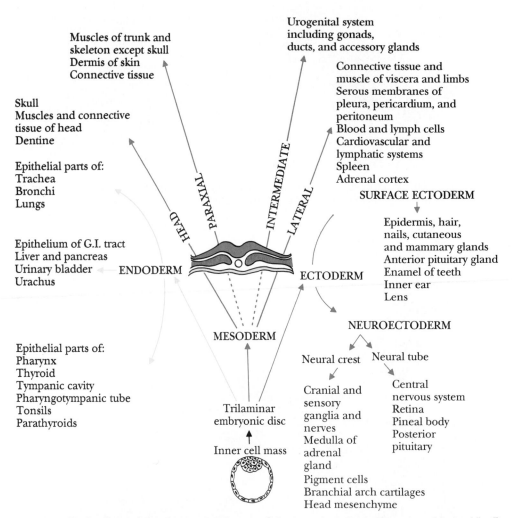

Figure 4.31. Derivatives of the three germ layers. *G.I.,* gastrointestinal. (Based on Moore KL, Persaud TVN: *The Developing Human,* 5th ed. Philadelphia, WB Saunders, 1993, p 74.)

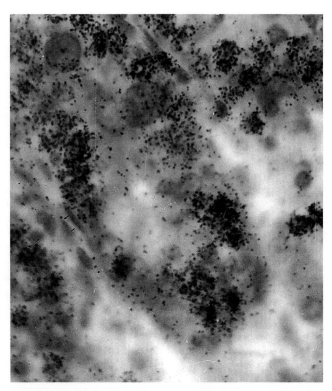

Figure 4.32. Autoradiograph of crypts in the jejunum of a rabbit that had been injected with tritiated thymidine 8 hours prior to death and fixation. Nearly all of the epithelial cells in this replicative zone of the intestinal mucosa are labeled, indicating that they were synthesizing DNA at the time the animal was injected. X600. (From Parker FG, Barnes EN, Kaye GI: *Gastroenterology* 67:607, 1974.)

MUCOUS AND SEROUS MEMBRANES

In two general locations, surface epithelium and its underlying connective tissue are regarded as a functional unit called a **membrane.** The two types of membrane are mucous membrane and serous membrane. The term *membrane* as used here is not to be confused with the biologic membranes of cells, nor are the designations *mucous* and *serous* to be confused with the nature of the secretion as discussed previously.

Mucous membrane, also called **mucosa,** lines those cavities that connect with the outside of the body, namely, the alimentary canal, the respiratory tract, and the genitourinary tract. It consists of surface epithelium (with or without glands), a supporting connective tissue called the **lamina propria,** a basal lamina separating the epithelium from the lamina propria, and, sometimes, a layer of smooth muscle called the **muscularis mucosae** as the deepest layer.

Serous membrane, also called **serosa,** lines the peritoneal, pleural, and pericardial cavities. These cavities are usually described as closed cavities of the body, although in the female the peritoneal cavity communicates with the exterior via the genital tract. Structurally, the serosa consists of a lining epithelium, the **mesothelium,** a supporting connective tissue, and a basal lamina between the two. Serous membranes do not contain glands, but the fluid on their surface is watery.

PLATE 1. Simple Squamous and Simple Cuboidal Epithelia

Selected examples of epithelia of different organs are presented here and on the next several pages. For each example, note the shape and arrangement of the epithelial cells, the location of their free surfaces, and the location of the underlying or adjacent connective tissue.

FIGURE 1, intestine, monkey, H&E ×640. This shows the *simple squamous epithelium* (mesothelium) covering the outer surface of the intestine. The epithelium overlies a well-defined layer of connective tissue *(CT)* containing several small blood vessels *(BV)*; deeper is a layer of smooth muscle *(SM)*. The epithelial cells are very flat, as judged by the shape of their nuclei *(N)*. Note that cell boundaries are not evident and the nuclei are unevenly spaced. The uneven spacing is because the sectioning knife passes through some cells without including the nucleus. This phenomenon can be understood better and visualized more easily in a nonsectioned (whole mount), silver-impregnated preparation of a piece of a very thin mesentery (the structure that holds the intestines in place), as in Figure 2.

FIGURE 2, mesentery, monkey, silver ×640. The mesentery is lying on the slide, and the microscope is focused on its upper surface to reveal the surface epithelial cells. Cell boundaries are revealed by a deposition of reduced silver along the intercellular spaces. The nuclei *(N)* appear oval or round when viewed from the surface, as opposed to flat or elongate when seen on edge, as in a section. If one were to draw a line representing a knife cut across the cells as revealed in this figure, it would be possible to envision why the epithelial nuclei are unevenly spaced in sectioned material; the knife would pass through the cytoplasm of each cell but would not necessarily cut across the nucleus of each cell. Some of the more ovoid nuclei in the preparation belong to fibroblasts *(F)* in the underlying connective tissue. Because of the thinness of the mesentery, they are in the same focal plane as the epithelial cells and are thus superimposed.

FIGURE 3, kidney, human, H&E ×640. This micrograph, another example of a *simple squamous epithelium,* reveals a sectioned renal corpuscle and adjacent kidney tubules. The renal corpuscle consists of a special capillary bed, the glomerulus, that is enclosed by Bowman's capsule, part of which (the visceral layer) is directly adjacent to the capillaries and part of which (the parietal layer) forms a thin-walled spherical structure composed of simple squamous epithelium. The nuclei *(N)* of the cells forming the parietal layer appear as flattened bodies that show the same uneven spacing as in Figure 1. The free surface of the epithelium faces Bowman's space. The cross sections of tubules, marked with an *asterisk* (lower left), provide a good example of a *simple cuboidal epithelium.* Although the cell boundaries are not evident, one can judge that the height of each cell approximates its width by the spacing of the nuclei. Thus, it is a cuboidal epithelium.

FIGURE 4, ovary, monkey, H&E ×640. This example of a *simple cuboidal epithelium (Ep)* shows the cells that cover the surface of the ovary. The epithelium rests on a highly cellular connective tissue *(CT)*. The surface epithelial cells are approximately square or cuboidal in three dimensions. The free surfaces of these cells face the abdominal cavity and are a modification of the simple squamous epithelium or mesothelium shown in Figures 1 and 2.

FIGURE 5, liver, human, H&E ×400. These cells also approximate a cube, but they are arranged in sheets separated by blood vessels *(BV)* called sinusoids. The epithelium is unusual, in that several surfaces of the cell possess a groove that represents the free surface. Where a grooved surface is present on one cell, the adjoining cell possesses a mirror-imaged grooved surface. The opposing grooves form a small lumen or *canaliculus* through which the bile produced by the cells reaches a bile duct. The canaliculi are not visible at this magnification but are located at the points of the *arrows* (see bile canaliculus, Plate 84).

KEY		
AV, arteriole, vessel supplying glomerulus	**Ep,** epithelium	**arrow,** site of bile canaliculus
BV, blood vessel	**F,** fibroblast nucleus	**asterisk,** tubule possessing simple cuboidal epithelium
CT, connective tissue	**N,** nucleus	
	SM, smooth muscle	

PLATE 1

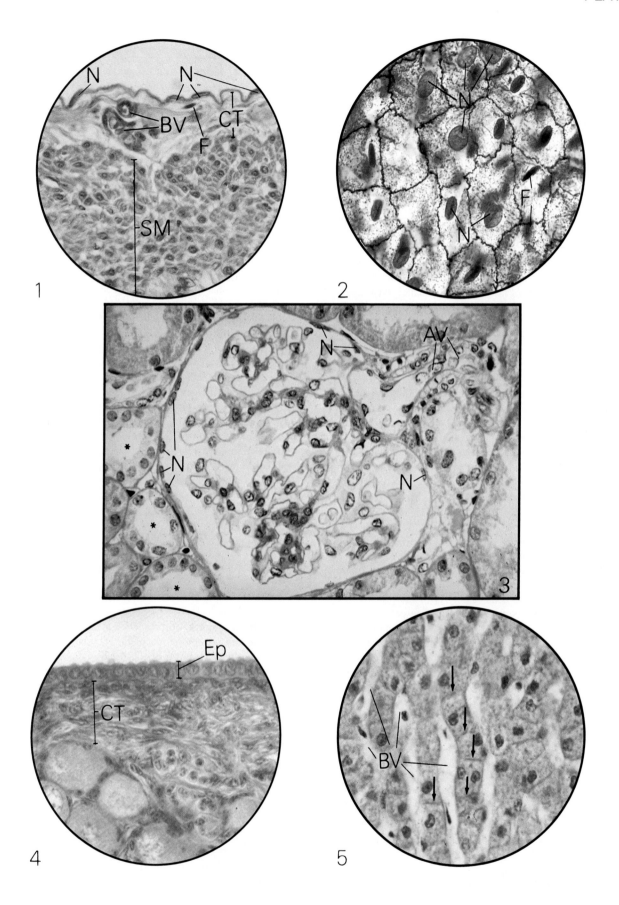

PLATE 2. Simple and Stratified Epithelia

FIGURE 1, exocrine pancreas, monkey, H&E ×450.
This shows three epithelial forms. In the *circle* is a well-oriented acinus, a functional group of secretory cells, each of which is pyramidal in shape. The secretory cells form a spherical or tubular structure. The free surface of the cells and the lumen are located in the center of the *circle*. (The lumen is not clearly evident, but in a similar cell arrangement in Figure 4 (see *circle*), the lumen and secretory surface can be seen.) Because the height of the cells (the distance from the edge of the *circle* to the lumen) is greater than the width, the epithelium is **simple columnar**. The second epithelial type is represented by a small, longitudinally sectioned duct *(arrows)* extending across the field. It is composed of flattened cells (note the nuclear shape), and on this basis, the epithelium is **simple squamous**. Finally, there is a larger cross-sectioned duct *(asterisk)* into which the smaller duct enters. The nuclei of this larger duct tend to be round, and the cells tend to be square in profile. Thus, these duct cells are a **simple cuboidal epithelium**.

FIGURE 3, stomach, monkey, H&E ×450. The simple columnar lining epithelium of the stomach forms a sheet of mucus-secreting cells. The epithelial cells are extremely tall, with a mucus-containing apical region just above the elongated nuclei, and extend down to the highly cellular connective tissue *(CT)*. Two round cells or lymphocytes *(arrows)* have wandered into the epithelium from the underlying connective tissue, a frequent finding in the digestive tract.

FIGURE 5, epididymis, human, H&E ×450. This is another example of pseudostratified columnar epithelium. Again, two layers of nuclei are evident, those of basal cells *(BC)* and those of columnar cells *(CC)*. As in the previous example, however, although not evident, the columnar cells rest on the basement membrane; thus, the epithelium is pseudostratified. Note that where the epithelium is vertically oriented, on the right of the micrograph, there appear to be more nuclei, and the epithelium is thicker. This is a result of a tangential plane of section. As a rule, always examine the thinnest area of an epithelium to visualize its true organization.

FIGURE 2, kidney, human, H&E ×450. This section shows cross-sectioned tubules of several types. Those that are labeled with the *arrows* provide another example of a simple cuboidal epithelium. The *arrows* point to the lateral cell boundaries; note that cell width approximates cell height. The cross-sectioned structures marked with *asterisks* are another type of tubule; they are smaller in diameter but are also composed of a simple cuboidal epithelium.

FIGURE 4, trachea, monkey, H&E ×450. In addition to the tall columnar cells *(CC)* in this columnar epithelium, there is a definite layer of basal cells *(BC)*. The columnar cells, which contain elongate nuclei and possess cilia *(C)*, extend from the surface to the basement membrane (clearly evident in the trachea as a thick, homogeneous region that is part of the connective tissue *(CT)*). The basal cells are interspersed between the columnar cells. Because all of the cells rest on the basement membrane, they are regarded as a single layer, as opposed to two discrete layers, one over the other. Because the epithelium appears to be stratified but is not, it is called **pseudostratified columnar epithelium**. The *circle* in the micrograph delineates a tracheal gland similar to the acinus in Figure 1 *(circle)*. Note that the lumen of the gland is clearly visible and the cell boundaries are also evident. The gland epithelium is simple columnar.

FIGURE 6, vagina, human, H&E ×225. This is the **stratified squamous epithelium** of the vaginal wall. The deeper cells, particularly those of the basal layer, are small, with little cytoplasm, and thus the nuclei appear closely packed. As the cells become larger, they tend to flatten out, forming disc-like squames. Because the surface cells retain this shape, the epithelium is called stratified squamous.

KEY

BC, basal cell
C, cilia
CC, columnar cell
CT, connective tissue

arrows: Fig. 1, tubule composed of simple squamous epithelium; Fig. 2, lateral boundaries of cuboidal tubule cells; Fig. 3, lymphocytes in epithelium

asterisk, duct or tubule of simple cuboidal epithelium

PLATE 2

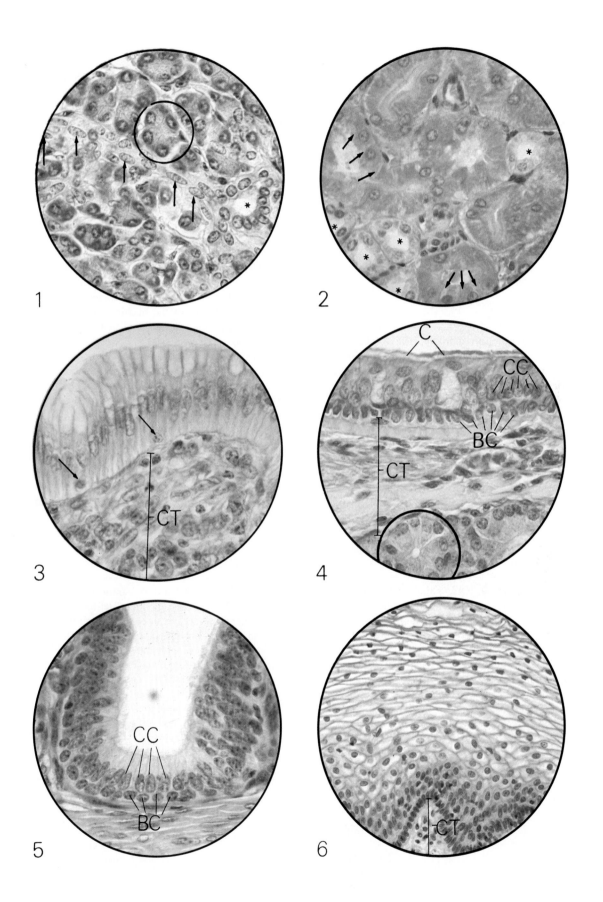

PLATE 3. Stratified Epithelia and Epithelioid Tissues

FIGURE 1, esophagus, monkey, H&E ×250. This part of the wall of the esophagus reveals two different epithelia. On the left is the lining epithelium of the esophagus. It is multilayered with squamous surface cells; therefore, it is a *stratified squamous epithelium (SS)*. On the right is the duct of an esophageal gland cut in several planes due to its tortuous path through the connective tissue. By examining a region where the plane of section is at a right angle to the surface, usually the thinnest area, the true character of the epithelium becomes apparent. In this case, the epithelium consists of two cell layers with cuboidal surface cells; thus, it is *stratified cuboidal epithelium (SC)*.

FIGURE 2, skin, human, H&E ×450. This shows a portion of the duct of a sweat gland just before the duct enters the stratified squamous epithelium *(SS)* (epidermis) of the skin. The *dashed line* traces the duct within the epidermis. This duct also consists of a stratified cuboidal epithelium *(SC)* in two layers; the cells of the inner layer (the surface cells) appear more or less square. Because the epidermal surface cells are not included in the field, the designation stratified squamous cannot be derived from the information offered by the micrograph.

FIGURE 3, anorectal junction, monkey, H&E ×450. This shows a crypt or fold in this terminal portion of the intestine. The area shows a transition zone where the epithelium changes from a *stratified cuboidal (SC)* to a *stratified columnar (SCol)* epithelium. Note how the surface cells along the lower part of the fold change in shape. Neither the cuboidal cells nor the columnar surface cells reach the basement membrane, but each represents a distinct cell layer occupying a surface position; therefore, the epithelia are stratified. Continuing along the columnar surface toward the right, to just beyond the field, would reveal a further change to a stratified squamous epithelium at the anal opening. (See Plate 82 for an orientation micrograph of this area.)

FIGURE 4, urinary bladder, monkey, H&E ×400. The epithelium of the urinary bladder is actually a stratified epithelium, but it changes in appearance according to the degree of distension of the bladder; thus, it is called *transitional epithelium*. In the nondistended state, as here, it is about four or five cells deep. The surface cells are large and dome shaped *(asterisks)*; occasionally, two nuclei are present in a single cell. The cells immediately under the surface cells are pear shaped and slightly smaller. The deepest cells are the smallest, and their nuclei appear more crowded. When the bladder is distended, the superficial cells are stretched into squamous cells, and the epithelium is reduced in thickness to about three cells deep. The bladder wall usually contracts when it is removed unless special steps are taken to preserve it in a distended state. Thus, its appearance is usually like that in Figure 4. Transitional epithelium is also present on the surface of the renal pelvis, the ureters, and part of the urethra.

FIGURE 5, testis, monkey, H&E ×350. This shows the interstitial (Leydig) cells *(IC)* of the testis, present in clumps between the seminiferous tubules. These cells possess certain epithelial characteristics. They do not possess a free surface, however, nor do they develop from a surface; instead, they develop from mesenchymal cells. They are referred to as *epithelioid* cells because they contact similar neighboring cells much the same as epithelial cells contact each other. The Leydig cells are endocrine in nature.

FIGURE 6, endocrine pancreas, human, H&E ×450. Cells of the endocrine islet (of Langerhans) *(En)* of the pancreas also have an epithelioid arrangement. The cells are in contact but lack a free surface, although they have developed from an epithelial surface by invagination. In contrast, the surrounding alveoli of the exocrine pancreas *(Ex)*, which developed from the same epithelial surface, are made up of cells with a free surface onto which the secretory product is discharged. Capillaries *(C)* are prominent in endocrine tissues. Similar examples of epithelioid tissue are seen in the adrenal (mesenchymal origin) and the parathyroid and pituitary (epithelial origin) glands, all of which are endocrine glands.

KEY

C, capillary
CT, connective tissue
En, endocrine cells
Ex, exocrine cells
IC, interstitial (Leydig) cells
SC, stratified cuboidal epithelium
SCol, stratified columnar epithelium
SS, stratified squamous epithelium
asterisks, dome-shaped cells

PLATE 3

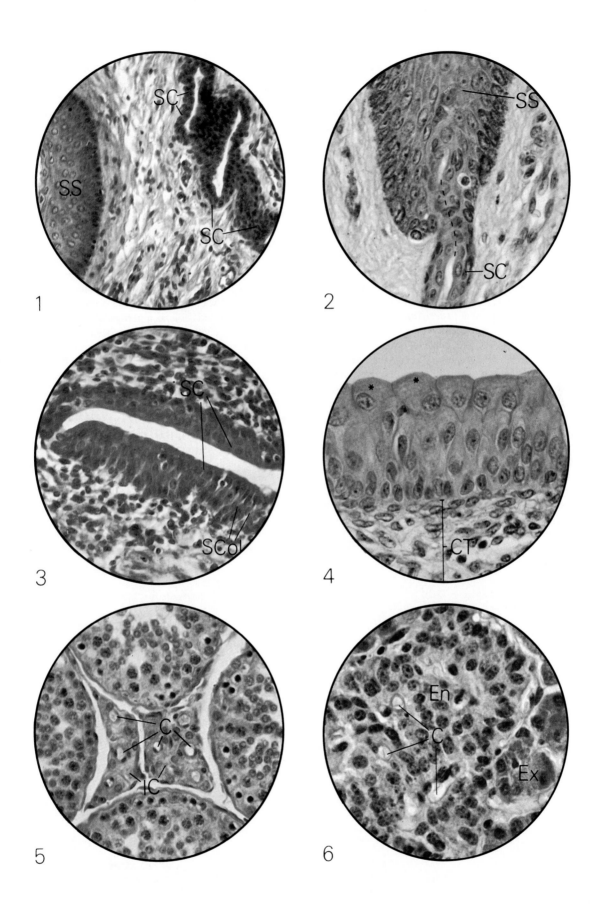

PLATE 4. Columnar Epithelium, Electron Microscopy

Small intestine, rat, electron micrograph ×**4100.** This electron micrograph illustrates some of the salient features of epithelium, particularly as they relate to the light microscopic image. It includes some of the underlying connective tissue, which in this instance is almost entirely occupied by a capillary containing a number of red blood cells *(RBC)*.

The epithelium is simple columnar. All of the cells are absorptive; no goblet cells are included. The two round cells at the base of the epithelium are lymphocytes *(Lym)* that migrated from the connective tissue. Similar lymphocyte invasion of the epithelium, a typical occurrence, is seen in Figure 3 of Plate 2.

In studying the electron micrograph, note first the relationship between the cells above the level of the nuclei. The cytoplasm of each cell comes into intimate apposition to its neighbors, and consequently, the cell boundaries at this magnification are difficult to discern. Below this level, prominent intercellular spaces are present *(asterisks)*. Here, it is easy to define the limits of the individual cells. Next, examine the very basal aspect of the epithelium. Note that each cell extends by means of lateral cytoplasmic processes *(arrows)* to meet with its neighbors, thus, again, providing intimate cell apposition. At some sites, these basal processes are discontinuous *(circles)*. This is probably due to the recent migration of the lymphocytes from the connective tissue into the epithelium. The basal cytoplasmic extensions rest on the basal lamina. (The basal lamina is not recognizable at this low magnification but can be seen in Plate 5.) The intercellular spaces, in effect, form a continuous compartment surrounding the epithelial cells; the compartment is bounded above by the apical cytoplasm, where adjoining cells meet, and below by the lateral basal processes, which also join with one another. The visualization of this intercellular space is also possible with the light microscope (see Plate 78, Fig. 3). The presence of intercellular spaces of this type is characteristic of epithelia actively engaged in fluid transport, i.e., the active movement of fluid across an epithelium from a lumen to the underlying connective tissue and, thus, may be observed not only in the intestine but also in many other epithelia where fluid is actively transported. The essential point, however, is that despite the intercellular spaces, these cells as an epithelium do maintain intimate apposition with one another. Thus, as a continuous epithelial layer, they can function as a selective barrier.

Two other features pertinent to epithelial cells as they relate to light microscopy are also evident in this micrograph. One concerns the apical contacts between neighboring cells, namely, the junctional complexes *(curved arrows)*. Each complex appears as a short, thin dark line in the electron micrograph. The complexes provide strong adhesion between adjoining cells and serve as a permeability barrier. Their unit structure and functional aspects are dealt with in the text that accompanies Plate 5. The junctional complexes are comparable to the fine, dot-like structures seen in the light microscope, where they are referred to as terminal bars (see text, Fig. 4.9).

The other feature worthy of mention here relates to the microvilli that extend from the apical surface of the epithelial cells. In the small intestine, the microvilli appear as closely packed, finger-like cytoplasmic projections, extremely uniform in size and shape. Because of their uniformity, at the light microscope level, they have a finely striped or striated appearance, hence the term ***striated border***. Examination of Plate 78, Figure 3, reveals the striated border as seen at medium-power magnification in the light microscope.

KEY

Lym, lymphocyte
RBC, red blood cell
arrows, basal lateral process

asterisks, intercellular spaces
circles, discontinuity between basal processes

curved arrows, junctional complexes

PLATE 4

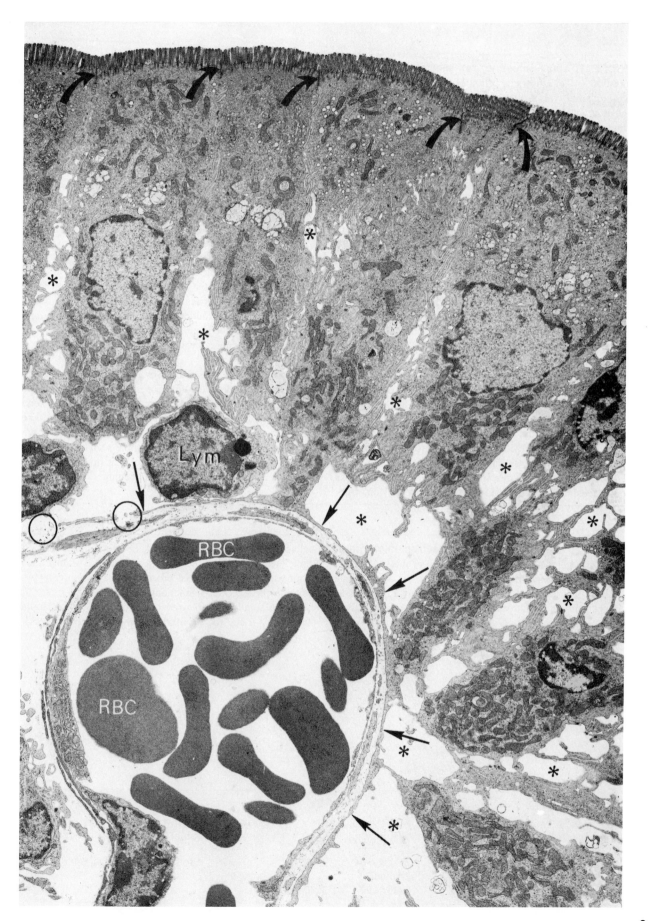

FIGURE 1, small intestine, rat, electron micrograph ×26,000. This shows a portion of the apical cytoplasm of two epithelial cells from the same specimen as in Plate 4. The micrograph reveals the microvilli *(M)*, the junctional complex *(JC)*, and, below this, the nonspecialized region of cell apposition *(NS)*.

Microvilli of the intestinal absorptive cell are uniform in size and shape. They display numerous fine actin filaments *(arrows)* that course the length of the microvilli and enter the underlying cytoplasmic region of the cell to become part of the terminal web *(TW)*. The latter is a narrow layer of actin filaments that extends across the most apical region of the cell. There is evidence indicating that the actin filaments are functionally joined by myosin to constitute a contractile apparatus. (Myosin is usually lost during the routine preparation of the tissue.) Other cell organelles are excluded from the terminal web (or may only transiently pass through it, as in the case of pinocytotic vesicles that originate from the plasma membrane at the base of adjacent microvilli). At the light microscope level, the terminal web appears as a slightly darker staining region in contrast to the striated border above and the cytoplasm immediately below. The staining of the terminal web is undoubtedly due to the numbers of filaments *(double arrows)* aggregated in this region of the cell.

Two of the three functionally important components of the junctional complex can be seen in Figure 1. One is the zonula occludens *(ZO)*, a surface specialization involving the membranes of adjacent cells. The outer leaflets of the opposing cell membranes within this specialization are in very close contact, essentially eliminating the intercellular fluid from the area. (The points of contact are actually in the form of rows or lines of membrane particles that can be seen in freeze fracture preparations.) The contact between the cells results in a narrow zone in which the intercellular space is functionally obliterated. The contact zone forms a band around the cell, thus preventing the free passage of substances across the epithelium via the intercellular space.

Immediately below the zonula occludens is the second structural component of the junctional complex, namely, the zonula adherens *(ZA)*. It, too, is a modification of the cell surface. Here, the plasma membranes of the adjacent cells diverge slightly, leaving a uniform intercellular space of 15–20 nm. The fine filaments of the terminal web converge and insert into dense material bordering the cytoplasmic side of the plasma membrane of the zonula adherens. The zonula adherens is probably the main element that contributes to the visualization of the terminal bar seen in the light microscope. Although the zonula adherens appears relatively electron lucent, with no apparent structural content, it is thought to serve as a zone of strong adhesion, as the name implies, between adjacent cells.

The *macula adherens* also serves as a strong attachment site, but it occurs as focal or spot-like (macular) attachments between adjacent cells, in contrast to the band-like zonula adherens that rings the cell. The macula adherens is not present in Figure 1 but may be seen in Figure 4.10*b*. The macula adherens corresponds to the desmosome seen by the light microscopist. When discernible in the light microscope, it appears as a fine dot or fusiform thickening.

FIGURE 2, small intestine, rat, electron micrograph ×15,000. This shows the basal portion of the epithelium. The epithelial compartment extends as far as the basal lamina *(arrows)*. The lamina has been cut on edge and appears as a delicate linear structure so thin that it cannot be resolved with the light microscope. Note that the basal processes of adjacent epithelial cells meet and, in effect, close off the intercellular epithelial space. The basal closure is simply a close approximation of the basal processes of adjacent cells without the presence of a junctional complex. The figure also shows a small part of a red blood cell *(RBC)*, a capillary lumen *(CL)*, and the capillary endothelium *(arrowheads)*.

KEY

CL, capillary lumen
F, fibroblast process
JC, junctional complex
M, microvilli
NS, nonspecialized region of cell apposition

RBC, red blood cell
TW, terminal web
ZA, zonula adherens
ZO, zonula occludens
arrows: Fig. 1, core filaments of microvilli; Fig. 2, basal lamina

arrowheads, capillary endothelium
asterisk, oblique cut of plasma membrane
double arrows, filaments of terminal web

PLATE 5

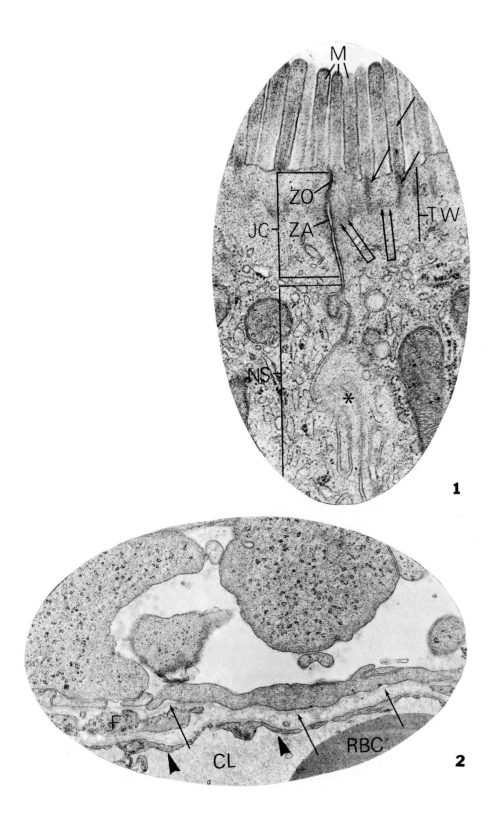

Connective Tissue

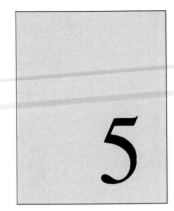

Connective Tissue Comprises a Diverse Group of Tissues With a Variety of Functions

Connective tissue consists of *cells* and an extracellular matrix that includes *extracellular fibers, ground substance,* and *tissue fluid.* It forms a vast and continuous compartment throughout the body, bounded by basal lamina of the various epithelia and by the basal or external lamina of muscle, nerve, and vascular endothelium.

The role and function of the various connective tissues is reflected in the

- Kinds of cells present
- Types of fibers
- Character of the ground substance

For example, in what is described as "loose connective tissue," a relatively large number of different cell types is present. One type, the fibroblast, is responsible for producing the extracellular fibers that serve a structural role in the tissue and for producing and maintaining the ground substance. Other cell types, such as plasma cells, macrophages, and eosinophils, to name a few, are associated with the body's defense system; they function within the ground substance of the tissue. In contrast, bone, another variety of connective tissue, contains a single cell type that is associated with the production of the fibers that make up the bulk of the bone tissue. A feature that makes bone unique or special as a connective tissue is that its fibers are organized in a very specific pattern and become calcified to create the hardness associated with bone.

Similarly, in tendons and ligaments the fibers are the prominent feature of the tissue. They are arranged in parallel array and are densely packed to provide maximum strength. The cells that produce the fibers are relatively few in number, and there is a paucity of ground substance.

CLASSIFICATION OF CONNECTIVE TISSUE

Classification Is Based on the Composition and Organization of the Cellular and Extracellular Components and on Special Functions

The term "connective tissue" includes a variety of tissues with differing functional properties but with certain common characteristics that allow them to be grouped together. For convenience of description they are classified in a manner that reflects these features. Thus, Table 5.1 provides a classification including subtypes of the principal connective tissues. *Connective tissue proper,* the first category listed in the table, is presented in this chapter. The connective tissues of the embryo are also included in this chapter. An understanding of mesenchyme is particularly relevant to the basic understanding of connective tissue, including the specialized connective tissues in the chapters that follow.

CONNECTIVE TISSUE PROPER

The tissues that belong to this category are divided into two general subtypes:

- Loose connective tissue
- Dense connective tissue

Loose Connective Tissue

Loose Connective Tissue, Also Called Areolar Tissue, Is Characterized by Loosely Arranged Fibers and an Abundance of Cells

Loose connective tissue, also sometimes called *areolar tissue,* is a cellular connective tissue. The fibers are thin and relatively sparse, and the ground substance is abundant. The latter occupies more volume than the fibers. It has a viscous to gel-like consistency and is important in the dif-

TABLE 5.1. Classification of Connective Tissue

Connective tissue proper
  Loose connective tissue
  Dense connective tissue
    Irregular
    Regular
Specialized connective tissue[A]
  Adipose tissue (Chapter 6)
  Blood (Chapter 9)
  Bone (Chapter 8)
  Cartilage (Chapter 7)
  Hemopoietic tissue (Chapter 9)
  Lymphatic tissue (Chapter 13)
Embryonic connective tissue
  Mesenchyme
  Mucous connective tissue

[A]The designations elastic tissue and reticular tissue have, in the past, been listed as separate categories of specialized connective tissue. The tissues usually cited as examples of elastic tissue are certain ligaments associated with the spinal column and the tunica media of elastic arteries. The identifying feature of reticular tissue is the presence of reticular fibers and reticular cells together forming a three-dimensional stroma. Reticular tissue serves as the stroma for hemopoietic tissue (specifically the red bone marrow) and lymphatic tissue organs (lymph nodes and spleen, but not the thymus).

fusion of oxygen and nutrients from the small vessels that course through this connective tissue as well as in the diffusion of metabolites back to the vessels (a more complete description of ground substance is provided later in this chapter).

The primary location of loose connective tissue is beneath those epithelia that cover the body surfaces and line the internal surfaces of the body. It is also present in association with the epithelium of glands and surrounds the smallest vessels. The location of this tissue thus represents the initial site in which antigens and other foreign substances, such as bacteria, having breached an epithelial surface can be challenged and destroyed. Most cell types present in loose connective tissue are transient wandering cells that migrate from the local blood vessels in response to specific stimuli. It is, thus, the site of inflammatory and allergic or immune reactions. Under such circumstances, loose connective tissue can undergo considerable swelling. In many areas of the body the continued presence of invasive foreign substances results in constantly large populations of these defending cells. This is particularly true of the *lamina propria,* the loose connective tissue of mucous membranes, such as those of the respiratory and alimentary systems.

Dense Connective Tissue

Dense connective tissue can be further subclassified into

- Dense irregular connective tissue
- Dense regular connective tissue

The distinction between these two tissues is simply the arrangement of the fibers. In the former the fibers exhibit variability in their orientation, whereas in the latter the fibers are arranged in a very orderly manner. Examples of dense regular connective tissue include ligaments, tendons, and aponeuroses.

Dense Irregular Connective Tissue Is Characterized by an Abundance of Fibers and Few Cells

The fibers make up the bulk of dense connective tissue (Fig. 5.1). The cell population is sparse and is typically of a single type, namely, the fibroblast. There is also relatively little ground substance. Because of the high proportion of collagenous fibers that constitute dense irregular connective tissue, it provides significant strength. Typically, the fibers are arranged in bundles oriented in various directions (thus, it is irregular) to withstand stresses to which an organ or structure may be subjected. In the case of hollow organs, e.g., the intestinal tract, there is a distinct layer of dense irregular connective tissue, referred to as the submucosa, in which the fiber bundles course in varying planes. This permits resistance to excessive stretching and distension of the intestinal tube. Similarly, skin contains a relatively thick layer of dense irregular connective tissue in the dermis. This is the reticular or deep layer of the dermis. It provides resistance to tearing as a consequence of stretching forces from different directions.

Dense Regular Connective Tissue Is Characterized by Ordered and Densely Packed Arrays of Fibers and Cells

Dense regular connective tissue is the main functional component of *tendons, ligaments,* and *aponeuroses.*

- *Tendons* are cord-like structures that join muscle to bone. They consist of parallel bundles of collagenous fibers between which are rows of fibroblasts, also referred to as *tendinocytes* (Fig. 5.2). In hematoxylin and eosin (H&E)-stained paraffin sections, the fibroblasts appear stellate when the tendon is cut in cross section; the cytoplasmic projections of the cell lie between the fibers and appear as thin cytoplasmic sheets in this plane. In longitudinal sections, fibroblasts appear in rows. They are identified by the staining of the nucleus. The nuclei are typically flattened. They appear as less intensely stained oval profiles. The cytoplasmic sheets that extend from the body of the fibroblasts are not usually evident in longitudinal sections because they are so thin and blend in with the collagen fibers.
- The substance of the tendon is surrounded by a thin connective tissue capsule, the *epitendineum,* in which the collagen fibers are not nearly as orderly. Typically, the tendon is subdivided into fascicles by *endotendineum,* a connective tissue extension of the epitendineum. It contains the small blood vessels and nerves of the tendon.
- A *ligament* is similar to a tendon, in that it also consists

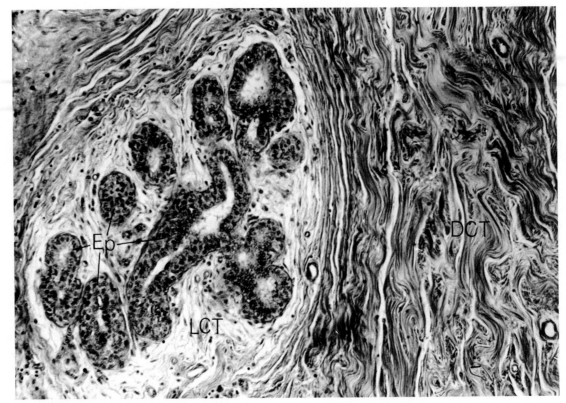

Figure 5.1.   Light micrograph comparing loose and dense connective tissue from the mammary gland stained with hematoxylin and eosin (H&E). On the left, surrounding the epithelium (*Ep*) of the gland, is loose connective tissue. On the right and upper left of the figure is dense irregular connective tissue (*DCT*). The loose connective tissue (*LCT*) is composed of a wispy arrangement of collagen fibers with many cells. Note the large number of nuclei as seen at this low magnification. In contrast, the dense connective tissue reveals a relative paucity of nuclei. However, the collagen is considerably more abundant and is composed of very thick fibers. ×200.

of fibers and fibroblasts arranged in parallel. The fibers, however, are less regularly arranged than those of tendons. Ligaments join bone to bone, and in some locations, such as in the spinal column, this requires some degree of elasticity. Thus, although collagen is the major extracellular fiber of most ligaments, some of the ligaments associated with the spinal column contain considerable numbers of elastic fibers and fewer collagen fibers. These ligaments are called ***elastic ligaments.***

• *Aponeuroses* are much like broad flattened tendons. Instead of all of the fibers lying in parallel arrays, the fibers of aponeuroses are arranged in multiple layers. The bundles of collagen fibers in one layer tend to be arranged at 90° angles to the neighboring layers. The fibers within each of the layers are arranged in regular arrays; thus it is a dense regular connective tissue.

CONNECTIVE TISSUE FIBERS

Connective Tissue Fibers Are of Three Principal Types

Connective tissue fibers are present in varying amounts, depending on the structural needs or function of the tissue.

Each of the fiber types is produced by the fibroblast and is composed of protein formed by long peptide chains. Depending on their character and composition they are referred to as

• Collagen fibers
• Reticular fibers
• Elastic fibers

Collagen Fibers and Fibrils

Collagen Forms the Most Abundant Fibers of Connective Tissue

Collagen fibers are flexible and have a remarkably high tensile strength. With the light microscope, collagen fibers typically appear as wavy structures of variable width and indeterminate length. They stain readily with eosin and other acid dyes, and they can be colored differentially with the dye aniline blue, used in Mallory's connective tissue stain, or with the dye light green, used in Masson's stain.

When examined in the electron microscope, the collagen fiber appears as a bundle or bundles of fine, thread-like subunits, the ***collagen fibrils*** (Fig. 5.3). The collagen fibrils within a fiber are relatively uniform in diameter. In

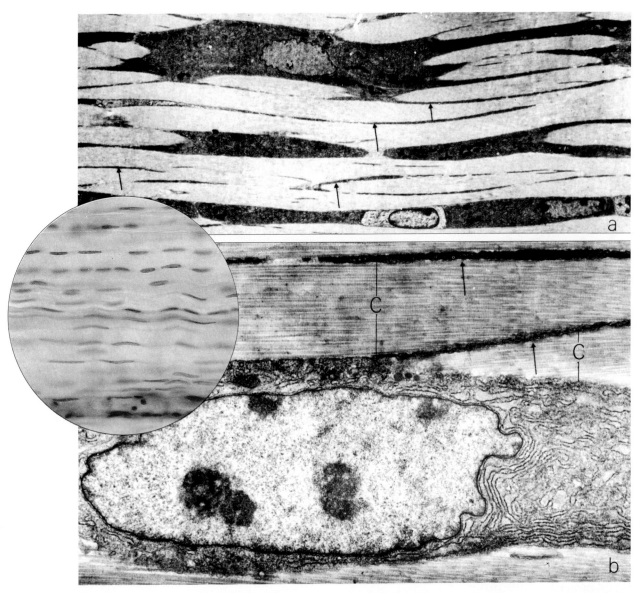

Figure 5.2. Inset. Light micrograph of a tendon. Note the orderly and regular alignment of the bundles of collagen fibers. The tendinocytes (fibroblasts) are aligned in rows between the collagen fibers. ×200. **a.** Electron micrograph of a tendon at low power, showing the tendinocytes (fibroblasts) and their thin processes (*arrows*) lying between the collagen bun-dles. ×1600. **b.** A tendon fibroblast with prominent profiles of rER is shown at higher magnification. The collagen fibers (*C*) can be resolved as consisting of very tightly packed collagen fibrils. ×9500. (Electron micrographs modified from Rhodin J: *Histology.* New York, Oxford University Press, 1974, p 165.)

different locations and in different stages of development, however, the fibrils differ in size. In developing or immature tissues, the fibrils may be as small as 15 or 20 nm in diameter, whereas those in dense regular connective tissue of tendons or in other tissues that are subject to considerable stress may measure up to 200 nm in diameter.

Collagen Fibrils Have a 68-nm Banding Pattern

The collagen fibril, when stained with osmium or other heavy metals, exhibits a sequence of closely spaced trans-verse bands that repeat every 68 nm along the length of the fibril (Fig. 5.3, *inset*). This banding pattern is a reflection of the fibril's subunit structure, specifically, the size and shape of the collagen molecule and the arrangement of the molecules in forming the fibril (Fig. 5.4). The collagen molecule, also called **tropocollagen,** measures about 300 nm long × 1.5 nm thick with a head and a tail. In forming a fibril, the collagen molecules become aligned head to tail in overlapping rows with a gap between the molecules within each row. The strength of the fibril is due to covalent bonds between the collagen molecules of adjacent rows—not by head to tail attachment of the molecules in a row. The banding pattern observed in the elec-

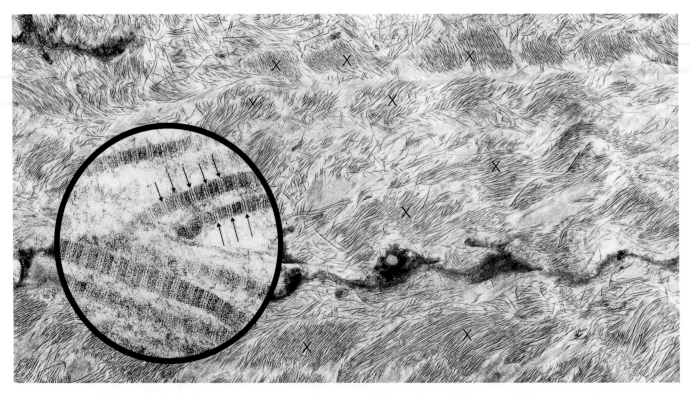

Figure 5.3. Electron micrograph of a dense connective tissue from the capsule of the testis of a young boy. The thread-like collagen fibrils are aggregated in some areas (*X*) to form relatively thick bundles; in other areas, the fibrils are more dispersed. The **inset** shows, at higher magnification, a longitudinal array of collagen fibrils from the same specimen. Note the banding pattern. The spacing of the *arrows* indicates the 68-nm repeat pattern.

tron microscope is caused largely by osmium deposition in the space between the heads and tails of the molecules in each row.

Differences in Collagen

The Collagen Molecule (Tropocollagen) Is Composed of Three Intertwined Polypeptide Chains

Each of the polypeptides that constitutes the collagen molecule is designated as an **α chain.** They intertwine, forming a right-handed triple helix (Fig. 5.4*d*). Every third amino acid in the chain is a glycine molecule, except at the ends of the α chains. A hydroxyproline frequently precedes each glycine in the chain, and a proline frequently follows each glycine in the chain. The glycine, along with proline and hydroxyproline, is essential for the triple-helix conformation (Fig. 5.4*e*). Associated with the helix are sugar groups that are joined to hydroxylysyl residues. Because of these sugar groups, collagen is properly described as a **glycoprotein.**

The α chains that constitute the helix are not all alike, and according to differences in α chains, as many as 16 different types of collagen have been identified. These various collagens are classified by Roman numerals on the basis of chronology of discovery. Type I collagen, the most prevalent kind of collagen occurs in loose and dense connective tissue. In type I collagen, two of the α chains (α1) are identical, and one is different (α2). Thus, in collagen nomenclature it is designated $[\alpha1(I)]_2\alpha2(I)$ (Table 5.2).

Type II collagen is present in hyaline and elastic cartilage. It occurs as very fine fibrils. The collagen molecules that make up the fibril in this case are composed of three identical α chains, but they differ from those of other collagens and are thus designated as $[\alpha1(II)]_3$.

Not only are there differences in the polypeptides of the various collagens, but the organization and arrangement of the molecules also differ. For example, the molecules of collagen types I, II, and III aggregate to form 68-nm-banded fibrils (as diagramed in Fig. 5.4*a*). In contrast, type IV collagen, a major constituent of the basal lamina, forms a nonfibrillar network that provides structural cohesion of the basal lamina. Similarly, another nonfibrillar collagen, type IX binds and interacts with type II collagen of cartilage at the intersections of the fibrils. It serves in a stabilizing capacity. Table 5.2 lists the collagens that have been best characterized to date. A perusal of the table shows their structural variations and some of the roles that are presently known for the various collagens.

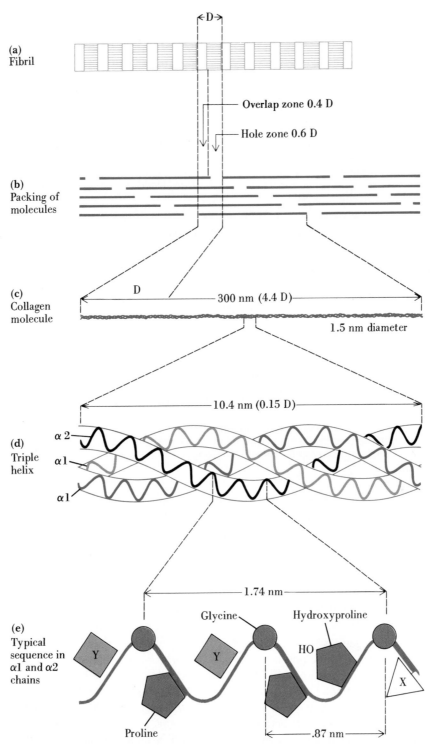

Figure 5.4. Diagram showing the molecular character of a collagen fibril in increasing order of structure. A collagen fibril **(a)** displays periodic banding with a distance (*D*) of 68 nm between repeating bands. It is made up of staggered collagen molecules **(b)**, each of which is about 300 nm long and 1.5 nm in diameter **(c)**. The collagen molecule consists of a triple helix **(d)**; the three components of the triple helix consist of α chains. Each third amino acid of the α chain is a glycine. The X position following glycine is frequently a proline, and the Y position preceding the glycine is frequently a hydroxyproline **(e)**. (Based on Prockop DJ, Guzman NA: *Hospital Practice* 12:2, Dec. 1977.)

TABLE 5.2. Types of Collagen

TYPE	COMPOSITION[A]	LOCATION OF ANALYZED TISSUES	FUNCTIONS
COLLAGENS THAT FORM FIBRILS WITH UNIFORM CROSS-STRIATIONS			
I	$[\alpha 1(I)]_2 \alpha 2(I)$	Connective tissue of skin, bone, tendon, ligaments, dentine, sclera, fascia, and organ capsules (accounts for 90% of body collagen)	Provide resistance to force, tension, and stretch
II	$[\alpha 1(II)]_3$	Cartilage (hyaline and elastic), notochord, and intervertebral disc	Provide resistance to pressure
III	$[\alpha 1(III)]_3$	Connective tissue of organs (uterus, liver, spleen, kidney, lung, etc.), smooth muscle, endoneurium, blood vessels, and fetal skin	Provide structural support and elasticity
COLLAGENS OF LESSER ABUNDANCE, NON-FIBRIL-FORMING			
IV	$[\alpha 1(IV)]_3$ or $[\alpha 2(IV)]_3$	Basal laminae of epithelial and endothelial cells; kidney glomeruli and lens capsule	Provide support and filtration barrier
V	$[\alpha 1(V)]_2 \alpha 2(V) \alpha 3(V)$	Distributed uniformly throughout connective tissue stroma; may be related to reticular network	Provide support and may be involved in other roles not yet defined
VI	$[\alpha 1(VI)]_2 \alpha 2(VI)$	Appears to originate from a microfibrillar component of connective tissues similar to those found at the interface between elastic and collagen fibrils	Not determined
VII	$[\alpha 1(VII)]_3$	Isolated from human skin and amniotic epithelial cells; present in anchoring fibrils	Secures basal lamina to connective tissue
VIII	$[\alpha 1(VIII)]_3$	Product of aortic endothelial cells (initially described as EC collagen) and a variety of normal cell and tumor cell lines; presumably broadly distributed	Not determined
IX	$\alpha 1(IX) \alpha 2(IX) \alpha 3(IX)$	Obtained as synthetic product of in vitro cartilage organ culture; associated with type II collagen of cartilage	Contributes to stabilization of network of cartilage collagen fibers by interaction at their intersections

[A] Each collagen molecule is composed of three polypeptide α chains intertwined in helical configuration. The Roman numerals in the parentheses under Composition indicate that the α chains have a distinctive structure that differs from the chains with different numerals. Thus, collagen type I has two identical α1 chains and one α2 chain; collagen type II has three identical α1 chains.

Collagen Fiber Synthesis

Fiber Formation Involves Events That Occur Both Within and Outside the Fibroblast

The production of fibrillar collagen involves a series of events within the fibroblast that leads to the production of **procollagen,** the precursor of the collagen molecule. These events are all associated with membrane-bounded organelles within the cell. The production of the actual fibril occurs outside of the cell and involves enzymatic activity at the plasma membrane to produce the collagen molecule, followed by the assembly of the molecules into fibrils under guidance of the cell (Fig. 5.5).

Collagen Synthesis Involves a Number of Intracellular Events

- *Polypeptide chains are produced by polyribosomes of the rough endoplasmic reticulum (rER).* This synthesis (trans-

lation) is directed by information provided by messenger RNA (mRNA), and newly synthesized polypeptides are simultaneously discharged into the cisternae of the rER.

- *Within the cisternae of the rER and the Golgi, a number of posttranslational modifications of the polypeptide chains occur.* These include *(a)* cleavage of the signal peptide (see page 29), *(b)* hydroxylation of proline and lysine residues while the polypeptides are still in the nonhelical conformation, *(c)* addition of O-linked sugar groups (glycosylation) to some hydroxylysine residues and N-linked sugars to the two terminal portions, *(d)* formation of a triple helix by three polypeptide chains except at the terminals where the polypeptide chains remain uncoiled, and *(e)* formation of intrachain and interchain hydrogen bonds that influence the shape of the molecule and stabilize the interactions of the polypeptides. The resultant molecule is called **procollagen.** Note that ascorbate or vitamin C is required for the function

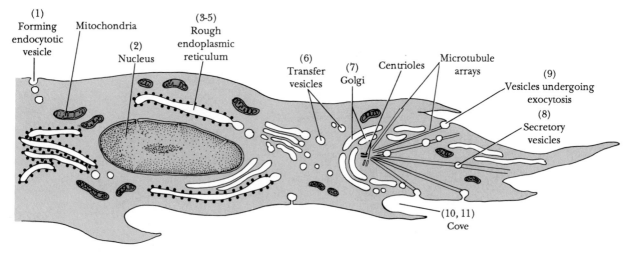

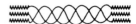

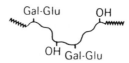

EVENTS IN COLLAGEN SYNTHESIS

Intracellular Events

(1) Uptake of amino acids (proline, lysine, etc.) by endocytosis
(2) Formation of mRNA

(3) Synthesis of alpha chains with registration peptides by ribosomes

(4) Hydroxylation of proline and lysine residues and cleavage of signal sequence in rER

(5) Glycosylation of specific hydroxylysyl residues in rER

(6) Formation of procollagen triple helix molecules in rER and movement into transfer vesicle

(7) Packaging of the procollagen by the Golgi into secretory vesicles
(8) Movement of vesicles to plasma membrane assisted by microfilaments and microtubules
(9) Exocytosis of procollagen

Extracellular Events

(10) Cleavage of registered, nonhelical ends of the procollagen to form tropocollagen

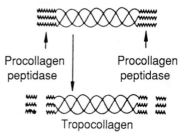

(11) Polymerization of tropocollagen into collagen fibril (in coves initially)

Figure 5.5. Schematic representation of the biosynthetic events and the organelles participating in collagen synthesis. (Modified from Junqueira LC, Carneiro J, Kelley RO: *Basic Histology*, 7th ed. Norwalk, CT, Appleton & Lange, 1992, p 103.)

of prolylhydroxylase and lysylhydroxylase; without the posttranslational hydroxylation of proline and lysine, the hydrogen bonds essential to the final structure of the collagen molecule cannot form. This explains why wounds fail to heal and bone formation is impaired in vitamin C deficiency (scurvy).

• *The procollagen moves to the exterior of the cell by means of exocytosis of secretory vesicles.* Microtubules are involved in the movement of the secretory vesicles from the region of the Golgi to the cell surface; if the microtubules are disrupted with agents such as colchicine or vinblastine, the secretory vesicles accumulate in the Golgi region.

Collagen Synthesis Also Involves Extracellular Events

• *The procollagen, on secretion from the cell, is converted to collagen molecules by procollagen peptidase, which cleaves the uncoiled ends of the molecule (Fig. 5.6).*
• *The aggregated collagen molecules then align to form the final collagen fibrils.* The manner in which the cell controls the orderly array of the newly formed fibrils is

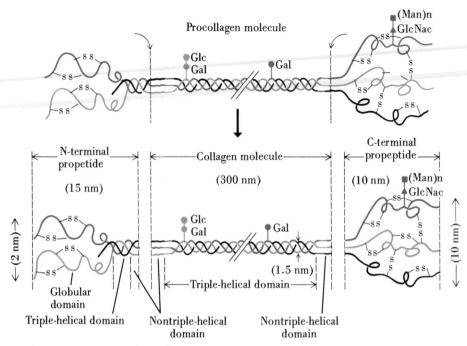

Figure 5.6. Illustration showing procollagen molecule with N- and C-terminals. *Small curved arrows* in upper part of illustration show where terminals are split from the procollagen molecule to form the collagen molecule (tropocollagen molecule). On the C-terminal of the diagram, the sugar subunit is GlcNac (*N*-acetylglucosamime) attached to [Man]n (mannose). (Based on Prockop DJ, et al: Reprinted with permission from *The New England Journal of Medicine* 30:18, 1979.)

by directing the secretory vesicles to a localized surface site for discharge. The cell simultaneously creates a "cove" or indentation at its surface to allow concentration of the secreted molecules where assembly will occur (Fig. 5.5). The collagen self-assembles within the cove as the molecules become aligned in rows and then cross-link.

Reticular Fibers

Reticular Fibers Provide a Supporting Framework for the Cellular Constituents of Various Tissues and Organs of the Body

Reticular fibers are closely related to collagenous fibers, in that they both consist of collagen fibrils. Unlike the collagen fiber, however, the reticular fiber is composed of type III collagen (type IV collagen may also be associated with reticular fibers). The individual fibrils that constitute the reticular fiber are always of narrow diameter (about 20 nm), and typically, the fibrils do not bundle to form thick fibers.

In routinely stained H&E preparations, reticular fibers cannot be positively identified. When made visible in the light microscope with special techniques, the reticular fiber has a thread-like appearance. Because they contain a greater relative content of sugar groups than collagen fibers, reticular fibers are readily displayed by means of the periodic acid-Schiff (PAS) reaction. They are also displayed with special silver-staining procedures, such as the Gomori and Wilder methods. After silver treatment, the fibers appear black; thus, they are said to be *argyrophilic* (Fig. 5.7). The thicker collagen fibers in such preparations are colored brown.

Reticular Fibers Are So Called Because They Are Arranged in a Mesh-Like Pattern or Network

In loose connective tissue, networks of reticular fibers are found at the boundary of connective tissue with epithelium and around adipocytes, small blood vessels, nerves, and muscle cells. Reticular fibers are also present as a supporting stroma in hemopoietic and lymphatic tissues (but not in the thymus). In these tissues, the collagen of the reticular fiber is produced by a special cell type, the *reticular cell*. This cell maintains a unique relationship to the fiber, surrounding it with its cytoplasm; the fiber is thus isolated from its environment.

In most other locations, the reticular fiber is produced by fibroblasts. Important exceptions to this general rule include the endoneurium of peripheral nerves, where Schwann cells secrete reticular fibers, and the reticular and other collagenous fibers secreted by smooth muscle cells of the tunica media of blood vessels and the muscularis of the alimentary canal.

Elastic Fibers

Elastic Fibers Provide Tissues With the Ability to Respond to Stretch and Distension

Elastic fibers are typically thinner than collagen fibers and are arranged in a branching pattern to form a three-

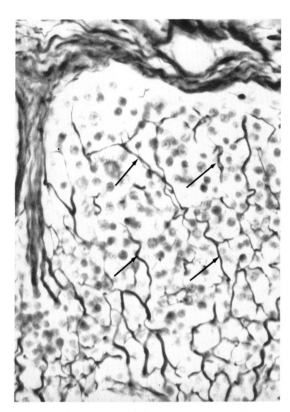

Figure 5.7. Photomicrograph of a lymph node silver preparation showing the connective tissue capsule at the top and a trabecula extending from it at the left. The reticular fibers (*arrows*) form an irregular anastomosing network.

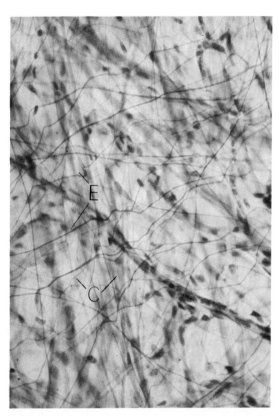

Figure 5.8. Photomicrograph of a mesentery spread stained with resorcin-fuchsin. The mesentery is very thin, and the microscope can be focused through the entire thickness of the tissue. The delicate thread-like branching strands are the elastic fibers (*E*). Collagen fibers (*C*) are also evident. They are much thicker, and although they cross one another, they do not branch.

dimensional network. The fibers are interwoven with collagen fibers to limit the distensibility of the tissue and to prevent tearing from excessive stretching.

Elastic fibers stain with eosin, but not well; thus, they cannot always be distinguished from collagen fibers in routine H&E preparations. Because elastic fibers become somewhat refractile with certain fixatives, they may be distinguished from collagen fibers in specimens stained with H&E when they display this characteristic. However, elastic fibers can be selectively stained with special dyes such as orcein or resorcin-fuchsin, as shown in Figure 5.8.

Elastic fibers are produced by most of the same cells that produce collagen and reticular fibers, particularly fibroblasts and smooth muscle cells. In contrast to the collagen-containing fibers, however, elastic fibers are composed of two structural components, elastin and microfibrils.

- *Elastin,* a protein that, like collagen, is rich in proline and glycine but, unlike collagen, is poor in hydroxyproline and completely lacks hydroxylysine
- *Microfibrils*[1], a fibrillar glycoprotein that is relatively straight and thin, measuring 12 nm in diameter

---

[1]The microfibril is an extracellular structure and should not be confused with the microfilament, an intracellular structure composed of actin.

The Elastic Property of the Elastin Molecule Is Due to Its Unusual Polypeptide Backbone That Produces a Random-Coiled Molecule

The random coiling of the elastin molecule gives the elastic fiber its ability to be stretched and then recoil back to its original state. Elastin also uniquely contains desmosine and isodesmosine. These large amino acids are responsible for the covalent bonding of the elastin molecules to one another. Figure 5.9 illustrates, in separate panels, *(a)* the randomly coiled elastin molecules, *(b)* the covalently bound elastin molecules joined together to form the elastin matrix, and *(c)* the effect of stretching the matrix with the ensuing straightening and alignment of the uncoiled molecules.

With the electron microscope, elastin appears as an amorphous structure of low electron density. The microfibrils, in contrast, are electron dense and are readily apparent even within the elastin matrix (Fig. 5.10). In developing tissues where elastic fibers are being formed, the microfibrils appear first. They are believed to serve as an organizing structure for the growing elastic fiber. The elastin material is deposited later as a secondary component of

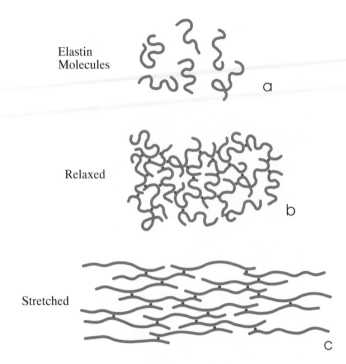

Elastin Molecules

a

Relaxed

b

Stretched

c

Figure 5.9. Schematic diagram of elastin molecules and their interaction. In **a,** the molecules are depicted in their individual and random-coiled conformation. The configuration of the individual molecules continuously changes, oscillating from one form to another. In **b,** the elastin molecules are shown joined by covalent bonding (red) to form a cross-linked network. In **c,** the effect of stretching is shown. When the force is withdrawn, the network reverts to the relaxed state as in **b.** (Redrawn after Alberts B, et al: *Molecular Biology of the Cell,* 2nd ed. New York, Garland Publishing, 1989, p 817.)

the fiber. In mature fibers, the microfibrils are located within the elastic fiber and at the periphery of the fiber. The presence of the microfibrils within the fiber is associated with the growth process; thus, as the fiber is formed and thickens, the microfibrils become entrapped within the newly deposited elastin[2].

A known component of the microfibril is the protein, *fibrillin.* It is of interest that in Marfan's syndrome, a complex, autosomal dominant, connective tissue disorder, there is a defect in the fibrillin gene. One of the consequences of the disease is abnormal elastic tissue.

---

[2]Elastic fibers as described here belong to a larger "system" of fibers with certain related characteristics. For example, *oxytalan* fibers, found in the dermis, in tooth sockets, and in the suspensory ligaments of the lens, are formed of microfibrils with little or no amorphous material. *Elaunin* fibers, found in the dermis, exhibit microfibrils and relatively small amounts of elastin. These fibers possess less elasticity than the elastic fibers. Studies have shown that the three types of fibers contain similar microfibrils but varying amounts of amorphous material. It was once thought that these types of fibers represented different stages in elastic fiber formation.

Elastic Material Is a Major Extracellular Substance in Vertebral Ligaments, Larynx, and Elastic Arteries

In the elastic ligaments, the elastic material is in the form of thick fibers interspersed with collagenous fibers. Examples are found in the ligamenta flava of the vertebral column and the ligamentum nuchae of the neck; also, finer fibers are present in elastic ligaments of the vocal folds of the larynx.

In the elastic arteries, the elastic material is in the form of fenestrated lamellae, sheets of elastin with gaps or openings. The lamellae are arranged in concentric layers between layers of smooth muscle cells. Like the collagenous fibers in the tunica media of the vessel wall, the elastic material is, in this case, produced by smooth muscle cells, not by fibroblasts. In contrast to elastic fibers, microfibrils are not found in the lamellae. Only the amorphous elastin component is seen in electron micrographs. The microfibrils are associated with the role of organizing elastin into fibers; their absence is associated with formation of elastin sheets or lamellae.

Elastin Is Synthesized by Means of the Same Pathway as Collagen

Elastic fibers, as already noted, are produced by the fibroblast. The synthetic process parallels collagen production; in fact, both processes can occur simultaneously in a cell. The orderly modification and assembly of procollagen and proelastin and the simultaneous synthesis of other protein and glycoprotein components of connective tissue are controlled by signal peptides that are built into the beginning of the polypeptide chains of each of the molecules.

As airline tags on luggage ensure that baggage moves correctly from one aircraft to another at airports, so the signal regions of polypeptides ensure that the components of procollagen and proelastin remain separate and properly identified as they pass one another during their transit through the organelles of the cell. During this transit, a series of synthetic events and posttranslational modifications occur before the polypeptides arrive ultimately at their proper destination.

GROUND SUBSTANCE

Ground Substance Is the Component That Occupies the Space Between the Cells and Fibers

In life, *ground substance* is a viscous, clear substance that has a slippery feel. It has a high water content and that, combined with its structureless nature, at least above the macromolecular level, offers little in terms of morphologic characterization. In the light microscope, ground substance has an amorphous appearance in sections of tissue pre-

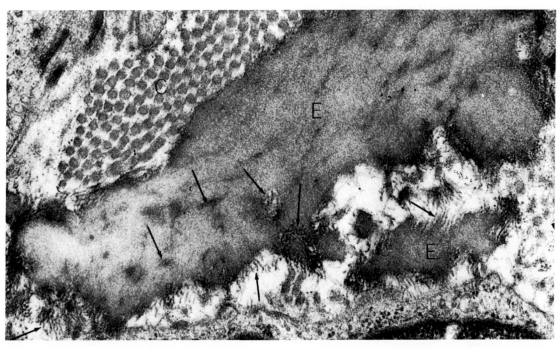

Figure 5.10. Electron micrograph of an elastic fiber. The elastin (*E*) has a relatively amorphous appearance. The microfibrils (*arrows*) are present at the periphery and within the sub- stance of the fiber. A number of collagen fibrils (*C*) are also present in the micrograph.

served by freeze drying or in frozen sections stained with basic dyes or by the periodic acid-Schiff (PAS) method. In routine H&E preparations the ground substance is always lost due to extraction during fixation and dehydration of the tissue. The result is an empty background; only the cells and fibers are evident. Thus, in most histologic prepara- tions, the appearance of ground substance belies its func- tional importance.

Ground Substance Consists Largely of Proteoglycans and Hyaluronic Acid

The physical properties of ground substance, whether it be its viscous nature in loose connective tissue or its more turgid character in cartilage, and its ability to permit dif- fusion of oxygen and nutrients between the microvascula- ture and adjacent tissues is due to the proteoglycans that it contains. *Proteoglycans* are very large macromolecules comprised of a core protein to which many glycosamino- glycan molecules are covalently bound. *Glycosaminogly- cans (GAGs),* formerly referred to as mucopolysacchar- ides, are long-chained polysaccharides made up of repeating disaccharide units. One of the sugars in each disaccharide is a hexosamine (glycosamine), hence the name. GAGs are highly negatively charged due to sulfate and carboxyl groups located on many of the sugars, thus the propensity for stain- ing with basic dyes. The high density of negative charges attracts water, forming a hydrated gel. It is this property

that permits rapid diffusion of water-soluble molecules in the ground substance but inhibits movement of large molecules and bacteria. Due to differences in specific sugar residues, the nature of their linkages, and the degree of sul- fation, a family of some seven distinct GAGs is recognized. They are listed below and partially characterized in Table 5.3:

- Hyaluronic acid
- Chondroitin 4- and 6-sulfate
- Dermatan sulfate
- Heparan sulfate
- Heparin
- Keratan sulfate

Several of these proteoglycans are modified in connective tissue cells or in the connective tissue after their synthesis; heparin is formed by enzymatic cleaving of heparan sulfate; dermatan sulfate is similarly modified from chondroitin sul- fate.

Hyaluronic acid (HA), one of the GAGs, requires spe- cial note. It differs from the others in several respects. It is an exceedingly long, rigid molecule composed of a car- bohydrate chain of thousands of sugars compared with sev- eral hundred or less in other GAGs. Also, HA is not bound to protein to form a proteoglycan. By means of special *linker proteins,* however, proteoglycans indirectly bind to HA, forming giant macromolecules as in cartilage ground sub- stance (Fig. 5.11). The swelling pressure or turgor that oc- curs with these giant hydrophilic macromolecules accounts for the ability of cartilage to resist compression without inhibiting flexibility.

EXTRACELLULAR MATRIX

The Extracellular Matrix Is a Complex Structural Network That Includes the Fibrous Proteins, Proteoglycans, and Several Glycoproteins

The current view of the extracellular components of connective tissue and their functional role reveals a dynamic system in which fibers, proteoglycans, some belonging to the ground substance and others associated with surfaces, and specific glycoproteins such as fibronectin and laminin interact with the other components. They comprise the *extracellular matrix.*

FIBROBLAST RELATION TO EXTRACELLULAR MATRIX

It is not evident, from the view afforded by microscopy, whether the fibroblasts passively rest in spaces in the matrix (i.e., ground substance and fibers) or are mechanically attached and integrated with it. Our understanding of the role of the fibroblast in forming, maintaining, and turning over extracellular matrix does not require a physical attachment to it. However, tissue culture studies reveal that fibroblasts are anchored tightly to matrix elements and that these attachments are important to the cell as it extends cytoplasmic processes and moves. The attachments made by the fibroblasts involve several mechanisms that may be divided into two classes (some of the mechanisms are understood better than others). The first class of mechanisms requires the presence of receptors for proteins of fibrils, such as collagen, and receptors for glycoproteins, such as fibronectin, that are attached to the fibrils. A second class appears to involve the covalent association of GAGs with specific integral plasma membrane proteins. The attachments established between the fibroblasts and the matrix involve proteins that are distinct from proteins that mediate cell-cell contacts. In terms of function, these proteins are similar to those involved in attachments of epithelial cells to the basal lamina. Small variations in the structure of the proteins involved in these contacts confer an individuality to the different cell and matrix types with which they are associated. These differences may establish molecular specificity and, presumably, assist in specialization of function found in different tissue sites.

CONNECTIVE TISSUE CELLS

The types of cells found in loose connective tissue as well as their relative numbers reflect the tissue's functional activity. In addition to its structural role through its fibers and other matrix components, loose connective tissue serves as an important site of the body's defense mechanisms, as

in inflammatory and immune reactions, and in surveillance of antigenic substances that have gained access to the body. Consequently, the types of cells present may exhibit significant differences according to functional response.

Connective Tissue Cells Can Be Categorized as Fixed or Wandering

The cells that comprise the *fixed cell population* are relatively stable; they normally exhibit little movement and can be regarded as permanent residents of the tissue. They include

- *Fibroblasts* and a closely related cell type, the *myofibroblast*
- *Macrophages*
- *Adipose cells*
- *Mast cells*
- *Undifferentiated mesenchymal cells*

The cells that comprise the wandering or transient population are mostly those that have migrated into the tissue from the blood in response to specific stimuli. They include

- *Lymphocytes*
- *Plasma cells*
- *Neutrophils*
- *Eosinophils*
- *Basophils*
- *Monocytes*

Fibroblasts and Myofibroblasts

The Fibroblast Is the Principal Cell of Connective Tissue

Fibroblasts are responsible for the synthesis of collagenous, elastic, and reticular fibers and the complex carbohydrates of the ground substance. It is believed that a single fibroblast has the capacity to produce all of the extracellular matrix components, both sequentially and simultaneously.

Fibroblasts reside in close proximity to the collagen fibers. In routine H&E preparations, however, only the nucleus tends to be visible. It appears as an elongated or discoid structure with a nucleolus sometimes evident. The thin, pale-staining, flattened processes that form the bulk of the cytoplasm are usually not visible, largely due to their blending with the collagenous fibers. In certain specially prepared specimens it is possible to distinguish the cytoplasm of the cell from the fibrous components (Fig. 5.12). When examined in the electron microscope, the fibroblast cytoplasm exhibits profiles of rER and a prominent Golgi apparatus (Fig. 5.13). Where active production of extracellular matrix material is in progress during active growth or in wound repair, the cytoplasm of the fibroblast is more extensive and

TABLE 5.3. Glycosaminoglycans

NAME	APPROXIMATE MOLECULAR WEIGHT (IN DALTONS)	DISACCHARIDE COMPOSITION
Hyaluronic acid	1,000,000	D-Glucuronic acid + N-acetylglucosamine
Chondroitin 4-sulfate	25,000	D-Glucuronic acid + N-acetylgalactosamine 4-sulfate
Chondroitin 6-sulfate	25,000	D-Glucuronic acid + N-acetylgalactosamine 6-sulfate
Dermatan sulfate	35,000	L-Iduronic acid + N-acetylgalactosamine 4-sulfate
Keratan sulfate	10,000	Galactose or galactose 6-sulfate + N-acetylglucosamine 6-sulfate
Heparan sulfate	15,000	Glucuronic acid or L-iduronic acid 2-sulfate + N-sulfamylglucosamine or N-acetylglucosamine
Heparin	40,000	Glucuronic acid or L-iduronic acid 2-sulfate + N-sulfamylglucosamine or N-acetylglucosamine 6-sulfate

displays a slight basophilia as a result of increased amounts of rER associated with protein synthesis.

Fibroblasts in some locations, e.g., those immediately beneath the epithelium of the intestine, under the epidermis, and around tubular and glandular epithelia, constitute a *replicating population* of cells that have a particularly close physical relationship to the overlying epithelium. They are believed to *interact with* the *epithelium* in normal renewal and differentiation in the adult organism (epithelial-mesenchymal interaction; see page 467).

The Myofibroblast Displays Properties of Both Fibroblast and Smooth Muscle Cell

The myofibroblast is an elongate spindly connective tissue cell that is not readily identifiable in routine H&E preparations. With the electron microscope, it displays cytologic characteristics of the fibroblast. In addition to the rER and Golgi profiles, the myofibroblast contains bundles of longitudinally disposed actin filaments and dense bodies similar to those observed in smooth muscle cells (Fig. 5.14). Like the smooth muscle cell, the nucleus often shows an undulating surface profile, a phenomenon associated with cell contraction. The myofibroblast differs from the smooth muscle cell in that there is no basal lamina surrounding it (smooth muscle cells are surrounded by a basal or external lamina). Also, it is usually seen as an isolated cell, although its processes may contact the process of other myofibroblasts. Such points of contact exhibit gap junctions, thus indicating intercellular communication.

The myofibroblast is implicated in wound contraction, a natural process that tends to close a wound in which actual loss of tissue has occurred. Electron microscopy studies have shown that myofibroblasts are numerous in such wound sites, particularly in the granulation tissue of these wounds. The possibility that these cells represent modified fibroblasts that have responded to stimuli associated with tissue damage and repair is very likely.

Macrophages

Macrophages Are Phagocytic Cells Derived From Monocytes

Connective tissue *macrophages,* also known as tissue *histiocytes,* are derived from monocytes of the blood. On migration into the connective tissue, the monocyte undergoes a maturation process. At this stage it is then referred to as a macrophage.

With the light microscope, using conventional stains, tissue macrophages are difficult to identify unless they display obvious evidence of phagocytic activity, i.e., the inclusion of visible ingested material within their cytoplasm. Another feature that assists in identifying the macrophage is the presence of an indented or kidney-shaped nucleus. Lysosomes are abundant in the cytoplasm and can be demonstrated by staining for acid phosphatase activity (at both the light microscope and the transmission electron microscope level); a positive reaction is a further aid in identification of the macrophage.

At the transmission electron microscope level, the surface of the macrophage exhibits numerous folds and finger-like projections (Fig. 5.15a). The surface folds are active in phagocytosis in that they engulf substances to be phagocytosed. In the case of large objects, such as other cells, the folds spread over and surround the object to be phagocytosed.

The Macrophage Contains a Large Golgi, Rough and Smooth Endoplasmic Reticulum, Mitochondria, Secretory Vesicles, and Lysosomes

The lysosomes of the macrophage, along with the surface cytoplasmic projections, are the structures most indicative of the specialized phagocytic capability of the cell (Fig.

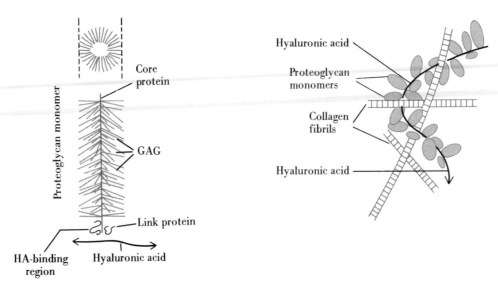

Figure 5.11. Schematic drawing showing, on the left, a proteoglycan monomer and its relationship to the HA molecule as represented in ground substance of cartilage. The proteoglycan monomer is composed of a core protein to which GAGs are covalently bound. The proteoglycan monomer consists of approximately 100 GAG units (*GAG*) joined to the core protein. The end of the core protein contains an HA-binding region; interaction with the HA is strengthened by a link protein. On the right, a HA molecule forming a linear aggregate with many proteoglycan monomers (pink ellipses) is interwoven with a network of collagen fibrils. (Based on Hascall VC, Lowther DA: In: Nancollas GH, et al (eds): *Biological Mineralization and Demineralization.* New York, Springer, 1982, p 181.)

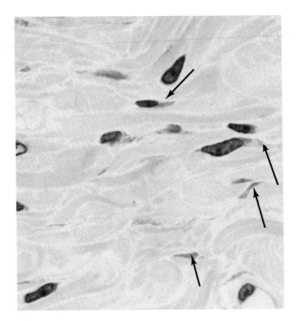

Figure 5.12. Light micrograph of a connective tissue specimen fixed with glutaraldehyde, embedded in plastic, and stained with H&E. Thin strands of fibroblast cytoplasm (*arrows*) belonging to a few preferentially oriented cells can just barely be recognized between collagen fibers. In routine H&E paraffin preparations, it is usually impossible to distinguish the attenuated and poorly preserved fibroblast cytoplasm from the collagen fibers. Typically, only the nuclei of these cells are evident.

5.15*b*). In addition, there may be endocytic vacuoles, secondary lysosomes, and other evidence of phagocytosis. The rER and Golgi support the synthesis of proteins involved in the phagocytotic and lysosomal systems as well as in the cell's secretory system. The secretory products leave the cell by both the constitutive and regulated exocytotic pathways (see page 24). Regulated secretion can be activated by phagocytosis, immune complexes, complement, and signals from lymphocytes (including the release of *lymphokines,* biologically active molecules that influence the activity of other cells). The secretory products released by the macrophage include a wide variety of substances related to the immune response, anaphylaxis, and inflammation. The release of neutral proteases and GAGases (enzymes able to break down GAGs) facilitates the migration of the macrophages through the connective tissue.

Although the main function of the macrophage is phagocytosis, either as a defense activity (as in phagocytosis of bacteria) or as a cleanup operation (as in phagocytosis of cell debris), the macrophage also plays a role in immune reactions by presenting lymphocytes with concentrated antigens derived from phagocytosed foreign cells or proteins.

It is noteworthy that when macrophages encounter large foreign bodies, they may fuse to form a large cell with up to 100 nuclei that engulfs the foreign body. These multinucleated cells are called *foreign body giant cells* (Langhans' cells).

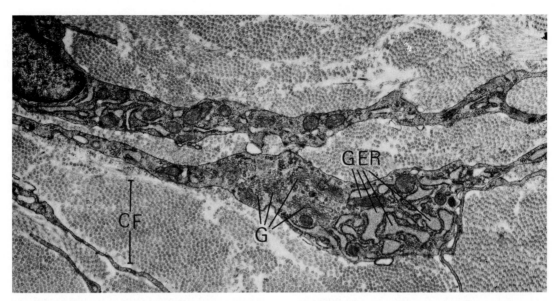

Figure 5.13. Electron micrograph of processes of several fibroblasts. The nucleus of one is in the upper left of the micrograph. The cytoplasm shows conspicuous profiles of granular (rough) endoplasmic reticulum (*GER*). The cisternae of the reticulum are distended, a reflection of active synthesis. In proximity to the reticulum is a Golgi profile (*G*). Surrounding the cells are collagen fibrils (*CF*); almost all have been cut in cross section and, thus, appear as small dots at this magnification.

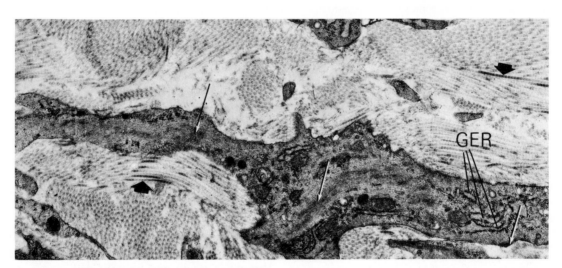

Figure 5.14. Electron micrograph showing a portion of the cytoplasm of a myofibroblast. The cell exhibits certain features of a fibroblast, such as areas with a moderate amount of granular or rough endoplasmic reticulum (*GER*). (Compare with Figure 5.13.) There are other areas, however, that contain aggregates of fine filaments and cytoplasmic densities (*arrows*), features characteristic of smooth muscle cells. The *arrowheads* indicate longitudinal profiles of collagen fibrils. A low-power micrograph of this cell is shown in Atlas Plate 8, page 121, in relation to other connective tissue cells. ×11,000.

MONONUCLEAR PHAGOCYTIC SYSTEM

The Mononuclear Phagocytic System Comprises a System of Cells Characterized by Their Avid Phagocytic Capability and Common Derivation From Monocytes

The cells that are included in the mononuclear phagocytic system (MPS) have the ability to phagocytize avidly vital dyes such as trypan blue and India ink. Such cells engulf and accumulate vital dyes within their cytoplasm, so that they are visible with the light microscope. Some of these cells were earlier described as constituting the reticuloendothelial system. This was a misconception based on the inability to distinguish, at the light microscope level, between the endothelial cells and perisinusoidal macrophages in the liver and between the reticular cells and fixed macrophages in lymph nodes and spleen. Certain cells not belonging to this group, e.g., fibroblasts, can also engage in phagocytoses, but such activity is not avid, nor is it enhanced by immunologic stimulation. It is now known that nearly all cells that functionally engage in the avid phagocytosis of injected vital dyes are derived from monocytes. This common origin serves as the major distinguishing feature of the system as it is currently perceived, and the system is now called the **mononuclear phagocytic system (MPS)**. However, certain functionally important phagocytic cells are not monocyte derived. The various cells of the MPS are listed below in Table 5.4.

Microglia, small stellate-shaped cells located mostly along capillaries of the central nervous system, function as phagocytic cells. They are generally thought to arise from mesectoderm of the neural crest and not from monocytes; nevertheless, they are included in the MPS. Similarly, fibroblasts of the subepithelial sheath of the lamina propria of the intestine (page 467) and fibroblasts of the uterine endometrium have been shown to differentiate into cells having the morphologic, enzymatic, and functional characteristics of connective tissue macrophages.

Mast Cells

The mast cell is a large ovoid connective tissue cell with a spherical nucleus and cytoplasm filled with large granules (Fig. 5.16). It is related to, but not identical with, the basophil of the blood, which contains similar granules. The cell surface exhibits numerous microvilli and folds. The cytoplasm displays only small amounts of rER, mitochondria, and a Golgi zone.

Mast cells are not easily identified in human tissue sections unless special fixatives are used to preserve the granules. After glutaraldehyde fixation, mast cell granules can be displayed with basic dyes, such as toluidine blue. It stains the granules intensely and metachromatically due to the content of heparin, a sulfated proteoglycan (Fig. 5.17).

Several Vasoactive and Immunoreactive Substances Are Contained in Mast Cell Granules

Mast cell granules are released from the cell on appropriate stimulation, such as exposure to an antigen to which the individual has already been sensitized. Sensitization develops when an individual is exposed to a foreign substance, an antigen, that the body recognizes as nonself and against which the body produces antibodies. On initial exposure to the antigen, cells of the immune system, which on their surface express antibody molecules that recognize and are specific for the antigen *(cognate antibodies)*, are induced to proliferate, thereby resulting in the production of more antibody specific to the original antigen. Several major classes of antibodies, referred to as immunoglobulins, are produced (page 336). The mast cells do not produce antibodies but are dependent on plasma cells to produce antibodies that bind to their surface. When stimulated by the presence of foreign antigen, the plasma cells produce antibodies that are released into the connective tissue. Immunoglobulins of the IgE class, which are specific to individual antigens, bind to receptors located in the plasma membrane of the mast cells. On subsequent exposure to the same antigen, an antigen-antibody reaction occurs that causes the discharge of mast cell granules.

The Secretions of Mast Cell Granules Can Result in Immediate Hypersensitivity Reactions, Allergy, and Anaphylaxis

Four substances known to be released by mast cells are

- *Histamine*
- *Slow-reacting substance of anaphylaxis (SRS-A)*
- *Eosinophil chemotactic factor of anaphylaxis (ECF-A)*
- *Heparin*

In the immune response, histamine and SRS-A increase the permeability of small blood vessels, thereby causing edema in the surrounding tissue. Heparin is an anticoagulant. The ECF-A stimulates eosinophils to migrate to the sites where mast cells have released their agents; the eosinophils counteract the effects of the histamine and SRS-A.

Mast Cells Are Especially Numerous in Connective Tissues of Skin and Mucous Membranes but Are Not Present in Brain and Spinal Cord

Mast cells are distributed chiefly in the vicinity of small blood vessels, a target of histamine and SRS-A. Mast cells are also present in the capsules of organs and, to a lesser degree, within the organs, e.g., in the connective tissue that surrounds the blood vessels of the organ. A notable exception is the central nervous system. Whereas the meninges

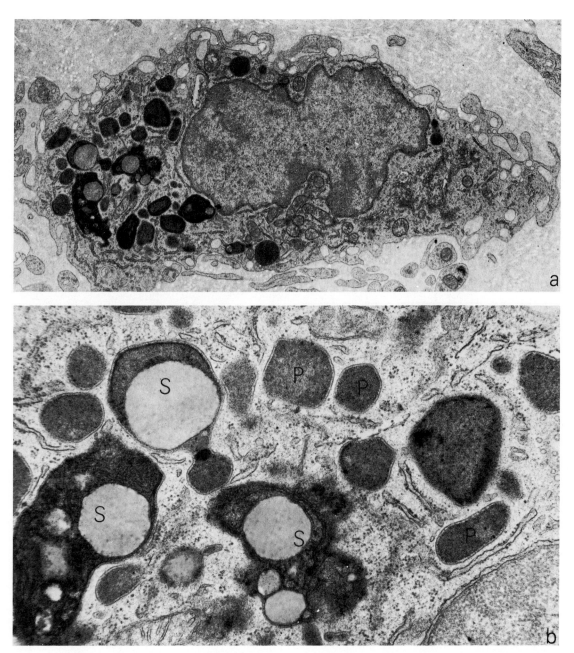

Figure 5.15. **a.** Electron micrograph of a macrophage. The most distinctive feature is the population of granules. Those that have a homogeneous matrix are primary lysosomes. Those that have a heterogeneous appearance represent second-ary lysosomes. The surface of the cell reveals a number of finger-like projections, some of which may be sections of sur-face folds. ×10,000. **b.** Higher magnification of the lysosomes. *P*, primary lysosomes; *S*, secondary lysosomes. ×45,000.

(sheets of connective tissue that surround the brain and spinal cord) contain mast cells, the connective tissue around the small blood vessels within the substance of the brain and spinal cord is devoid of mast cells, thereby protecting the brain and spinal cord from the potentially disrupting effects of the edema characteristic of allergic reactions. Mast cells are also numerous in the thymus and, to a lesser degree, in other lymphatic organs, but they are not present in the spleen.

Adipose Cells

The Adipose Cell Is a Connective Tissue Cell Specialized to Store Neutral Fat

Adipose cells differentiate from fibroblasts and from un-differentiated mesenchymal cells and gradually accumulate fat in their cytoplasm. They are found throughout the loose connective tissue as individual cells and groups of cells.

TABLE 5.4. Cells of the Mononuclear Phagocytic System

NAME OF CELL	LOCATION
Macrophage (histiocyte)	Connective tissue
Perisinusoidal macrophage (Kupffer cell)	Liver
Alveolar macrophage	Lungs
Macrophage	Spleen, lymph nodes, bone marrow, and thymus
Pleural and peritoneal macrophage	Serous cavities
Osteoclast	Bone
Microglia	Central nervous system
Langerhans' cell	Epidermis
Fibroblast-derived macrophage	Lamina propria of intestine, endometrium of uterus

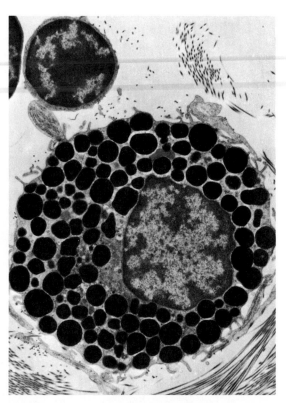

Figure 5.16. Electron micrograph of a mast cell. The cytoplasm is virtually filled with granules. Note a small lymphocyte is present in the upper left of the figure. ×6000.

When they accumulate in very large numbers, they are called adipose tissue. This specialized connective tissue is presented in Chapter 6.

Undifferentiated Mesenchymal Cells and Pericytes

Many histologists have postulated the existence of cells in loose connective tissue of the adult that retain the multiple potentials of embryonic mesenchymal cells. These cells, called undifferentiated mesenchymal cells, were thought to give rise to differentiated cells that would serve in repair and formation of new tissue, as in wound healing, and in development of new blood vessels (neovascularization). Some histologists believed that the cells that gave rise to new fibroblasts and blood vessels in healing wounds came from the blood, leaving the circulation to enter the connective tissue.

The Pericyte Is a Cell That Serves as an Undifferentiated Mesenchymal Cell

Pericytes, also called *adventitial cells* and *perivascular cells,* are found around capillaries and venules (Fig. 5.18). They are surrounded by basal lamina material that is directly continuous with the basal lamina of the capillary endothelium; thus, they are not truly in the connective tissue compartment. The pericyte is typically wrapped, at least partially, around the capillary, and its nucleus takes a shape corresponding to that of the endothelial cells, i.e., flattened but curved to conform to the tubular shape of the vessel.

Electron microscope studies of pericytes have shown that those surrounding the smallest venules have cytoplasmic characteristics almost identical with the endothelial cells of the same vessel. When pericytes associated with larger ve-

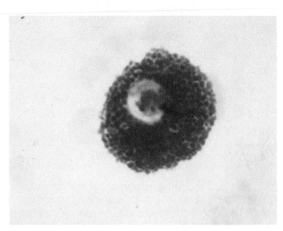

Figure 5.17. Photomicrograph of a mast cell stained with toluidine blue. The granules stain intensely and, because of their numbers, tend to appear as a solid mass in some areas. The nucleus of the cell is represented by the pale-staining area.

nules are examined, they are found to have characteristics of the smooth muscle cells of the tunica media of small veins. In fortuitous sections cut parallel to the long axis of venules, the distal portions and proximal portions of the same pericyte can be shown to have characteristics of endothelial cells and smooth muscle cells, respectively. This suggests that in the development of new vessels, cells hav-

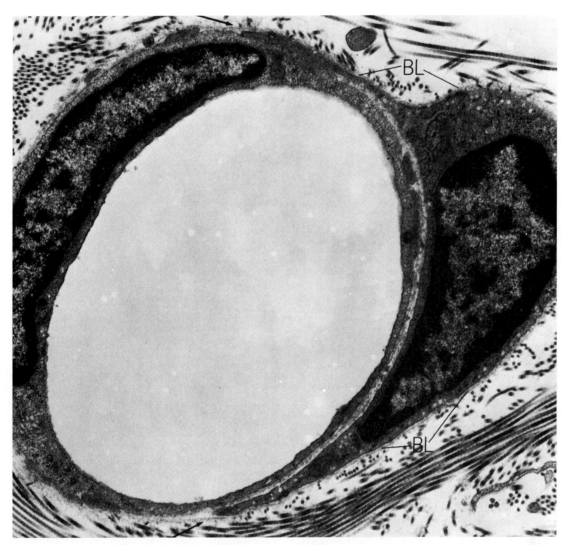

Figure 5.18. Electron micrograph of a small blood vessel. The nucleus at the left belongs to the endothelial cell that forms the wall of the vessel. At the right is another cell, a peri-cyte, that is in intimate relation to the endothelium. Note that the basal lamina (*BL*) covering the endothelial cells divides (*arrows*) also to surround the pericyte.

ing characteristics of pericytes may differentiate into the smooth muscle of the vessel wall.

The Fibroblasts and Blood Vessels of Healing Wounds Develop From Undifferentiated Mesenchymal Cells Associated With the Tunica Adventitia of Venules

Autoradiographic studies of healing wounds, using parabiotic (crossed-circulation) pairs of animals, have now established that undifferentiated mesenchymal cells located in the tunica adventitia of venules and small veins are the primary source of new cells in healing wounds. In addition, fibroblasts, pericytes, and endothelial cells in portions of the connective tissue adjacent to the wound divide and give rise to additional cells that form the new connective tissue and blood vessels. No cells derived from the circulating blood give rise to the fibroblasts, pericytes, or endothelial cells in the healing wound.

Lymphocytes

Lymphocytes Are Principally Involved in Immune Responses

Connective tissue lymphocytes are the smallest of the free cells in the connective tissue, having a diameter of 6–8 μm (see Fig. 5.16). They have a thin rim of cytoplasm surrounding a deeply staining, heterochromatic nucleus. In many instances, the cytoplasm of connective tissue lymphocytes may not be visible.

Normally, small numbers of lymphocytes are found in the connective tissue throughout the body. The number increases dramatically, however, at sites of tissue inflammation caused by infectious agents and foreign bodies. Lymphocytes are most numerous in the lamina propria of the respiratory and gastrointestinal tracts, where they are

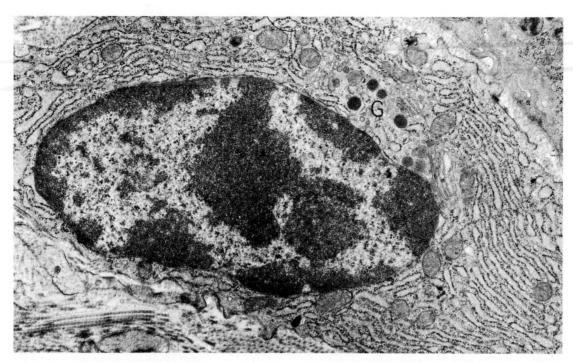

Figure 5.19. Electron micrograph of a plasma cell. A very extensive rER occupies most of the cytoplasm. The Golgi apparatus (*G*) is also relatively large, a further reflection of the cell's secretory activity. ×15,000.

involved in the immunosurveillance against pathogens and foreign substances that enter the body through these routes.

Lymphocytes are a heterogeneous population of two functional cell types:

- *T lymphocytes,* which have a long life span and are involved in cell-mediated immunity
- *B lymphocytes,* which have variable life spans and are involved in the production of antibodies

In response to the presence of antigens, *B lymphocytes* may divide several times, producing more B lymphocytes as well as large clones of cells that mature into *plasma cells.*

Plasma Cells

Plasma Cells Are Antibody-Producing Cells Derived From B Lymphocytes

Plasma cells are a prominent constituent of loose connective tissue where antigens are most capable of entering the body, i.e., the gastrointestinal and respiratory tracts. They are also a regular component of salivary glands, lymph nodes, and hemopoietic tissue. The plasma cell, once derived from its precursor, the B lymphocyte, has only limited migratory ability and a somewhat short life of 10–30 days.

The plasma cell is a relatively large (20 μm) ovoid cell with considerable cytoplasm. The cytoplasm displays strong basophilia due to the presence of an extensive rER (Fig.

5.19). The Golgi is usually prominent due to its relatively large size and lack of staining. It appears as a clear area in contrast to the basophilic cytoplasm.

The nucleus is spherical and typically offset or eccentrically positioned. It is small, not much larger than the nucleus of the lymphocyte. It exhibits large clumps of peripheral heterochromatin alternating with clear areas of euchromatin. This arrangement has traditionally been described as resembling a cartwheel or clock face, with the heterochromatin giving the illusion of the spokes of the wheel or the numbers on a clock.

Despite the fact that the plasma cell is synthesizing very large amounts of protein, it has a largely heterochromatic nucleus. This is explained by the fact that it is making large amounts of *only one protein,* a specific antibody. Therefore, only a small segment of the genome must be exposed for transcription.

Eosinophils, Monocytes, and Neutrophils

Eosinophils, Monocytes, and Neutrophils May Also Be Observed in Connective Tissue

As a result of immune responses and tissue injury, certain cells rapidly migrate from the blood to enter the connective tissue, particularly neutrophils and monocytes. Their presence generally reflects an acute inflammatory reaction. In such cases the neutrophils migrate into the connective tissue in substantial numbers, followed by large numbers of monocytes. As already noted, the monocytes then dif-

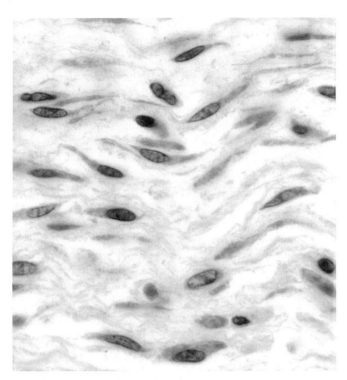

Figure 5.20. Photomicrograph of mesenchymal tissue from a developing fetus. Morphologically, the mesenchymal cells appear as a homogeneous population, even though they may be committed to give rise to cells that differentiate into various cell types. They exhibit cytoplasmic processes, which often give the cell a tapering or spindle appearance. The extracellular component of the tissue contains a sparse arrangement of reticular fibers and abundant ground substance.

ferentiate into macrophages. A description of these cells and their role is deferred to the chapter on blood. Similarly, the eosinophil, whose role is served in allergic reactions and parasitic infections, is also presented in the chapter on blood. In the meantime, it should be pointed out that eosinophils may be observed in normal connective tissue, particularly the lamina propria of the intestine as the result of the chronic low-level immunologic responses occurring there.

Basophils

In Certain Immune Responses, Basophils Leave the Circulation and Function in the Connective Tissue

The release of histamine (and, in some species, serotonin) from the secretory granules of basophils enhances the vascular response in dermal hypersensitivity reactions such as those in insect bites.

Immunoglobulins (IgE) are passively bound on the surface of the basophil. When an antigen binds to these receptors, the basophil granules release their contents. In some highly sensitive individuals the response to bee and wasp stings, for example, can be so violent and so extensive as to be life-threatening.

HISTOGENESIS OF CONNECTIVE TISSUE

Connective Tissue Mostly Arises from Mesoderm; Some Comes From Ectoderm

The mesoderm gives rise to almost all of the connective tissues of the body. An exception is in the head region where certain progenitor cells are derived from ectoderm by way of the neural crest cells. Through proliferation and migration of the mesodermal and specific neural crest cells, a primitive connective tissue referred to as *mesenchyme* (in the case of the head region it is sometimes referred to as *ectomesenchyme*) is established in the early embryo. Maturation of this primitive connective tissue or mesenchyme gives rise not only to the various connective tissues of the adult but also to muscle, the vascular and urogenital systems, and the serous membranes of the body cavities.

Mesenchyme contains relatively uniform appearing, small, spindle-shaped cells (Fig. 5.20). Processes of these cells extend and contact similar processes of neighboring cells, forming a three-dimensional cellular network. Where the processes make contact, gap junctions are present. The extracellular space is occupied by a viscous, almost jelly-like ground substance. Collagen (reticular) fibers are present, but they are very fine and relatively sparse in number. The paucity of collagen fibers is consistent with the limited physical stress on the growing fetus.

The manner in which the mesenchymal cells proliferate and organize sets the stage for the kind of connective tissue that will form at any specific site. When differentiation of the mesenchymal cells is initiated, the cytoplasm increases in amount and exhibits basophilia, a reflection of collagen synthesis. As development proceeds, the pattern in which the collagen is laid down and the orientation of the cells reflect the type of connective tissue being formed. Thus, in the area where a tendon will arise, the cells aggregate and align themselves to form the parallel arrays of collagen fibers.

PLATE 6. Loose and Dense Connective Tissue

The tissues surrounding the epithelial elements of inactive mammary gland lobules (Figures 1 and 2) serve as an excellent example of loose and dense connective tissue, particularly for the purpose of comparing them within the same field of view. The light microscopic appearance of loose connective tissue includes the presence of several cell types; the cells are not organized in any special pattern; the collagen fibers are fine and wispy; and the tissue usually stains lightly with eosin due to the relative paucity of collagen fibers and loss of ground substance during fixation. In contrast, dense connective tissue is composed of thick collagen bundles that stain deeply with eosin and has relatively few cells, most of which are fibroblasts. Both connective tissues also contain elastic fibers, but the fibers are not discernible without special staining methods (see Plate 10).

FIGURE 1, mammary gland, human, H&E ×160. This micrograph shows, at low magnification, loose connective tissue (*LCT*) immediately surrounding the gland epithelium (*Ep*). It is relatively less stained with eosin, compared with the dense connective tissue (*DCT*) that occupies much of the field. The dense connective tissue, with its numerous thick fibers, is in contrast to the loose connective tissue that has a relative paucity of fibers. The typical wispy nature of the collagen fibers found in loose connective tissue is seen more clearly in Figure 2, which shows one of the lobules at higher magnification.

The most conspicuous components of loose connective tissue are the numerous cells interspersed singly and in small groups between the delicate collagen fibers and the small blood vessels (*BV*) that supply the connective tissue and adjacent epithelium.

FIGURE 3, vagina, human, H&E ×250. This is another example of loose connective tissue, this time from the wall of the vagina just below the epithelial surface. Again, note the myriad nuclear profiles. The area immediately to the right of the upper marked blood vessel (*BV*) is shown at higher magnification in Figure 4.

FIGURE 2, mammary gland, human, H&E ×250. Although the magnification of this figure is not sufficiently high to explore cytologic detail, two general cell types are recognized in the loose connective tissue, based on nuclear shape. One population of cells contains elongate nuclei (*arrows*); these most likely belong to fibroblasts. The other population contains round nuclei; most of these nuclei represent lymphocytes (*L*), although some are of plasma cells. The significant feature, however, is that the loose connective tissue is highly cellular, considerably more so than the surrounding dense connective tissue. Typically, the cells of dense connective tissue are fibroblasts. They are usually not present in appreciable numbers; under normal conditions, few if any other cell types are present.

FIGURE 4, vagina, human, H&E ×480. Here the wispy nature of the fine collagen fibers is evident, and the variation of nuclear profiles is even more apparent. Identification of the cell type represented by each nucleus is not possible; however, certain cells of the total population can be identified with assurance. Thus, the small, dense, round nuclei without visible surrounding cytoplasm belong to lymphocytes (*L*). Some of the round nuclei exhibit a surrounding but eccentric mass of cytoplasm. These are plasma cells (*PC*). Sometimes, the cytoplasm of a plasma cell may be obscured partially by the nucleus, making identity less certain. Such is the case of the cell indicated by the question mark (*?*). Because the size, density, and chromatin pattern of its nucleus are similar to those of the more readily identifiable plasma cells, it too is probably a plasma cell. With respect to the fibroblasts, the nuclei are typically elongate. Two fibroblast nuclei (*F*) are indicated in the micrograph; both are elongate, but one appears quite narrow. It is being viewed on edge, whereas the broader nucleus profile represents a fibroblast in face view. This nucleus also shows prominent nucleoli, typical of active fibroblasts. Usually, the thin cytoplasmic processes of the fibroblasts are obscured by blending in with the collagen. Some of the nuclei seen here may represent macrophages or mast cells, but without identifiable cytoplasmic inclusions, these cells cannot be identified.

KEY

AT, adipose tissue
BV, blood vessel
DCT, dense connective tissue
Ep, epithelium
F, fibroblast nucleus
L, lymphocyte
LCT, loose connective tissue
PC, plasma cell
arrow, elongate nucleus

PLATE 6

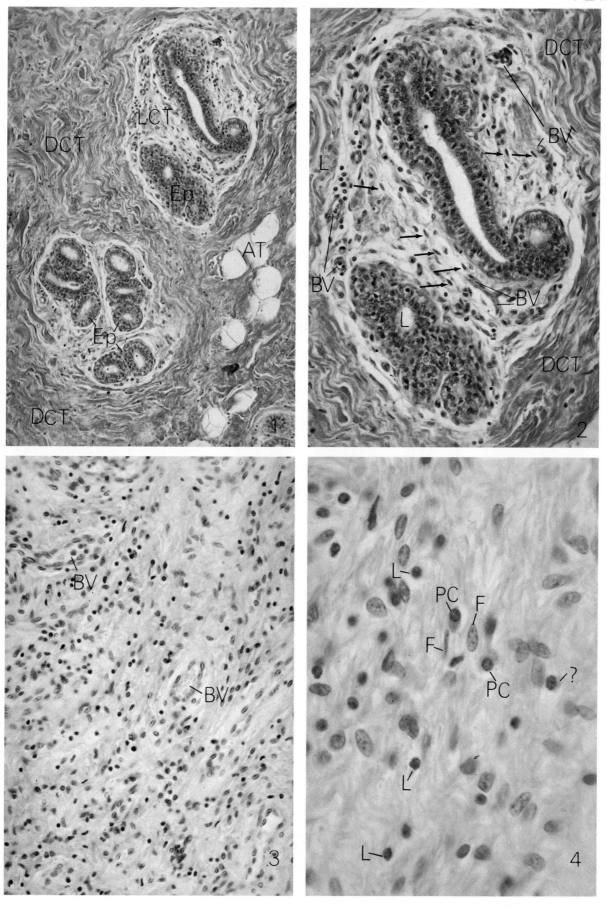

PLATE 7. Connective Tissue, Electron Microscopy

Oviduct, human, electron micrograph ×4100. The formed elements that constitute a connective tissue, namely, the fibers and cells, are readily characterized by transmission electron microscopy. The specimen shown here is from a section through the wall of an oviduct. The tissue is rather cellular, but it also contains a considerable amount of fibrous material. In terms of its constituent elements, it is comparable to the connective tissue shown in Figure 3 of Plate 6. With the electron microscope, the morphologic character of the tissue constituents becomes immediately apparent. The fibroblasts (*F*), which constitute the bulk of the connective tissue cell population, usually exhibit long cytoplasmic processes that pass between the collagen bundles. The processes extend for indeterminate distances and may become so attenuated (*arrowheads*) that their thinness precludes the possibility of being visualized with the light microscope.

In addition to the fibroblast population, there are at least two other connective tissue cell types present in this specimen (see *rectangles*). One is a cell with both myoid and fibroblast-like features. This we refer to as a myofibroblast (*My*). The other is a cell that has certain features that suggest it is a monocyte (*M*) or a closely related cell type. These two cell types, along with a fibroblast, are illustrated at higher magnification in Plate 8.

The collagen fibers (*CF*), between which the fibroblast processes pass, have a stippled appearance at this relatively low magnification. This is due to the cut, end-on profiles of the individual collagen fibrils. It is these thread-like units, the fibrils, that aggregate into bundles to form the fiber that is visualized at the light microscope level.

In the specimen shown here, almost all of the collagen fibers have been cross-sectioned, and consequently, it is possible to discern their variable size and shape. During the fixation and dehydration stages of preparation of the routinely prepared light microscopic specimen, there may be considerable initial hydration and then, with subsequent dehydration, shrinkage of the tissue. One consequence of this is the artificial separation of the collagen fibers. The fibers are then discerned in the light microscope as wispy, isolated, thread-like elements, rather than the more evenly distributed fibers seen in the electron microscope.

Typically, one finds small blood vessels passing through the substance of the connective tissue; in this view, there is a capillary (*Cap*) as well as a longitudinally sectioned venule (*V*). The latter contains a number of red blood cells (*RBC*).

KEY		
Cap, capillary	**M**, monocyte	**V**, venule
CF, collagen fiber	**My**, myofibroblast	**arrowhead**, attenuated fibroblast process
F, fibroblast	**RBC**, red blood cell	

PLATE 7

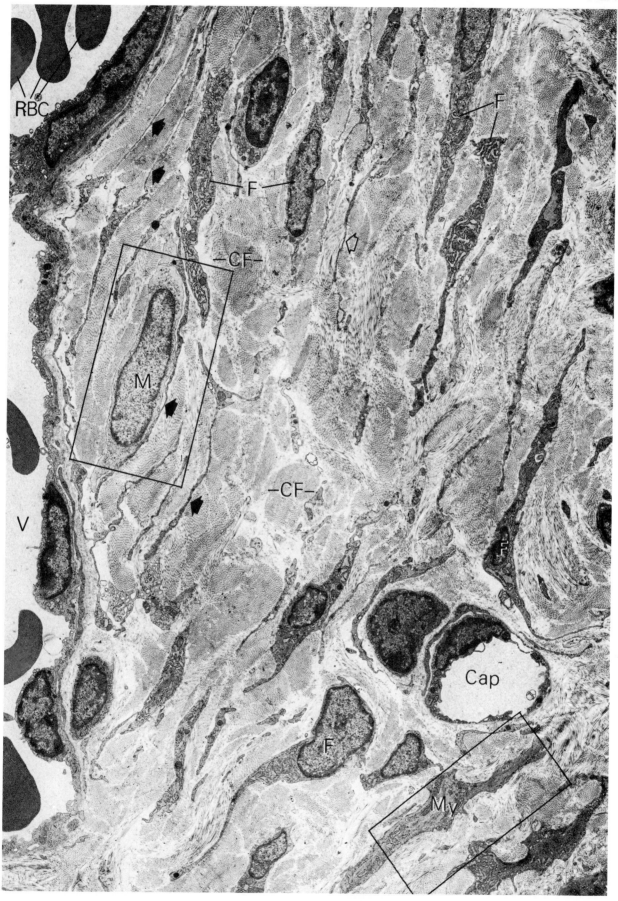

PLATE 8. Connective Tissue Cells, Electron Microscopy

As noted previously, the cytologic features displayed by the various connective tissue cell types at the electron microscopic level serve as an accurate fingerprint that allows one, with few exceptions, to identify readily the cell type in question.

FIGURE 1, fibroblasts, electron micrograph ×11,000. This figure reveals portions of two adjacent fibroblasts. Despite the fact that only a small portion of each cell is evident, they can be identified readily as fibroblasts on the basis of the presence of a moderate amount of granular (rough) endoplasmic reticulum (*GER*) and by the elongate processes that both cells exhibit.

The cisternae of the endoplasmic reticulum are notably dilated, as seen in the lower cell, and contain a homogeneous substance of moderate density. This substance is a product of the synthetic activity of the ribosomes on the surface of the endoplasmic reticulum and, having been released into the cisternae, mostly represents a precursor of the collagen seen in the extracellular space. In this same cell, the section reveals a portion of the Golgi apparatus (*G*). The Golgi consists of a multitude of small vesicles and flattened sac-like profiles.

FIGURE 2, myofibroblast, electron micrograph ×11,000. The portion of the cell shown here is, in many respects, similar to the fibroblasts just described and, at the light microscopic level, would probably be indistinguishable from them. Note that in one area profiles of granular (rough) endoplasmic reticulum (*GER*) are evident and their contents exhibit the same texture and density as that of the fibroblast. However, the cell differs from the fibroblast in that the cytoplasm reveals an extensive filamentous component, just barely visible at this magnification. Associated with these filaments are cytoplasmic densities (*arrows*); the combination of these dense areas and a high concentration of cytoplasmic filaments is a feature characteristic of smooth muscle cells. Evidently, this cell type, designated as a ***myofibroblast,*** functions as both a fibroblast and a contractile cell. Other examples of this kind of cell can be found in the testis, ovary, spleen, and nerve (perineurium) and are common in healing skin wounds.

FIGURE 3, mononuclear cell, electron micrograph ×11,000. The last cell type on this plate is one that would probably also be recognized as a fibroblast if viewed in the light microscope. As seen here, the cell exhibits a flattened nucleus with only a little cytoplasm about it. The cytoplasm is somewhat nondescript, the most notable feature being the small vesicular profiles of smooth endoplasmic reticulum (*SER*). Presumably, this cell is a monocyte that may be in transition to a tissue macrophage. Again, the essential point here is that we are viewing a cell type cytologically different from a fibroblast, although with the light microscope, in a routinely stained H&E section, the distinction between these two cells is not possible.

In all three figures, the collagen fibrils can be clearly identified as the subunits of the collagen fibers (*CF*). In most locations, the fibrils have been cross-sectioned and appear as closely packed circular profiles; in locations where the fibrils have been sectioned more longitudinally (*arrowheads*), the typical cross-banded pattern is evident. Again, it is indicated that individual fibrils cannot be identified with the light microscope; rather, one sees a bundle of fibrils, and this bundle is then referred to as a collagen fiber. One can also ascertain from these illustrations that the diameter of the collagen fiber depends on how many fibrils are within the bundle.

KEY

CF, collagen fiber
GER, granular (rough) endoplasmic reticulum

G, Golgi apparatus
SER, smooth endoplasmic
reticulum

arrow, cytoplasmic densities
arrowhead, longitudinally sectioned collagen fibrils

PLATE 8

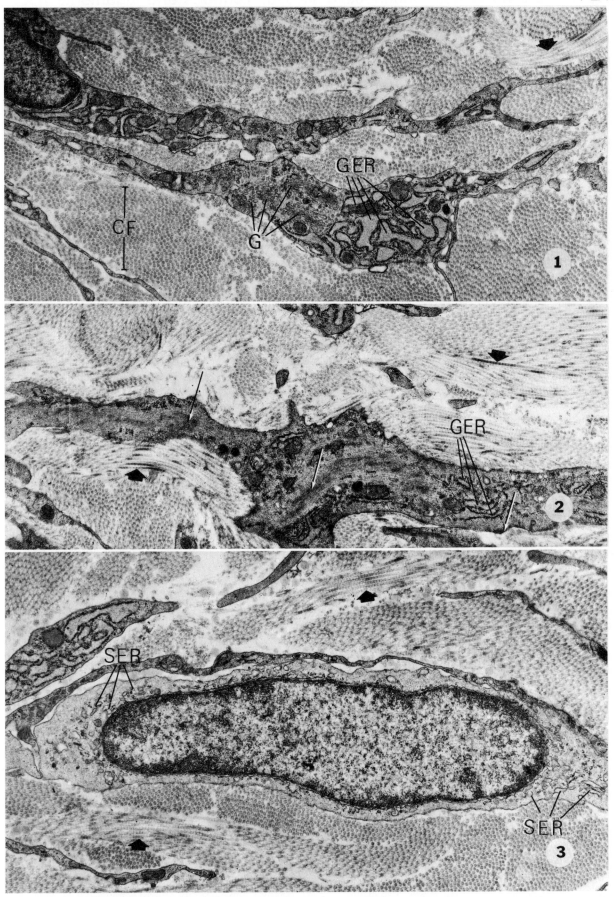

PLATE 9. Dense Regular Connective Tissue, Tendons and Ligaments

Dense *regular connective tissue,* such as tendons and ligaments, is distinctive in that its fibers are very densely packed and are organized in parallel array into fascicles. The collagen fibrils that make up the fibrils are also arranged in an ordered parallel array. *Tendons,* which attach muscle to bone, and *ligaments,* which attach bone to bone, are examples of this type of tissue. Ligaments are similar to tendons in most respects, but their fibers and the organization of the fascicles tend to be less ordered. Both are composed of collagen fibrils in very orderly array.

In tendons as well as ligaments, the fascicles are separated from one another by dense irregular connective tissue, the *endotendineum,* through which travel vessels and nerves. Also, a fascicle may be partially divided by connective tissue septa from the *endotendineum,* which contain the smallest vessels and nerves. Some of the fascicles may be grouped into larger functional units by a thicker, surrounding connective tissue, the *peritendineum.* Finally, the fascicles and groups of fascicles are surrounded by the dense irregular connective tissue of the epitendineum.

The fibroblasts, also called tendon cells in tendons, are elongated cells that possess exceedingly thin, sheet-like cytoplasmic processes that reside between and embrace adjacent fibers. The margins of the cytoplasmic processes contact those of neighboring tendon cells, thus forming a syncytium-like cytoplasmic network.

FIGURE 1, tendon, longitudinal section, human, H&E ×100. The specimen includes the surrounding dense irregular connective tissue of the tendon, the epitendineum (*Ept*). The tendon fascicles (*TF*) that make up the tendon are surrounded by a less dense connective tissue than that associated with the epitendineum. In longitudinal sections such as this, the connective tissue that surrounds the individual fascicles, the endotendineum (*Ent*), seems to disappear at certain points, with the result that one fascicle appears to merge with a neighboring facscicle. This is due to an obliqueness in the plane of section rather than an actual merging of fascicles. The collagen that makes up the bulk of the tendon fascicle has a homogeneous appearance due to the orderly packing of the individual collagen fibrils. The nuclei of the tendon cells appear as elongate profiles arranged in linear rows. The cytoplasm of these cells blends in with the collagen, leaving only the nuclei as the representative feature of the cell.

FIGURE 2, tendon, longitudinal section, human, H&E ×400. This higher magnification micrograph shows the ordered single-file array of the tendon cell nuclei (*TC*) along with the intervening collagen. The latter has a homogeneous appearance. The cytoplasm of the cells is indistinguishable from the collagen, as is typical in H&E paraffin specimens. The variation in nuclear appearance is due to the plane of section and the position of the nuclei within the thickness of the section. A small blood vessel (*BV*) coursing within the endotendineum is also present in the specimen.

FIGURE 3, tendon, cross section, human, H&E ×400. This specimen is well preserved, and the densely packed collagenous fibers appear as a homogeneous field, even though the fibers are viewed on their cut ends. The nuclei appear irregularly scattered, as opposed to their more uniform pattern in the longitudinal plane. This is explained by examining the *dashed line* in Figure 2, which is meant to represent an arbitrary cross-sectional cut of the tendon. Note the irregular spacing of the nuclei that are in the plane of the cut. Lastly, several small blood vessels (*BV*) are present within the endotendineum (*Ent*) within a fascicle.

KEY

BV, blood vessel	**Ept,** epitendineum	**TF,** fascicle of tendon
Ent, endotendineum	**TC,** tendon cell nuclei	**dashed line,** arbitrary cross-sectional cut of tendon

PLATE 9

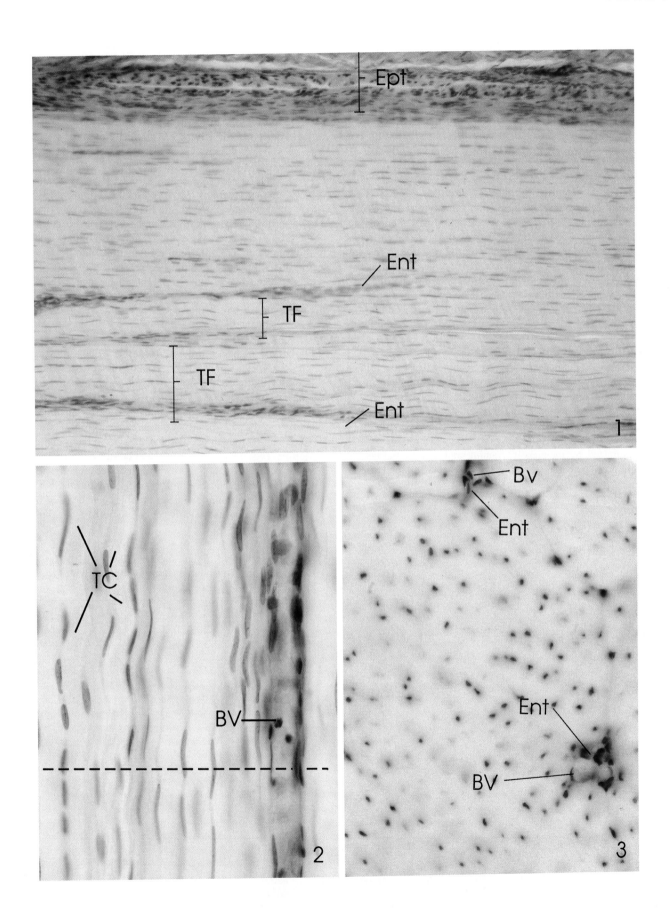

PLATE 10. Elastic Fibers and Elastic Lamellae

Elastic fibers are present in loose and dense connective tissue throughout the body, but in lesser amounts than collagenous fibers. Elastic fibers are not conspicuous in routine H&E sections but may be readily visualized with special staining methods. (The following selectively color elastic material: Weigert's elastic tissue stain, purple-violet; Gomori's aldehyde fuchsin stain, blue-black; Verhoeff's hematoxylin elastic tissue stain, black; and modified Taenzer-Unna orcein stain, red-brown.) By using a combination of the special elastic stains and counterstains, such as H&E, not only the elastic fibers but also the other tissue components may be revealed.

FIGURE 1, dermis, monkey, Weigert's ×160. This shows the connective tissue of the skin, referred to as the dermis, stained to show the nature and distribution of the elastic fibers (*E*), which appear purple. The collagen fibers (*C*) have been stained by eosin, and the two fiber types are easily differentiated. The connective tissue at the top of the figure, close to the epithelium (the papillary layer of the dermis), contains thin elastic fibers (see upper left of figure) as well as less coarse collagen fibers. The lower portion of the figure shows considerably heavier elastic and collagen fibers. Also note that many of the elastic fibers appear as short rectangular profiles. These profiles simply represent fibers traveling through the thickness of the section at an oblique angle to the path of the knife. Careful examination will also reveal a few fibers that appear as dot-like profiles. They represent cross-sectioned elastic fibers. Overall, the elastic fibers of the dermis have a three-dimensional interlacing configuration, thus the variety of forms.

FIGURE 2, mesentery, rat, Weigert's ×160. This is a whole mount specimen of mesentery, similar to Figure 2 in Plate 1 but prepared to show the connective tissue elements and differentially stained to reveal elastic fibers. The elastic fibers (*E*) appear as thin, long, crisscrossing and branching threads without discernible beginnings or endings and with a somewhat irregular course. Again, the collagen fibers (*C*) are contrasted by their eosin staining and appear as long, straight profiles that are considerably thicker than the elastic fibers.

FIGURE 3, artery, monkey, Weigert's ×80. Elastic material also occurs in sheets or lamellae rather than string-like fibers. This figure shows the wall of an elastic artery (pulmonary artery) that was stained to show the elastic material. Each of the wavy lines is a lamella of elastic material that is organized in the form of a fenestrated sheet or membrane. The plane of section is such that the elastic membranes are seen on edge. This specimen was not subsequently stained with H&E. The empty-appearing spaces between elastic layers contain collagen fibers and smooth muscle cells, but they remain essentially unstained. In the muscular layer of blood vessels, both elastin and collagen are secreted by the smooth muscle cells.

Tissues of the body containing large amounts of elastic material are limited in distribution to the walls of elastic arteries and some ligaments that are associated with the spinal column.

KEY		
BV, blood vessel	**D,** duct of sweat gland	**E,** elastic fibers
C, collagen fibers		

PLATE 10

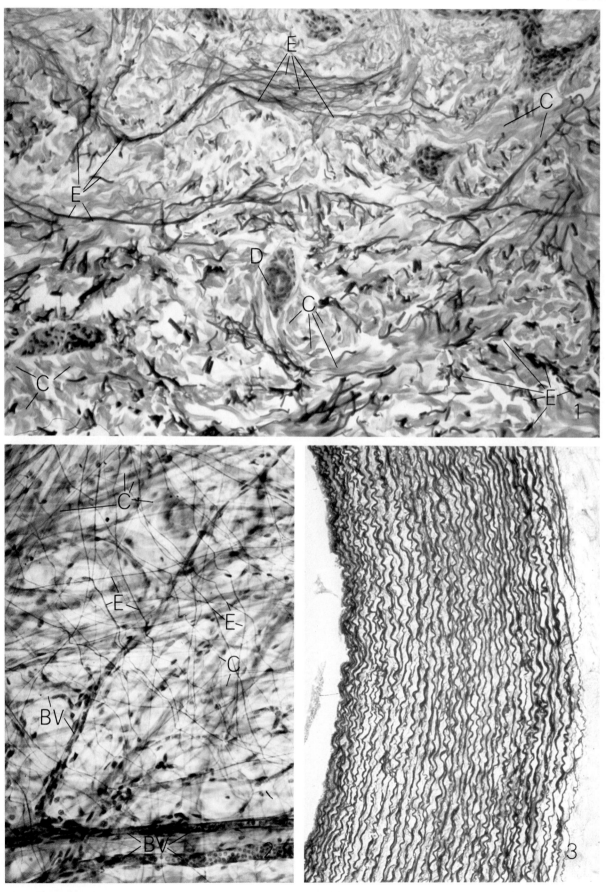

Adipose Tissue

6

Adipose Tissue Is a Specialized Form of Connective Tissue Consisting of Fat-Storing Cells (Adipocytes) Associated With a Rich Blood Supply

Individual fat-storing cells or *adipocytes* and groups of adipocytes are found throughout the loose connective tissue. When adipocytes are the primary cell type present in a tissue, we designate it as adipose tissue.

The body has a limited capacity to store carbohydrate and protein; the fat contained within the adipocytes represents the storage of nutritional calories in excess of what is utilized. Fat is an efficient form of calorie storage because it has about twice the calorie density of carbohydrate and protein. The metabolism of fat can also be an essential source of water for the body in extreme conditions. In fact, the hump of a camel consists largely of fat and is a source of both energy and water for this animal in the desert.

There Are Two Types of Adipose Tissue: White (or Unilocular) and Brown (or Multilocular)

The two types of adipose tissue are so named because of their color in the living state.

- *White adipose* tissue is the predominant type in adult humans.
- *Brown adipose* tissue is present in humans during fetal life but diminishes during the first decade after birth.

WHITE ADIPOSE TISSUE

Functions of White Adipose Tissue Include Energy Storage, Insulation, and Cushioning of Vital Organs

Unilocular adipose tissue forms a layer called the *panniculus adiposus* in the connective tissue under the skin. This subcutaneous layer of connective tissue is also referred to as the *hypodermis.* It has a significant insulating function in the skin. Concentrations of adipose tissue are found in the connective tissue under the skin of the abdomen, buttocks, axilla, and thigh. Sex differences in the thickness of the fatty layer in the skin of different parts of the body account, in part, for the difference in body contour between females and males. In both sexes, the breast is a preferential site for the accumulation of adipose tissue; the non-lactating female breast is composed primarily of this tissue.

Internally, adipose tissue is preferentially located in the omentum, mesentery, and retroperitoneal space and is usually abundant around the kidneys. It is also found in bone marrow and between other tissues, where it appears to fill in spaces. In the palms of the hands and the soles of the feet, beneath the visceral pericardium (around the outside of the heart), and in the orbits around the eyeballs, adipose tissue serves a structural function as a cushion. It retains this structural function even during reduced caloric intake; when the adipose tissue elsewhere becomes depleted of lipid, this structural adipose tissue remains undiminished.

Histogenesis of Fat Cells

Early histologists were undecided as to whether adipose tissue was a specific organ, distinct from connective tissue, or whether it was merely ordinary connective tissue in which fibroblasts stored fat globules. The current consensus is that adipocytes are a specific cell type and that most of them derive from undifferentiated mesenchymal cells that are associated with the adventitia of small venules. This is the same stem cell population from which fibroblasts and myofibroblasts (page 112) in healing wounds originate. Morphologically, even with the transmission electron microscope (TEM), it is still nearly impossible to distinguish the *lipoblast* or *preadipocyte* from a fibroblast. Many investigators describe a cell that is indistinguishable from a fibroblast between the undifferentiated mesenchymal stem cell and the lipoblast.

White Adipose Tissue Begins to Develop in Miduterine Life

The lipoblasts that develop along the small blood vessels in the fetus are free of fat. Nevertheless, these cells are committed to becoming fat cells at this early stage and are sometimes called primitive fat organs. In some rodents, e.g., mice and rats, adipose tissue starts to form at about the time of birth.

The primitive fat organ is characterized by the presence of proliferating lipoblasts and proliferating capillaries. Lipid accumulation in lipoblasts produces the typical morphology of the adipocytes.

Early Lipoblasts Look Like Fibroblasts With Small Lipid Inclusions and a Thin Basal Lamina

In the earliest stages, the lipoblasts are indistinguishable from fibroblasts. They have an elongated configuration, multiple cytoplasmic processes, and abundant endoplasmic reticulum and Golgi membranes. As lipoblastic differentiation begins, smooth-surfaced vesicles increase in number, with a corresponding decrease in rough endoplasmic reticulum (rER). Small lipid inclusions start to appear at one pole of the cytoplasm. Pinocytotic vesicles and basal lamina also start to appear. Cells having these features are designated as *early lipoblasts* or preadipocytes.

Midstage Lipoblasts Become Ovoid as Lipid Accumulation Changes the Cell Dimensions

With further development, the cells assume an oval configuration. The most characteristic feature at this stage is the extensive concentration of smooth vesicles and small lipid droplets, generally around the nucleus toward both poles of the cell. Glycogen particles start to appear at the periphery of the lipid droplets, and pinocytotic vesicles and basal lamina become more apparent. Collagen fibrils are in intimate contact with the cells. These cells are designated *midstage lipoblasts*.

The Mature Adipocyte Is Characterized by a Single, Large Lipid Inclusion Surrounded by a Thin Rim of Cytoplasm

In the late stage of differentiation, the cells increase in size and become more spherical. Large lipid vacuoles are formed by coalescence of smaller droplets and occupy the central portion of the cytoplasm. Smooth vesicles of varying sizes are abundant, whereas rER is less prominent. These cells are referred to as *late lipoblasts*.

Eventually, the lipid mass compresses the nucleus to an eccentric position, producing a *signet-ring* appearance. These cells are designated *adipocytes* or *mature lipocytes*.

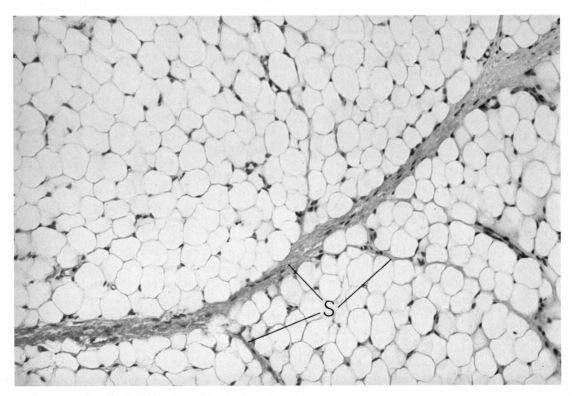

Figure 6.1. Photomicrograph of a mass of unilocular adipose tissue showing its characteristic meshwork appearance in a hematoxylin and eosin preparation. Each space represents the site of the single large drop of lipid before its dissolution from the cell during preparation of the tissue. The surrounding eosin-stained material represents the cytoplasm of the adjoining cells and some intervening connective tissue. Heavier connective tissue septa (S) create lobules of varying size.

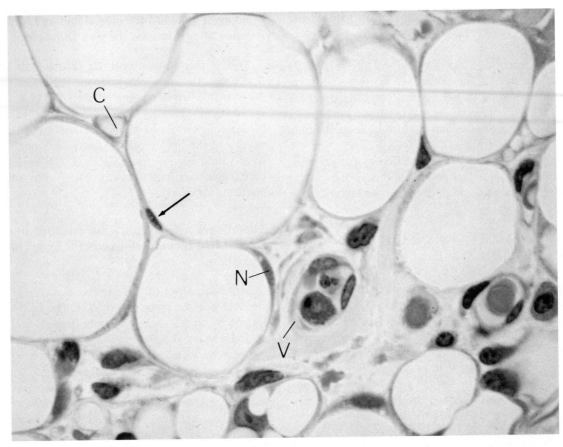

Figure 6.2.   High-power photomicrograph of a well-preserved plastic-embedded specimen of unilocular adipose tissue. The cytoplasm of the individual adipose cells is recognizable in some areas, and part of the nucleus (N) of one of the cells is included in the plane of section. A second nucleus (arrow), which appears intimately related to one of the adipose cells, may actually belong to a fibroblast; it is difficult to tell with assurance. Because of the large size of the adipose cells, the nucleus is infrequently observed in a given cell. A capillary (C) and a venule (V) are also evident in the photomicrograph.

Structure of Adipocytes and Adipose Tissue

Unilocular Adipocytes Cells Are Large, Sometimes 100 µm or More in Diameter

Adipocytes are spherical when isolated, but they are polyhedral or oval when crowded together as adipose tissue (Fig. 6.1). The large size of the fat cell is due to the accumulated lipid mass in the cell. The nucleus is flattened and displaced to one side of the lipid mass; the cytoplasm forms a thin rim around the lipid. In routine histologic sections, the lipid is lost through extraction by organic solvents, such as xylene, and consequently, the adipose tissue has the appearance of a delicate meshwork of irregular polygonal profiles (Figs. 6.1 and 6.2). The thin strand of the meshwork separating adjacent adipocytes represents the cytoplasm of both cells and the components of the extracellular matrix. The strand is usually so thin, however, that it is not possible to resolve its component parts with the light microscope.

Adipose tissue is richly supplied with blood vessels; capillaries are found at many of the angles of the meshwork where adjacent adipocytes meet. Silver stains show that the adipocytes are surrounded by reticular fibers, a product of the adipocytes. Special stains also show that there are unmyelinated nerve fibers and numerous mast cells in adipose tissue.

The Lipid Mass in the Adipocyte Is Not Membrane Bounded

The interface between the contained lipid and surrounding cytoplasm of the adipocyte appears in the TEM to have two distinct components, a 5-nm-thick condensed layer of the lipid reinforced by parallel microfilaments measuring 5 nm in diameter. This layer separates the hydrophobic contents of the lipid droplet and the hydrophilic cytoplasmic matrix.

The perinuclear cytoplasm of the adipocyte contains a small Golgi complex, free ribosomes, short profiles of rER, microfilaments and intermediate filaments, and *filamentous* mitochondria. Filaments, mitochondria, and profiles of smooth endoplasmic reticulum are also found in the thin rim of cytoplasm surrounding the lipid droplet (Fig. 6.3).

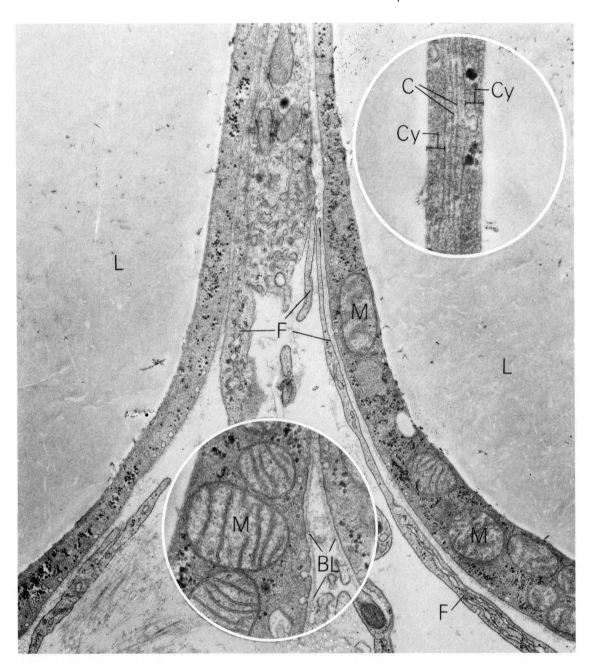

Figure 6.3. Electron micrograph showing portions of two adjacent adipose cells. The cytoplasm of the adipose cells reveals mitochondria *(M)* and glycogen, with the latter appearing as the very dark particles. The **upper inset** shows the attenuated cytoplasm *(Cy)* of two adjoining adipose cells. Each cell is separated by a narrow space containing basal lamina material and an extremely attenuated process of a fibroblast *(C)*. The **lower inset** shows the basal lamina *(BL)* of the adipose cells as a discrete layer where the cells are adequately separated from one another. *F,* fibroblast processes; and *L,* lipid. ×15,000; **upper inset,** ×65,000; **lower inset,** ×30,000.

Regulation of Adipose Tissue

The Amount of Adipose Tissue in an Individual Is Determined by Heredity and Caloric Intake

Identical twins usually have the same or close to the same amount of body fat. Even when the *amount* of body fat in identical twins varies, however, the *patterns of distribution* are always the same.

Studies with genetically obese rodents show that the obesity is associated with an *increased efficiency* of food utilization. Obese rodents use a larger proportion of their food calories for the formation of adipose tissue; i.e., the body weight per gram of food consumed is greater in obese rodents than in littermate controls. The factors that account for the positive caloric balance in the obese rodents are, probably, diminished heat production and diminished activity.

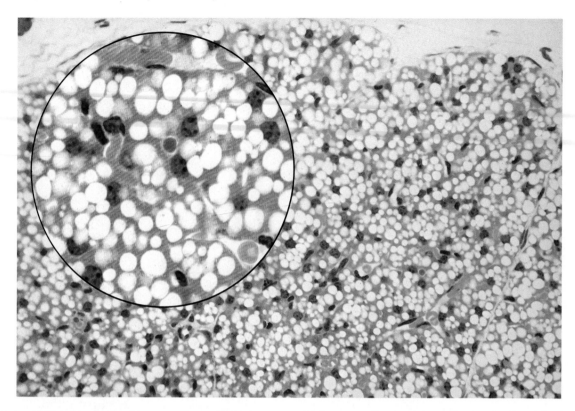

Figure 6.4. Photomicrograph of brown adipose tissue from a newborn. The cells contain fat droplets of varying size. The **inset** shows the cells and their populations of droplets at a higher magnification. The cells are closely packed, and the cell boundaries are difficult to discern.

Mobilization and Deposition of Lipid Are Influenced by Neural and Hormonal Factors

During early stages of experimental starvation in rodents, adipose cells in a denervated fat pad continue to *deposit* fat. Adipose cells in the intact contralateral fat pad *mobilize* fat.

It is now known that norepinephrine (which is liberated by the endings of nerve cells of the sympathetic nervous system) initiates a series of metabolic steps that lead to the activation of lipase. This enzyme splits triglycerides, which constitute over 90% of the lipid in the fat droplets. The enzymatic activity is an early step in the mobilization of the lipid. The neural mobilization of lipid is particularly important during periods of fasting and exposure to severe cold.

The pancreatic hormone insulin enhances the conversion of glucose into the triglycerides of the lipid droplet by the adipocyte. Other hormones also modify various steps in the metabolism of adipose tissue. These include thyroid hormone, glucocorticoids, and hormones of the pituitary gland.

An unusual form of obesity is due to injury of the hypothalamus, the portion of the base of the brain where neurosecretions that control pituitary function are synthesized. Although clinical manifestations of hypothalamic obesity are associated with increased food consumption, experiments with laboratory animals subjected to hypothalamic injury show that caloric intake is not the only factor leading to obesity. Lesioned rats deposit more body fat than control animals fed the same amounts of food.

BROWN ADIPOSE TISSUE

Adipocytes of Brown, Multilocular Adipose Tissue Contain Numerous Fat Droplets

The cells of brown adipose tissue are smaller than those of white adipose tissue. The nucleus of a mature multilocular adipocyte is typically in an eccentric position within the cell, but it is not flattened, as is the nucleus of a unilocular adipocyte.

In routine hematoxylin and eosin-stained sections, the cytoplasm of the multilocular adipocyte consists largely of empty vacuoles because the lipid that ordinarily occupies the vacuolated spaces is lost during preparation (Fig. 6.4). The multilocular adipocyte contains numerous mitochondria, a small Golgi zone, and only small amounts of rER and smooth endoplasmic reticulum. The mitochondria are unique in that they do not contain elementary particles (which contain many of the enzymes for ATP production); i.e., the energy produced by the mitochondria is dissipated or used as heat rather than stored as ATP. However, they contain large amounts of cytochrome oxidase, which imparts the brown color to the cells.

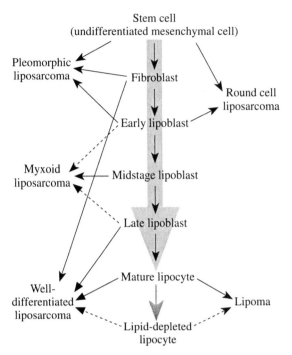

Figure 6.5. Diagram summarizing the relationships between differentiation of normal adipose tissue (midcolumn) and several types of adipose tissue tumors (lateral columns). Each type of adipose tissue tumor exhibits a predominant cell type that resembles one of the stages of differentiation of normal adipose cells. *Solid line arrows* indicate the most frequently occurring cell type in each kind of tumor. *Dotted line arrows* indicate the less frequently occurring cell type in that tumor. (After Fu et al: *Pathology Annual* 15(Part 1):85, 1980.)

Brown adipose tissue is subdivided into lobules by partitions of connective tissue, but the connective tissue stroma between individual cells within the lobules is sparse. The tissue has an exceedingly rich supply of blood capillaries that enhance its color. Numerous unmyelinated nerve fibers are present among the fat cells. Multilocular adipocytes de-

pleted of their lipid bear a closer resemblance to epithelial cells than to connective tissue cells.

Brown adipose tissue is present in large amounts in hibernating animals. It serves as a ready source of lipid, the oxidation of which produces heat that is used by the animal to warm the blood flowing through the brown fat on arousal from hibernation. It is also present in nonhibernating animals, again serving as a source of heat. In humans, multilocular adipose tissue is present in large amounts in the newborn. This is related to the high surface-to-mass ratio in the newborn that results in excessive heat loss. The amount gradually decreases as the body grows, but it remains widely distributed through the first decade of life. It then disappears from most sites except for regions around the kidney and aorta and regions in the neck and mediastinum. As in the mobilization of lipid in white fatty tissue, lipid is mobilized and heat is generated by multilocular adipocytes on stimulation by the sympathetic nervous system.

ADIPOSE TISSUE TUMORS

The study of the numerous varieties of benign and malignant adipose tissue tumors provides further insight into and confirmation of the sequence of adipose tissue differentiation described above.

Adipose tissue tumors are classified by the morphology of the predominant cell in the tumor (Fig. 6.5). As with epithelial tumors and tumors of fibroblast origin, adipose tissue tumors recapitulate in their variety the normal pattern of adipose tissue differentiation. That is, discrete tumor types can be described that consist primarily of cells resembling a single stage in the differentiation of adipose tissue.

Although Figure 6.5 relates primarily to white adipose tissue tumors, tumors of brown adipose tissue are also found. Not surprisingly, these are called ***hibernomas.***

Cartilage

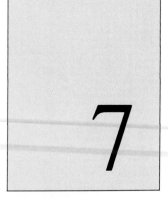

7

Cartilage Is a Form of Connective Tissue Composed of Cells Called Chondrocytes and a Highly Specialized Extracellular Matrix

Cartilage is an ***avascular tissue*** that consists of chondrocytes and an extensive matrix that is produced and maintained by the chondrocytes. The matrix of cartilage is solid and firm but also somewhat pliable. This accounts for its resilient nature. The large amount of glycosaminoglycans in the matrix permits diffusion of substances between blood vessels in the surrounding connective tissue and the chondrocytes, thereby maintaining the viability of the tissue. The presence of large amounts of hyaluronic acid in cartilage matrix makes it well adapted to serve in a weight-bearing capacity, especially at points of movement, as in synovial joints. Because it is able to maintain this property even during internal growth of the cartilage itself, cartilage is a key tissue in most growing bones.

Cartilage is found in specific locations in the body and forms structures that have characteristic shapes. In the ***fetus,*** most ***long bones*** are initially represented by ***cartilage models*** that resemble the shape of the adult bone. In the adult, the only remnants of the hyaline cartilage models are the articular cartilages of joints, the tracheal ring cartilages, and the knee cartilages, which retain their characteristic shapes.

Three different kinds of cartilage are distinguished on the basis of characteristics of the matrix:

- ***Hyaline cartilage,*** characterized by a homogeneous amorphous matrix
- ***Elastic cartilage,*** whose matrix contains elastic fibers and elastic lamellae
- ***Fibrocartilage,*** whose matrix contains large bundles of type I collagen

HYALINE CARTILAGE

Hyaline Cartilage Is Distinguished by a Homogeneous, Amorphous Matrix

The matrix of hyaline cartilage appears glassy in the living state, hence the name hyaline from the Greek, *hyalos,* meaning glassy. Throughout the cartilage matrix are spaces called ***lacunae.*** Within these lacunae are the ***chondrocytes.*** The matrix consists of two components, collagen fibrils (predominantly type II) and ground substance. In developing bone, the matrix calcifies before it is replaced by bone matrix.

Cartilage Matrix

The collagen component of the matrix is in the form of relatively thin fibrils, ≈20 nm in diameter. The fibrils do not normally display the characteristic 68-nm banding. In some locations, however, the collagen fibrils are thicker and may display banding. The collagen fibrils are generally arranged in a three-dimensional felt-like pattern.

Chemical analysis of the ground substance of hyaline cartilage reveals the presence of three kinds of glycosaminoglycans:

- ***Hyaluronic acid***
- ***Chondroitin sulfate***
- ***Keratan sulfate***

As in loose connective tissue matrix, the chondroitin and keratin sulfates of cartilage matrix are joined to a core protein to form a ***proteoglycan monomer*** (Fig. 7.1). Within the tissue, each hyaluronic acid molecule is associated with about 80 proteoglycan units to form large aggregates whose structure is reinforced by ***link proteins.*** The large ***hyaluronate proteoglycan aggregates*** are bound to the thin collagen fibrils by electrostatic interactions and by cross-link-

132

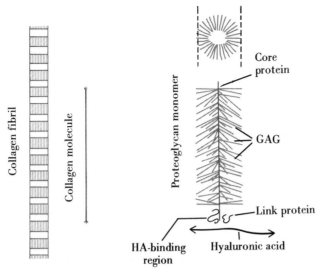

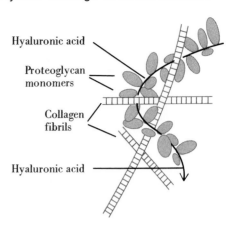

Figure 7.1. Schematic diagram showing a model for the organization of ground substance of cartilage. On the left, a collagen fibril and a collagen molecule are depicted for size reference. The next diagram shows a proteoglycan monomer, hyaluronic acid *(HA),* and a link protein. The proteoglycan monomer consists of approximately 100 glycosaminoglycan *(GAG)* units joined to a core protein. The end of the core protein contains a hyaluronic acid-binding region that is joined to the hyaluronic acid by a link protein. On the right, a hyaluronic acid molecule forming a linear aggregate with many proteoglycan monomers *(pink ellipses)* is interwoven with a network of collagen fibrils. (Based on Hascall VC, Lowther DA: In: Nancollas GH, et al (eds): *Biological Mineralization and Demineralization.* New York, Springer, 1982, p 181.)

ing glycoproteins. The cartilage matrix also contains other proteoglycans that do not form aggregates and contains noncollagenous and nonproteoglycan-linked glycoproteins.

Like other connective tissue matrices, cartilage matrix is highly hydrated. From 60% to 78% of the net weight of hyaline cartilage is water. Much of this water is bound tightly to the proteoglycan aggregates, which explains the resilience of cartilage. Some of the water is bound loosely enough, however, to allow the essential diffusion of small metabolites to and from the chondrocytes.

In articular cartilage, there are both transient and regional changes in water content. These changes occur during joint movement and when the joint is subjected to pressure. The high degree of hydration and the movement of water in the matrix are factors that allow the cartilage matrix to respond to varying pressure loads; they also contribute to cartilage's weight-bearing capacity.

Ground Substance Components of Hyaline Cartilage Matrix Are Not Uniformly Distributed

Because of the large numbers of bound sulfate groups, the proteoglycans of hyaline cartilage ground substance stain with basic dyes and with hematoxylin. Thus, the basophilia and metachromasia seen in stained sections of cartilage provide information on the distribution and relative concentration of sulfated proteoglycans. The highest concentration of these substances is immediately around the lacunae. This ring of intensely staining matrix has been designated as the *capsule* by classical histologists (Fig. 7.2). This high concentration of sulfated proteoglycans in the immediate vicinity of cells and cell clusters is designated as the *territorial matrix.* Sulfated proteoglycans are in their lowest concentration in regions of the matrix farthest removed from the cells. These areas are designated as the *interterritorial matrix.* Aside from these regional differences in the distribution of sulfated proteoglycans, there are staining differences that occur because the proteoglycan content in the matrix diminishes as cartilage ages.

Cartilage Chondrocytes

Chondrocytes Vary in Appearance According to Their Activity

Chondrocytes that are active in matrix production display areas of cytoplasmic basophilia, indicative of protein synthesis, and clear areas, due to the large Golgi apparatus (Fig. 7.3) The cells secrete not only the collagen of the matrix but also all of the glycosaminoglycans and proteoglycans. In older, less active cells, the Golgi is reduced in size; clear areas of cytoplasm, when evident, usually indicate sites of extracted lipid droplets and glycogen stores. In such specimens, chondrocytes also display considerable distortion due to shrinkage after the glycogen and lipid are lost during the preparation of the tissue.

With the electron microscope, the active chondrocyte is seen to contain numerous profiles of rough endoplasmic reticulum (rER), a large Golgi apparatus, secretory granules, vesicles, intermediate filaments, microtubules, and actin microfilaments (Fig. 7.4). In old cartilage cells, there are numerous intermediate filaments.

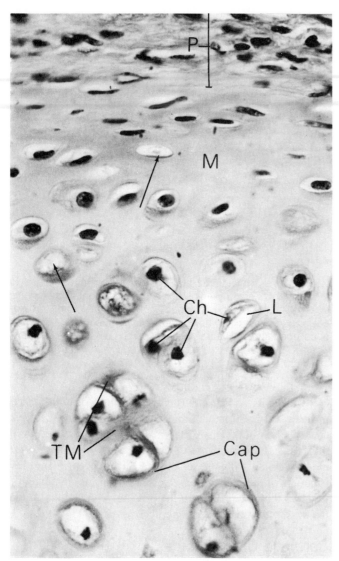

Figure 7.2. Photomicrograph of a typical hyaline cartilage specimen stained with hematoxylin and eosin (H&E). The chondrocytes *(Ch)* are poorly preserved and display little more than the nucleus residing in an empty-appearing lacuna *(L)*. In some instances, the cells have dropped out of the lacunae *(arrows)*. The cartilage matrix shows the darker-staining capsule *(Cap)* immediately around the lacunae and the territorial matrix *(TM)* between chondrocytes in a cluster. The matrix between the single and clustered chondrocytes is the interterritorial matrix *(M)*. The upper portion of the figure shows the perichondrium *(P)*, from which new cartilage cells are derived (appositional growth). Growth from within the cartilage (interstitial growth) is reflected by the chondrocyte pairs and clusters in the lower part of the micrograph. ×640.

Hyaline Cartilage Forms Most of the Initial Skeleton of the Fetus

Hyaline cartilage is the precursor to bones that will develop by the process of **endochondral ossification** (Fig. 7.5). While endochondral bone development is in progress, hyaline cartilage serves as a epiphyseal growth site. This cartilaginous **epiphyseal growth plate (epiphyseal disc)** re-

mains functional as long as the bone grows in length (Fig. 7.6). In bones of the adult, hyaline cartilage is present only at articular surfaces (Fig. 7.7). Hyaline cartilage is also present in the adult as the skeletal unit in the trachea, bronchi, larynx, nose, and the ends of the ribs (costal cartilages).

Perichondrium

Hyaline Cartilage Is Surrounded by a Firmly Attached Connective Tissue, the *Perichondrium*

The **perichondrium** consists of dense connective tissue whose cells are indistinguishable from fibroblasts. In many respects, the perichondrium resembles the capsule that surrounds glands and many organs. It is more than simply a covering capsule, however, because it serves as the source of new cartilage cells. When actively growing, the perichondrium appears to be divided into an *inner cellular layer*, which gives rise to cartilage cells, and an *outer fibrous layer*. This division is not always evident, especially in perichondrium that is inactive with respect to producing new cartilage. The changes that occur during the differentiation of

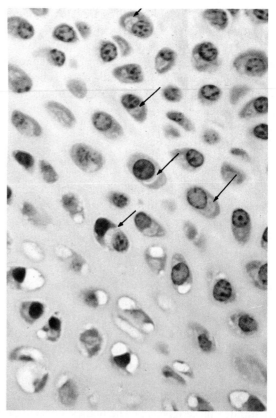

Figure 7.3. Photomicrograph of a young, growing cartilage from a glutaraldehyde-fixed, plastic-embedded specimen stained with H&E. The cartilage cells are well preserved. The cytoplasm is deeply stained, exhibiting a distinct and relatively homogeneous basophilia. The clear areas *(arrows)* represent sites of the Golgi apparatus. ×500.

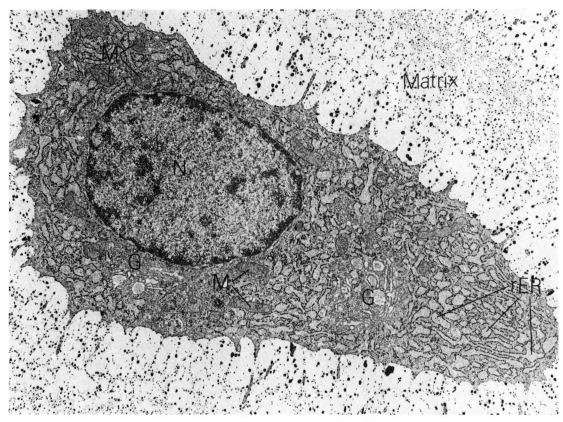

Figure 7.4. Electron micrograph of a young, active chondrocyte and surrounding matrix. The nucleus *(N)* of the chondrocyte is eccentrically located, like those seen in Figure 7.3, and the cytoplasm displays numerous and somewhat dilated profiles of rER, Golgi profiles *(G)*, and mitochondria *(M)*. The large amount of rER and the extensive Golgi area indicate that the cell is actively engaged in the production of cartilage matrix. Within the matrix, there are numerous dark particles. They contain proteoglycans of the matrix. The particles adjacent to the cell are particularly large. They are in the region of the matrix that is identified as the capsule of the lacuna with the light microscope. ×15,000. (Courtesy of Dr. H. Clarke Anderson.)

new chondrocytes in a growing cartilage are illustrated and described in Plate 13.

Exceptions to the general rule that hyaline cartilage is surrounded by a perichondrium occur where cartilage forms a free surface, as in the articular surfaces in joints, and where cartilage makes direct contact with bone, as in the nasal and costal cartilages and in forming bone. In these sites, proliferation of chondrocytes within the cartilage lacunae provides the new cells for *interstitial growth*. The process is described later.

ELASTIC CARTILAGE

Elastic Cartilage Is Distinguished by the Presence of Elastin in the Cartilage Matrix

In addition to the normal components of hyaline cartilage matrix, elastic cartilage matrix contains elastic fibers and interconnecting sheets of elastic material. These fibers and lamellae are best demonstrated in paraffin sections with special stains such as resorcin-fuchsin and orcein. The elastic material gives the cartilage elastic properties in addition to the resilience and pliability that are characteristic of hyaline cartilage.

Elastic cartilage is found in the external ear, in the walls of the external auditory canal and the auditory (Eustachian) tube, in the epiglottis, and in the larynx. In all of these locations there is surrounding perichondrium, such as that found around most hyaline cartilage. Unlike hyaline cartilage, however, the matrix of elastic cartilage does not calcify.

FIBROCARTILAGE

Fibrocartilage Consists of Chondrocytes and Their Territorial Matrix in Combination With Dense Connective Tissue

It is often difficult to distinguish fibrocartilage from dense regular connective tissue, particularly in hematoxylin and eosin (H&E)-stained sections. The presence of aggregates of rounded cells *(isogenous groups)* among bundles of collagen and of basophilic staining in the capsular matrix and territorial matrix, when present, aids in its identification.

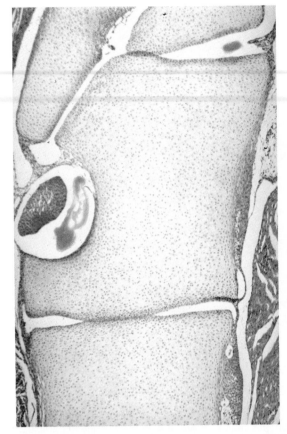

Figure 7.5. Photomicrograph of several of the cartilages forming the initial skeleton of the foot. The hyaline cartilage of the fetal skeleton will be replaced by bone as development proceeds (endochondral ossification). A developing tendon is evident in the indentation of the cartilage seen on the left side of the micrograph.

Fibrocartilage is typically present in the intervertebral discs, the symphysis pubis, the articular discs of the sternoclavicular and temporomandibular joints, the menisci of the knee joint, and certain places where tendons attach to bones. Usually, the presence of fibrocartilage indicates that resistance to both compression and shear forces is required of the tissue.

HISTOGENESIS AND GROWTH OF HYALINE CARTILAGE

Cartilage Arises From Mesenchyme

In areas where cartilage develops, excluding the head, mesenchymal cells aggregate and form a mass of rounded, closely apposed cells. In the head, most of the cartilage arises from aggregates of ectomesenchyme derived from neural crest cells. These aggregates, called a *blastema* of precartilage *(protochondral tissue)*, mark the site of hyaline cartilage formation. The cells of the blastema, although in close apposition, begin to secrete cartilage matrix and are then referred to as *chondroblasts.* They progressively

move apart as they deposit matrix. When they have become completely surrounded by matrix material, the cells are then called *chondrocytes.* During this process the mesenchymal tissue immediately surrounding the chondrogenic blastema gives rise to perichondrium.

Cartilage Is Capable of Two Kinds of Growth, Appositional and Interstitial

With the onset of matrix secretion, cartilage growth will continue by a combination of two processes:

- *Appositional growth,* the process that forms new cartilage at the surface of preexisting cartilage
- *Interstitial growth,* the process that forms new cartilage within the cartilage mass (see Fig. 7.2)

The new cartilage cells produced in the process of *appositional growth* derive from the inner portion of the surrounding perichondrium. The cells have the appearance of fibroblasts and function as such in producing the collagenous component of the perichondrium (type I collagen). When cartilage growth is initiated, however, the cells undergo a change; the cytoplasmic processes disappear, the nucleus becomes rounded, and the cytoplasm increases in amount and becomes more prominent. These changes result in the cell becoming a chondroblast; the cells are now associated with cartilage matrix production and secrete the type II collagen characteristic of cartilage matrix. The new matrix in-

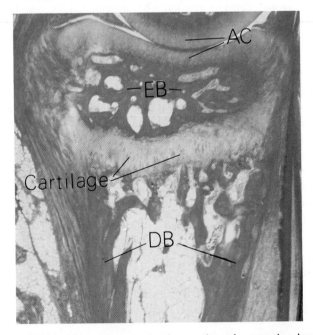

Figure 7.6. Photomicrograph of a portion of a growing long bone. The spaces in the bone are occupied by marrow. A disc of cartilage—the epiphyseal disc—separates the epiphyseal bone *(EB)* from the diaphyseal bone *(DB).* The articular surface of the bone is also composed of cartilage *(AC).* Whereas the epiphyseal cartilage disappears with the cessation of lengthwise growth of the bone, the articular cartilage remains throughout life.

creases the cartilage mass while at the same time new fibroblasts are produced to maintain the perichondrium.

The new cartilage cells produced in the process of *interstitial growth* arise from division of chondrocytes within their lacunae. This is possible only because the chondrocytes retain the ability to divide and the surrounding matrix is distensible, thus permitting further secretory activity. The daughter cells of the dividing chondrocytes temporarily occupy the same lacuna, but they become separated as each secretes new matrix material. As the matrix is secreted, a partition is formed between the cells, and at this point each cell occupies its own lacuna. With continued secretion of matrix, the cells become even further removed from each other. The overall growth of the cartilage is thus a reflection of the new matrix material that has been secreted by the chondrocytes, both interstitially and appositionally.

In adult cartilage, chondrocytes are frequently situated in compact groups or may be aligned in rows. These groups of chondrocytes are formed as a consequence of several successive divisions during the last phase of growth, without significant additional matrix production. Consequently, the chondrocytes remain in close apposition. Such groups of chondrocytes are called *isogenous groups*.

CARTILAGE REPAIR

The Ability of Damaged Cartilage to Repair Itself Is Limited

When cartilage is damaged and repair does occur, it is due to activity of the perichondrium mainly and usually only during the period of growth in young individuals. In the adult, typically, the cells of the perichondrium proliferate to initiate repair, but few cartilage cells, if any, are produced. In this case, the repair mostly involves the production of dense connective tissue. However, not infrequently in adults the development of new blood vessels at the site of the healing wound stimulates the growth of bone rather than actual cartilage repair. The limited ability of cartilage to repair itself can cause significant problems in cardiothoracic surgery when costal cartilage must be cut to enter the chest cavity, as in coronary artery bypass surgery.

The reason that bone is produced in favor of cartilage in many repairing sites may, in part, be related to the fact that chondrocytes normally reside in an environment with low oxygen concentration. It has been shown experimentally that in cultures of mesenchymal tissue that would ordinarily produce bone, cartilage develops if the oxygen tension is lowered. However, other factors may also play a role.

CALCIFICATION OF CARTILAGE AND REPLACEMENT BY BONE

Hyaline Cartilage, When Calcified, Is Generally Replaced by Bone

Hyaline cartilage is prone to calcification, a process in which calcium phosphate crystals become impregnated in

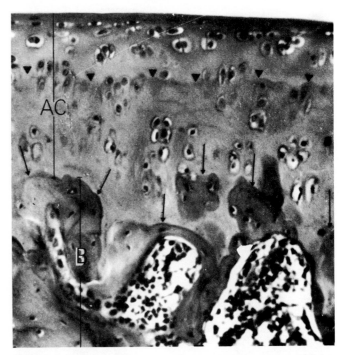

Figure 7.7. Photomicrograph of the epiphysis of a long bone. The articular surface is composed of hyaline cartilage. *Arrows* indicate the boundary between the articular cartilage *(AC)* and the underlying bone *(B)*. The deeper part of the articular cartilage—the portion below the *arrowheads*—appears darker than the more superficial portion. This deeper portion is characteristically calcified. Although the calcium salt has been removed during preparation of the specimen, its previous location is marked by a deeper staining than seen in the noncalcified matrix.

the cartilage matrix. The matrix of hyaline cartilage undergoes calcification as a regular occurrence in three well-defined situations:

- The portion of articular cartilage that is in contact with bone tissue, but not the surface portion, is calcified.
- Calcification always occurs in cartilage that is about to be replaced by bone (endochondral ossification) during the growth period of an individual.
- Hyaline cartilage throughout the body calcifies with time as part of the aging process.

In most of these cases and given sufficient time, cartilage, when calcified, will be replaced by bone. For example, in older individuals it is not uncommon to find portions of the cartilage rings in the trachea replaced by bone tissue (Fig. 7.8). Chondrocytes normally derive all their nutrients and dispose of wastes by diffusion of materials through the matrix. When the matrix becomes heavily calcified, diffusion is impeded and the chondrocytes swell and die. The ultimate consequence of this event is removal of the calcified matrix and its replacement by bone.

Some investigators have described a cell type, a *chondroclast,* that resembles an osteoclast (page 158) in both morphology and function and that appears to play a role in the digestion of calcified cartilage that is being replaced by carried out on the developing mandible, in which true endochondral ossification does not take place. It is still unclear whether chondroclasts are cells found wherever bone is replacing cartilage or whether they are limited to cartilages and bones that derive from the ectomesenchyme that originates from neural crest cells.

CARTILAGE CANALS

Although cartilage is an avascular tissue, many cartilages are penetrated by small canals containing blood vessels, nerves, and surrounding connective tissue within the canal (Fig. 7.9). Although these canals are variable in terms of their location and appearance, nevertheless they do persist until old age in some cartilages. They are most frequently found in laryngeal and nasal cartilages. The significance of cartilage canals is not yet clear.

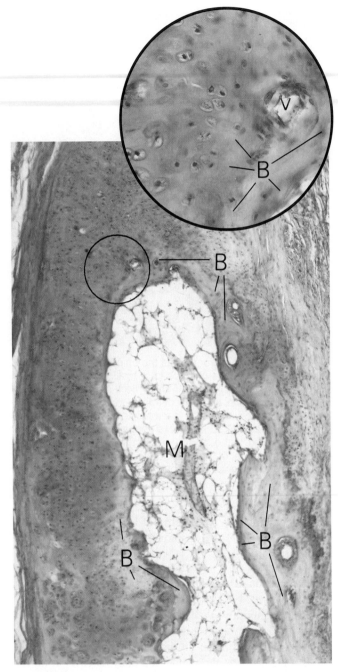

Figure 7.8. Photomicrograph showing part of a tracheal ring. A marrow cavity *(M)* has formed within the cartilage structure. The darker areas are normal cartilage matrix. The lighter and more eosinophilic areas are bone *(B)* that has replaced the original cartilage matrix. ×75. **Inset.** A higher magnification from the *circled area* showing the normal cartilage and the adjacent new bone tissue *(B)* for comparison. A blood vessel *(V)* is present in the bone tissue. ×250.

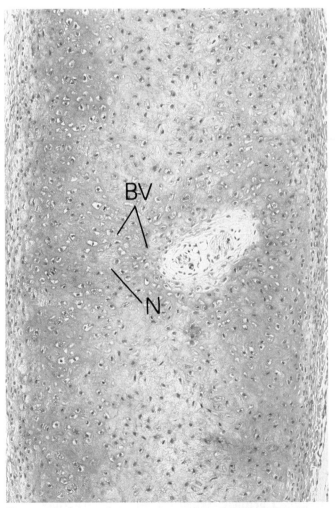

Figure 7.9. A cartilage canal containing a nerve *(N)* and several small blood vessels *(BV)*. The canal is lined by connective tissue. ×100.

bone. These cells appear to enter the cartilage along with newly sprouting blood vessels and may, in fact, derive from perivascular cells. Prechondroclasts resemble fibroblasts when seen in the transmission electron microscope. Most studies of chondroclast structure and function have been

ATLAS PLATES

11–15

PLATE 11. Cartilage I, Light and Electron Microscopy

Hyaline cartilage is found in the adult as the structural framework for the larynx, trachea, and bronchi; it is found on the anterior ends of the ribs and on the surfaces of synovial joints. In addition, hyaline cartilage constitutes much of the fetal skeleton and plays an important role in the growth of many bones.

FIGURE 1, cartilage, human, H&E ×450. This figure shows hyaline cartilage from the trachea. It appears as an avascular expanse of a matrix material and a population of cells referred to as chondrocytes *(Ch)*. The chondrocytes produce the matrix; the space each chondrocyte occupies is called a lacuna *(L)*. Surrounding and in immediate apposition to the cartilage is a cover of connective tissue, the perichondrium *(P)*. The perichondrium is more than a simple capsule in that it also serves as a source of new chondrocytes during *appositional growth* of the cartilage. Often, the perichondrium reveals two layers: an outer, more fibrous layer and an inner, more cellular layer. It is this inner, more cellular layer that is chondrogenic.

Cartilage matrix contains collagenous fibrils masked by the ground substance; thus, the fibrils are not evident in routine H&E preparations. The matrix also contains, among other components, sulfated glycosaminoglycans that exhibit basophilia with hematoxylin or other basic dyes. If the sulfated material is not adequately retained, however, as is usually the case in routine H&E preparations, the matrix stains predominately with eosin and to a minimal extent with hematoxylin. Also, the matrix material immediately surrounding a lacuna tends to stain more intensely with basic dyes. This region is referred to as a capsule *(Cap)*. Not uncommonly, the matrix may stain deeply in localized areas *(asterisks)* and appear much like capsule matrix. This is the result of a capsule being included within the thickness of the section, but not the lacuna it surrounds.

Frequently, two or more chondrocytes are extremely close, separated only by a thin partition of matrix. These are said to be isogenous cell clusters because they arise from a single predecessor cell. The proliferation of cells by this means, with the consequent addition of matrix, results in *interstitial growth* of the cartilage, i.e., growth within the substance of the cartilage.

FIGURE 2, cartilage, mouse, electron micrograph ×3000. This low-magnification electron micrograph shows to advantage the nature and relationship of the cartilage and perichondrium. The perichondrial cells *(P)* extend long, flat cytoplasmic processes between the collagen fibers. Their nuclei are flattened and are surrounded by scant cytoplasm. Although these cells constitute the cellular component of the perichondrium and, thus, are referred to as perichondrial cells, morphologically they are typical fibroblasts. In contrast, the fully differentiated, mature chondrocytes exhibit round to ovoid nuclei with a moderate amount of cytoplasm. Not being subject to the shrinkage encountered in routine light microscopic preparations, the chondrocyte in electron microscopic preparations does not separate from its surrounding matrix. Consequently, one does not see an empty or partially empty lacuna.

Because the cartilage shown is in a growing state, it is possible to point to the changes that occur during the process of appositional growth. The cells labeled *A, B,* and *C* represent transitional stages in the differentiation of a fibroblast to a chondrocyte. Cell *A* is already in the process of transforming into a chondrocyte. Cell *B* is similar to *A* in shape, but it exhibits a slightly scalloped surface on its upper left side (this is just barely discernible at the low magnification of the micrograph). In addition, the matrix along this surface shows a greater density than that seen on the opposite side of the cell. The more dense material represents cartilage matrix. Cell *C* represents a further transition; this cell is now a young chondrocyte. The entire surface of the cell is scalloped and is completely surrounded by cartilage matrix. Also, the nucleus of the cell has become ovoid, and the cell has become more polygonal in shape. With time, the nucleus will assume the more rounded shape of the mature cartilage cells. The areas in the *rectangles* are described in Plate 12.

KEY		
A, B, C, progressive stages in chondrocyte differentiation	**Ch,** chondrocytes	**P,** perichondrium
Ca, calcium deposits	**G,** glycogen	**asterisk,** capsule of a lacuna, but with lacuna and contained chondrocyte not included within the thickness of the section
Cap, capsule	**L,** lacuna	
	Li, lipid	

PLATE 11

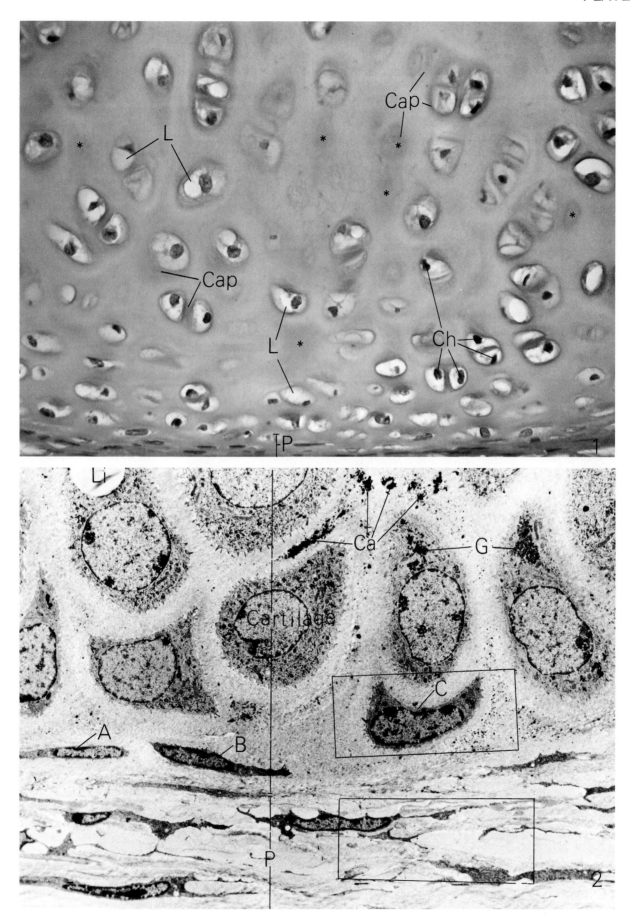

PLATE 12. Cartilage II, Electron Microscopy

These electron micrographs depict the cells and extracellular matrix contained in the rectangles on Figure 2 of Plate 11. The greater resolution of the electron microscope allows more detailed comparison of the perichondrium and cartilage.

FIGURE 2, cartilage, mouse, electron micrograph ×16,000; inset ×31,000. Small, irregular projections on the surface of this differentiated chondrocyte give the cell a ruffled or scalloped appearance *(arrowheads)*. These projections first appear when cartilage matrix formation is initiated. Other than the accumulation of lipid and glycogen, the cytoplasm of the cartilage cell does not appear appreciably different from the cytoplasm of the fibroblast. Because of the particular region through which the cell was sectioned, the chondrocyte in this figure does not reveal its granular (rough) endoplasmic reticulum. This organelle is particularly well developed in the active chondrocyte. The cell seen here, however, does display a fairly prominent portion of its Golgi apparatus *(GA)*. Also note that the glycogen *(G)* within the cell can just be resolved as a particulate component at this magnification. The other very electron dense, *extracellular* material represents calcium deposits *(Ca)*.

In contrast to the perichondrial connective tissue matrix, the cartilage matrix, exclusive of the calcium deposits, appears almost homogeneous, particularly when observed at lower magnifications. It contains extremely fine (5–20 nm) matrix fibrils. These fibrils consist primarily of type II collagen, which forms a fibril with a smaller diameter and a less discernible periodic banding pattern than is seen in type I collagen. The **lower inset** shows the cartilage matrix from the area included in the *circle* of this figure. Note the fineness of the fibrils and the absence of typical banded collagen fibrils. The relative homogeneity of the cartilage matrix, as seen here, accounts for its amorphous appearance when observed in the light microscope.

FIGURE 1, cartilage, mouse, electron micrograph ×16,000; inset ×31,000. The perichondrium in this figure reveals portions of two fibroblasts or perichondrial cells. One of the cells displays multiple arrays of rough-surfaced or granular endoplasmic reticulum *(GER)*, a feature characteristic of the fibroblast. The surface of the cell is relatively smooth. Also characteristic of the fibroblast are the long, tenuous cytoplasmic processes *(F)* that extend between the bundles of collagen fibrils *(CF)*. During the process of its differentiation and maturation into a chondrocyte, the fibroblast changes from a flat elongate cell to one that is ovoid to round. The extracellular formed elements of the perichondrial matrix consist mostly of collagen fibrils that are aggregated into bundles, i.e., collagen fibers *(CF)*, oriented in varying directions. The **upper inset** shows bundles of cross and obliquely sectioned collagen fibrils from the area included within the *circle* of this figure. These collagen fibers belong to the perichondrium. Note the very tight packing of the fibrils. Elastic fibers *(E)* are also evident in the perichondrium. They are composed of an electron-lucent core material and numerous surrounding, electron-dense microfibrils. The microfibrils *(arrows)* are just perceptible at this magnification.

KEY

Ca, calcium deposits	**F,** fibroblast process	**GER,** granular endoplasmic reticulum
CF, collagen fibrils	**G,** glycogen	**arrowheads,** scalloped surface of chondrocyte
E, elastic fibers	**GA,** Golgi apparatus	**arrows,** microfibrils of elastic fibers

PLATE 12

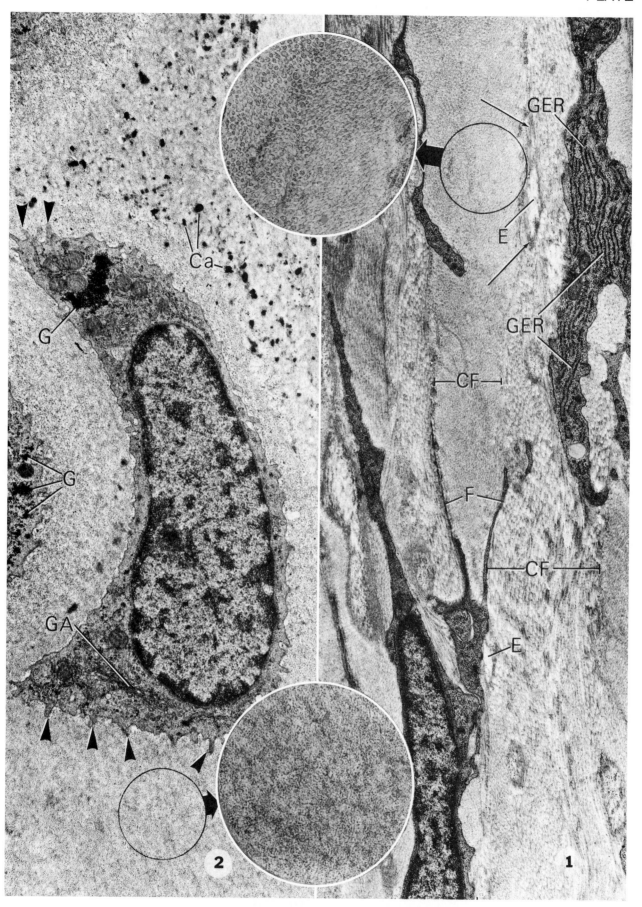

PLATE 13. Cartilage and the Developing Skeleton

Hyaline cartilage is present as a precursor to bones in the fetus. This cartilage is replaced by bone tissue except where one bone contacts another bone, as in a joint. In these locations, cartilage persists and covers the bone as articular cartilage. In addition, cartilage, being capable of interstitial growth, persists in weight-supporting bones as a growth plate so long as growth in length occurs. The role of hyaline cartilage in bone growth is considered below.

FIGURE 1, fetal foot, rat, H&E ×85. This section shows the cartilages that will ultimately become the bones of the foot. In several places, developing ligaments *(L)* can be seen where they join the cartilages. The nuclei of the fibroblasts within the ligaments are just barely perceptible. They are aligned in rows and are separated from other rows of fibroblasts by collagenous material. The hue and intensity of color of the cartilage matrix, except at the periphery, is due to the combined uptake of the H&E. The collagen of the matrix stains with eosin; however, the presence of sulfated glycosaminoglycans results in staining by hematoxylin. The matrix of cartilage that is about to be replaced by bone, such as that shown here, becomes impregnated with calcium salts, and the calcium is also receptive to staining with hematoxylin. The many enlarged lacunae (seen as light spaces within the matrix where the chondrocytes have fallen out of the lacunae) are due to hypertrophy of the chondrocytes, an event associated with calcification of the matrix. Thus, where these large lacunae are present, i.e., in the center region of the cartilage, the matrix is heavily stained.

This figure also shows that the cartilage is surrounded by perichondrium, except where it faces a joint cavity *(JC)*. Here, the bare cartilage forms a surface. Note that the joint cavity is a space between the cartilages whose boundaries are completed by connective tissue *(CT)*. The connective tissue at the surface of the cavity is special. It will constitute the synovial membrane in the adult and contribute to the formation of a lubricating fluid (synovial fluid) that is present in the joint cavity. Therefore, all the surfaces that will enclose the adult joint cavity are derived originally from the mesenchyme. Synovial fluid is a viscous substance containing, among other things, glycosaminoglycans; it can be considered an exudate of interstitial fluid. The synovial fluid could be considered an extension of the extracellular matrix, as the joint cavity is not lined by an epithelium.

FIGURE 2, fetal finger, human, thionine-picric acid ×30. This figure shows a developing long bone of the finger and its articulation with the distal and proximal bones. Before the stage shown here, each bone consisted entirely of a hyaline cartilaginous structure similar to the cartilages seen in Figure 1 but shaped like the long bones into which they would develop. Here, only the ends or epiphyses of the bone remain as cartilage, the epiphyseal cartilage *(C)*. The shaft or diaphysis has become a cylinder of bone tissue *(B)* surrounding the marrow cavity *(MC)*. The dark region at the ends of the marrow cavity is calcified cartilage *(arrowheads)* that is being replaced by bone. The bone at the ends of the marrow cavity constitutes the metaphysis. With this staining method, the calcified cartilage appears dark brown. The newly formed metaphyseal bone, which is admixed with this degenerating calcified cartilage and is difficult to define at this low magnification, has the same yellow-brown color as the diaphyseal bone. By the continued proliferation of cartilage, the bone grows in length. Later, the cartilage becomes calcified; bone is then produced and occupies the site of the resorbed cartilage. With the cessation of cartilage proliferation and its replacement by bone, growth of the bone stops and only the cartilage at the articular surface remains. The details of this process are explained under endochondral bone formation (Plates 19 and 20).

KEY

B, bone
C, cartilage
CT, connective tissue
JC, joint cavity
L, ligament
MC, marrow cavity
arrowhead, calcified cartilage

PLATE 13

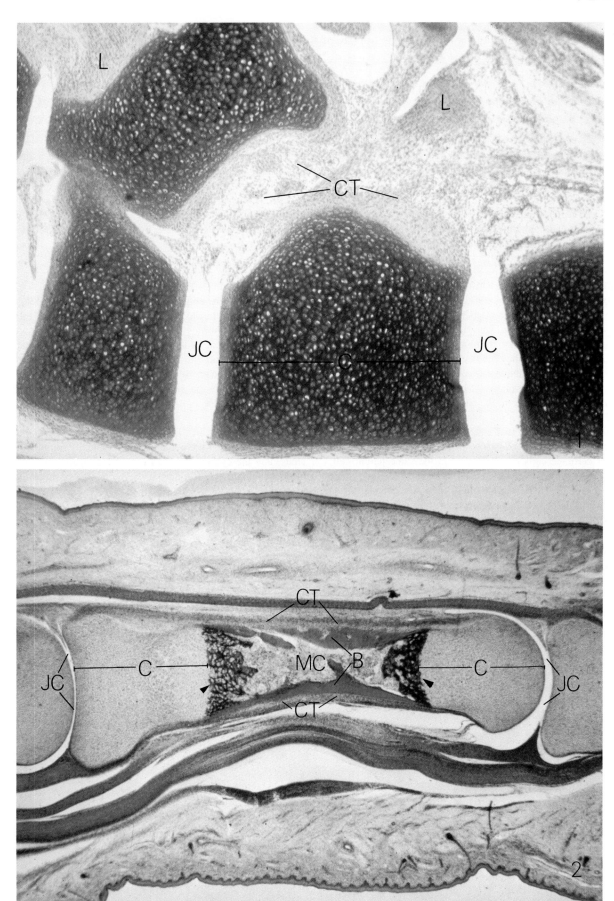

PLATE 14. Elastic Cartilage

Elastic cartilage is found in the auricle of the external ear, in the auditory tube, in the epiglottis, and in part of the larynx. It differs from hyaline cartilage in that the matrix contains elastic material, either as fibers or as interconnecting sheets, in addition to the other constituents of cartilage matrix. The elastic material imparts properties of elasticity to the cartilage that are not shared by hyaline cartilage.

FIGURE 1, epiglottis, human, H&E ×80. This section of the epiglottis contains elastic cartilage *(EC)* as the centrally located structure. The essential components of the cartilage, namely, the matrix that stains deep blue and the light, unstained lacunae surrounded by matrix, are evident in this low-magnification micrograph. The perimeter of the cartilage is covered by perichondrium; its fibrous character is just barely visible in this figure. Also to be noted is the adipose tissue *(AT)* within the boundaries of the elastic cartilage.

Both above and below the elastic cartilage there is connective tissue, and each surface of the epiglottis is formed by stratified squamous epithelium. Mucous glands *(MG)* are in the connective tissue in the bottom of this figure.

FIGURE 2, epiglottis, human, H&E ×250; inset ×400. This shows an area of the elastic cartilage at higher magnification. The elastic fibers appear as the blue, elongate profiles within the matrix. They are most evident at the edges of the cartilage, but they are obscured in some deeper parts of the matrix, where they blend with the elastic material that forms a honeycomb about the lacunae. Elastic fibers *(E)* are also in the adipose tissue *(AT)*, between the adipocytes.

Some of the lacunae in the cartilage are arranged in pairs separated by a thin plate of matrix. The plate of matrix appears as a bar between the adjacent lacunae. This is a reflection of interstitial growth by the cartilage, in that the adjacent cartilage cells are derived from the same parent cell. They have moved away from each other and secreted a plate of cartilage matrix between them to form two lacunae. Most chondrocytes shown in this figure occupy only part of the lacuna. This is, in part, due to shrinkage, but it is also due to the fact that older chondrocytes contain lipid in large droplets that is lost during the processing of the tissue. The shrinkage of chondrocytes within the lacunae or their loss due to dropping out of the section during preparation cause the lacunae to stand out as light, unstained areas against the darkly stained matrix

The **inset** shows the elastic cartilage at still higher magnification. Here, the elastic fibers *(E)* are again evident as elongate profiles chiefly at the edges of the cartilage. Most of the chondrocytes in this part of the specimen show little shrinkage. Many of the cells display a typically rounded nucleus, and the cytoplasm is evident. Note, again, that some lacunae contain two chondrocytes, indicative of interstitial growth.

KEY

AT, adipose tissue
E, elastic fiber
EC, elastic cartilage
MG, mucous gland

PLATE 14

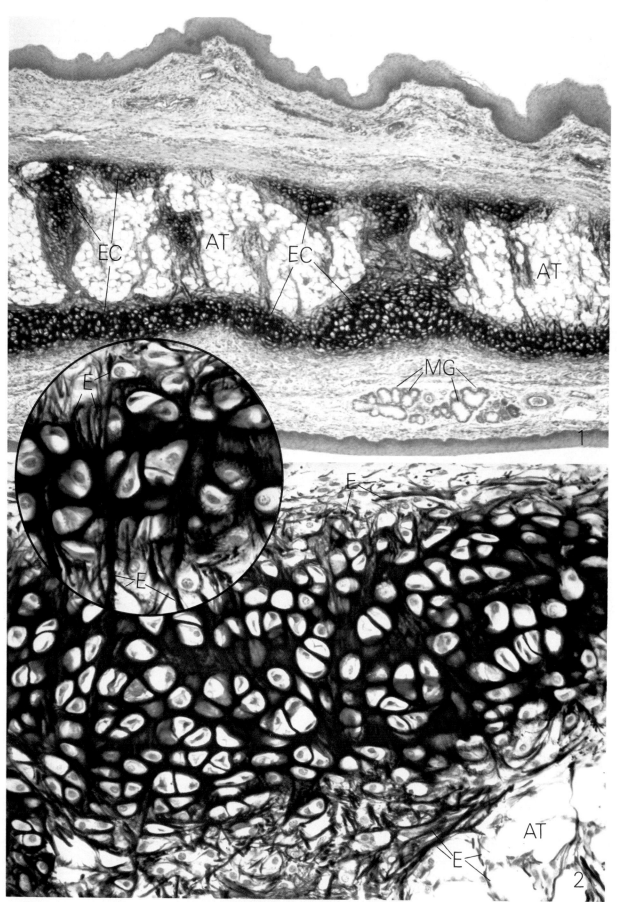

PLATE 15. Fibrocartilage

Fibrocartilage is a combination of dense connective tissue and cartilage. The amount of cartilage varies, but in most locations the cartilage cells and their matrix occupy a lesser portion of the tissue mass. Fibrocartilage is found at the intervertebral discs, the symphysis pubis, the knee joint, the mandibular joint, the sternoclavicular joint, and the shoulder joint. It may also be present along the grooves or insertions for tendons and ligaments. Its presence is associated with sites where resilience is required in dense connective tissue to help absorb sudden physical impact. Histologically, fibrocartilage appears as small fields of cartilage blending almost imperceptibly with regions of fibrous tissue. No perichondrium is present.

FIGURE 1, intervertebral disc, human, Mallory's trichrome ×160. This is a low-magnification view of fibrocartilage. The Mallory method stains collagen light blue. The tissue has a fibrous appearance, and at this low magnification the nuclei of the fibroblasts *(F)* appear as small, elongate or spindle-shaped bodies. There are relatively few fibroblasts present, as is characteristic of dense connective tissue. The cartilage cells *(C)* are more numerous and exhibit close spatial groupings, i.e., *isogenous groups.* Some of the cartilage cells appear as elongate clusters of cells, whereas others appear in single-file rows. The matrix material immediately surrounding the cartilage cells has a homogeneous appearance and is, thereby, distinguishable from the fibrous connective tissue.

FIGURE 2, intervertebral disc, human, Mallory's trichrome ×700. This figure shows the area circumscribed by the *rectangle* in Figure 1 at higher magnification. The cartilage cells are contained within lacunae *(arrows),* and their cytoplasm stains deeply. The surrounding cartilage matrix material is scant and blends into the dense connective tissue. The presence of cartilage matrix material can be detected best by observing the larger group of cartilage cells at the left of this figure and then observing this same area in Figure 1. Note the light homogeneous area around the cell nest in the lower-power view. This is the region of cartilage matrix. At the greater magnification of Figure 2, it is possible to see that some of the collagen fibers are incorporated in the matrix, where they appear as wispy bundles.

KEY		
C, cartilage	**F**, fibroblast	**arrow**, lacuna

PLATE 15

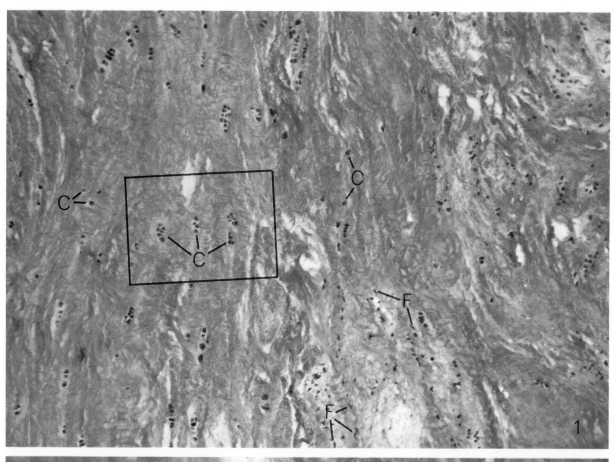

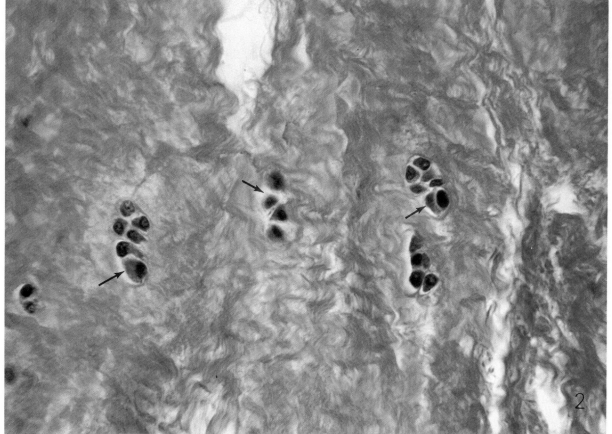

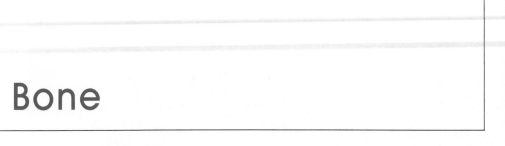

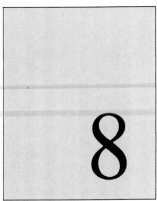

Bone

Bone Is a Connective Tissue Characterized by a Mineralized Extracellular Matrix

Bone is a specialized form of connective tissue that, like the other connective tissues, consists of cells and extracellular matrix. The feature that distinguishes bone from other connective tissues is the mineralization of the matrix. This produces an extremely hard tissue capable of providing support and protection. The mineral is calcium phosphate, in the form of **hydroxyapatite crystals** $[Ca_{10}(PO_4)_6(OH)_3]$.

By virtue of its mineral content, bone also serves as a *storage site* for calcium and phosphate. Both calcium and phosphate can be mobilized from the bone matrix and taken up by the blood, as needed, to maintain appropriate levels throughout the body. Thus, in addition to support and protection, bone has an important secondary role in the homeostatic regulation of blood calcium levels.

Bone matrix consists of type I collagen and ground substance containing proteoglycans and noncollagenous glycoproteins. Both the collagen and the ground substance components are mineralized. Within the bone matrix are spaces called **lacunae,** each of which contains a bone cell, the **osteocyte.** The osteocyte extends numerous processes into little tunnels called **canaliculi.** These run through the mineralized matrix, connecting adjacent lacunae and allowing contact between the cell processes of neighboring osteocytes. In this manner, a continuous network of canaliculi and lacunae containing the cells and their processes is formed throughout the entire mass of mineralized tissue. Electron micrographs have shown that the processes of osteocytes communicate by gap junctions.

In addition to the osteocyte, there are three other designations for the cells present in bone:

- *Osteoprogenitor cells:* These cells can give rise to the osteoblast.
- *Osteoblasts:* These cells secrete the extracellular matrix

of bone; once the cell has surrounded itself with its secreted matrix, it is referred to as an osteocyte.
- *Osteoclasts:* These are bone resorbing cells present on bone surfaces where bone is being removed.

Each of these cells is described more fully below.

The osteoprogenitor cell and the osteoblast are developmental precursors of the osteocyte. The osteoclast is a phagocytic cell derived from the bone marrow.

BONES AND BONE TISSUE

Bones Are the Organs of the Skeletal System; Bone Tissue Is the Structural Component of Bones

Typically, a bone consists of bone tissue, other connective tissues of various sorts, including hemopoietic tissue, fat tissue, blood vessels, nerves, and, if the bone forms a freely movable (synovial) joint, hyaline cartilage. The ability of the bone to perform its skeletal function is due to the bone tissue and, where present, the articular cartilage.

Classification of Bone Tissue

Bone Tissue Is Classified as Either Compact (Dense) or Spongy (Cancellous)

If one makes a cut through a bone, two distinct structural arrangements of the bone tissue can be recognized (Fig. 8.1). One arrangement appears as a compact, dense layer that forms the outside of the bone. The other arrangement has the appearance of a sponge, with trabeculae (thin anastomosing spicules) of bone tissue forming a meshwork in the interior of the bone. The spaces of the meshwork are continuous and, in a living bone, are occupied by marrow and blood vessels.

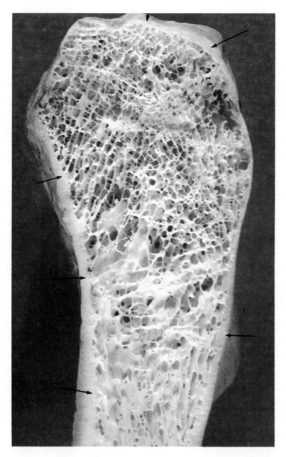

Figure 8.1. Gross specimen of a longitudinally sliced long bone. The outer portion of the bone has a solid structure *(arrows)* and represents compact bone. The interior of the bone exhibits a spongy configuration and consists of numerous interconnecting marrow spaces bounded by bony trabeculae.

Classification and General Structure of Bones

Spongy and compact bone tissue are located in specific parts of bones. It is useful, then, to outline briefly the kinds of bones and survey where the two kinds of bone tissue are located. On the basis of shape, bones can be classified into four groups:

- *Long bones* are longer in one dimension than the other and consist of a shaft and two ends, e.g., the tibia and the metacarpals. A schematic diagram of a long bone sectioned longitudinally through the shaft is shown in Figure 8.2.
- *Short bones* are nearly equal in length and diameter, e.g., the carpal bones of the hand.
- *Flat bones* are thin and plate-like, e.g., the bones of the calvarium (the skull cap) and the sternum. They consist of two layers of relatively thick compact bone with an intervening layer of spongy bone.
- *Irregular bones* have a shape that does not fit into any one of the three groups just described; the shape may

be complex, e.g., a vertebra, or the bone may contain air spaces or sinuses, as in the ethmoid.

Long bones, have a shaft called the *diaphysis* and two expanded ends, each called an *epiphysis* (Fig. 8.2). The flared portion of the bone between the diaphysis and the epiphysis is called the *metaphysis.* It extends from the diaphysis to the epiphyseal line. A large cavity filled with bone marrow, called the *marrow* or *medullary cavity,* forms the inner portion of the bone. In the shaft, almost the entire thickness of the bone tissue is compact; at most, only a small amount of spongy bone faces the medullary cavity. At the ends of the bone, the reverse is true. Here, the spongy bone is extensive, and the compact bone is little more than a thin outer shell (Fig. 8.1).

Short bones possess a shell of compact bone on the outside and have spongy bone and a marrow space on the inside. Short bones usually form movable joints with their neighbors, and as with long bones, the articular surfaces are covered with hyaline cartilage. Elsewhere, *periosteum,* a fibrous connective tissue capsule, covers the outer surface of the bone.

Surfaces of Bone

Bones Are Covered by Periosteum, a Sheath of Dense Connective Tissue Containing Osteoprogenitor Cells

The periosteum that covers an actively growing bone consists of an outer fibrous layer that resembles other dense connective tissues and an inner, more cellular layer that contains the *osteoprogenitor cells.* If active bone formation is not in progress on the bone surface, the fibrous layer is the main component of the periosteum, and few cells are seen in the inner layer. The relatively few cells that are present, the *periosteal cells,* are, however, capable of undergoing division and becoming osteoblasts under appropriate stimulus.

Generally, the collagen fibers of the periosteum are arranged parallel to the surface of the bone in the form of a capsule. The character of the periosteum is different where ligaments and tendons attach to the bone. Collagen fibers from these structures extend directly, but at an angle, into the bone tissue, where they are continuous with the collagen fibers of the bone tissue extracellular matrix. These fibers are called *Sharpey's fibers.*

Some Bones Articulate With Neighboring Bones to Form Movable (Synovial) Joints

The contact area of the bone, referred to as the *articular surface,* is covered with hyaline cartilage, also called *articular cartilage* because of its location and function. The articular cartilage is exposed to the joint cavity. This cartilage is not covered with perichondrium.

Lining of Bone Cavities

Bone Cavities Are Lined by Endosteum, a Layer of Connective Tissue Cells Containing Osteoprogenitor Cells

The lining tissue of both the compact bone facing the medullary cavity and the trabeculae of spongy bone within the cavity is referred to as *endosteum.* The endosteum, often only one cell thick, consists of cells that have the capacity to differentiate into osteoblasts in response to appropriate stimuli. These osteoprogenitor cells are flattened cells that resemble fibroblasts but are called *endosteal cells.*

The Medullary Cavity and the Spaces in Spongy Bone Contain Bone Marrow

Red bone marrow consists of developing blood cells in different stages of development (see page 202) and a network of reticular cells and fibers that serve as a supporting framework for the developing blood cells and blood vessels. As an individual grows, the amount of red marrow does not increase in proportion to bone growth. In later stages of growth and in the adult, when the rate of blood cell formation has diminished, the tissue in the medullary cavity consists mostly of fat cells; it is then called *yellow marrow.* Under appropriate stimuli, such as extreme blood loss, the yellow marrow can revert to red marrow. In the adult, red marrow is normally restricted to the spaces of spongy bone in a few locations such as the sternum and the iliac crest. Diagnostic bone marrow samples and marrow for transplantation are obtained from these sites.

ADULT BONE

Structure

Mature Bone Is Composed of Structural Units Called Osteons (Haversian Systems)

Mature compact bone is largely composed of cylindrical units of bone structure called *osteons* or *Haversian systems* (Fig. 8.3). The osteons consist of *concentric lamellae* of bone matrix surrounding a central canal, the *osteonal canal (Haversian canal),* that contains the vascular and nerve supply of the osteon. Canaliculi containing the processes of osteocytes are arranged mostly in a radial pattern with respect to the canal. The system of canaliculi that open to the osteonal canal also serves for the passage of substances between the osteocytes and the blood vessels. Between the osteons are remnants of previous osteonal lamellae, now called *interstitial lamellae* (Fig. 8.3). This form of matrix organization is called *lamellar bone.*

The long axis of an osteon is usually parallel to the long axis of the bone. The collagen fibers in the concentric lamellae in an osteon are laid down parallel to one another in any given lamella but in different directions in adjacent lamellae, giving the cut surface of lamellar bone the appearance of a plywood and giving great strength to the osteon.

Lamellar bone is also found at sites other than the osteon. *Circumferential lamellae* follow the entire inner and outer circumferences of the shaft of a long bone, appearing much like the growth rings of a tree (Fig. 8.3). *Perforating canals (Volkmann's canals)* are channels in lamellar bone through which blood vessels and nerves travel from the periosteal and endosteal surfaces to reach the osteonal canal; Volkmann's canals also connect osteonal canals to one another. They usually run at approximately right angles to the long axis of the osteons and of the bone (Fig. 8.3). The Volkmann's canal is not surrounded by concentric lamellae, a key feature in its histologic identification.

Lamellar bone may be compared with woven bone, in which the collagen fibers and bundles are at random orientations and are loosely intertwined, giving a woven appearance. Spongy bone may be either woven or lamellar bone; compact bone is almost entirely lamellar bone.

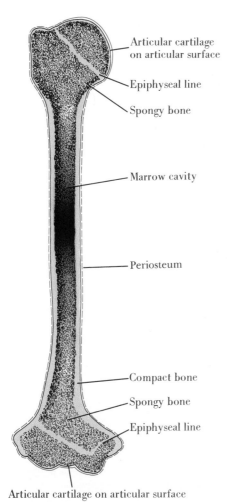

Articular cartilage
on articular surface

Epiphyseal line

Spongy bone

Marrow cavity

Periosteum

Compact bone

Spongy bone

Epiphyseal line

Articular cartilage on articular surface

Figure 8.2. Structure of a typical long bone. The shaft of the long bone, the diaphysis, contains a large marrow or medullary cavity surrounded by a thick-walled tube of compact bone. A small amount of spongy bone may line the inner surface of the compact bone. The ends or epiphyses of the long bone consist chiefly of spongy bone with a thin outer shell of compact bone. An additional term, the metaphysis, refers to the expanded or flared part of the bone at the extremities of the diaphysis. Except for the articular surfaces that are covered by hyaline (articular) cartilage, indicated by the *solid blue line,* the outer surface of the bone is covered by a fibrous connective tissue capsule called the periosteum, indicated by the *dashed blue line.*

Adult Spongy Bone

Adult spongy bone is very similar to adult compact bone except that the tissue is arranged as trabeculae or spicules; numerous interconnecting marrow spaces of various size are present between the bone tissue. The matrix of the bone is lamellated. If the trabeculae are sufficiently thick, they will contain osteons.

Blood Supply of Adult Bone

The blood supply to the shaft of a long bone is chiefly by arteries that enter the marrow cavity through nutrient

foramina. The greatest numbers of nutrient foramina are in the diaphysis and epiphysis (Fig. 8.4). Metaphyseal arteries provide a supplementary blood supply to the bone. Drainage of the bone is by veins that leave through the nutrient foramina or through the bone tissue of the shaft and out through the periosteum.

The nutrient arteries that supply the diaphysis and epiphysis arise developmentally as the principal vessel of the periosteal buds from which the primary and secondary centers of ossification develop (see page 163). The metaphyseal arteries, in contrast, arise developmentally from periosteal vessels that become incorporated into the metaphysis during the growth process, i.e., through the widening of the bone.

The Blood Supply to Bone Tissue Is Essentially Centrifugal

The blood that nourishes bone tissue moves from the marrow cavity into and through the bone tissue and out via periosteal veins. With respect to nourishment of the bone tissue itself, Volkmann's canals provide the major route of entry into the compact bone where they anastomose. The smaller blood vessels enter into the Haversian canals wherein one may find a single arteriole and a venule. In others, there may be only a single capillary. A much smaller supply to the bone tissue arises from periosteal vessels, but these usually provide for only the very outermost portions of the compact bone. Bone tissue lacks lymphatics; only the periosteal tissue is provided with lymphatic drainage.

MATURE AND IMMATURE BONE

Most samples of compact and spongy bone from an adult skeleton display the patterns of lamellar bone described above. Such bone may also be classified as *adult* or *mature bone.* On the other hand, the bone tissue initially deposited in the skeleton of the developing fetus is called *immature bone.* It differs from adult bone in several aspects (Fig. 8.5).

- Immature bone does not display an organized lamellated appearance, and on the basis of collagen fiber arrangement, such bone is designated as *nonlamellar.* Nonlamellar bone may also be referred to as *bundle* or *woven bone* because of the interlacing arrangement of the collagen fibers.
- Immature bone contains relatively more cells per unit area than does mature bone.
- The cells in immature bone tend to be randomly arranged, whereas cells in mature bone tend to have their long axis in the same direction as the lamellae.
- The matrix of immature bone has more ground substance than does the matrix of mature bone. The matrix in immature bones stains more intensely with hematox-

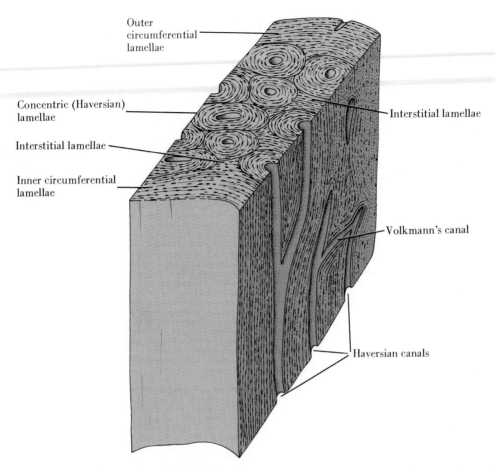

Figure 8.3. Three-dimensional diagram of a dried sample of compact bone. The concentric lamellae and the osteonal (Haversian) canal that they surround constitute an osteon (Haversian system). Between the osteons are interstitial lamellae, remnants of old osteons. The inner and outer surfaces of the compact bone in the figure show additional lamellae—the outer and inner circumferential lamellae—that are arranged in broad layers. (Based on Tandler J: *Lehrbuch der Systematischen Anatomie.* Leipzig, Vogel, 1926.)

ylin, whereas the matrix of mature bone stains more intensely with eosin.

Although not evident in typical histologic sections, immature bone is heavily mineralized when it is initially formed, whereas mature bone undergoes a prolonged secondary mineralization. The secondary mineralization of mature bone is evident in microradiographs of ground sections that show younger Haversian systems to be less mineralized than older Haversian systems (see Fig. 8.15).

Immature bone forms more rapidly than mature bone. Although mature bone is clearly the major bone type in the adult and immature bone is the major bone type in the developing fetus, areas of immature bone are regularly seen in the adult, especially where bone is being remodeled. Areas of immature bone are also seen regularly in the alveolar sockets of the adult oral cavity and where tendons insert into bones. It is the presence of this immature bone in the alveolar sockets that makes it possible to undertake orthodontic corrections even in adults.

CELLS OF BONE TISSUE

As noted earlier in this chapter, four designated cells are associated with bone tissue:

- *Osteoprogenitor cell*
- *Osteoblast*
- *Osteocyte*
- *Osteoclast*

With the exception of the osteoclast, each of these cells may be regarded as a differentiated form of the same basic cell type because each undergoes transformation from a less mature form to a more mature form in relation to functional activity (growth of bone). In contrast, the osteoclast has as its origin a different cell line and is responsible for bone resorption, an activity associated with bone remodeling.

Figure 8.4. Diagram showing the blood supply of a mature long bone. The nutrient artery and the epiphyseal arteries enter the bone through nutrient foramina. These openings in the bone arose developmentally as the pathways of the principal vessels of periosteal buds. Metaphyseal arteries arise from periosteal vessels that become incorporated into the metaphysis as the bone grows in diameter.

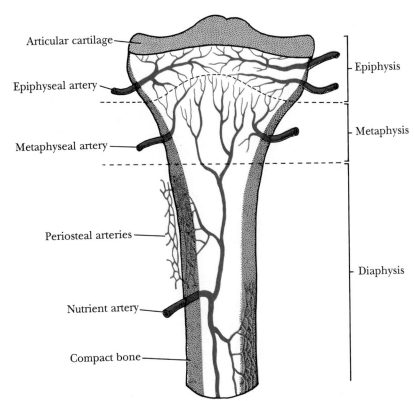

Osteoprogenitor Cell

The Osteoprogenitor Cell Is a Resting Cell That Can Transform Into an Osteoblast and Secrete Bone Matrix

Osteoprogenitor cells are found on the external and internal surfaces of bones. They comprise the ***periosteal cells*** that form the innermost layer of the periosteum and the ***endosteal cells*** that line the marrow cavities, the osteonal (Haversian) canals, and the perforating (Volkmann's) canals. The osteoprogenitor cells have the capacity to divide and proliferate, as shown by autoradiographic studies. In growing bones, the osteoprogenitor cells appear as flattened cells with lightly staining, elongate or ovoid nuclei and inconspicuous acidophilic or slightly basophilic cytoplasm (see Fig. 8.8). Electron micrographs reveal profiles of rough endoplasmic reticulum (rER) and free ribosomes as well as a small Golgi apparatus and other organelles. The morphology of the osteoprogenitor cell is consistent with the finding that its stimulation leads to differentiation into a more active secretory cell, the osteoblast.

In the mature individual, where remodeling of bone is not occurring, the bone surfaces are covered by a layer of extremely flat cells with very attenuated cytoplasm and a paucity of organelles beyond the perinuclear region (Fig. 8.6a). They do not form a complete cellular lining on the bone surface, but where the lining cell processes contact one another, gap junctions can be found (Fig. 8.6b). These cells, designated simply as ***bone-lining cells,*** are analogous

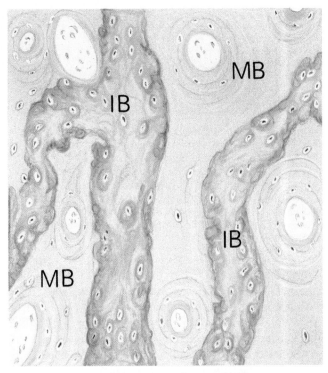

Figure 8.5. Drawing of a low-magnification view of immature bone *(IB)* and mature bone *(MB)* in a hematoxylin and eosin (H&E)-stained section of decalcified bone. The immature bone has more cells, and the matrix is not layered in osteonal arrays.

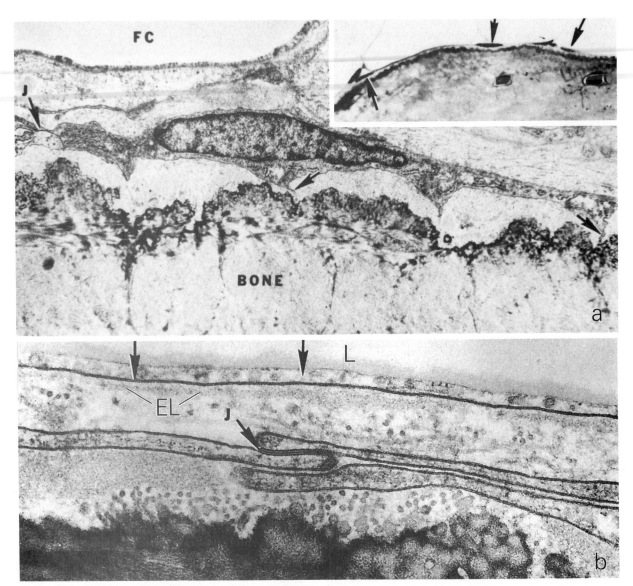

Figure 8.6.   a. Electron micrograph showing portions of two bone-lining cells on the surface of a spicule of mature bone. The cytoplasm is very attenuated and contains small amounts of rER and free ribosomes. A gap junction *(J)* is seen between the two bone-lining cells. In addition, cytoplasmic processes *(arrows)* are clearly seen where they pass through the non-calcified bone matrix (osteoid). A fat cell of the marrow is also present *(FC)*. The **inset** is a high-power light micrograph of a similar bone spicule and is included for orientation purposes. The bone-lining cells on the surface of the spicule are indicated by the *arrows.* Electron micrograph, ×8900; light micrograph, ×700. (From Miller SC, Bowman BM, Smith JM, Jee WSS: *Anatomical Record* 173:163–173, 1980.) **b.** Higher-power electron micrograph of the cytoplasm of two bone-lining cells. The gap junction *(J)* is clearly seen where the two cells come in apposition. The edge of a fat cell is seen at the top of the micrograph; its lipid *(L)*, the thin rim of cytoplasm and plasma membrane *(arrows)*, and external lamina *(EL)* are also evident.

to the osteoprogenitor cells but are probably in a more quiescent state than those located at sites where bone growth is occurring. They are also thought to function in the maintenance and nutritional support of the osteocytes embedded in the underlying bone matrix. This suggested role is based on the observation that cell processes of the bone-lining cells extend into the canalicular channels of the adjacent bone and communicate by means of gap junctions with processes of osteocytes.

The degree of differentiation of the osteoprogenitor cell is not entirely clear. Their derivation from mesenchymal cells and their apparent ability to differentiate into three kinds of cells other than osteoblasts (adipose cells, chondroblasts, and fibroblasts), suggest that they, like the fibroblast, are able to modify their morphologic and functional characteristics in response to specific stimuli. This question is of importance because the healing of fractures of bone involves the formation of new connective tissue and cartilage in the callus that develops around the bone as part of the repair process (see Fractures and Bone Repair, below). Although the precise origin of the cells in healing bone may still be unclear, some evidence indicates that the periosteal cells and the endosteal cells participate in all stages of the healing process.

Osteoblast

The Osteoblast Is the Differentiated Bone-Forming Cell That Secretes Bone Matrix

The osteoblast resembles its close relatives, the fibroblast and the chondroblast, in being a very versatile secretory cell while retaining the ability to divide. It secretes both the collagen and the ground substance that constitutes the initial unmineralized bone or *osteoid.* The osteoblast is also responsible for the calcification of the matrix. The calcification process appears to be initiated by the osteoblast through the secretion into the matrix of small, 50–250-nm, membrane-limited *matrix vesicles.* The vesicles are rich in alkaline phosphatase and are actively secreted only during the period in which the cell is producing the bone matrix. The role of these vesicles is discussed on page 168 under biologic mineralization.

With the light microscope, osteoblasts are recognized by their cuboidal or polygonal shape and their aggregation as a single layer of cells lying in apposition to the forming

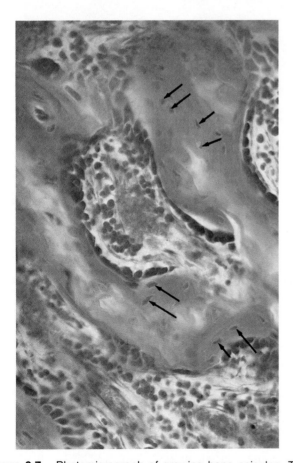

Figure 8.7. Photomicrograph of growing bone spicules. The osteocytes are the small, relatively inconspicuous cells within the bone matrix *(arrows).* The osteoblasts are larger and are on the surfaces of the bone tissue.

bone (Fig. 8.7). Because the newly deposited matrix is not immediately calcified, it stains lightly or not at all, compared with mature mineralized matrix, which stains heavily with eosin. Because of this staining property of the newly formed matrix, the osteoblasts appear to be separated from the bone by a light band. This band represents the osteoid; it is nonmineralized matrix. The cytoplasm of the osteoblast is markedly basophilic, and the Golgi complex, because of its size, is sometimes observed as a clear area adjacent to the nucleus. Small periodic acid-Schiff (PAS)-positive granules are observed in the cytoplasm, and a strong alkaline phosphatase reaction associated with the cell membrane can be detected by appropriate histochemical staining.

Osteoblast Processes Communicate With Other Osteoblasts and With Osteocytes by Gap Junctions

At the electron microscope level, the osteoblast exhibits very thin cytoplasmic processes that penetrate through the adjacent osteoid that the cell has produced and are joined by gap junctions to similar processes of adjacent osteocytes. It is by this method, i.e., by the early establishment of junctions between the osteoblast and the adjacent osteocyte (as well as between adjacent osteoblasts), that the neighboring cells within the bone tissue communicate.

The cytoplasm of the osteoblast is characterized by abundant rER and free ribosomes (Fig. 8.8). This is consistent with its basophilia, as observed in the light microscope, as well as with its role in the production of collagen and proteoglycans for the extracellular matrix. The Golgi apparatus and surrounding regions of the cytoplasm contain numerous vesicles with a flocculent content that is presumed to be matrix precursors. It is these vesicles that are seen as the PAS-staining granules by light microscopy. The matrix vesicles, also produced by the osteoblast, appear to arise by a different pathway, originating as sphere-like outgrowths that pinch off from the plasma membrane to become free in the matrix. Other cell organelles include numerous rod-shaped mitochondria and occasional dense bodies and lysosomes.

Osteocyte

The Osteocyte, the Mature Bone Cell, Is Enclosed by Bone Matrix That It Previously Secreted as an Osteoblast

The osteocyte is a differentiated osteoblast. Osteocytes are responsible for maintaining the bone matrix. They have the capacity to synthesize matrix, as well to resorb it, at least to a limited extent. Such activities are important in contributing to the homeostasis of blood calcium. Death of the *osteocytes,* either through trauma, e.g., a fracture, or cell senescence, results in resorption of the bone matrix by *osteoclast* activity, followed by repair or remodeling of the bone tissue by osteoblast activity.

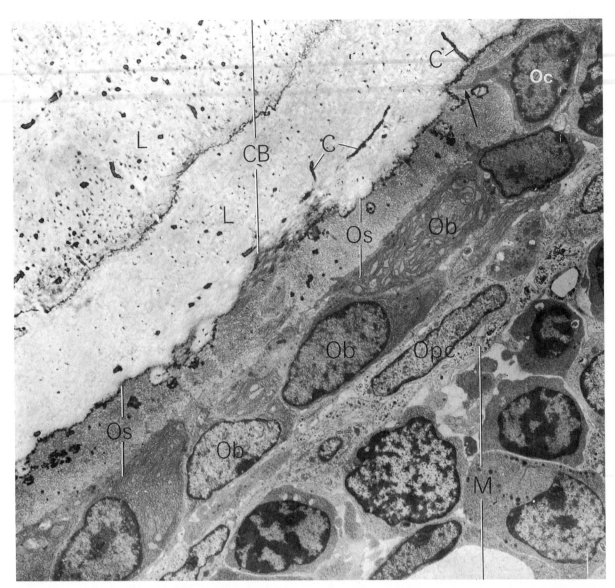

Figure 8.8. Electron micrograph showing active bone formation comparable with that seen in the preceding light micrograph, Figure 8.7. The marrow cavity *(M)* with its developing blood cells is seen in the lower right corner of the micrograph. Osteoprogenitor cells *(Opc)* are evident between the marrow and the osteoblasts *(Ob)*. They exhibit elongate or ovoid nuclei. The osteoblasts are aligned along the growing portion of the bone, which is composed of osteoid *(Os)*. In this same region, one of the cells (upper right corner) embedded within the osteoid exhibits a small process *(arrow)*. This cell, because of its location within the osteoid, can now be called an osteocyte *(Oc)*. The remainder of the micrograph (upper left) is composed of calcified bone matrix *(CB)*. Within the matrix are canaliculi *(C)* containing osteocyte processes. The boundary between two adjacent lamellae *(L)* of previously formed bone is evident as an irregular dark line. ×9000.

Each osteocyte occupies a space or *lacuna* that conforms to the lenticular shape of the cell. The osteocytes extend cytoplasmic processes through the fine tunnels or canaliculi in the matrix to contact, by means of gap junctions, processes of neighboring cells. In hematoxylin and eosin (H&E)-stained sections, the canaliculi and the processes they contain are not discernible; in ground sections, the canaliculi are evident. The osteocyte is typically smaller than its precursor, due to its reduced perinuclear cytoplasm. Often, in routinely prepared microscopic specimens, the cell is highly distorted due to shrinkage and other artefacts that result from

decalcifying the bone matrix in order to section the bone. In such instances, the nucleus may be the only prominent feature.

In well-preserved specimens, osteocytes usually exhibit less cytoplasmic basophilia than osteoblasts, but little additional cytoplasmic detail can be seen. By means of electron microscopy, variations in the functional state of the cell are recognized. Indeed, there is evidence that the osteocyte is able to modify the surrounding bone matrix through synthetic and reabsorptive activities. Three functional states, each with a characteristic morphology, can be described:

- *Quiescent osteocytes* exhibit a paucity of rER and a markedly diminished Golgi complex (Fig. 8.9a). An osmiophilic lamina representing mature calcified matrix is seen in close apposition to the cell membrane.
- *Formative osteocytes* show evidence of matrix deposition and exhibit certain characteristics similar to osteoblasts. Thus, the rER and Golgi are more abundant, and there is evidence of osteoid in the pericellular space within the lacuna (Fig. 8.9b).
- *Resorptive osteocytes,* like formative osteocytes, contain numerous profiles of endoplasmic reticulum and a well-developed Golgi. Moreover, secondary lysosomes are conspicuous (Fig. 8.9c).

The concept that the resorptive osteocyte is removing matrix is supported by the observation that the pericellular space is devoid of collagen fibrils and may contain a flocculent material suggestive of a breakdown product. The more peripheral nonresorbed matrix is bounded by an osmiophilic lamina, which presumably represents the boundary of the intact mature calcified matrix. It has been clearly shown that resorption of bone by this mechanism, a process designated as *osteocytic osteolysis,* with the concomitant release of calcium ions, allows for increase of blood calcium to maintain appropriate levels. The stimulus for the resorption of bone is increased secretion of parathyroid hormone.

Osteoclast

The Osteoclast Is a Large Multinucleated Cell Whose Function Is to Resorb Bone

When active, the osteoclast rests directly on the surface of the bone where resorption is to take place (Fig. 8.10). As a result of its activity, a shallow bay called a *Howship's lacuna* or a *resorption bay* is formed in the bone directly under the osteoclast. The cell is conspicuous not only because of its size but also because of its marked acidophilia. It also exhibits a strong histochemical reaction for acid phosphatase due to the numerous lysosomes that it contains.

The portion of the cell directly in contact with the bone can be divided into two parts: a central region containing numerous plasma membrane infoldings forming microvillous-type structures, called the *ruffled border,* and a ring-like perimeter of cytoplasm, the *clear zone,* that more or less demarcates the limits of the bone area being resorbed. The clear zone contains abundant microfilaments but is essentially lacking in other organelles. The ruffled border stains less intensely than the remainder of the cell and often appears as a light band adjacent to the bone at the resorption site (Fig. 8.10).

At the electron microscopic level, hydroxyapatite crystals from the bone substance are observed between the processes of the ruffled border (see Plate 24, page 187). Internal to the ruffled border, but in close proximity, are numerous mitochondria and lysosomes. The nuclei are typically in the part of the cell more removed from the bone surface. In this same region are profiles of rER, multiple stacks of Golgi saccules, and many vesicles.

Osteoclasts Release Lysosomes Into the Extracellular Space

Some, if not most, of the vesicles in the osteoclast are lysosomes that arise from the Golgi. They are released into the extracellular space in the clefts between the cytoplasmic processes of the ruffled border; this is a clear example of lysosomal hydrolases functioning outside of the cell. Once liberated, the hydrolytic enzymes, which include collagenase, digest the organic components of the bone matrix. Before this can occur, however, it is necessary to decalcify the bone matrix. Current evidence indicates that the dissolution of the calcium salts occurs through secretion of organic acids by the membranes of the ruffled border. Moreover, a low pH favors the action of acid hydrolyses. Accordingly, a local acidic environment is created in the extracellular space between the bone and the osteoclast. The clear zone adjacent to the ruffled border seems to create a seal against the bone, thus creating a compartment at the site of the ruffled border where the focal decalcification and degradation of the matrix occurs. Support for the concept of acid secretion by the osteoclast comes, in part, from the finding that carbonic anhydrase, an enzyme associated with carbonic acid production, is present in the region of the ruffled border.

Osteoclasts Are Phagocytic

In addition to the ruffled border being the site of hydrolytic enzyme release and acid secretion, numerous coated pits and coated vesicles are also present at this site, suggesting endocytic activity. Osteoclasts are observed at sites where bone remodeling is in progress. (The process or remodeling is described in more detail shortly.) Thus, in sites where osteons are being altered or where a bone is undergoing change during the growth process, osteoclasts are relatively numerous and are easily found. As already noted, an increase in parathyroid hormone level promotes bone resorption and has a demonstrable effect on osteoclast activity, in addition to its effects on osteocytes, described above. In contrast, calcitonin, secreted by parafollicular cells of the thyroid gland (see page 606), has a counterbalancing effect, reducing osteoclast activity. Little is known, however, concerning the role of endocrine activity in normal bone remodeling during growth.

Osteoclasts are unrelated to the bone-forming cells, contrary to what was once thought. They arise from monocytes and acquire their multinucleate form either by repeated DNA replications and nuclear divisions without subsequent cell divisions or by the fusion of many monocytes or developing osteoclasts. In both their origin and their function, they are

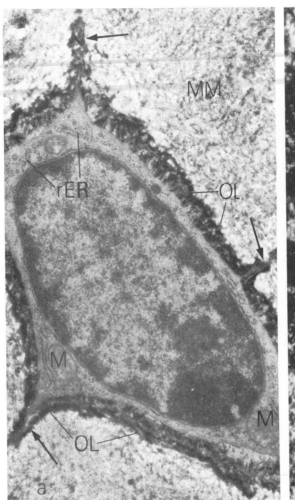

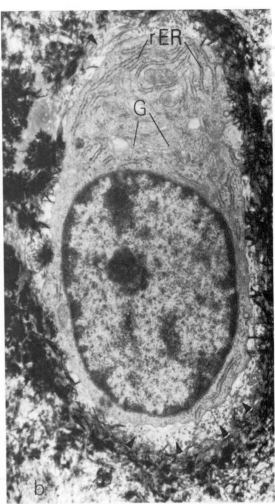

Figure 8.9. Electron micrographs of three osteocytes representing different functional states. In **a,** the osteocyte is relatively quiescent. It exhibits only a few profiles of rER and a few mitochondria *(M).* The cell virtually fills the lacuna that it occupies; the *arrows* indicate where cytoplasmic processes extend into canaliculi. Hydroxyapatite crystals have been lost from the matrix, which is ordinarily mineralized *(MM),* but some hydroxyapatite crystals fill the pericellular space. The hydroxyapatite crystals obscure the other substances within the peri- cellular space. The dark band marking the boundary of the lacuna is the osmiophilic lamina *(OL).* In **b,** the cell is a formative osteocyte. It shows larger amounts of rER and a large Golgi profile *(G).* Of equal importance is the presence of a small amount of osteoid in the pericellular space within the lacuna. The osteoid shows profiles of collagen fibrils *(arrowheads, lower right of figure)* not yet mineralized. The lacuna of a formative osteocyte is not bounded by an osmiophilic lamina.

closely related to other macrophages. Morphologically, they resemble the Langhans' giant cells formed by fusion of tissue macrophages (histiocytes) in loose connective tissue.

BONE FORMATION

Bone formation is a complex process that is sometimes difficult to understand if an adequate distinction is not made between the development of bone as an organ and the histogenesis of bone tissue.

The Development of a Bone Is Traditionally Classified as Endochondral or Intramembranous

The distinction between endochondral and intramembranous formation rests on whether a cartilage model serves as the precursor of the bone (endochondral ossification) or whether the bone is formed by a simpler method, without the intervention of a cartilage precursor (intramembranous ossification). The bones of the extremities and those parts of the axial skeleton that bear weight (e.g., vertebrae) develop by endochondral ossification. The flat bones of the skull and face, the mandible, and the clavicle develop by intramembranous ossification.

The separate labels for types of bone or bone tissue should not be taken to mean existing bone is either membrane bone or endochondral bone. These names refer *only* to the mechanism by which a bone is initially formed. Because of the remodeling that occurs later, the initial bone tissue that was laid down by endochondral formation or by intramembranous formation is soon replaced. The replacement bone is established on the preexisting bone by appositional growth

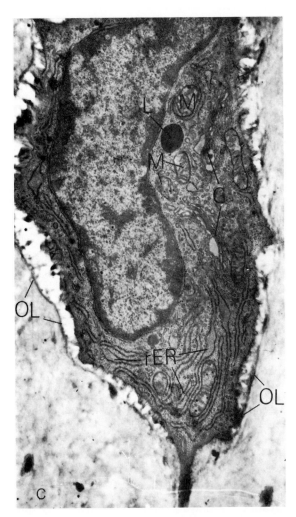

Figure 8.9. c. In **c**, the cell is a resorptive osteocyte. It contains a substantial amount of rER, a large Golgi *(G)*, mitochondria *(M)*, and lysosomes *(L)*. The pericellular space is devoid of collagen fibrils and may contain some flocculent material. The lacuna containing a resorptive osteocyte is bounded by an osmiophilic lamina *(OL)*.

and is identical in both cases. Although the long bones are classified as forming by endochondral formation, their continued growth involves the histogenesis of endochondral bone and the histogenesis of intramembranous bone, with the latter occurring through the activity of the periosteal (membrane) tissue.

Intramembranous Ossification

In Intramembranous Ossification, Bone Is Formed by Differentiation of Mesenchymal Cells Into Osteoblasts

The first evidence of intramembranous ossification occurs around the eighth week of gestation in the human. Some of the pale-staining elongate mesenchymal cells within the mesenchyme migrate and aggregate in specific areas, the sites where bone is destined to form. This condensation of cells within the mesenchymal tissue is the membrane referred to in the term intramembranous ossification (Fig.

8.11). As the process continues, the newly organized tissue at the presumptive bone site becomes more vascularized, and the aggregated mesenchymal cells become larger and rounded. The cytoplasm of the mesenchymal cells changes from eosinophilic to basophilic, and a clear Golgi area becomes evident. These cytologic changes result in the differentiated osteoblast, which then secretes the collagen and proteoglycans of the bone matrix (osteoid). The osteoblasts within the bone matrix become increasingly separated from one another as the matrix is produced, but they remain attached by thin cytoplasmic processes. Because of the abundant collagen content, the bone matrix appears more dense than the surrounding mesenchyme in which the intercellular spaces reveal only delicate connective tissue fibers.

Newly Formed Bone Matrix Appears in Histologic Sections as Small, Irregularly Shaped Spicules and Trabeculae

With time, the matrix becomes calcified, and the interconnecting cytoplasmic processes of the bone-forming cells, now termed osteocytes, are contained within canaliculi.

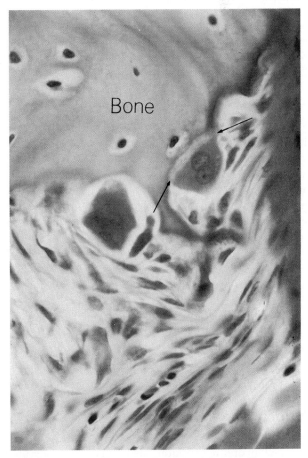

Figure 8.10. Photomicrograph of bone tissue where resorption is taking place. Two osteoclasts are evident. Note that each cell exhibits several nuclei. One of the osteoclasts is in close apposition to the bone, and the site of the ruffled border can be seen between the *arrows*. Also, note the osteocytes in the bone tissue in the region.

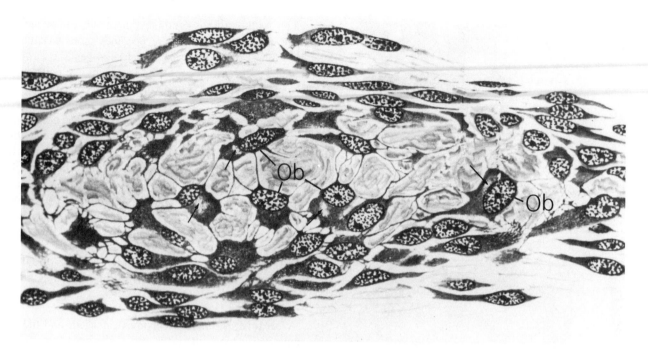

Figure 8.11. Initial stage in the development of intramembranous bone as seen in the skull of a cat embryo. The *central area* shows densely aggregated collagenous fibers (osteoid) that will become the bone matrix on later calcification. The cells in the middle of this matrix are osteoblasts *(Ob)*. They are relatively large cells that exhibit basophilic cytoplasm and a large Golgi area *(arrows)*. The osteoblasts exhibit fine cytoplasmic processes that join with the processes of their neighbors. Peripheral to these cells are other more elongate cells that are in the process of differentiating into osteoblasts. At the very periphery are those cells that have much smaller elongate nuclei with very thin cytoplasmic processes extending from each end of the nucleus of the cell. They are the least differentiated cells and resemble a fibroblast. The extracellular fibers in the vicinity of these cells are delicate and sparse. (Modified from a drawing by A. A. Maximow.)

Concomitantly, more of the surrounding primitive cells in the membrane proliferate, giving rise to a population of what may now be regarded as osteoprogenitor cells. Some of the osteoprogenitor cells come into apposition with the initially formed spicules, become osteoblasts, and add more matrix. By this method, *appositional growth,* the spicules enlarge and become joined in a trabecular network having the general shape of the developing bone.

Through continued mitotic activity, the osteoprogenitor cells maintain their numbers and thus provide a constant source of osteoblasts for growth of the bone spicules. The new osteoblasts, in turn, lay down bone matrix in successive layers, giving rise to woven bone. This immature bone, discussed on page 153, is characterized internally by interconnecting spaces occupied by connective tissue and blood vessels. Bone tissue formed by the method just described is referred to as *membrane bone* or *intramembranous bone.*

Endochondral Ossification

Endochondral ossification, also, begins with the proliferation and aggregation of mesenchymal cells at the site of the future bone. However, the mesenchymal cells differentiate into chondroblasts that, in turn, produce cartilage matrix.

The Hyaline Cartilage Produced at This Early Stage Acquires the General Shape of the Bone That Will Be Formed; i.e., It Is a Cartilage Model

The cartilage model, once established, grows by interstitial as well as appositional growth. Most of the increase in length of the cartilage model can be attributed to interstitial growth. The increase in its width is largely by addition of cartilage matrix produced by new chondrocytes that differentiate from the chondrogenic layer of perichondrium surrounding the cartilage mass. Illustrations *1* and *1a* of Figure 8.12 show an early cartilage model.

The First Sign of Ossification Is the Appearance of a Cuff of Bone Around the Cartilage Model

The perichondral cells in the midregion of the cartilage model no longer give rise to chondrocytes. Instead, bone-forming cells or osteoblasts are produced. Thus, the connective tissue surrounding the middle of the cartilage is no longer functionally a perichondrium; rather, because of its altered role, it is now called periosteum. Moreover, we may now describe an osteogenic layer within the periosteum because the cells within this layer are differentiating into osteoblasts. As a result of these changes, a thin layer of bone is formed around the cartilage model. We may describe this

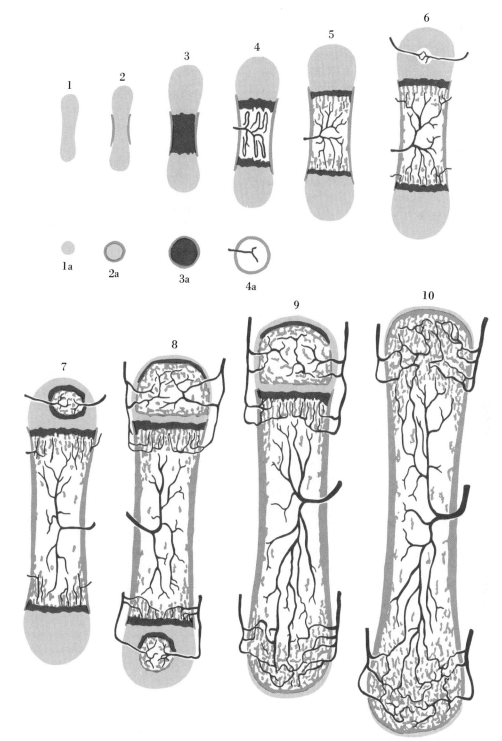

Figure 8.12. Schematic diagram of development of a long bone. Illustrations **1–10** depict longitudinal sections; **1a–4a** depict cross sections through the shaft of the bone. The process begins with the formation of a cartilage model (**1** and **1a**); next, a periosteal (perichondrial) collar of bone forms about the diaphysis (shaft) of the cartilage model (**2** and **2a**); then, the cartilaginous matrix in the diaphysis begins to calcify (**3** and **3a**). Blood vessels and connective tissue cells then erode and invade the calcified cartilage (**4** and **4a**), creating a primitive marrow cavity in which remnant spicules of calcified cartilage remain at the two ends of the cavity. Endochondral bone forms on these spicules of calcified cartilage. The bone at the ends of the developing marrow cavity constitutes the metaphysis. Periosteal bone continues to form; the periosteal bone is intramembranous bone. It can be recognized histologically be-

cause it is not accompanied by local cartilage erosion, nor is the bone deposited on spicules of calcified cartilage. Blood vessels and perivascular cells invade the upper epiphyseal cartilage **(6)**, and a secondary center of ossification is established in the upper epiphysis **(7)**. A similar epiphyseal ossification center forms at the lower end of the bone **(8)**, and an epiphyseal disc or plate is thus formed between each epiphysis and the diaphysis. With continued growth of the long bone, the lower epiphyseal plate disappears **(9)**, and finally, with cessation of growth, the upper epiphyseal plate disappears **(10)**. The metaphysis then becomes continuous with the epiphysis. Epiphyseal lines remain where the epiphyseal plate last existed. (From Bloom W, Fawcett DW: *A Textbook of Histology,* 10th ed. Philadelphia, WB Saunders, 1975, p 266.)

bone as either periosteal bone, because of its location, or as intramembranous bone, because of its method of development. In the case of a long bone, a distinctive cuff of periosteal bone, the bony collar, is established around the cartilage model in what can be described as the diaphyseal portion of the developing bone. This is shown in illustrations 2 and 2a of Figure 8.12.

With the Establishment of the Periosteal Bony Collar, the Chondrocytes in This Midregion of the Cartilage Model Become Hypertrophic

As the chondrocytes enlarge, their surrounding cartilage matrix becomes compressed, forming thin irregular cartilage plates between the hypertrophic cells. The hypertrophic cells begin to synthesize alkaline phosphatase, and concomitantly, the surrounding cartilage matrix undergoes calcification; see illustrations 3 and 3a of Figure 8.12. The calcification of the cartilage matrix is not to be confused with calcification that occurs in bone tissue.

The Calcified Cartilage Matrix Inhibits Diffusion of Nutrients, Causing Death of the Chondrocytes in the Cartilage Model

With the death of the chondrocytes, much of the matrix breaks down, and neighboring lacunae become confluent, producing an increasingly large cavity. While these events are occurring, one or several blood vessels grow through the thin diaphyseal bony collar to vascularize the cavity; see illustrations 4 and 4a of Figure 8.12.

Periosteal Cells Migrate Into the Cavity Along With Growing Blood Vessels

Cells from the periosteum migrate with the penetrating blood vessels and some of the primitive periosteal cells to become osteoprogenitor cells in the cavity. Other primitive cells also gain access to the cavity via the new vasculature, leaving the circulation to give rise to the marrow. As the calcified cartilage breaks down and is partially removed, some remains as irregular spicules. When the osteoprogenitor cells come in apposition to the remaining calcified cartilage spicules, they become osteoblasts and begin to lay down bone (osteoid) on the spicule framework. Thus, the bone formed in this manner is endochondral bone. The combination of the bone, which is initially only a thin layer, and the underlying calcified cartilage is described as a *mixed spicule.*

Histologically, mixed spicules can be recognized by virtue of their staining characteristics. Calcified cartilage tends to be basophilic, whereas bone is distinctly eosinophilic. Such spicules persist for a short time before the calcified cartilage component is removed. The remaining bone component of the spicule may continue to grow by appositional growth, thus becoming larger and stronger, or it may undergo resorption as new spicules are being formed.

Growth of Endochondral Bone

Endochondral Bone Growth Begins in the Second Trimester of Fetal Life and Continues Into Early Adulthood

The events described above represent the early stage of endochondral bone formation as seen in the fetus, beginning at about the 12th week of gestation. The continuing growth process, which takes place throughout the growing period of the individual into early adulthood, is now described.

The Continued Growth of Long Bones Is Dependent on the Presence of *Epiphyseal Cartilage* Throughout the Growth Period

As the diaphyseal marrow cavity enlarges (see illustration 5 of Fig. 8.12), a distinct zonation can be recognized in the cartilage at either end of the cavity. This remaining cartilage, referred to as *epiphyseal cartilage,* exhibits distinct zones as illustrated in Figure 8.13. The zones in the epiphyseal cartilage, beginning with that most distal to the diaphyseal center of ossification and proceeding toward that center, are

- **Zone of reserve cartilage,** which exhibits no cellular proliferation or active matrix production.
- **Zone of proliferation,** which is adjacent to the zone of reserve cartilage in the direction of the diaphysis. In this zone, the cartilage cells undergo division and are organized into distinct columns. These cells are larger than those in the reserve zone and are actively producing matrix.
- **Zone of hypertrophy,** which contains cartilage cells that are greatly enlarged. Their cytoplasm is clear, a reflection of the glycogen that they normally accumulate (and that is lost during fixation), and the matrix is compressed into linear bands between the columns of hypertrophied cartilage cells.
- **Zone of calcified cartilage,** in which the enlarged cells begin to degenerate and the matrix becomes calcified.
- **Zone of resorption,** which is the zone nearest the diaphysis. The cartilage here is in direct contact with the connective tissue of the marrow cavity.

In the zone of resorption, small blood vessels and accompanying connective tissue invade the region occupied by the dying chondrocytes. They form a series of spearheads, leaving the calcified cartilage as longitudinal spicules, at least as seen in a longitudinal section of the bone. Actually, in a cross section of the bone the cartilage would appear as a honeycomb because the invading vessels and connective tissue migrate into the sites previously occupied by the cartilage cells.

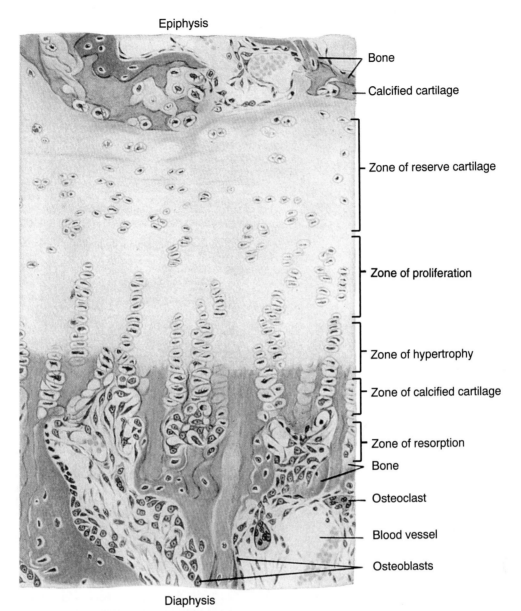

Epiphysis

Bone
Calcified cartilage
Zone of reserve cartilage
Zone of proliferation
Zone of hypertrophy
Zone of calcified cartilage
Zone of resorption
Bone
Osteoclast
Blood vessel
Osteoblasts

Diaphysis

Figure 8.13. Longitudinal section through the distal end of a metatarsal bone of a 2-month infant. The epiphyseal (secondary) ossification center is well formed. Bone formation is taking place at both the epiphyseal and the diaphyseal surface of the epiphyseal plate. The zonation is apparent on the diaphyseal side because the growth rate there is so much greater than the epiphyseal ossification center. Because both centers are active, the zone of reserve cartilage is relatively normal. H&E ×256. (From Copenhaver WM (ed): *Bailey's Textbook of Histology,* 15th ed. Baltimore, Williams & Wilkins, 1964, fig. 6.24.)

Bone Deposition Occurs on the Cartilage Spicules in the Same Manner as Described for the Formation of the Initial Ossification Center

As bone is laid down on the calcified spicules, the cartilage is resorbed, ultimately leaving a primary spongy bone. This spongy bone undergoes reorganization through osteoclastic activity and addition of new bone tissue, thus accommodating to the continued growth and physical stresses placed on the bone.

Shortly after birth, a secondary ossification center develops in the upper epiphysis. The cartilage cells hypertrophy and degenerate. As in the diaphysis, calcification of the matrix occurs, and blood vessels and osteogenic cells from the perichondrium invade the region, creating a new marrow cavity; see illustrations *6* and *7* of Figure 8.12. Later, a similar epiphyseal ossification center forms at the lower end of the bone; see illustration *8* of Figure 8.12. This, too, is regarded as a secondary ossification center, although it develops later. With the development of the secondary ossification centers, the only cartilage that remains from the original model is the articular cartilage at the ends of the bone and a transverse disc, known as the ***epiphyseal plate,*** that separates the epiphyseal and diaphyseal cavities.

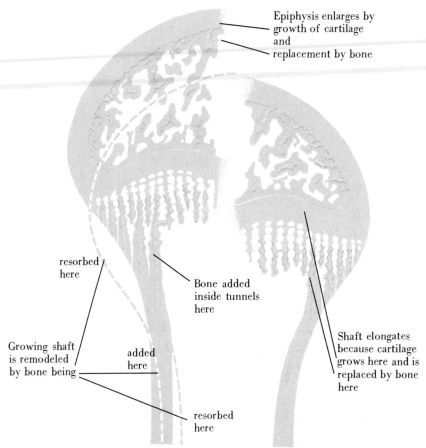

Epiphysis enlarges by
growth of cartilage
and
replacement by bone

resorbed
here

Bone added
inside tunnels
here

Shaft elongates
because cartilage
grows here and is
replaced by bone
here

Growing shaft
is remodeled
by bone being

added
here

resorbed
here

Figure 8.14.   Diagram of external remodeling of a long bone, showing two periods during the growth of the bone. The younger bone profile is shown on the right; the older, on the left. Superimposed on the left side of the figure is the shape of the bone (left half only) as it appeared at the earlier time. The bone is now longer, but it has retained its general shape. To grow in length and retain the general shape of the particular bone, bone resorption occurs on some surfaces, and bone deposition occurs on other surfaces, as indicated in the diagram. (Based on Ham AW: *The Journal of Bone and Joint Surgery* 34A:701, 1952.)

The Cartilage of the Epiphyseal Plate Is Responsible for Maintaining the Growth Process

For a bone to retain proper proportions and its unique shape, external as well as internal remodeling must occur as the bone grows in length. The proliferative zone of the epiphyseal plate gives rise to the cartilage on which bone is later laid down.

• The thickness of the epiphyseal plate remains relatively constant during growth.
• The amount of new cartilage produced (zone of proliferation) equals the amount resorbed (zone of resorption).
• The resorbed cartilage is, of course, replaced by spongy bone.

In reviewing the growth process, it is important to realize that

• *Actual lengthening of the bone occurs when new cartilage matrix is produced at the epiphyseal plate.* This has the effect of pushing the epiphysis away from the diaphysis, thus causing elongation of the bone. The events that follow this incremental growth, namely, hypertrophy, calcification, resorption, and ossification, simply involve the mechanism by which the newly formed cartilage is replaced by bone tissue during development.
• *Increase in width or diameter of the bone occurs when appositional growth of new bone occurs between the cortical lamellae and the periosteum.* The marrow cavity then enlarges by resorption of bone on the endosteal surface of the cortex of the bone.

As Bones Elongate, Remodeling Is Required

Remodeling consists of preferential resorption of bone in some areas and deposition of bone in other areas, as described above and outlined in Figure 8.14. The histologic features of intramembranous and endochondral bone formation are considered further in Plates 19–23, pages 176–185.

Брянск

Cessation of Growth

When an Individual Achieves Maximal Growth, Proliferation of New Cartilage Within the Growing Bones Terminates

When proliferation of new cartilage ceases, the cartilage that has already been produced in the epiphyseal plate continues to undergo the changes that lead to the deposition of new bone until, finally, there is no remaining cartilage. At this point, the epiphyseal and diaphyseal marrow cavities become confluent. The elimination of the epiphyseal plate is referred to as *epiphyseal closure.* In illustration *9* of Figure 8.12, the lower epiphyseal cartilage is no longer present, and in illustration *10,* both epiphyseal cartilages are gone. Growth is now complete, and the only remaining cartilage is found on the articular surfaces of the bone. Vestigial evidence of the site of the epiphyseal plate is reflected by an *epiphyseal line,* consisting of bone tissue (see Fig. 8.2).

NUTRITIONAL FACTORS IN BONE FORMATION

Both nutritional and hormonal factors affect the degree of bone mineralization. It has long been known that calcium deficiency during growth causes **rickets,** a condition in which the bone matrix does not calcify normally. Rickets may be due to insufficient amounts of dietary calcium or to insufficient vitamin D (a steroid prohormone), which is needed for absorption of calcium by the intestines. In the adult, the same nutritional or vitamin deficiency leads to **osteomalacia.**

Although rickets and osteomalacia are no longer major problems where nutrition is adequate, another form of insufficient bone mineralization is regularly seen in the condition known as **osteoporosis.** In this condition, bone tissue (both mineral and matrix) is diminished, presumably because resorption by osteoclasts exceeds deposition by osteoblasts. Osteoporosis develops as a consequence of immobilization (as in a bedridden patient) and in postmenopausal women. The factors that bring on the imbalance in cellular activity are not known, although some relief appears to result from maintaining hormonal (estrogen) levels and dietary fluoride levels.

In addition to its influence on intestinal absorption of calcium, vitamin D is also needed for normal calcification. Other vitamins long known to affect bone are A and C. Vitamin A deficiency results in a suppression of endochondral growth of bone; vitamin A excess leads to fragility and subsequent fractures of long bones. Vitamin C is essential for syntheses of collagen, and its deficiency leads to scurvy. The matrix produced in scurvy is not calcifiable.

Development of the Osteonal System (Haversian System)

Osteons Typically Develop in Preexisting Compact Bone

The compact bone might have formed from fetal spongy bone by continued deposition of bone on the spongy bone spicules, it might have been deposited directly as adult compact bone, e.g., the circumferential lamellae of an adult bone, or it might be older compact bone consisting of osteons and interstitial lamellae.

In the Development of New Osteons, a Tunnel Is Bored Through the Compact Bone by Osteoclasts

When the osteoclasts have produced an appropriately sized cylindrical tunnel by resorption of compact bone, blood vessels and their surrounding connective tissue occupy the tunnel. As the tunnel is occupied, new bone deposition on its wall begins almost immediately. These two aspects of cellular activity, namely, osteoclast resorption and osteoblast synthesis, constitute a *bone-remodeling* unit. There are two distinct parts to the bone-remodeling unit: an advancing *cutting cone* (also called a *resorption canal*) and a *closing cone.* The cutting cone consists of active osteoclasts followed by an advancing capillary loop and pericytes. It also contains numerous cells in mitosis. These give rise to osteoblasts, additional pericytes, and endothelial cells. (Recall that the osteoclasts derive from blood-borne monocytes.) The osteoclasts cut a canal about 200 μm in diameter. This canal establishes the diameter of the future osteonal (Haversian) system. The cutting cone constitutes only a small fraction of the length of the bone-remodeling unit; thus, it is seen much less frequently than the closing cone of the developing osteon.

After the diameter of the future Haversian system is established, osteoblasts begin to deposit the organic matrix (osteoid) of bone on the walls of the canal in successive lamellae. With time, the bone matrix in each of the lamellae becomes mineralized. As the successive lamellae of bone are deposited, *from the periphery inward,* the canal ultimately attains the relatively narrow diameter of the adult osteonal canal. This process in which new osteons are formed is referred to as *internal remodeling.*

Compact Adult Bone Contains Haversian Systems of Varying Age and Size

If a ground section of bone is examined microradiographically, it can be seen that younger Haversian systems are less completely mineralized than older systems (Fig. 8.15). They undergo a progressive secondary mineralization that continues (up to a point) even after the osteon has been fully formed. Figure 8.15 also illustrates the dynamic internal remodeling of compact bone. In the adult, deposition balances resorption. In the aged, resorption often exceeds deposition. If this imbalance becomes excessive, osteoporosis develops (see Nutritional Factors in Bone Formation, page 166).

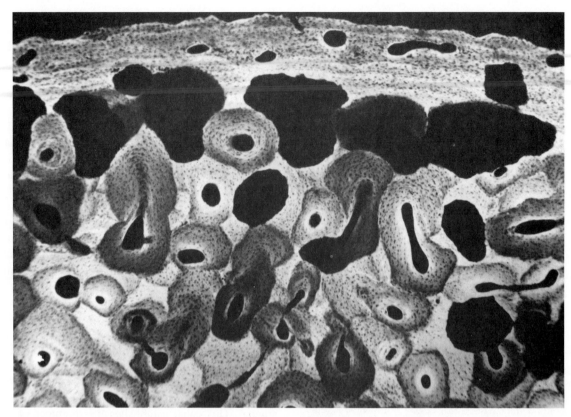

Figure 8.15. Microradiograph of a 200-μm-thick cross section of bone from a normal 19-year-old male. Secondary Haversian bone is actively replacing non-Haversian bone, which is seen on the periosteal (upper) surface. The degree of mineralization is reflected by the shade of light and dark in the microradiograph. Thus, *very light areas* represent the highly mineralized tissue that deflects the x-rays and prevents them from striking the photographic film. Conversely, *dark areas* contain less mineral and, thus, are less effective in deflection of the x-rays. Note how the interstitial areas (the older bone) are very light, whereas some of the Haversian systems are very dark (these are the most newly formed). The Haversian canals appear black, as they represent only soft tissue. ×57. (Courtesy of Dr. J. Jowsey.)

BIOLOGIC MINERALIZATION AND MATRIX VESICLES

Biologic Mineralization Is an Extracellular Event

Mineralization occurs in the extracellular matrices of bone and cartilage and in the dentin, cementum, and enamel of teeth. All of these except enamel contain collagen fibrils and ground substance within the matrix, and mineralization occurs both within the collagen fibrils and external to the collagen fibrils, presumably in relation to components of the ground substance. Enamel mineralization occurs within the extracellular organic matrix secreted by the enamel organ (see page 410). Despite the extracellular location of biologic mineralization and the fact that physicochemical factors are basic to the process, *biologic mineralization is a cell-regulated event.*

In places where mineralization of immature bone, cartilage, dentin, and cementum is initiated, small vesicles called matrix vesicles are seen in the matrix. These vesicles are typically located at some distance from the cells where mineralization is to occur. The vesicles measure about 100 nm in diameter; they are formed by exocytosis from the cells that secrete the mineralized matrix tissue (osteoblasts, chondrocytes, odontoblasts, etc.). Matrix vesicles contain alkaline phosphatase and other enzymes that are responsible for loading the vesicle with calcium and phosphate. Subsequently, the loaded matrix vesicle ruptures, producing an increase in local concentration of mineral sufficient to initiate mineralization.

BONE AS A CALCIUM RESERVOIR

Bone Serves as a Reservoir for Body Calcium

The maintenance of normal blood calcium levels is critical to health and life. Calcium may be removed from the bone matrix to the blood if the circulating levels of calcium fall. Conversely, excess blood calcium may be removed from the blood and stored in the bone.

These processes are regulated by *parathormone (parathyroid hormone),* secreted by the parathyroid gland (see page 608), and by *calcitonin,* secreted by the parafollicular cells of the thyroid gland (see page 606).

- *Parathormone* acts on the bone to *raise low blood calcium levels* to normal.
- *Calcitonin* acts to *reduce elevated blood calcium levels* to normal.

Parathormone stimulates both osteocytes and osteoclasts to resorb bone, thus releasing calcium to the blood. As described earlier, resorption of bone by osteocytes constitutes *osteocytic osteolysis.* Parathormone also reduces excretion of calcium by the kidney and stimulates absorption of calcium by the small intestine. Parathormone further acts to maintain homeostasis by stimulating the kidney to excrete the excess phosphate produced by bone resorption. Calcitonin inhibits bone resorption, specifically inhibiting the parathyroid hormone effects on osteoclasts.

HORMONAL REGULATION OF BONE GROWTH

Hormones other than parathyroid hormone and calcitonin have major effects on bone growth. One of these is *somatotropin* (pituitary growth hormone). This hormone stimulates growth in general and, especially, growth of epiphyseal cartilage and bone. Oversecretion in childhood leads to gigantism, which is an abnormal increase in the length of bones; absence or hyposecretion of somatotropin in childhood leads to a failure of growth of the long bones, resulting in pituitary dwarfism.

Oversecretion of growth hormone in an adult leads to *acromegaly,* an abnormal thickening and selective overgrowth of hands, feet, mandible, nose, and intramembranous bones of the skull. Absence or severe hyposecretion of thyroid hormone during development and infancy (cretinism) also leads to failure of bone growth and dwarfism.

FRACTURES AND BONE REPAIR

The initial response to a fracture is similar to the response to any injury that produces tissue destruction and hemorrhage. Neutrophils are the first cells to arrive on the scene, followed by macrophages that clean up the site of injury. Fibroblasts and capillaries then proliferate and grow into the site o f injury. New loose connective tissue, **granulation tissue,** is formed, and as this tissue becomes denser, cartilage forms in parts of it. Both fibroblasts and periosteal cells participate in this phase of the healing process. The dense connective tissue and newly formed cartilage grow, covering the bone at the fracture site and producing what is known as a ***callus.*** A callus will form whether or not the fractured parts of the bone are in apposition to each other, either because they were not displaced or because they were reapproximated, i.e., *set* by a physician. The callus helps stabilize and bind together the fractured bone.

Even while the callus is forming, osteoprogenitor cells of the periosteum divide and differentiate into osteoblasts. The newly formed osteoblasts begin to deposit new bone on the outer surface of the bone at some distance from the fracture.

This new formation of bone progresses toward the fracture site until new bone forms a bony sheath over the fibrocartilaginous callus. Osteogenic buds from the new bone invade the callus and begin to deposit new bone within the callus, gradually replacing the original fibrous and cartilaginous callus with a **bony callus.** The cartilage in the original callus calcifies and is replaced by bone as in endochondral ossification.

Endosteal proliferation and differentiation also occur in the marrow cavity, and medullary bone grows from both ends of the fracture toward the center. When this bone unites, the bony union of the fractured bone produced by the osteoblasts derived from both the periosteum and endosteum is spongy bone. As in normal bone formation, the spongy bone is gradually replaced by compact bone. While this is taking place, the bony callus is removed by the action of osteoclasts, and gradual remodeling restores the bone to its original shape.

In healthy individuals, this process usually takes from 6–12 weeks, depending on the severity of the break and the particular bone that is broken. Setting the bone, i.e., reapproximating the normal structure, and holding the parts in place by internal fixation (pins, screws, or plates) or by external fixation (by a cast or by pins and screws) will speed the healing process and will usually result in superior structural and functional restoration.

PLATE 16.   Bone, Ground Section

Ground sections are prepared by removing as much soft tissue and organic matter from the bone as possible and allowing the bone to dry. Thin slices of bone are then cut with a saw. The slices are ground to adequate thinness to be viewed through the microscope. The specimen may be treated with India ink to define the spaces that were formerly occupied by organic matter, e.g., cells and other soft tissue components. A simpler method involves mounting the ground specimen on the slide with a viscous balsam medium that keeps air imprisoned in the spaces. In the specimen in this plate, prepared by this method, some of the Haversian canals and the Volkmann's canal are filled with the mounting medium, making them translucent instead of black. Specimens prepared in this manner are of value chiefly to display the architecture of the compact bone.

FIGURE 1, ground bone, human, ×80. This figure reveals a cross-sectioned area of a long bone at low power and includes the outer or peripheral aspect of the bone, identified by the presence of circumferential lamellae *(CL)*. (The exterior or periosteal surface of the bone is not included in the micrograph.) To their right are the osteons *(O)* or Haversian systems that appear as circular profiles. Between the osteons are interstitial lamellae *(IL)*, the remnants of previously existing osteons.

Osteons are essentially cylindrical structures. In the shaft of a long bone, the long axes of the osteons are oriented parallel to the long axis of the bone. Thus, a cross section through the shaft of a long bone would reveal the osteons in cross section, as in this figure. At the center of each osteon is an osteonal (Haversian) canal *(HC)* that contains blood vessels, connective tissue, and cells lining the surface of the bone material. Because the organic material is not retained in ground sections, the Haversian canals and other spaces will appear black, as they do here, if filled with India ink or air. Concentric layers of mineralized substance, the concentric lamellae, surround the Haversian canal and appear much the same as growth rings of a tree. The canal is also surrounded by concentric arrangements of lacunae. These appear as the small, dark, elongate structures.

During the period of bone growth and during adult life, there is constant internal remodeling of bone. This involves the destruction of osteons and formation of new ones. The breakdown of an osteon is usually not complete, however; part of the osteon may remain intact. Moreover, portions of adjacent osteons may also be partially destroyed. The space created by the breakdown process is reoccupied by a new osteon. The remnants of the previously existing osteons become the interstitial lamellae.

Blood vessels reach the Haversian canals from the marrow through other tunnels called perforating (Volkmann's) canals. In some instances, Volkmann's canals travel from one Haversian canal to another *(VC)*. Volkmann's canals can be distinguished from Haversian canals in that they pass through lamellae, whereas Haversian canals are surrounded by concentric rings of lamellae.

FIGURE 2, ground bone, human, ×300. This figure shows a higher power of the labeled osteon from the upper left of Figure 1. It includes some of the circumferential lamellae (here labeled *IL*) that are now seen at the bottom of the micrograph (the micrograph has been reoriented). Note the lacunae *(L)* and the fine thread-like profiles emanating from the lacunae. These thread-like profiles represent the canaliculi, spaces within the bone matrix that contained cytoplasmic processes of the osteocyte. The canaliculi of each lacuna communicate with canaliculi of neighboring lacunae to form a three-dimensional channel system throughout the bone.

FIGURE 3, ground bone, human, ×400. In a still higher magnification, the circumferential lamellae are found around the shaft of the long bone at the outer as well as the inner surface of the bone. The osteoblasts that contribute to the formation of circumferential lamellae at these sites come from the periosteum and endosteum, respectively, whereas the osteons are constructed from osteoblasts in the canal of the developing Haversian system. This figure reveals not only the canaliculi but also the lamellae of the bone. The latter are just barely defined by the faint lines *(arrows)* that extend across the micrograph. Collagenous fibers in neighboring lamellae are oriented in different directions. This change in orientation accounts for the faint line or interface between adjacent lamellae.

KEY

CL, circumferential lamellae	**L**, lacuna	**VC**, Volkmann's canal
HC, Haversian canal	**O**, osteon	**arrow**, lamellar boundary
IL, interstitial lamellae		

PLATE 16

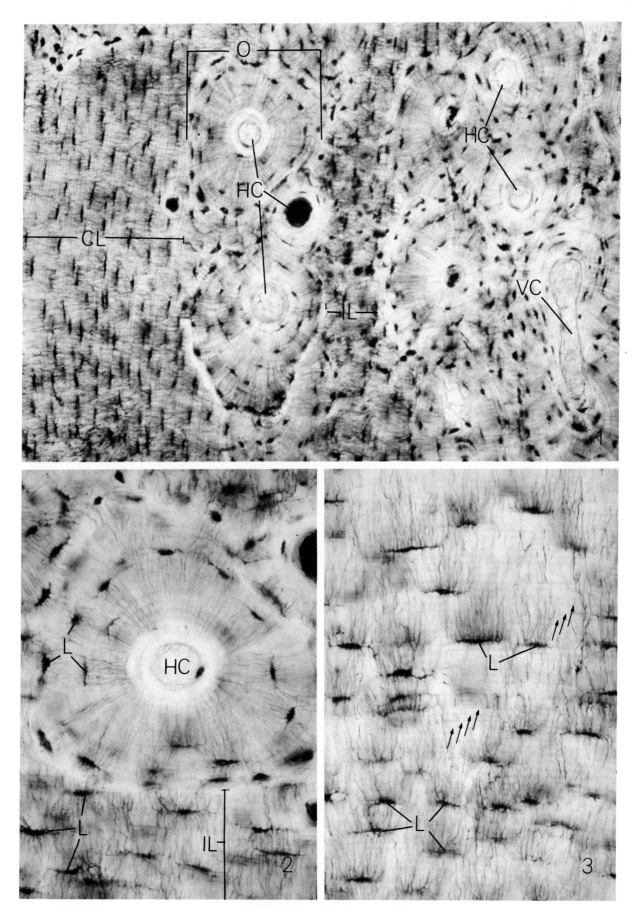

PLATE 17. Cortical Bone, Electron Microscopy

Cortical bone, rabbit femur, electron micrograph ×3000. The bone shown in this figure was decalcified, leaving the cells and extracellular soft tissue components (collagen) essentially intact. The particular osteon illustrated here consists of three complete lamellae, numbered *1–3*, and, immediately surrounding the osteonal (Haversian) canal *(HC)*, a fourth lamella that is incomplete *(asterisks)*. The outer limit of the osteon is marked by a cement line *(CL)*, and beyond this is an interstitial lamella *(IL)*.

The most apparent structures in the Haversian canal are the blood vessels. Both are capillaries *(Cap)*. The smaller vessel is surrounded by pericytes, whereas the larger one does not possess this additional cellular investment. Note that with the light microscope the closely packed preosteoblasts around the capillaries can be mistaken easily for smooth muscle cells of larger blood vessels. Examination with the electron microscope, however, shows that veins and arteries are not present in Haversian canals but, rather, that there are two types of capillaries. The cells within the Haversian canal (other than those associated with the capillaries) are either osteo-blasts or preosteoblasts. The osteoblasts *(Ob)* line the Haversian canal. The remainder of the cells are regarded as preosteoblasts *(POb)*. They are less differentiated cells but are in the process of transforming into osteoblasts in order to replace those that will become incorporated into the bone matrix that they produce. In examining the osteoblasts, note that one of them exhibits a process extending into a canaliculus *(double arrow)* of the incomplete lamella. Similarly, the osteocyte *(Oc)* in the lower portion of the figure also shows cytoplasmic processes entering canaliculi *(arrows)*.

The canaliculi *(C)* within the lamellae and those extending across the lamellae appear less numerous than those seen in a light micrograph (see Plate 16). The difference is a reflection of the relative thickness of the sections, with more canaliculi being included in the thick light microscope section than in the thin section utilized in the electron microscope. (Micrograph provided courtesy of Luk SC, Nopajaroonsri C, Simon GT: *Journal of Ultrastructure Research* 46:184, 1974.)

KEY

C, canaliculus
Cap, capillary
CL, cement line (of von Ebner)
HC, Haversian canal
IL, interstitial lamella
L, lacuna

Ob, osteoblast
Oc, osteocyte
POb, preosteoblast
arrow, osteocyte process in canaliculus extending from lacuna, lower left

asterisks, inner, forming lamella
double arrow, osteoblast process in canaliculus
1, 2, 3, lamellae

PLATE 17

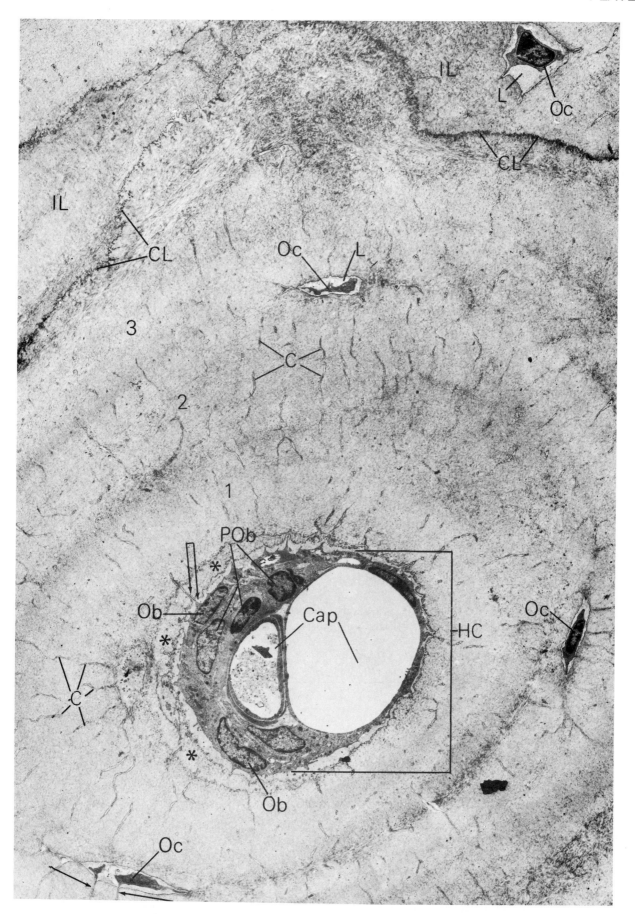

PLATE 18. Spongy and Compact Bone

The second method for viewing bone with the light microscope is the examination of demineralized tissue sections. This procedure involves steps that are essentially similar to those employed for the routine preparations of histologic sections except that after fixation the tissue is placed in a demineralizing solution (acid or chelating agent). Once the mineral has been removed, the tissue is treated just as any other tissue sample (as described in Chapter 1). The demineralized section retains all of the formed soft tissue components that are normally seen in a hematoxylin and eosin (H&E) section.

FIGURE 1, bone, monkey, H&E ×80; upper inset ×175. This figure shows a demineralized section of two bones framing a joint cavity. Articular cartilage *(AC)* covers the surfaces that contact the neighboring bone. The free surface of each cartilage presents a relatively smooth contour, whereas the junction between the cartilage and the bone *(SB)* is irregular.

The articular cartilage is hyaline **(upper inset).** It shows the characteristic features of hyaline cartilage seen in Plate 11, page 141, namely, chondrocytes in lacunae, a homogeneous avascular matrix (homogeneous in that it presents no formed elements visible with the light microscope), and variable staining of the matrix. At least some of the cartilage cells are in lacunae that are close to each other, suggesting that they are daughter cells of the same parent cell.

The bone under the articular cartilage is spongy bone. It consists of spicules or trabeculae of bone tissue as well as marrow spaces *(M)*. In this sample, the marrow consists pri-marily of adipose tissue. In addition to the marrow spaces, the bone tissue also contains space or tunnels for blood vessels *(BV);* in this respect, bone differs fundamentally from the hyaline cartilage on the articular surface, which is avascular. The essential features of the bone tissue are seen at higher magnification in the **upper inset.** These are osteocytes *(Oc)* in lacunae, an eosinophilic matrix, and blood vessels *(BV)*. The spongy bone shown in this figure is nonlamellar; i.e., the matrix is not organized as lamellae, but rather, the collagen fibers are in the form of interwoven bundles. Certain features of woven nonlamellar bone are also displayed in the **upper inset;** namely, the cells are unevenly and randomly dispersed and are not arranged in an oriented pattern around the blood vessels. For comparison, note how the lacunae (and, therefore, also the osteocytes) display an oriented pattern about the Haversian canal in Figure 2 of Plate 16.

FIGURE 2, bone, monkey, ×80; lower inset ×350. This figure shows the shaft of a long bone. The center of the bone consists of a large marrow cavity *(M)* filled chiefly with adipose tissue; surrounding the marrow cavity is the bone tissue of the shaft. It is compact bone *(CB)*. Although the compact bone tissue contains tunnels for blood vessels *(BV)*, it does not contain marrow spaces. On its outer surface, the bone tissue is covered by a periosteum *(Po)*, and its inner surface is covered by endosteum *(Eo,* **lower inset)**. The endosteum consists of several layers of cells (nuclei of these cells are evident) and collagenous fibers. The endosteal cells have the potential to develop into osteoblasts (as do periosteal cells) if the need should arise, e.g., in fracture repair.

Histologically, the compact bone shown in this figure displays three characteristics: an eosinophilic matrix; lacunae in which osteocytes are located; and vascular tunnels *(BV)*. The osteocytes *(Oc)* are identified chiefly by their nuclear staining, which stands out in contrast to the surrounding eosinophilic matrix. The boundaries of the lacunae and the canaliculi radiating from them (see Plate 16) are not evident.

In the adult human, compact bone is organized chiefly as Haversian systems or as other forms of lamellar bone. Although this form of bone tissue is readily seen in well-oriented ground sections, it is not always easy to identify in decalcified sections. It is particularly difficult to make this identification in longitudinal decalcified sections of a long bone as shown in this figure.

KEY

AC, articular cartilage	**Eo,** endosteum	**Po,** periosteum
BV, blood vessel	**M,** marrow spaces	**SB,** spongy bone
CB, compact bone	**Oc,** osteocyte	

PLATE 18

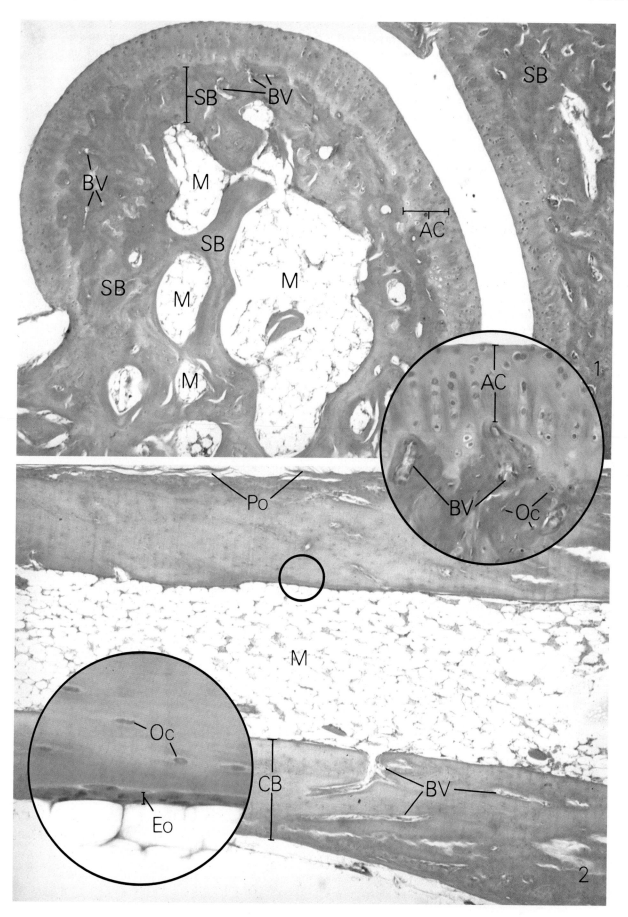

PLATE 19. Endochondral Bone Formation I

Endochondral bone formation involves the continuing growth of a cartilage precursor, which serves as a fetal skeleton, and the simultaneous removal of the cartilage and its replacement with bone tissue. In addition, as a bone grows, some of the bone tissue is removed while newer bone tissue is being laid down, a process called remodeling. Remodeling that alters the shape of the bone is called *external remodeling;* that which does not alter the shape of the bone, as in the formation of Haversian systems, is called *internal remodeling.*

Two specialized cell types have been identified with the process of bone growth and remodeling. The *osteoblast* is engaged in the formation of bone. Although the removal of bone is not as well understood, it has been established that multinucleated cells, called *osteoclasts*, are engaged in the removal of bone. Osteocytes, also, can alter and resorb bone in their immediate vicinity. The process is called osteocytic osteolysis; although it is important in calcium homeostasis, its role in bone remodeling, if any, is not clear.

FIGURE 1, developing bone, monkey, H&E ×240. The early steps of endochondral bone formation are shown in this figure. The structure seen here is the cartilage model of the bone about to be formed. The steps of bone formation are

1. The cartilage *(C)* cells in the center of the cartilage model become hypertrophic *(HC)*.

2. The matrix of the cartilage becomes calcified *(CM)*. (The calcified matrix stains intensely with hematoxylin and appears as the darker condensed matrix material between the enlarged cartilage cells.)

3. A collar of bone forms around the circumference of the center of the cartilage model. This bone is called *periosteal bone (PB)* because the osteoblasts that have produced the bone material develop from the periosteum. (Note that the periosteal bone is, in fact, intramembranous bone [see Plate 21, page 181] because it develops within the connective tissue membrane that immediately surrounds the developing bone and not on a spicule of calcified cartilage.)

FIGURE 2, developing bone, human, H&E ×60. The bone in this figure shows later events and a continuation of the earlier ones just described. A vascular bud (not shown) and accompanying perivascular cells from the periosteum have invaded the shaft of the cartilage model, resulting in the formation of a cavity *(Cav)*. Examination at higher power would reveal that the cavity contains fat cells, hematopoietic tissue (the dark-blue-staining component), and other connective tissue elements. While the new steps of bone formation occur, the earlier steps continue.

1. Cartilage *(C)* cells proliferate at the epiphyses. They are responsible for production of new matrix material. It is this process that creates lengthening of the bone.

2. Periosteal bone *(PB)* continues to form.

3. Cartilage cells facing the cavity become hypertrophic.

4. Cartilage matrix becomes calcified.

5. Erosion of cartilage occurs, creating spicules of cartilage.

6. Bone forms on the spicules of the calcified cartilage at the erosion front; this bone is *endochondral bone (EB)*.

As these processes continue in the shaft of the bone, one end of the cartilage model (the epiphysis) is invaded by blood vessels and connective tissue from the periosteum (periosteal bud), and it undergoes the same changes that occurred earlier in the shaft (except that no periosteal bone forms). This same process then occurs at the other end of the bone. Consequently, at each end of the developing long bone, a cartilaginous plate (epiphyseal plate) is created that lies between two sites of bone formation.

FIGURE 3, developing bone, human, H&E ×60. This shows an early stage after the invasion of the epiphysis. A secondary ossification center *(Os°)* has formed, and along with this event, the head of the long bone will develop a cavity similar in its content to that of the diaphysis. The cartilage separating the two cavities is the epiphyseal plate *(EP)*. At the early stage shown in this figure, the plate is not well defined. Despite the enlargement of the epiphyseal cavity, the remaining cartilage between the two cavities persists as a disc or plate until growth ceases. The **inset** shows some calcified cartilage *(CC)* as well as the deposition of endochondral bone *(EB)* within the secondary ossification center. *JC*, joint cavity.

KEY

C, cartilage
Cav, marrow cavity
CC, calcified cartilage
CM, calcified matrix

EB, endochondral bone
EP, epiphyseal plate
HC, hypertrophic cartilage cell

JC, joint cavity
Os°, secondary ossification center
PB, periosteal bone

PLATE 19

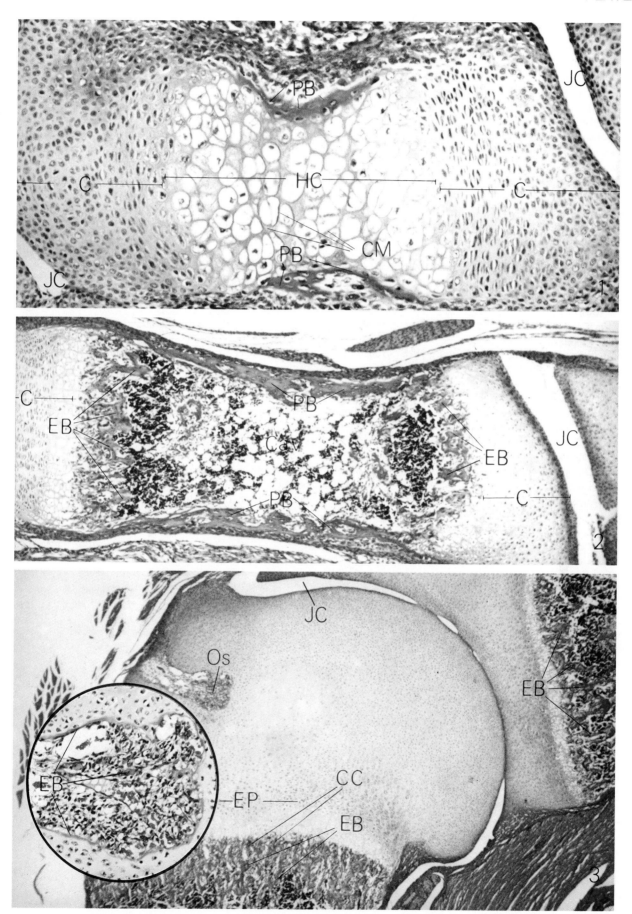

PLATE 20. Endochondral Bone Formation II

FIGURE 1, developing bone, human, H&E ×80; inset ×380. This is a photomicrograph of an epiphysis at higher magnification than that seen in Figure 3 of Plate 19. Different zones of the cartilage of the epiphyseal plate reflect the progressive changes that occur in active growth of endochondral bone. These zones are not sharply delineated, and the boundaries between them are somewhat arbitrary. They lead toward the marrow cavity *(M)*, so that the first zone is furthest from the cavity. The zones are

• *Zone of reserve cartilage (RC).* The cartilage cells of this zone have not yet begun to participate in the growth of the bone; thus, they are reserve cells. These cells are small, usually only one to a lacuna, and not grouped. At some time, some of these cells will proliferate and undergo the changes outlined for the next zone.

• *Zone of proliferating cartilage (PC).* The cells of this zone are increasing in number; they are slightly larger than the reserve cells and close to their neighbors; they begin to form rows.

• *Zone of hypertrophic cartilage (HC).* The cells of this zone are aligned in rows and are significantly larger than the cells in the preceding zone.

• *Zone of calcified matrix (C).* In this zone the cartilage matrix is impregnated with calcium salts.

• *Zone of resorption.* This zone is represented by eroded cartilage that is in direct contact with the connective tissue of the marrow cavity. Spicules (actually a honeycomb at the level of the advancing blood vessels) of cartilage are formed because the pericapillary cells invade and resorb in spearheads rather than along a straight front. Specifically, the pericapillary cells break into the rows of hypertrophied chondrocytes temporarily leaving the calcified cartilage between the rows of cells. In this manner, spicules of calcified cartilage are formed. Endochondral bone *(EB)* deposition then occurs on the surfaces of these calcified cartilage spicules, forming *mixed spicules.*

FIGURE 2, developing bone, human, H&E ×150; inset ×380. This is a higher magnification of the lower middle area of Figure 1. It shows calcified cartilage spicules on which bone has been deposited. In the lower portion of the figure, the spicules have already grown to create anastomosing bone trabeculae. These initial trabeculae still contain remnants of calcified cartilage, as shown by the blue color of the cartilage matrix (compared with the red staining of the bone). Osteoblasts *(Ob)* are aligned on the surface of the spicules where bone formation is active.

The **upper inset** in Figure 1 shows the surface of several spicules from the *left circle* in Figure 2, at higher magnification. Note the osteoblasts *(Ob),* some of which are just beginning to produce bone in apposition to the calcified cartilage *(C).* The lower right of the **inset** shows bone *(EB)* with an osteocyte *(Oc)* already embedded in the bone matrix.

The **lower inset,** an enlargement of the *right circle* in Figure 2, reveals several osteoclasts *(Ocl).* They are in apposition to the spicule, which is mostly cartilage. A small amount of bone is evident, based on the red-staining material in this **inset.** Note the light area *(arrow)* representing the ruffled border of the osteoclast. Examination of Figure 2 reveals a number of other osteoclasts *(Ocl).*

KEY

C, calcified cartilage matrix	**Ob,** osteoblast	**PC,** proliferating cartilage
EB, endochondral bone	**Oc,** osteocyte	**RC,** reserve cartilage
HC, hypertrophic cartilage	**Ocl,** osteoclast	**arrow,** ruffled border of osteoclast
M, marrow		

PLATE 20

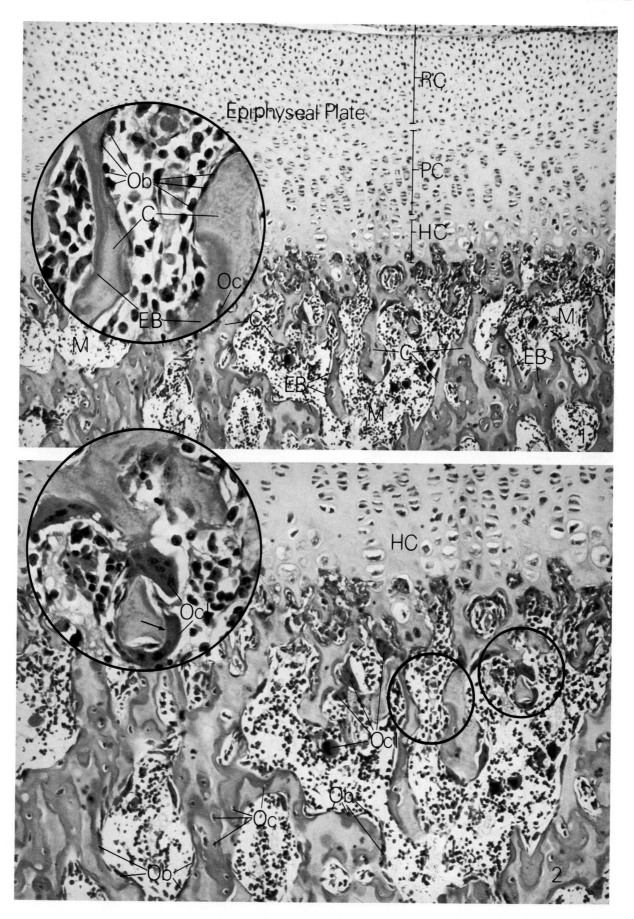

Epiphyseal Plate

PLATE 21. Intramembranous Bone Formation

Intramembranous bone formation is limited to those bones that are not required to perform an early supporting function, e.g., the flat bones of the skull. This process requires the proliferation and differentiation of cells within mesenchyme to become *osteoblasts*, the bone-forming cells. They produce ground substance and collagen. This initial matrix, called *osteoid*, calcifies to form bone.

As the osteoblasts continue to secrete their product, some are entrapped within their matrix and are then known as *osteocytes*. They are responsible for maintenance of the newly formed bone tissue. The remaining osteoblasts continue the bone deposition process at the bone surface. They are capable of reproducing to maintain an adequate population for continued growth.

These newly formed *bone spicules* enlarge and interconnect as growth proceeds, creating a three-dimensional trabecular structure similar in shape to the future mature bone. The interstices contain blood vessels and connective tissue (mesenchyme). As the bone continues to grow, remodeling occurs. This involves resorption of localized areas of bone tissue by *osteoclasts* in order to maintain appropriate shape in relation to size and to permit vascular nourishment during the growth process.

FIGURE 1, fetal head, pig, H&E. A cross section of the developing lower jaw bone, as seen at this relatively early stage of development, consists of bone spicules *(BS)* of various sizes and shapes. Other structures present that will assist in orientation include a developing tooth *(DT)*, Meckel's cartilage *(MC)*, also referred to as the mandibular process, oral cavity *(OC)*, oral cavity epithelium *(Ep)*, and a small portion of the tongue *(T)*. The bone spicules *(BS)* interconnect and, in three dimension, form a trabecula having the general shape of the mandible. Peripheral to the bone spicules, the connective tissue is very cellular; this is the early periosteum *(P)*. Beyond the limits of the developing bone are regions in which developing muscle fibers *(DM)* are present.

FIGURE 3, fetal head, pig, H&E. High magnification of a bone spicule that is elongating through the deposition of new matrix material or osteoid *(Os)*. The older calcified portion of the spicule is stained more deeply than the new osteoid and contains an osteocyte *(OC)*, surrounded by bone matrix. A recently trapped osteoblast is indicated by the *arrow*. It is partly associated with the calcified bone matrix and partly associated with osteoid matrix. The newly deposited osteoid, by comparison, stains poorly and has a dense fibrous appearance due to the unmasked collagen that makes up the osteoid matrix. The numerous osteoblasts *(Ob)* responsible for this growing region of the spicule are seen at the periphery of the newly deposited osteoid.

FIGURE 2, fetal head, pig, H&E. Higher magnification of the *lower boxed area* in Figure 1. Osteoblasts *(Ob)* are present on much of the surface of the bone spicules *(BS)*. Where these bone-forming cells are large and in close apposition, active bone matrix deposition is occurring. The new matrix is recognized by the light-staining band of osteoid *(Os)* between the osteoblasts and the calcified bone matrix. Where the osteoblasts are flattened or attenuated *(single arrows)*, matrix deposition is not occurring, and the osteoid is absent. Within the interstices of the trabeculae is connective tissue with blood vessels *(BV)*. Haversian systems are not formed until much later when bone remodeling occurs.

KEY		
BS, bone spicule	**MC,** Meckel's cartilage	**Os,** osteoid
BV, blood vessels	**Ob,** osteoblast	**P,** developing periosteum
DT, developing tooth	**Oc,** osteocyte	**arrow,** partly entrapped osteoblast

PLATE 21

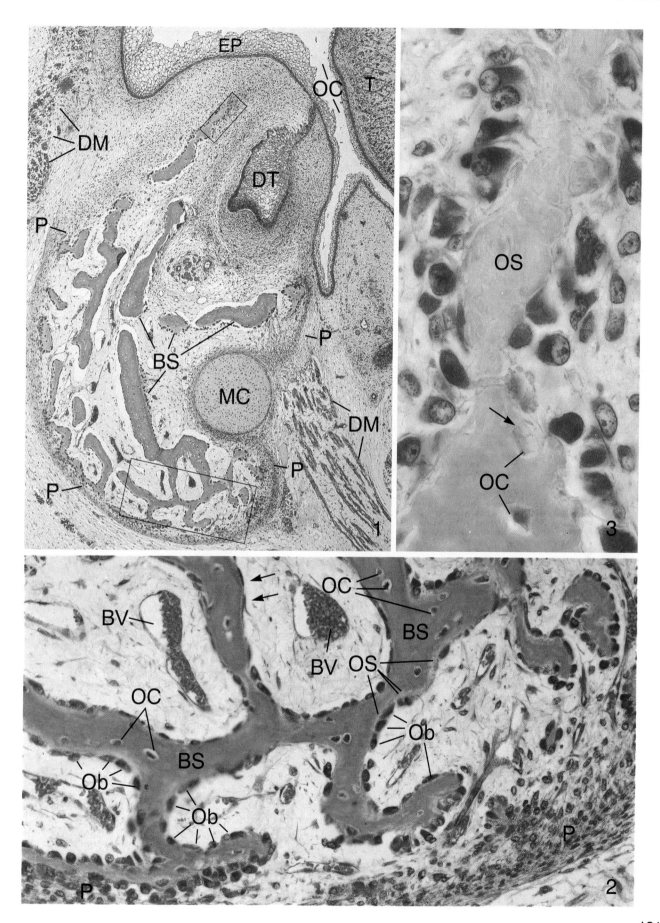

PLATE 22. Developing Bone I, Electron Microscopy

Developing bone, electron micrograph ×5000. This electron micrograph reveals the *periosteal surface* of a growing long bone. It is from the midportion of the shaft, a region of the bone that develops by intramembranous ossification. Accordingly, no cartilage is present. The upper part of the illustration reveals typical fibroblasts *(Fib)* and bundles of collagen fibers *(CF)*. This constitutes the layer that, with the light microscope, is referred to as the *fibrous portion of the periosteum (FP)*. Below is the *cellular layer of the periosteum* that contains, sequentially, the preosteoblasts *(POb)* and osteoblasts *(Ob)*.

The osteoblasts are aligned on the surface of the developing bone. They appear more or less cuboidal in shape. The lateral boundaries of adjacent osteoblasts are not very conspicuous, but the distinction between adjacent cells is somewhat enhanced by differences in electron density of the cytoplasmic matrix. The osteoblasts contain large amounts of rough-surfaced endoplasmic reticulum *(RER)* and an extensive Golgi apparatus (see Plate 23), features indicative of cells highly active in protein synthesis and secretion. Note that the preosteoblasts possess more cytoplasm than the fibroblasts, but the preosteoblast's rough-surfaced endoplasmic reticulum *(RER)* is not yet as extensive at the reticulum in the osteoblasts.

Below the osteoblasts is the osteoid *(Os)*, the material that in the light microscope appears as the poorly staining homogeneous band between the osteoblasts and the bone. The osteoid consists principally of collagen, ground substance, and some processes from the osteoblasts that extend between the collagen fibrils. These are shown at higher magnification in Plate 23.

To understand the biology of bone growth, it is necessary to realize that the osteoblasts move away from the bone as they secrete their product, the osteoid. Shortly after the osteoid is produced, it becomes calcified by a wave of mineralization that follows the movement of the osteoblasts, with the osteoid always intervening. The calcium is in the form of hydroxyapatite crystals. In this specimen, most of the calcium salts have been lost from the bone *(B)*; consequently, it has a relatively electron-lucent appearance. However, calcium salts remain at the mineralization front where it appears as a black electron-opaque material *(asterisks)*.

At intervals, certain osteoblasts no longer continue to move away from the bone, and as a consequence, the cell is surrounded by the osteoid it has produced. As the mineralization front progresses, the cell becomes surrounded by bone. It is then contained within a lacuna and referred to as an osteocyte. A recently formed osteocyte *(Oc)* can be seen in the micrograph. Note that the bone matrix that borders the lacuna has retained its calcium salts. The processes of the osteocyte are contained in canaliculi *(C)*.

Other osteocytes also arise in the same manner as just described. Thus, as the bone thickens, the osteoblast layer tends to become depleted as the osteoblasts become transformed into osteocytes. The depletion is balanced, however, by the proliferation of connective tissue cells that differentiate first into preosteoblasts and then into osteoblasts.

KEY		
B, bone	**FP,** fibrous periosteum	**POb,** preosteoblast
C, canaliculus	**Ob,** osteoblast	**RER,** rough-surfaced endoplasmic reticulum
CF, collagen fibers	**Oc,** osteocyte	
Fib, fibroblast	**Os,** osteoid	**asterisk,** mineralization front

PLATE 22

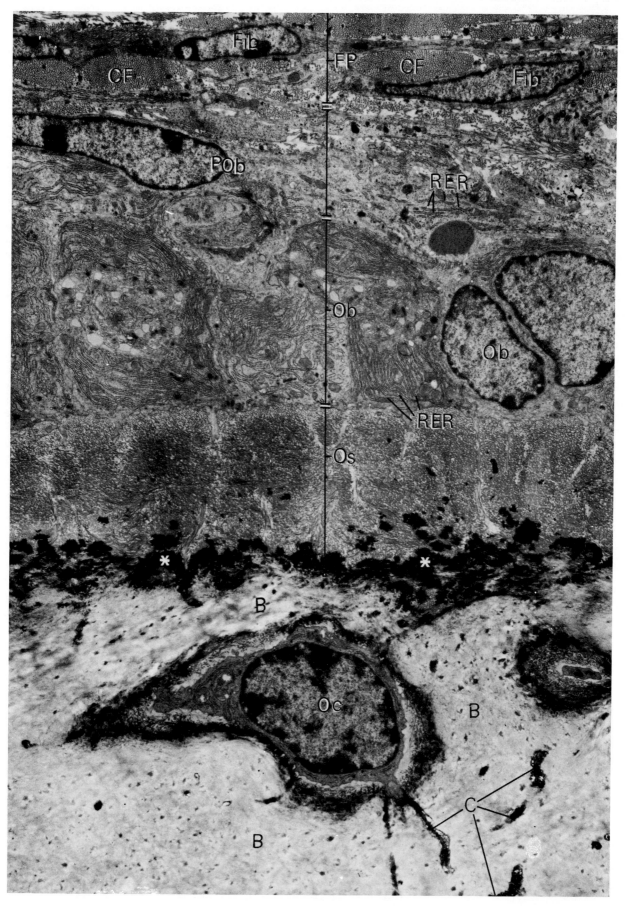

PLATE 23.   Developing Bone II, Electron Microscopy

FIGURE 1, osteoblast, electron micrograph ×14,000.
The osteoblasts shown in this figure are comparable to those seen in the preceding plate. The higher magnification shows to advantage the cytologic detail of the cells.

In characterizing the osteoblast as well as understanding the nature of its product, it is important to realize that osteoblasts are derived from connective tissue cells that are indistinguishable from fibroblasts. They retain much of the cytologic morphology of the fibroblasts, and this is evident in this electron micrograph. In active fibroblasts, there is a large amount of rough-surfaced endoplasmic reticulum and an extensive Golgi apparatus. The osteoblasts pictured here also contain a large amount of rough-surfaced endoplasmic reticulum *(RER)* and a prominent Golgi apparatus *(GA)*, indicative of their role in the production of osteoid. The Golgi apparatus shown in the osteoblast contains typical flattened sacs and transport vesicles. It also shows enlarged vesicles that contain material of various densities. Two of the large elongated Golgi vesicles *(arrows)* contain a filamentous component. On the basis of special staining techniques for electron microscopy, such filaments are considered to be collagen precursors.

The osteoblasts in this figure (and those in the preceding plate) are cuboidal and, because of their close apposition, bear a resemblance to cuboidal cells in an epithelial sheet. Although the osteoblasts are, indeed, arranged on the surface of the developing bone in a sheet-like manner, they nevertheless exhibit properties of connective tissue cells, not epithelial cells. No basal lamina surrounds the osteoblasts. Moreover, although no collagen fibrils are pictured here, they are occasionally observed between osteoblasts. The osteoblast is highly polar, secreting onto the bone surface. Thus, the surface of the osteoblast that faces the osteoid *(Os)* can be regarded to be the secretory face or secretory pole of the cell.

FIGURE 2, osteoblast, electron micrograph ×30,000. The secretory face of the osteoblast is shown adjacent to the osteoid at higher magnification in this figure. Both the round and the somewhat larger, irregularly shaped profiles in the osteoid are collagen fibrils *(C)*. Ground substance occupies the space between the collagen fibrils. Recall that the osteoblast is moving away from the bone, leaving its product behind. The collagen fibrils closest to the cell are of small diameter and represent the most recently formed fibrils. With time, as the cell recedes and as the mineralization front approaches, the collagen fibrils increase in diameter. This is thought to occur by the accretion of additional collagen onto the fibrils already present. It is not unlikely that some large, irregularly shaped fibrils *(arrowheads)* arise by a combination of accretion and the fusion of smaller fibrils. By the time the mineralization front reaches the fibrils, they have achieved their greatest diameter. Mineralization results in an impregnation of both the collagen fibrils as well as the ground substance with calcium hydroxyapatite.

The figure also shows a process of the bone-forming cell *(arrow)*. Such processes will be contained in canaliculi after the osteoblast is transformed into an osteocyte.

	KEY	
C, collagen fibrils	**POb,** preosteoblast	**curved arrows (Fig. 1):** elongate Golgi vesicles with collagen precursor
GA, Golgi apparatus	**RER,** rough-surfaced endoplasmic reticulum	
M, mitochondria		**straight arrow (Fig. 2):** process of osteoblast
N, nucleus of osteoblast	**arrowheads,** large collagen fibrils	
Os, osteoid		

PLATE 23

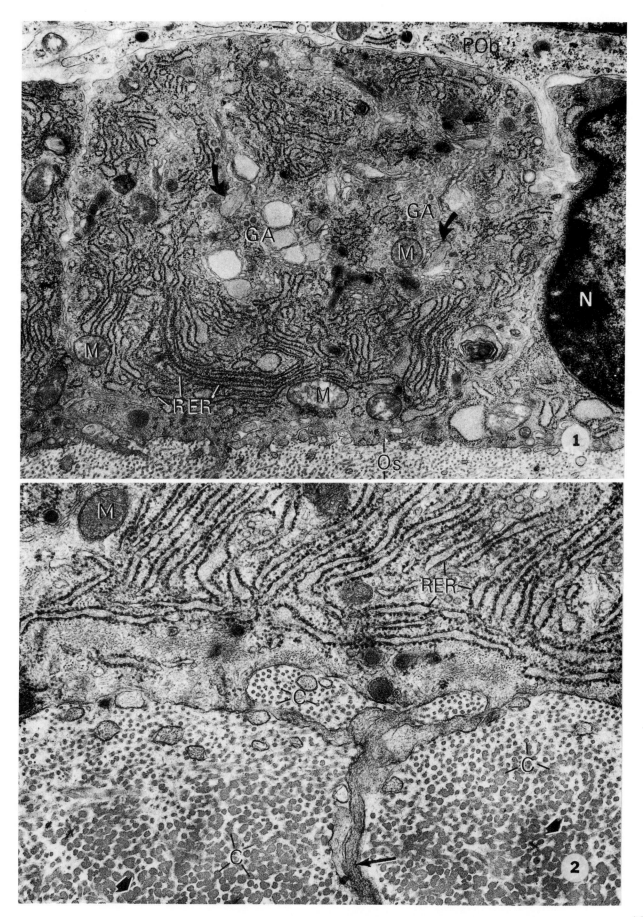

PLATE 24. Osteoclast, Electron Microscopy

Osteoclast, electron micrograph ×10,000; **inset** ×25,000. This figure shows a segment of bone surface *(B)* and, adjacent to the bone, portions of two cells, an osteoblast *(Ob)* and an osteoclast *(Oc)*. The difference between these two cell types is reflected not only in their cytologic appearance but also in the character of the adjacent extracellular matrix. The osteoblast is typically separated from the mineralization front of the bone by osteoid *(Os)*. The portion of the cell seen in relation to the osteoid is readily identified as an osteoblast by its extensive rough-surfaced endoplasmic reticulum. Similarly, the osteoid is recognized by the presence of the numerous collagen fibrils.

In contrast, the osteoclast is adjacent to a mixture of collagen fibrils and hydroxyapatite crystals. In effect, at this site, bone is being broken down. The portion of the osteoclast that is in apposition to this partially digested bone possesses numerous infoldings of the plasma membrane **(inset)**. When viewed with the light microscope, the infoldings are evident as the ruffled border. When the plane of section is at right angles to the infoldings, they resemble microvilli. They are, however, folds, not finger-like microvillous projections. When they are sectioned in a plane paralleling a fold *(asterisks)*, a broad, nonspecialized expanse of cytoplasm is seen. This is the cytoplasm within the fold of the ruffled border *(Rb)*; it is free of organelles except for fine filaments. Hydroxyapatite crystals *(arrowheads)* can often be seen in the extracellular space of the infoldings.

The cytoplasm of the osteoclast contains numerous mitochondria *(M)*, lysosomes, and Golgi profiles, all of which are functionally linked with the resorption and degradation of the bone substance. Electron micrographs show that the hydroxyapatite crystals are ingested by the cell. After the hydroxyapatite crystals are ingested, the calcium is mobilized for passage into the bloodstream. The organic matrix (collagen and ground substance) is also resorbed by the osteoclast. There is evidence that the osteoclast secretes hydrolytic enzymes into the area of bone where actual resorption is in progress.

As in Plate 22, the bone, except at the mineralization front *(MF)* and the resorption front *(RF)*, appears unusually light because the mineral component has been lost during the preparation of the specimen. In the lower left of the figure, some collagen fibrils are evident; the *arrows* indicate where 68-nm cross-banding is visible.

The proximity of osteoblasts and osteoclasts on the bone surface is not atypical. It highlights the fact that the bone surface is subject to continuous localized change, especially in growing individuals.

KEY

B, bone	**Os,** osteoid	**arrows,** collagen fibrils
M, mitochondria	**RB,** ruffled border	**asterisk,** cytoplasm within folds of
MF, mineralization front	**RF,** resorption front	ruffled border
Ob, osteoblast	**arrowheads,** hydroxyapatite crys-	
Oc, osteoclast	tals	

PLATE 24

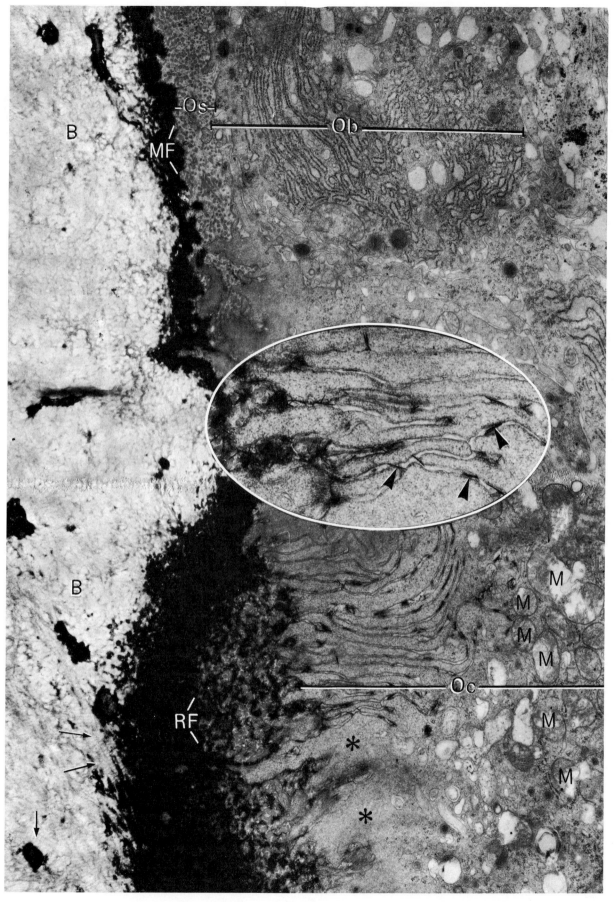

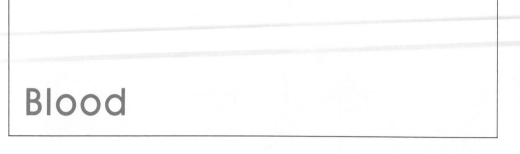

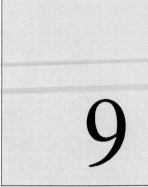

Blood

Blood Is a Fluid Connective Tissue That Circulates Through the Cardiovascular System

Like the other connective tissues, blood consists of cells and an extracellular matrix whose volume exceeds that of the cells. It is propelled throughout the body by the pumping action of the heart and reaches all of the other body tissues. Its many functions include

- Conveying *nutrients* and *oxygen* directly or indirectly to cells
- Carrying *wastes* and *carbon dioxide* away from the cells
- Carrying *hormones* and other *regulatory agents* to and form the cells and tissues of the body
- Having a major *homeostatic* role based on its *thermoregulatory* and *buffering* capacity
- Transporting *humoral agents* and *cells* that protect the body from infections, foreign cells, foreign proteins, and transformed cells, i.e., cancer cells

Blood Consists of *Formed Elements,* Cells and Their Derivatives, and a Protein-Rich Matrix Called *Plasma*

The formed elements include

- *Red blood cells,* also called erythrocytes
- *White blood cells,* also called leukocytes
- *Platelets*

Plasma is the liquid intercellular material or matrix that imparts to the blood its fluid properties. The relative volume of cells and plasma is about 45% and 55%, respectively. This value is called a *hematocrit.* It is obtained by centrifuging a blood sample with anticoagulants added. The hematocrit reading is then obtained by measuring the percent volume in the centrifuge tube occupied by the red cells compared with the whole blood volume. A normal reading is about 45; thus, 45% consists of red cells.

The cell fraction consists mainly of packed *erythrocytes.* At the upper part of the packed cells is a narrow layer called the *buffy coat.* It constitutes only about 1% of the entire sample but contains all of the *leukocytes* and *platelets.* There are far more red blood cells (5×10^6/mm^3 of blood) than white blood cells ($6-9 \times 10^3$/mm^3 of blood). Although the cells are the major object of interest in histology, a brief examination of plasma is also useful.

PLASMA

The composition of plasma is summarized in Table 9.1. As the table indicates, most of the plasma consists of water. It serves as the solvent for a variety of solutes, including proteins, dissolved gases, electrolytes, nutrients, waste materials, and regulatory substances. The proteins are the largest fraction of the solutes.

Plasma Proteins Consist Primarily of *Fibrinogens, Globulins,* and *Albumins*

Fibrinogens, the largest proteins, are made in the liver and function in blood clotting.

Albumins, also made in the liver, are the smallest proteins. They are responsible for exerting the major osmotic pressure on the blood vessel wall, what physiologists call the *colloid osmotic pressure.* If albumins leak out of the

TABLE 9.1. Composition of Blood Plasma

COMPONENT	%
Water	91–92
Protein (fibrinogens, globulins, albumin)	7–8
Other solutes	1–2
Electrolytes (Na$^+$, K$^+$, Ca^{2+}, Mg^{2+}, Cl$^-$, HCO$_3^-$, PO$_4^{3-}$, SO$_4^{2-}$)	
Nonprotein nitrogen substances (urea, uric acid, creatine, creatinine, ammonium salts)	
Nutrients (glucose, lipids, amino acids)	
Bood gasses (oxygen, carbon dioxide, nitrogen)	
Regulatory substances (hormones, enzymes)	

blood vessels, as in the case of albumin being lost from the blood to the urine in the kidneys, the osmotic pressure of the blood decreases, and fluid accumulates in the tissues. (This increase in tissue fluid is most readily noted by swelling of the ankles at the end of a day.)

Globulins include the *immunoglobulins,* by far the largest component of the globulin fraction. The immunoglobulins are antibodies, a class of functional molecules of the immune system that are secreted by plasma cells (see page 114). (Antibodies are discussed in Chapter 13.) Nonimmune globulins are secreted by the liver and include glycoproteins such as fibronectin and other molecules that may exchange between the blood and the other connective tissues.

Plasma proteins are generally large molecules and react with the common fixatives; they are often retained within the blood vessels in tissue sections. Plasma proteins do not possess structural form above the molecular level; thus, when they are retained in the tissue block, they appear in blood vessels as a homogeneous substance staining evenly with eosin in hematoxylin and eosin (H&E)-stained sections.

Aside from these large proteins and the regulatory substances, which are small proteins or polypeptides, most of the other plasma constituents under physiologic conditions are sufficiently small to pass easily through the blood vessel wall into the extracellular spaces of the adjacent connective tissue.

The Interstitial Fluid of the Connective Tissues Is Derived From Blood Plasma

Interstitial fluid, not surprisingly, has an electrolyte composition reflective of that of blood plasma, from which it is derived. The composition of extracellular fluid in non-connective tissues, however, is subject to considerable modification by the absorptive and secretory activities of epithelia. Epithelia may create special microenvironments reflective of or conducive to their function. For example, it has long been known that a blood-brain barrier exists between the blood and nerve tissue. Barriers also exist between the blood and the parenchymal tissue in the testis, thymus gland, eye, and other epithelial compartments. In these instances, the nature of the interstitial fluid, the nature of the barriers, and their effects are discussed in subsequent chapters that describe these particular organs.

BLOOD CELLS AND CELLULAR ELEMENTS

Red blood cells perform their functions only within the bloodstream. Their role is restricted to binding oxygen for delivery to the tissues and, in exchange, binding carbon dioxide for removal from the tissues.

White blood cells, in contrast, leave the blood through the walls of capillaries and venules to enter the connective tissues, lymphatic tissues, and bone marrow, where they perform their specific functions. Therefore, whereas red blood cells must be considered essential components for the normal functions of blood, white blood cells must be regarded as transients within the blood. That is, they use the bloodstream as a vehicle for transport to specific sites within the body. The formed elements of the blood and their relative numbers are summarized in Table 9.2.

HISTOLOGIC METHOD FOR EXAMINING BLOOD CELLS— BLOOD SMEARS

The method that best displays the cell types of peripheral blood is the blood smear. This differs from the usual preparation seen in the histology laboratory in that the specimen is not embedded in paraffin and sectioned. Rather, a drop of blood is placed directly on a slide and spread thinly over the surface of the slide, i.e., "smeared," with the edge of another slide to produce a monolayer of cells (see below). This preparation is air dried and stained. Another difference in the preparation of a blood smear is that instead of H&E, special mixtures of dyes are used for staining blood cells. The resulting preparation may then be examined with a high-power oil-immersion lens with or without a coverslip.

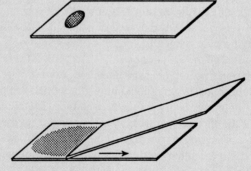

The modified Romanovsky-type stain commonly used for blood smears consists of a mixture of methylene blue (a basic dye), related azures (also basic dyes), and eosin (an acid dye). On the basis of their appearance after staining, white blood cells are divided into granulocytes and agranulocytes. Although both cell types may contain granules, the granulocytes possess obvious, specifically stained granules in their cytoplasm. In principle, the basic dyes stain nuclei, granules of basophils, and the RNA of the cytoplasm, whereas the acid dye stains the red blood cells and the granules of eosinophils. It was originally thought that the neutrophil granules were stained by a "neutral dye" that formed when methylene blue and its related azures were combined with eosin. However, the mechanism whereby the **specific neutrophil granules** are stained is not clear. To complicate matters further, some of the basic dyes (the azures) are metachromatic and may impart a violet to red color to the material they stain.

Red Blood Cells

Red Blood Cells Constitute the Largest Number of Cells in the Blood

Circulating erythrocytes are biconcave discs with a diameter of 7.8 μm, an edge thickness of 2.6 μm, and a central thickness of 0.8 μm.

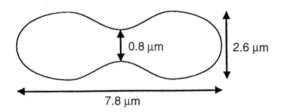

In H&E-stained sections, erythrocytes range from 6 to 10 μm in diameter but are usually 7–8 μm in diameter. Because of the remarkable consistency of their size in fixed tissue, they provide a useful internal gauge for estimating the size of other cells and structures in histologic sections.

Red Blood Cells Do Not Have a Nucleus

Because erythrocytes are biconcave discs and usually display this appearance, they tend to give the impression that their form is rigid and inelastic (Fig. 9.1). They are, in fact, extremely elastic and deform readily, if necessary, in passing through the smallest blood vessels. They stain uniformly with eosin. In thin sections viewed with the electron microscope, they are devoid of organelles; the interior of an erythrocyte is seen to consist of a dense, finely granular material (Fig. 9.2).

A plasma membrane surrounds the erythrocyte. This membrane is an enzyme-containing functional component of the red blood cell and not just a container. The biconcave shape of the mature erythrocyte is maintained by the presence of a specific intermediate protein filament, *spectrin*, that binds to the inner side of the plasma membrane.

Erythrocytes Are Specialized for the Transport of Oxygen and Carbon Dioxide

Oxygen and carbon dioxide are transported bound to a *hemoglobin* protein that fills the red cells and is responsible for their uniform staining with eosin. The disc shape of the erythrocyte facilitates gas exchange because more hemoglobin molecules are closer to the plasma membrane than they would be in a spherical cell. Thus, the gases have less distance to diffuse within the cell to reach a binding site on the hemoglobin.

Hemoglobin consists of four polypeptide chains complexed to iron-containing *heme* groups (Fig. 9.3). There is variation in the structure of the polypeptide chains, and depending on the particular polypeptides present, hemoglobin is designated as HbA, HbA₂, and HbF. Adult hemoglobin is about 96% HbA, 2% HbA₂, and 2% HbF. HbF is the principal form of hemoglobin in the fetus, and its persistence in high percentages in the adult is indicative of certain forms of anemia. Hemoglobin is similar in composition and structure to myoglobin, the oxygen-binding protein found in striated muscle (see page 216).

ANEMIA

When hemoglobin is not present in sufficient amounts, either because the normal amount in each cell is decreased or because the amount in each cell is sufficient but the cells are reduced in number, the condition is manifested clinically as **anemia.** Anemia has a variety of causes, including the loss of blood, insufficient iron for hemoglobin synthesis, vitamin deficiencies, and genetic factors.

Sickle Cell Anemia

In **sickle cell anemia** (thalassemia major), a recessive single point mutation in the gene that codes for the globin of hemoglobin produces a hemoglobin (HbS) in which there is a single amino acid difference from normal HbA. In HbS, a valine is substituted for glutamic acid in position 6 of the β chain of globin. The substitution of the hydrophobic valine for the hydrophilic glutamic acid causes the HbS to aggregate in the red blood cell, leading to a loss of plasticity in the cell. Instead of the normal biconcave disc shape, many of the red blood cells become comma-shaped at low oxygen tension, giving rise to the name, sickle cell.

Sickled red blood cells are more rigid than normal red blood cells and do not pass easily through the finest capillaries. Therefore, the capillaries may be damaged, leading to bleeding into the tissues, causing inflammation and pain. Further, portions of tissues and organs may be deprived of normal circulation because of packing of the sickled cells in the smallest vessels. Finally, sickled red blood cells are more fragile and break down or are destroyed more quickly than normal red blood cells, producing an anemia.

Platelets

Platelets Are Membrane-Bounded, Enucleate Cytoplasmic Fragments

Platelets derive from large polyploid cells (multiple sets of chromosomes) in the bone marrow, called *megakaryocytes* (Fig. 9.4). In the formation of platelets, small bits of cytoplasm are separated from the peripheral regions of the megakaryocyte by extensive *platelet demarcation channels.* The membrane that lines these channels arises by invagination of the plasma membrane; therefore, the channels are in continuity with the extracellular space. The continued development and fusion of the platelet demarcation membranes result in the complete partitioning of cytoplasmic fragments to form individual platelets.

Human platelets have a life span of about 10 days; they are seen in a peripheral blood smear either singly or in clusters (see Plate 25, page 211). They are about 2 μm in diameter and exhibit an intensely stained core, the *granulomere,* and a less intensely stained periphery, the *hyalomere.*

TABLE 9.2. Formed Elements of the Blood

FORMED ELEMENT	NO. OR %
Red blood cells (erythrocytes)	4–5 million/mm³
White blood cells (leukocytes)	6000–9000/mm³
Agranulocytes	
Lymphocytes	30–35%[A]
Monocytes	3–7%[A]
Granulocytes	
Neutrophils	55–60%[A]
Eosinophils	2–5%[A]
Basophils	0–1%[A]
Platelets	200,000–400,000/mm³

[A]Percentage of white cells.

Microtubules and actin filaments are the major components of the hyalomere. The prominent circumferential band of microtubules in the hyalomere is probably responsible for maintaining the biconvex (lens-like) shape of the platelet.

Platelets Function in Blood Clotting, Clot Retraction, and Clot Dissolution

Cytoplasmic constituents of platelets include two types of granules, *α lysosomal granules* and ***very dense granules*** (containing serotonin); two systems of tubules, one connecting to the surface and another containing an electron-dense material; microtubules; and filaments (Fig. 9.5). The dense tubules appear to be similar to the tubular cisternae of the smooth endoplasmic reticulum.

When the wall of a blood vessel is cut or broken, platelets adhere to the ruptured end of the vessel and to exposed tissue components such as collagen. The platelets will aggregate into a platelet clot at the site of vessel injury and will release, among other substances, *serotonin* and ***thromboplastin***. Serotonin, a potent vasoconstrictor, causes the vascular smooth muscle cells to contract, thereby reducing

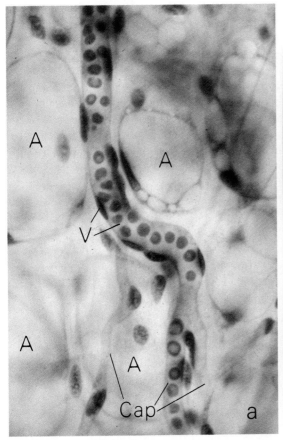
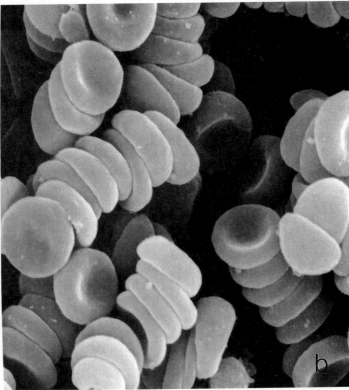

Figure 9.1. **a**. Photomicrograph of several capillaries *(Cap)* joining to form a venule *(V)*, as observed in a full-thickness mesentery spread. The red blood cells appear in single file in one of the capillaries. The light center area of some of the red blood cells is due to their biconcave shape. Examination of in vivo preparations similar to this shows that the red blood cells are highly plastic and can fold on themselves when passing through very narrow capillaries. The large round structures *(A)* are adipose cells. **b**. Scanning electron micrograph of erythrocytes collected in a blood tube. Note the concave shape of the cells. The stacks of erythrocytes in these preparations are not unusual and are referred to as ***rouloux.*** Such formations in vivo indicate an increased level of immunoglobulin. ×2800.

for their lack of characteristic cytoplasmic staining, but they are also readily identified by the multilobed shape of their nucleus; thus, they are also called *polymorphonuclear neutrophils* or *polymorphs*. The mature neutrophil possesses three to five lobes of nuclear material joined by thinner nuclear strands. The arrangement is not static; rather, in vivo the lobes and connecting strands can change their shape, position, and even number.

The chromatin of the polymorph has a characteristic arrangement. Wide regions of heterochromatin are located chiefly at the periphery of the nucleus, in contact with the nuclear envelope. Regions of euchromatin are chiefly at the center of the nucleus, with relatively smaller regions contacting the nuclear envelope (Fig. 9.6). In females, the Barr body (page 46) forms a drumstick-shaped appendage to one of the nuclear lobes.

The Neutrophil Is an Active Phagocyte

The cytoplasm of the neutrophil contains two kinds of granules, *specific granules* and *azurophilic granules,* both reflective of the functions of the cell. There is sparse representation of membrane-bounded organelles other than the granules. Small Golgi profiles are evident in the center of the cell; mitochondria are few and may not be evident in a section.

- *Specific granules* are small and most numerous. They contain bacteriostatic and bacteriocidal agents, such as *lysozyme,* as well as alkaline phosphatases.
- *Azurophilic granules* are larger and less numerous. They contain a dense core in addition to other finely stippled material in the granule.

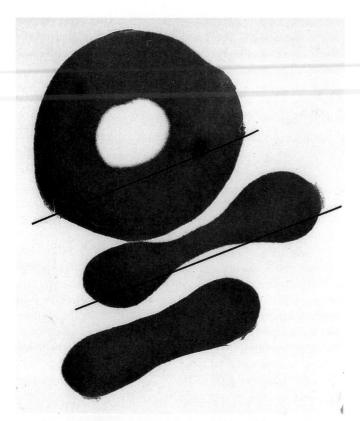

Figure 9.2. Electron micrograph of some erythrocytes seen in different planes. The donut-shaped erythrocyte represents a section cut in a plane paralleling the diameter of the cell but missing its center. The plane of section is represented by the *black line* in the adjacent erythrocyte; thus, the "hole in the donut" is that area represented by the segment of the *line* that is exterior to the cell. The third erythrocyte has a smaller diameter than its neighbor. This is because the section passed in a plane represented by the *line* passing through the donut-shaped erythrocyte. ×8000.

local blood flow at the site of injury. Thromboplastin, also secreted by the damaged blood vessel cells, initiates the series of reactions that leads to the formation of a fibrin clot. These components are released from the platelet granules into the surface-connected tubular system from which they diffuse into the plasma and tissue spaces.

After the definitive clot is formed, platelets bring about clot retraction, probably as a function of the actin in the hyalomere. Finally, after the clot has served its function, platelets are presumably responsible for clot dissolution, probably by release of the contents of the α lysosomal granules into the clot.

White Blood Cells

Neutrophils Are the Most Numerous of the White Blood Cells as Well as the Most Common of the Granulocytes

Neutrophils. Neutrophils measure 10–12 μm in diameter, obviously larger than an erythrocyte. They are named

Figure 9.3. Conventional structural diagram of the heme molecule. Four of these constitute the iron-containing portion of the hemoglobin molecule.

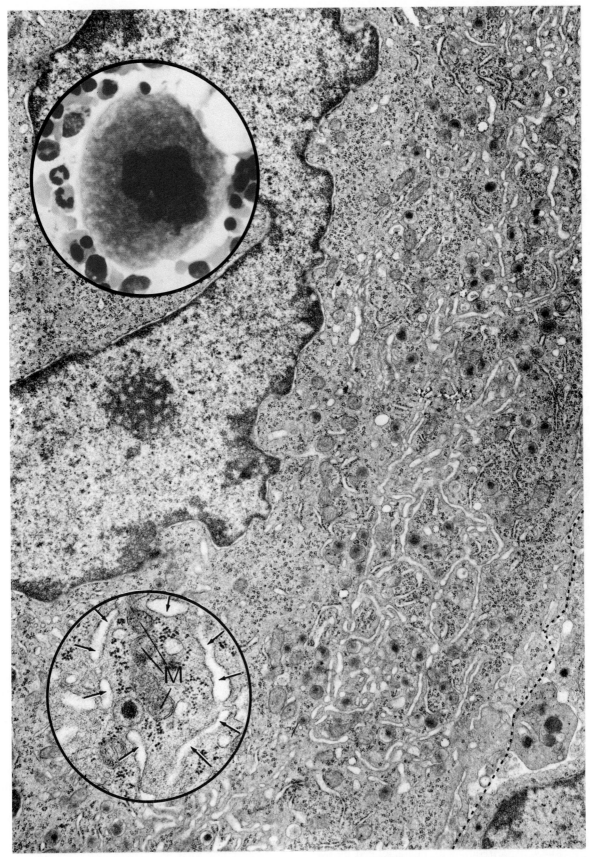

Figure 9.4. Electron and light micrographs of megakaryocytes. The **upper inset** is a light micrograph revealing an entire megakaryocyte from a marrow smear. Its nucleus is multilobed and folded on itself, giving an irregular outline. The "foamy" peripheral cytoplasm of the megakaryocyte represents areas in which segmentation to form platelets is occurring. The smaller surrounding cells are developing blood cells. The **central figure** is an electron micrograph that shows a portion of a megakaryocyte from a bone marrow section that includes two lobules of the nucleus and some of the surrounding cytoplasm. The limit of the cell is defined by the *dotted line* (lower right). The cytoplasm reveals evidence of platelet formation as indicated by the extensive platelet demarcation channels. The **lower inset** is a higher-power electron micrograph that shows a segment of cytoplasm that is almost fully partitioned by the platelet demarcation channels *(arrows)*. It also shows mitochondria *(M)*, a maturing very dense granule, and glycogen particles. A mature circulating platelet is shown in Figure 9.5 for comparison. **Upper inset,** ×1,000; **central figure,** ×15,000; **lower inset,** ×30,000.

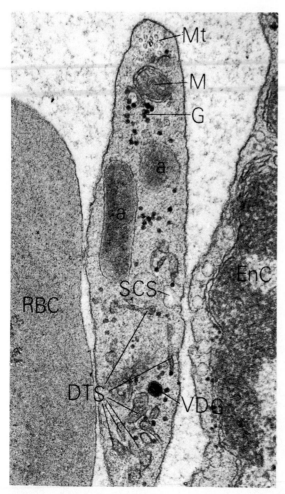

Figure 9.5. High-magnification electron micrograph of a platelet. The cell coat does not show to advantage, but the inclusions and organelles are revealed. They include a mitochondrion *(M)*, microtubules *(Mt)*, a single profile of the surface-connecting system *(SCS)*, profiles of the dense tubular system *(DTS)*, the moderately dense α granules *(a)*, a single very dense granule *(VDG)*, and glycogen particles *(G)*. The microfilaments are not evident against the background matrix of the platelet. *EnC*, endothelial cell; and *RBC*, red blood cell.

The azurophilic granules, which appear early in granulopoiesis and occur in all granulocytes as well as in monocytes and lymphocytes, are the lysosomes of the neutrophil and contain peroxidase and lysosomal enzymes.

Neutrophils Function Extravascularly in the Early Phases of Acute Inflammation

Acute inflammation is the local tissue response at and near the site of injury. It is traditionally characterized by *heat, redness, swelling, pain,* and *loss of function.* The inflammatory response occurs in the connective tissue into which plasma and formed elements of the blood leak from blood vessels damaged by the injury or from vessels that become more permeable in response to the injury, particularly the postcapillary venules. The neutrophils are the most

numerous of the first wave of cells to enter the inflammatory site except, of course, for extravasated red blood cells. They engage in active phagocytosis of bacteria and other foreign organisms and passive phagocytosis of damaged connective tissue cells, red blood cells, and fibrin.

When a bacterium is phagocytosed, the specific granules fuse with the membrane of the phagosome within 30–60 seconds, and their bacteriocidal content is emptied into the phagosome. Azurophilic granules fuse with the phagosome-specific granule complex somewhat later; the hydrolytic enzymes of the lysosomal azurophilic granules digest the microorganism. Many neutrophils die in this process; the accumulation of dead bacteria and dead neutrophils constitutes the thick yellowish exudate called *pus.*

Phagocytosis of Some Bacteria by Neutrophils Is Receptor Mediated

If a person has developed antibodies for the particular bacterium present at the site of injury, the bacterium becomes coated with the specific immunoglobulin (IgG) as well as with a derivative of the complement system of the plasma, both of which act as **ligands** to bind the bacterium to receptors on the surface of the neutrophil. This specific binding triggers a zipper-like closing of the neutrophil membrane around the bacterium. Plasma components that enhance phagocytosis in this manner are called **opsonins.**

Inflammation and Wound Healing Also Involve Monocytes, Lymphocytes, Eosinophils, Basophils, and Fibroblasts

Monocytes also enter the connective tissue during inflammation and transform into *macrophages* that phagocytose cell and tissue debris, fibrin, remaining bacteria, and even the spent neutrophils. For normal wound healing to occur, it is essential that macrophages participate in the inflammatory response; they become the major cell type present in the inflammatory site after the neutrophils are spent. At the same time that the macrophages are becoming active at the site of inflammation, fibroblasts near the site and undifferentiated mesenchymal cells in the adventitia of small vessels at the site begin to divide and differentiate into the fibroblasts that will secrete the fibers and ground substance of the healing wound. Neutrophils and monocytes are attracted to the inflammatory site by chemical factors, a process referred to as **chemotaxis.** Lymphocytes, eosinophils, and basophils also play a role in inflammation, but they are more associated with the immunologic aspects of the process (see page 114). Eosinophils and lymphocytes are more commonly found at sites of **chronic inflammation.**

White Blood Cells Are Motile Cells; They Leave the Circulation and Migrate to Their Site of Activity in the Connective Tissue

An important property of neutrophils and other leukocytes is motility. The neutrophil is rounded while circulat-

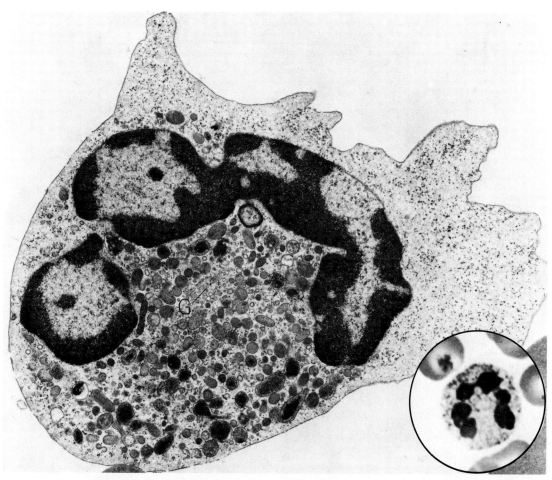

Figure 9.6. Electron micrograph of a human mature neutrophil. The nucleus shows the typical multilobed configuration with the heterochromatin at the periphery and the euchromatin more centrally located. A small Golgi apparatus *(G)* is present, and other organelles are sparse. The punctate appearance of the cytoplasm adjacent to the convex aspect of the nuclear profile is due to glycogen particles. Adjacent to the concave aspect of the nuclear profile are numerous granules. Specific granules appear less dense and more rounded than the azurophilic granules. The latter are fewer in number and appear extremely electron dense. For comparison, a neutrophil from a blood smear observed in the light microscope (LM) is shown in the **inset.** (Electron micrograph courtesy of Dorothea Zucker-Franklin.)

ing through the blood vessels. When it contacts a substratum, it tends to flatten somewhat and extend pseudopods from the main body of the cell. In thin sections, the cytoplasmic content of a pseudopod appears as an expanse of finely granular cytoplasmic matrix with no membranous organelles (Fig. 9.6). The finely granular appearance is due to the presence of actin filaments, some microtubules, and glycogen. These are involved in the extension of the cytoplasm to form the pseudopod and the subsequent contraction that pulls the cell forward through the connective tissue.

Basophils Are the Least Numerous of the White Blood Cells, Less Than 0.5% of the Total Leukocytes

Basophils. Often, several hundred white blood cells must be examined in a blood smear before one basophil is found. A basophil is about the same size as a neutrophil and is so designated because the numerous large granules in its cytoplasm stain with basic dyes. The lobulated basophil nucleus is usually obscured by the granules in stained blood smears, but its characteristics are evident in electron micrographs (Fig. 9.7). Heterochromatin is chiefly in a peripheral location, and euchromatin is chiefly centrally located; typical cytoplasmic organelles are poorly represented.

The large, membrane-bounded granules are those seen with the light microscope (LM) as the basophilic granules. These granules exhibit a grainy texture and myelin figures. The granules contain a variety of substances, namely, hydrolytic enzymes, heparan sulfate, histamine, and slow-reacting substance (SRS) of anaphylaxis.

- *Histamine* and the *SRS of anaphylaxis* are vasoactive agents that, among other actions, bring on the dilation of small blood vessels.

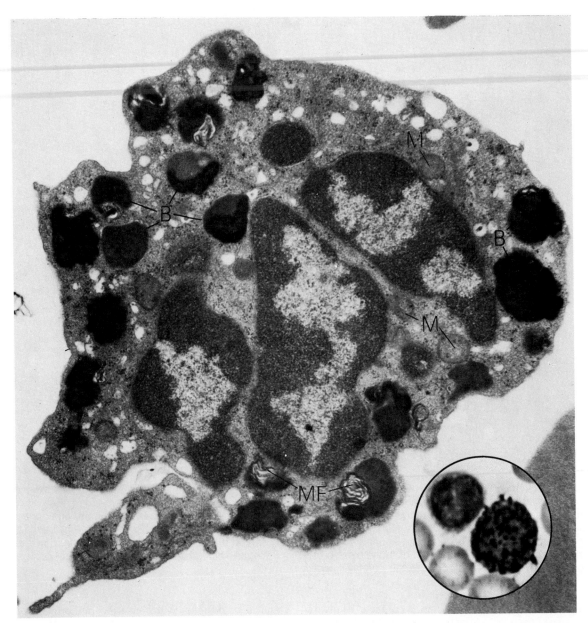

Figure 9.7. Electron micrograph of a human basophil. The nucleus appears as three separate bodies; the connecting strands are not in the plane of section. The basophil granules (B) are very large and have an irregular morphology. Some granules reveal myelin figures (MF). The small, spherical, less dense profiles are mitochondria (M). **Inset.** A blood smear demonstrating the LM appearance of a basophil and an adjacent small lymphocyte. (Electron micrograph courtesy of Dorothea Zucker-Franklin.)

- *Heparan sulfate* is a sulfated glycosaminoglycan that is closely related to the heparin found in the granules of tissue mast cells (page 110). The amount of sulfate in this molecule accounts for the intense basophilia of the specific granules of the basophil. No role for heparan sulfate in inflammation has yet been elucidated.

It is now clear, however, that basophils are functionally related but not identical with mast cells of the connective tissue. Both the mast cell and basophil bind an antibody secreted by plasma cells (page 114), immunoglobulin E (IgE), that on subsequent exposure to and reaction with its allergen results in the release of the vasoactive agents from the basophil (and mast cell) granules. These substances cause the severe vascular disturbances associated with hypersensitivity and anaphylaxis (see page 115). It is likely that these two cell types developed independently during mammalian evolution.

Eosinophils Are So Designated Because of the Large Eosinophilic Refractile Granules in Their Cytoplasm

Eosinophils. An eosinophil, too, is about the same size as a neutrophil; the nucleus of an eosinophil is typically bilobed (Fig. 9.8). As with neutrophils, the compact heterochromatin is chiefly adjacent to the nuclear envelope, whereas the euchromatin is chiefly in the center. The cytoplasm contains numerous large elongated granules measuring 1 μm or more in their largest dimension. The center of the granules contains a **crystalloid body** that is readily seen with the electron microscope. Otherwise, the eosinophil contains only a sparse representation of membranous organelles.

The large granules with their **crystalloid inclusions** are the lysosomes of the eosinophil; it is the crystalloid that is responsible for the refractility of the granules in the LM. It contains an arginine-rich protein called **major basic protein** that probably accounts for the intense acidophilia of the granule. The granules contain peroxidase, histaminase, arylsulfatase, and other hydrolytic enzymes.

- Histaminase neutralizes the activity of histamine.
- Arylsulfatase neutralizes the action of SRS; thus, release of eosinophilic granules counteracts the action of the basophils.

The eosinophil is known to release arylsulfatase and his-

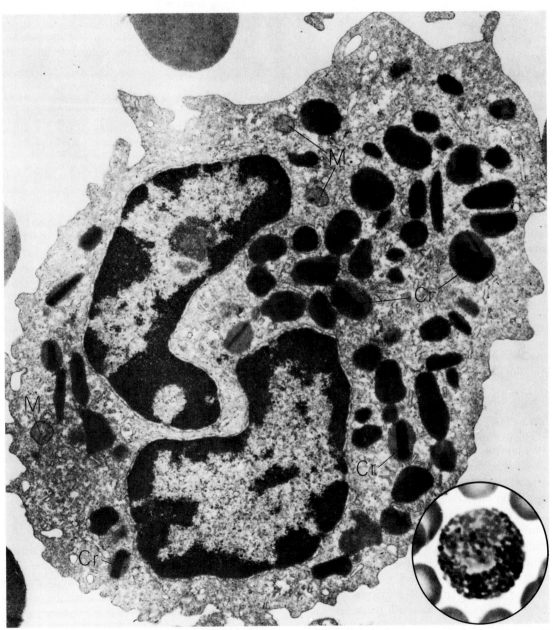

Figure 9.8. Electron micrograph of a human eosinophil. The nucleus is bilobed, but again, the connecting segment is not within the plane of section. The granules are moderate in size, compared with those of the basophil, and show a crystalline body *(Cr)* within the substance of the granule. Careful examination shows the extreme density of a region within the granules to be due to the crystalline body; the remainder of the granule is less dense. A few mitochondria *(M)* are also evident. **Inset.** LM appearance of an eosinophil from a blood smear. (Electron micrograph courtesy of Dorothea Zucker-Franklin.)

taminase at sites of allergic reaction, thereby moderating the potentially deleterious effects of the inflammatory vasoactive agents. The eosinophil is also known to participate in other immunologic responses. It engages in the phagocytosis of antigen-antibody complexes. Thus, the count of eosinophils in blood samples of individuals suffering from allergies and parasitic infections is usually high. They are also found in large numbers in the lamina propria of the intestinal tract (see pages 462 and 468) and at other sites of potential chronic inflammation.

Lymphocytes Are the Main Functional Cells of the Lymphatic or Immune System

Lymphocytes. In the tissues associated with the *immune system* (see Chapter 13), three groups of *lymphocytes* can be identified according to size: small, medium, and large, ranging in diameter from 6 to 18 μm. In the bloodstream, most lymphocytes are small or medium in size, 6–12 μm, with the vast majority being small lymphocytes (more than 90%).

Lymphocytes are the most common agranulocytes and account for about 30% of the total blood leukocytes. In understanding the function of the lymphocytes, it is important to realize that the majority of the lymphocytes found in blood or lymph represent *recirculating immunocompetent cells,* i.e., cells that have developed the capacity to recognize and respond to foreign antigen and are in transit from one site of lymphatic tissue to another.

In Blood Smears, the Small Lymphocyte Approximates the Size of a Red Blood Cell

The small lymphocyte, when observed in a blood smear, has an intensely staining, slightly indented, spherical nucleus. The cytoplasm appears as a very thin pale blue rim surrounding the nucleus. In general, there are no recognizable cytoplasmic organelles.

Electron microscopy reveals that the cytoplasm primarily contains free ribosomes and a few mitochondria. Other organelles are so sparse that they are usually not seen in a thin section. Small dense lysosomes that correspond to the azurophil granules seen in the LM are occasionally seen; a pair of centrioles and a small Golgi complex are located in the area of the indentation of the nucleus, known as the cell center. In the medium lymphocyte, the cytoplasm is more abundant, the nucleus is larger and less heterochromatic, and the Golgi complex is somewhat more developed (Fig. 9.9). Greater numbers of mitochondria and polysomes and small profiles of rough endoplasmic reticulum are also seen in these medium-sized cells. The ribosomes are the basis for the slight basophilia displayed by medium lymphocytes in stained blood smears.

Two Functionally Distinct Types of Lymphocytes Are Present in the Body: T Lymphocytes and B Lymphocytes

Functional Classification of Lymphocytes. The characterization of the lymphocyte types is independent of their size and general morphologic characteristics. The two types are called *T lymphocytes* (*T cells,* thymus-dependent lymphocytes) and *B lymphocytes* (B cells, so named because they were first recognized as a separate population in the *bursa* of Fabricius in birds).

- *T lymphocytes* have a long life span and are involved in cell-mediated immunity.
- *B lymphocytes* have variable life spans and are involved in the production of the several varieties of circulating antibodies.

These two cell types are indistinguishable in blood smears or tissue sections; immunocytochemical staining for different types of receptors on their cell surface must be used to identify them (see below)].

Lymphocytes Are Primed During Their Maturation to Respond to a Specific Antigen

When lymphocytes first encounter a specific antigen that they have been programmed to recognize through the molecules on their plasma membranes, they are stimulated to undergo several mitotic cell divisions. Some of the resulting lymphocytes differentiate into *effector cells,* i.e., cells that have specific functions. For example,

- B lymphocytes may divide several times, producing more B lymphocytes and large clones of cells that differentiate into *plasma cells* involved in the production of antibodies.
- T lymphocytes may undergo several rounds of cell division, producing cells that differentiate into *cytotoxic T lymphocytes* [killer T lymphocytes, helper T lymphocytes, or suppressor T lymphocytes (see below)].
- Some B and T cells do not undergo differentiation into effector cells but serve as long-lived *memory cells,* circulating lymphocytes that are primed to respond more rapidly and to a greater extent to subsequent exposure to their specific antigen.

Although the T and B cells cannot be distinguished on the basis of their morphology, they do have distinctive surface proteins that can be used to identify the cells by using immunolabeling techniques. B cells have intramembrane immunoglobulin molecules that function as antigen receptors. In contrast, T cells have unique cell surface proteins (not antibodies) that appear during discrete stages in the maturation of the cells within the thymus. These surface molecules mediate or augment specific T-cell functions and are required to facilitate the recognition or binding of T cells to foreign antigens.

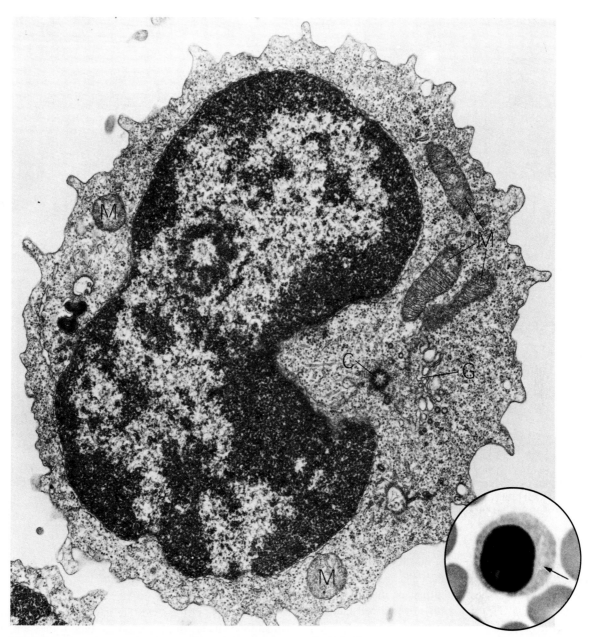

Figure 9.9. Electron micrograph of a medium-sized lymphocyte. The punctate appearance of the cytoplasm is due to the presence of numerous free ribosomes. Several mitochondria *(M)* are evident. The cell center or centrosphere region of the cell (the area of the nuclear indentation) also shows a small

Golgi apparatus *(G)* and a centriole *(C)*. **Inset.** LM appearance of a medium-sized lymphocyte from a blood smear. The Golgi-containing centrosphere region is indicated by the *arrow*. (Electron micrograph courtesy of Dorothea Zucker-Franklin.)

In human blood, it has been found that approximately 90% of the lymphocytes are mature T cells, and 4–10% are mature B cells. Approximately 5% of the cells are identified as **null lymphocytes** and do not demonstrate the presence of the surface markers associated with T or B cells. The null lymphocytes may include cells that are circulating hemopoietic stem cells (see below) or that are natural killer cells (see below). The size differences described above may have functional significance; some of the large lymphocytes may be cells that have been stimulated to divide, whereas others may be plasma cell precursors that are undergoing differentiation in response to the presence of antigen.

Three Fundamentally Different Types of T Lymphocytes Have Been Identified: Cytotoxic, Helper, and Suppressor Lymphocytes

Cytotoxic, Helper, and Suppressor T Lymphocytes. The activities of these cell types are mediated by molecules located on their surface. By employing immunolabeling techniques, it has been possible to identify specific types of T cells and study their function.

- *Cytotoxic T cells* or *killer T lymphocytes (CTLs)* serve as the primary effector cells in cell-mediated immunity.

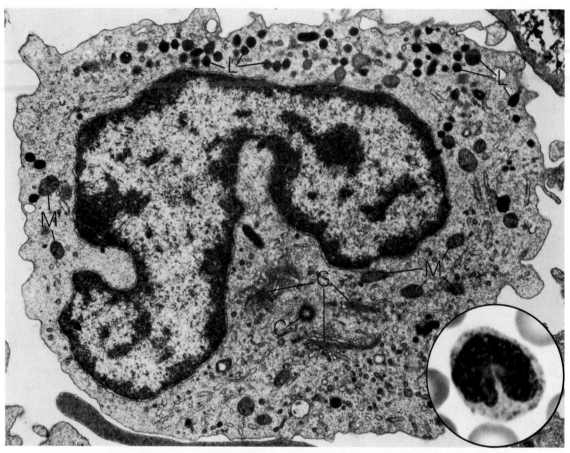

Figure 9.10. Electron micrograph of a human mature monocyte. The nucleus is markedly indented, and the cell center shows several Golgi profiles *(G)* as well as a centriole *(C)*. The small dark granules are the lysosomes *(L)* of the cell. The slightly larger and less dense profiles are mitochondria *(M)*. **Inset.** LM appearance of a monocyte from a blood smear. (Electron micrograph courtesy of Dorothea Zucker-Franklin.)

The CTLs recognize other cells that have foreign antigens on their surfaces and kill the cells by causing them to lyse (by creating holes in the plasma membrane). A classic target of a CTL is a virus-infected cell that displays viral glycoproteins on its surface.

• *Helper T lymphocytes (T_H cells)* assist B cells as well as macrophages in their response to antigens. The interaction between most foreign antigens and the antibodies on the surface of B cells is insufficient to stimulate B-cell growth, differentiation, and secretion of soluble antibody. A major function of the T_H cell is to recognize foreign antigens, usually presented by macrophages, and then to secrete factors (such as lymphokines) that stimulate B cells or other cells that participate in immune reactions, such as CTLs and macrophages.

• *Suppressor T cells (T_S cells)* suppress the activity of B cells. T_S cells appear to dampen the response to foreign antigens and may play a role in suppressing the immune response to self molecules (those normally present in an individual). The T_S cells may also function in the regulation of erythroid cell maturation in the bone marrow.

Monocytes Are the Precursor of the Cells of the *Mononuclear Phagocytic System*

Monocytes. Monocytes are the largest of the white cells in a blood smear. In the peripheral blood, they are in transit from the bone marrow to the body tissues, where they will differentiate into the various phagocytes of the mononuclear phagocytic system, i.e., the connective tissue macrophages (histiocytes), osteoclasts, alveolar macrophages, perisinusoidal macrophages in the liver (Kupffer cells), and macrophages of lymph nodes, spleen, and bone marrow, among others. Monocytes remain in the blood only for about 3 days.

The nucleus of the monocyte is typically more indented than that of the lymphocyte (Fig. 9.10). The indentation is the site of the cell center where there are a well-developed Golgi apparatus and centrioles. The monocyte also contains smooth and rough endoplasmic reticulum and small mitochondria. Although classified as agranular, there are often numerous small, dense azurophilic granules (lysosomes) in the cytoplasm of the monocyte.

As already indicated, during inflammation, the monocyte leaves the blood vessel at the site of inflammation, transforms into a tissue macrophage, and participates in the phagocytosis of bacteria, other cells, and tissue debris. The monocyte-macrophage also plays an important role in immune responses by concentrating antigen and presenting this to lymphocytes (see page 339).

FORMATION OF BLOOD CELLS (HEMOPOIESIS)

Each blood cell has a life cycle of limited duration; during only part of that cycle is the cell a component of the peripheral blood. Blood cell production and destruction go on constantly.

In the adult, red blood cells, granulocytes, monocytes, and platelets are formed in the red bone marrow; lymphocytes are formed both in the marrow and in the lymphatic tissues. To study the stages of blood cell formation, a sample of bone marrow is prepared as a stained smear in a manner similar to that described above for the preparation of a smear of peripheral blood.

Hemopoiesis in Embryonic and Fetal Life

During fetal life, both red and white cells are formed in several organs before the differentiation of the bone marrow. The first phase of *hemopoiesis* or *hematopoiesis* in the developing individual occurs in "blood islands" in the wall of the yolk sac. In the second or hepatic phase, still early in development, hemopoietic centers appear in the liver (and lymphatic tissues); for a time, the liver is the major blood-forming organ in the fetus. The third phase of fetal hemopoiesis involves the bone marrow (and other lymphatic tissues). After birth, hemopoiesis occurs in the red bone marrow and in lymphatic tissues as in the adult. It is interesting that the precursors of the blood cells as well as the precursors of the germ cells (see page 679) both arise in the yolk sac.

Colony-Forming Unit: Monophyletic Theory of Hemopoiesis

The long-standing controversy over whether all blood cells arise from a common stem cell, the unitarian or monophyletic theory, or whether each blood cell type has its own stem cell, the dualistic or polyphyletic theory, has recently been settled with the description of the colony-forming unit (CFU).

The Colony-Forming Unit Is a Pleuripotential Stem Cell That Gives Rise to All of the Blood Cell Lines Found in the Bone Marrow

The CFU was first described after an elegant series of experiments on the restoration of hemopoiesis in lethally irradiated animals, leading to their survival.

If nonirradiated, genetically compatible bone marrow cells are transfused into a lethally irradiated animal, the spleen and bone marrow become colonized by the injected cells. In some of these colonies, called nodular colonies, all of the hemopoietic cell lines (erythrocytic, granulocytic, megakaryocytic, and mononuclear) are found. Experimental studies show that all of the blood cells in a particular nodule are the progeny of one *pleuripotential CFU.*

Other experimental evidence suggests that the CFU is morphologically indistinguishable from a small lymphocyte. Only one in several thousand nucleated bone marrow cells is a CFU. CFUs are even less common in peripheral blood; only one in a million nucleated cells in peripheral blood is believed to be a CFU. Older descriptions of the monophyletic theory suggested that a *hemocytoblast,* a large cell with a euchromatic nucleus and a slightly basophilic cytoplasm, might be the pleuripotential hemopoietic stem cell. It is now believed that the CFU gives rise to a hemocytoblast-like cell that is, at best, short lived. There is, however, reason to question whether it is in any way different from the proerythroblast and the myeloblast described below.

The easiest way to begin the histologic study of blood cell development is to refer to an illustration such as the one in Figure 9.11. The figure outlines those stages in blood cell development that can be recognized by an experienced individual in a section or smear of bone marrow.

Development of Erythrocytes (Erythropoiesis)

The First Recognizable Cell That Begins the Process of Erythropoiesis Is Called the *Proerythroblast;* It Derives From the Colony-Forming Unit

The *proerythroblast* is a relatively large cell, measuring 12–15 μm in diameter. It contains a large spherical nucleus with one or two visible nucleoli. The cytoplasm shows mild basophilia due to the presence of free ribosomes. The proerythroblast, though recognizable, is not easily identified in routine marrow smears.

The Basophilic Erythroblast Is Smaller Than the Proerythroblast, From Which It Arises by Mitotic Division

The nucleus of the basophilic erythroblast becomes smaller and progressively more heterochromatic with repeated mitoses. The cytoplasm shows strong basophilia due to the large number of free ribosomes (polyribosomes) that synthesize the intracellular protein, hemoglobin. The accumulation of hemoglobin in the cell gradually changes the staining reaction of the cytoplasm so that it stains with eosin. At the stage when the cytoplasm displays both eosinophilia, due to the staining of hemoglobin, and basophilia, due to

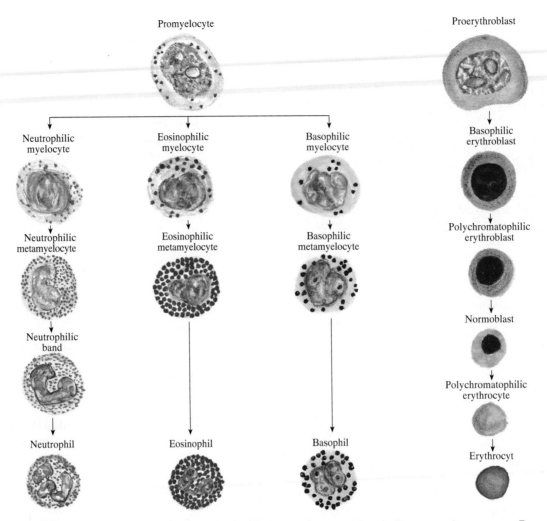

Promyelocyte

Proerythroblast

Neutrophilic myelocyte

Eosinophilic myelocyte

Basophilic myelocyte

Basophilic erythroblast

Neutrophilic metamyelocyte

Eosinophilic metamyelocyte

Basophilic metamyelocyte

Polychromatophilic erythroblast

Neutrophilic band

Normoblast

Polychromatophilic erythrocyte

Neutrophil

Eosinophil

Basophil

Erythrocyt

Figure 9.11. Illustration of the morphologically recognizable stages of erythrocytic and granular leukocytic differentiation in myeloid tissue. Drawn are normal human bone marrow cells as they would typically appear in a smear. Romanovsky-type stain.

the staining of the ribosomes, the cell is called a ***polychromatophilic erythroblast.*** The staining reactions may blend to give an overall gray or lilac color to the cytoplasm, or distinct pink (acidophilic) and purple (basophilic) regions may be resolved in the cytoplasm.

The nucleus of the polychromatophilic erythroblast is smaller than that of the basophilic erythroblast, and coarse heterochromatin granules form a checkerboard pattern that is of help in identifying this cell type. The next named stage in erythropoiesis is the ***normoblast.*** This cell has a small, compact, intensely stained nucleus. The cytoplasm is eosinophilic due to the large amount of hemoglobin (Fig. 9.12). It is only slightly larger than a mature erythrocyte.

The normoblast next loses its nucleus by extruding it from the cell; it is then ready to pass into a blood sinus of the red marrow. Some polyribosomes, still able to synthesize hemoglobin, are retained in the cell. These polyribosomes impart a slight degree of basophilia to the otherwise eosinophilic cells, and because of this, these new red blood cells are called ***polychromatophilic erythrocytes*** (Fig. 9.13). The

polyribosomes of the new red blood cells can also be demonstrated with special stains that cause the polyribosomes to clump and form a reticular network. Because of this, the polychromatophilic erythrocytes are also, and more frequently, called ***reticulocytes.*** In normal blood, reticulocytes (new red blood cells) constitute about 1–2% of the red blood cells. If, however, increased numbers of red blood cells enter the bloodstream (as during increased erythropoiesis to compensate for loss of blood), the number of reticulocytes increases.

Kinetics of Erythropoiesis

Mitoses Occur in Proerythroblasts, Basophilic Erythroblasts, and Polychromatophilic Erythroblasts

At each of these stages of development, the erythroblast will divide several times. It takes about a week for the progeny of a newly formed basophilic erythroblast to reach the circulation. Nearly all erythrocytes are released into the

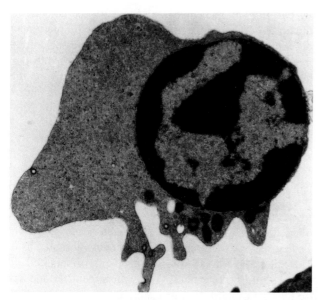

Figure 9.12. Electron micrograph of a normoblast just before extrusion of the nucleus. The cytoplasm reveals mitochondria, a few small vacuoles, a coated pit, and some coated vesicles. The latter are recognizable by their dense outline, a reflection of the coat. The fine dense particles in the cytoplasm are polysomes. ×10,000. (Courtesy of Dorothea Zucker-Franklin.)

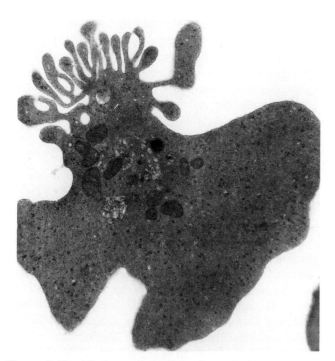

Figure 9.13. Electron micrograph of a reticulocyte. The nucleus is no longer present, and the cytoplasm shows the characteristic fimbriated processes that occur just after nuclear extrusion. Mitochondria are still present, as are degradation vacuoles and polysomes. ×16,500. (Courtesy of Dorothea Zucker-Franklin.)

circulation as soon as they are formed; bone marrow is not a storage site for red blood cells. Virtually all of the apparently mature erythrocytes observed in bone marrow smears are reticulocytes; a few may be intravascular cells that were passing through the marrow at the time of biopsy. Red blood cell formation and release are under the regulation of *erythropoietin,* a glycoprotein hormone secreted by the kidney in response to decreased tissue oxygen tension.

Red Blood Cells Have a Life Span of About 120 Days in Humans

When erythrocytes are about 4 months old, they become fragile and subject to breakage. The macrophage system of the spleen, bone marrow, and liver phagocytoses the red blood cells undergoing degradation. The iron is separated from the hemoglobin and stored as *ferritin* in the spleen for reuse in hemoglobin synthesis. The rest of the *heme* moiety of the hemoglobin molecule binds to albumin and is transported to the liver where it is partially degraded, conjugated, and excreted via the gallbladder as the bilirubin of bile

---

HEMOGLOBIN BREAKDOWN AND JAUNDICE

Bilirubin and other breakdown products of hemoglobin are pigmented. If the conjugation of bilirubin or its excretion into the bile by the hepatocytes are inhibited or if blockage of the bile duct system occurs, the bile pigments may reenter the blood, giving rise to the appearance of yellow in the white of the eye, in the skin, and, finally, systemically. This condition is called jaundice. Some degree of jaundice is common in newborn infants as the fetal hemoglobin (HbF) is broken down and replaced with adult hemoglobins (HbA and HbA$_2$).

Development of Granulocytes (Granulopoiesis)

The First Recognizable Cell That Begins the Process of Granulopoiesis Is the *Promyelocyte;* It, Too, Derives From the Colony-Forming Unit

The *promyelocyte* has a large spherical nucleus, and there are azurophilic (primary) granules in the cytoplasm. Azurophilic granules are produced only in promyelocytes; cells in subsequent stages of granulopoiesis do not make azurophilic granules. For this reason, the number of azurophilic granules is reduced with each division of the promyelocyte and its progeny. Promyelocytes do not exhibit subtypes. Recognition of the neutrophil, eosinophil, and basophil lines becomes possible only in the next stage, the *myelocyte,* when specific granules begin to form.

Specific Granules, With Their Characteristic Staining Reactions, First Appear in Myelocytes

Myelocytes begin with a more or less spherical nucleus that becomes increasingly heterochromatic and acquires a distinct indentation during subsequent divisions. Specific granules emerge from the convex surface of the Golgi complex, whereas azurophilic granules appear at the concave side. The significance of this separation is unclear. Myelocytes continue to divide and give rise to *metamyelocytes.*

The Metamyelocyte Is the First Stage That Is Clearly Divided Into Neutrophil, Eosinophil, and Basophil Lines

A few hundred granules are present in the cytoplasm of each metamyelocyte, and the specific granules of each variety outnumber the azurophilic granules by about 4:1. The nucleus becomes more heterochromatic, and the indentation deepens to form a horseshoe-shaped structure. In the eosinophil and basophil lines, the next stage of development is the *mature eosinophil* and *mature basophil,* respectively.

In the Neutrophil Line, One Last Immature Stage, the Band (Stab) Cell, Precedes Development of First Distinct Nuclear Lobes

The nucleus of the band cell is elongated and of nearly uniform width. Nuclear constrictions then develop in the band neutrophil and become more prominent until three to five nuclear lobes are recognized; the cell is then considered a mature neutrophil, also called a *polymorphonuclear neutrophil.* Band cells are sometimes seen in the circulation along with mature granulocytes, particularly in states of chronic infection.

Kinetics of Granulopoiesis

Cell Division in Granulopoiesis Stops by the Late Myelocyte Stage

The mitotic phase lasts about a week. The postmitotic phase, from metamyelocyte to mature granulocyte, also lasts about a week. The mature granulocytes circulate in the peripheral blood for about 8–12 hours, after which they leave the blood to enter the perivascular connective tissue.

Neutrophils live for 1–2 days in the connective tissue, after which they are destroyed by macrophages. The life span of eosinophils and basophils in the connective tissue has not yet been determined unequivocally. "Mature" neutrophils are divided into a peripheral fraction and a marrow fraction. About 15 times as many mature and near-mature neutrophils are found in the marrow as in the peripheral blood. Neutrophils stored in the marrow enter the circulation in response to infection. The hematopoietic process is summarized in Table 9.3.

A partition of neutrophils also occurs in the vascular compartment. There is a circulating pool and a marginated pool, with the latter contained in small blood vessels through which the blood is not actively circulating. The neutrophils adhere to the endothelium, i.e., marginate, much as they do immediately prior to leaving the vasculature at sites of injury or infection.

A Truly Pluripotential Stem Cell Gives Rise to Colony-Forming Units

Refinements on the original experiments that demonstrated the existence of the CFU as a pluripotential cell have shown that the process is even more complex than described above. A *pluripotential stem cell* that precedes even cells that may be identified as CFUs is now accepted as the basic cell in hematopoiesis. Descendants of this cell differentiate into both general (i.e., pluripotential) and *specific CFUs* (Table 9.4). For example, a descendant of the stem cell may differentiate into a lymphoid stem cell or a myeloid stem cell.

Colony-Forming Units Give Rise to Specific Colony-Forming Cells

The lymphoid stem cell will produce progeny that differentiate into *colony-forming cells (CFC)* that give rise either to T lymphocytes, designated *CFC-T,* or to B lymphocytes, designated *CFC-B.*

The myeloid stem cell, a CFU, will produce progeny that may differentiate into CFC that give rise to several types of blood cells or to single types of blood cells. *Eventually, CFC for each mature blood cell type are produced.* These are designated *CFC-E* for erythrocytes (see above), *CFC-Meg* for megakaryocytes, *CFC-GM* for monocyte- and/or neutrophil-producing cells, *CFC-Bas* for basophils, and *CFC-Eosin* for eosinophils.

Glycoprotein Hormones and Stimulating Factors Regulate All Stages of Hematopoiesis

In addition to identifying the various types of CFC, recent studies have identified and begun to characterize numerous glycoproteins that act both as circulating hormones and as local mediators to regulate hematopoiesis and the differentiation of specific cell types (Table 9.5). The first of these (described more than 30 years ago) is *erythropoietin,* discussed above, which regulates erythrocyte development. The other factors are collectively called *colony-stimulating factors (CSFs)* and are subclassified by the specific cell or groups of cells whose development they affect. The best characterized of the recently isolated factors are several that stimulate granulocyte and macrophage formation, viz., *GM-CSF, G-CSF,* and *M-CSF.* Erythropoietin is now also called *E-CSF. Interleukin-3 (IL-3)* is a CSF that appears to affect the pluripotent stem cell, most CFUs, and, even, terminally differentiated cells. Any par-

TABLE 9.3. Hematopoietic Cell Development[A]

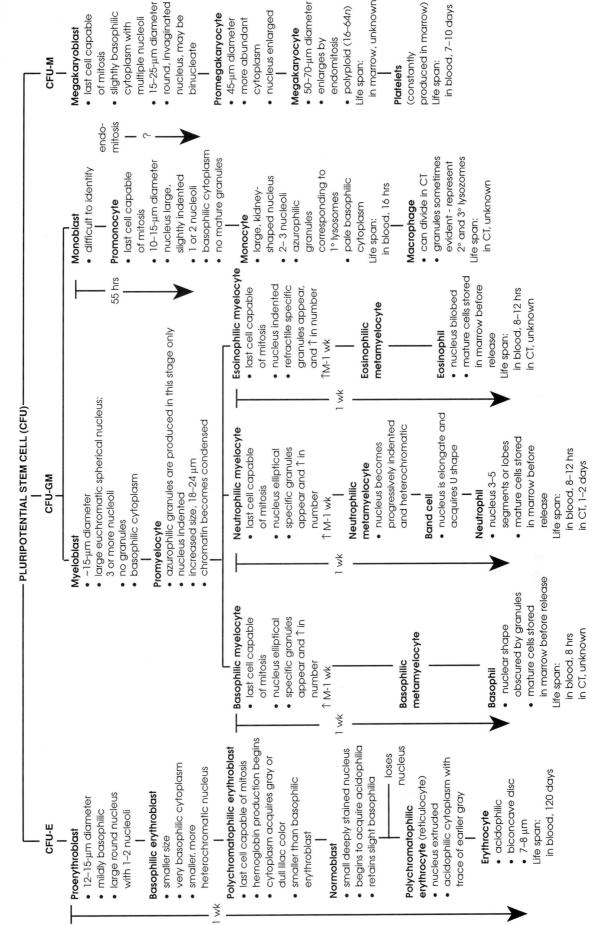

[A]This table shows the maturation of blood cells with histologic characteristics at the various stages, maturation time, and life span after leaving the marrow. Times indicated along vertical lines are the approximate time between recognizable stages. ↑M–1 wk indicates increase in number by mitosis for 1 week before differentiation begins, and CT means connective tissue.

TABLE 9.4.   Hematopoiesis[A]

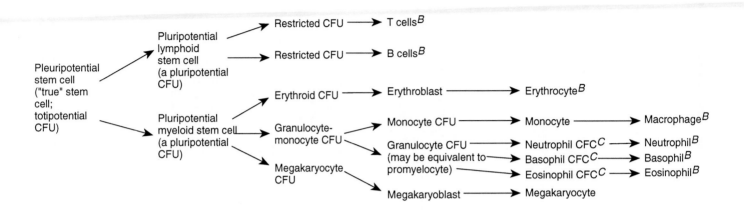

[A]This table includes the most recent concepts of a totipotential stem cell, pluripotential colony-forming units (CFUs), restricted CFUs, and colony-forming cells (CFC). Hematopoietic growth factors [colony-stimulating factors (CSFs)] may and do act individually and severally at any point in the process from the first stem cell to the mature blood cell.
[B]Mature functional cell in blood, bone marrow, or connective tissue.
[C]May be equivalent to myelocyte.

TABLE 9.5.   Hematopoietic Growth Factors and Their Target Cells[A]

FACTOR	SYMBOL	TARGET
Multipotential colony-stimulating factor (CSF) and Interleukin-3	MultiCSF and IL-3	Multipotential progenitor cell, stem cells, granulocyte, monocyte-macrophage, eosinophil, megakaryocyte, and tissue mast cells
Granulocyte-macrophage CSF	GM-CSF	Granulocyte, monocyte-macrophage, eosinophil, megakaryocyte, multipotential progenitor cells
Granulocyte CSF	G-CSF	Granulocyte-macrophage
Macrophage CSF	M-CSF	Monocyte-macrophage, granulocyte
Erythropoietin	Epo	Erythroid
Interleukin-1	IL-1	Stem cells
Interleukin-2	IL-2	T lymphocytes, B lymphocytes
Interleukin-4	IL-4	B lymphocytes, T lymphocytes, tissue mast cells
Interleukin-5	IL-5	B lymphocytes, eosinophil
Interleukin-6	IL-6	B lymphocytes, T lymphocytes, granulocyte, multipotential progenitor cells
Leukemia inhibitory factor	LIF	Monocyte-macrophage

[A]Hematopoietic growth factors include colony-stimulating factors (CSFs), interleukins, and inhibitory factors. They are almost all glycoproteins with a basic polypeptide chain of about 20,000 Daltons. Nearly all of them act on stem cells, colony-forming units (CFUs), colony-forming cells (CFC), committed cells, maturing cells, and mature cells. Therefore, the targets listed above are target lines rather than individual target cells. (Modified from Metcalf D: *Nature* 339:27–30, 1989. Reprinted with permission from *Nature*. Copyright 1989, Macmillan Magazines Limited.)

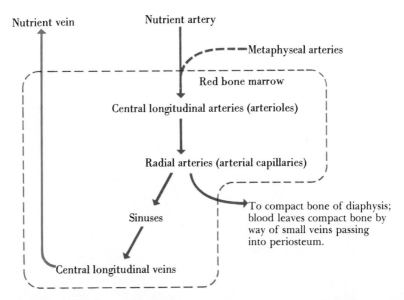

Nutrient vein   Nutrient artery

Metaphyseal arteries

Red bone marrow

Central longitudinal arteries (arterioles)

Radial arteries (arterial capillaries)

To compact bone of diaphysis; blood leaves compact bone by way of small veins passing into periosteum.

Sinuses

Central longitudinal veins

Figure 9.14. Schematic diagram of blood vessels in the bone marrow of a young long bone. The *black dashed line* surrounds vessels within the marrow cavity. A nutrient artery enters the cavity through a large nutrient foramen in the shaft of the bone. Other arteries typically enter the cavity near the ends of the bone. These are designated as metaphyseal arteries.

At least one large nutrient vein leaves the marrow cavity through the nutrient foramen in company with the nutrient artery. Blood vessels also pass from the narrow cavity into the compact bone of the shaft. The vessels leaving the compact bone of the shaft exit as periosteal vessels (see Fig. 8.4, page 155).

ticular CSF may act at one or more stages in hematopoiesis, affecting cell division, differentiation, or cell function. These factors are synthesized by many different cell types, including kidney cells (erythropoietin), T lymphocytes and epidermal cells (IL-3), endothelial cells, fibroblasts, macrophages, and even stromal cells in the bone marrow (the several CSFs that affect granulocyte and macrophage development).

The isolation, characterization, manufacture, and clinical testing of the various CSFs in treatment of human disease is a major activity of the burgeoning biotechnology industry around the world.

Monocyte Development

The Pleuripotential Colony-Forming Unit Also Gives Rise to the Cells That Develop Along the Monocyte-Macrophage Pathway

Promonocytes that are *rapidly dividing* constitute about half of the progenitor cells of this line in the marrow. The other half appear to be promonocytes that divide slowly and serve as a *reserve population of near stem cells*. The stem cell-to-monocyte transformation takes about 55 hours, and the monocytes remain in the circulation only about 16 hours before emigrating to the tissues in which they will differentiate into macrophages. The subsequent life span is not yet elucidated fully.

Megakaryocyte Development

The Fourth Line of Development From the Stem Cell Colony-Forming Unit Is a Colony-Forming Unit Committed to Developing Into a Megakaryocyte

The *megakaryoblast (megakaryocytoblast)* that develops from this CFU is a large cell (about 30 μm in diameter) with a nonlobulated nucleus. No evidence of platelet formation is seen at this stage. Successive *endomitoses* occur in the megakaryoblast; i.e., chromosomes replicate, but there is neither karyokinesis nor cytokinesis. Ploidy increases to 16–64n before chromosomal replication ceases and the cell becomes a megakaryocyte, a cell measuring 50–70 μm in diameter and having a complex multilobulated nucleus and scattered azurophilic granules. Both the nucleus and the cell have increased in size in proportion to the ploidy of the cell. With the transmission electron microscope (TEM), multiple centrioles and multiple Golgi complexes are also seen in these cells.

When bone marrow is examined in a smear, single platelets and clusters of platelets are often seen at the edge of the megakaryocyte. When examined with the TEM, the peripheral cytoplasm of the megakaryocyte is seen to be divided into small compartments by invagination of the plasma membrane. As described on page 190, these invaginations are called *platelet demarcation channels.* The portion of the cytoplasm defined by adjacent channels will be a platelet that will subsequently be released from the cell (see page 193).

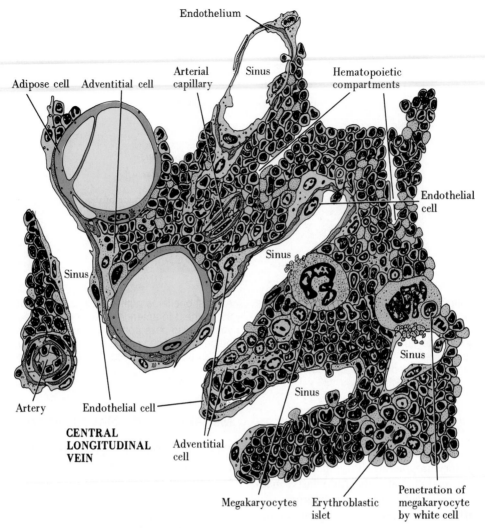

Figure 9.15. Schematic diagram of a cross section through the marrow of a young long bone showing active hemopoiesis. To be noted are the erythroblastic islets engaged in the formation of red blood cells, megakaryocytes discharging platelets into the sinuses, endothelial cells adjacent to a basal lamina that is sparse in places and absent where blood cells are entering the sinuses, and adventitial or reticular cells extending from the basal lamina into the hemopoietic compartment. (Redrawn from a black and white figure in Weiss L (ed): *Cell and Tissue Biology: A Textbook of Histology*, 6th ed. Baltimore, Urban & Schwarzenberg, 1988, p 471.)

Lymphopoiesis

Lymphopoietic Stem Cells Also Originate in the Bone Marrow

Although there is constant proliferation of lymphocytes in the peripheral lymphatic organs during life, the marrow also remains a source of lymphocytes. Those progeny of the *lymphopoietic stem cells* that are destined to become T cells leave the marrow and travel to the thymus where they complete their differentiation. They then enter the circulation as long-lived small lymphocytes. In mammals, cells destined to become B cells originate in several sites including the marrow, the gut-associated lymphatic tissue, and the spleen. The bone marrow, however, remains the primary site of lymphopoiesis in mammals. Lymphocytes constitute as much as 30% of all nucleated cells in the bone marrow.

The precursors of the small lymphocytes in the marrow are called *transitional cells.* They are slightly larger than small lymphocytes but also have a thin rim of cytoplasm and few organelles. The nucleus has a fine, lightly staining chromatin network. Although no figures are available for humans, it is calculated that as many as 10^8 small lymphocytes/day are produced in the mouse bone marrow. The production and differentiation of lymphocytes are discussed in more detail in Chapter 13.

BONE MARROW

Red Bone Marrow Lies Entirely Within the Spaces of Bone, in the Medullary Cavity of Young Long Bones and the Spaces of Spongy Bone

The marrow consists of blood vessels, specialized units of blood vessels called *sinuses,* and a sponge-like network of hemopoietic cells. In sections, the hemopoietic cells appear to lie in "cords" between sinuses or between sinuses and bone.

The sinus of red bone marrow is a unique vascular unit. Its relationship to other blood vessels in the medullary cavity of a long bone is shown schematically in Figure 9.14. The sinus occupies the position normally occupied by a capillary; i.e., it is interposed between arteries and veins. It is believed to derive from vessels that have just nourished the cortical osseous tissue. The sinuses arise from these vessels at the corticomedullary junction. The sinus wall consists of an endothelial lining, a basal lamina, and an outer adventitial cell layer (Fig. 9.15). The endothelium consists of simple squamous epithelium.

The *adventitial cell,* also called a *reticular cell,* sends sheet-like extensions into the substance of the hemopoietic cords, and these thin cellular sheets provide some degree of support for the developing blood cells. In addition to providing support, the adventitial cell produces the reticular fibers. It also plays a role in stimulating the differentiation of stem cells into blood cells by secreting several CSFs. When blood cell formation and the passage of mature blood cells into the sinuses are active, the adventitial cell and the basal lamina become displaced by the mature blood cells as they approach the endothelium to enter the sinus from the marrow cavity.

The Marrow Sinusoidal System Is a Closed Circulation; Newly Formed Blood Cells Must Penetrate the Endothelium to Enter the Circulation

As a maturing blood cell or a megakaryocyte process pushes against an endothelial cell, the abluminal plasma membrane is pressed against the luminal plasma membrane until they fuse, thus forming a transitory opening or *aperture.* The migrating cell or the megakaryocyte process literally pierces the endothelial cell. Each blood cell must squeeze through such an aperture in order to enter the lumen of a sinus. This process may be the mirror image of the mechanism by which the same cells subsequently leave the small venules to enter the peripheral connective tissue. Similarly, a megakaryocyte process must protrude through an aperture so that the platelets can be released directly into the sinus lumen. The aperture is lined by the fused plasma membrane, thus maintaining the integrity of the endothelial cell during the transcellular passage. As the blood cell completes its passage through the aperture or the megakaryocyte that has extruded its platelets withdraws its process, the endothelial cell "repairs itself," and the aperture disappears.

In active red bone marrow, the cords of hemopoietic cells contain chiefly developing blood cells and megakaryocytes. The cords also contain macrophages, mast cells, and some fat cells. Although the cords of hemopoietic tissue appear to be unorganized, specific types of blood cells develop in nests or clusters. Each nest in which red blood cells develop contains a macrophage. These nests are located near the sinus wall. Megakaryocytes are also adjacent to the sinus wall, and they discharge their platelets directly into the sinus through apertures in the endothelium. Granulocytes develop in cell nests farther from the sinus wall. When mature, the granulocyte migrates to the sinus and enters the bloodstream.

Marrow Not Active in Blood Cell Formation Chiefly Contains Fat Cells, Giving It the Appearance of Adipose Tissue

Inactive marrow is called *yellow bone marrow.* It is the chief form of marrow in the medullary cavity of bones in the adult. The yellow marrow retains its hemopoietic potential, however, and when necessary, as after severe loss of blood, it can revert to red marrow, a sign that hemopoiesis has resumed.

PLATE 25. Erythrocytes and Agranulocytes

In examining a blood smear, it is useful to survey the smear with a low-power objective in order to ascertain which parts of the preparation show an even distribution of blood cells. In general, the periphery of a blood smear should be avoided, the cells being either distorted, too close to each other (at the end where the drop of blood was placed), or too widely dispersed (at the opposite end, where the smear ended). Furthermore, the edges of a blood smear do not show a true percent distribution of white cells.

FIGURE 1, blood smear, human, Wright's stain ×400. This figure shows a low-power view of a smear with the blood cells well distributed. Most of the cells are erythrocytes (RBC). They are readily identified because of their number and lack of a nucleus. Scattered among the red cells are four white blood cells that can be distinguished from the erythrocytes without difficulty by their larger size and their staining characteristics. Interspersed among the cells are numerous small speck-like objects. These are blood platelets that have aggregated into small groups and, thus, can be readily observed even at this low magnification. They can be visualized better at higher magnification in Figures 2–4 (arrows).

Erythrocytes have a biconcave shape. They measure about 8.0 μm in diameter in the circulating blood, about 7.5 μm in blood smears, and 6–10 μm, depending on the method used for preserving the tissue, in sectioned material. (A size of 7 μm for the erythrocyte in sectioned material is useful to remember. It enables one to estimate the size of other structures in a histologic section by comparison with the RBC without resorting to a micrometer.) Erythrocytes stain uniformly with eosin, a component of the usual dye mixture (e.g., Wright's) used to stain blood smears. Because of the biconcave form of the erythrocyte, however, its center is thinner and appears lighter than the periphery.

To distinguish the different kinds of leukocytes in a blood smear, it is advantageous to use the highest available magnification, usually an oil-immersion lens. This enables one to use the morphologic features of the cytoplasm in addition to nuclear morphology and cytoplasmic staining in identifying the cell type.

FIGURES 2–6, blood smear, white blood cells, human, Wright's stain ×1800. Figures 2–4 illustrate characteristic features of lymphocytes. The nucleus stains intensely, generally has a rounded shape, and, as illustrated in Figure 2, may possess a slight indentation. These cells measure about 8, 10, and 12 μm in diameter, respectively (circulating lymphocytes range from 6 to 12 μm). In a small lymphocyte (Figure 2), only a small amount of cytoplasm is evident, and the nucleus seems to constitute most of the cellular volume. In large lymphocytes of circulating blood (Figures 3 and 4), there is a larger amount of cytoplasm. (Large lymphocytes of circulating blood are equivalent to the medium-sized lymphocytes of lymphatic tissue. The large lymphocytes of lymphatic tissue are not a characteristic feature of circulating blood except in certain abnormal conditions.) The cytoplasm of lymphocytes may stain a pale blue; sometimes, a distinct, lightly stained Golgi area is evident. In addition, lymphocyte cytoplasm may contain azurophilic granules, as shown in Figures 3 and 4.

Figures 5 and 6 show characteristic features of monocytes. These cells measure approximately 12 and 15 μm in diameter, respectively (monocytes range from 9 to 18 μm). The nucleus is somewhat less "compact" than the nucleus of lymphocytes. The cytoplasm, like that of lymphocytes, stains lightly but tends to have a grayer or duller blue tint. Azurophilic granules are also present in the cytoplasm. Lymphocytes and monocytes are classified as agranulocytes; i.e., they are usually free of specific cytoplasmic granules. Moreover, their nuclei are nonlobed. Thus, they are distinguished from granulocytes, which possess specific cytoplasmic granules as well as a lobed or segmented nucleus.

KEY

arrows, blood platelets

PLATE 25

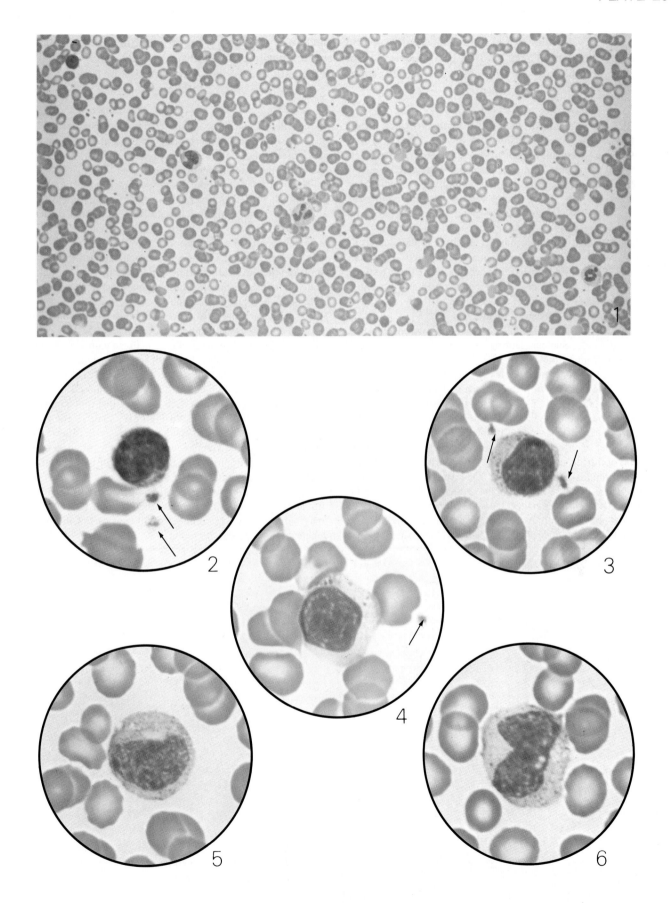

PLATE 26. Granulocytes

Granulocytes are characterized by a lobed nucleus and specific granules within the cytoplasm. Three kinds of granulocytes are present in a peripheral blood smear: *neutrophils*, 55–60% of the white blood cell count; *eosinophils*, about 2–5%, and *basophils*, 1% or less.

FIGURES 1–7, blood smears, human, Wright's stain ×1800. Eosinophils are shown in Figures 1 and 2. These cells measure about 13 μm in diameter (eosinophils range from 10 to 14 μm). The most conspicuous feature of eosinophils is the presence of numerous cytoplasmic granules that stain with eosin. The granules virtually fill the cytoplasm. The eosinophilic granules have specific morphologic characteristics that can be used in the identification of the cells. They are relatively uniform in size within a particular cell; they are about 0.6 μm in diameter, significantly larger than granules of neutrophils; and they are typically closely packed. In going "through focus," eosinophilic granules often display a marked refractility. The nucleus of the eosinophil is usually bilobed, as seen in Figure 2.

Neutrophils develop in the red bone marrow from cells that have a rounded nucleus. During their maturation, the nucleus changes from a rounded to a segmented or lobed form. A fully developed neutrophil nucleus may have as many as five lobes. The configuration and number of lobes vary from one cell to another (Figs. 3–5), and on the basis of the variable nuclear morphology, these cells are sometimes called polymorphonuclear leukocytes. It should be understood, however, that each cell has only one nucleus, with each lobe being joined to its neighbor by a strand of nuclear material.

Neutrophils usually measure 9–14 μm in diameter. The cytoplasm of these cells contains granules that range from 0.1 to 0.4 μm in diameter and stain variably, either azure, light blue, or violet. Although neutrophils contain specific granules, the identification of these cells can usually be accomplished on the basis of the distinctive lobulation of the nucleus. Moreover, because these cells are the most numerous of the leukocytes in a smear of normal blood, their number is an aid in their identification.

The neutrophil in Figure 5 shows a small projection from one of the nuclear lobes *(arrow)*. This is referred to as a drumstick. It is the inactive female X chromosome. Its presence is sufficient to identify the blood as having come from a female, assuming that the normal complement of chromosomes is present. Because the visualization of the drumstick requires a fortuitous orientation of the nuclear lobes, many cells usually need to be examined before a recognizable drumstick profile is found.

Basophils are shown in Figures 6 and 7. They measure about 8 and 14 μm in diameter, respectively (this represents the range in basophil size). These cells contain cytoplasmic granules of variable size that stain intensely with the methylene blue of the blood stain. The granules are randomly distributed throughout the cell, usually superimposed over the nucleus and obscuring it to such a degree that its boundaries barely can be distinguished. In Figure 7, some of the granules are larger than the eosinophilic granules, others are smaller than the eosinophilic granules, and some are as small as those found in the neutrophils. The range in size of basophil granules (in contrast to the more uniform size of granules in eosinophils) is another characteristic that may aid in the identification of these cells. Because the basophil is so rare, it may be necessary to examine a significant part of the blood smear before one can be found.

KEY

arrow, drumstick (inactive X chromosome)

PLATE 26

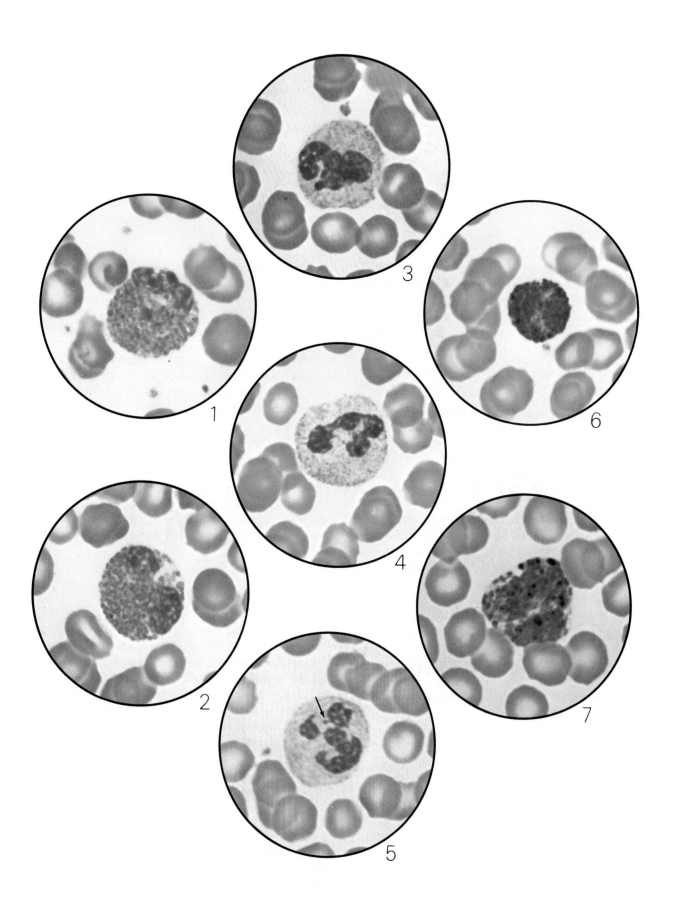

Muscle Tissue

10

Muscle tissue is responsible for movements of the body and for changes in the size and shape of its internal organs. It is characterized by aggregates of specialized cells whose primary role is contraction. Muscle cells are typically elongate and arranged in parallel array, allowing them to work together effectively (Fig. 10.1).

Myofilament Interaction Is Responsible for Muscle Cell Contraction

Two types of myofilaments are associated with cell contraction. They are

- *Thin filaments (6–8 nm in diameter),* composed primarily of the protein *actin*
- *Thick filaments (~15 nm in diameter),* composed of the protein *myosin*

The two types of myofilaments occupy the bulk of the muscle cell cytoplasm. Actin and myosin are also demonstrable in most other cell types, though in considerably lesser amounts, where they play a role in cellular activities such as cytokinesis, exocytosis, and cell migration. Compared with other cells, however, the muscle cell has an enormous number of aligned contractile filaments that it utilizes for the single purpose of producing mechanical work.

CLASSIFICATION OF MUSCLE

Muscle Is Classified on the Basis of the Appearance of the Contractile Cells

Two principal types of muscle are recognized:

- *Striated muscle,* in which the cells exhibit cross-striations at the light microscope (LM) level
- *Smooth muscle,* in which the cells do not exhibit cross-striations

Striated muscle tissue is, however, further subclassified on the basis of its location; thus,

- *Skeletal muscle* is attached to bone and responsible for movements of the axial and peripheral skeleton.

- *Visceral striated muscle* is identical with skeletal muscle, but it is restricted to the soft tissues, namely, the tongue, pharynx, diaphragm, and upper part of the esophagus.
- *Cardiac muscle* is, of course, the muscle of the heart.

The arrangement of the myofilaments is the same in the several types of striated muscle cells. The chief differences between skeletal muscle cells and cardiac muscle cells are in their size and shape and their arrangement relative to one another.

It is largely the specific cytoarchitectural arrangement of the two myofilament types that gives rise to the cross-striations in striated muscle. Smooth muscle cells do not exhibit cross-striations because the myofilaments do not achieve the same degree of order in their arrangement. In addition, the myosin-containing myofilaments are highly labile. Smooth muscle is restricted to the viscera and vascular system.

SKELETAL MUSCLE

Skeletal muscle tissue is the major muscle component of the body. It is organized into muscles that are responsible for the gross and fine movements of limbs and digits and for the maintenance of body position and posture. Similarly, the extraocular muscles of the eye provide precise eye movement. The muscles of the tongue, pharynx, diaphragm, and upper part of the esophagus (visceral striated muscle) play essential roles in speech, breathing, and swallowing.

A Skeletal Muscle Cell Is a Multinucleated Syncytium

In a skeletal muscle, each muscle cell, more commonly called a *muscle fiber,* actually consists of a multinucleated syncytium. It is formed by the fusion of small, individual muscle cells, *myoblasts,* during development. The multinucleated cylindrical fiber may have a diameter of 10–100 μm. (A muscle fiber should not be confused with a connective tissue fiber; muscle fibers are cellular elements, connective tissue fibers are extracellular products of connective tissue cells.)

The nuclei of the muscle fiber are located immediately under the plasma membrane (also called the **sarcolemma**). Traditional histologic descriptions of skeletal muscle used the term **sarcolemma** to describe a thick ''membrane'' as the cytoplasmic boundary of the muscle cell. It is now known that the thick sarcolemma actually represents the plasma membrane of the cell, its **basal** or **external lamina,** and the surrounding **reticular lamina** (see page 63).

A Skeletal Muscle Consists of Striated Muscle Fibers Held Together by Connective Tissue

The connective tissue that surrounds both individual muscle fibers and bundles of muscle fibers is essential for force transduction. At the end of the muscle, the connective tissue continues as a tendon or some other arrangement of collagenous fibers that attaches the muscle, usually, to bone. A rich blood supply and a rich supply of nerves travel in the connective tissue.

The connective tissue associated with muscle is given a specific set of names describing its relationship with the muscle fibers:

- **Endomysium** is the delicate layer of reticular fibers that immediately surrounds individual muscle fibers. Only small diameter capillaries and the finest neuronal branches are present within the endomysium, running in parallel with the muscle fibers.
- **Perimysium** is a thicker connective tissue layer that surrounds a group of fibers to form a bundle or **fascicle.** Larger blood vessels and nerves travel in the perimysium.
- **Epimysium** is the sheath of dense connective tissue that surrounds the collection of fascicles that constitute the muscle. The major vascular and nerve supply of the muscle penetrates through the epimysium.

Red, White, and Intermediate Fibers

Skeletal muscle fibers differ in diameter and in their natural color. The color differences are not conspicuous or ev-

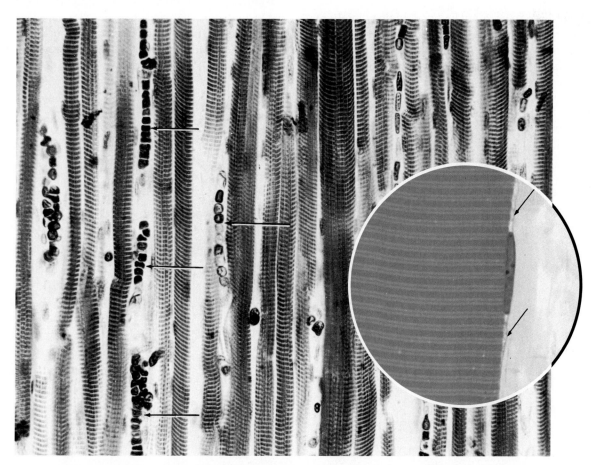

Figure 10.1. Photomicrograph of a longitudinally sectioned skeletal muscle. The muscle cells are arranged in parallel with the capillaries *(arrows)* between the fibers. The length of each fiber or cell extends far beyond the top and bottom limits of the micrograph. The cross-striations of the muscle fibers are readily apparent. The **inset** shows a portion of a single muscle cell at higher magnification. The sarcolemma and adherent substances *(arrows)* can be seen overlying a clear area of sarcoplasm. The visible striations include the Z line, the thin dark lines; the I band, the lighter-staining areas on each side of the Z line; and the A band, the wide darker-staining bands.

ident in hematoxylin and eosin (H&E)-stained sections. However, special cytologic and histochemical reactions based on oxidative enzyme activity (Fig. 10.2), as well as examination of fresh tissue, enable one to distinguish several types of fibers. The most obvious of these are *red fibers, white fibers,* and an intermediate type of fiber. The histochemical staining and enzyme activity of these three types of muscle fibers directly reflect their functional differences.

Fiber Type Is Attributable to Myoglobin and Mitochondrial Content

- *Red fibers* are small fibers with large amounts of myoglobin and cytochromes and many mitochondria.
- *White fibers* are large fibers with less myoglobin and cytochromes and fewer mitochondria.
- *Intermediate fibers* are of intermediate size and have pigment contents and mitochondrial numbers between the two extremes of red and white fibers.

Myoglobin is an oxygen-binding protein that closely resembles hemoglobin (see page 190) and occurs in widely varying amounts in muscle. It is the content of myoglobin and the number of mitochondria with their constituent cy-

tochrome system that is involved in the terminal oxidation reactions that allow skeletal muscle fibers to be classified into the three types, red, white, and intermediate, as described above.

Red fibers make up *slow-twitch* motor units. They have a great resistance to fatigue but generate relatively less muscle tension than white fibers. Myosin adenosine triphosphatase (ATPase) activity (see below) is greatest in red muscle fibers. The large numbers of mitochondria in red fibers are characterized by strong succinic dehydrogenase and nicotinamide adenine dinucleotide-tetrazolium (NADH-TR) histochemical staining reactions (Fig. 10.2). Red fibers are typically found in the limb muscles of mammals and in the breast muscle of migrating birds. More importantly, they are the principal fibers of the long muscles of the back in humans and other higher primates, where they are particularly adapted to the long, slow contractions needed to maintain erect posture.

White fibers make up *fast-twitch* motor units, fatigue rapidly, and generate a large peak muscle tension. Thus, they are adapted for rapid contraction and precise fine movements. They constitute the principal fibers of the extraocular muscles and the muscles that control the movements of the digits. White fibers in these muscles have both greater and more precise innervation than do red fibers.

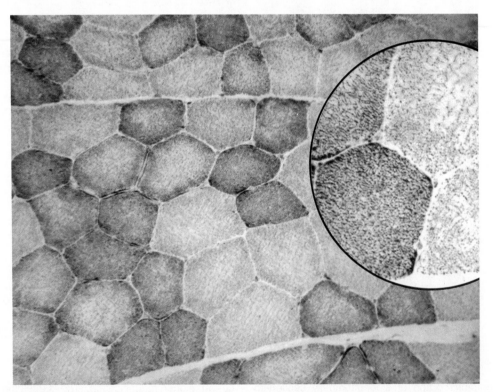

Figure 10.2. Cross section of muscle fibers demonstrating two fiber types with the NADH-TR. The deeply stained, smaller muscle fibers exhibit a strong reaction and correspond to the red muscle fibers. The lighter-staining larger fibers correspond to the white fibers. The **inset** shows portions of the two fiber types at higher magnification. The reaction enables one to visualize the mitochondria that contain the enzymes. The contractile components, the myofibrils, are unstained. (Original slide specimen courtesy of W. Ballinger.)

Fatty Acids Are Broken Down in Mitochondria to Produce ATP

Oxidative phosphorylation occurs primarily in muscle recovering from contraction and in resting muscle. Oxidative phosphorylation follows closely the β-oxidation of fatty acids in mitochondria to liberate two carbon fragments. The oxygen needed for oxidative phosphorylation and other terminal metabolic reactions is derived from the *hemoglobin* in circulating red blood cells and from oxygen stored in the muscle cells bound to myoglobin.

Myofibrils and Myofilaments

The structural and functional subunit of the muscle fiber is the *myofibril.* Muscle fibers are filled with these longitudinally arrayed subunits (Fig. 10.3). Myofibrils are visible in favorable histologic preparations and are best seen in cross sections of muscle fibers in which, collectively, they give the fiber a stippled appearance. The organization of a skeletal muscle from the gross level to the molecular level is illustrated in Figure 10.3.

Myofibrils Are Composed of Bundles of *Myofilaments*

Myofilaments are the individual filamentous polymers of myosin (thick filaments) and actin and its associated proteins (thin filaments). They are the actual contractile elements of striated muscle. The bundles of myofilaments that constitute the myofibril are surrounded by a well-developed smooth endoplasmic reticulum (sER), also called *sarcoplasmic reticulum.* This reticulum forms a highly organized tubular network around the contractile elements in all striated muscle, i.e., skeletal, visceral, and cardiac. Mitochondria and glycogen deposits are located between the myofibrils in association with the sER.

Cross-striations Are the Principal Histologic Feature of Striated Muscle

Cross-striations. Cross-striations are evident in H&E-stained preparations of longitudinal sections of muscle fibers. They may also be seen in unstained preparations of living muscle fibers examined with phase contrast or polarization microscopy. In stained sections and in phase contrast microscopy, alternating light and dark bands are evident; these are termed the *A band,* the *I band,* and the *Z line* (Fig. 10.3).

In polarizing microscopy, the dark bands are *birefringent;* i.e., they alter the plane of polarized light. The dark bands are, therefore, *anisotropic* and are given the name *A band.* The light bands are *monorefringent;* i.e., they do not alter the plane of polarized light. They are, therefore, *isotropic* and are given the name *I band.* Each of the major bands, the A band and the I band, is bisected by a narrow zone of contrasting density (Fig. 10.3).

- The *Z line,* actually *Z disc* (fr. Ger. *Zwischenscheibe,* a between disc), is a dense zone that bisects the I band.
- The *H zone* (fr. Ger. *Helle,* light) is a light zone that bisects the A band.
- An *M line* can be seen in the middle of the H band in ideal preparations.

The H band and M line are demonstrated best in electron micrographs, such as that shown in Plate 28, page 239. As noted above, the cross-banding pattern of striated muscle is largely due to the arrangement of the two kinds of myofilaments. This arrangement now needs to be considered in more functional terms in order to understand the mechanism of contraction.

The Functional Unit of the Myofibril Is the Sarcomere, the Segment of the Myofibril Between Two Z Discs

Sarcomere. The sarcomere is the basic contractile unit of striated muscle. It measures 2–3 μm in relaxed mammalian muscle, may be stretched to more than 4 μm, and, in extreme contraction, may measure as little as 1 μm (Fig. 10.4). The entire muscle exhibits cross-striation because sarcomeres in adjacent myofibrils and in adjacent myofibers are in register.

The Arrangement of Thick and Thin Filaments Gives Rise to the Density Differences That Produce the Cross-striations

The thick filaments are about 1.5 μm long and are restricted to the central portion of the sarcomere, i.e., the A band (Figs. 10.3 and 10.4). The thin filaments attach to the

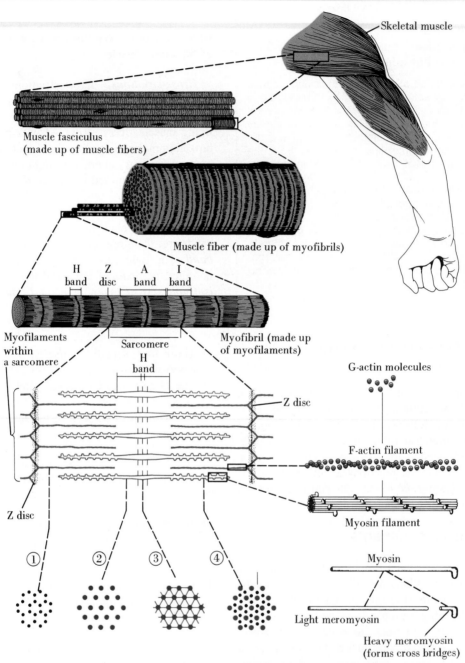

Figure 10.3. Organization of a skeletal muscle. A skeletal muscle consists of bundles of muscle fibers called fascicles. In turn, each fascicle consists of a bundle of elongate muscle fibers (cells). Within the muscle cell are longitudinal units, the myofibrils, which, in turn, are made up of myofilaments of two types: myosin (thick) filaments and actin (thin) filaments. The myofilaments are organized in a specific manner that imparts to the myofibril and, in turn, to the fiber, a cross-striated appearance. The functionally significant repeating unit of the myofibril is the sarcomere; it extends from one Z disc to the next Z disc. The A band marks the extent of the myosin filaments. Actin filaments extend from the Z band into the region of the A band, where they interdigitate with the myosin filaments as shown in the illustration. Items ①–④ show cross sections through different regions of the sarcomere: ①, through actin filaments of the I band; ②, through myosin filaments of the H band; ③, through the center of the A band where adjacent myofilaments are linked to form the M line; and ④, where actin and myosin filaments interdigitate in the A band, each myosin filament is within the center of an hexagonal array of actin filaments. Actin filaments can be broken down into globular actin molecules. Myosin filaments consist of myosin molecules; each one can be further broken down to a light and heavy meromyosin. (From Bloom W, Fawcett DW: *A Textbook of Histology,* 10th ed. Philadelphia, WB Saunders, 1975, p 306.)

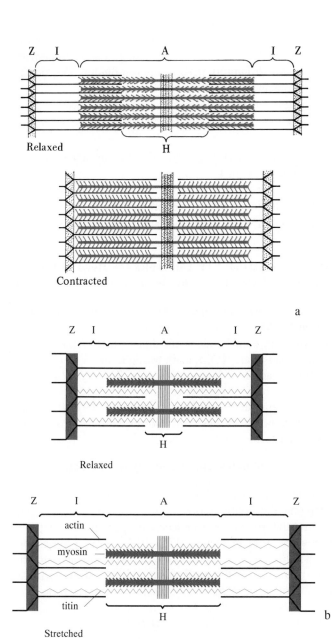

Figure 10.4. **a.** Relaxed and contracted sarcomere. In the relaxed state, interdigitation of actin and myosin filaments is not complete; the H and I bands are relatively wide. During contraction, the interdigitation of the actin and myosin filaments is increased according to the degree of contraction. The length of the A band remains the same; the length of the H and I bands is diminished, again in proportion to the degree of contraction. (Based on E. Schultz, and C. P. Leblond.) **b.** Titin, a large elastic molecule shown in *blue,* anchors the thick myosin filaments, shown in *brown,* to the Z disc. This elastic network maintains the centering of the myosin filaments in the sarcomere and accommodates to extreme stretching that may even eliminate the overlap of thick and thin filaments, as indicated in the lower diagram. (From Alberts B, et al: *Molecular Biology of the Cell,* 2nd ed. New York, Garland Publishing, 1989, p 624.)

Z line and extend into the A band to the edge of the H zone (Figs. 10.3 and 10.4). Portions of two sarcomeres, on either side of a Z disc, constitute the I band and contain only thin filaments (Figs. 10.3 and 10.4).

Thin filaments are composed of *actin, tropomyosin,* and *troponin* and are associated with *α-actinin* at the Z disc. Thick filaments are composed of *myosin* and are held in register in the center of the H zone by fine, transversely oriented filaments of *myomesin* that constitute the M line.

· In a longitudinal section of a sarcomere, the Z disc appears as a zigzag line with a matrix material, the Z matrix, bisecting the zigzag (Figs. 10.3 and 10.4a). The Z disc and its matrix material are cytoskeletal structural elements, and the thin filaments are anchored to the angles of the zigzag by *α-actinin.*

The primary protein components of skeletal muscle fibrils, myosin and actin, and the tropomyosin and troponins associated with actin constitute more than 75% of the total protein of the muscle fiber and are visible as the thick and thin filaments. The remaining proteins are essential in regulating the spacing, attachment, and precise alignment of the myofilaments. These structural proteins include

- *Titin,* a very large elastic protein that connects the *thick* filaments to the Z disc (Fig. 10.4b). The spring-like function of this protein helps to stabilize the centering of the thick myosin filaments in the sarcomere.
- *Nebulin,* an elongated inelastic protein that is attached to the Z discs and runs parallel to the thin (actin) myofilaments.
- *α-Actinin,* a short, bipolar, rod-shaped molecule that bundles actin filaments into parallel arrays at the level of the Z disc and helps to anchor the thin filaments at the Z disc.
- *Myomesin,* a myosin-binding protein that serves to hold thick myosin filaments in register at the M line.
- *C protein,* one of possibly several myosin-binding proteins that serve the same function as myomesin and form several distinct stripes on either side of the M line.

More than 20 other presumably structural or regulatory proteins found in the myofibril have not been functionally characterized as fully as those noted above. Some of these are intermediate filaments that connect the Z discs of adjacent myofibrils to keep them in register; others connect the peripheral myofibrils to the plasma membrane of the muscle fiber.

Cross sections through different parts of the sarcomere provide additional morphologic information regarding the three-dimensional organization of myofilaments. Thus,

- A section through the I band region shows only thin filaments, and they are arranged in an hexagonal pattern (① in Fig. 10.3).
- A section through the H portion of the A bands shows only thick filaments, also in an hexagonal array (② in Fig. 10.3).

- A section through the M band shows a network of fine filaments connecting the myosin filaments. These are the transversely oriented filaments of myomesin that bind the thick filaments together (③ in Fig. 10.3).
- A section at the site where the thick and thin filaments interact in the sarcomere, namely, the A band, reveals the spatial relationship between the two filaments (④ in Fig. 10.3).

Thick and Thin Filaments Overlap in the Lateral Portions of the A Band; Each Thick Filament Is Surrounded by Six Thin Filaments

In the lateral portions of the A band, i.e., the portions closest to the Z disc, cross-bridges can be seen between the thick myosin filaments and the thin actin filaments (Figs. 10.3 and 10.4). These cross-bridges constitute the morphologic and functional basis of the contractile mechanism that is now described.

Contractile Mechanism: Sliding Filament Model

When a Muscle Contracts, Each Sarcomere Shortens and Becomes Thicker, *But the Myofilaments Remain the Same Length*

For the muscle and sarcomere to shorten without the length of the myofilaments changing, the shortening of the sarcomere must be due to an increase in the overlap of the thick and thin filaments in the sarcomere. The I band shortens during contraction, whereas the A band is unchanged in length. The H zone becomes narrower, and the thin filaments penetrate the H zone during contraction. All of these observations indicate that the *thin filaments slide past the thick filaments* during contraction.

Actin and Myosin Structure. The *F-actin* (filamentous actin) of the thin filaments is composed of two strands of *G-actin* (globular) monomers that form a double helix (Fig. 10.3). The monomers have polymerized in a head-to-tail manner similar to that described for tropocollagen in Chapter 5. *Each G-actin molecule has a binding site for myosin.*

Myosin is also composed of two polypeptide chains arranged as a double helix. Each chain has a small globular head that projects at approximately a right angle at one end of the long rod-like molecule (Fig. 10.3). *This globular head has both a specific adenosine triphosphate (ATP)-binding site and the ATPase activity of myosin.*

The myosin molecules aggregate *tail to tail* to form the thick filaments; the rod-like segments overlap, leaving the globular heads projecting from the thick filament. The "bare" zone in the middle of the filament, i.e., the portion of the filament that does not have globular projections, is the *H band*. The projecting globular heads of the myosin molecules form the cross-bridges between the thick filaments and the thin filaments on either side of the H band (Figs. 10.3 and 10.4).

Tropomyosin and the Troponins. *Tropomyosin* also consists of a double helix of two polypeptides to form filaments that run in the groove between the F-actin molecules in the thin filament. In the resting muscle, tropomyosin and *the troponins* mask a myosin-binding site on the actin molecule (Fig. 10.5).

There is one *troponin complex,* consisting of three globular subunits, for each tropomyosin molecule.

- *Troponin-T* (TnT) binds to tropomyosin, anchoring the troponin complex.
- *Troponin-C* (TnC) binds calcium ions, the essential step in the initiation of contraction (see below).
- *Troponin-I* (TnI) usually inhibits the actin-myosin interaction.

The Hydrolysis of ATP Uncouples the Head of the Myosin Molecule From the Actin Filament

Actin-Myosin Interaction: The Basis of the Sliding Filament Model. In the resting muscle, the breakdown products of ATP, namely adenosine diphosphate (ADP) and inorganic phosphate (P_i), remain bound to the ATPase of the globular head of the myosin molecule. Binding between actin and myosin is needed for the ATPase to release the breakdown products and for the energy of the high-energy phosphate bond that has been hydrolyzed by ATPase to be converted to mechanical work.

Calcium Stimulates Binding of Myosin to Actin

When Ca^{2+} is added to the system, it binds to the TnC, changing the configuration of the troponin subunits and driving the tropomyosin molecule deeper into the cleft between the F-actin chains (Fig. 10.5). This exposes the myosin-binding site on the G-actin. Myosin binds to the actin filament, ADP and P_i are released, and the terminal portion of the myosin rod bends toward the H zone. *Because this portion of the myosin is now bound to the actin, the actin filament is driven in the same direction.*

ATP Binding by Myosin Is Essential for the Release of Actin From Myosin

The bending of the myosin head that drives the actin filament also reexposes the ATP-binding site in the head. ATP binds to the ATPase, thus releasing the myosin head from the actin filament. The ATP is split, and the myosin head resumes its original conformation; *it is recocked for the next stroke.* Because the myosin heads are a mirror image about the H zone, this action pulls the thin filaments into the A band, thus shortening the sarcomere. So long as there is both Ca^{2+} and ATP present, this process will keep repeating itself, and the sarcomere will continue to shorten until one of the two components is exhausted. If no ATP is present, the binding will not release, and the muscle cannot relax; this is the basis of *rigor mortis,* the muscular rigidity that develops after death.

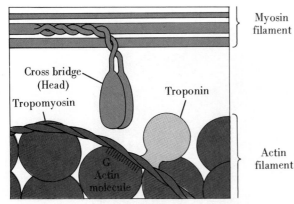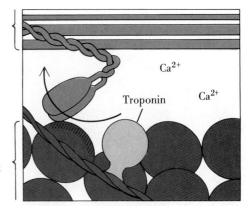

Figure 10.5. Diagram of the sliding filament mechanism of contraction. During relaxation **(left panel)**, tropomyosin blocks the active site on actin *(hatched area)* and prevents interaction with the myosin cross-bridge. During contraction **(right panel)**, the configuration of the troponin is altered by calcium ions. This causes tropomyosin to move away from the active site on actin and allows the actin and myosin head to interact at the now-exposed active site on actin. The movement of many cross-bridges (only one is shown) causes the actin filament to slide along the length of the myosin filaments. The ratcheting process is repeated many times during a single contraction, thereby causing a shortening of the individual sarcomeres. (From Ganong WF: *Review of Medical Physiology,* 15th ed. Norwalk, CT, Appleton & Lange, 1991, p 61.)

SLIDING FILAMENT MODEL

The sliding filament model postulated that ratchet-like movements of the heads of myosin molecules bound to actin produced the movement of the thin filaments relative to the thick filaments, which, in turn, produced the shortening of the sarcomere. Although the sliding filament model could explain contraction in a single sarcomere, it could not adequately explain the shortening of a myofibril of a muscle fiber. It should be obvious that if the activity just described were to occur precisely simultaneously in adjacent sarcomeres, no contraction could occur. Equal and opposite forces would be exerted on either side of the Z disc, and the contraction of any given sarcomere would be prevented by the contraction of its two immediate serial neighbors. Recent studies with ultrahigh-speed photography have demonstrated that there is an extremely small temporal delay in the contraction of adjacent sarcomeres, so that a wave-like contraction actually occurs in each muscle fibril and, consequently, in each muscle fiber.

Regulation of Contraction: Calcium, Sarcoplasmic Reticulum, and the T System. Calcium must be available for the reaction between actin and myosin; i.e., it must be available for contraction to occur. After contraction, the calcium must be removed. This rapid delivery and removal of calcium is accomplished by the combined work of the sarcoplasmic reticulum and a *transverse tubular system* or *T system* derived from the plasma membrane. The sarcoplasmic reticulum is arranged in networks around or between a group of myofilaments (such a group of myofilaments is recognized as a myofibril with the LM). In the most highly developed arrangements, one network of sarcoplasmic reticulum surrounds the A band, and another network surrounds the I band (Fig. 10.6). Where the two networks meet, at the junction between A and I bands, the sarcoplasmic reticulum forms a slightly more regular ring-like channel, called the *terminal cisterna* or *sac,* around the filaments of the myofibril.

Invaginations of the plasma membrane of the muscle cell form the T system. The *T tubules* penetrate to all levels of the muscle fiber. They are located between the adjacent terminal cisternae.

The Sarcoplasmic Reticulum Serves as the Reservoir and Regulator of the Ca^{2+}

The complex of T tubule and two terminal cisternae seen with the transmission electron microscope (TEM) is called the *triad.* The T tubules provide for the rapid transmission of the surface membrane excitation to the terminal sacs throughout the thickness of the muscle fiber. In turn, the terminal sacs release and then reaccumulate calcium. Thus, they serve as a reservoir for this essential ion.

Also located around the myofibrils, in association with the sarcoplasmic reticulum, are large members of mitochondria and glycogen storage granules, both of which are involved in providing the energy for the reactions involved in contraction.

Membrane Depolarization and Ca^{2+} Release. When a nerve impulse arrives at the muscle membrane, the plasma membrane depolarizes, and there is a rush of Na^+ ions into the muscle cell. The depolarization is transmitted into the depths of the cell along the membranes of the T system.

The Influx of Na^+ Ions Into the Cell Across the T-Tubule Membrane Triggers the Release of Ca^{2+} Ions From the Terminal Cisternae of the Sarcoplasmic Reticulum

It is still unclear how the influx of Na^+ ions signals the sarcoplasmic reticulum to release Ca^{2+}. However, large Ca^{2+} release channels in the membrane of the sarcoplasmic reticulum open, and Ca^{2+} rushes into the cytosol, initiating contraction in each myofibril.

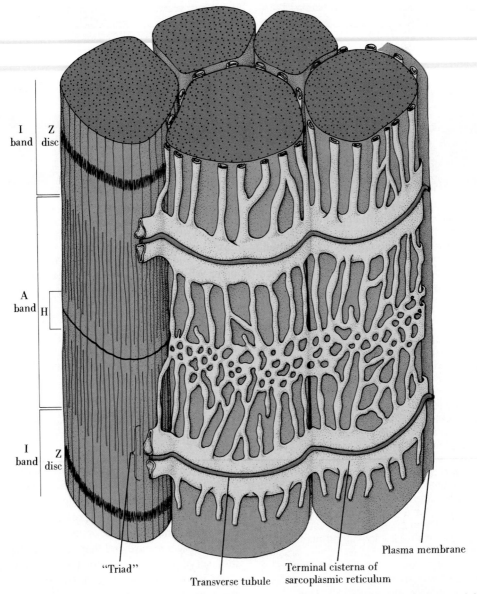

I band | Z disc

A band | H

I band | Z disc

"Triad"

Transverse tubule

Terminal cisterna of sarcoplasmic reticulum

Plasma membrane

Figure 10.6. Diagram of part of a mammalian striated muscle fiber, illustrating the organization of the sarcoplasmic reticulum and its relationship to the myofibrils. In the myofibril at the left, the A, I, and H bands and the Z lines are indicated. The sarcoplasmic reticulum is shown surrounding the myofibrils at the middle and right of the illustration. Note that in mammalian striated muscle fibers two transverse (T) tubules supply a sar- comere. Each T tubule is located at an A-I band junction, where it is associated with two terminal cisternae of the sarcoplasmic reticulum, one cisterna on either side of the T tubule. The triple structure as seen in cross section, where the two terminal cisternae flank a transverse tubule at the A-I junction, is referred to as a triad. (Courtesy of C. P. Leblond.)

- The Ca^{2+} ions interact with the TnC portion of the troponin complex to initiate contraction.
- Simultaneously, a Ca^{2+}-activated ATPase in the membrane of the sarcoplasmic reticulum begins to transport Ca^{2+} back into the terminal cistern.
- The resting concentration of Ca^{2+} is restored in the cytosol in *less than 30 msec.*

This restoration of resting Ca^{2+} concentration near the myofilaments normally leads to the cessation of contraction. Contraction will continue, however, so long as a nerve impulse continues to depolarize the membrane of the muscle cell and T tubules (see Fig. 10.9 for a diagrammatic summary of these events).

Motor Innervation

Skeletal muscle fibers are richly innervated by *motor neurons* that originate in the spinal cord or brain stem. The axons of the neurons branch as they near the muscle, giving rise to twigs that end on individual muscle fibers (Fig. 10.7).

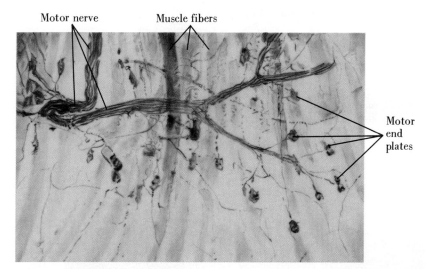

Motor nerve   Muscle fibers

Motor
end
plates

Figure 10.7. Drawing of a silver preparation showing a motor nerve and its final branchings that lead to the motor end plates. The skeletal muscle fibers are oriented vertically in the field. The motor nerve is vertically disposed where it enters the field in the upper left; it then turns and is horizontally disposed.

The *Motor End Plate* Is the Contact Made by the Terminal Branches of the Axon With the Muscle

At the motor end plate on the muscle fiber, the *myelin sheath* of the axon (neurilemma) ends, and the terminal portion of the axon is covered only by a thin portion of the *neurilemmal (Schwann) cell,* here also called *teloglia,* and its basal lamina. At this site, the end of the axon ramifies into a number of end branches, each of which lies in a shallow depression on the surface of the muscle fiber (Fig. 10.8), the receptor region. The axon ending is a typical presynaptic structure and contains numerous mitochondria and synaptic vesicles that contain the transmitter, acetylcholine.

The Synaptic Cleft Is the Space Between the Plasma Membrane of the Axon Ending and the Muscle Fiber

The myoneural junction is a modified synaptic cleft. The muscle fiber plasma membrane that underlies the synaptic cleft has many deep *junctional folds* (subneural folds). Specific receptors are limited to the plasma membrane immediately bordering the clefts and at the top of the folds. The basal lamina extends into the subneural folds.

The synaptic vesicles of the nerve terminal release acetylcholine into the cleft; it reacts with specific acetylcholine receptors on the sarcolemma and initiates the processes leading to muscle contraction. Acetylcholinesterase quickly inactivates the acetylcholine to prevent continued stimulation.

The muscle fiber cytoplasm that underlies the folds contains nuclei, many mitochondria, rough endoplasmic reticulum (rER), free ribosomes, and glycogen. These cytoplasmic organelles are believed to be involved in the synthesis of the specific receptor protein in the membrane of the cleft and of the acetylcholinesterase that breaks down the neurotransmitter.

The *Motor Unit* or *Neuromotor Unit* Is the Name Given to a Neuron and the Specific Muscle Cells It Innervates

A single neuron may innervate from several to a hundred or more muscle fibers. Muscles capable of the most delicate movements have the fewest muscle cells per motor neuron in their motor units. Eye muscles have an innervation ratio of about one neuron to three muscle cells; in the postural muscles of the back, a single neuron may innervate hundreds of muscle cells.

The precise characteristics of any given contraction in a muscle are determined by the specific number of motor neuron endings that depolarize and by the specific numbers of each type of fiber in a mixed muscle that are depolarized. Although depolarization of a single motor end plate is characterized as an ''all-or-none'' phenomenon, not all end plates discharge at once, thus allowing a graded response to the contractile stimulus. Loss of innervation produces fiber (and muscle) *atrophy* as well as total loss of function in the denervated muscle. A summary diagram relating the motor unit to the process of contraction is presented in Figure 10.9.

MYASTHENIA GRAVIS

Myasthenia gravis is an autoimmune disease characterized by extreme muscular weakness. In this disease, the acetylcholine receptors on the sarcolemma become blocked by antibodies to the receptor protein. Thus, the number of functional receptor sites is reduced, and the muscle fiber can respond to the nerve stimulus in only a feeble manner.

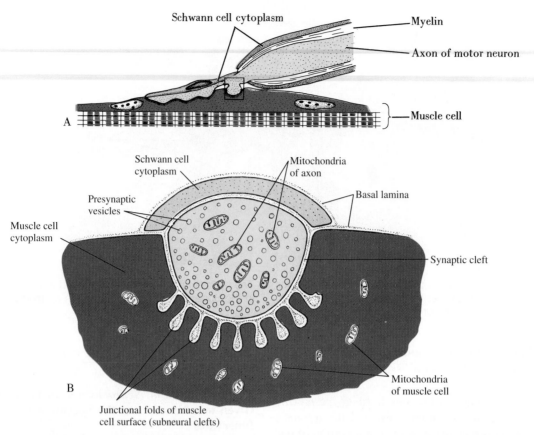

Schwann cell cytoplasm

Myelin

Axon of motor neuron

Muscle cell

A

Schwann cell cytoplasm

Mitochondria of axon

Presynaptic vesicles

Basal lamina

Muscle cell cytoplasm

Synaptic cleft

Mitochondria of muscle cell

B

Junctional folds of muscle cell surface (subneural clefts)

Figure 10.8.   A. Diagram of neuromuscular junction. An axon is shown making contact with the muscle cell. An area similar to the one shown in the *small rectangle* in **A** is diagramed at higher magnification in **B. B.** Note how the junctional folds of the muscle cell augment the surface area within the synaptic cleft. The basal lamina extends throughout the cleft area. The cytoplasm of the Schwann cell is shown covering the axon terminal. (**B** is from Copenhaver WM (ed): *Bailey's Textbook of Histology,* 15th ed. Baltimore, Williams & Wilkins, 1964, p 225.)

Continued Innervation Is Necessary for Muscle Cells to Maintain Their Structural Integrity

The motor nerve cell not only instructs the muscle cells to contract but also exerts a trophic influence on the muscle cells. If the nerve supply to a muscle is disrupted, the muscle cell undergoes regressive changes known as *disuse atrophy.* The most conspicuous indication of this atrophy is the thinning of the muscle and its cells. If the innervation is reestablished surgically or by the slower process of natural regeneration of the nerve, the muscle will regain normal shape and strength.

Sensory Innervation

Encapsulated sensory receptors in muscles and tendons provide information on the degree of tension in a muscle.

The Muscle Spindle Is the Receptor in the Two-Neuron Stretch Reflex, e.g., Knee-Jerk Reflex

The neuromuscular spindle is a specialized receptor unit in muscle that consists of two types of modified muscle fibers and neuron terminals surrounded by a capsule (Fig. 10.10). A fluid-filled space separates the modified muscle cells and the capsule. One type of modified muscle cell, called a *nuclear bag fiber,* contains an aggregation of nuclei in an expanded midregion; the other type, a *nuclear chain fiber,* has many nuclei arranged in a chain.

Primary afferent neuron terminals (terminals of nerves carrying information from the muscle to the spinal cord) are arranged in a spiral around the nuclear region of both fiber types and also make contact with the ends of the nuclear chain fibers. Both fiber types also receive *efferent innervation by γ efferent fibers;* it is believed that the γ efferents regulate the sensitivity of the receptor.

Recent real-time studies using computed tomography (CT) scans of living muscles in different states of contraction suggest that neuromuscular spindles may also represent the axes of functional units within large skeletal muscles. This thus allows precisely regulated contractions of only portions of the muscle by creating ''fixation points'' within the substance of the muscle.

Similar encapsulated receptors, *tendon organs,* are found

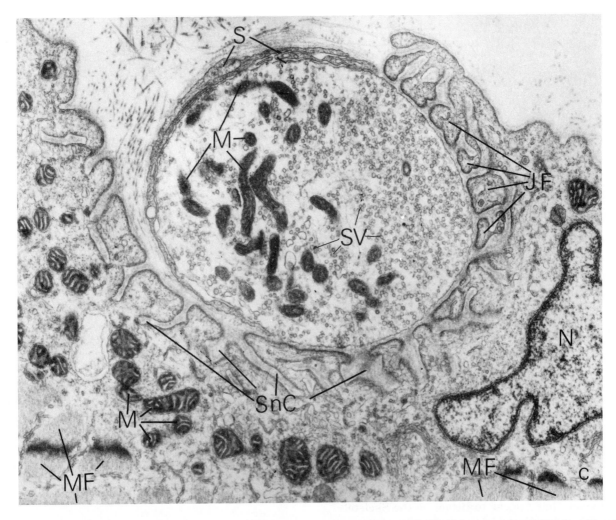

Figure 10.8. C. Electron micrograph of a motor end plate. The axon ending is shown here within the synaptic cleft of a skeletal muscle fiber. It reveals an aggregation of mitochondria *(M)* and numerous synaptic vesicles *(SV)*. The portion of the motor axon ending that is not in apposition to the muscle fiber is covered by Schwann cell cytoplasm *(S)*, but no myelin is present. The muscle fiber shows the junctional folds *(JF)* and the subneural clefts *(SnC)* between them. The basal lamina of the muscle fiber is barely evident within the subneural clefts. Other structures present are the aggregated mitochondria of the muscle fiber *(M)* in the region of the end plate, a nucleus *(N)* of the muscle fiber, and some myofibrils *(MF)*. (Courtesy of George D. Pappas.)

in the tendons of muscle and also respond to stretch. These receptors contain only afferent fibers.

Summary of Events Leading to Contraction of Skeletal Muscle

The event that leads to the contraction of a skeletal muscle fiber is the arrival of a nerve impulse at the neuromuscular junction, i.e., at the motor end plate (see Fig. 10.9). The nerve cell conducting these impulses is called a ***motor neuron.*** The cell body of this neuron is within the spinal cord (or in the brain stem). It sends a long cytoplasmic process, called the ***axon*** or ***nerve fiber,*** to the skeletal muscle, where the axon branches to innervate one or more muscle fibers (see Fig. 10.7).

The events involved in contraction can be summarized as follows (the numbers in parentheses refer to the numbers in Fig. 10.9): The nerve impulses are measured as an action potential of the nerve fiber *(1)*. The nerve impulses are transmitted to the muscle cell *(2)*, and this results in a depolarization of the plasma membrane and in the generation of an action potential by the membrane of the muscle cell *(3)*. The depolarization action potential spreads over the muscle cell and continues via membranes of the T tubules into the substance of the muscle cell *(4)*. At the muscle cell triads, the T tubules are in close contact with the lateral enlargements of the sarcoplasmic reticulum, and at this point, the excited (depolarized) T-tubule membrane *(5)* causes calcium to be released from the sarcoplasmic reticulum into the cytoplasmic matrix *(6)*. The calcium then

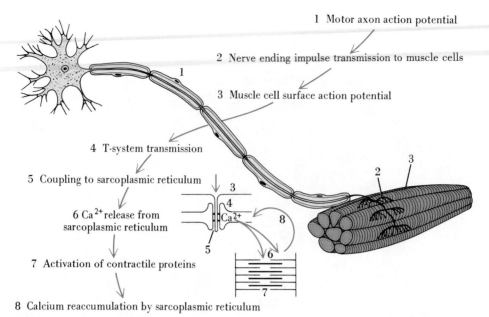

1 Motor axon action potential

2 Nerve ending impulse transmission to muscle cells

3 Muscle cell surface action potential

4 T-system transmission

5 Coupling to sarcoplasmic reticulum

6 Ca²⁺ release from sarcoplasmic reticulum

7 Activation of contractile proteins

8 Calcium reaccumulation by sarcoplasmic reticulum

Figure 10.9. Diagram showing summary of events leading to contraction of skeletal muscle and the site where these occur. See the text for a description of the events indicated by the numerals. (Based on Peachey LD: In: *Bicore* XVIII. New York, McGraw-Hill, 1974.)

activates the contractile proteins *(7)*, as described above, and contraction ensues. The calcium is returned to the cisterns of the sarcoplasmic reticulum *(8)* at the end of these events.

Repair, Healing, and Renewal

Some Nuclei That Appear to Belong to the Skeletal Muscle Fiber Are Nuclei of Small Satellite Cells

Satellite cells are interposed between the plasma membrane of the muscle fiber and its basal lamina. They are stem cells that may proliferate after minor injury to give rise to new myoblasts.

So long as the basal lamina remains intact, the myoblasts fuse within the basal lamina to form myotubes, which then mature into a new fiber. In contrast, disruption of the basal lamina results in fibroblast repair of the injured site with scar tissue formation.

CARDIAC MUSCLE

Cardiac muscle is the type of striated muscle found in the wall of the heart and in the base of the large veins that empty into the heart. It consists of long fibers that appear to branch and anastomose with neighboring fibers. Unlike skeletal muscle fibers, the fibers of cardiac muscle are formed by individual, mononucleated cardiac muscle cells that are joined to one another in linear array.

Cardiac muscle has the same types and arrangement of contractile filaments as described above for skeletal muscle. Therefore, the cardiac muscle cells as well as the fibers

they form exhibit cross-striations that are evident in routine histologic sections. In addition, cardiac muscle fibers exhibit densely staining cross-bands, called *intercalated discs*, that cross the fibers in a linear fashion or in a fashion that resembles the risers of a set of steps (Fig. 10.11). The intercalated discs represent the site of attachment of a cardiac muscle cell to its neighbors.

Nuclei of Cardiac Muscle Cells Are Located in the Center of the Cell

The central location of the nucleus in cardiac muscle cells helps to distinguish them from multinucleated skeletal muscle fibers, whose nuclei lie immediately under the sarcolemma. With the TEM, it can be seen that the myofibrils of cardiac muscle separate to pass around the nucleus, thus outlining a biconical juxtanuclear region in which the cell organelles are concentrated. This region is rich in mitochondria and contains the Golgi apparatus, lipofuscin pigment granules, and glycogen. In the atria, *atrial granules* measuring 0.3–0.4 μm in diameter, are also concentrated in the juxtanuclear cytoplasm. These granules contain two polypeptide hormones. Each hormone affects urinary excretion of sodium and contraction of vascular smooth muscle. The hormones are called *atrial natriuretic factor (ANF)* (fr. L. *natrium*, sodium) and *brain natriuretic factor (BNF)*, with the latter being identical with a hormone first isolated from the brain. Both hormones are diuretics and inhibit renin secretion in the kidney and aldosterone secretion in the adrenal gland (see pages 570 and 613). Both hormones also stimulate relaxation of vascular smooth muscle. In congestive heart failure, circulating BNF increases. There is evi-

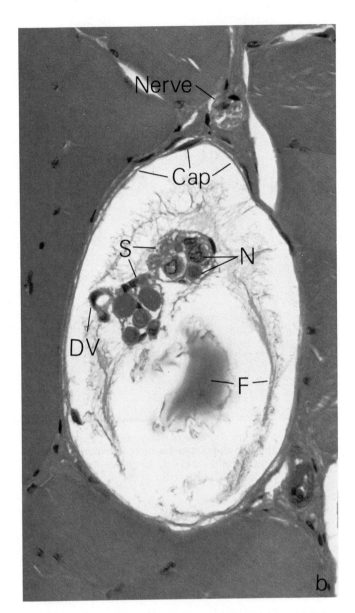

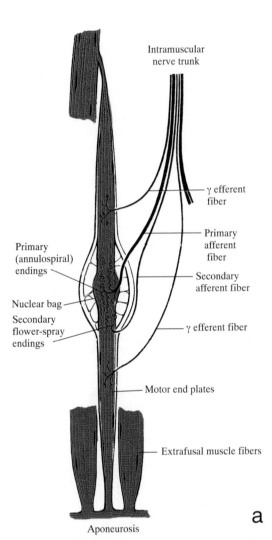

Intramuscular
nerve trunk

γ efferent
fiber

Primary
afferent
fiber

Secondary
afferent fiber

γ efferent fiber

Motor end plates

Extrafusal muscle fibers

Primary
(annulospiral)
endings

Nuclear bag

Secondary
flower-spray
endings

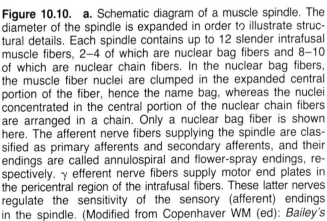

Aponeurosis

a

Figure 10.10. **a.** Schematic diagram of a muscle spindle. The diameter of the spindle is expanded in order to illustrate structural details. Each spindle contains up to 12 slender intrafusal muscle fibers, 2–4 of which are nuclear bag fibers and 8–10 of which are nuclear chain fibers. In the nuclear bag fibers, the muscle fiber nuclei are clumped in the expanded central portion of the fiber, hence the name bag, whereas the nuclei concentrated in the central portion of the nuclear chain fibers are arranged in a chain. Only a nuclear bag fiber is shown here. The afferent nerve fibers supplying the spindle are classified as primary afferents and secondary afferents, and their endings are called annulospiral and flower-spray endings, respectively. γ efferent nerve fibers supply motor end plates in the pericentral region of the intrafusal fibers. These latter nerves regulate the sensitivity of the sensory (afferent) endings in the spindle. (Modified from Copenhaver WM (ed): *Bailey's*

Textbook of Histology, 15th ed. Baltimore, Williams & Wilkins, 1964, p 231.) **b.** Light micrograph of a cross section of a muscle spindle, showing two bundles of spindle cells in the encapsulated, fluid-filled receptor. In one bundle, several of the spindle cells are cut at an angle that exhibits their nuclei *(N)*. The capsule of the spindle *(Cap)* can be seen as a faint boundary separating it from the adjacent muscle fibers. Immediately above and outside of the spindle is a nerve that may be supplying the spindle. The complex nerve endings associated with the spindle cells cannot be distinguished in this H&E-stained section. In close proximity to one of the bundles of spindle cells is a small blood vessel *(BV)*. The flocculent material *(F)* within the capsule is precipitated proteoglycans and glycoproteins from the fluid that filled the spindle before fixation.

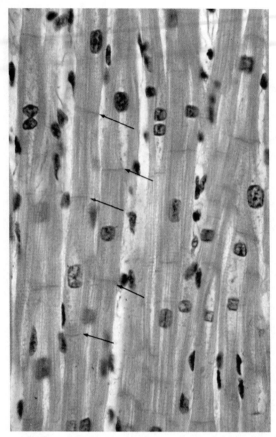

Figure 10.11. Photomicrograph of longitudinally sectioned cardiac muscle. The *arrows* point to the intercalated discs. The discs represent specialized end-to-end junctions of adjoining cells. Also note the apparent branching of the muscle fibers.

dence that the increased level of BNF in this pathologic condition comes from secretory granules induced in *ventricular* cardiac muscle cells.

In addition to the juxtanuclear mitochondria, cardiac muscle cells are characterized by very large mitochondria that are densely packed between the myofibrils. These large mitochondria often extend for the full length of a sarcomere and have numerous, closely packed cristae (Fig. 10.12). There are, also, associated concentrations of glycogen granules between the myofibrils. Thus, the structures that store energy (glycogen granules) and the structures that release and recapture energy (mitochondria) are located adjacent to the structures (myofibrils) that use the energy to drive contraction.

Intercalated Discs

The intercalated discs represent the major site of attachment between cardiac muscle cells. When examined with the TEM, the step-like appearance of the intercalated discs seen in the LM appears to be due to the presence of a *transverse component* that crosses the fibers at a right angle to the myofibrils and a *lateral component* that runs parallel to the myofibrils.

The junctions between the cardiac muscle cells to form the fibers are composed of three components:

- *Fasciae adherentes*
- *Maculae adherentes,* desmosomes
- *Gap junctions*

These three components are found in different parts of the intercalated discs and have different functions.

Fasciae Adherentes Are the Major Portion of the *Transverse* Component of the Intercalated Discs

The adhering plates serve to hold cardiac muscle cells together at their ends to form the functional fiber. They are equivalent in structure, both in the presence of a space between the plasma membranes and in the presence of dense material in this space, to the zonulae adherentes of epithelia.

They also serve as the site at which the thin filaments in the terminal sarcomere anchor onto the plasma membrane. Thus, they are also *functionally* similar to the zonulae adherentes of epithelial cells, which serve as anchoring sites for actin filaments of the terminal web.

Some cardiac muscle cells in a fiber may join with two or more cells through intercalated discs, thus creating a branched fiber.

Maculae Adherentes (Desmosomes) Bind the Individual Myocytes to One Another

The desmosomes help to prevent the cells from pulling apart under the strain of regular repetitive contractions. They are found in both the transverse and lateral components of the intercalated disc.

Gap Junctions Constitute the Major Structural Element in the *Lateral* Component of the Intercalated Disc

The gap junctions provide ionic continuity between adjacent myocytes, thus allowing contractile signals to pass from cell to cell. They allow cardiac muscle to **behave as a syncytium** while retaining cellular integrity and individuality.

Smooth Endoplasmic Reticulum and the T System

The smooth endoplasmic reticulum (sER) of cardiac muscle is not as well organized as that of skeletal muscle. It does not usually separate bundles of myofilaments into discrete cylindrical myofibrils.

The Smooth Endoplasmic Reticulum in Cardiac Muscle Is Organized Into a Single Network per Sarcomere, Extending From Z Disc to Z Disc

The T tubules in cardiac muscle penetrate into the myofilament bundles at the level of the Z disc, between the ends

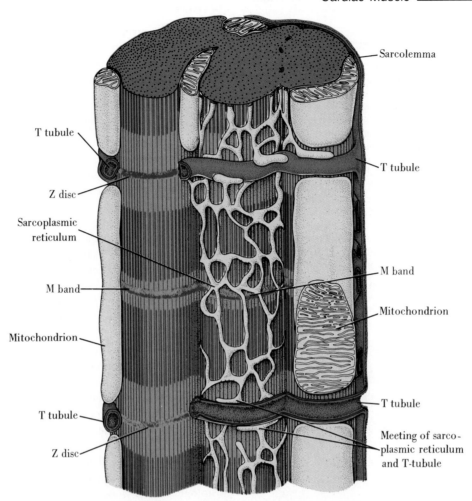

Figure 10.12. Organization of mammalian ventricular cardiac muscle fiber. The transverse tubules are much larger than the T tubules of skeletal muscle and carry an investment of basal lamina material into the cell. They also differ in that they are located at the level of the Z disc. The portion of the sarco- plasmic reticulum adjacent to the T tubule is not in the form of an expanded cisterna, but rather, it is organized as an anastomosing network. (Redrawn from Fawcett DW, McNutt S: *The Journal of Cell Biology* 42:1, 1969, by copyright permission of The Rockefeller University Press.)

of the sER network. Thus, there is only one T tubule per sarcomere in cardiac muscle. The small terminal cisternae of the sER at the level of the Z disc interact with the T tubules to form a *diad* (Fig. 10.12). The basal lamina adheres to the invaginated plasma membrane of the T tubule as it penetrates into the cytoplasm of the muscle cell.

The T tubules are larger and more numerous in mammalian cardiac ventricular muscle than in mammalian skeletal muscle. They are less numerous, however, in cardiac atrial muscle.

Spontaneous Contraction Versus Neural Control

All Cardiac Muscle Cells Exhibit a Spontaneous Rhythmic Contraction or Beat

The intrinsic spontaneous beat is evident in embryonic cardiac muscle cells as well as in cardiac muscle cells in tissue culture. In the heart, this beat is initiated, locally

regulated, and coordinated by specialized, modified cardiac muscle cells that are organized into nodes and bundles to transmit the contractile impulse to various parts of the myocardium in a precise sequence. These cells, called *cardiac conducting cells (Purkinje cells),* and their functions are described in Chapter 12 (see, also, Plate 33, page 249.)

Many unmyelinated nerves, mostly derived from the vagus nerve (cranial nerve X), end near the nodes. The impulses carried by these nerves do not initiate contraction but only modify the rate of intrinsic cardiac muscle contraction.

Injury and Repair

Mature Cardiac Muscle Cells Do Not Divide

Destroyed cardiac muscle cells are not replaced by muscle cells. An injury to cardiac muscle tissue that results in the death of cells is repaired by the formation of fibrous connective tissue with consequent loss of cardiac function at the site of injury. This is the pattern of injury and repair

COMPARISON OF THE THREE MUSCLE TYPES

Cardiac muscle can be described as resembling both skeletal muscle and smooth muscle in its structural and functional characteristics. As in skeletal muscle, the contractile elements of cardiac muscle, i.e., thick and thin filaments, are organized into sarcomeres surrounded by sER and mitochondria and are in communication with the cell surface via T tubules, and the adult cells do not divide. Cardiac muscle cells retain their individuality, however, as do smooth muscle cells, although they are in functional communication with their neighbors through gap junctions. Cardiac muscle cells have, as do smooth muscle cells, a spontaneous beat that is regulated but not initiated by autonomic and hormonal stimuli, and a centrally located nucleus and perinuclear organelles. These common characteristics suggest that cardiac muscle may have evolved in the direction of skeletal muscle from the smooth muscle of primitive circulatory systems.

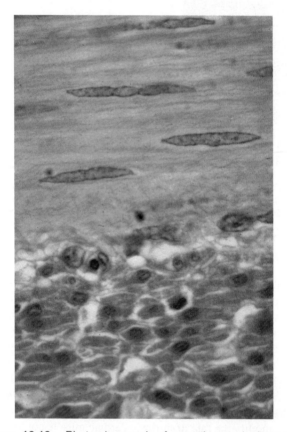

Figure 10.13. Photomicrograph of smooth muscle from the small intestine. The muscle is arranged in two layers. The upper portion of the micrograph shows the muscle cells cut in longitudinal section. Where the cells are cross-sectioned, some have the nucleus included in the plane of section, whereas others do not. This is a reflection of the much greater length of the cell compared with its width. Note that it is usually the smaller cross-section profiles that lack the nucleus. They represent the tapering ends of the muscle cells. Also note that the longitudinal smooth muscle cells are not easily delineated from one another. This is due to the way they lie over one another within the thickness of the section.

in nonfatal *myocardial infarction* (commonly, heart attack). The buildup of scar tissue due to repeated small myocardial infarctions can be as dangerous as the damage from a single large infarction.

SMOOTH MUSCLE

Smooth muscle is the simplest appearing muscle tissue. Smooth muscle is the intrinsic muscle of the *alimentary canal, blood vessels, genitourinary tract, respiratory tract,* and other hollow and tubular organs. It is also found as organized muscle bundles in the *iris* and *ciliary body of the eye,* as a thin sheet in the skin of the scrotum (the dartos muscle), and as isolated fibers in association with hair follicles (arrector pili muscles).

Smooth muscle generally occurs as bundles or sheets of elongate fusiform cells (Fig. 10.13). The cells, also called fibers, range in length from 20 μm in the walls of small blood vessels to about 200 μm in the wall of the intestine; they may be as large as 500 μm in the wall of the uterus during pregnancy. Smooth muscle cytoplasm stains rather evenly with eosin in routine H&E preparations due to the concentration of *actin* and *myosin* that they contain.

The nuclei of smooth muscle cells are located in the center of the cell and often have a corkscrew appearance in longitudinal section. This is due to contraction of the cell during fixation. This characteristic is often of help in distinguishing smooth muscle cells from fibroblasts in routine histologic sections.

In the TEM, it is evident that the cytoplasmic organelles are concentrated at each end of the nucleus. The rest of the cytoplasm is seen to be filled with 6–8-nm actin filaments interspersed with 8–10-nm intermediate filaments (Fig. 10.14). *Cytoplasmic densities* are seen among the filaments and in relation to the plasma membrane. Special techniques are needed to demonstrate 16-nm myosin filaments in smooth muscle cells.

The *Cytoplasmic Densities or Dense Bodies* Contain the Protein α-*Actinin*

α-Actinin is found in the Z discs of striated muscle where it helps to anchor the actin myofilaments. Together, the intermediate filaments and dense bodies in smooth muscle are thought to serve a skeletal function akin to that of the Z disc of striated muscle. In support of this concept is the finding that the dense bodies, when observed in the TEM, sometimes appear as linear structures. In some fortuitous sections, they exhibit a branching configuration consistent with a three-dimensional anastomosing network that extends from the sarcolemma into the interior of the cell (Fig. 10.15).

A modified version of the sliding filament model described above can explain contraction in both striated and smooth muscle. In smooth muscle, bundles of contractile

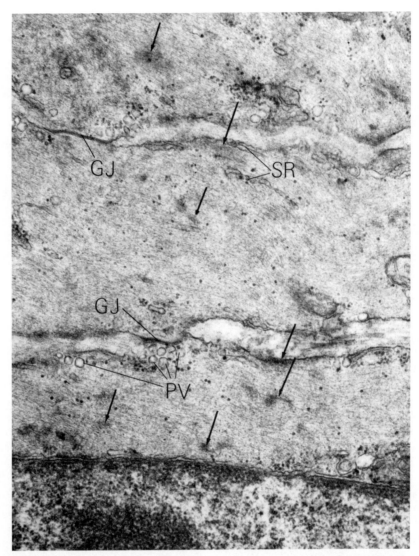

Figure 10.14. Electron micrograph of a portion of three smooth muscle cells. The nucleus of one cell is in the lower part of the micrograph. The bulk of the cytoplasm is occupied by actin filaments, which are just recognizable at this magnification. The α-actinin-containing dense areas are indicated by the *arrows*. Elements of the sarcoplasmic reticulum *(SR)* and the pinocytotic vesicles *(PV)* are also indicated. The small dark particles are glycogen. Lastly, the presence of a gap junction *(GJ)* or nexus between adjacent cells can also be seen. ×30,000.

filaments containing both actin and myosin are thought to be anchored to dense bodies on the plasma membrane at one end and to dense bodies associated with bundles of intermediate filaments of the cytoskeleton at the other (Fig. 10.16*a*). As in striated muscle, the contraction is initiated by a rise in Ca^{2+} in the cytosol, but this does not act through a troponin-tropomyosin complex on the actin filament. Rather, a rise in Ca^{2+} stimulates a ***myosin light-chain kinase*** to phosphorylate one of the two light chains of myosin. When this chain is phosphorylated, the myosin head can react with actin and produce contraction (Fig. 10.16*b*). When it is dephosphorylated, the myosin head dissociates from actin. This phosphorylation occurs rather slowly, with maximum contraction often taking up to a second to achieve.

Smooth muscle cell myosin hydrolyzes ATP at about 10% of the rate in skeletal muscle, producing a slow cross-bridg-

ing cycle that gives a slow contraction in these cells. However, smooth muscle cells and nonmuscle cells that contract by this same mechanism can produce sustained contractions over long periods of time while using only 10% of the ATP that would be used by a striated muscle cell performing the same job.

Smooth Muscle Cells Have No T System

Large numbers of pinocytotic vesicles are associated with the sarcolemma and the sER. The vesicles and the sER sequester the calcium that is released to stimulate contraction.

In the sarcoplasm adjacent to each nuclear pole, there are numerous mitochondria, some cisternae of rER, free ribosomes, glycogen granules, and a small Golgi apparatus. Smooth muscle cells make contact with neighboring cells

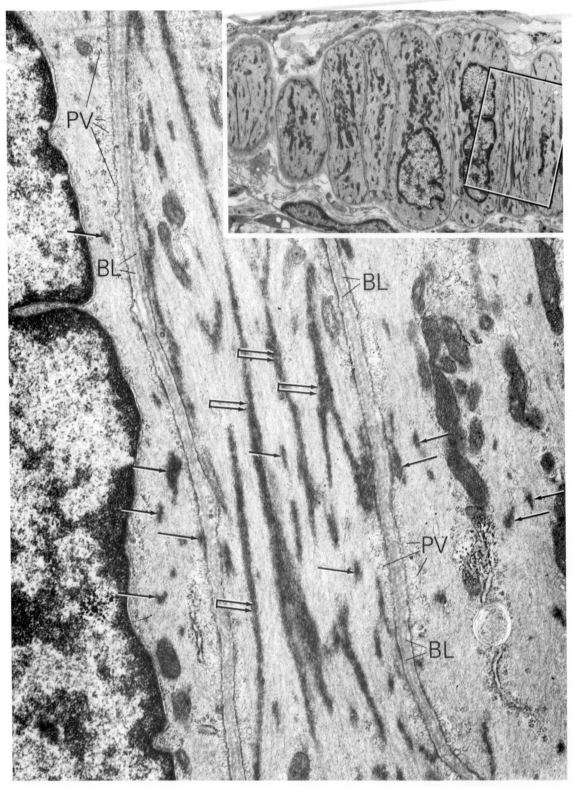

Figure 10.15. Electron micrographs showing the cytoplasmic densities in vascular smooth muscle cells. The plane of section includes only the smooth muscle cells in the wall of the vessel (see **inset**). The *rectangle* in the **inset** shows portions of three smooth muscle cells that appear at higher magnification in the large micrograph. The α-actinin-containing cytoplasmic densities *(single arrows)* usually appear as irregular masses, some of which are in contact with and attached to the plasma membrane. The cell in the center of the micrograph has been cut in a plane closer to the cell surface and reveals these same densities as a branching structure *(double arrows)*. A three-dimensional model of the cytoplasmic densities would reveal an anastomosing network. *BL,* basal (external) lamina; and *PV,* pinocytotic vesicles. ×30,000; **inset,** ×4,000.

by gap junctions. The gap junction between two smooth muscle cells was originally designated as a *nexus;* that term is still in use.

Contraction and Its Control

Smooth Muscle Is Specialized for *Slow, Prolonged Contraction*

As noted above, smooth muscle cells may remain contracted for long periods of time without fatigue. Smooth muscle may contract in a wave-like manner, producing peristaltic movements as in the gastrointestinal tract and the male genital tract, or it may contract throughout, producing extrusive movements as in the urinary bladder, the gallbladder, and the uterus. Smooth muscle has *spontaneous contractile activity* in the absence of nerve stimuli.

Contraction of smooth muscle is usually under the reg-

ulatory control of postganglionic neurons of the *autonomic nervous system (ANS)* (see page 276); most smooth muscle is directly innervated by both sympathetic and parasympathetic nerves. In the gastrointestinal tract, however, the third component of the ANS, the enteric branch, is the primary source of nerves to the muscular layers.

Smooth muscle contraction may also be stimulated by hormones released by the posterior pituitary gland (oxytocin and, to a lesser extent, vasopressin; see page 600) and may be stimulated or inhibited by hormones secreted by the adrenal medulla (the biogenic amines, i.e., epinephrine and norepinephrine; see page 620).

Oxytocin is a potent stimulator of smooth muscle contraction, and its release by the posterior pituitary plays an essential role in uterine contraction during parturition. It is often used as an exogenous inducer or enhancer of labor.

Many of the peptide secretions of the enteroendocrine cells (see page 449) also stimulate or inhibit smooth muscle

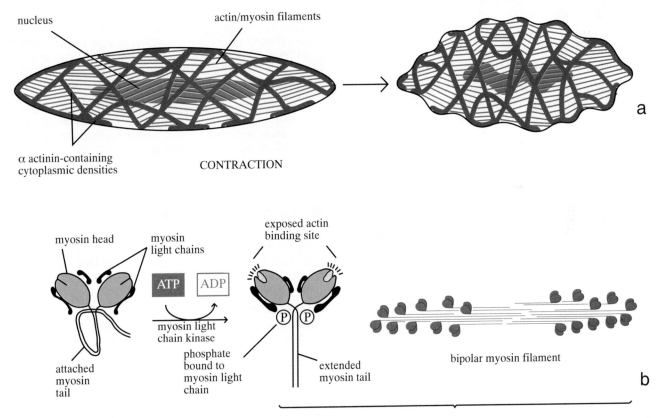

Figure 10.16. **a.** A suggested model for smooth muscle cell contraction. Bundles of filaments containing both actin and myosin, shown in *red,* anchor on cytoplasmic densities shown in *gray.* The densities are associated with the plasma membrane and with cytoplasmic intermediate filaments. Because the contractile filament bundles are oriented obliquely to the long axis of the cell, their contraction shortens the cell and produces the "corkscrew" shape of the nucleus. (Adapted from Alberts B, et al: *Molecular Biology of the Cell,* 2nd ed. New York, Garland Publishing, 1989, p 615.) **b.** A suggested model for the molecular events of smooth muscle contraction. For con-

traction to occur in smooth muscle myosin and nonmuscle myosin, the myosin light chains associated with the head of the molecule must be phosphorylated. Phosphorylation produces a conformational change in the myosin head, exposing the actin-binding site. Phosphorylation also releases the tail of the myosin molecule from its attachment to a "sticky patch" on the head, thus allowing the myosin molecules to self-assemble into short, bipolar filaments that then resemble the thick filaments of striated muscle. (Adapted from Alberts B, et al: *Molecular Biology of the Cell,* 2nd ed. New York, Garland Publishing, 1989, p 627.)

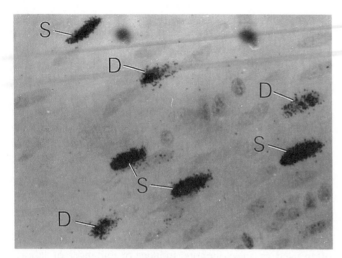

Figure 10.17. Autoradiograph of rabbit colon muscularis externa from an animal that had been injected with tritiated thymidine 21 days before the tissue was sampled. In this nest of labeled cells, both heavily labeled stem cells *(S)* and lightly labeled daughter cells *(D)* can be seen. These are frequently adjacent to each other. ×700.

contraction, particularly in the alimentary canal and its associated organs.

Nerve Terminals in Smooth Muscle Are Observed Only in the Connective Tissue Adjacent to the Muscle Cells

The nerve fibers pass through the connective tissue within the bundles of smooth muscle cells; enlargements in the passing nerve fiber (*bouton en passant;* see page 262) occur adjacent to those muscle cells that are to be innervated. The enlargements contain synaptic vesicles with neuromuscular transmitters. However, the neuromuscular contact is not comparable to the motor end plate of striated muscle. Rather, a considerable distance, usually 10–20 μm (in some locations, up to 200 μm), may separate the nerve terminal and the smooth muscle. The neurotransmitter released by the nerve terminal must diffuse across this distance in order to reach the muscle.

Not all smooth muscle cells are exposed directly to the transmitter, however. As in cardiac muscle, contraction is propagated from cell to cell via gap junctions, thus producing coordinated activity within a smooth muscle bundle or layer.

Secretion

Smooth Muscle Cells Also Secrete Connective Tissue Matrix

Smooth muscle cells have organelles typical of secretory cells. A well-developed rER and large Golgi complex are found in the perinuclear zone. Smooth muscle synthesizes both type IV (basal lamina) collagen and type III (reticular) collagen as well as laminin, elastin, and proteoglycans. Except at the gap junctions, smooth muscle cells are surrounded by a basal lamina. In some locations, such as the walls of blood vessels and the uterus, smooth muscle cells secrete large amounts of collagen and elastin.

In the wall of the afferent arteriole of the glomerulus in the kidney (see page 570), modified smooth muscle cells, the *juxtaglomerular cells,* secrete the hormone *renin,* an essential component in the renin-angiotensin regulatory control of blood pressure.

COMPLEXITY OF SMOOTH MUSCLE INNERVATION

The description of autonomic innervation of smooth muscle according to the sympathetic and parasympathetic classification and their respective **adrenergic** and **cholinergic** transmitters may be more complex than traditionally thought. Viewed in the TEM, nerve terminals with empty-appearing synaptic vesicles are interpreted to be cholinergic, secreting the neurotransmitter acetylcholine; those nerve terminals with dense granular material in the synaptic vesicles are interpreted to be adrenergic, secreting the neurotransmitter norepinephrine. Other transmitters have also been identified, but they are not as well understood as the two mentioned. They have been collectively grouped under the heading **purinergic,** and they are likely to be contained in large vesicles with an opaque content. Nerve endings in smooth muscle tissue that contain primarily mitochondria and no vesicles are construed to be sensory. Both sympathetic and parasympathetic fibers innervate smooth muscle, and it is most difficult to distinguish between the fibers. Autonomic fibers are efferent. In some smooth muscle, the adrenergic transmitters stimulate and the cholinergic transmitters inhibit contraction; in other smooth muscle, the reverse is true.

Renewal, Repair, and Differentiation

Smooth Muscle Cells Are *Not Postmitotic;* i.e., They Are Still Capable of Dividing to Maintain or Increase Their Number

Smooth muscle cells may respond to injury by undergoing mitosis. In addition, there are regularly replicating populations of smooth muscle cells. Smooth muscle in the uterus proliferates during the normal menstrual cycle and during pregnancy, both activities being under hormonal control. The smooth muscle cells of blood vessels have also been shown to divide regularly in the adult, presumably to replace damaged or senile cells; the smooth muscle of the muscularis externa of the stomach and colon regularly replicates and may even slowly thicken during life (Fig. 10.17).

New smooth muscle cells have been shown to develop from undifferentiated mesenchymal cells in the adventitia of blood vessels. Smooth muscle cells have also been shown to develop from the division and differentiation of endothelial cells and *pericytes* in developing vessels. Pericytes are stellate cells located within the basal lamina of capillaries and postcapillary venules that make contact with the adluminal surface of the vascular endothelial cells via fine processes and maculae occludentes. In capillaries, they have a cytoplasmic morphology difficult to distinguish from that of the endothelial cell. In postcapillary venules and pericytic venules, they may form a nearly complete investment of the vessel with cells that resemble smooth muscle cells (see Chapter 12).

Fibroblasts in healing wounds may develop morphologic and functional characteristics of smooth muscle cells (*myofibroblasts,* see page 107). Epithelial cells in numerous locations, particularly sweat glands, mammary glands, salivary glands, and the iris of the eye, may take on the characteristics of smooth muscle cells *(myoepithelial cells). Myoid cells of the testis* have a contractile function in the seminiferous tubules; and even the cells of the perineurium, a concentric layer of connective tissue that surrounds groups of nerve fibers and partitions peripheral nerves into distinct fascicles, function as contractile cells as well as transport barrier cells.

PLATE 27. Skeletal Muscle

Skeletal muscle cells, also called fibers, are long multinucleated protoplasmic units arranged in parallel with their neighbors. Their multiple nuclei are at the periphery of the cell, just under the plasma membrane (sarcolemma). The main volume of the cell is occupied by the contractile elements. The organization of contractile filaments is particularly well ordered, and their specific arrangement accounts for the cross-striations seen in a longitudinal section of the skeletal muscle fibers; this is the basis for the name, *striated muscle*. Skeletal muscle is richly supplied with blood, and each fiber is usually in proximity to several capillaries.

FIGURE 1, skeletal muscle, H&E ×400. A section of skeletal muscle fibers in longitudinal profile is shown in this figure. Note the parallel alignment of the fibers *(M)*; they are vertically oriented in the illustration. The fibers appear to be of different thickness. This is largely a reflection of the plane of section through the muscle fibers. For example, note the polygonal shape of the fibers when cross-sectioned, as in Figures 2 and 3. By drawing a random imaginary line across either micrograph, as if the line were the plane of a longitudinal section, considerable variation would occur with respect to the width of each fiber included in the section. Some fibers might be sectioned along their broadest dimension; some, at their narrowest dimension; and others, at some intermediate dimension.

The cross-striations are the bands that appear at right angles to the long axis of the fibers. They are seen at higher magnification in the **inset**. Two major bands, the darker or more heavily stained *A* band and the lighter *I* band, have been labeled. In addition, the **inset** shows a thin line that bisects the I band; this is the Z line. The other bands, i.e., the M and H bands, are not evident despite the relaxed state of the muscle fibers. The relatively wide I band is an indicator of the relaxed state of the muscle.

Examination of the cytoplasm about the nucleus in the **inset** reveals that the cross-striations do not extend into the areas adjacent to the nuclear poles. This cytoplasm stains lightly *(asterisks)* and contains a concentration of organelles not directly involved in the contractile process.

Between the muscle fibers is a small amount of delicate connective tissue, the *endomysium.* There are also two capillaries *(C)* within the endomysium. Although they do not display the structural features of the vessel walls, they can be identified by virtue of the red blood cells in the lumen. The nuclei directly associated with the capillary belong to endothelial cells. Note how they appear to bulge into the lumen **(inset).**

FIGURE 2, skeletal muscle, H&E ×260. A cross section of striated muscle cells is shown here. As already noted, the muscle fibers *(M)* appear as polygonal profiles. They are partially outlined by numerous nuclei; at the relatively low magnification shown in this figure, however, it is not easy to ascertain if these nuclei belong to the muscle cells, to the capillary endothelial cells, to satellite cells, or to fibroblasts in the endomysium that surrounds the individual muscle cells. A larger amount of connective tissue *(CT)* separates bundles of muscle fibers; this connective tissue is called *perimysium;* it contains small arteries and veins *(BV).*

FIGURE 3, skeletal muscle, H&E ×640. Several cross-sectioned muscle cells are shown at higher magnification in this figure. The nuclei *(N)* that bulge into the cytoplasm belong to the muscle cell. (However, some nuclei in this position may belong to satellite cells. These undifferentiated cells on the muscle side of the basal lamina cannot be identified definitely in H&E sections.) Numerous ring-like structures *(asterisks)* are seen in the endomysium; these are "empty" capillaries. Other capillaries have been cut more obliquely or longitudinally; these contain red blood cells *(arrows).* During maximal muscular activity, the capillaries are all patent; in a less active state, only some of the capillaries are patent at a particular time. The striated muscle cell contains longitudinal units called *myofibrils* (see Plate 29, page 241). The cut ends of the myofibrils (sarcostyles) account for the stippled appearance often seen in cross-sectioned muscle cells, as in this figure.

KEY

A, A band
BV, blood vessels (small artery and vein)
C, capillary
CT, connective tissue (perimysium surrounding muscle fascicles)
I, I band
M, muscle fiber
N, nuclei of muscle cells
Z, Z line
arrows, red blood cells in capillaries
asterisks: Fig. 1, myofibril free region of cytoplasm; Fig. 3, empty capillaries

PLATE 27

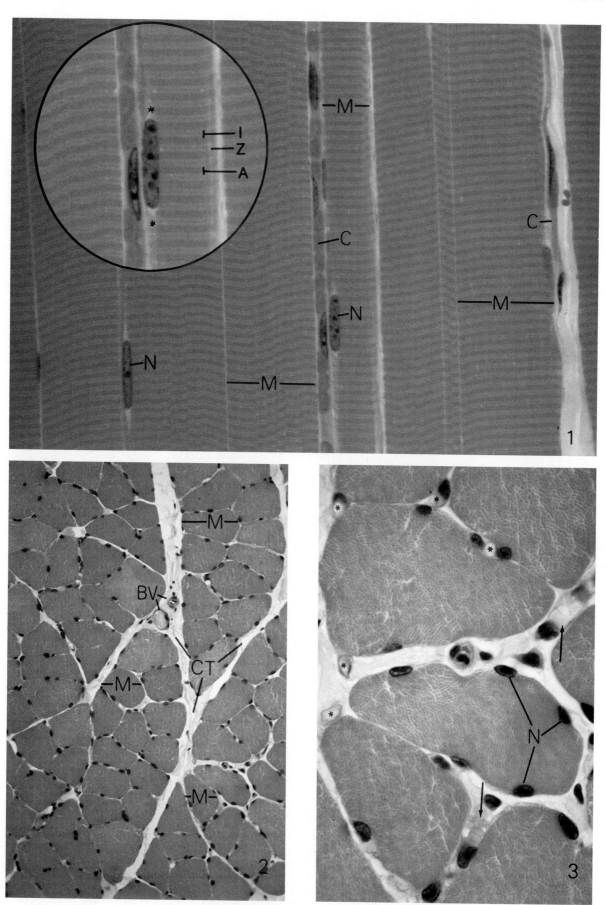

PLATE 28. Skeletal Muscle I, Electron Microscopy

Skeletal muscle, electron micrograph ×6,500; **inset** ×30,000. The cytologic organization and functional units of the skeletal muscle cell are revealed in this low-power electron micrograph. For purposes of orientation, note that only small portions of two muscle cells (fibers) are included in the micrograph. Both are seen in longitudinal profile. One of the sectioned muscle cells occupies the upper two-thirds of the figure and reveals a nucleus *(N)* at its periphery. Below and largely covered by the **inset** is part of the second muscle cell. The connective tissue in the extracellular space between the two cells, i.e., the collagen fibrils *(Col)* and fibroblast *(Fib),* constitutes the endomysium of the muscle.

The individual myofibrils *(Myf),* which were not perceptible in the light micrograph (Plate 27), are clearly seen here in longitudinal profile. The myofibrils, which are more or less cylindrical structures, extend across the micrograph. Each is separated from neighboring myofibrils by a thin sheath of surrounding sarcoplasm *(Sp).*

Each repeating part of the myofibril between adjacent Z lines (fr. Ger. *Zwischenscheibe,* between disc) is a sarcomere. In the electron micrograph shown here, two sarcomeres *(S),* one following the other but in adjacent myofibrils, have been marked. The essential features of a sarcomere are shown at higher magnification in the **inset.** Here, the filamentous nature of the myofibrils is evident. For example, the *I* (isotropic) band, which is bisected by the Z line, is seen to consist of thin, 6–8-nm, barely visible filaments. These thin filaments, which are composed of actin, are joined to the Z line and extend across the I band into the *A* (anisotropic) band. The thick filaments, composed of myosin, account for the full width of the A band.

In the A band there are additional bands or lines. One of these, the *M* line (fr. Ger. *mitte,* middle), is seen at the middle of the A band. This line appears to be due to the presence of a substance that binds the thick filaments to one another. A second subband within the A band is the *H* band (fr. Ger. *Helle,* light). This band appears as the less dense segment within the A band and consists of only myosin filaments. The lateral segments *(double-headed arrows)* of the A band are rather dense. This more dense-appearing area is a reflection of the extent to which the actin filaments have extended into the A band and interdigitated with the thick filaments. Because contraction involves the interdigitation of the thick and thin filaments, increasing degrees of contraction result in continued narrowing of the I and H bands. Inasmuch as the individual thick filaments do not change in length, the width of the A band is always the same.

The cross-banded pattern that characterizes the striated muscle fiber is a reflection of the arrangement, in register, of the individual myofibrils. Additionally, the cross-banded pattern of the myofibril is a reflection of the arrangement, in register, of the myofilaments **(inset).** The in-register arrangement of myofibrils is an important feature relating to impulse propagation within the cell; this is considered in Plate 29.

KEY

A, A band
CM, cell membrane (sarcolemma)
Col, collagen fibrils
Fib, fibroblast
H, H band

I, I band
M, M line
Myf, myofibril
N, nucleus
S, sarcomere

Sp, sarcoplasm between adjacent myofibrils
Z, Z line
arrowhead, glycogen
double-headed arrow, overlap in A band of thick and thin filaments

PLATE 28

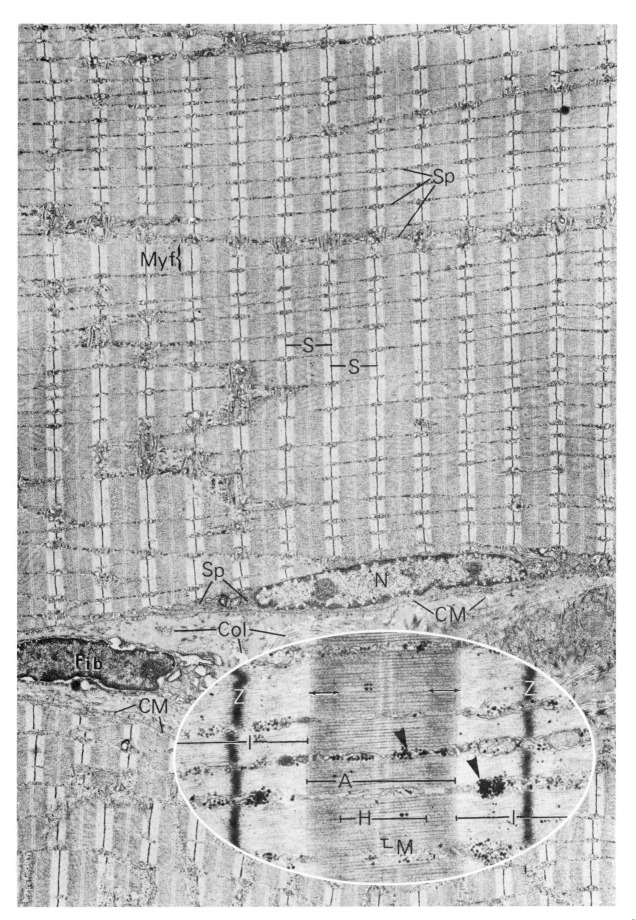

PLATE 29. Skeletal Muscle II, Electron Microscopy

Skeletal muscle, electron micrograph ×45,000; insets ×52,000. The electron micrograph shown here illustrates the nature of the sarcoplasm, especially the membrane system that pervades it. It also demonstrates the filamentous components that make up the myofibril.

The muscle fiber is longitudinally sectioned but has been turned so that the direction of the fiber has a vertical orientation. The various bands and lines of a single sarcomere are labeled in the myofibril on the left of the illustration. The thin actin filaments are especially well resolved in the *I* band in the lower left corner and can easily be compared with the thicker myosin filaments of the *A* band. The point of juncture or insertion of the actin filaments into the *Z* line is also readily apparent.

In contrast to the relatively nondescript character of the sarcoplasm as seen in the light microscope, the electron microscope reveals a well-developed membrane system called the sarcoplasmic reticulum *(SR)*. The reticulum consists of segments of anastomosing tubules that form a network around each myofibril. The electron micrograph here fortuitously depicts a relatively wide area of sarcoplasm in a plane between two myofibrils. Prominent in this area are numerous glycogen particles *(G)*. Somewhat less apparent but nevertheless evident are the anastomosing tubules of the sarcoplasmic reticulum. Near the junction of the A and I bands the tubules of the reticulum become confluent, forming flattened, sac-like structures, the terminal cisternae. These cisternae come in proximity to another membrane system, the T (transverse tubular) system.

The *T system* consists of tubular structures *(T)*, with each tubule originating as an invagination of the sarcolemma. The tubules course transversely through the muscle fiber. Because of the uniform register of the myofibrils, each T tu-

bule comes to surround the myofibrils in proximity to the juncture of the A and I bands. In effect, the T system is not simply a straight tubule but, rather, is a grid-like system that surrounds each myofibril at the level of the A-I junction. Thus, in a section passing tangentially to a myofibril, as is seen in the center of the micrograph and in the **upper inset,** the lumen of the T tubules may appear as elongate channels *(arrows)* bounded by a pair of membranes. The inner, facing pair of membranes belongs to the T tubule. The outer membranes, on either side, belong to the terminal cisternae of the sarcoplasmic reticulum. The communication between a terminal cisterna and the tubular portion of the sarcoplasmic reticulum is marked by an *arrowhead* in the **upper inset.** In contrast, a longitudinal section passing through two adjacent myofibrils **(lower inset)** reveals the T tubule to be flattened with the terminal elements of the sarcoplasmic reticulum *(SR)* on either side. The combination of the T tubule and the adjoining dilated terminal cisternae of the sarcoplasmic reticulum on either side is referred to as a ***triad.***

The nature and geometric configuration of the triad helps explain the rapid and uniform contraction of a muscle fiber. The depolarization of the sarcolemma continues along the membranes of the T tubules and, thereby, results in an inward spread of excitation to reach each myofibril at the A-I junction. This initiates the first stage in the contraction process, i.e., the release of calcium ions from the immediately adjacent terminal cisternae. Relaxation occurs through the recapture of calcium ions by the sarcoplasmic reticulum. In terms of energetics, it is also of interest that the mitochondria *(Mi)* occupy a preferential site in the sarcoplasm, being oriented in a circular fashion around the myofibrils in the region of the I band.

KEY

A, A band	**Mi,** mitochondria	**arrow,** longitudinal profile of T tubule
G, glycogen	**SR,** sarcoplasmic reticulum	**arrowhead,** junction between tubular component of sar-
I, I band	**T,** T tubule	coplasmic reticulum and terminal cisterna
M, M line	**Z,** Z line	

PLATE 29

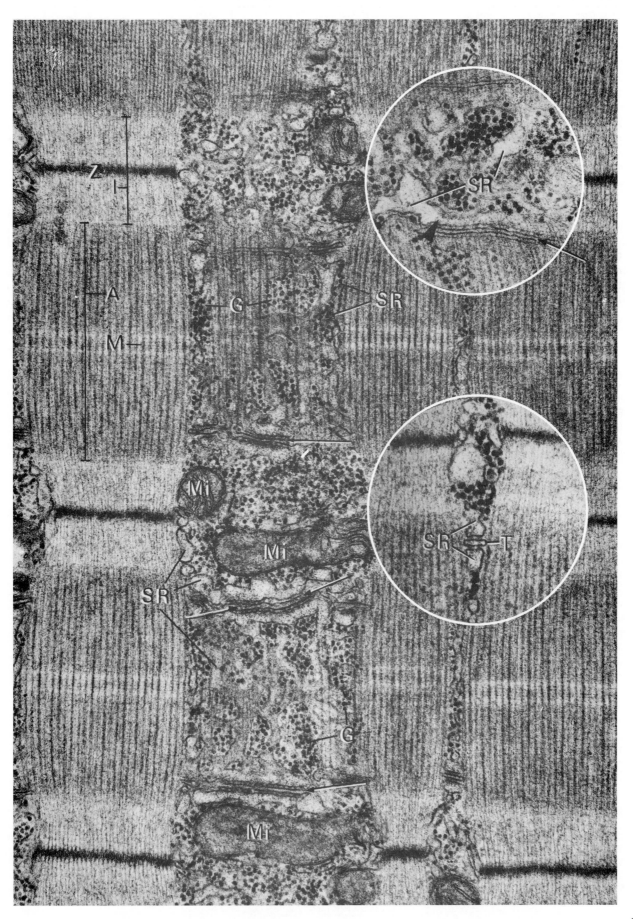

PLATE 30. Musculotendinous Junction and Neuromuscular Junction

Skeletal muscle fibers attach at their ends to collagen fibers. The latter may be part of a tendon, a fibrous sheet (aponeurosis), the periosteum, or a raphe.

FIGURE 1, musculotendinous junction, H&E ×350. In this figure, the muscle fibers appear to terminate directly on the tendon. The muscle fibers *(M)* are in the left half of the figure. They stain redder than the tendon *(T)*, which typically stains a pale pink with eosin. The skeletal muscle fibers have been cut obliquely, and the boundaries between individual muscle cells are not distinct. In many places, however, there is a slight separation of the muscle fibers, and along with the orientation of the muscle cell nuclei, this separation tends to show their general direction. Cross-striations can be identified at right angles to the direction of the fibers. In contrast, the tendon gives no obvious indication of how the collagen fibers are arranged. This needs to be surmised from the orientation of the fibroblast nuclei, which usually have their long axis parallel to the direction of the fibers. Although the nuclei of the fibroblasts are readily identified, the cytoplasm of these cells is not distinguishable from the collagen of the tendon.

FIGURE 2, musculotendinous junction, electron micrograph ×24,600. At the actual junction between the muscle cell and tendon, the end of the cell becomes serrated, and the cytoplasmic projections of the muscle cell interdigitate with the collagen fibrils of the tendon. This arrangement is, at best, only suggested in Figure 1, but it is clearly evident in an electron micrograph of the junction, such as that shown in here.

This figure shows four finger-like projections of the muscle cell. The basal lamina *(BL)* is directly adjacent to the plasma membrane *(PM)* of the muscle cell and follows the finger-like projections. Actin filaments *(arrows)* of the terminal sarcomeres extend into the finger-like projections and insert into densities on the inner face of the plasma membrane *(arrowheads)*. Note that the terminal sarcomeres possess only one Z disc *(ZD)*. Also to be seen within the muscle cell cytoplasm are triads *(Tr)*, glycogen granules *(G)*, and mitochondria *(Mi)*. External to the cell are fibrils of the tendon *(T)*.

FIGURE 3, neuromuscular junction, Golgi stain ×280. In the neuromuscular junction shown here, a special stain has been used to visualize the neural elements. In this staining procedure, the skeletal muscle cells are not revealed to best advantage. They are horizontally disposed in the illustration; cross-striations *(arrows)* are visible in some muscle fibers. The nerve *(N)* enters the field from the left; initially, it dips downward; then it turns in an upward direction. As it does, it can be seen to divide into smaller branches, and finally, as it nears the muscle cells, the nerve fiber branches to make contact with several muscle cells. At the terminal between nerve fiber and each muscle cell, the nerve fiber arborizes to form a disc-like structure, the motor end plate *(MEP)*, on the surface of the muscle cells. The motor end plate is the physiologic contact between nerve and muscle; it is, in fact, a neuromuscular synapse station at which the neurotransmitter acetylcholine is liberated. This transmitter initiates a sequence of muscle membrane events that lead to contraction of the muscle.

KEY		
BL, basal lamina	**N,** nerve	**ZD,** Z disc
G, glycogen	**PM,** plasma membrane (sarco-	**arrowheads,** attachment of actin
M, striated muscle	lemma)	filaments into plasma membrane
MEP, motor end plate	**T,** tendon	**arrows,** actin filaments
Mi, mitochondria	**Tr,** triad	

PLATE 30

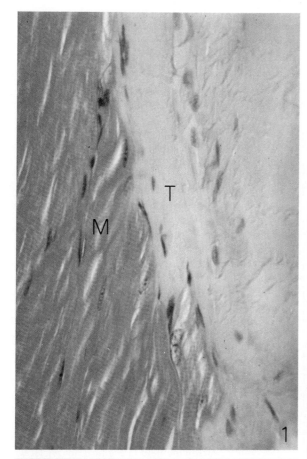

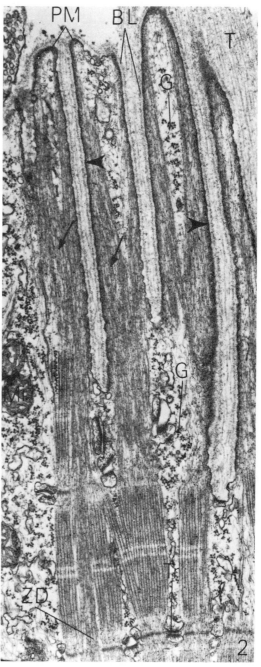

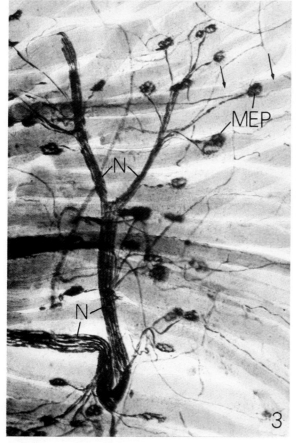

PLATE 31. Cardiac Muscle

Cardiac muscle consists of fibers that possess the same cross-banding patterns as are present in striated skeletal muscle. Thus, it is also striated. However, cardiac muscle differs in many other respects from skeletal muscle. The histologically obvious differences are the presence of intercalated discs, the location of the cardiac cell nuclei in the center of the fiber, and the branching nature of the muscle fiber. All of these are evident in a well-prepared longitudinal section of the muscle.

FIGURE 1, heart, H&E ×160. This figure shows a longitudinal section of cardiac muscle. The muscle fibers are disposed horizontally in the illustration and show cross-striations. In addition to the regular cross-striations (those of greater frequency), however, there is another group of very pronounced cross-bands, namely, the intercalated discs *(ID)*. Intercalated discs most often appear as a straight band, but sometimes they are arranged in a stepwise manner (see also Fig. 2 and Plate 32). These discs are not always displayed in routine H&E sections; therefore, one may not be able to depend on these structures for identifying cardiac muscle. Intercalated discs are opposing cell-to-cell contacts. Thus, cardiac muscle fibers differ in a very fundamental respect from fibers of skeletal muscle. The cardiac muscle fiber consists of an end-to-end alignment of individual cells; in contrast, the skeletal muscle fiber is a single multinucleated protoplasmic unit. In examining a longitudinal section of cardiac muscle, it is useful to scan specific fibers along their long axis. By doing so, one can find places where the fibers obviously branch. Two such branchings are indicated by the *arrows* in this figure.

FIGURE 3, heart, H&E ×160. This figure shows cross-sectioned cardiac muscle fibers. Many have rounded or smooth-contoured polygonal profiles. Some fibers, however, are generally more irregular and elongate in profile. These probably reflect a profile of both a fiber and a branch of the fiber. The more lightly stained region in the center of many fibers represents the myofibril-free region of the cell already referred to above and indicated by the *asterisks* in Figure 2. Delicate connective tissue surrounds the individual muscle fibers. This contains capillaries and sometimes larger vessels, such as the venule *(V)* in the center of the bundle of muscle fibers. Larger amounts of connective tissue *(CT)* surround bundles of fibers, and this tissue contains larger blood vessels, such as the arteriole *(A)* marked in the figure.

FIGURE 2, heart, H&E ×400. Like skeletal muscle, the cardiac muscle is composed of linear contractile units, the *myofibrils*. These are evident in this figure as the longitudinally disposed linear structures that extend through the length of the cell. The myofibrils separate to bypass the nuclei and, in doing so, they delineate a perinuclear region of cytoplasm that is free of myofibrils and their cross-striations. These perinuclear cytoplasmic areas *(asterisks)* contain the cytoplasmic organelles that are not directly involved in the contractile process. Many cardiac muscle cells are binucleate; both nuclei typically occupy the myofibril-free region of cytoplasm, as shown in the cell marked by the *asterisks*. The third nucleus in this region appears to belong to the connective tissue either above or below the "in-focus" plane of section. Often, the staining of muscle cell nuclei in a specific specimen is very characteristic, especially when seen in face view as here. Notice, in the nucleus between the *asterisks,* the well-stained nucleolus and the delicate pattern of the remainder of the nucleus. Once such features have been characterized for a particular specimen, it becomes easy to identify nuclei having a similar staining character throughout the specimen. For example, survey the field in Figure 1 for nuclei with similar features. Having done this, it is substantially easier to identify nuclei of connective tissue cells *(CT)*, which display different staining properties and are not positioned in the same relationship to the muscle cells.

FIGURE 4, heart, H&E ×400. At higher magnification, it is possible to see the cut ends of the myofibrils. These appear as the numerous red areas that give the cut face of the muscle cell a stippled appearance. The nuclei *(N)* occupy a central position surrounded by myofibrils. Remember, in contrast, that nuclei of skeletal muscle fibers are located at the periphery of the cell. Note, also, that as already mentioned, the nuclear free central area of the cell, devoid of myofibrils, shows areas of perinuclear cytoplasm similar to that marked with *asterisks* in Figure 2.

KEY		
A, arteriole	**ID,** intercalated discs	**arrows,** sites where fibers branch
C, capillaries	**N,** nuclei of cardiac muscle cells	**asterisks,** perinuclear cytoplasmic
CT, connective tissue	**V,** venule	areas

PLATE 31

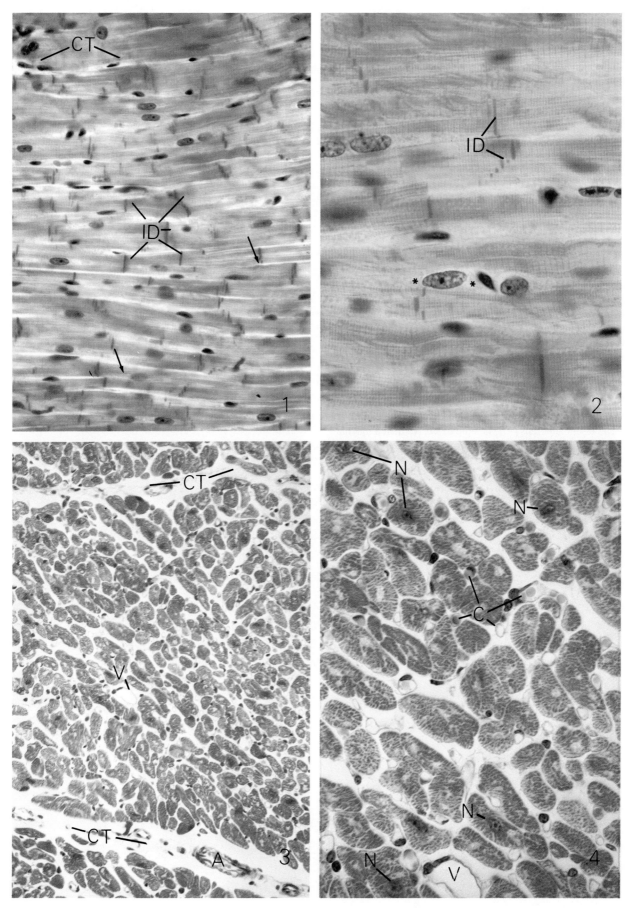

PLATE 32. Cardiac Muscle, Intercalated Disc, Electron Microscopy

Heart, electron micrograph ×30,000; insets ×62,000.

This electron micrograph reveals portions of two cardiac muscle cells, including the site where they join in end-to-end apposition. The apposition between the two cells can be followed in its entirety across the micrograph. It takes an irregular, step-like course, making a number of near right-angle turns, so that part of the junction is disposed crosswise, part is disposed longitudinally, and part is disposed obliquely. In its course, different junctional specializations of the intercalated disc are evident. These include the macula adherens, fascia adherens, and gap junction. It is principally the fascia adherens and, to some extent, the macula adherens that correspond to the intercalated disc of light microscopy.

The macula adherens *(MA)* in the upper left of the illustration has been enlarged in **inset 1.** It displays the typical features seen in maculae adherentes in other tissues (referred to as desmosomes when seen with the light microscope), namely, a thickening of the inner leaflet of the plasma membrane, a condensation of the adjacent cytoplasm, and an intermediate dense line seen in the middle of the intercellular space. Typically, intermediate filaments form loops in the adjacent cytoplasmic condensation, and although the loops are not evident, the intermediate filaments *(arrow)* can be seen in the macula adherens *(MA)* that has been sectioned obliquely on the right side of the illustration. As in other tissues, the macula adherens is a plaque-like site of contact between cells that provides adhesion between the two cells.

The fascia adherens *(FA)* is more extensive than a macula, being disposed in a larger area of irregular outline. Thin sections showing the fascia adherens on edge **(inset 3)** reveal the plasma membranes of the neighboring cells to be separated by a space of 15–20 nm. In each cell, the fascia adherens is typified by a condensation of the subplasmalemmal cytoplasm. The thin actin filaments of the myofibril are anchored in the cytoplasmic density. The fascia adherens of the intercalated disc corresponds to the zonula adherens of other tissues (see Plate 5, page 93).

The gap junctions *(GJ)* are seen in those portions of the intercalated disc that are disposed longitudinally with respect to the direction of the myofilaments. (This orientation may not be significant because gap junctions also appear crosswise in some electron micrographs.) In electron micrographs of routinely prepared tissues **(inset 2),** the gap junction appears as two dense lines, with each representing a thickened inner layer of plasma membrane, and a barely discernible intermediate line. The intermediate line represents the outer layers of the plasma membranes of the two adjacent cells. Gap junctions are sites where excitation spreads from one cell to another and where small molecules or ions pass readily from one cell to another.

Other features typical of striated muscle are also revealed in the illustration, namely, mitochondria *(Mi)*, sarcoplasmic reticulum *(SR)*, and components of the sarcomere, including Z lines *(Z)*, M line *(M)*, and myofilaments. This particular specimen is in a highly contracted state, and consequently, the *I* band is practically obscured.

KEY

FA, fascia adherens	**Mi,** mitochondria	**Inset 1,** macula adherens
GJ, gap junctions	**SR,** sarcoplasmic reticulum	**Inset 2,** gap junction
M, M line	**Z,** Z lines	**Inset 3,** fascia adherens
MA, macula adherens	**arrow,** intermediate filaments	

PLATE 32

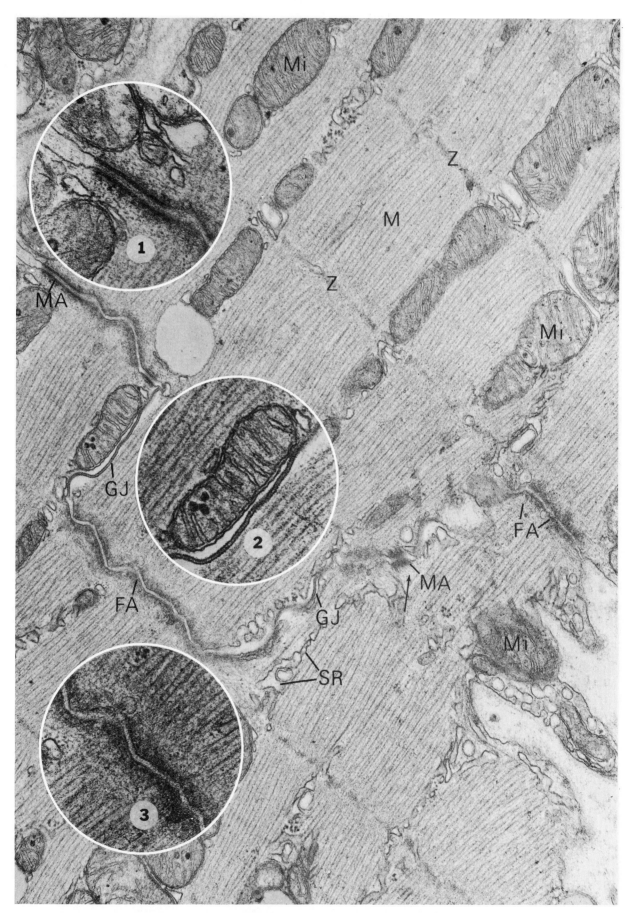

PLATE 33.   Cardiac Muscle, Purkinje Fibers

Some of the muscle cells within the heart are specialized to conduct impulses from the atrioventricular (AV) node through the ventricular septum into the ventricles. Within the ventricular septum, the cells are grouped into a bundle, the AV bundle. The bundle quickly branches into two main components, one going into each ventricle. These special conducting fibers are responsible for the final distribution of the electrical stimulus to the myocardium. As the bundles ramify in the ventricle, the specialized conducting cells are given the name *Purkinje fibers*.

FIGURE 1, heart, sheep, H&E ×160.   A section of cardiac muscle and Purkinje fibers is shown in a relatively low power view in this figure. The cardiac muscle fibers *(CM)* appear in the left of the figure; the Purkinje fibers *(PF)* occupy much of the remainder of the field. Connective tissue separates groups of Purkinje fibers from each other and from the cardiac muscle. Small blood vessels *(BV)* and nerves *(NF)* are also present within the connective tissue.

FIGURE 2, heart, sheep, H&E ×350.   The nature of the Purkinje fibers and their architecture are seen more advantageously here at higher magnification. The fibers are made up of individual cells of irregular shape that maintain extensive contact with one another. Intercalated discs are not observed, but desmosomes are present joining adjacent cells of the fiber.

The cytoplasm of a Purkinje cell contains a large amount of glycogen. The glycogen-rich areas *(G)* appear as homogeneous, pale-staining regions that usually occupy the center portion of the cell. The periphery of the cell contains the myofibrils *(Mf)*. The nucleus *(N)* is round and much larger than the nucleus of the cardiac muscle cell. Because of the considerable size of the Purkinje cells, the nuclei are often not included in the section, and one may get a misleading impression as to the disposition and number of cells that make up a fiber. On the other hand, because the myofibrils tend to be located at the periphery of the cell, they can be used to locate the cell boundaries and, thus, help delineate the individual cells of the bundle. The Purkinje fibers ultimately terminate by joining cardiac muscle fibers, thereby permitting direct passage of the impulse to the cardiac muscle fiber.

The connective tissue *(CT)* through which the Purkinje fibers course may also contain nerves *(NF)* and ganglion cells *(GC)*. These neural elements belong to the autonomic nervous system, which regulates the activity of the Purkinje fibers and heart muscle.

KEY

BV, blood vessel	**G,** glycogen-rich area	**N,** nucleus of Purkinje cell
CM, cardiac muscle fibers	**GC,** ganglion cell	**NF,** nerve fibers
CT, connective tissue	**Mf,** myofibrils	**PF,** Purkinje fibers

PLATE 33

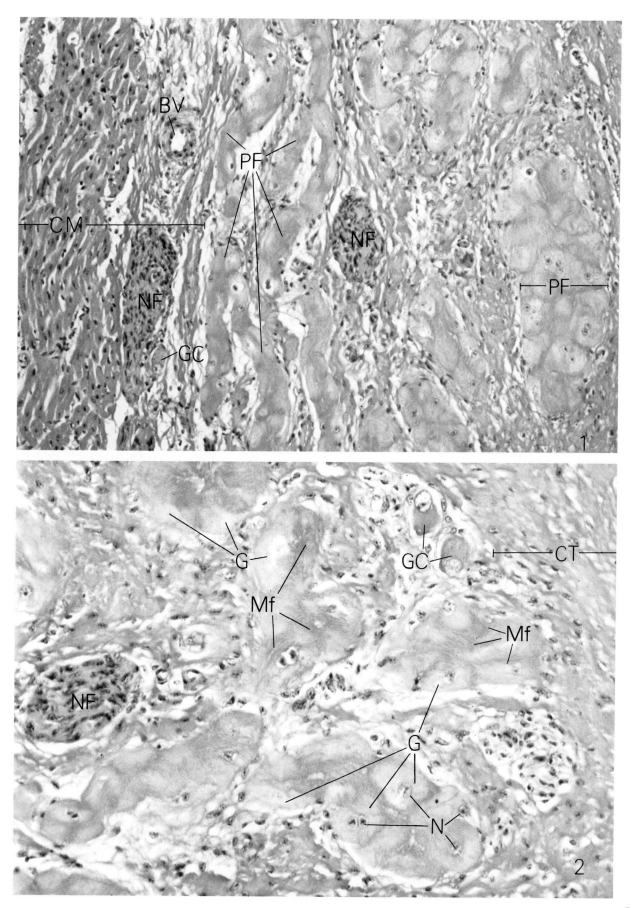

PLATE 34. Smooth Muscle

FIGURE 1, intestine, monkey, H&E ×900. Smooth muscle tissue is composed of cells that are typically fusiform or spindle-shaped and organized in parallel arrangements. In this longitudinal section, smooth muscle cells appear elongate. Their nuclei *(N)* are also elongated and conform to the general shape of the cell. In this preparation the nuclei appear slightly twisted, like a corkscrew; this is a characteristic of contracted cells. In this specimen, the cells are sufficiently separated from one another to allow one to delineate the cell boundaries. However, the boundaries cannot always be seen in H&E sections (see Fig. 4).

FIGURE 3, artery, human, H&E ×425. The smooth muscle cells *(SM)* of a blood vessel (arterial) wall are shown here. These cells are arranged in a circular pattern, forming part of the vessel wall. When the blood vessel is bisected longitudinally, as it is in the upper part of the figure, the smooth muscle cells are cut in cross section, and the nuclei appear rounded *(arrows)*, as they are in Figure 2. In addition, most of the cells display cross-sectioned profiles of only cytoplasm, for the reasons given above. In the bottom of the figure, the blood vessel presents a different profile. It has turned and is leaving the plane of section. Here, the blood vessel is cut in essentially a cross section. The smooth muscle cells are now seen as longitudinal curved profiles, as evidenced by the elongate profiles of the nuclei *(arrowheads)*. The vertically disposed nuclei between the two luminal profiles *(L)* are nuclei of endothelial cells. Connective tissue *(CT)* is external to the smooth muscle cells.

FIGURE 2, intestine, monkey, H&E ×900. This is a cross section through smooth muscle cells from the same specimen as shown in Figure 1. The cells now appear as circular or polygonal profiles with variations in size. The nuclei *(N)* also appear as circular profiles and are included in some cells. In most of the cells, however, the nuclei have not been included in the section, and only the eosinophilic cytoplasm appears. Because the cells are staggered, some are cut through the thick central portion, in which case the nucleus is included, whereas others are cut through the tapering ends, in which case only the cytoplasm is seen *(asterisks)*. The differences in diameter between neighboring cells and the variable nuclear profiles are characteristic features of cross-sectioned smooth muscle. Typically, smooth muscle cells are grouped in ill-defined bundles. Note the connective tissue *(CT)* surrounding part of the bundle. Small amounts of extracellular connective tissue fibers and, occasionally, a fibroblast *(F)* are seen between the individual muscle cells within a bundle.

FIGURE 4, uterus, human, H&E ×160. Interlacing bundles of smooth muscle cells from the uterus are shown here. These bundles are separated from each other by connective tissue. However, it is not always easy to distinguish between connective tissue and the smooth muscle. Three bundles of smooth muscle cells have been delineated by the *interrupted lines*. In each, there are smooth muscle cells that are arranged in predominately one direction: longitudinal, oblique, and cross section. Careful examination of these areas will reveal nuclei whose profile can be used to determine the orientation of the cells. Having noted the orientation of the cells and the nuclei, now note their number per given area of tissue. Comparing the smooth muscle with the connective tissue *(CT)*, note that the connective tissue shows far fewer nuclear profiles per given area of tissue. The lumen in the upper part of the figure belongs to a blood vessel *(BV)* whose mural components blend imperceptibly with the surrounding connective tissue.

	KEY	
BV, blood vessel	**SM,** smooth muscle cell	**asterisks,** cytoplasm of smooth muscle cell
CT, connective tissue	**arrow,** nucleus of cross-sectioned smooth muscle cell	**interrupted lines,** boundaries of bundles of smooth muscle cell
F, nucleus of fibroblast	**arrowhead,** nucleus of longitudinally sectioned smooth muscle cell	
L, lumen of arteriole		
N, nucleus of smooth muscle cells		

PLATE 34

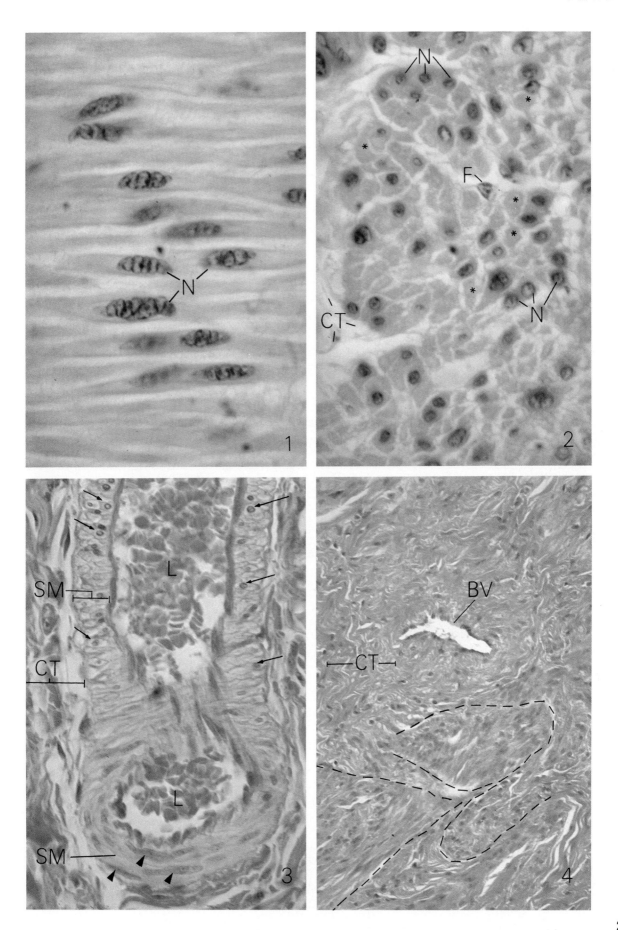

PLATE 35. Smooth Muscle, Longitudinal Section, Electron Microscopy

Oviduct, monkey, electron micrograph ×5,500; insets ×20,000. This electron micrograph shows smooth muscle comparable with that shown in the light micrograph in Figure 1 of Plate 34. The muscle cells are longitudinally oriented and are seen in a relatively relaxed state, as evidenced by the smooth contour of their nuclei. The intercellular space is occupied by abundant collagen fibrils *(C)* that course in varying planes between the cells.

At the low magnification utilized here, much of the cytoplasmic mass of the muscle cells has a homogeneous appearance. This homogeneous appearance is due to the contractile components of the cell, namely, the thin (6–8-nm) actin filaments that are oriented in parallel array in the direction of the long axis of the cell. (The thicker myosin filaments of mammalian smooth muscle cells are extremely labile and tend to be lost during tissue preparation.) The nonhomogeneous-appearing portions of the cytoplasm contain mitochondria and other cell organelles. To illustrate these differences, the area within the *lower right small circle* is shown at higher magnification in the **upper inset** of the micrograph. The particular site selected for the **upper inset** reveals a filamentous area *(F)* as well as a region containing mitochondria *(M)*, a few profiles of rER *(arrows)*, and numerous dense particles, most of which are glycogen. Although the distinction between the filament-containing regions of cytoplasm and those areas containing the remaining organelles are clearly evident in the electron microscope, the routine H&E preparation of light microscopy reveals only a homogeneous eosinophilic cytoplasm.

Fibroblasts and other connective tissue cells, when present, are also readily discernible in electron micrographs among the smooth muscle cells of various organs. In this micrograph, several fibroblasts *(Fib)* are evident. In contrast to the smooth muscle cell, their cytoplasm exhibits numerous profiles of rER as well as other organelles throughout all but the very attenuated cytoplasmic processes. For comparison, the area of the fibroblast in the *lower left small circle* is shown at higher magnification in the **lower inset.** Note the more numerous dilated profiles of endoplasmic reticulum *(arrows)* and the multitude of small particles (ribosomes), most of which are associated with the membranes of the reticulum. The ribosomes are slightly smaller and stain less intensely than the glycogen particles of the smooth muscle cells. The presence of rER in both the fibroblast and the smooth muscle cell is consistent with the finding that in addition to their contractile role, smooth muscle cells have the ability to produce and maintain collagen and elastic fibers.

The tissue utilized in this micrograph is from a young animal and contains fibroblasts in a relatively active state, hence, the well-developed endoplasmic reticulum and abundant cytoplasm. With the light microscope, it is not likely that one would be able to distinguish readily between the fibroblasts shown here and the smooth muscle cells. Less active fibroblasts, as in a more mature tissue or in an older individual, however, have less extensive cytoplasm and, accordingly, are more easily distinguished from the smooth muscle cells.

KEY		
C, collagen fibrils	**Fib,** fibroblast	**N,** nucleus of smooth muscle cell
F, filamentous area of cytoplasm	**M,** mitochondria	**arrows,** endoplasmic reticulum

PLATE 35

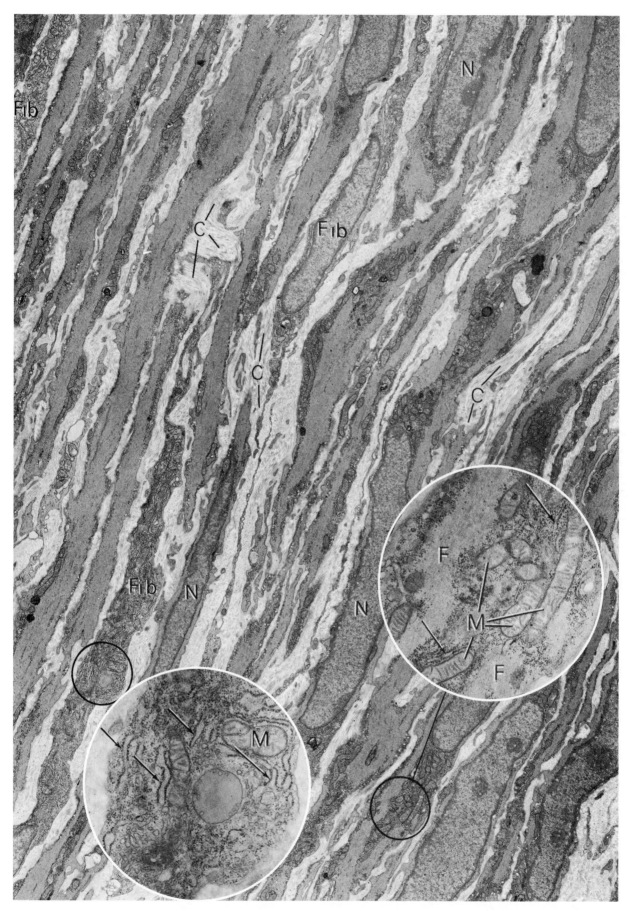

PLATE 36. Smooth Muscle, Cross Section, Electron Microscopy

Oviduct, monkey, electron micrograph ×5,500; inset ×30,000. The specimen from which this micrograph was obtained is the same as that shown in Plate 35. It is an electron micrograph of cross-sectioned smooth muscle cells and shows, at higher resolution, many of the features of smooth muscle cells seen already with the light microscope. For example, the muscle cells can be seen to be arranged in bundles comparable with those seen with the light microscope in Figures 2 and 4 of Plate 34, page 251. The bundle arrangement is not readily apparent, even in electron micrographs, when the muscle cells are longitudinally sectioned as in the preceding plate. The cross-sectioned profiles of the greatest diameter depict the midportion of the muscle cells and show nuclei; the profiles of lesser diameter depict the tapered ends of the cell and show cytoplasm only. The smooth muscle cells display cytoplasmic areas that appear homogeneous due to the presence of myofilaments. The homogeneous areas are evident, but the individual myofilaments are not. Also seen within the cytoplasm are mitochondria. Other cytoplasmic constituents are not resolved at this relatively low magnification.

Generally, the cross-sectioned smooth muscle cells (SM) show an irregular contour when seen at the electron microscopic level. This is, in part, due to the better resolution obtained with the electron microscope but, even more so, reflects the extreme thinness of the section. At this low magnification, numerous sites are seen where a cell appears to contact its neighbor. Most of these sites do not reflect true cell-to-cell contacts. There are, however, places where the smooth muscle cells do make contact by means of a nexus or gap junction (inset). These junctions are similar to gap junctions in other cells. They are the structural sites for easy ion movement from cell to cell and for the spread of exci-

tation from one cell to another. Usually, special staining procedures are employed to demonstrate the nature of the junction. When seen in face view, the special stains reveal hexagonal patterns on the opposing plasma membranes. In routinely prepared electron micrographs of a gap junction (arrow, inset), it appears as though the adjacent plasma membranes make contact (see, also, Plate 32, page 247).

The electron micrograph shows connective tissue cells associated with the bundles of smooth muscle cells. Fibroblasts are the most numerous of the connective tissue cells. The processes of the fibroblasts tend to delineate and define the limits of the bundles. Note the very thin fibroblast processes (Fib) coursing along the periphery of the two muscle bundles (one bundle occupying the left half of the micrograph, the other occupying the right half). Although the nuclei of the fibroblasts would be evident with the light microscope, the cellular processes would not. In addition to fibroblasts, cells of another type are also seen about or between the bundles of smooth muscle cells. These are macrophages (M), readily identified with the electron microscope by the presence of lysosomal bodies within the cytoplasm. With the light microscope, these cells would be difficult to identify because the lysosomes are not evident without the use of special histochemical staining procedures. If, however, the macrophages contain phagocytosed particles of large size or of distinctive coloration (e.g., hemosiderin), their identification with the light microscope becomes easier.

In the electron micrograph shown here, the macrophages appear to have taken up a preferential position, lying in immediate apposition to the fibroblasts. The relationship is so close that, at this magnification, the intercellular space is difficult to discern. The dashed line indicates the boundary between the two cell types.

KEY		
Fib, fibroblast	**SM,** smooth muscle cells	**dashed line,** boundary between fibroblast and macrophage
M, macrophages	**arrow,** gap junction	

PLATE 36

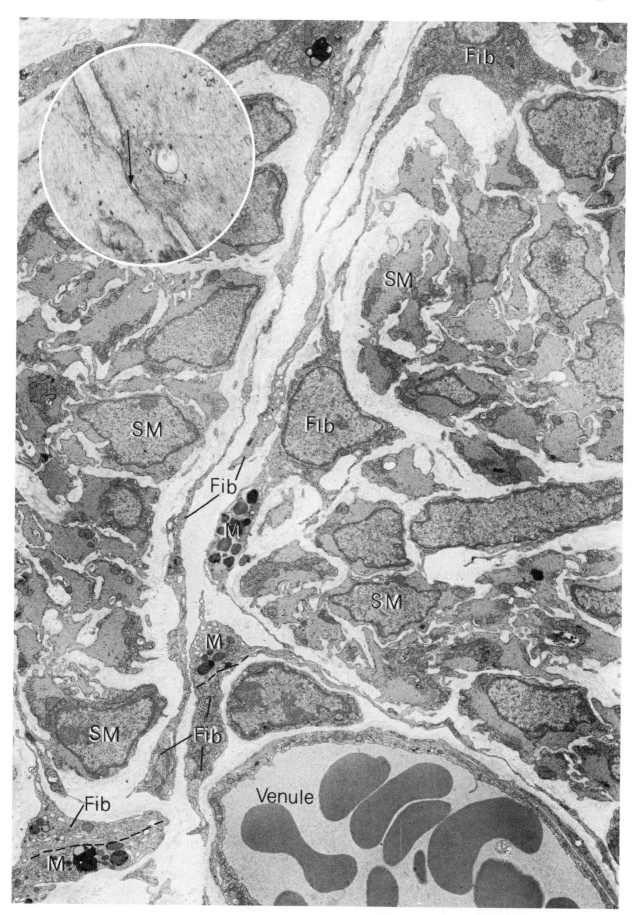

Nervous Tissue

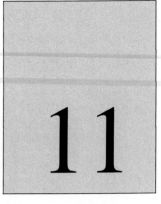

11

The nervous system consists of all the nervous tissue in the body. It can be divided into the

- *Central nervous system (CNS),* consisting of the brain and the spinal cord, located in the cranial cavity and spinal canal, respectively
- *Peripheral nervous system (PNS),* consisting of cranial and spinal nerves (both motor and sensory), ganglia (collections of nerve cells outside the CNS), and motor nerve endings and sensory nerve endings (receptors)

COMPOSITION OF NERVOUS TISSUE

Nervous Tissue Consists of Two Principal Types of Cells: *Nerve Cells (Neurons)* and *Supporting Cells*

The *neuron* or *nerve cell* is the functional unit of the nervous system. Nerve cells are

- Specialized to receive stimuli and to conduct electrical impulses to other parts of the system
- Arranged as an integrated communications network, with several neurons in a chain-like fashion typically involved in sending impulses from one part of the system to another

The specialized contacts between neurons that provide for the transmission of information from one neuron to the next in the chain are called *synapses.*

Supporting cells are nonconducting cells that are in intimate physical contact with neurons. In the CNS, they are called *neuroglia* or, simply, *glia;* in the PNS, *Schwann cells* surround nerve cell *processes,* and *satellite cells* surround nerve cell bodies in ganglia. Supporting cells provide

- *Physical support* (protection) for delicate neuronal processes
- *Electrical insulation* for nerve cell bodies and processes
- *Metabolic exchange* pathways between the vascular system and the nervous system

In addition to nerve cells and supporting cells, there are many blood vessels in both the CNS and the PNS. The blood vessels are separated from the nervous tissue by the interposition of basal laminae and variable amounts of connective tissue, depending on vessel size. In the CNS, the boundary between blood vessels and nervous tissue has long been recognized as special, in that many substances that readily leave blood vessels to enter other tissues do not normally enter the nervous tissue. This selective restriction of blood-borne substances in the CNS is designated as the *blood-brain barrier.* The barrier has been shown to reside in the elaborate tight junctions between the endothelial cells of brain capillaries.

The Nervous System Allows for Rapid Response to External Stimuli

The nervous system evolved from the simple neuroeffector system of lower animals. In primitive nervous systems, only simple receptor-effector reflex loops exist to respond to external stimuli. In higher animals, the nervous system retains the capability of responding to stimuli from the external environment through the action of effector cells (such as skeletal muscle), but the neuronal responses are infinitely more varied. They range from simple reflexes that require only the spinal cord, to complex operations of the brain that bring to bear the memory of past experiences.

In Higher Animals, the Nervous System Also Regulates the Function of Internal Organs

The specific effectors in the organs that respond to the information carried by neurons include

- *Smooth muscle,* the contraction of which can modify the diameter or shape of tubular or hollow viscera such as blood vessels, gut, gallbladder, and urinary bladder
- *Cardiac muscle,* in which only the rate and intensity of the inherent contractions can be modified
- *Glandular epithelium,* in which the synthesis, composition, and release of secretions can be modified

The part of the PNS that innervates these effectors is the *autonomic nervous system (ANS)*.

The regulation of the function of internal organs involves close cooperation between the nervous system and the endocrine system (see Chapter 20). Nerve cells in several parts of the brain and in other sites behave as secretory cells and are referred to as *neuroendocrine tissue.* The varied roles of neurosecretions in regulating the functions of the endocrine system, the digestive system, the respiratory system, the urinary system, and the reproductive system are described in the subsequent chapters concerned with those systems.

THE NEURON (NERVE CELL)

The Neuron or Nerve Cell Is the Structural and Functional Unit of the Nervous System

There are more than 10 billion neurons in the human nervous system. Although nerve cells show the greatest variety of sizes and shapes of any group of cells in the body, they fall into three general categories:

- *Sensory neurons* convey impulses from receptors to the CNS.
- *Motor neurons* convey impulses from the CNS or from ganglia to effector cells (Fig. 11.1).
- *Interneurons,* also called *internuncial neurons, intercalated neurons,* or *central neurons,* form a communicating and integrating network between the sensory and motor neurons. It is estimated that more than 99.9% of all neurons belong to this integrating network.

All Neurons Have a *Cell Body* and Processes, the *Axon* and *Dendrites*

The cell body of a neuron contains the nucleus and those organelles that maintain the nerve cell. The processes extending from the cell body constitute the single common structural characteristic of all neurons. Most neurons have only **one axon,** usually the longest process extending from the cell; some axons may be more than 1 meter long. A neuron usually has **many dendrites,** processes that are shorter and, usually, thicker than an axon.

Neurons are classified on the basis of the number of processes extending from the cell body (Fig. 11.2). Thus,

- *Multipolar* neurons have one axon and two or more dendrites.
- *Bipolar* neurons have one axon and one dendrite.
- *Unipolar* (actually pseudounipolar) neurons have one process, the axon, that divides close to the cell body into two long processes.

Motor Neurons and Interneurons Are Multipolar

In interneurons, which constitute most of the neurons in the nervous system, the physiologic direction of impulses is from dendrite to cell body to axon or from cell body to axon. Thus, functionally, the dendrites and cell body of multipolar neurons are the receptor portions of the cell, and their plasma membrane is specially adapted for impulse generation. The axon is the conducting portion of the cell, and its plasma membrane is specialized for impulse conduction. The terminal portion of the axon, the transmitter or effector portion of the nerve cell, contains various transmitter substances that affect other nerve cells as well as muscles and glands.

Sensory Neurons Are Unipolar

The cell body of a sensory neuron is situated in a dorsal root ganglion close to the CNS (Fig. 11.3); one axonal branch extends to the periphery, and one extends to the CNS. The two axonal branches are the conducting units. Functionally, impulses are generated in the peripheral arborizations of the neuron; those arborizations are the receptor portion of the cell. Unipolar neurons are also sometimes called *pseudounipolar* because during development they exist as bipolar neurons that then become unipolar as they differentiate into their mature form.

True Bipolar Neurons Are Limited to the Retina and the Ganglia of the Vestibulocochlear Nerve (Cranial Nerve VIII)

Neurons associated with the receptors for the special senses (taste, smell, hearing, sight, and equilibrium) often do not fit the generalizations made above. For example, the amacrine cells of the retina have no axons; and the olfactory receptors resemble neurons of primitive neural systems, in that they retain a surface location and remain a slowly renewing cell population (see Chapter 2).

Cell Body

The Cell Body of the Neuron Has the Characteristics of a Protein-Secreting Cell

The cell body or *perikaryon* is the usually large, dilated region of the cell that contains a large, euchromatic nucleus with a prominent nucleolus. Nerve cell perikarya contain inclusions, *Nissl bodies,* that stain intensely with basic dyes and metachromatically with thionine dyes. Each Nissl body corresponds to a stack of rough endoplasmic reticulum (rER). The perikaryon also contains numerous mitochondria, a large perinuclear Golgi apparatus, lysosomes, microtubules, neurofilaments, vesicles, and inclusions (Fig. 11.4). Nissl bodies, free ribosomes, and, occasionally, the Golgi complex extend into the dendrites *but not into the axon.* In both light microscope (LM) and transmission electron microscope (TEM) preparations, this distinction helps to distinguish between axons or dendrites.

The combination of euchromatic nucleus, large nucleolus, prominent Golgi apparatus, and Nissl substance is in-

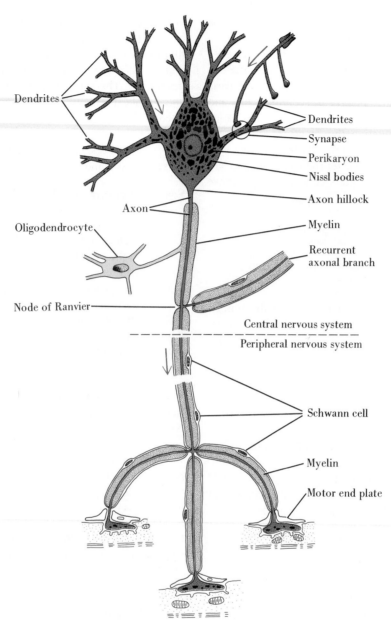

Figure 11.1. Diagram of a motor neuron. The perikaryon, dendrites, and initial part of the axon are within the CNS. The axon leaves the CNS and, while in the PNS, is part of a nerve (not shown) as it courses to its effectors (striated muscle). In the CNS, the myelin for the axon is produced by and is ac-tually part of an oligodendrocyte; in the PNS, the myelin is produced by and is actually part of a Schwann cell. (From Junqueira LC, Carneiro J, Kelley RO: *Basic Histology,* 7th ed. Norwalk, CT, Appleton & Lange, 1992, p 164.)

dicative of the high level of anabolic activity needed to maintain these large, postmitotic cells.

Neurons Do Not Divide; They Must Last for a Lifetime

Although neurons do not replicate, the subcellular components of the neurons turn over regularly, having molecular life spans measured in hours, days, and weeks. The constant need to replace enzymes, transmitter substances, membrane components, and other complex molecules explains the presence of morphologic features characteristic of a high level of synthetic activity. Newly synthesized molecules also need to be transported to distant locations within the neuron; that is accomplished by a process referred to as *axonal transport.*

Dendrites and Axons

Dendrites Are Neuronal Processes That Receive Stimuli From Other Nerve Cells or From the Environment

Generally, dendrites are located in the vicinity of the cell body. They have a greater diameter than axons, are un-

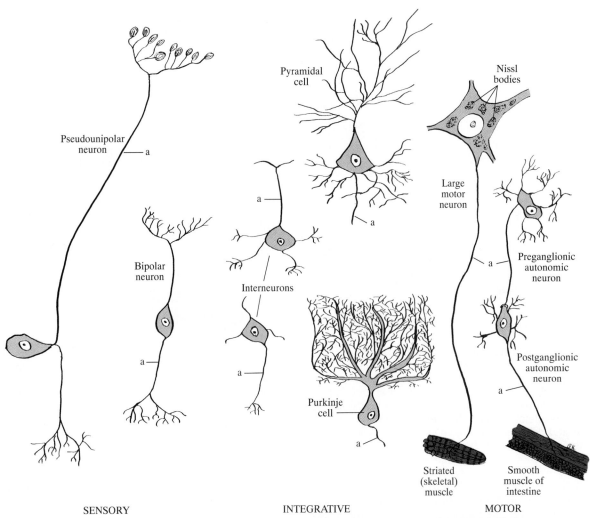

Figure 11.2. Diagram illustrating several of the many different types and shapes of neurons. Pseudounipolar (unipolar), bipolar, and post-ganglionic autonomic neurons have their cell bodies outside of the CNS. Integrative neurons are restricted to the CNS; many of them have elaborate dendritic arborizations that allow easy identification. *a*, axon.

myelinated, are usually tapered, and form extensive arborizations called *dendritic trees.* Dendritic trees significantly increase the receptor surface of a neuron. Many neuron types are characterized by the extent and shape of their dendritic trees (see Fig. 11.2). There is generally no sharp delineation between the contents of the cell body and those of the dendrites. Whereas the Golgi network remains close to the nucleus, other organelles characteristic of the cell body proper, including ribosomes and rER, are found in the dendrites, especially in the base of the dendrites.

Axons Are Neuronal Processes That Transmit Stimuli to Other Neurons or to Effector Cells

There is only *one axon for each neuron,* and it may be extremely long. Axons that originate from neurons in the motor nuclei of the CNS *(Golgi type I neurons)* may travel more than a meter to reach their effector targets, i.e., skeletal muscle. Interneurons of the CNS *(Golgi type II neu-*

rons), in contrast, have a short axon. Although an axon may give rise to a *recurrent branch* near the cell body (i.e., one that turns back toward the cell body; see Fig. 11.1) and to other collateral branches, the branching of the axon is most extensive in the vicinity of its targets.

The axon originates from a conical projection of the cell body known as the *axon hillock.* It is usually devoid of large cytoplasmic organelles such as Nissl bodies and Golgi cisternae. Microtubules, neurofilaments, mitochondria, and vesicles, however, pass through the axon hillock into the axon. It is here that molecules synthesized in the cell body and destined for transport to distant portions of the neuron enter the *axonal transport systems.* These systems are described later.

The region of the axon between the apex of the axon hillock and the beginning of the myelin sheath (see below) is called the *initial segment.* The initial segment is the site at which an *action potential* is generated in the axon. The action potential is stimulated by impulses carried to the axon

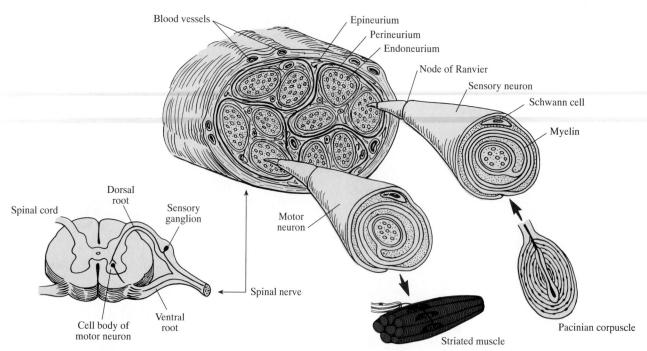

Figure 11.3. Schematic diagram showing arrangement of motor and sensory neurons. The motor neuron has its cell body in the ventral gray matter of the spinal cord. The axon, surrounded by myelin, leaves the cord via a ventral root and becomes part of a spinal nerve that carries it to its destination on a striated (skeletal) muscle. The sensory neuron originates in the skin and continues as a component of a spinal nerve, entering the spinal cord via the dorsal root. Note the location of the cell body in the sensory ganglion of the dorsal root. A segment of the spinal nerve is enlarged to show the relationship of the nerve fibers to the endoneurium and the location of perineurium and epineurium. In addition, segments of the sensory and motor neurons have been enlarged to show the relationship of the axons to the Schwann cells and myelin. (Autonomic nerve fibers are not shown in the diagram.)

hillock in the membrane of the cell body after other impulses are received on the dendrites or the cell body itself.

Axons in the CNS may be insulated by a ***myelin sheath (myelinated),*** especially in the tracts that constitute the ***white matter,*** or may be ***bare (unmyelinated),*** as in the integrative portions that constitute the ***gray matter.*** Axons in the PNS are never completely bare. Although they are described as myelinated or unmyelinated, even the unmyelinated axons are embedded in invaginations of the Schwann cell.

Synapses

Neurons Communicate With Other Neurons and With Effector Cells by Means of Synapses

Synapses are specialized junctions between neurons that facilitate transmission of impulses from one neuron to another. Synapses also occur between axons and effector cells, such as muscle and gland cells. Synapses between neurons may be classified morphologically as

- ***Axodendritic,*** occurring between axons and dendrites
- ***Axosomatic,*** occurring between axons and the cell body
- ***Axoaxonic,*** occurring between axons and axons

- ***Dendrodendritic,*** occurring between dendrites and dendrites (Fig. 11.5)

Synapses may also be classified as ***chemical or electrical.*** In chemical synapses, neurons and their processes are closely apposed; usually, only a 20–30-nm intercellular space separates them. At a typical chemical synapse, there is a

- ***Presynaptic knob (presynaptic component),*** which is the end of the neuron process from which neurotransmitter is released
- ***Synaptic cleft,*** the 20–30-nm space that the neurotransmitter must cross
- ***Postsynaptic membrane (postsynaptic component),*** which has receptor sites on the plasma membrane with which the neurotransmitter interacts

Electrical synapses, which are common in lower vertebrates and invertebrates, are gap junctions that permit movement of ions between cells and, consequently, permit direct spread of current from one cell to another. Mammalian equivalents of electrical synapses include the

- ***Nexus*** in smooth muscle (see page 234)
- ***Gap junctions*** of cardiac muscle (see page 229)

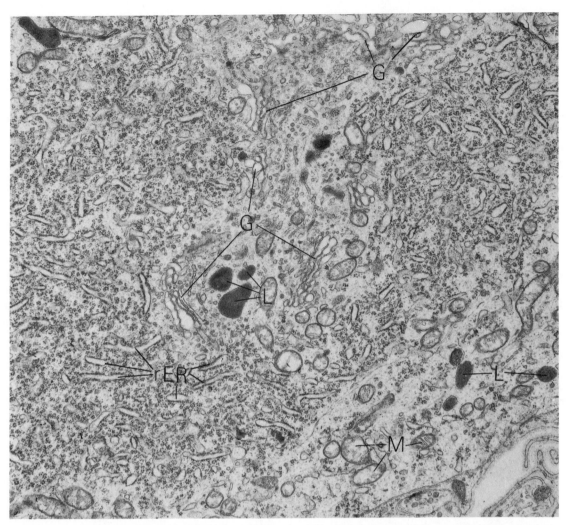

Figure 11.4. Electron micrograph showing a portion of a nerve cell body. The cytoplasm is occupied by masses of free ribosomes and profiles of rough endoplasmic reticulum *(rER)* that constitute the Nissl bodies of light microscopy. The Golgi apparatus *(G)* is arranged as a network but appears in an ul-trathin tissue section as isolated areas containing profiles of flattened sacs, vesicles, and anastomosing tubules. Other characteristic organelles include mitochondria *(M)* and lysosomes *(L)*. The neurofilaments and neurotubules are difficult to discern at this relatively low magnification. ×15,000.

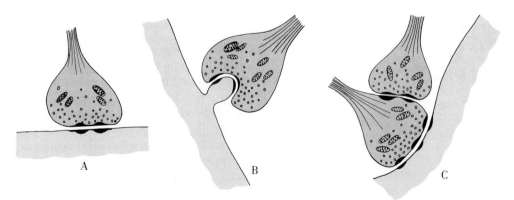

Figure 11.5. Schematic diagram of different types of synapses: **A,** axodendritic or axosomatic; **B,** axodendritic, in which an axon terminal synapses with a dendritic spine; and **C,** axoaxonic. The axoaxonic synapse may enhance or inhibit the axodendritic (or axosomatic) synapse also shown in **C.** (From Barr ML: *The Human Nervous System,* 3rd ed. New York, Harper & Row, 1979, p 18.)

Synapses are not resolvable in routine LM preparations. Silver precipitation staining methods (e.g., Golgi method) not only demonstrate the overall shape of some neurons but also show synapses as oval bodies on the surface of the receptor neuron (Fig. 11.6). Typically, an axon makes several of these button-like contacts with the receptor portion of the neuron. Often, the incoming neuron travels along the surface of the neuron, making several synaptic contacts called **boutons en passant** (Fr. for buttons in passing). The axon then continues, to end finally as a terminal twig with an enlarged tip, a **bouton terminal** (Fr. for terminal button) or **end bulb.** The number of synapses on a neuron or its processes, which may vary from just a few to **tens of thousands** per neuron, appears to be directly related to the number of impulses that neuron is receiving and processing.

Synaptic Transmission

The presynaptic component, i.e., the bouton ending of the axon, is characterized by the presence of **synaptic vesicles,** membrane-limited structures that range from 30 to 100 nm in diameter and contain neurotransmitter. There are also numerous small mitochondria and a layer of dense ma-

terial, the **presynaptic density,** on the cytoplasmic side of the plasma membrane.

The synaptic cleft separates the presynaptic component from the postsynaptic component. This component, a portion of the plasma membrane of the second neuron (Fig. 11.7), is characterized by the presence of a layer of dense material, the **postsynaptic density,** on the cytoplasmic side of the membrane.

Calcium Channels in the Membrane of the Bouton Regulate Transmitter Release

When a nerve impulse reaches the bouton, the voltage reversal across the membrane produced by the impulse (colloquially called depolarization) causes voltage-gated calcium channels to open in the plasma membrane of the bouton. The influx of calcium from the extracellular space causes the synaptic vesicles to migrate to and fuse with the presynaptic membrane, thereby releasing the transmitter into the synaptic cleft by exocytosis. The transmitter then diffuses across the synaptic cleft. Receptors on the postsynaptic membrane bind neurotransmitter, causing channels to open in that membrane that allow ions to enter the neuron. This ion flux causes voltage reversal (''depolarization'') in the postsynaptic membrane, thereby generating a second nerve impulse. The firing of impulses in the postsynaptic neuron is due to the action of hundreds of synapses.

The release of neurotransmitter by the presynaptic component can cause either **excitation** or **inhibition** at the postsynaptic membrane.

- In **excitatory synapses,** neurotransmitter causes local reversal of voltage of the postsynaptic membrane to a threshold level that leads to the initiation of a nerve impulse.
- In **inhibitory synapses,** release of neurotransmitter hyperpolarizes the postsynaptic membrane, making the generation of a nerve impulse more difficult.

The ultimate generation of a nerve impulse in a postsynaptic neuron (firing) is dependent on the summation of excitatory and inhibitory impulses reaching that neuron. In this manner, the reaction of a postsynaptic neuron (or muscle or gland cell) may be very precisely regulated. The function of synapses is not simply to transmit impulses in an unchanged manner from one neuron to another. Rather, synapses allow for the processing of neuronal input. Typically, the impulse passing from the presynaptic to the postsynaptic neuron is modified at the synaptic station by other neurons that, although not in the direct pathway, nevertheless have access to the synaptic station (see Fig. 11.5C). These other neurons may influence the membrane of the presynaptic neuron or the postsynaptic neuron and facilitate or inhibit the transmission of impulses.

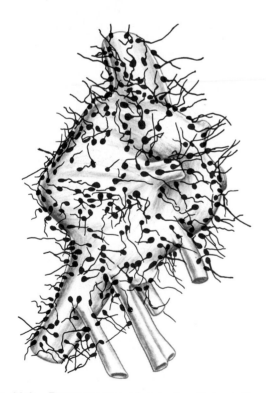

Figure 11.6. Reconstruction of axon terminals making contact on a neuron cell body and its dendrites. The axon terminals appear as the numerous ovoid bodies with a tail-like appendage. This tail is the terminal segment of the axon, which is also stained by the special procedure. The remainder of the axon is unstained and, therefore, not visible. (Based on Hagger RA, Barr ML: *Journal of Comparative Neurology* 93:17, 1950.)

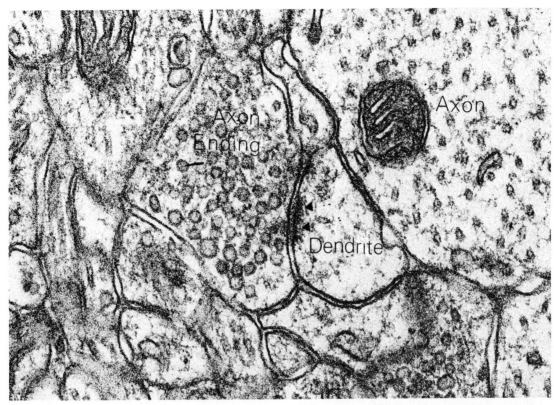

Figure 11.7. Electron micrograph of nerve processes in the cerebral cortex. A synapse can be seen in the center of the micrograph, where an axon ending is apposed to a dendrite. The ending of the axon exhibits numerous transmitter-containing vesicles that appear as circular profiles. The postsynaptic membrane of the dendrite characteristically shows a dense material *(arrowheads)*. A substance of similar density is also present in the synaptic cleft (intercellular space) at the synapse. ×76,000. (Courtesy of Dr. George D. Pappas and Virginia Kriho.)

Neurotransmitters

A number of molecules that serve as transmitters have been identified in various parts of the nervous system. The most common transmitters are

- *Acetylcholine (ACh)*
- *Norepinephrine (NE)*

Both act as transmitters between nerve cells themselves and between nerve cells and effector cells.

ACh is the transmitter between axons and striated muscle at the neuromuscular junction (see page 223). ACh and NE also serve as transmitters between axons and effectors in the ANS. Other commonly found transmitters are γ-aminobutyric acid (GABA), dopamine, serotonin, glutamic acid, and glycine.

Recently, several small peptides also have been shown to act as synaptic transmitters. Among these are *substance P* (so named because it was originally found in a *p*owder of acetone extracts of brain and intestine), *hypothalamic releasing hormones, enkephalins, vasoactive intestinal peptide (VIP), cholecystokinin (CCK)*, and *neurotensin.* Many of these same substances are synthesized and released by the enteroendocrine cells of the intestinal tract. They may act immediately on neighboring cells *(paracrine secretion)* or be carried in the blood, as *hormones,* to act on distant target cells *(endocrine secretion).* They are also synthesized and released by endocrine organs and by the *neurosecretory neurons* of the *hypothalamus* (see page 601).

Neurotransmitter Released Into the Synaptic Cleft May Be Degraded or Recaptured

Acetylcholinesterase (AChE) and *catechol o-methyltransferase (COMT)* associated with the postsynaptic membrane rapidly degrade ACh and NE, respectively. These and other transmitters may also be reincorporated into vesicles in the presynaptic component by endocytosis. The degradation or recapture of neurotransmitters is necessary in order to limit the duration of stimulation or inhibition of the postsynaptic membrane.

Normally, membrane added to the plasma membrane of the nerve ending by exocytosis when synaptic vesicles fuse with it is retrieved by endocytosis and is reprocessed into synaptic vesicles by the smooth endoplasmic reticulum (sER) located in the nerve ending.

Axonal Transport Systems

Substances Needed in the Axon and Dendrites Are Synthesized in the Cell Body and Require Transport to Those Sites

Because the synthetic activity of the neuron is concentrated in the perikaryon, *axonal transport* is required to convey newly synthesized material to all parts of the axon. Axonal transport also serves as a mode of intercellular communication, carrying molecules and information from the axon terminal to the perikaryon. Axonal transport is a bidirectional mechanism. It may be described as

- *Anterograde transport,* which carries material from the perikaryon to the periphery
- *Retrograde transport,* which carries material from the axon terminal and the dendrites to the perikaryon

The transport systems may also be distinguished by the rate at which substances are transported.

- A *slow transport system* conveys substances from the cell body to the terminal button at the speed of 0.2–4 mm/day. It is only an anterograde transport system.
- A *fast transport system* conveys substances in both directions at a rate of 20–400 mm/day. Thus, it is both an anterograde and a retrograde system.

Structural elements such as tubulin molecules (microtubule precursors) and the proteins that will form neurofilaments are carried away from the perikaryon by the slow transport system. So, too, are cytoplasmic matrix proteins, such as actin, calmodulin, and various metabolic enzymes.

Membrane-limited organelles, such as sER tubules, synaptic vesicles, and some mitochondria, and low-molecular-weight materials, such as sugars, amino acids, nucleotides, some neurotransmitters, and calcium, are carried to the axon terminal by the fast anterograde transport system. The fast retrograde transport system carries to the perikaryon many of the same materials as well as proteins and other molecules endocytosed at the axon terminal. Fast transport in either direction requires ATP and is dependent on individual microtubules that extend from the perikaryon to the termination of the axon.

Retrograde transport is the pathway followed by toxins and viruses that enter the CNS at nerve endings. Retrograde transport of exogenous enzymes, such as horseradish peroxidase, and of radiolabeled or immunolabeled tracer materials is now used to trace neuronal pathways and to identify the perikarya related to specific nerve endings.

Dendritic transport has not been studied as extensively as axonal transport. It appears to have the same characteristics and to serve the same functions for the dendrite as axonal transport does for the axon.

SUPPORTING CELLS OF NERVOUS TISSUE

Schwann Cells and the Myelin Sheath

Axons in the Peripheral Nervous System May Be Described as Myelinated or Unmyelinated

The myelinated axons are surrounded by a lipid-rich layer called the *myelin sheath*. External to and contiguous with

the myelin sheath is a layer of Schwann cell cytoplasm called the *sheath of Schwann* or the *neurilemma* (Fig. 11.8). This layer contains the nucleus and most of the organelles of the *Schwann cell*. The Schwann cell, itself, is surrounded by its basal or external lamina. Functionally, it is the myelin sheath and the neurilemma that *insulate* the axon from the surrounding extracellular compartment. Only the axon hillock and the terminal arborizations where the axon synapses with its target cells are completely devoid of the myelin sheath.

The Myelin Sheath Is Composed of Multiple Layers of Schwann Cell Membrane Wrapped Concentrically Around the Axon

To produce the myelin sheath, each Schwann cell wraps in a spiral around a short (0.08–0.1-mm) segment of myelin on an axon. During the wrapping of the axon, cytoplasm is squeezed out of the concentric layers of the Schwann cell. The inner leaflets of the plasma membrane then fuse. With the TEM, these fused inner leaflets are electron opaque, appearing as the *major dense lines* of myelin. These concentric dense lamellae alternate with the slightly less dense *intraperiod lines* that are formed by fusion of the outer membrane leaflets (Fig. 11.9).

The myelin sheath is segmented because it is formed by numerous Schwann cells arrayed sequentially along the axon. The junction where two adjacent Schwann cells meet is devoid of myelin. This site is called the *node of Ranvier.* Therefore, the myelin between two sequential nodes of Ranvier is called an *internodal segment.*

In the formation of the myelin sheath, the axon initially lies in a groove on the surface of the Schwann cell (Fig. 11.9*a*). Fusion of the edges of the groove to enclose the axon produces the *inner mesaxon,* the narrow intercellular space of the innermost rings. The first few lamellae are not compactly arranged; i.e., some cytoplasm is left in the first few concentric layers (Fig. 11.9*b*). Similarly, the outermost layer contains some cytoplasm as well as the Schwann cell nucleus (Fig. 11.9*c*). The apposition of the plasma membrane of the last layer to itself as it closes the ring produces the *outer mesaxon,* the narrow intercellular space adjacent to the basal lamina.

The myelin is lipid rich because, as the Schwann cell winds around the axon, its cytoplasm, as just noted, is extruded from between the opposing layers of the plasma membranes. Electron micrographs, however, typically show small amounts of cytoplasm in several locations (Figs. 11.10 and 11.11): the *inner collar of Schwann cell cytoplasm,* between the axon and the myelin; the *Schmidt-Lanterman clefts,* small islands within successive lamellae of the myelin; *perinodal cytoplasm,* at the node of Ranvier; and the *outer collar of perinuclear cytoplasm,* around the myelin (Fig. 11.12). This is what light microscopists identified as the Schwann sheath. If one conceptually unrolls the Schwann cell, as shown in Figure 11.13, its full extent can be ap-

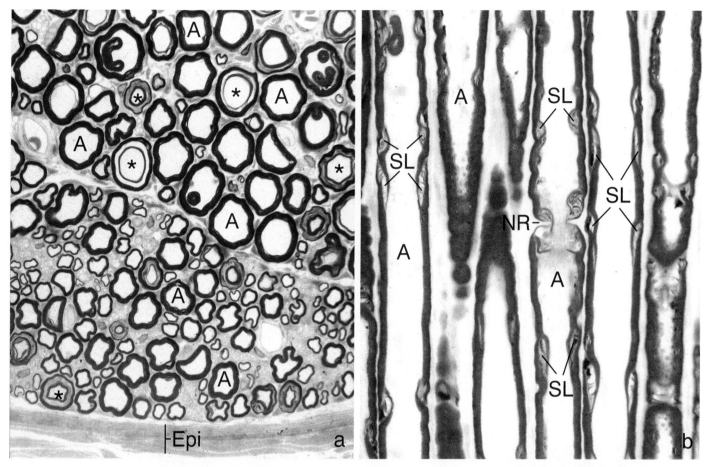

Figure 11.8. **a**. Photomicrograph of an osmium-fixed, toluidine blue-stained peripheral nerve cut in cross section. The axons *(A)* appear clear. The myelin is represented by the dark ring surrounding the axons. Note the variation in diameter of the individual axons. In some of the nerves the myelin appears to consist of two separate rings *(asterisks)*. This is due to the section passing through a Schmidt-Lanterman cleft. *Epi,* epineurium. **b**. Light micrograph showing longitudinally sectioned myelinated nerve axons. A node of Ranvier *(NR)* is seen near the center of the micrograph. In the same axon, a Schmidt-Lanterman cleft *(SL)* is seen on each side of the node. In addition, a number of Schmidt-Lanterman clefts can be seen in the adjacent axons. The perinodal cytoplasm of the Schwann cell at the node of Ranvier and the Schwann cell cytoplasm at the Schmidt-Lanterman cleft appear virtually unstained in this osmium-fixed, plastic-embedded specimen.

preciated, and the inner collar of Schwann cell cytoplasm can be seen to be continuous with the body of the Schwann cell through the Schmidt-Lanterman clefts and through the perinodal cytoplasm.

Unmyelinated Axons in the Peripheral Nervous System Are Enveloped by Schwann Cells and Their Basal Lamina

The nerves in the PNS that are described as *unmyelinated* are, nevertheless, enveloped by Schwann cell cytoplasm as shown in Figure 11.14.

The Schwann cells are elongated in parallel to the long axis of the axons, and the axons fit into grooves in the surface of the cell. The lips of the groove may be open, exposing a portion of the axolemma to the adjacent basal lamina of the Schwann cell, or the lips may be closed, forming a mesaxon.

A single axon or a group of axons may be enclosed in a single invagination of the Schwann cell surface. Large Schwann cells in the PNS may have 20 or more grooves, with each containing one or more axons. In the ANS, it is common for bundles of unmyelinated axons to occupy a single groove.

Satellite Cells

The neuronal cell bodies of ganglia are surrounded by a layer of small cuboidal cells called *satellite cells*. Although they form a complete layer around the cell body, only their nuclei are visible in routine hematoxylin and eosin (H&E) preparations (Fig. 11.15, *a* and *b*). In paravertebral and peripheral ganglia, neural cell processes must penetrate between the satellite cells to establish a synapse (there are no synapses in sensory ganglia).

Like Schwann cells, satellite cells also originate from neural crest cells. They help to establish and maintain a controlled microenvironment around the neuronal body in

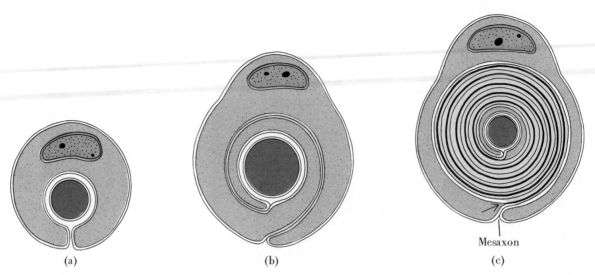

Mesaxon

(a)   (b)   (c)

Figure 11.9. Schematic diagrams showing the successive stages in the formation of myelin by a Schwann cell. **a.** The axon is initially surrounded by a Schwann cell. **b.** The Schwann cell then wraps around the axon, forming multiple Schwann cell layers. **c.** During the process the cytoplasm is extruded from between the two apposing plasma membranes, which then fuse, inner leaflet to inner leaflet, to form the major dense line *(arrow)*. The outer opposing leaflets also fuse to form the less conspicuous intraperiod line. The outer mesaxon represents invaginated plasma membrane extending from the outer surface of the Schwann cell to the myelin. The inner mesaxon extends from the inner surface of the Schwann cell (the part facing the axon) to the myelin. (From Barr ML, Kiernan JA: *The Human Nervous System,* 4th ed. New York, Harper & Row, 1983, p 45.)

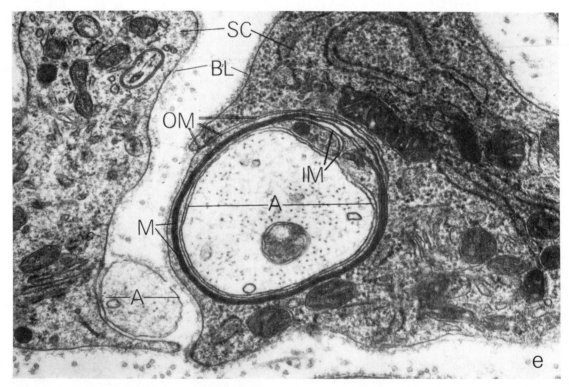

Figure 11.10. Electron micrograph of an axon (see *central A)* in the process of being myelinated. At this stage of development, the myelin *(M)* consists of about six membrane layers. The inner mesaxon *(IM)* is represented by the apposition of the internal opposing processes of the Schwann cell *(SC).* Similarly, the outer mesaxon *(OM)* is represented by the outer fold or lip of the Schwann cell where it meets itself. Another axon (see *lower left A)* is present that has not yet been enwrapped by a Schwann cell. Other features of note include the Schwann cell basal lamina *(BL)* and the considerable amount of Schwann cell cytoplasm associated with the myelination process. ×50,000. (Courtesy of Dr. Stephen G. Waxman.)

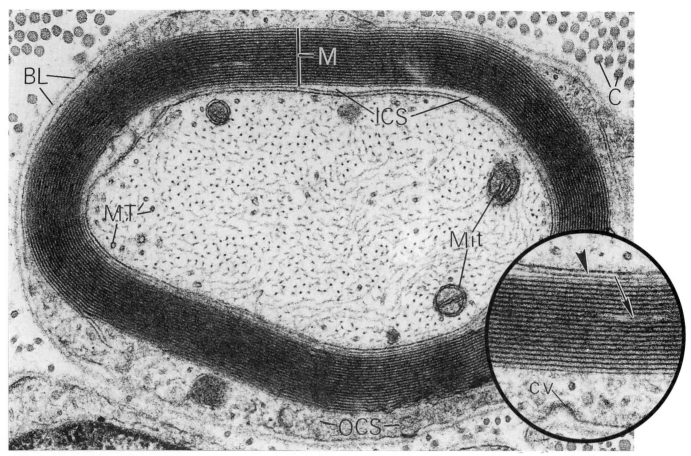

Figure 11.11. Electron micrograph of a mature myelinated axon. The myelin sheath *(M)* shown here consists of 19 paired layers of Schwann cell membrane. The pairing of membranes in each layer is due to the extrusion of the Schwann cell cytoplasm. The axon displays an abundance of neurofilaments, most of which have been cross-sectioned, giving the axon a stippled appearance. Also evident in the axon are microtubules *(MT)* and several mitochondria *(Mit)*. The outer collar of Schwann cell cytoplasm *(OCS)* is relatively abundant, compared with the inner collar of Schwann cell cytoplasm *(ICS)*. The collagen fi-brils *(C)* constitute the fibrillar component of the endoneurium. *BL,* basal lamina. ×70,000. **Inset.** Higher magnification of the myelin. The *arrow* points to cytoplasm within the myelin that would contribute to the appearance of the Schmidt-Lanterman cleft as seen in the light microscope. It appears as an isolated region here due to the thinness of the section. The intercellular space between axon and Schwann cell is indicated by the *arrowhead.* The early stage in the formation of a coated vesicle *(CV)* appears in the outer collar of Schwann cell cytoplasm. ×130,000. (Courtesy of Dr. George D. Pappas.)

the ganglion, providing electrical insulation as well as a pathway for metabolic exchanges. Thus, in both its origin and functional role the satellite cell is analogous to the Schwann cell except that it does not make myelin.

Neuroglia

Within the CNS, the supporting cells are designated *neuroglia* or *glial cells.* The three types of glial cells are

- *Oligodendrocytes,* the myelin-forming cells of the CNS
- *Astrocytes,* the cells that provide physical and metabolic support for the neurons of the CNS
- *Microglia,* the phagocytic cells of the CNS

Only the nuclei of glial cells are seen in routine histologic preparations of the CNS. It is necessary to use heavy-metal staining or immunocytochemical methods to demonstrate the shape of the entire glial cell.

Although glial cells have long been described as supporting cells of nerve tissue in the purely physical sense, current concepts emphasize the functional interdependence of neuroglial cells and nerve cells. The most obvious example of physical support occurs during development. The brain and spinal cord develop from the embryonic neural tube. In the head region, the neural tube undergoes remarkable thickening and folding, leading ultimately to the final structure, which is the brain. During the early stages of the process, embryonic glial cells extend through the entire thickness of the neural tube in a radial manner. These radial glial cells serve as a physical substrate for the migration of neurons to their appropriate position in the brain.

Microglia. Microglia are phagocytic cells. They are normally present only in small numbers in the adult CNS

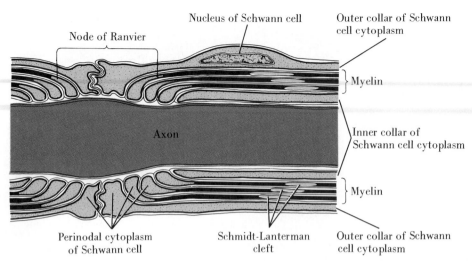

Nucleus of Schwann cell

Outer collar of Schwann cell cytoplasm

Node of Ranvier

Myelin

Axon

Inner collar of Schwann cell cytoplasm

Myelin

Perinodal cytoplasm of Schwann cell

Schmidt-Lanterman cleft

Outer collar of Schwann cell cytoplasm

Figure 11.12. Diagram of an axon and its covering sheaths in longitudinal section to show the relationship between the axon, the myelin, and the cytoplasm of the Schwann cell and the node of Ranvier. Schwann cell cytoplasm is present at four locations. These are (1) the inner and (2) the outer cytoplasmic collar of the Schwann cell, (3) the perinodal location, and (4) the Schmidt-Lanterman clefts. Note that the cytoplasm throughout the Schwann cell is continuous; it is not a series of cytoplasmic islands as it appears in the diagram (see Fig. 11.13). The node of Ranvier is where successive Schwann cells meet. The adjacent plasma membranes of the Schwann cells are not tightly apposed at the node, and extracellular fluid has free access to the neuronal plasma membrane. Also, the node is where depolarization of the neuronal plasma membrane occurs during the transmission of the nerve impulse. (Courtesy of C. P. Leblond.)

but proliferate and become actively phagocytic in regions of injury and disease. They are considered part of the mononuclear phagocytic system (see page 110) and are believed to originate in the bone marrow and enter the CNS parenchyma from the blood. There is also evidence that they remove debris of cells that die during development of the nervous system.

Microglia are the smallest of the neuroglial cells and have relatively small nuclei. When stained with heavy metals, microglia exhibit short, twisted processes. Both the processes and the cell body are covered with numerous spikes. The spikes may be the equivalent of the ruffled border seen on other phagocytic cells. The TEM reveals numerous lysosomes, inclusions, and vesicles. However, there is little rER, and there are few microtubules or microfilaments.

Astrocytes. Astrocytes are the largest of the neuroglial cells. Two kinds of astrocytes are identified:

• *Protoplasmic astrocytes,* which are more prevalent in the gray matter
• *Fibrous astrocytes,* which are more common in white matter

Both types of astrocytes contain prominent bundles of intermediate filaments composed of **glial fibrillary acidic protein (GFAP).** The filaments are much more numerous in the fibrous astrocytes, however, hence the name. Antibodies to GFAP are used as specific stains for astrocytes in sections and in tissue cultures.

Astrocytes have elaborate processes that extend between blood vessels and neurons. The ends of the processes expand, forming **end feet** that may cover large areas of the outer surface of a blood vessel or of the axolemma. It is now thought that astrocytes play a role in the movement of metabolites and wastes to and from neurons and regulate ionic concentrations in the intercellular compartment, thus maintaining the microenvironment of the neurons. They may also have a role in regulating the function of the tight junctions of the brain capillaries and venules that form the blood-brain barrier.

Astrocytes also provide a covering for the "bare areas" of myelinated axons, e.g., at the nodes of Ranvier and at synapses. Perisynaptic astrocytes may confine neurotransmitters to the synaptic cleft and may remove excess neurotransmitters by pinocytosis.

Oligodendrocytes. The oligodendrocyte is the cell responsible for producing CNS myelin. The myelin sheath in the CNS is formed by concentric layers of oligodendrocyte plasma membrane. The formation of the sheath in the CNS is more complex, however, than the simple wrapping that occurs in the PNS.

The oligodendrocytes appear in specially stained preparations in the LM as small cells with relatively few processes, compared with the astrocytes. They are often aligned in rows between the axons. Each oligodendrocyte gives off several tongue-like processes that find their way to the axons, where each process wraps itself around a portion of an axon, forming an internodal segment of myelin. The internodal myelin segments formed by the multiple processes of a single oligodendrocyte may be on one axon or on several nearby axons (Fig. 11.16). The nucleus-containing region of the oligodendrocyte may be at some distance from the axons it is myelinating.

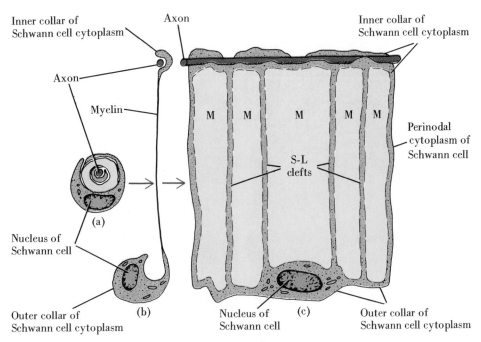

Figure 11.13. Diagrams to aid in conceptualizing the relationship of myelin and cytoplasm of a Schwann cell. **a.** Cross section of a myelinated axon. **b.** Hypothetically uncoiled Schwann cell viewed on edge. **c.** The same uncoiled Schwann cell viewed *en face.* Note how the cytoplasm of the Schwann cell is continuous. *S-L clefts,* Schmidt-Lanterman clefts; and *M,* myelin. (Modified from Webster HdeF: *The Journal of Cell Biology* 48:348, 1971, by copyright permission of The Rockefeller University Press.)

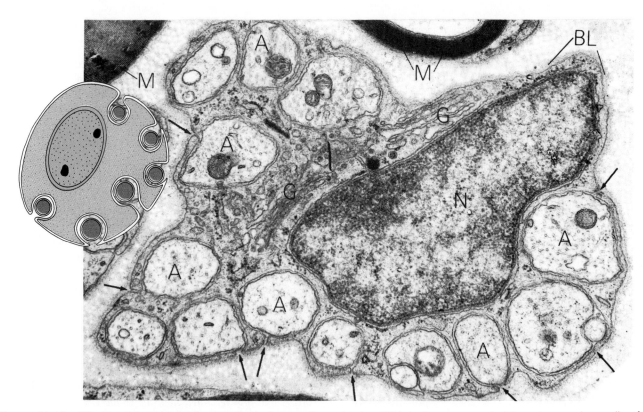

Figure 11.14. Electron micrograph of unmyelinated nerve fibers. The individual fibers or axons *(A)* are engulfed by the cytoplasm of the Schwann cell. The *arrows* indicate the site of the mesaxon. In effect, each axon is enclosed by the Schwann cell cytoplasm, except for the intercellular space of the mesaxon. Other features evident in the Schwann cell are its nucleus *(N),* the Golgi apparatus *(G),* and the surrounding basal lamina *(BL).* In the upper part of the micrograph, myelin of two myelinated nerves *(M)* is also evident. ×27,000. **Inset.** Schematic diagram showing the relationship of axons engulfed by the Schwann cell. (From Barr ML, Kiernan JA: *The Human Nervous System,* 4th ed. New York, Harper & Row, 1983, p 45.)

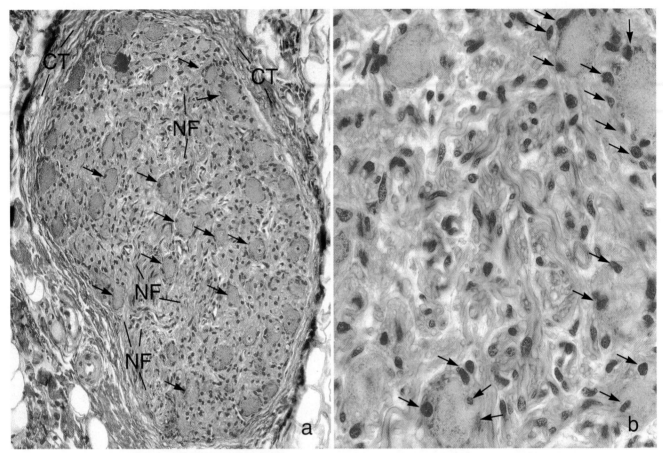

Figure 11.15. **a.** Photomicrograph of a ganglion showing the large neuronal cell bodies *(arrows)* and a central region that contains numerous nerve fibers *(NF)*. The satellite cells are represented by the very small nuclei at the periphery of the neuronal cell bodies. The ganglion is surrounded by a dense connective tissue capsule *(CT)* that is comparable to and con- tinuous with the epineurium of the nerve. ×200. **b.** Higher magnification of the ganglion showing individual axons and a few neuronal cell bodies with their satellite cells *(arrows)*. The nuclei in the region of the axons are mostly Schwann cell nuclei. Mallory-Azan stain. ×640.

The precise manner by which oligodendrocyte plasma membrane becomes concentrically wrapped around a portion of a CNS neuron is not yet as clearly understood as the parallel process in the PNS. Because a single oligodendrocyte myelinates several nearby axons simultaneously, the cell cannot spiral around each axon in an independent manner, as the Schwann cell does in the PNS. Instead, each tongue-like process appears to spiral around the axon, always staying in proximity to it, until the myelin sheath is formed. Thus, PNS myelin may be described as forming centrifugally by the movement of the Schwann cell around the outer surface of the newly formed myelin. CNS myelin, on the other hand, may be described as forming centripetally by the continued insinuation of the leading edge of the growing process between the inner surface of the newly formed myelin and the axon.

There are several other important differences between the myelin sheath in the CNS and that in the PNS. Myelin in the CNS exhibits fewer Schmidt-Lanterman clefts be- cause the astrocytes provide metabolic support for the CNS neurons. Unlike the Schwann cell of the PNS, the oligodendrocyte does not have a basal lamina. Thus, where myelin sheaths of adjacent axons touch, they may share an intraperiod line. Further, because of the manner in which oligodendrocytes form CNS myelin, there may be little or no cytoplasm in the outermost layer of the myelin sheath, allowing the myelin of adjacent axons to come into contact. Finally, the nodes of Ranvier in the CNS are larger than those in the PNS; i.e., there is more exposed axolemma, thus making *saltatory conduction* (see below) even more efficient in the CNS.

Another difference between the CNS and the PNS in regard to the relationships between supporting cells and neurons is that *unmyelinated neurons in the CNS are truly bare;* i.e., they are not embedded in glial cell processes. The bare unmyelinated axons as well as the absence of basal lamina material and connective tissue within the substance of the CNS help to distinguish the CNS from the PNS in histologic sections and in TEM specimens.

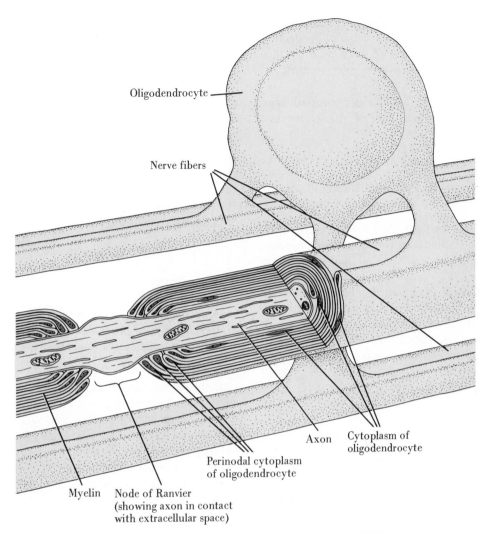

Oligodendrocyte

Nerve fibers

Axon

Cytoplasm of
oligodendrocyte

Perinodal cytoplasm
of oligodendrocyte

Myelin   Node of Ranvier
(showing axon in contact
with extracellular space)

Figure 11.16. Three-dimensional view of an oligodendrocyte as it relates to three axons. Cytoplasmic processes from the oligodendrocyte cell body form flattened cytoplasmic sheaths that wrap around each of the axons. The relationship of cytoplasm and myelin is essentially the same as that found in Schwann cells. (Based on Bunge et al: Reproduced from *The Journal of Cell Biology* 10:67, 1961, by copyright permission of The Rockefeller University Press.)

Impulse Conduction, Myelin, and the Node of Ranvier

The nerve impulse, an electrochemical process propagated along the nerve fiber, can be measured as a rapid sweep of an *action potential* along an axon, much as a flame travels along the fuse of a firecracker. The action potential is due to changes in permeability of the axolemma, resulting in an influx of sodium ions into the axoplasm and the consequent voltage reversal across the membrane. Initially, the charge internal to the resting membrane is negative (-70 mV). After the influx of the sodium ions, it is briefly positive ($+30$ mV). This voltage reversal (''depolarization'') constitutes the action potential.

A return to the original polarity is associated with a rapid efflux of potassium ions from the axon. The original state is then restored by the subsequent action of the Na^+-K^+- activated ATPase of the axolemma that pumps sodium from the axoplasm in exchange for potassium.

Rapid Conduction of the Action Potential Is Due to the Presence of the Nodes of Ranvier

Myelinated axons conduct impulses more rapidly than unmyelinated axons. Physiologists describe the nerve impulse as ''jumping'' from node to node along the myelinated axon. This is called *saltatory* or *discontinuous conduction.* Furthermore, large-diameter myelinated axons conduct impulses more rapidly than small-diameter myelinated axons because they have longer internodal lengths of myelin than do small-diameter axons.

In myelinated nerves, the voltage reversal can *only* occur at the nodes of Ranvier, where the axolemma is exposed to extracellular fluids via the intercellular space (see Figs. 11.12 and 11.16). Because of this, the voltage reversal (and, thus, the impulse) jumps as "current flow" from one node of Ranvier to the next. The speed of saltatory conduction is related not only to the thickness of the myelin but also to the thickness of the axon, being more rapid in thick axons than in thin ones.

In unmyelinated axons, the impulse is conducted more slowly, moving as a continuous wave of voltage reversal along of the axon.

Ependyma

Ependymal Cells Form the Epithelial Lining of the Ventricles of the Brain and of the Spinal Canal

Ependymal cells line the fluid-filled cavities of the CNS. They are cuboidal to columnar cells that have the morphologic and physiologic characteristics of fluid-transporting cells (Fig. 11.17).

In several locations in the brain, this lining epithelium is further modified to produce cerebrospinal fluid by transport and secretion of materials derived from adjacent capillary loops. The modified ependymal cells and associated capillaries are called the *choroid plexus.*

ORIGIN OF CELLS OF NERVOUS TISSUE

Central Nervous System Neurons Derive From Neuroectodermal Cells of the Neural Tube

After the developing nerve cells have migrated to their predestined location in the neural tube and have differentiated into mature neurons, they no longer divide. Astrocytes and oligodendrocytes also derive from cells of the neural tube, but studies with tritiated thymidine indicate that these neuroglial cells may undergo a slow turnover.

As noted above, microglia derive from the mononuclear cells of blood along with other macrophages of the body. There is still some question, however, as to whether they are able to divide after they have reached the CNS.

Peripheral Nervous System Ganglion Cells Derive From the Neural Crest

Development of the ganglion cells of the PNS, in order of occurrence, involves

- *Proliferation* of ganglion precursor cells in the neural crest
- *Migration* of cells from the neural crest to their future ganglionic site
- A *second wave of mitosis* at the site
- *Development of processes* that reach the cells' target tissues (e.g., glandular tissue for smooth muscle cells) and sensory territories

In the second mitotic wave, more cells are produced than are needed. Those that do not make functional contact with a target tissue undergo cell death.

Schwann cells also arise originally from the neural crest but they undergo mitosis along the developing nerve. Most Schwann cells are formed by mitosis of parent Schwann cells in the peripheral nerves rather than by the migration of cells from the neural crest.

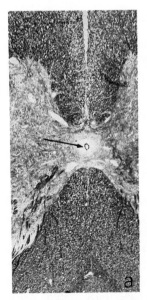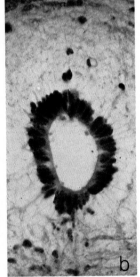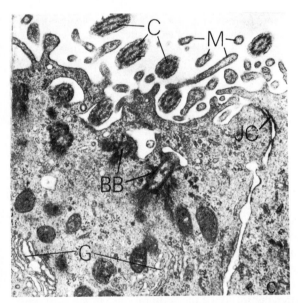

Figure 11.17.   a. Light micrograph of center region of the spinal cord, with an *arrow* pointing to the central canal. **b.** At higher magnification, the ependyma, which lines the canal, can be seen to consist of columnar cells. **c.** Transmission electron micrograph showing a portion of the apical region of two columnar ependymal cells. They are joined by a junctional complex *(JC)* that separates the lumen of the canal from the lateral intercellular space. The apical surface of the ependymal cells has both cilia *(C)* and microvilli *(M)*. Basal bodies *(BB)* and a Golgi apparatus *(G)* within the apical cytoplasm are also marked. (**a** and **b,** courtesy of Dr. George D. Pappas; **c,** courtesy of Dr. Paul Reier.)

ORGANIZATION OF THE PERIPHERAL NERVOUS SYSTEM

A Peripheral Nerve Is a Bundle of Nerve Fibers Held Together by Connective Tissue

The nerves of the PNS are made up of many nerve fibers that carry sensory and motor (effector) information between the organs and tissues of the body and the brain and spinal cord. Unfortunately, the term, *nerve fiber,* is used in different ways that can be confusing. It can be used to mean the axon with all of its covers (myelin and Schwann cell), as used above, or it can mean the axon alone. It is also used to refer to any process of a nerve cell, either dendrite or axon, especially if insufficient information is available to identify the process as either an axon or a dendrite.

The cell bodies of peripheral nerves may be located in the CNS or in paravertebral or peripheral *ganglia.* Ganglia contain clusters of neuronal cell bodies and nerve fibers leading to and from them (see Fig. 11.15). The cell bodies in ganglia may belong to sensory neurons (somatic and visceral afferents), and their distribution is restricted to specific locations (Table 11.1 and Fig. 11.3), or they may belong to postsynaptic "motor" neurons (visceral efferents) of the ANS (see Table 11.1 and Figs. 11.15 and 11.21).

To understand the PNS, it is necessary to describe, also, some parts of the CNS.

Motor Neurons Cell Bodies of the Peripheral Nervous System Lie in the Central Nervous System

The cell bodies of motor neurons that innervate skeletal muscle *(somatic efferents)* are located in the brain, the brain stem, and the spinal cord. The axons leave the CNS and travel in peripheral nerves to the skeletal muscles that they innervate. A *single neuron* conveys impulses from the CNS to the effector organ.

In the ANS, a chain of *two neurons* connects the CNS to smooth muscle, cardiac muscle, and glands *(visceral efferents).* The **preganglionic neurons** of the ANS have their cell bodies in specific locations in the CNS. Their axons leave the CNS and travel in peripheral nerves to synapse with the **postganglionic** neurons in peripheral ganglia (see Table 11.1).

Sensory Neuron Cell Bodies Are Located in Ganglia Outside of but Close to the Central Nervous System

In the sensory system, both the *somatic* and the *visceral afferent* components, a single neuron connects the receptor, through a sensory ganglion, to the spinal cord or brain stem.

TABLE 11.1. Peripheral Ganglia[A]

Ganglia that contain cell bodies of sensory neurons; these are *not* synaptic stations.
    Dorsal root ganglia of all spinal nerves
    Sensory ganglia of cranial nerves
        Trigeminal (semilunar, Gasserian) ganglion of trigeminal (V) nerve
        Geniculate ganglion of facial (VII) nerve
        Spiral ganglion (contains bipolar neurons) of vestibulocochlear (VIII) nerve
        Vestibular ganglion (contains bipolar neurons) of vestibulocochlear (VIII) nerve
        Superior and inferior ganglia of glossopharyngeal (IX) nerve
        Superior and inferior ganglia of vagus (X) nerve

Ganglia that contain cell bodies of autonomic (postsynaptic) neurons; these *are* synaptic stations.
    Sympathetic ganglia
        Sympathetic trunk (paravertebral or vertebral chain) ganglia (the highest of these is the superior cervical ganglion)
        Prevertebral ganglia (adjacent to origins of large branches of abdominal aorta), including celiac, superior mesenteric, inferior mesenteric, and aorticorenal ganglia
        The adrenal medulla (p. 000), which may be considered a modified sympathetic ganglion (each of the secretory cells of the medulla, as well as the recognizable ganglion cells, is innervated by cholinergic sympathetic nerves)
    Parasympathetic ganglia
        Head ganglia
            Ciliary ganglion of oculomotor (III) nerve
            Geniculate ganglion of facial (VII) nerve
            Submandibular ganglion of facial (VII) nerve
            Pterygopalatine (sphenopalatine) ganglion of facial (VII) nerve
            Otic ganglion of glossopharyngeal (IX) nerve
        Terminal ganglia (near or in wall of organs), including ganglia of the submucosal (Meissner's) and myenteric (Auerbach's) plexuses of the gastrointestinal tract (these are also ganglia of the *enteric* division of the ANS) and isolated ganglion cells in a variety of organs

---

[A]*Practical note:* Neuron cell bodies seen in tissue sections such as tongue, pancreas, urinary bladder, and heart are invariably terminal ganglia or "ganglion cells" of the parasympathetic nervous system.

Sensory ganglia are located along the dorsal roots of the spinal nerves and in association with cranial nerves V, VII, VIII, IX, and X (see Table 11.1).

Organization of the Spinal Cord

A brief description of the spinal cord will help to elucidate the structural relationships between the CNS and the PNS. The spinal cord is a flattened cylindrical structure that is directly continuous with the brain. It is divided into 31 segments (8 cervical, 12 thoracic, 5 lumbar, 5 sacral, and 1 coccygeal), and each segment is connected to a pair of spinal nerves. Each spinal nerve is joined to its segment of the cord by a number of roots or rootlets grouped as posterior (dorsal) or anterior (ventral) roots (Fig. 11.18; see also Fig. 11.3 and Plate 44, page 301).

In cross section, the spinal cord exhibits a butterfly-shaped grayish-tan inner substance, the *gray matter* surrounding the central canal, and a whitish peripheral substance, the *white matter*. The *white matter* (see Fig. 11.3) contains only myelinated and unmyelinated axons traveling to and from other parts of the spinal cord and to and from the brain. Functionally related bundles of axons in the white matter are called *tracts*.

The *gray matter* contains neuronal cell bodies and their dendrites, along with axons and neuroglia. Functionally related groups of nerve cell bodies in the gray matter are called *nuclei*. In this context, the term, nucleus, means a cluster or group of neuronal cell bodies plus fibers and neuroglia.

Nuclei of the CNS are the morphologic and functional equivalents of the ganglia of the PNS. Synapses occur only in the gray matter.

Motor Neurons That Innervate Striated Muscle Have Their Cell Bodies in the *Ventral (Anterior) Horn* of the Gray Matter

Ventral motor neurons, also called *anterior horn cells,* are very large basophilic cells and are easily recognized in routine histologic preparations (see Plate 44, page 301). Because the motor neuron conducts impulses away from the CNS, it is called an *efferent neuron.*

The axon of a motor neuron leaves the spinal cord, passes through the anterior (ventral) root, becomes a component of the spinal nerve of that segment, and, as such, is conveyed to the muscle. The axon is myelinated except at its origin and termination. Near the muscle cell, the axon divides into numerous terminal branches that form neuromuscular synapses with the muscle cell (see page 223).

Sensory Neurons Have Their Cell Bodies in Ganglia That Lie on the Dorsal (Posterior) Root of the Spinal Nerve

Sensory neurons in the dorsal root ganglia are pseudounipolar. They have a single process that divides into a peripheral segment that brings information from the periphery to the cell body and a central segment that carries information from the cell body into the gray matter of the

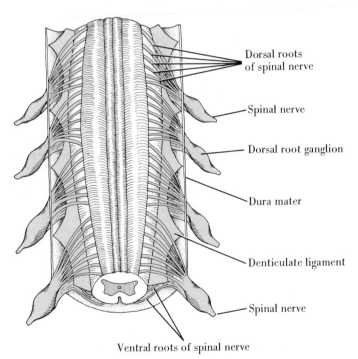

Dorsal roots
of spinal nerve

Spinal nerve

Dorsal root ganglion

Dura mater

Denticulate ligament

Spinal nerve

Ventral roots of spinal nerve

Figure 11.18. Dorsal view of exposed spinal cord showing that each spinal nerve joins the cord by a number of dorsal and ventral roots. Also shown are the dura mater and the denticulate ligaments. The former is the outer layer of the meninges covering the cord; the latter is a delicate connective tissue sheet that aids in anchoring the cord. (Based on Barr ML, Kiernan JA: *The Human Nervous System,* 4th ed. New York, Harper & Row, 1983, p 62.)

spinal cord. Because the sensory neuron conducts impulses to the CNS, it is called an **afferent neuron.** Impulses are generated in the terminal receptor arborization of the peripheral segment.

Afferent (Sensory) Receptors

Afferent Receptors Are Specialized Structures Located at the Distal Tips of the Peripheral Processes of Sensory Neurons

Although **receptors** may have many different structures, they have one basic characteristic in common: They are able to initiate a nerve impulse in response to a stimulus. The many types of receptors may be classified as

- **Exteroceptors,** which react to stimuli from the external environment, e.g., temperature, touch, smell, sound, or vision
- **Enteroceptors,** which react to stimuli from within the body, e.g., the degree of filling or stretch of the alimentary canal, bladder, and blood vessels
- **Proprioceptors,** which also react to stimuli from within the body, providing sensation of body position and muscle tone and movement

The simplest receptor is a bare axon, called a **nonencapsulated (free) ending.** This ending is found in epithelia, in connective tissue, and in close association with hair follicles.

Most Sensory Nerve Endings Acquire Connective Tissue Capsules or Sheaths of Varying Complexity

Sensory nerve endings with connective tissue sheaths are called **encapsulated endings.** Many of these encapsulated endings are mechanoreceptors in the skin and joint capsules (end bulb of Krause, Ruffini corpuscles, Meissner's corpuscles, and Pacinian corpuscles) and are described in Chapter 14, Integumentary System (page 380).

Neuromuscular spindles are encapsulated sensory endings in skeletal muscle; they are described in Chapter 10, Muscle Tissue (page 224). Functionally related Golgi tendon organs are encapsulated tension receptors found at muscle-tendon junctions.

Connective Tissue Components of a Peripheral Nerve

The bulk of a peripheral nerve consists of nerve fibers and their supporting Schwann cells. The individual nerve fibers and their associated Schwann cells are held together by connective tissue that is organized into three distinctive components, with each having specific morphologic and functional characteristics (Fig. 11.19; also, see Fig. 11.3). They are designated as

- **Endoneurium**
- **Perineurium**
- **Epineurium**

Endoneurium Constitutes the Connective Tissue Associated With Individual Nerve Fibers

The endoneurium is not conspicuous in routine LM preparations, but special connective tissue stains permit its demonstration. At the electron microscope level, collagen fibrils that constitute the endoneurium are readily apparent (see Figs. 11.10 and 11.11). They are longitudinally disposed, paralleling the nerve fibers but functionally binding them together into a fascicle or bundle. Because fibroblasts are relatively sparse in the interstices of the nerve fibers, it is likely that most of the collagen fibrils are secreted by the Schwann cells. This conclusion is supported by tissue culture studies in which collagen fibrils are formed in pure cultures of Schwann cells and dorsal root neurons. Other than occasional fibroblasts, the only other connective tissue cell normally found within the endoneurium is the mast cell.

Perineurium Is the Specialized Connective Tissue Surrounding a Nerve Fascicle

Surrounding the nerve bundle is a sheath of unique connective tissue cells, the **perineurium.** It serves as a semipermeable barrier. It may be one or more cell layers thick, depending on the nerve diameter. The cells that comprise this layer are squamous in shape; each layer exhibits an external (basal) lamina on both surfaces (Fig. 11.19b). The cells are contractile and contain an appreciable number of actin microfilaments, a characteristic of smooth muscle cells and other contractile cells. Moreover, in those instances where there are two or more perineurial cell layers (as many as five of six layers may be present in larger nerves), collagen fibrils are present between the perineurial cell layers, but fibroblasts are typically absent. In effect, the arrangement of these cells to form a barrier and the presence of basal lamina material liken them to an epithelioid tissue. On the other hand, their contractile nature and the apparent ability to produce collagen fibrils also liken them to smooth muscle cells as well as to fibroblasts. The limited number of connective tissue cell types within the endoneurium is undoubtedly a reflection of a protective role that the perineurium plays. It excludes the need for the presence of cells belonging to the immune system (other than the mast cell) within the endoneurial compartment.

Epineurium Consists of Dense Connective Tissue That Surrounds and Binds Together Nerve Fascicles Into a Common Bundle

The epineurium forms the outermost tissue of the peripheral nerve. It is a typical dense connective tissue that binds together the fascicles formed by the perineurium.

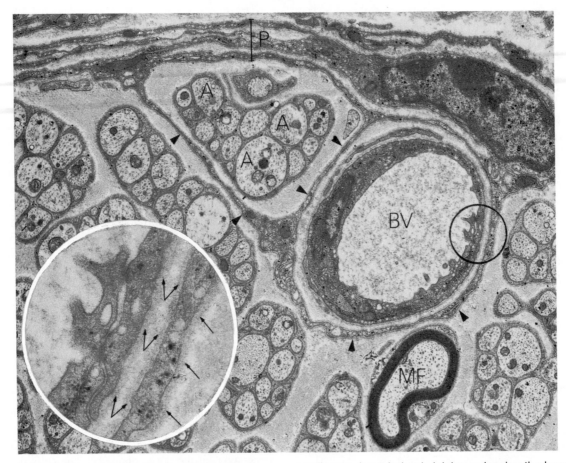

Figure 11.19.   a. Electron micrograph of unmyelinated nerve fibers and a single myelinated fiber *(MF)*. The perineurium *(P)*, consisting of several cell layers, is seen in the upper portion of the micrograph. Perineurial cell processes *(arrowheads)* have also extended into the nerve to surround a group of axons *(A)* and their Schwann cell, as well as a small blood vessel *(BV)*. The enclosure of this group of axons represents the root of a small nerve branch that is joining or leaving the larger fascicle. The area within the *circle* encompassing the endothelium of the vessel and the adjacent perineurial cytoplasm is shown in the **inset** at higher magnification. Note the basal laminae of the vessel and the perineurial cell *(arrows)*. The junction between endothelial cells of the blood vessel is also apparent *(double-arrows)*. ×10,000; **inset,** ×46,000.

Adipose tissue is often associated with the epineurium in the larger nerves.

The blood vessels that supply the nerves travel in the epineurium, and their branches penetrate into the nerve and travel within the perineurium. Tissue at the level of the endoneurium is poorly vascularized, to a large extent depending for metabolic exchanges of substrates and wastes on diffusion from and to the blood vessels through the perineurial sheath (Fig. 11.19).

Autonomic Nervous System

Although the existence of the ANS was introduced early in this chapter, it will be useful here to describe some of the salient features of its organization and distribution. The ANS is classified into three divisions:

- *Sympathetic division*
- *Parasympathetic division*
- *Enteric division*

The ANS is that portion of the PNS that conducts impulses to smooth muscle, cardiac muscle, and glandular epithelium. These effectors are the functional units in the organs that respond to regulation by nervous tissue. The term, visceral, is sometimes used in referring to the ANS or its neurons, which are, therefore, called *visceral efferent neurons.*

Sensory neurons also leave the organs to convey impulses to the CNS. These *visceral afferent neurons* have the same arrangement as other sensory neurons; i.e., their cell bodies are in sensory ganglia, and they possess long peripheral and central axons, as already described.

The main organizational difference between the efferent flow of impulses to skeletal muscle (the somatic effectors) and the efferent flow to smooth muscle, cardiac muscle, and glandular epithelium (the visceral effectors) is that one neuron conveys the impulses from the CNS to the somatic effector (Fig. 11.20*a*), whereas a chain of two neurons conveys the impulses from the CNS to the visceral effectors (Fig. 11.20*b*). Thus, there is a synaptic station in a ganglion outside of the CNS where a *preganglionic* or *presynaptic* neuron makes contact with *postganglionic* or *post-*

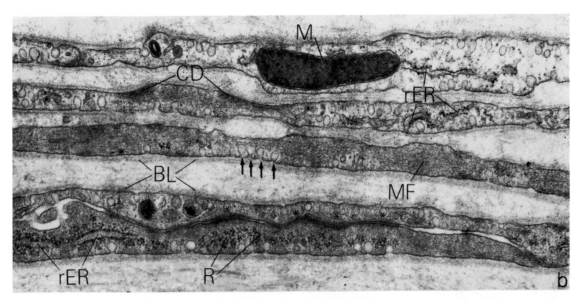

Figure 11.19. b. Electron micrograph showing the perineurium of a nerve. Four cellular layers of the perineurium are present. Each layer has a basal lamina *(BL)* associated with it on both surfaces. Other features of the perineurial cell include an extensive population of microfilaments *(MF)* known to consist of actin, pinocytotic vesicles *(arrows)*, and cytoplasmic densities *(CD)*. These features are characteristic of smooth muscle cells. The cytoplasm of the peripheral cell layer is less electron dense due to a paucity of microfilaments. The presence of basal lamina in association with this cell indicates, however, that it is a perineurial cell. The innermost perineurial cell layer exhibits a junctional specialization *(asterisks)* where one cell is overlapping a second cell in forming the sheath. Such junctions (fasciae adherentes) are associated with strong adhesion between neighboring cells. Other features seen in the cytoplasm are mitochondria *(M)*, rough endoplasmic reticulum *(rER)*, and free ribosomes *(R)*. ×27,000.

synaptic neurons. Each presynaptic neuron synapses with several postsynaptic neurons.

The Presynaptic Neurons of the *Sympathetic* Division Are Located in the Thoracic and Upper Lumbar Portions of the Spinal Cord

The presynaptic neurons send axons from the thoracic and upper lumbar spinal cord to the vertebral and paravertebral ganglia. The ganglia in the paravertebral and vertebral *sympathetic chain* contain the cell bodies of the postsynaptic effector neurons of the *sympathetic division* (Figs. 11.20*b* and 11.21).

The Presynaptic Neurons of the *Parasympathetic Division* Are Located in the Brain Stem and Sacral Spinal Cord

The presynaptic neurons send axons from the brain stem, i.e., the midbrain, pons, and medulla, and the sacral spinal cord to visceral ganglia. The ganglia in or near the wall of abdominal and pelvic organs and the visceral motor ganglia of cranial nerves III, VII, IX, and X contain cell bodies of the postsynaptic effector neurons of the *parasympathetic division* (Figs. 11.20*c* and 11.21).

The sympathetic and parasympathetic divisions of the ANS often supply the same organs. In these cases, the actions of the two are usually antagonistic. An obvious example of this is that sympathetic stimulation brings on increased activity of cardiac muscle, whereas parasympathetic stimulation inhibits activity.

Many functions of the sympathetic nervous system are similar to those of the adrenal medulla, an endocrine gland. This is partly explained by the fact that the cells of the adrenal medulla are related to postganglionic sympathetic neurons. Both derive from the neural crest, are innervated by preganglionic sympathetic neurons, and produce closely related physiologically active agents, epinephrine and norepinephrine (NE). The difference is that the sympathetic neurons deliver the agent directly to the effector, whereas the cells of the adrenal medulla deliver the agent indirectly through the bloodstream. The innervation of the adrenal medulla may constitute an exception to the rule that autonomic innervation consists of a two-neuron chain from CNS to an effector; for the adrenal medulla, it is only one neuron, unless the adrenal medullary cell is considered the functional equivalent of the second neuron, in effect, a neurosecretory neuron.

The *Enteric Division* of the Autonomic Nervous System Consists of the Ganglia and Postganglionic Neuronal Networks of the Alimentary Canal

Ganglia and postganglionic neurons of the enteric division are located in the lamina propria, muscularis mucosae, submucosa, muscularis externa, and subserosa of the alimentary canal from the esophagus to the anus (see page 441). The enteric division can function independently of preganglionic input from the vagus nerve and sacral outflow; e.g., the intestine will continue peristaltic movements even after the vagus nerve is cut. There are many millions

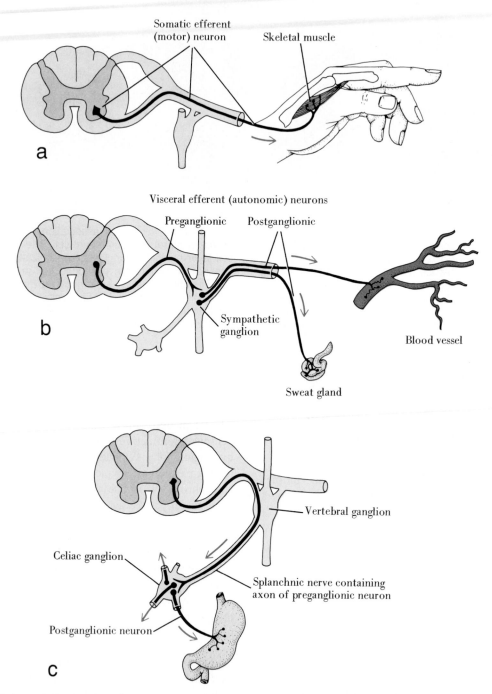

Figure 11.20. Schematic comparison between arrangement of efferent neurons of the somatic system supplying skeletal muscle **(a)** and efferent neurons of the autonomic (sympathetic) nervous system supplying smooth muscle (as in a blood vessel) or glandular epithelium (as in a sweat gland) **(b)**. In the somatic system **(a)**, one neuron conducts the impulses from CNS to the effector (skeletal muscle); in the autonomic system **(b)**, the impulses are conducted by a chain of two neurons. Moreover, each preganglionic neuron makes synaptic contact with more than one postganglionic neuron. Neurons of the autonomic (sympathetic) nervous system supplying organs of the abdomen reach the abdominal organs by way of the splanchnic nerves **(c)**. In the case shown, the splanchnic nerve joins with the celiac ganglion where most of the synapses of the two-neuron chain occur. Note that one preganglionic neuron makes contact with several postganglionic neurons. (From Reith EJ, Breidenbach M, Lorenc M, et al: *Textbook of Anatomy and Physiology*, 2nd ed. St. Louis, CV Mosby, 1978, pp 201 and 202.)

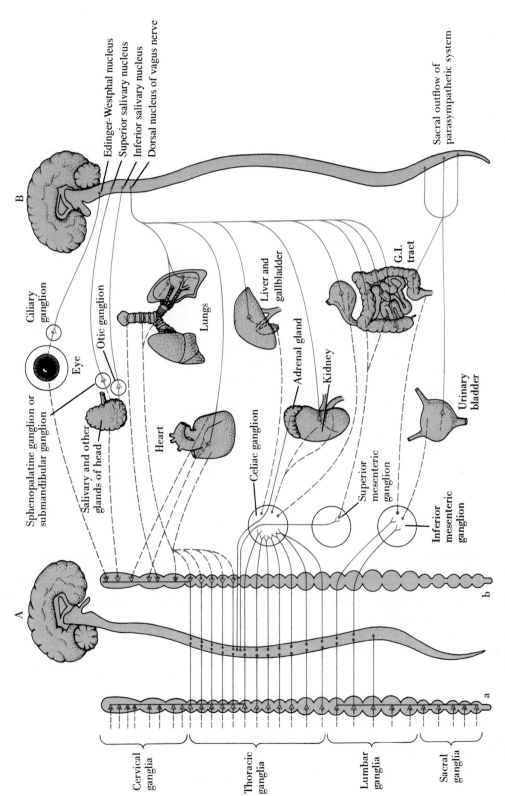

Figure 11.21. Schematic diagram showing the general arrangement of sympathetic and parasympathetic neurons of the ANS. The sympathetic outflow is shown in **A.** There are two chains of vertebral ganglia: **a** and **b.** Both contain the same neuronal components, but **a** shows only the outflow destined for the smooth muscle and glands in somatic territories (e.g., smooth muscle in blood vessels of the limbs), whereas **b** shows the outflow to the viscera of the body. The sympathetic outflow leaves the CNS from the thoracic and upper lumbar segments of the spinal cord. The parasympathetic outflow **(B)** leaves the CNS from the brain stem and sacral spinal cord segments and is distributed to the viscera. The viscera, thus, contain both sympathetic and parasympathetic innervation. Note that a two-neuron chain carries impulses to all effectors except the adrenal medulla. (From Reith EJ, Breidenbach M, Lorenc M, et al: *Textbook of Anatomy and Physiology*, 2nd ed. St. Louis, CV Mosby, 1978, p 203.)

more ganglion cells in the enteric division than could be supplied by the preganglionic neurons of the vagal and sacral outflows.

A Summarized View of Autonomic Distribution

Figures 11.20 and 11.21 summarize diagrammatically the origins and distribution of the ANS. Please refer to those figures as you read the following descriptive sections. Note that the diagrams indicate both the paired innervation (parasympathetic and sympathetic) common to the ANS as well as the important exceptions to this general characteristic.

Head

- *Parasympathetic preganglionic* outflow to the head leaves the brain with the cranial nerves, as indicated in Figure 11.21, but the routes are quite complex. Cell bodies may also be found in structures other than head ganglia listed in Table 11.1 and Figure 11.21, e.g., in the tongue. These are "terminal" ganglion cells of the parasympathetic system.
- *Sympathetic preganglionic* outflow to the head comes from the thoracic region of the spinal cord. The *postganglionic neurons* have their cell bodies in the superior cervical ganglion; the axons leave the ganglion in a nerve network that hugs the wall of the internal carotid artery. The nerve is called the **internal carotid nerve** or the **internal carotid plexus.** Some postganglionic fibers also reach the head by a much smaller **external carotid nerve** and **plexus.**

Thorax

- *Parasympathetic preganglionic* outflow to the thoracic viscera is via the vagus nerve (X). The *postganglionic neurons* have their cell bodies in the walls or in the substance of the organs of the thorax.
- *Sympathetic postganglionic* neurons for the heart are mostly in the cervical ganglia; their axons make up the **cardiac nerves. Postganglionic sympathetic neurons** for the other thoracic viscera are in ganglia of the thoracic part of the sympathetic chain. The axons are in small **splanchnic nerves** that travel from the sympathetic chain to the organs.

Abdomen and Pelvis

- *Parasympathetic preganglionic* outflow to the abdominal viscera is via the vagus (X) and pelvic nerves. *Postganglionic neurons* of the parasympathetic system to abdominopelvic organs are in terminal ganglia that generally are in the walls of the organs, such as the ganglia of the submucosal (Meissner's) plexus and the myenteric (Auerbach's) plexus in the alimentary canal.
- *Sympathetic preganglionic* outflow to the abdominopelvic organs is from the thoracic and upper lumbar segments of the spinal cord. *Postganglionic neurons* have their cell bodies mostly in the prevertebral ganglia (see Fig. 11.20c), although some are in the vertebral chain, and their neurons enter the splanchnic nerves.

Extremities and Body Wall. There is no parasympathetic outflow to the body wall and extremities. Anatomically, the autonomic innervation in the body wall is only sympathetic (see Fig. 11.20b). Each spinal nerve contains postganglionic sympathetic fibers, i.e., unmyelinated visceral efferents, of neurons whose cell bodies are in the vertebral chain of ganglia. For sweat glands, the neurotransmitter released by the "sympathetic" neurons is ACh instead of the usual NE.

ORGANIZATION OF THE CENTRAL NERVOUS SYSTEM

The organization of the spinal cord into a central, butterfly-shaped core of gray matter and a peripheral, surrounding white matter has been described above (see Figs. 11.3 and 11.20). The brain (**cerebrum** and **cerebellum**) also contains gray matter and white matter but in a different arrangement.

In the Brain, the Gray Matter Forms an Outer Covering or *Cortex;* the White Matter Forms an Inner Core or Medulla

The cortex of gray matter in the brain contains nerve cell bodies, axons, dendrites, and glial cells and is the site of synapses. In addition to the gray matter of the cortex, islands of gray matter, **nuclei** (see page 274), are found in the deep portions of the cerebrum and cerebellum.

The white matter contains only axons of nerve cells plus the associated glial cells and blood vessels. These axons travel from one part of the nervous system to another. Whereas many of the axons going to or coming from a specific location are grouped into bundles called **tracts,** the tracts themselves do not stand out as delineated bundles. The demonstration of a tract in white matter of the CNS requires some special procedure, such as the destruction of cell bodies that contribute fibers to the tract. The damaged fibers can be displayed by the use of appropriate staining or labeling methods and then traced. Even in the spinal cord, where the grouping of tracts is most pronounced, there are no sharp boundaries between adjacent tracts.

Cells of the Gray Matter

The kinds of cell bodies found in the gray matter vary according to which part of the brain or spinal cord is being examined.

Each Functional Region of the Gray Matter Has a Characteristic Variety of Cell Bodies Associated With a Meshwork of Axonal, Dendritic, and Glial Processes

The meshwork of axonal, dendritic, and glial processes associated with the gray matter is called the **neuropil.** The organization of the neuropil is not demonstrable in H&E-stained sections. It is necessary to use methods other than H&E histology to decipher the cytoarchitecture of the gray matter.

Although general histology programs usually do not deal with the actual arrangements of the nerve cells in the CNS, the presentation of two examples will add to the appreciation of H&E sections that students usually examine. These examples present a region of the cerebral cortex (Fig. 11.22) and the cerebellar cortex (Fig. 11.23), respectively. These figures refer to neuron types illustrated in Plates 42 and 43, pages 297 and 299. The figures should be correlated with the description of those plates.

The **brain stem** is not clearly separated into regions of gray matter and white matter. The nuclei of the cranial nerves located in the brain stem, however, appear as islands surrounded by more or less distinct tracts of white matter. The nuclei contain the cell bodies of the motor neurons of the cranial nerves and are both the morphologic and functional counterparts of the anterior horns of the spinal cord. In other sites in the brain stem, as in **reticular formation,** the distinction between white matter and gray matter is even less evident.

- Many of the nuclei in the brain stem contain cell bodies of motor neurons of the cranial nerves.
- These motor nuclei are both morphologic and functional counterparts of the anterior horns of the spinal cord.

Connective Tissue of the Central Nervous System

Three sequential connective tissue membranes, the **meninges,** cover the brain and spinal cord:

- The **dura mater** is the outermost layer.
- The **arachnoid** layer lies beneath the dura.
- The **pia mater** is a delicate layer resting directly on the surface of the brain and spinal cord.

The *Dura Mater* (Literally, Tough Mother) Is a Relatively Thick Sheet of Dense Connective Tissue

In the cranial cavity, the thick layer of connective tissue that forms the dura mater is continuous at its outer surface

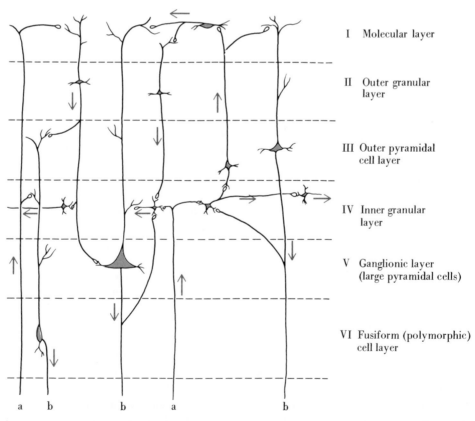

I Molecular layer

II Outer granular layer

III Outer pyramidal cell layer

IV Inner granular layer

V Ganglionic layer (large pyramidal cells)

VI Fusiform (polymorphic) cell layer

a b   b a   b

Figure 11.22. Simple scheme of intracortical circuits: *a,* cortical afferent fibers; and *b,* cortical efferent fibers. The interneurons are unlabeled. The *arrows* show direction of impulses. The *Roman numbers* and the *labels* on the right correspond to the layers of the cerebral cortex in Plate 42, page 297. (Based on Barr ML, Kiernan JA: *The Human Nervous System,* 4th ed. New York, Harper & Row, 1983, p 227.)

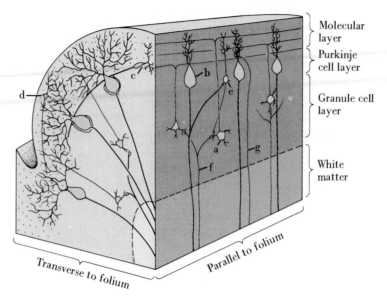

Figure 11.23. Cytoarchitecture of the cerebellar cortex: *a,* granule cell; *b,* Purkinje cell; *c,* basket cell; *d,* stellate cell; *e,* Golgi cell; *f,* mossy fiber; and *g,* climbing fiber. A folium is a narrow leaf-like gyrus typical of the cerebellar cortex. (Based on Barr ML, Kiernan JA: *The Human Nervous System,* 4th ed. New York, Harper & Row, 1983, p 162.)

with the periosteum of the skull. Within the dura mater, there are spaces lined by endothelium (and backed by periosteum and dura mater, respectively) that serve as the principal channels for blood returning from the brain. These *venous sinuses* receive blood from the principal cerebral veins and carry it to the internal jugular veins.

Sheet-like extensions of the inner surface of the dura mater form partitions between parts of the brain, supporting these parts within the cranial cavity and carrying the arachnoid to some of the deeper parts of the brain. In the spinal canal, the vertebrae have their own periosteum, and the dura mater forms a separate tube surrounding the spinal cord (see Fig. 11.18).

The *Arachnoid* Is a Delicate Sheet of Connective Tissue Loosely Joined to the Inner Surface of the Dura

The arachnoid abuts on the inner surface of the dura and extends delicate trabeculae to the pia mater on the surface of the brain and spinal cord. The space bridged by these trabeculae is the *subarachnoid space;* it contains *cerebrospinal fluid* (Fig. 11.24).

The *pia mater* is also a delicate connective tissue layer. It lies directly on the surface of the brain and spinal cord and is continuous with the perivascular connective tissue sheath of the blood vessels of the brain and spinal cord. Both surfaces of the arachnoid, the inner surface of the pia

mater, and the trabeculae are covered with a thin squamous epithelial layer.

Blood-Brain Barrier

The Blood-Brain Barrier Restricts Passage of Some Substances From the Circulation to the Parenchyma of the Central Nervous System

Studies with the TEM, using electron-opaque tracers, have shown that complex tight junctions exist between the endothelial cells of the blood vessels of the brain. These junctions prevent passage of solutes and fluid from the lumen to the extravascular space via the intercellular space of the endothelium (see Fig. 12.5, page 308). Also, few pinocytotic vesicles are seen in the capillaries of the CNS, thus further restricting transendothelial transport.

Evidence also suggests that the perineurium constitutes a blood-neural barrier, regulating the microenvironment within fascicles of nerve fibers in peripheral nerves.

Some parts of the CNS, however, are not isolated from substances carried in the blood. The barrier is ineffective or absent in the neurohypophysis (posterior pituitary; see page 599), substantia nigra, and locus ceruleus. These may be areas of the brain in which sampling of materials circulating in the blood is necessary to regulate neurosecretory control of parts of the nervous system and of the endocrine system.

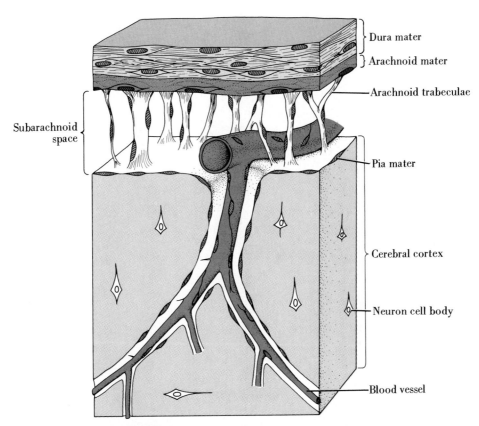

Figure 11.24. Schematic diagram of the cerebral meninges. The outer layer, the dura mater, is joined to adjacent bone of the cranial cavity (not shown). The inner layer, the pia mater, rests directly on the neural tissue. The intervening layer, the arachnoid mater, is attached to the dura mater and sends delicate trabeculae to the pia mater. Between the arachnoid and the pia mater is the subarachnoid space; it contains cerebrospinal fluid. The space also contains the larger blood vessels that send branches into the substance of the brain. A sheath of cells that is continuous with the pia mater and surrounds the branches of the blood vessels supplying the brain is indicated by the nuclei of the cells located on the external surface of the vessels. (Based on Junqueira LC, Carneiro J, Long JA: *Basic Histology,* 5th ed. Norwalk, CT, Appleton-Century-Crofts, 1986, p 198.)

RESPONSE OF NEURONS TO INJURY

The Portion of a Nerve Fiber Distal to a Site of Injury Undergoes Degeneration Due to Interrupted Axonal Transport

Degeneration of an axon distal to a site of injury is called *anterograde (Wallerian) degeneration.* In the PNS, the axon distal to the injury becomes beaded and fragments into discontinuous segments within a few days (Fig. 11.25, *a* and *b*). In the CNS, breakdown of the isolated axon segments takes several weeks.

The myelin sheath also fragments, and the myelin fragments enclose the axon fragments. Phagocytic cells, derived from the Schwann cells in the PNS, from microglia in the CNS, and from blood monocytes that migrate to the site of injury, remove the myelin and axon fragments. Some retrograde degeneration also occurs, but this extends for only a few internodal segments. In the PNS, the Schwann cells and their basal laminae remain as tubular structures distal to the injury (Fig. 11.25*c*).

The Cell Body of an Injured Nerve Swells, Its Nucleus Moves Peripherally, and There Is Loss of Nissl Substance

Nerve injury leads to a loss of Nissl substance from the cell body, called *chromatolysis.* This is seen within 1–2 days after injury. Chromatolysis reaches a peak at about 2 weeks (Fig. 11.25*b*). The changes in the cell body are proportionate to the amount of axoplasm lost by the injury; extensive loss of axoplasm can lead to death of the cell. When a motor fiber is cut, the muscle innervated by that fiber undergoes atrophy (Fig. 11.25*c*).

Before the development of modern dye and radioisotope tracer techniques, Wallerian degeneration and chromatolysis were used as research tools. This allowed tracing of the pathways and destination of axons and the localization of the cell bodies of experimentally injured nerves.

Scar Formation

In the PNS, connective tissue and Schwann cells form scar tissue in the gap between the ends of a severed or crushed nerve. If the amount of scar tissue is not too great or if

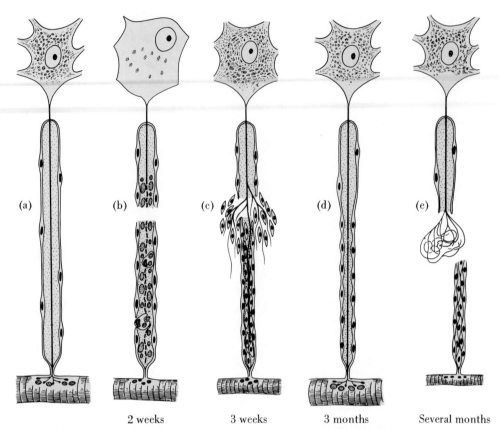

2 weeks   3 weeks   3 months   Several months

Figure 11.25.   Main changes that take place in an injured nerve fiber. **a.** Normal nerve fiber, with its perikaryon and the effector cell (striated skeletal muscle). Note the position of the neuron nucleus and the number and distribution of Nissl bodies. **b.** When the fiber is injured, the neuronal nucleus moves to the cell periphery, and Nissl bodies become greatly reduced in number. The nerve fiber distal to the injury degenerates along with its myelin sheath. Debris is phagocytosed by macrophages. **c.** The muscle fiber shows a pronounced disuse atrophy. Schwann cells proliferate, forming a compact cord pen- etrated by the growing axon. The axon grows at a rate of 0.5– 3 mm/day. **d.** In this example, the nerve fiber regeneration was successful. Note that the muscle fiber was also regenerated after receiving nerve stimuli. **e.** When the axon does not penetrate the cord of Schwann cells, its growth is not organized. (Based on Willis RA, Willis AT: *The Principles of Pathology and Bacteriology,* 3rd ed. Woburn, MA, Butterworth, 1972; from Junqueira LC, Carneiro J, Kelley RO: *Basic Histology,* 7th ed. Norwalk, CT, Appleton & Lange, 1992, p 188.)

surgical apposition of the cut ends of the nerve is possible, the severed nerve will probably regenerate.

In the CNS, scar tissue derived from proliferating glial cells appears to prevent regeneration. Current research on CNS regeneration is, therefore, focused on preventing or inhibiting glial scar formation.

Regeneration

In the Peripheral Nervous System, Schwann Cells Divide and Develop Cellular Bands That Bridge a Newly Formed Scar

Division of Schwann cells is the first step in the regeneration of a severed or crushed peripheral nerve. The Schwann cells then bridge the scar. As the second step in regeneration, large numbers of new nerve processes *(neurites)* sprout from the proximal stump (Fig. 11.25c). The Schwann cell bridges then serve as guides for the regenerating axons to grow across the scar, thus maintaining the normal pathways of the growing axons.

Although many of the new nerve processes degenerate, their large number increases the probability of reestablishing sensory and motor connections. Successful sprouts grow at about 3 mm/day. After crossing the scar, neurites enter the surviving Schwann tubes in the distal stump. These tubes will then guide the neurites to their destination as well as provide the microenvironment for continued growth (Fig. 11.25d).

If Functional Contact Is Reestablished Between a Motor Neuron and Its Muscle, Function Is Reestablished

Microsurgical techniques that rapidly reestablish intimate apposition of severed nerve and vessel ends have made reattachment of severed limbs and digits, with subsequent reestablishment of function, a relatively common procedure.

If the axonal sprouts do not reestablish contact with the bridge of Schwann cells, the sprouts grow in a disorganized manner, and the muscle remains atrophic (Fig. 11.25e).

ATLAS PLATES

37–44

PLATE 37. Sympathetic and Dorsal Root Ganglia

Sympathetic ganglia constitute a major subclass of autonomic ganglia (parasympathetic ganglia and enteric ganglia constitute the other subclasses). Autonomic ganglia are peripheral motor ganglia containing cell bodies of postsynaptic neurons. These neurons conduct nerve impulses to smooth muscle, cardiac muscle, and glands. Synapses between presynaptic neurons (all of which have their cell body in the CNS) and postsynaptic neurons occur in autonomic ganglia.

FIGURE 1, ganglion, human, silver stain ×160. A sympathetic ganglion stained with silver and counterstained is illustrated here. Shown to advantage in the preparation are several discrete bundles of nerve fibers *(NF)* and numerous large circular structures, namely, the cell bodies *(CB)* of the postsynaptic neurons. In addition to the organized nerve fibers, more random patterns of nerve fibers are also seen. Moreover, careful examination of the cell bodies shows that some display several processes joined to them. Thus, these are multipolar neurons, one of which is contained within the *rectangle* that is shown at higher magnification in Figure 2. Generally, the connective tissue is not conspicuous in a silver preparation, although it can be identified by virtue of its location about the larger blood vessels *(BV)*, particularly in the upper part of this figure.

FIGURE 2, ganglion, human, silver stain ×500. The cell bodies of the sympathetic ganglion are typically large, and the one labeled here shows several processes *(P)*. In addition, the cell body contains a large, pale-staining spherical nucleus *(N)*; this, in turn, contains a spherical, intensely staining nucleolus *(Nl)*. These features, namely, a large pale-staining nucleus (indicative of much extended chromatin) and a large nucleolus, reflect a cell that is metabolically active in protein synthesis. Also shown in the cell body are accumulations of pigment; this is lipofuscin *(L)*, a yellow pigment that is darkened by the silver. Because of the large size of the cell body, the nucleus is not always included in the section; in that case, the cell body appears as a rounded cytoplasmic mass. Whereas the silver preparation displays the multipolar cell bodies and nerve fibers to great advantage, other methods need to be used to display satellite cells and myelin adequately.

FIGURE 3, ganglion, cat, H&E ×160. Dorsal root ganglia differ from autonomic ganglia in a number of ways. Whereas the latter contain multipolar neurons and have synaptic connections, dorsal root ganglia contain unipolar sensory neurons and have no synaptic connections.

Part of a dorsal root ganglion stained with H&E is shown in this figure. The specimen includes the edge of the ganglion, where it is covered with connective tissue *(CT)*. The dorsal root ganglion contains large cell bodies *(CB)* that are typically arranged as closely packed clusters. Also, between and around the cell clusters, there are bundles of nerve fibers *(NF)*. Most of the fiber bundles indicated by the label have been sectioned longitudinally.

FIGURE 4, ganglion, cat, H&E ×350. At higher magnification of the same ganglion, the constituents of the nerve fiber show their characteristic structure, namely, a centrally located axon *(A)* surrounded by a myelin space (not labeled), which, in turn, is bounded on its outer border by the thin cytoplasmic strand of the neurilemma *(arrowheads)*.

The cell bodies of the sensory neurons display large, pale-staining spherical nuclei *(N)* and intensely staining nucleoli *(Nl)*. Also seen in this H&E preparation are the nuclei of satellite cells *(Sat C)* that completely surround the cell body. Note how much smaller these cells are than the neurons. In effect, the satellite cells form a sheath around the nerve cell body. They are continuous with the Schwann cells that invest the axon. Clusters of cells *(asterisks)* within the ganglion that have an epithelioid appearance are *en face* views of satellite cells where the section tangentially includes the satellite cells but barely grazes the adjacent cell body.

KEY

A, axon	**L,** lipofuscin	**P,** processes of nerve cell body
BV, blood vessels	**N,** nucleus of nerve cell	**Sat C,** satellite cells
CB, cell body of neuron	**NF,** nerve fibers	**arrowheads,** neurilemma
CT, connective tissue	**Nl,** nucleolus	**asterisks,** clusters of satellite cells

PLATE 37

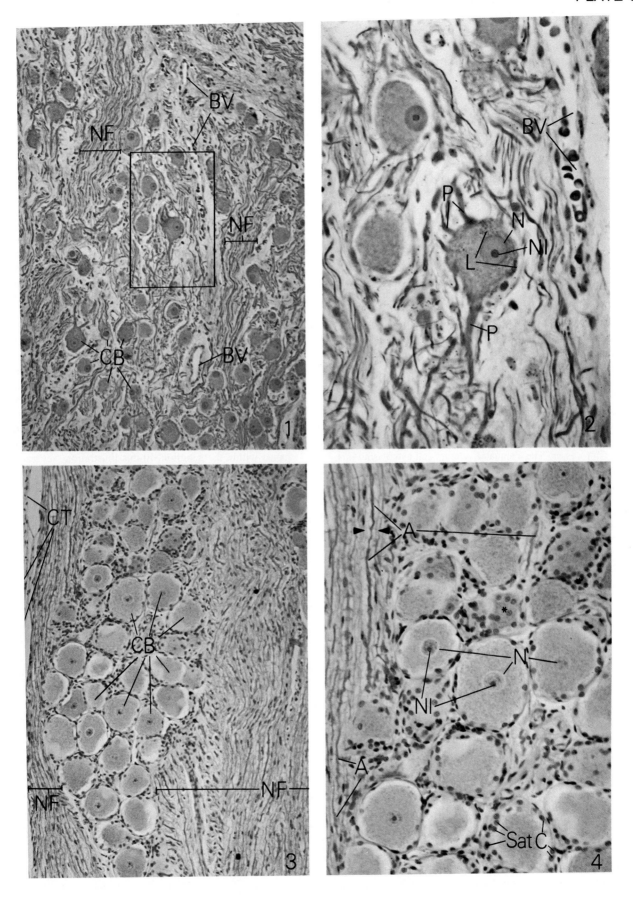

PLATE 38.   Sympathetic Ganglion I, Electron Microscopy

Ganglion, human, electron micrograph ×4200. This electron micrograph depicts a sympathetic ganglion similar to that seen in the light micrographs of the preceding plate. At the magnification used here, the neuron cell bodies *(CB)* along with a myriad of nerve fibers *(NF)* can be identified readily. Two of the cell bodies were sectioned in a plane that includes the nucleus *(N)*, and one also reveals the nucleolus *(Nu)*. A neuron cell body and one of its processes (within the *rectangle*) are shown at higher magnification in Plate 39. Other cells within the ganglion that are somewhat less easy to identify at this magnification include fibroblasts *(F)*, Schwann cells *(SCN)*, and satellite cells *(Sat; Sat N)*. Surrounding the ganglion is a specialized connective tissue, the perineurium *(P)*, part of which can be seen in the upper left corner of the micrograph. It is continuous with the connective tissue covering of the nerve bundles that enter the ganglion. Perineurium is considered in some detail with respect to nerve in Plate 40 and at the electron microscopic level in Plate 41. Also seen in the ganglion is a small blood vessel *(BV)*. The intercellular matrix consists largely of collagen that, together with the fibroblasts, comprises the endoneurium of the ganglion.

A feature not appreciated with the light microscope but evident in electron micrographs is the relationship of the satellite cells to the neuron cell bodies. Each cell body is surrounded by a thin sheath of satellite cell cytoplasm that not only covers the cell body but may extend for a short distance onto its processes. The attenuated satellite cell cytoplasm *(Sat)* is just barely recognizable at this low magnification. It can be seen best around the two cell bodies in the lower part of the micrograph. The cytoplasm of the satellite cell has slightly greater electron density than the neuron and, thus, gives the appearance of a thin rim around the neuron cell body. In the thin sections employed in electron microscopy, the nuclear region of the satellite cell is infrequently included in the plane of section; in the preparation shown here, only one satellite cell nucleus *(Sat N)* is present.

Typically, both myelinated and unmyelinated fibers are present in sympathetic ganglia. Only one of the many fibers included in the portion of the ganglion seen here is myelinated, however; it is just to the left of the blood vessel. The myelin sheath *(My)* surrounding the nerve fiber appears as the ovoid black ring. External to the myelin, one can identify the nucleus of the associated Schwann cell *(SCN)*. All of the unmyelinated nerve fibers are also enclosed by Schwann cell cytoplasm. Instead of a single axon being surrounded by Schwann cell cytoplasm as in the case of the myelinated fibers, however, the Schwann cells related to the unmyelinated nerve fibers will usually ensheathe more than a single fiber. Generally, a number of sectioned fibers can be seen included within a Schwann cell. In effect, the Schwann cell has the same relationship to the nerve fiber as the satellite cell has to the cell body. Both are disposed as an intimate cellular sheath around the neural element. Although Schwann and satellite cells are designated by different names, they probably have the same function and may differ only in terms of location. Both satellite cells and Schwann cells are even designated by some neurobiologists as peripheral neuroglia.

Connective tissue occupies the interstices of the neural elements within the ganglion. In this illustration, several fibroblasts *(F)* are evident. Some fibroblasts are located in close apposition to the neuron cell bodies. With the light microscope, it would be most difficult, if not impossible, to distinguish such a fibroblast nucleus from that of a satellite cell.

KEY		
BV, blood vessel	**N,** nucleus	**Sat,** satellite cell cytoplasm
CB, neuron cell body	**NF,** nerve fibers	**Sat N,** satellite cell nucleus
F, fibroblast (endoneurial cell)	**Nu,** nucleolus	**SNC,** Schwann cell nucleus
My, myelin	**P,** perineurium	

PLATE 38

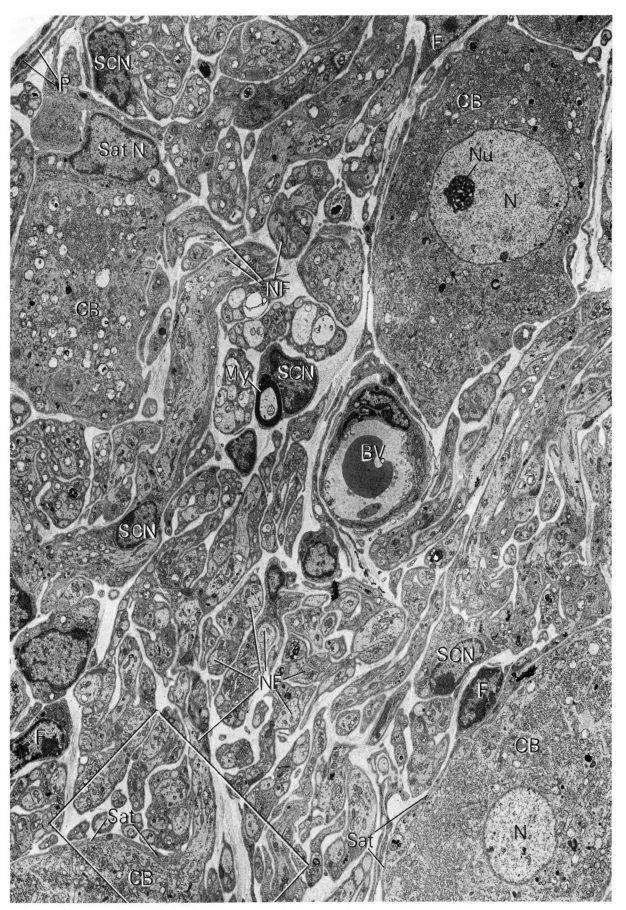

PLATE 39. Sympathetic Ganglion II, Electron Microscopy

Ganglion, human, electron micrograph ×22,000; inset ×46,000. The electron micrograph shown here presents, at higher magnification, the *rectangular area* from Plate 38. The cytoplasm of the neuron cell body exhibits numerous mitochondria *(M)*, clusters of polyribosomes *(R)*, and profiles of rough-surfaced endoplasmic reticulum *(RER)*. The ribosomes and elements of the endoplasmic reticulum tend to aggregate in recognizable masses. The limits of these ribosome-rich areas are not sharply defined. One such concentration, however, is outlined by the *broken line* (left). These localized regions of ribosome-rich cytoplasm may be visualized with the light microscope after staining with a basic dye such as toluidine blue. The staining reaction results in the appearance of small basophilic bodies, referred to as Nissl bodies (see Plate 44, Fig. 3, page 301). Between the ribosome-rich areas, microtubules, neurofilaments, and mitochondria predominate, as they do throughout the cell process.

The satellite cell *(Sat C)* can be distinguished from the neuron cell body simply by differences in cytoplasmic density; it appears conspicuously more electron-dense than the neuron. The satellite cell provides a complete covering sheath about the cell body. In some areas, it may be extremely attenuated *(arrowheads)*. Similarly, the nerve process emanating from the cell body is ensheathed by cytoplasm, identical in appearance with that covering the cell body. The neuronal process is covered by cytoplasm of the Schwann cell *(SC)*. (The site at which the satellite cell terminates and the Schwann cell investment begins is not evident in the example shown here.)

The unmyelinated nerve fibers *(NF)* are sectioned in various planes. Each nerve fiber is surrounded by Schwann cell cytoplasm *(SC)* that displays the same electron density as the cytoplasm of the satellite cells. A few of these nerve fibers appear as single profiles covered by Schwann cell cytoplasm *(asterisks)*. Most of the nerve fibers, however, are embedded in groups within the confines of the Schwann cell. Both the satellite cell and Schwann cell are surrounded by basal lamina *(BL)* (see **inset**). Thus, the neuron, by means of its associated cell cover, is isolated from the collagen *(C)* of the extracellular matrix.

With respect to the individual fibers, it is not always possible to distinguish an axon from a dendrite. A general rule, however, is that if the fiber displays synaptic vesicles (the small round profiles), it is identified as an axon terminal *(A)*; if it displays profiles of granular endoplasmic reticulum, it is identified as a dendrite *(D)*. Fibers that do not exhibit these specific characteristics are best referred to simply as nerve fibers. The axon *(A')* that has entered the satellite sheath of the neuron cell body contains numerous synaptic vesicles. Presumably, it will make synaptic contact with the cell body in this vicinity (an axosomatic synapse).

The *small circle* encloses an axodendritic synapse that is shown at higher magnification in the **inset.** The axon *(A)* of this synapse reveals numerous synaptic vesicles, most of which appear empty; however, they contain the neurotransmitter acetylcholine. The vesicles with granules, several of which are seen in the **inset,** contain catecholamines. The space *(arrow)* between the axon and dendrite *(D)* is the synaptic cleft. It is across this space that the neurotransmitter substance passes to stimulate the membrane of the postsynaptic cell. The presence of ribosomes in the postsynaptic cytoplasm indicates a dendrite; thus, the synapse is an axodendritic synapse.

KEY

A, axon terminal
A′, axon terminal of axosomatic synapse
BL, basal lamina
C, collagen
D, dendrite
L, lysosome
M, mitochondria
NF, nerve fiber
R, ribosome clusters
RER, rough-surfaced endoplasmic reticulum
Sat C, satellite cell
SC, Schwann cell
arrow, synaptic cleft
arrowhead, attenuated satellite cell sheath
asterisk, nerve fiber covered by Schwann cell cytoplasm

PLATE 39

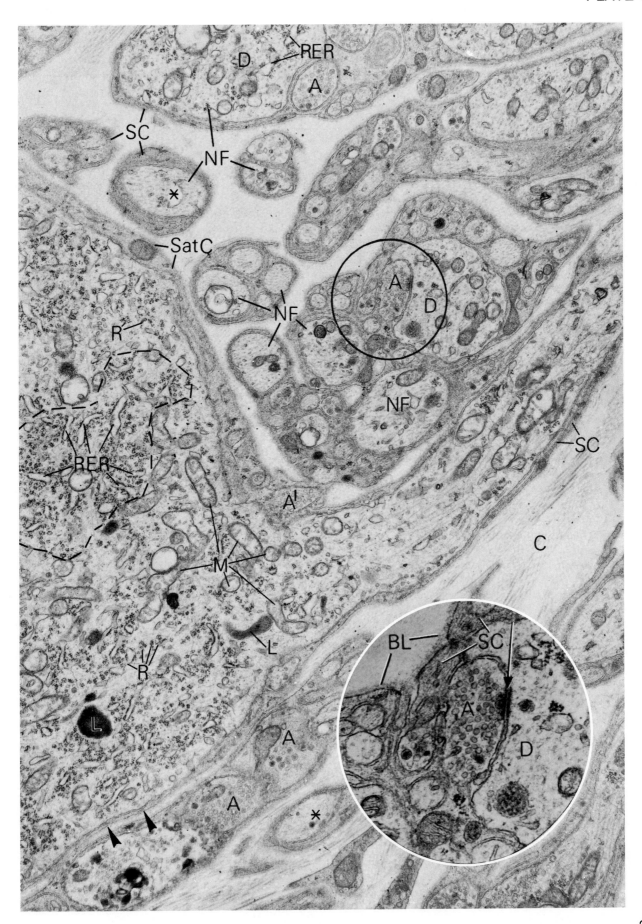

PLATE 40.   Peripheral Nerve

Nerves are composed of bundles of nerve fibers held together by perineurium and connective tissue. Each nerve fiber consists of an axon that is surrounded by a cellular investment called the neurilemma or the sheath of Schwann. In addition, the fiber may be myelinated or unmyelinated. The myelin, if present, is immediately around the axon and is, in turn, surrounded by the neurilemma.

FIGURES 1 and 2, femoral nerve, H&E. This cross section shows several bundles of nerve fibers *(BNF)*. The external cover for the entire nerve is the epineurium *(Epn)*, the layer of dense connective tissue that one touches when a nerve has been exposed during a dissection. The epineurium also serves as the outermost cover of the individual bundles. The epineurium contains blood vessels *(BV)* and may contain some fat cells. Typically, adipose tissue *(AT)* is found about the nerve.

Figure 2 shows, at higher magnification, an area from the upper left of Figure 1. The illustration has been rotated, and the septum (marked with *arrows* in Fig. 1) is now vertically disposed *(arrows)*.

The layer under the epineurium that directly surrounds the bundle of nerve fibers is the perineurium *(Pn)*. As seen in the cross section through the nerve, the nuclei of the perineurial cells appear flat and elongate; they are actually being viewed on edge and belong to flat cells that are also being viewed on edge. Again, as noted by the distribution of nuclei, it can be ascertained that the perineurium is only a few cells thick. The perineurium is a specialized layer of cells and extracellular material whose arrangement is not evident in H&E sections. It is shown in more detail in the following

electron micrograph (Plate 41). The perineurium *(Pn)* and epineurium *(Epn)* are readily distinguished in the triangular area formed by the diverging perineurium of the two adjacent nerve bundles.

The nerve fibers included in Figure 2 are mostly myelinated, and because the nerve is cross-sectioned, the nerve fibers are also seen in this plane. They have a characteristic cross-sectional profile. Each nerve fiber shows a centrally placed axon *(A)*; this is surrounded by a myelin space *(M)* in which some radially disposed precipitate may be retained, as in this specimen. External to the myelin space is a thin cytoplasmic rim representing the neurilemma. On occasion, a Schwann cell nucleus *(SS)* appears to be perched on the neurilemma. As shown in the illustration, the upper edge of the nuclear crescent appears to occupy the same plane as that occupied by the neurilemma *(N)*. These features enable one to identify the nucleus as belonging to a Schwann (neurilemma) cell. Other nuclei are not related to the neurilemma but, rather, appear to be between the nerve fibers. Such nuclei belong to the rare fibroblasts of the endoneurium. The latter is the delicate connective tissue between the individual nerve fibers; it is extremely sparse and contains the capillaries *(C)* of the nerve bundle.

FIGURES 3 and 4, femoral nerve, H&E. The edge of a longitudinally sectioned nerve bundle is shown here; a portion of the same nerve bundle is shown at higher magnification in Figure 4. The boundary between the epineurium *(Epn)* and perineurium is ill defined. Within the nerve bundle, the nerve fibers show a characteristic wavy pattern. Included among the wavy nerve fibers are nuclei belonging to Schwann cells and to cells within the endoneurium. Higher magnification allows one to identify certain specific components of the nerve. Note that the nerve fibers *(NF)* are now shown in longitudinal profile. Moreover, each myelinated

nerve fiber shows a centrally positioned axon *(A)*, surrounded by a myelin space *(M)*, which, in turn, is bordered on its outer edge by the thin cytoplasmic band of the neurilemma cell *(Nl)*. Another diagnostic feature of myelinated nerve fibers is also seen in longitudinal section, namely, the node of Ranvier *(NR)*. This is where the ends of the two Schwann cells meet. Histologically, the node appears as a constriction of the neurilemma, and sometimes, the constriction is marked by a cross-band, as in Figure 4. It is difficult to determine whether the nuclei *(N)* shown in Figure 4 belong to Schwann cells or to endoneurial fibroblasts.

KEY

A, axon
AT, adipose tissue
BNF, bundle of nerve fibers
BV, blood vessels
C, capillary

Epn, epineurium
M, myelin
N: Fig. 2, neurilemma; Fig. 4, nucleus of Schwann cell
NF, nerve fiber
Nl (Fig. 4), neurilemma

NR, node of Ranvier
Pn, perineurium
SS, Schwann cell nucleus
arrows (Figs. 1 and 2), septum formed by perineurium

PLATE 40

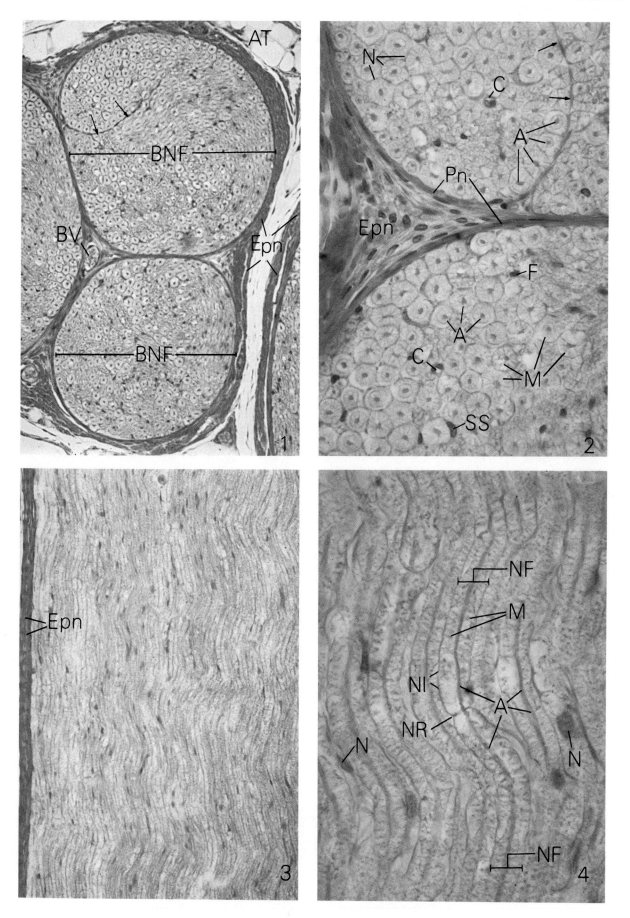

PLATE 41. Perineurium, Electron Microscopy

Perineurium has special characteristics that distinguish it from the connective tissue that comprises epineurium and endoneurium. Unlike epineurial and endoneurial cells, which are typical fibroblasts, perineurial cells exhibit epithelioid as well as myoid features.

Peripheral nerve, human, electron micrograph ×7,000; insets ×26,000. This electron micrograph reveals the outer portion of a small nerve that has been sectioned longitudinally; an axon (A) that has been cut obliquely and its covering myelin sheath (M) are present in the upper right corner. The perineurium (Per) is to the left of the axon and appears as an orderly series of cellular layers. To the left of the perineurium is the epineurium, which contains a moderate amount of collagen (C), epineurial fibroblast processes (Epi F), and elastic material (E). The epineurium, unlike the perineurium, is not well defined. It tends to blend with the connective tissue more removed from the nerve. Thus, there is no discrete boundary between the epineurium and the surrounding connective tissue.

In examining the perineurium at this low magnification, the most notable feature is the relative uniformity of the individual cellular layers or lamellae. The cells that constitute each layer, in effect, are contiguous with one another. Typically, the edge of one cell is in apposition to its neighbors, thus forming a series of uninterrupted concentric cellular sheaths, each of which completely surrounds the nerve bundle.

In contrast to the perineurial cells, a portion of another cell can be seen along the inner aspect of the perineurium. Although closely applied to the perineurium, this cell exhibits characteristics of a typical fibroblast and, as such, represents an endoneurial fibroblast (End F). Note that it does not form a continuous sheath-like structure but, rather, exhibits a lateral margin (arrowhead) that does not meet on edge with another cell to provide continuity. This endoneurial cell is morphologically identical with the epineurial cell (Epi F); both are typical fibroblasts.

The cytologic distinction between the fibroblasts of the epineurium and endoneurium and the specialized perineurial cell can be appreciated better at high magnification (**insets**). The **upper inset** reveals a small portion of the perineurial cell; the **lower inset** reveals an epineurial cell. The specific site from which each is taken is indicated by the *small ovals*. In comparing the two cells, note that the perineural cell exhibits basal lamina (BL) on both surfaces; the fibroblast typically lacks this covering material. Both cell types reveal pinocytotic vesicles as well as mitochondria (Mi). The remainder of the cytoplasm in these two micrographs, however, shows an important difference. The perineurial cell reveals numerous fine filaments, thought to represent myofilaments, and cytoplasmic densities (CD). Both are features characteristic of the smooth muscle cell. Again, the fibroblasts lack these elements. Although not evident here, the perineural cells also exhibit profiles of rough endoplasmic reticulum, but fewer than are seen in the fibroblast (RER). The presence of rough endoplasmic reticulum in the perineurial cell suggests that it, like the fibroblast, produces collagen and, thus, could be responsible for the deposition of collagen (C) between the cellular laminae. The myoid nature of the perineurial cells, as evidenced by the myofilaments and cytoplasmic densities, explains the shortening of a nerve when it is accidentally or surgically cut. Finally, the epithelial-like arrangement of the perineurial cells is regarded as a selective permeability barrier.

KEY

A, axon	**End F,** endoneurial fibroblast	**Per,** perineurium
BL, basal lamina	**Epi F,** epineurial fibroblast	**RER,** rough endoplasmic reticulum
C, collagen fibrils	**M,** myelin	**S,** Schwann cell
CD, cytoplasmic density	**Mi,** mitochondria	**arrowhead,** margin of fibroblast
E, elastic fibers		

PLATE 41

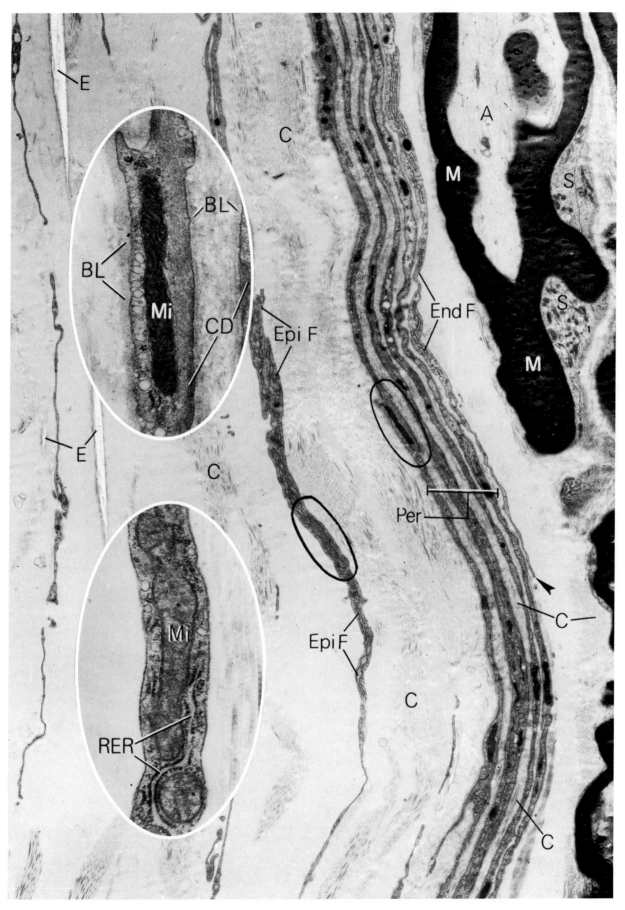

PLATE 42. Cerebrum

FIGURE 1, brain, human, H&E ×66. The cerebral cortex is described as containing six distinguishable layers. No sharp boundaries separate these layers; rather, they are distinguished on the basis of predominant cell type and fiber (axons and dendrites) arrangement. Although the various layers can be recognized in H&E preparations, these preparations do not provide information regarding the fiber arrangement.

This is a low-power view of the cerebral cortex and includes a small amount of white matter below the *lowest broken line.* It is possible to recognize the two areas at a glance, inasmuch as the white matter contains many more nuclei of neuroglial cells *(NN),* which are shown at higher magnification in Figure 5.

The six layers of the cortex are marked in this figure and are shown at higher magnification in Figures 2–5. None of the layers is sharply delineated; the *horizontal broken lines* represent only rough approximations. From the surface, the layers are

I: The plexiform or molecular layer consists largely of fibers, most of which travel parallel to the surface, and relatively few cells.

II: The layer of small pyramidal cells (or outer granular layer) consists mainly of small cells, many of which have a pyramidal shape.

III: The layer of medium pyramidal cells (or layer of outer pyramidal cells) is not sharply demarcated from *layer II.* However, the cells are somewhat larger and possess a typical pyramidal shape.

IV: The granular layer (or inner granular layer) is characterized by the presence of many small stellate cells (granule cells).

V: The layer of large pyramidal cells (or inner layer of pyramidal cells) contains pyramidal cells that, in many parts of the cerebrum, are smaller than the pyramidal cells of *layer III* but, in the motor area, are extremely large and are called Betz cells.

VI: The layer of polymorphic cells contains cells with diverse shapes, many of which have a spindle or fusiform shape. These cells are called fusiform cells.

Three cell types have been referred to above: pyramidal cells, stellate cells (or granule cells), and fusiform cells. Two other cell types are also present in the cerebral cortex but are not illustrated. They are the horizontal cells of Cajal, which are present only in *layer I* and send their processes laterally, and cells of Martinotti, which send their axons toward the surface (opposite to that of pyramidal cells).

FIGURES 2–5, brain, human, H&E ×640. FIGURE 2. *Layer 1* is illustrated at higher magnification in this figure and reveals a blood capillary *(Cap)* and several nuclei. Most of these nuclei belong to neuroglial cells *(NN).* This conclusion is based on the fact that the cytoplasm belonging to these nuclei cannot be distinguished. One nucleus, however, is surrounded by cytoplasm *(arrow)* and, thus, is identified as part of a neuron cell body.

FIGURE 3. The *rectangle* in Figure 1 is examined at higher magnification here. The pyramidal cells *(PC)* contain an oval nucleus in which a small, intensely staining, round nucleolus is located. The cytoplasmic limits of the cell body appear roughly triangular. The base of the cell faces the white matter and sends a single axon in that direction. This process, however, is not evident. The apex of each cell body shows a large dendritic process, the apical dendrite, that extends toward the surface of the gray matter.

FIGURE 4. This shows the small polymorphic cell bodies *(Pol C)* of *layer VI* and, again, neuroglial nuclei *(NN).*

FIGURE 5. This shows that the cytoplasm of the neuroglial cells is not distinguishable, and consequently, the cells appear as naked nuclei in a "no man's land," referred to as the neuropil *(Np).* Small blood vessels *(BV)* are also evident in the white matter.

KEY		
BV, blood vessel	**Np,** neuropil	**Pol C,** polymorphic cell body
Cap, capillary	**PC,** pyramidal cell	**arrow (Fig. 2),** cytoplasm of neuron
NN, neuroglial cell nucleus		

PLATE 42

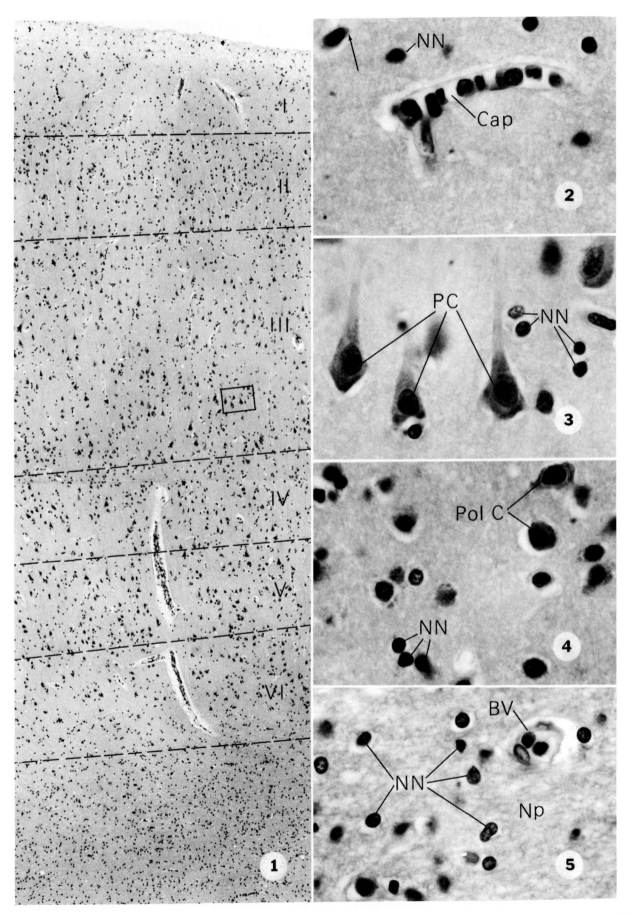

PLATE 43. Cerebellum

FIGURE 1, cerebellum, human, H&E ×40. The cerebellar cortex has the same appearance regardless of which region is examined. In this low-power view of the cerebellum, the outermost layer, the molecular layer *(Mol)*, is lightly stained with eosin. Under this is the granular layer *(Gr)*, which stains intensely with hematoxylin. Together, these two layers constitute the cortex of the cerebellum. Deep in the granular layer is another region that stains lightly with H&E and, except for location, shows no distinctive histologic features. This is the white matter *(WM)*. As in the cerebrum, it contains nerve fibers, supporting neuroglial cells, and small blood vessels, but no neuronal cell bodies. The fibrous cover on the cerebellar surface is the pia mater *(Pia)*. Cerebellar blood vessels *(BV)* travel in this layer. (Shrinkage artefact has separated the pia mater from the cerebellar surface). The *rectangular area* is shown at higher magnification in Figure 2.

FIGURE 2, cerebellum, human, H&E ×400. At the junction between the molecular and granular layers are the extremely large flask-shaped cell bodies of the Purkinje cells *(Pkj)*. These cells are characteristic of the cerebellum. Each possesses numerous dendrites *(D)* that arborize in the molecular layer. The Purkinje cell has a single axon that is not usually evident in H&E sections. This nerve fiber represents the beginning of the outflow from the cerebellum.

The illustration shows relatively few neuron cell bodies, the basket cells *(BC)*, in the molecular layer; they are widely removed from each other and, at best, show only a small amount of cytoplasm surrounding the nucleus. In contrast, the granular layer presents an overall spotted-blue appearance due to the staining of numerous small nuclei with hematoxylin. These small neurons, called granule cells, receive incoming impulses from other parts of the CNS and send axons into the molecular layer, where they branch in the form of a T, so that the axons contact the dendrites of several Purkinje cells and basket cells. Incoming (mossy) fibers contact granule cells in the lightly stained areas called glomeruli *(arrows)*. If one carefully examines the granular layer where it meets the molecular layer, there will be found a group of nuclei *(G)* that are larger than the nuclei of granule cells. These belong to Golgi type II cells.

FIGURE 3, cerebellum, human, silver stain ×40. The specimen in this figure has been stained with a silver procedure. Such procedures do not always color the specimen evenly, as do H&E. Note that the part of the molecular layer on the right is much darker than that on the left. A *rectangular area* on the left has been selected for examination at higher magnification in Figure 4. Even at the relatively low magnification shown here, however, the Purkinje cells can be recognized in the silver preparation because of their large size, characteristic shape, and location between an outer molecular layer *(Mol)* and an inner granular layer *(Gr)*. The main advantage of this silver preparation is that the white matter *(WM)* can be recognized as being composed of fibers; they have been blackened by the silver-staining procedure. The pia mater *(Pia)* and cerebellar blood vessels are also evident in the preparation.

FIGURE 4, cerebellum, human, silver stain ×400. At higher magnification, the Purkinje cell bodies *(Pkj)* stand out as the most distinctive and conspicuous neuronal cell type of the cerebellum, and numerous dendritic branches *(D)* can be seen. Note, also, the blackened fibers within the granular layer *(Gr)*, about the Purkinje cell bodies, and in the molecular layer *(Mol)* disposed in a horizontal direction (relative to the cerebellar surface). The *arrow* indicates a T turn characteristic of the turn made by axons of granule cells. As these axonal branches travel horizontally, they make synaptic contact with numerous Purkinje cells.

KEY

BC, basket cells
BV, blood vessels
D, dendrites
F, fibers
G, Golgi type II cells

Gr, granular layer
Mol, molecular layer
Pia, pia mater
Pkj, Purkinje cells
WM, white matter

arrows: Fig. 2, glomeruli; Fig. 4, T branching of axon in molecular layer
rectangular area (Figs. 1 and 3), areas shown at higher magnification in Figs. 2 and 4, respectively

PLATE 43

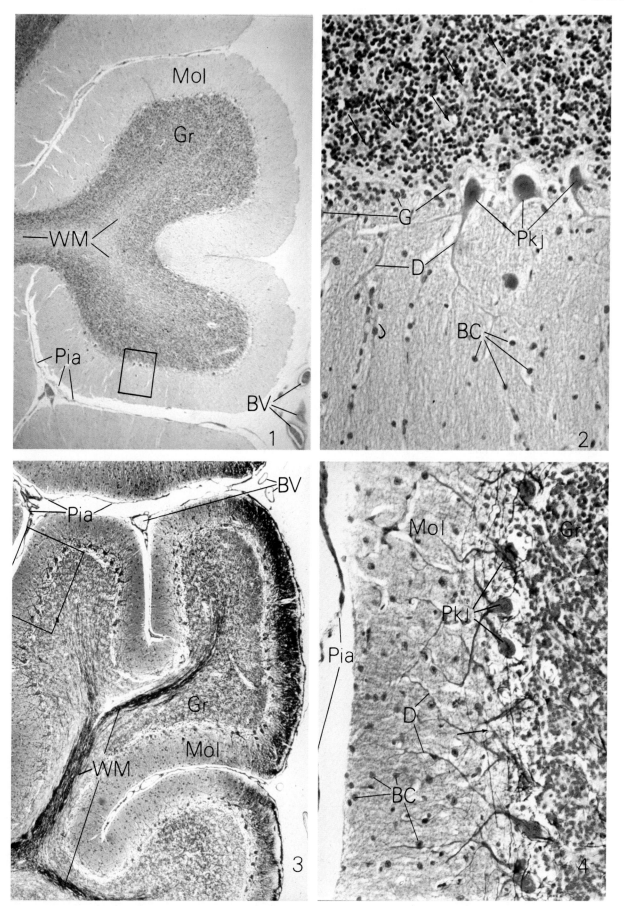

PLATE 44. Spinal Cord

The spinal cord is organized into two discrete parts. The outer part contains ascending and descending nerve fibers. This constitutes the white matter of the cord. The inner part contains cell bodies of neurons and nerve fibers. This is the gray matter of the spinal cord. Neuroglial cells are in both the white matter and the gray matter.

FIGURE 1, spinal cord, human, myelin stain ×16. A cross section through the cervical region of the spinal cord (human) is shown here. The preparation is designed to stain the myelin that surrounds the ascending and descending fibers. Although the fibers that have common origins and destinations in the physiologic sense are arranged in tracts, these tracts cannot be distinguished unless they have been marked by special techniques, such as causing injury to the cell bodies from which they arise or by using special dyes or radioisotopes to label the axons.

The gray matter of the spinal cord appears roughly in the form of a butterfly. The anterior and posterior prongs are referred to as anterior horns *(AH)* and posterior horns *(PH),* respectively. The connecting bar is called the gray commissure *(GC).* The neuron cell bodies that are within the anterior horns (anterior horn cells) are so large that they can be seen even at this extremely low magnification *(arrows).* The pale-staining fibrous material that surrounds the spinal cord is the pia mater *(Pia).* It follows the surface of the spinal cord intimately and dips into the large ventral fissure *(VF)* and into the shallower sulci. Blood vessels are present in the pia mater. Some ventral *(VR)* and dorsal *(DR)* roots of the spinal nerves are included in the section.

FIGURE 2, spinal cord, human, H&E ×640. This preparation shows a region of an anterior horn. The nucleus *(N)* of the anterior horn cell is the large, spherical, pale-staining structure within the cell body. It contains a spherical, intensely staining nucleolus. The anterior horn cell has many processes, two of which are obvious. A number of other nuclei *(NN)* belong to neuroglial cells. The cytoplasm of these cells is not evident. The remainder of the field consists of nerve fibers and neuroglial cells whose organization is hard to interpret. This is called the neuropil *(Np).* A capillary crosses through the field below the cell body.

FIGURE 3, spinal cord, human, toluidine blue ×640. This preparation of the spinal cord is from an area comparable with that of Figure 2. The toluidine blue reveals the Nissl bodies *(NB)* that appear as the large, dark-staining bodies in the cytoplasm. Nissl bodies do not extend into the axon hillock. The axon leaves the cell body at the axon hillock. The nuclei of neuroglial cells *(NN)* are also evident here, but their cytoplasm is not. The neuropil stains very faintly.

KEY

AH, anterior (ventral) horn
DR, dorsal root
GC, gray commissure
N, nucleus of anterior horn cell
NB, Nissl bodies
NN, nucleus of neuroglial cell
Np, neuropil
PH, posterior (dorsal) horn
Pia, pia mater
VF, ventral fissure
VR, ventral root
arrows (Fig. 1), cell body of anterior (ventral) horn cell

PLATE 44

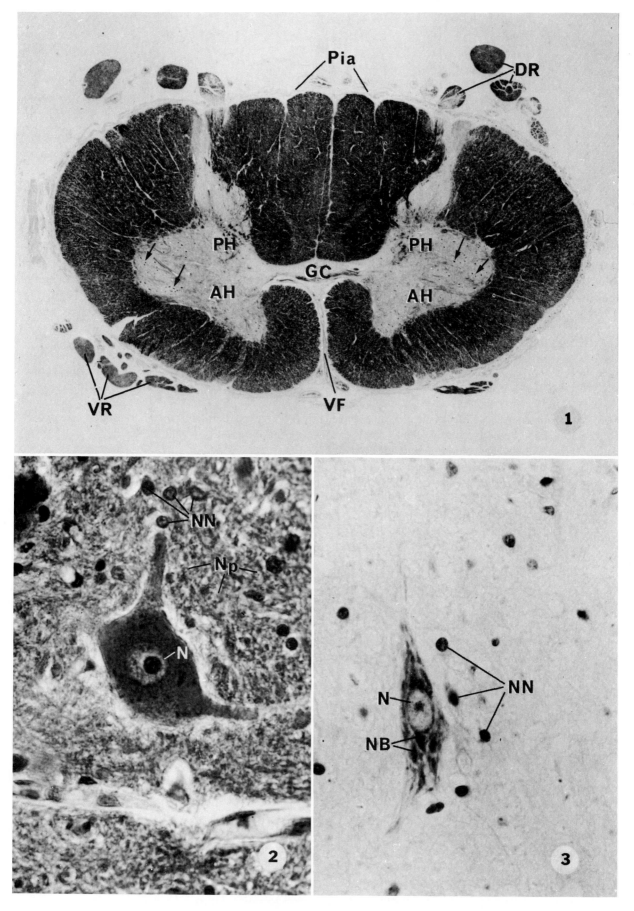

Cardiovascular System

12

The cardiovascular system is a transport system that carries blood and lymph to and from the tissues of the body. The constitutive elements of these fluids include cells, nutrients, waste products, hormones, and antibodies.

The Cardiovascular System Includes the Heart, Blood Vessels, and Lymphatic Vessels

Blood vessels provide the route by which blood circulates to and from all parts of the body. The heart pumps the blood. Lymphatic vessels carry tissue-derived fluid, called lymph, back to the blood vascular system. The blood vessels are arranged so that blood delivered from the heart quickly reaches a network of narrow, thin-walled vessels, the blood *capillaries,* within or in proximity to the tissues in every part of the body. Fluid usually leaves the blood vessels in the capillaries, whereas cells leave the blood in the *postcapillary venules.* The remainder of the vessels function as impermeable tubes to convey the blood.

In the capillaries, a two-directional exchange of fluid occurs between the blood and tissues. The fluid, called *blood filtrate,* carrying oxygen and metabolites, passes through the capillary wall. In the tissues, these products are exchanged for carbon dioxide and waste products. Most of the fluid reenters the distal or venous end of the blood capillaries. The remaining fluid enters lymphatic capillaries and is returned to the bloodstream through a system of lymphatic vessels that join the blood system at the junction of the internal jugular veins with the subclavian veins. Normally, many of the white blood cells conveyed in the blood leave the blood vessels to enter the tissues. This occurs at the level of the *postcapillary venules.* When pathologic changes occur in the body, as in the inflammatory reaction, large numbers of neutrophils, other granulocytes, and monocytes emigrate from these venules.

The vessels that deliver blood to the capillaries are the *arteries.* The smallest arteries, called *arterioles,* are functionally associated with networks of capillaries into which they deliver blood. The arterioles regulate the amount of blood going to these capillary networks. Together, the arterioles, associated capillary network, and postcapillary venules form a functional unit referred to as the *microcirculatory* or *microvascular bed* of that tissue (Fig. 12.1). Veins collect blood from the microvascular bed and carry it away.

Two Circuits Distribute Blood in the Body: the Systemic and the Pulmonary Circulation

There are actually two pathways of circulation formed by the blood vessels and the heart:

- *Pulmonary circulation* conveys blood from the heart to the lungs and from the lungs to the heart (Fig. 12.2).
- *Systemic circulation* conveys blood from the heart to other tissues of the body and from other tissues of the body to the heart.

Although the general arrangement of blood vessels in both circulations is from arteries to capillaries to veins, in some parts of the systemic circulation it is modified so that a vein or an arteriole is interposed between two capillary networks; this is called a *portal system.* Venous portal systems occur in vessels carrying blood to the liver, namely, the *hepatic portal system (portal vein),* and in vessels leading to the pituitary, the *hypothalamic-hypophyseal portal system.* An arterial portal system occurs in the kidney where an *efferent arteriole* carries blood from the glomerulus to the peritubular capillaries (see page 577).

GENERAL FEATURES OF ARTERIES AND VEINS

The Walls of Arteries and Veins Are Composed of Three Layers called Tunics

The three layers of the vascular wall, from the lumen outward (see Fig. 12.1), are

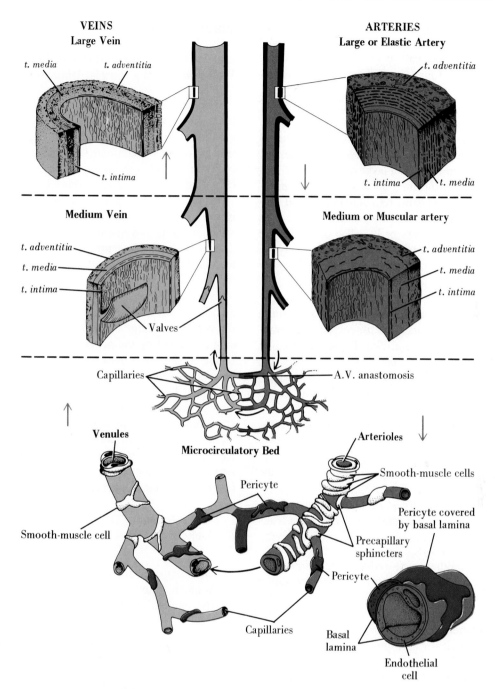

Figure 12.1. Schematic diagram of the major structural features of blood vessels. The layers or tunics of the blood vessel walls are marked in the **upper two panels.** The arrangement of the microcirculatory bed in certain parts of the body is shown in the **lowest panel.** Note that the microcirculation shows an arteriovenous *(A.V.)* anastomosis and a thoroughfare channel (arteriovenous shunt). *t.,* tunica. (Based on Rhodin JG: *Handbook of Physiology.* New York, Oxford University Press, 1980.)

- *Tunica intima,* the innermost layer that includes the endothelial lining
- *Tunica media,* the muscular middle layer
- *Tunica adventitia,* the outermost connective tissue layer

Histologically, the various types of arteries and veins are distinguished from each other on the basis of the thickness of the vascular wall and differences in the composition of the various layers, especially the tunica media.

Tunica Intima. The *tunica intima* consists of a single layer of squamous epithelial cells, the endothelium, resting on a basal lamina and the underlying connective tissue. This *subendothelial layer* consists of loose connective tissue and, in arteries and arterioles, a layer of fenestrated elastic tissue called the *internal elastic membrane or lamina*. The fenestrations enable substances to diffuse through the layer and reach cells deep within the wall of the vessel. Occasional smooth muscle cells are found in the loose connective tissue.

Tunica Media. The *tunica media* consists primarily of circumferentially arranged layers of smooth muscle cells. In arteries, it is relatively thick and extends from the *internal elastic membrane* to the *external elastic membrane.* The external elastic membrane is a layer of elastin that separates the tunica media from the tunica adventitia in arteries. Variable amounts of elastin, reticular fibers, and proteoglycans are interposed between the smooth muscle cells of the tunica media. The sheets or lamellae of elastin are fenestrated and are arranged in circular concentric layers. All of the extracellular components of the tunica media are secreted by the smooth muscle cells.

Tunica Adventitia. The *tunica adventitia* is composed mostly of longitudinally arranged collagenous tissue and a few elastic fibers. These connective tissue elements gradually merge with the loose connective tissue surrounding the vessels. The tunica adventitia ranges from relatively thin in most of the arterial system to quite thick in the venules and veins, where it is the major component of the vessel wall.

In addition to the three tunics, large arteries and veins may have

- A system of vessels, called *vasa vasorum,* to supply the vessels themselves
- A network of autonomic nerves, called *nervi vascularis,* to control contraction of the smooth muscle in the walls of the vessels

Contraction of smooth muscle reduces the luminal diameter of the vessel *(vasoconstriction),* whereas relaxation increases the luminal diameter *(vasodilation).* Generally, vasoconstriction is induced by nerve impulses or circulating hormones. Vasodilation is passive and may occur in the absence of nerve impulses or in response to inhibitory nerve impulses (see page 277).

Table 12.1 summarizes the features of the various types of blood vessels.

ARTERIES

Traditionally, arteries are classified into three types on the basis of size and the characteristics of the tunica media:

- *Large* or *elastic arteries*
- *Medium* or *muscular arteries* (most of the "named" arteries of the body)
- *Small arteries* and *arterioles*

In each type of artery, the wall is composed of the three layers defined above.

Elastic Arteries

Elastic Arteries Have Sheets of Elastic Tissue in Their Wall and Are the Largest Diameter Arteries

The largest elastic arteries, the aorta and pulmonary arteries, convey blood from the heart to the systemic and pulmonary circulations, respectively (Fig. 12.2). These arteries, as well as their main branches, the brachiocephalic, common carotid, subclavian, and common iliac arteries, are classified as elastic arteries (Fig. 12.3).

From a functional point of view, the elastic arteries serve primarily as conduction tubes; however, they also facilitate the continuous movement of blood along the tube. This occurs as follows: The ventricles of the heart pump blood into the elastic arteries during the contraction phase *(systole)* of the cardiac cycle. The pressure generated by contraction of the ventricles moves the blood through the elastic arteries and along the arterial tree. Simultaneously, it also causes the wall of the large elastic arteries to distend. The distension is limited by the network of collagenous fibers in the tunica media and tunica adventitia. During the relaxation phase *(diastole)* of the cardiac cycle, when no pressure is generated by the heart, the recoil of the distended elastic arteries serves to maintain arterial blood pressure and sustained flow of blood within the vessels. Initial elastic recoil forces blood both away from and back toward the heart. The flow of blood toward the heart causes the aortic and pulmonic valves to close. Continued elastic recoil then maintains continuous flow of blood away from the heart.

Tunica Intima. The tunica intima of elastic arteries is relatively thick and consists of

- An endothelial lining with its basal lamina
- A subendothelial layer of connective tissue
- The internal elastic membrane (lamina)

In elastic arteries, the internal elastic membrane is not conspicuous because it is one of many elastic layers in the wall of the vessel. It is usually identified only because it is the innermost of the layers in the arterial wall.

The endothelium is a simple squamous epithelium that functions in the control of the movement of substances from and to the vascular lumen. The cells are typically flat and elongate, with their long axis oriented parallel to the direction of blood flow in the artery (Fig. 12.4). In forming the epithelial sheet, the cells are joined by tight junctions (zonulae occludentes) and gap junctions (Fig. 12.5).

Endothelial Tight Junctions Serve as the Barrier to Transendothelial Diffusion

The movement of substance into and out of blood vessels is controlled by the endothelium. The endothelial cell tight junctions restrict diffusion between the cells to varying de-

TABLE 12.1. Characteristics of Blood Vessels

		ARTERIES		
VESSEL	DIAMETER	INNER LAYER (TUNICA INTIMA)	MIDDLE LAYER (TUNICA MEDIA)	OUTER LAYER (TUNICA ADVENTITIA)
Elastic artery	>1 cm	Endothelium Connective tissue Smooth muscle	Smooth muscle Elastic lamellae	Connective tissue Elastic fibers Thinner than tunica media
Muscular artery Large	2–10 mm	Endothelium Connective tissue Smooth muscle Prominent internal elastic membrane	Smooth muscle Collagen fibers Relatively little elastic tissue	Connective tissue Some elastic fibers Thinner than tunica media
Small	0.1–2 mm	Endothelium Connective tissue Smooth muscle Internal elastic membrane	Smooth muscle (8–10 cell layers) Collagen fibers	Connective tissue Some elastic fibers Thinner than tunica media
Arteriole	10–100 nm	Endothelium Connective tissue Smooth muscle	Smooth muscle (1–2 cell layers)	Thin, ill-defined sheath of connective tissue
Capillary	4–10 nm	Endothelium	None	None

		VEINS		
VESSEL	DIAMETER	INNER LAYER (TUNICA INTIMA)	MIDDLE LAYER (TUNICA MEDIA)	OUTER LAYER (TUNICA ADVENTITIA)
Postcapillary venule	10–50 nm	Endothelium Pericytes	None	None
Muscular venule	50–100 nm	Endothelium Pericytes	Smooth muscle (1 or 2 cell layers)	Connective tissue Some elastic fibers Thicker than tunica media
Small vein	0.1–1 mm	Endothelium Smooth muscle (2 or 3 layers)	Smooth muscle (2 or 3 layers continuous with tunica intima)	Connective tissue Some elastic fibers Thicker than tunica media
Medium vein	1–10 mm	Endothelium Connective tissue Smooth muscle Internal elastic membrane in some cases	Smooth muscle Collagen fibers	Connective tissue Some elastic fibers Thicker than tunica media
Large vein	>1 mm	Endothelium Connective tissue Smooth muscle	Smooth muscle (2–15 layers) Cardiac muscle near heart Collagen fibers	Connective tissue Some elastic fibers Much thicker than tunica media

grees. Pinocytotic vesicles, however, have been shown to transport experimental markers such as peroxidase through the endothelium. The vesicles move these substances from the vascular lumen to the basal surface of the endothelial cell and to the lateral surface of the cell. Thus, nutrients and regulatory substances pass via the pinocytotic vesicles to the cells of the tunica intima and tunica media. This is illustrated by the series of pinocytotic vesicles marked with *arrows* in Figure 12.5.

Rod-like inclusions, called Weibel-Palade bodies, are present in the cytoplasm of arterial endothelial cells. These specific endothelial organelles are electron-dense structures and contain a ***coagulating factor (factor VIII)***. Experimental studies indicate that the coagulating factor is syn-

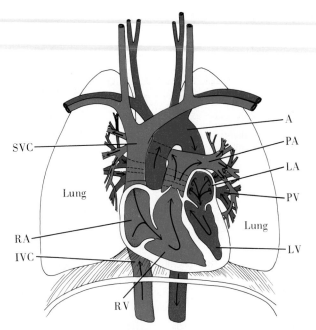

Figure 12.2. Diagram depicting circulations of blood through the heart. Blood returns from the tissues of the body via the superior vena cava *(SVC)* and inferior vena cava *(IVC)*. These two major venous vessels return the blood to the right atrium *(RA)*. Blood then passes into the right ventricle *(RV)*, and from this chamber, the blood is pumped into the pulmonary arteries *(PA)* that convey the blood to the lungs. The blood is aerated in the lungs and is then returned to the left atrium *(LA)* via the pulmonary veins *(PV)*. Blood then passes to the left ventricle *(LV)*, and from here, it is pumped into the aorta *(A)*, which conveys the blood to the tissues of the body. From the heart to the lungs and from the lungs to the heart constitutes the pulmonary circulation; from the heart to the tissues and from the tissues to the heart constitutes the systemic circulation.

thesized by the arterial endothelial cell and secreted into the blood. Thus, among other activities, the cell has a secretory function.

In the larger elastic arteries, the subendothelial layer consists of connective tissue with both collagen and elastic fibers. The main cell type of this layer is the smooth muscle cell. It is contractile and also secretes extracellular ground substance and both types of fibers. A few macrophages are also present.

Tunica Media. The tunica media is the thickest of the three layers of elastic arteries and consists of

- *Elastin* in the form of fenestrated sheets or lamellae between the muscle layers
- *Smooth muscle cells* arranged in layers
- *Collagen fibers* and *ground substance*

The elastic lamellae are arranged in concentric layers. Fenestrations in the lamellae facilitate the diffusion of sub-

stances through the arterial wall. The number and thickness of these lamellae are related to blood pressure and age. At birth, the aorta is almost devoid of lamellae; in the adult, the aorta has 40–70 lamellae. In individuals with hypertension, there are increases in both the number and the thickness of the lamellae.

The smooth muscle cells are arranged in a low-pitch spiral relative to the long axis of the vessel; thus, in cross sections of the artery they appear in a circular array. The cells are invested with an external (basal) lamina except where joined together by gap junctions. Note that fibroblasts are not present in the tunica media. The smooth muscle cells synthesize and secrete the collagenous and elastic components as well as the proteoglycans of this layer.

Tunica Adventitia. In elastic arteries, the tunica adventitia is a relatively thin connective tissue layer that is usually less than half the thickness of the tunica media. It consists of

- *Collagen fibers*
- *Elastic fibers* (not lamellae)
- *Fibroblasts* and *macrophages*

The extracellular components, the collagen fibers and a loose network of elastic fibers, are less well organized than in the tunica media. The fibers aid in preventing the expansion of the arterial wall beyond physiologic limits during the systolic period of the cardiac cycle. Fibroblasts and macrophages are the principal cells of the tunica adventitia.

The tunica adventitia contains blood vessels *(vasa vasorum)* and nerves *(nervi vascularis)*. Branches of each enter the tunica media to supply the blood vessel wall. These vessels supply only the outer portion of the arterial wall. The inner part is supplied from the lumen of the vessel via the pinocytotic transport across the endothelium.

Muscular Arteries

Muscular Arteries Have More Smooth Muscle and Less Elastin in the Tunica Media Than Do Elastic Arteries

There is no sharp dividing line between elastic arteries and the large muscular arteries (Fig. 12.6). Arteries are often difficult to classify because they have features that are intermediate between the two types. Generally, in the region of transition, the amount of elastic material decreases, and smooth muscle cells become the predominant constituent of the tunica media. Prominent *internal and external elastic membranes* help to distinguish muscular arteries from elastic arteries.

Tunica Intima. The tunica intima is thinner in muscular arteries than in elastic arteries and consists of an endothelial lining with its basal lamina, a sparse subendo-

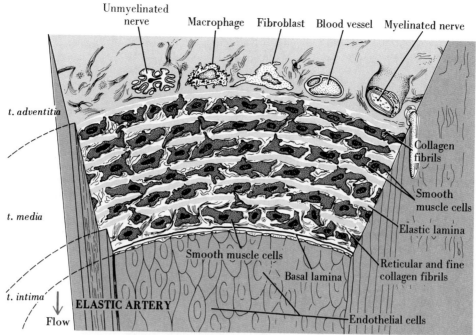

Figure 12.3. Schematic diagram of an elastic artery showing its cellular and extracellular components. *t.,* tunica.

(Based on Rhodin JG: *Handbook of Physiology.* New York, Oxford University Press, 1980.)

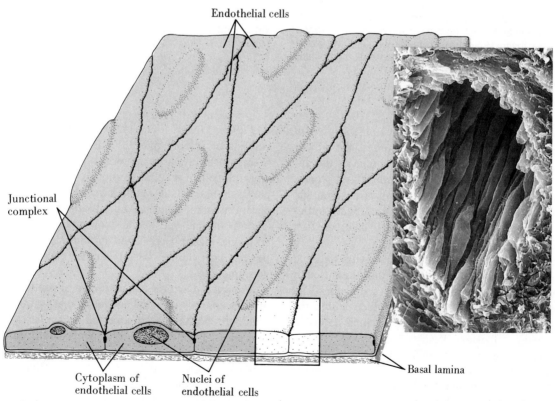

Figure 12.4. Diagram of luminal surface and cut edge of endothelium. The cells are elongate; their long axis is parallel to the direction of blood flow. Nuclei of endothelial cells are also elongated in the direction of blood flow. The *rectangular area* is shown in Figure 12.5. **Inset.** Scanning electron micrograph of a small vein, showing the cells of the endothelial lining. Note their spindle shape and their long axis running parallel to the vessel. ×1100. (Drawing based on Rhodin JG: *Handbook of Physiology.* New York, Oxford University Press, 1980.)

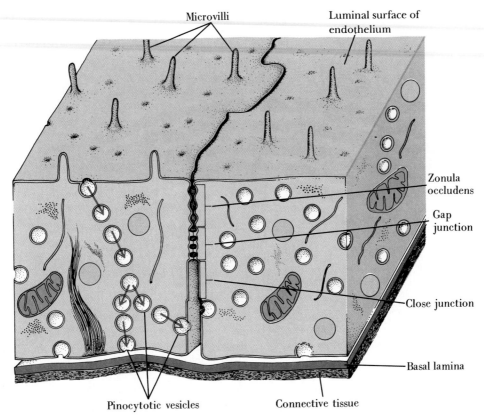

Microvilli

Luminal surface of
endothelium

Zonula
occludens

Gap
junction

Close junction

Basal lamina

Pinocytotic vesicles

Connective tissue

Figure 12.5. Diagram depicting segments of two adjacent endothelial cells in which a junctional complex joins the cells. Pinocytotic vesicles in the cell on the left have been positioned to suggest the pathway of vesicles from the lumen of the blood vessel to the base of the cell or to the basal-lateral intercellular space. Various markers have been traced through pinocytotic vesicles across the endothelial cell as suggested by the *arrows*. (Based on Rhodin JG: *Handbook of Physiology*. New York, Oxford University Press, 1980.)

thelial layer of connective tissue, and a prominent *internal elastic membrane.* In some muscular arteries, the subendothelial layer is so scant that the basal lamina of the endothelium makes contact with the internal elastic membrane. In histologic sections, the internal elastic membrane usually appears as a well-defined undulating or wavy structure due to contraction of the smooth muscle and reduction in the amount of elastin in the tunica media.

The thickness of the tunica intima varies with age and other factors. In young children, it is very thin. In muscular arteries of young adults, the tunica intima accounts for about one-sixth of the total wall thickness. In older adults, the tunica intima may be grossly expanded by lipid deposits, often in the form of irregular "fatty streaks."

An unusual feature of the endothelium of muscular arteries (and, often, elastic arteries) is that processes of the endothelial cells penetrate through the basal lamina and make junctional contacts with processes extending toward the lumen from smooth muscle cells of the media. The significance of these junctions is not yet determined.

Tunica Media. The tunica media of muscular arteries consists of smooth muscle cells amid collagen fibers and relatively little elastic material. The smooth muscle cells are arranged in a spiral fashion in the arterial wall. Their contraction assists in maintaining blood pressure. As in the elastic arteries, there are no fibroblasts in this layer. The smooth muscle cells here, too, produce the extracellular collagen, elastic fibers, and ground substance. They also possess an external (basal) lamina, except at the sites of gap junctions.

Tunica Adventitia. The tunica adventitia of muscular arteries consists of collagen fibers, elastic fibers, and scattered fibroblasts and adipose cells. Compared with elastic arteries, the tunica adventitia of muscular arteries is relatively thick, about the same thickness as the tunica media. Collagen fibers are the principal extracellular component. However, a concentration of elastic material immediately adjacent to the tunica media constitutes the *external elastic lamina* typical of muscular arteries. Nerves and tiny vessels of the vasa vasorum travel in the adventitia and give branches that penetrate into the tunica media.

Small Arteries and Arterioles

Small Arteries and Arterioles Are Distinguished from One Another by the Number of Smooth Muscle Layers in the Tunica Media

Arterioles have, by definition, only one or two layers of smooth muscle in the tunica media (Fig. 12.7); a small artery may have up to about eight layers. Typically, the tunica intima of a small artery has an internal elastic membrane, whereas this layer may or may not be present in the arteriole. The endothelium in both is essentially similar to endothelium in other arteries except that there are gap junctions between endothelial cells and the smooth muscle cells of the tunica media. Lastly, the tunica adventitia is a thin, ill-defined sheath of connective tissue that blends with the connective tissue in which these vessels travel.

Arterioles Control Blood Flow to Capillary Networks

The arterioles serve as flow regulators to the capillary beds. In the normal relationship between an arteriole and a capillary network, contraction of the smooth muscle in the wall of the arteriole reduces or shuts off the blood going to the capillaries. A slight thickening of the smooth muscle at the origin of a capillary bed from an arteriole is called the *precapillary sphincter.* In the absence of nerve impulses or hormonal stimulation, the muscle cells relax, and the blood pressure causes passive vasodilation. The regulation is important in directing blood where it may be needed most. When intense physical activity is taking place, for instance, blood flow to the skeletal muscle is increased by the dilation of arterioles, and blood flow to the intestine is reduced by contraction of arterioles. After ingestion of a large meal, however, the reverse may be true.

CAPILLARIES

Capillaries Are the Smallest Diameter Blood Vessels, Often Smaller than the Diameter of an Erythrocyte

Capillaries form blood vessel networks that allow fluids containing gases, metabolites, and waste products to move through their thin walls. They consist of a single layer of endothelial cells and their basal lamina. The endothelial cells form a tube just large enough to allow the passage of red blood cells one at a time. In cross sections, the tube may be seen to be formed by only one cell or portions of two or three cells. The margins of the endothelial cells are joined by tight junctions. Because of their thin wall and close physical association with metabolically active cells and tissues, capillaries are particularly well suited for the exchange of gases and metabolites between cells and the bloodstream. The ratios of capillary volume to endothelial surface area and thickness also favor movement of material across the vessel wall.

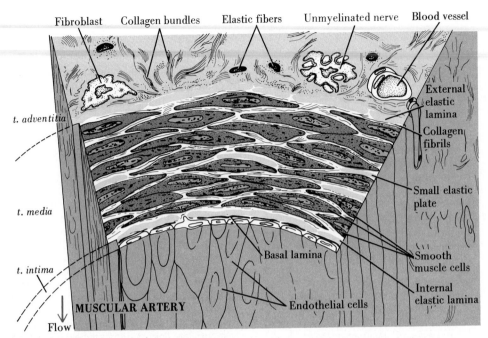

Figure 12.6. Schematic diagram of a muscular artery. In certain locations, muscle cells are shown to be in contact to represent the presence of a gap junction (nexus) between the cells. *t.*, tunica. (Based on Rhodin JG: *Handbook of Physiology*. New York, Oxford University Press, 1980.)

Continuous and Fenestrated Capillaries

Capillaries are described as

- *Continuous,* typically found in muscle, lung, and central nervous system (CNS)
- *Fenestrated,* typically found in endocrine glands and sites of fluid and metabolite absorption such as the gallbladder and intestinal tract
- *Discontinuous,* typically found in the liver, spleen, and bone marrow (also called *sinusoids*)

Continuous capillaries appear in cross sections in the transmission electron microscope (TEM) as two plasma membranes enclosing a ribbon of cytoplasm that may include the nucleus (Fig. 12.8). At least one occluding junction can be seen in a typical cross section of a continuous capillary.

Numerous pinocytotic vesicles underlie both the luminal and basal plasma membrane surfaces. The vesicles, approximately 70 nm in diameter, function in transport of materials between the lumen and the connective tissue and vice versa.

In certain continuous capillaries, *pericytes* may be found in association with the endothelium (Fig. 12.8). The pericyte, when present, is enclosed by a basal lamina that is continuous with that of the endothelium. The pericyte displays features of a relatively unspecialized cell. It is derived from the same precursor cell that forms endothelial cells in new vessels and can give rise to smooth muscle cells during vessel growth (as in development and wound healing).

Fenestrated capillaries are characterized by the presence of fenestrations, 80–100 nm in diameter, that provide channels across the capillary wall (Fig. 12.9). Fenestrated capillaries also have pinocytotic vesicles. One theory of how fenestrations are produced suggests that they occur when a forming pinocytotic vesicle spans the narrow cytoplasmic layer and opens, simultaneously, on the opposite surface. A fenestration may have a thin, monmembranous diaphragm across its opening. This diaphragm has a central thickening and may be the remnant of the glycocalyx formerly enclosed in the pinocytotic vesicle from which the fenestra may have formed.

Fenestrated capillaries in the gastrointestinal tract and gallbladder have fewer fenestrae and a thicker wall when no absorption is occurring. When absorption takes place, the walls thin, and both the number of pinocytotic vesicles and fenestrae increase rapidly. It is the ionic changes in the perivascular connective tissue due to the absorbed solutes that stimulates pinocytosis. These observations support the suggested mode of formation of the fenestrae described above.

Discontinuous capillaries (*sinusoidal capillaries* or *sinusoids*) are larger and more irregularly shaped than other capillaries. Structural features of these capillaries vary and include

- Presence of specialized cells, such as the stellate sinusoidal macrophages (Kupffer cells) and vitamin A storage cells (of Ito) in the liver, among the lining endothelial cells
- Unique shape of some endothelial cells as in the spleen

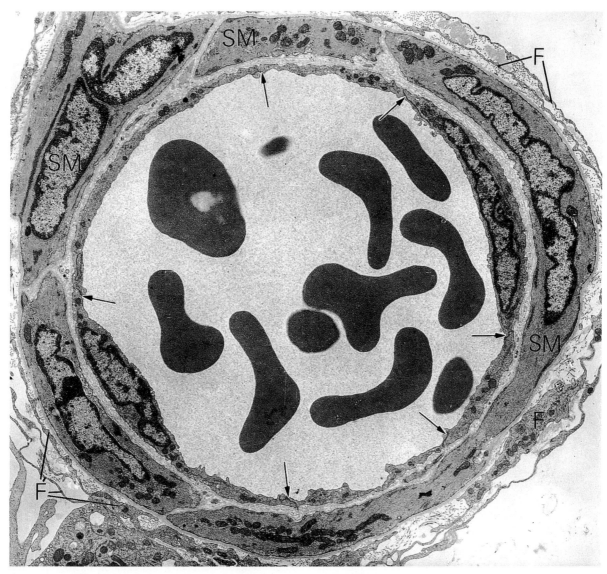

Figure 12.7. Electron micrograph of a relatively small arteriole. The tunica intima of the vessel is made up of an endothelium with a very thin layer of subendothelial connective tissue (collagen fibrils and ground substance only). The *arrows* indicate the site of junctions between adjoining endothelial cells. The tunica media consists of a single layer of smooth muscle cells *(SM)*. The tunica adventitia is composed of collagen fibrils and several layers of fibroblasts with extremely attenuated processes *(F)*. A number of red blood cells are visible in the lumen.

- Presence of unusually wide gaps between endothelial cells, as in the liver and spleen
- Partial or total absence of basal lamina underlying the endothelium

Correlation of Structure and Function in Capillaries

In considering the functioning of capillaries, two important points, blood flow and extent of the capillary network, should be considered. Blood flow or vasomotor state (vasodilation or vasoconstriction) is controlled through local and systemic signals. In response to low oxygen tension, the smooth muscle in the walls of the arterioles relax, resulting in vasodilation and increased blood flow. Systemic signals, through the autonomic nervous system, and release of norepinephrine by the adrenal gland cause the smooth muscle of the arterioles to contract (vasoconstriction), resulting in decreased blood flow, particularly to the skin and organs of the gastrointestinal tract.

The richness of the capillary networks is related to the metabolic activity of the tissue. Liver, kidney, cardiac muscle, and skeletal muscle have rich capillary networks. Dense connective tissue and smooth muscle are less metabolically active and have less extensive capillary networks.

Capillaries have three essential functions:

- *Selective permeability:* The movement of large molecules from the blood to the tissues and from the tissues

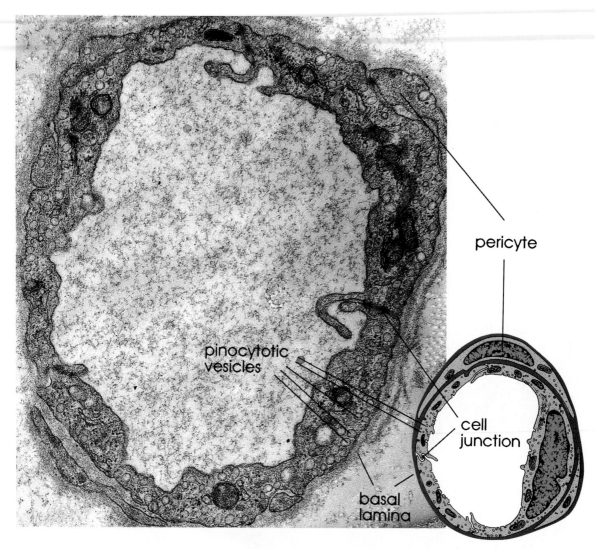

Figure 12.8. Electron micrograph of a continuous capillary with a schematic diagram. The endothelial cells that make up the capillary wall contain numerous pinocytotic vesicles. The cell junctions are frequently marked by cytoplasmic (marginal) folds that protrude into the lumen. The nuclei of the endothelial cells are not included within the plane of section in the electron micrograph, but an endothelial cell with its nucleus is shown in the diagram. Similarly, the electron micrograph shows only a small amount of pericyte cytoplasm that has been included in the section; see the upper right and lower left of the micrograph. Note, in both regions, the pericyte cytoplasm is enclosed by basal lamina. ×30,000.

to the blood is related to the size and charge of the molecules. The mechanisms by which this exchange occurs, however, remains unclear. Small hydrophilic and hydrophobic molecules (e.g., oxygen, carbon dioxide, glucose, amino acids, and electrolytes) can diffuse or be actively transported across the plasma membrane and be released into the extracellular space. Physiologists have postulated the existence in capillaries of "pores" of two sizes, small pores of 9–11 nm and large pores of 50–70 nm. Three possible morphologic equivalents to these postulated "pores" exist: the intercellular clefts and junctions between endothelial cells; the actual pores and diaphragms in the endothelial cells of fenestrated capillaries; and the pinocytotic vesicles of the endothelial cells of continuous and fenestrated capillaries.

The intercellular junctions are now believed to be the morphologic equivalent of the "small pores" and to allow passage of water and hydrophilic molecules with a diameter of less than 1.5 nm and a molecular weight of less than 10,000. The pinocytotic vesicles and the fenestrations of the endothelial cells are believed to be the morphologic equivalent of the "large pores" and allow the passage of large molecules through the endothelium.

• **Synthetic and metabolic activities:** Endothelial cells are involved in a number of synthetic activities, such as production of prostacyclin [prostaglandin I_2 (PGI_2), see below], plasminogen activator (a procoagulant factor), interleukin-1 (a mediator of the inflammatory response), and various growth factors (blood cell colony-stimulating factor, fibroblast growth factor, and platelet-derived growth factor). Endothelial cells also function in the conversion of angiotensin I to angiotensin II in the renin-

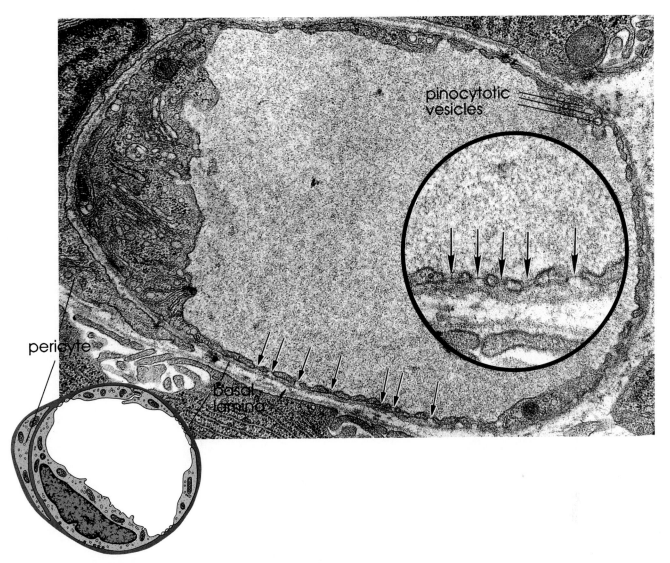

Figure 12.9. Electron micrograph of a fenestrated capillary with a schematic diagram. The cytoplasm of the endothelial cell contains numerous fenestrations *(small arrows).* The **inset** shows to advantage the fenestrations and the diaphragm that spans the openings *(large arrows).* In some of the thicker regions of the endothelial cell where the fenestrations are absent, pinocytotic vesicles are present. Part of a pericyte is seen on the left side of the electron micrograph, including its nucleus in the upper left corner of the micrograph. ×21,500; **inset,** ×55,000.

angiotensin system that controls blood pressure (see page 570), as well as in the inactivation or conversion of a number of compounds conveyed in the blood (norepinephrine, thrombin, prostaglandins, bradykinin, and serotonin) to inactive forms.

• *Antithrombogenic function:* Endothelial cells produce anticoagulants (thrombomodulin and others) and antithrombogenic agents (prostacyclin, PGI$_2$, an inhibitor of platelet aggregation and a powerful vasodilator). They also form a barrier between platelets of the blood and the subendothelial tissue. If the endothelial cells are damaged, substances released from the subendothelial tissue cause platelets to aggregate and release factors that result in the formation of clots or masses, called thrombi, that potentially prevent the loss of blood.

ARTERIOVENOUS SHUNTS

Arteriovenous Shunts Allow Blood to Bypass Capillaries by Providing Direct Routes Between Arteries and Veins

The general arrangement for a microvascular bed of a tissue is that arteries convey blood to the capillaries and that veins convey blood away from the capillaries. However, all the blood does not necessarily pass from arteries to capillaries and, thence, to veins. In many tissues, there are direct routes between the arteries and veins that can divert blood from the capillaries. These routes are called *arteriovenous (AV) anastomoses or shunts* (see Fig. 12.1). AV shunts are commonly found in the skin of the fingertips, nose, and lips and in the erectile tissue of the penis and clitoris. The arteriole of the AV shunts is often coiled, has a relatively thick smooth muscle layer, is enclosed in a connective tissue capsule, and is richly innervated. *Contrary to the ordinary precapillary sphincter, contraction of the arteriole smooth muscle of the AV shunt sends blood to a capillary bed; relaxation of the smooth muscle sends blood to a venule, bypassing the capillary bed.* AV shunts serve in thermoregulation at the body surface. Closing an AV shunt in the skin causes blood to flow through the capillary bed, enhancing heat loss. Opening an AV shunt in the skin reduces the blood flow to the skin capillaries, thereby conserving body heat. In erectile tissue, such as the penis, closing the AV shunt directs blood flow into the corpora cavernosa, initiating the erectile response (see page 665).

In addition, preferential thoroughfares, the proximal segment of which is called a *metarteriole* (Fig. 12.10), also exist that allow some blood to pass more directly from artery to vein. Capillaries arise from both arterioles and metarterioles. Although capillaries themselves have no smooth muscle in their wall, there is a sphincter of smooth muscle, called the *precapillary sphincter,* at their origin from either an arteriole or a metarteriole. These sphincters control the amount of blood passing through the capillary bed.

VEINS

The tunics of veins are not as distinct (well defined) as the tunics of arteries. Traditionally, veins are divided into three types on the basis of size:

- *Small veins* or *venules,* further subclassified as *postcapillary* and *muscular venules*
- *Medium veins*
- *Large veins*

Although large and medium veins have three layers, also designated tunica intima, tunica media, and tunica adventitia, these layers are not as distinct as they are in arteries.

Large- and medium-sized veins usually travel with large- and medium-sized arteries; arterioles and muscular venules also sometimes travel together, thus allowing comparison in histologic sections. Typically, veins have thinner walls than their accompanying arteries, and the lumen of the vein

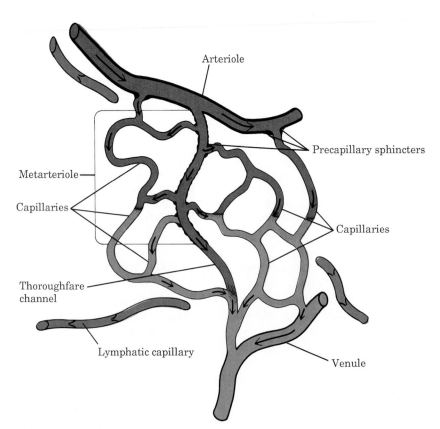

Figure 12.10. Diagram of microcirculation showing a metarteriole (initial segment of a thoroughfare channel) giving rise to capillaries. The precapillary sphincters of the arteriole and metarteriole control the entry of blood into the capillaries. The distal segment of the thoroughfare channel receives capillaries from the microcirculatory bed, but no sphincters are present where the afferent capillaries enter the thoroughfare channels. Blind-ending lymphatic vessels are shown in association with the capillary bed. (Courtesy of B. Zweifach.)

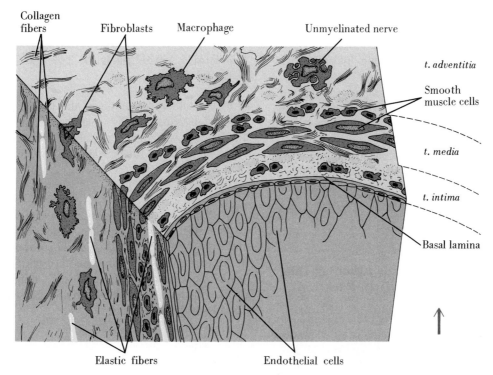

Collagen fibers   Fibroblasts   Macrophage   Unmyelinated nerve

t. adventitia

Smooth muscle cells

t. media

t. intima

Basal lamina

Elastic fibers   Endothelial cells

Figure 12.11. Schematic diagram of a medium-sized vein. *t.,* tunica. (Based on Rhodin JG: *Handbook of Physiology.* New York, Oxford University Press, 1980.)

is usually larger than that of the artery. The arteriole lumen is usually patent, whereas that of the vein is often collapsed. Many veins, especially those that convey blood against gravity, such as those of the limbs, contain valves that allow blood to flow only in one direction, back toward the heart. The valves are semilunar flaps consisting of a thin connective tissue core covered with endothelial cells in contact with the blood.

INFLAMMATION AND CELL MIGRATION

In inflammation, blood cells stick to the luminal plasma membrane of the endothelial cells *(marginate)* and migrate actively either along the intercellular space or through pores that open through the endothelial cell cytoplasm. Although neutrophils are the most common cell to leave the circulation in this manner, the other granulocytes, monocytes, and even erythrocytes may be observed traversing the endothelium of the postcapillary venules.

The apparent ameboid movement of these cells is called *diapedesis.* Precisely how the migrating cells cross the basal lamina of the endothelium, leaving it morphologically intact (at least at the TEM level), is still a subject of investigation. Although collagenases can be demonstrated in the white blood cells, the basal lamina does not appear to be digested during their passage across it. Contraction of endothelial cells and pericytes under the stimulus of the vasoactive agents histamine and serotonin may be responsible for tension needed to open intercellular junctions.

Venules

Muscular Venules Are Distinguished from Postcapillary Venules by the Presence of a Tunica Media

Postcapillary venules receive blood from capillaries and possess an endothelial lining with its basal lamina and pericytes. As previously noted, pericytes are enclosed by basal lamina material that is continuous with that of the endothelium. The endothelium of postcapillary venules is the principal site of action of vasoactive agents such as histamine and serotonin. The response to such agents results in the extravasation of fluid and the emigration of white blood cells from the vessel during inflammation and allergic reactions. Postcapillary venules of lymph nodes also participate in the transmural migration of lymphocytes from the vascular lumen into the lymphatic tissue.

Muscular venules are located distal to the postcapillary venules in the returning venous network. Whereas postcapillary venules have no true tunica media, the muscular venules have one or two layers of smooth muscle that constitute a tunica media and have a thin tunica adventitia.

Medium Veins

The three tunics of the venous wall are most evident in medium-sized veins (Fig. 12.11):

- The *tunica intima* consists of an endothelium with its basal lamina, a thin subendothelial layer with some smooth muscle cells scattered among connective tissue elements, and, in some cases, a thin internal elastic membrane.
- The *tunica media* of medium-sized veins is much thinner than the same layer in medium-sized arteries and contains circularly arranged smooth muscle cells and collagen fibers.
- The *tunica adventitia* is usually thicker than the tunica media and consists of longitudinally oriented bundles of smooth muscle cells, collagen fibers, and networks of elastic fibers.

Large Veins

In Large Veins, the Tunica Media Is Relatively Thin, and the Tunica Adventitia Is Relatively Thick

The tunica intima of large veins (Fig. 12.12) consists of an endothelial lining with its basal lamina, a small amount of subendothelial connective tissue, and some smooth muscle cells. Often, the boundary between the tunica intima and tunica media is not clear, and it is not always easy to decide if the smooth muscle cells close to the intimal endothelium should be classified as belonging to the tunica intima or to the tunica media.

The tunica media is relatively thin and contains smooth muscle cells, collagen fibers, and some fibroblasts. Cardiac muscle cells extend into the tunica media of the largest veins,

the venae cavae and the pulmonary veins, near their junction with the heart.

The Tunica Adventitia Is the Thickest Layer of the Wall of a Vein

In the tunica adventitia of the largest veins, e.g., the subclavian veins and the venae cavae, bundles of longitudinally disposed smooth muscle cells are found along with the usual collagen fibers, elastic fibers, and fibroblasts.

Atypical Veins

In several locations, veins are present that have a highly atypical structure. For example, venous channels in the cranial cavity, called **venous** or **dural sinuses,** are essentially spaces in the dura mater that are lined with endothelial cells. Veins in certain other locations (e.g., retina, placenta, trabeculae of the spleen) also have atypical walls and are discussed with those organs.

HEART

The Heart Is a Pump With Four Chambers With Valves That Maintain a One-Way Flow of Blood

The heart contains four chambers (two atria and two ventricles) through which the blood is pumped (Figs. 12.2 and 12.13). Valves guard the exits of the chambers, preventing the backflow of blood. An **interatrial septum** and

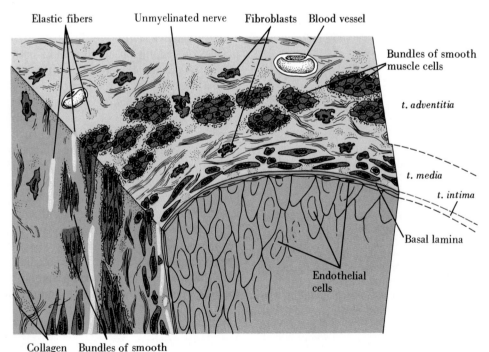

Figure 12.12. Schematic diagram of a large vein. *t.,* tunica. (Based on Rhodin JG: *Handbook of Physiology.* New York, Oxford University Press, 1980.)

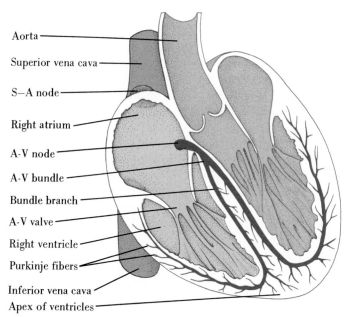

Aorta
Superior vena cava
S–A node
Right atrium
A-V node
A-V bundle
Bundle branch
A-V valve
Right ventricle
Purkinje fibers
Inferior vena cava
Apex of ventricles

Figure 12.13. Chambers of the heart and the impulse-conducting system. The heart has been cut open in the coronal plane to expose its interior and the main parts of its impulse-conducting system (indicated in *red*). Impulses are generated in the sinoatrial *(S-A)* node; they are transmitted through the atrial wall to the atrioventricular *(A-V)* node and then along the atrioventricular *(A-V)* bundle to the Purkinje fibers. The valve guarding the entrance to the aorta is a semilunar valve. (Based on Shepard RS: *Human Physiology.* Philadelphia, JB Lippincott, 1971, p 95.)

an *interventricular septum* separate the right and left sides of the heart. The *right atrium* receives blood returning from the body via the inferior and superior venae cavae, the two largest veins of the body. The *right ventricle* receives blood from the right atrium and pumps it to the lungs via the pulmonary arteries. The *left atrium* receives the oxygenated blood returning from the lungs via the four pulmonary veins. The *left ventricle* receives blood from the left atrium and pumps it into the aorta for distribution into the systemic circulation.

The wall of the heart includes

- A musculature of *cardiac muscle for contraction* to propel the blood
- A *fibrous "skeleton" for attachment* of the valves
- An *internal conducting system for synchronization* of muscle contraction

The fibrous skeleton, comprised of dense connective tissue, encircles the base of the two arteries leaving the heart (aorta and pulmonary trunk) and the openings between the atria and the ventricles [right and left atrioventricular (A-V) orifices] (Fig. 12.14). Each annular arrangement of fibrous tissue serves for the attachment of valves that allow blood to flow in only one direction through the openings. The fibrous skeleton also includes an extension into the interventricular septum. This small part of the interventricular

septum (the membranous portion) is devoid of cardiac muscle; it contains a short length of unbranched A-V bundle of the cardiac conduction system (see page 318). Elsewhere, the heart wall contains cardiac muscle.

The wall of the heart is organized in essentially the same manner in the atria and ventricles (see Plate 45, page 321). It consists of three layers:

- ***Epicardium*** consists of a layer of mesothelial cells on the outer surface of the heart and its underlying connective tissue. The blood vessels and nerves that supply the heart lie in the epicardium and are surrounded by adipose tissue that cushions the heart in the pericardial cavity.
- ***Myocardium,*** the cardiac muscle, is the principal component of the heart. The myocardium of the ventricles is substantially thicker than that of the atria because of the large amount of cardiac muscle in the walls of the two pumping chambers.
- ***Endocardium*** consists of an inner layer of endothelium and subendothelial connective tissue, a middle layer of connective tissue and smooth muscle cells, and a deeper layer, also called the ***subendocardial layer,*** of connective tissue that is continuous with the connective tissue of the myocardium. The impulse-conducting system of the heart (see below) is located in the subendocardial layer of the endocardium.

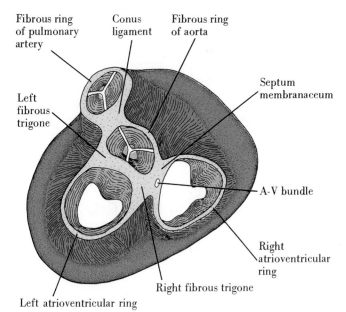

Fibrous ring of pulmonary artery
Conus ligament
Fibrous ring of aorta
Septum membranaceum
Left fibrous trigone
A-V bundle
Right atrioventricular ring
Right fibrous trigone
Left atrioventricular ring

Figure 12.14. Fibrous skeleton of the heart as seen with the two atria removed. This fibrous network serves for the attachment of the cardiac muscle; it also serves for the attachment of the cuspid valves between the atria and ventricles and for the semilunar valves of the aorta and the pulmonary artery. The atrioventricular *(A-V)* bundle passes from the right atrium to the ventricular septum via the membranous septum of the fibrous skeleton. (Based on Tandler J: *Lehrbuch der Systematischen Anatomie.* Leipzig, Vogel, 1926, vol. 3.)

The *interventricular septum* is the wall between the right and left ventricles. It contains cardiac muscle except in the membranous portion. Endocardium lines each surface of the interventricular septum. The *interatrial septum* is much thinner than the interventricular septum. Except for certain localized areas that contain fibrous tissue, it has a center layer of cardiac muscle, with a lining of endocardium facing each chamber.

The valves of the heart have a center sheet of fibrous tissue. The surfaces of the valve that are exposed to blood are covered with endothelium. Fibrous, thread-like cords called the *chordae tendineae,* also covered with endothelium, extend from the free edge of the A-V valves to muscular projections from the wall of the ventricles, called *papillary muscles.*

ISCHEMIC HEART DISEASE

The most common cause of ischemic heart disease is atherosclerosis. In atherosclerosis, the lumina of the coronary arteries progressively narrow due to the accumulation of proteoglycans, lipid, and collagen in the intima. The reduction in blood flow becomes critical when flow is reduced by 90%. A sudden occlusion of the narrowed lumen by a thrombus or clot released from the surface of an atheromatous plaque precipitates an acute ischemic event. The event is characterized by anginal pain associated with the loss of blood to the region of the heart supplied by the affected coronary vessel. Coronary artery thrombosis usually precedes and precipitates a myocardial infarct, i.e., a sudden insufficiency of blood supply that results in an area of muscle cell death. With time, a scar forms and replaces the damaged tissue. In the area of infarction, there is loss of contractile function. Multiple infarctions over time can produce sufficient loss of cardiac function to cause death. Infarction also commonly occurs in the brain, spleen, kidney, lung, intestine, testes, and tumors (especially of the ovaries and uterus).

Intrinsic Regulation of Heart Rate

Contraction of the Heart Is Synchronized by Specialized Cardiac Muscle Fibers

Cardiac muscle is capable of contracting in a rhythmic manner without any direct stimulus from the nervous system. The pace of this beating action is initiated at the *sinoatrial (SA) node,* a group of specialized cardiac muscle cells located near the junction of the superior vena cava and the right atrium (see Fig. 12.13). Because of this function, the SA node is referred to as the *pacemaker.* The SA node initiates an impulse that spreads along the cardiac muscle fibers of the atria and along internodal tracts composed of modified cardiac muscle fibers. The impulse is then picked up at the *atrioventricular (A-V) node* and conducted across the fibrous skeleton to the ventricles by the *atrioventricular (A-V) bundle (of His).* The bundle divides into smaller *right* and *left bundle branches* and then into *Purkinje fibers.*

The A-V bundle, the bundle branches, and the Purkinje fibers are modified cardiac muscle cells that are specialized to conduct impulses (see Plate 33, page 249). The nodes and A-V bundle and its branches are modified cardiac muscle fibers that are smaller than normal. The Purkinje fibers are modified cardiac muscle fibers that are larger than normal. The components of the conducting system convey the impulse at a rate approximately 4 times faster than the cardiac muscle fibers. The conducting elements are the only elements that can convey impulses across the fibrous skeleton and serve to coordinate the contractions of the atria and ventricles. The contraction is initiated in the atria, forcing blood into the ventricles. Then, a wave of contraction in the ventricles begins at the apex of the heart, forcing blood from the heart through the aorta and pulmonary trunk.

Systemic Regulation of Heart Function

The heart is innervated by both divisions of the autonomic nervous system. The autonomic nerves *do not initiate contractions of the cardiac muscle* but, rather, regulate the heart rate according to the body's immediate needs. The parasympathetic fibers terminate chiefly about the SA and A-V nodes but also extend into the myocardium. The sympathetic fibers supply the SA and A-V nodes, extend into the myocardium, and also pass through the epicardium to reach the coronary arteries that supply the heart. The autonomic fibers *only regulate the rate of impulses* emanating from the SA node. Under the influence of the sympathetic component of the autonomic nervous system, the rate of contractions increases; the parasympathetic component causes a decrease in the rate of contraction.

Specialized *Receptors* Monitor Heart Function

Specialized sensory nerve receptors for physiologic reflexes are located in the walls of large blood vessels near the heart. They function as

- *Baroreceptors,* which sense general blood pressure. These receptors are located in the carotid sinus and aortic arch.
- *Chemoreceptors,* which detect alterations in oxygen and carbon dioxide tension and in pH. These receptors are the *carotid* and *aortic bodies* located at the bifurcation of the carotid arteries and in the aortic arch, respectively.

The carotid body consists of cords and irregular groups of epithelioid cells. Associated with these cells is a rich supply of nerve fibers. The neural elements are both afferent and efferent. The structure of the aortic bodies is essentially similar to that of the carotid bodies. Both receptors function in neural reflexes that adjust cardiac output and respiratory rate.

LYMPHATIC VESSELS

Lymphatic Vessels Convey Fluids From the Tissues to the Bloodstream

In addition to blood vessels, there is a set of vessels that circulates fluid, called *lymph,* through certain parts of the body. These *lymphatic vessels* are an adjunct to the blood vessels. Unlike the blood vessels, which convey blood to and from tissues, the lymphatic vessels are unidirectional, conveying fluid only from tissues. The smallest lymphatic vessels are called *lymphatic capillaries.* They are especially numerous in the loose connective tissues under the epithelium of the skin and mucous membranes. The lymphatic capillaries begin as "blind-ending" tubes in the microcapillary beds (see Fig. 12.10). Lymphatic capillaries converge into increasingly larger vessels, called *lymphatic vessels,* that ultimately unite to form two main channels that empty into the blood vascular system by draining into the large veins in the base of the neck. They enter the vascular system at the junctions of the internal jugular and subclavian veins. The largest lymphatic vessel, draining most of the body and emptying into the veins on the left side, is the *thoracic duct.* The other main channel is the *right lymphatic duct.*

Lymphatic Capillaries

Lymphatic Capillaries Are More Permeable Than Blood Capillaries

Due to their greater permeability, lymphatic capillaries are more effective than blood capillaries in removing protein-rich fluid from the intercellular spaces. Lymphatic vessels also serve to convey large proteins and lipids that do not get across the fenestrae of the absorptive capillaries in the small intestine.

Before lymph is returned to the blood, it passes through *lymph nodes,* where it is exposed to the cells of the immune system. Thus, the lymphatic vessels serve not only as an adjunct to the blood vascular system but also as an integral component of the immune system.

Lymphatic capillaries are essentially tubes of endothelium that, unlike the typical blood capillary, lack a continuous basal lamina. The incomplete basal lamina can be correlated with their high permeability. Anchoring filaments extend between the incomplete basal lamina and the perivascular collagen. These filaments may help maintain the patency of the vessels during times of increased tissue pressure, as in inflammation.

As lymphatic vessels become larger, the wall becomes thicker. The increasing thickness is due to connective tissue and bundles of smooth muscle. Lymphatic vessels possess valves that prevent backflow of the lymph, thus aiding unidirectional flow. There is no central pump in the lymphatic system. Lymph moves sluggishly, driven primarily by the compression of the lymphatic vessels by adjacent skeletal muscles.

PLATE 45. Heart

FIGURE 1, heart, human, hematoxylin and eosin (H&E) ×44. A section through the wall of the atrium is shown here. The outermost part is the epicardium *(Epi)*, the thick middle portion is the myocardium *(Myo)*, and the inner part is the endocardium *(End)*. The myocardium is, by far, the thickest component. It consists of bundles of cardiac muscle. These do not all travel in the same direction; in most sections, therefore, cardiac muscle fibers may be cut longitudinally, in cross section, or obliquely. Connective tissue *(CT)* separates the bundles of cardiac muscle. Most connective tissue is in the vicinity of the blood vessel *(BV)* in the periphery of the myocardium.

The ventricles have essentially the same structure as the atria except that the myocardium is much thicker. In addition, the subendocardial layer of the ventricles contains special muscle fibers that belong to the intrinsic conducting system of the heart (Purkinje fibers).

The epicardium can be distinguished from endocardium in several ways. The larger blood vessels and nerves that supply the heart wall are in the epicardium; blood vessels in the endocardium are considerably smaller. The endocardium is layered and contains smooth muscle cells; the epicardium is not layered and contains large amounts of adipose tissue, particularly in the vicinity of the large vessels. Finally, Purkinje fibers, when included in the section, are found in or near the subendocardial layer of the endocardium (see Plate 33, page 249).

FIGURE 2, heart, human, H&E ×160. The epicardium *(Epi)* is shown at higher magnification in this figure. Its outer surface is covered by mesothelium. Under the mesothelium is the supporting connective tissue *(CT)*, the fibrous elements of which are loosely arranged. Elastic fibers are present in the connective tissue; however, they are not evident in routine H&E-stained preparations. A small nerve *(N)* that is entering the myocardium is present in the connective tissue between the muscle bundles. The nerve appears as a bundle of thin wavy fibers that are significantly thinner than the muscle fibers.

FIGURE 3, heart, human, H&E ×160. The endocardium *(End)* is shown at higher magnification in this figure. It can be divided into three layers: *(1)* an inner layer, i.e., the one closest to the lumen of the heart, that is composed of endothelial cells that rest on a subendothelial layer of delicate collagenous fibers; *(2)* a middle layer, which is somewhat thicker and contains not only collagenous fibers but also smooth muscle cells *(SM)* and elastic fibers (not evident); and *(3)* an outer layer, closest to the myocardium, that consists of loose connective tissue and is called the subendocardial layer. The subendocardial layer is continuous with the connective tissue of the myocardium. The subendocardial layer contains blood vessels *(BV)* and collagenous and elastic fibers but no smooth muscle.

KEY		
BV, blood vessel	**Myo,** myocardium	**1,** endothelium and subendothelial connective tissue
CT, connective tissue	**N,** nerve	**2,** middle layer of endocardium
End, endocardium	**SM,** smooth muscle	**3,** subendocardial layer
Epi, epicardium		

PLATE 45

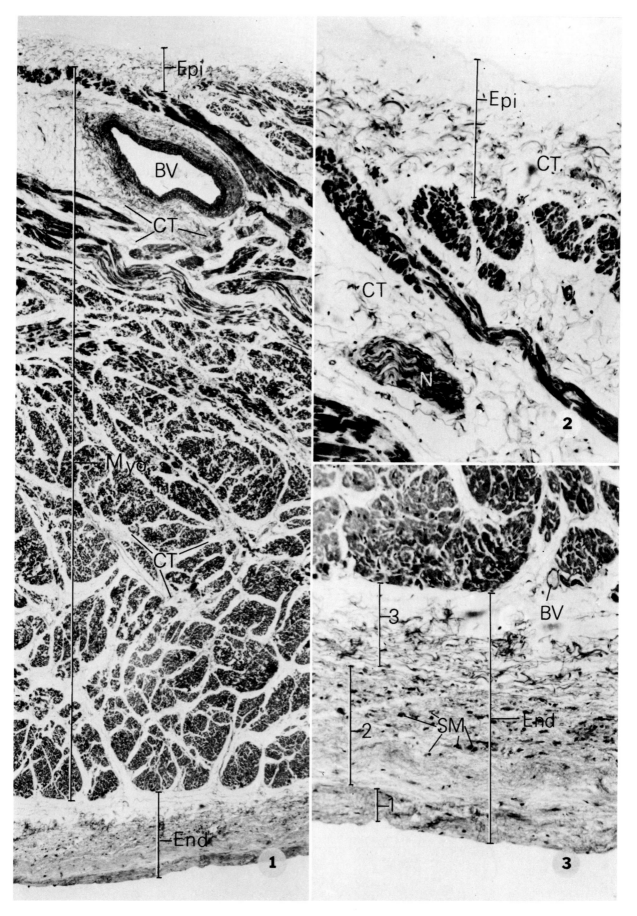

PLATE 46.   Aorta

The aorta is the artery that carries blood away from the left ventricle. Because of the large amount of elastic material it contains, it is referred to as an *elastic artery*. The elastic material is not readily evident, however, without special stains.

Other elastic arteries are the brachiocephalic, the subclavian, the beginning of the common carotid, and the pulmonary arteries. The elastic arteries are also called conducting arteries.

FIGURE 1, aorta, human, H&E ×65.   The layers that make up the wall of the aorta are shown in this figure. This is a longitudinal section through the entire thickness of the arterial wall. Three layers can usually be recognized: the tunica intima *(TI)*, tunica media *(TM)*, and tunica adventitia *(TA)*. The adventitia is the outermost part. It consists mainly of connective tissue and contains the blood vessels (vasa vasorum) and nerves (nervi vascularis) that supply the arterial wall.

FIGURE 3, aorta, human, resorcin-fuchsin ×65.   The tunica media contains an abundance of smooth muscle; the more distinctive feature, however, is its large amount of elastic material. The elastic material is present not in the form of fibers but, rather, as fenestrated membranes. This figure and the higher magnification (Fig. 5) are from a specimen stained to demonstrate elastic material. This figure reveals elastic laminae present in the media *(TM)* as well as the deep portion of the intima *(TI)*. The adventitia *(TA)*, however, essentially lacks these elastic laminae.

FIGURE 5, aorta, human, resorcin-fuchsin ×300.   Careful examination of the tunica media at higher magnification reveals what appear to be interruptions of some of the elastic lamellae. These are actually the fenestrations or openings in the elastic membranes.

FIGURE 2, aorta, human, H&E ×160.   The tunica intima is shown here at higher magnification. The boundary between it and the tissue below, the tunica media, is not sharply defined. Largely because of staining characteristics and degree of cellularity, the two tunics are more easily distinguished at low magnification (Fig. 1). The tunica intima consists of a lining of endothelial cells that rest on a layer of connective tissue. However, the endothelium is difficult to preserve in these vessels and is frequently lost. Both collagenous fibers and elastic lamellae are in the connective tissue. Smooth muscle cells are also present in the intima of the aorta *(arrows)*.

FIGURE 4, aorta, human, H&E ×160.   This figure shows a higher magnification of the tunica media of Figure 1. Here, the elastic lamellae are unstained, as is usually the case in H&E sections. (In some instances, the elastic material will stain lightly with eosin.) The *arrowheads* reveal the sites of some of the lamellae. Their presence is recognized by the apparent absence of structure, which, in turn, is due to the absence of staining of the elastic material. The smooth muscle cells of the media are arranged in a closely wound spiral between the elastic membranes. This arrangement, however, is difficult to recognize in sectioned material.

FIGURE 6, aorta, human, H&E ×160.   The outermost layer of the aorta, the tunica adventitia, is shown here. The tunica adventitia consists mostly of collagenous fibers that course in longitudinal spirals. (Their course, like that of the smooth muscle fibers, however, is unrecognizable in tissue sections.) There are no elastic lamellae in the adventitia, but elastic fibers are present, though relatively few in number. The cells of the adventitia, represented by the nuclei seen in the adventitia, are fibroblasts. Occasionally, ganglion cells are present as well as some scattered smooth muscle cells. The ganglion cells, when present, are quite conspicuous, whereas the smooth muscle may be overlooked.

KEY

TA, tunica adventitia	**TM,** tunica media	**arrowheads (Fig. 4),** elastic lamel-
TI, tunica intima	**arrows (Fig. 2),** smooth muscle cell	lae, unstained

PLATE 46

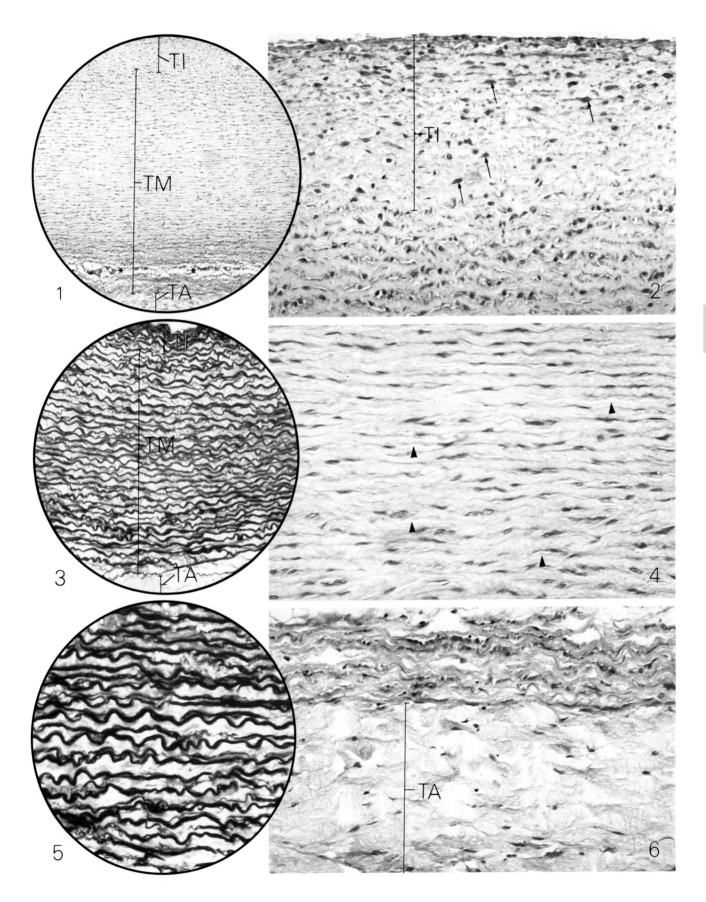

PLATE 47.   Muscular Arteries and Veins

As the arterial tree is traced further from the heart, the elastic tissue is considerably reduced in amount, and smooth muscle becomes the predominant component in the tunica media. The arteries are then called muscular arteries or arteries of medium caliber.

FIGURES 1 and 2, muscular artery, monkey, H&E ×160 (Fig. 1); ×640 (Fig. 2). A cross section through a muscular artery is shown here. Blood cells are in the lumen. The wall of the artery is divided into three layers: the tunica intima *(TI)*, tunica media *(TM)*, and tunica adventitia *(TA)*.

Figure 2 is a higher magnification of the *rectangular area* included in Figure 1. The tunica intima is composed of an endothelial lining, its basal lamina (not evident), an extremely small amount of connective tissue, and the internal elastic membrane *(IEM)*. The internal elastic membrane has a scalloped appearance and is highly refractile. The connective tissue is extremely scant, and the endothelial cells appear to rest directly on the internal elastic membrane. The agonal contraction of the artery causes the internal elastic membrane to assume its scalloped formation, and this contracts the endothelial cells, so that the endothelial nuclei [*E(N)*] appear rounded and perched on the internal elastic membrane.

The tunica media consists mainly of circularly arranged smooth muscle cells. The nuclei of the smooth muscle cells [*SM(N)*] are elongated and oriented in the same direction. Their twisted appearance indicates that the smooth muscle cells are in a contracted state. The material between the nuclei is mainly cytoplasm of the muscle cells; however, the cytoplasmic boundaries are not evident. The refractile undulating material in the tunica media is elastic material *(EM)*. Reticular fibers are also present, but they are not visualized in H&E preparations.

The tunica adventitia *(TA)* consists of connective tissue. The refractile scalloped sheet at the junction of the tunica media and tunica adventitia is the external elastic membrane *(EEM)*. The nuclei of some fibroblasts [*F(N)*] can be seen; the cytoplasm of these cells cannot be distinguished from the extracellular material.

FIGURE 3, artery and vein, monkey, H&E ×65; inset ×640. The walls of veins that accompany muscular arteries can also be divided into a tunica intima, tunica media, and tunica adventitia. Although there is elastic material in the wall of the vein, there is significantly less material than in the wall of the artery. This figure enables one to compare a muscular artery with its accompanying vein. The lumen of the vein is larger than that of the artery, but the wall is thinner, and the vessel frequently appears collapsed or flattened. The tunica intima *(TI)* is extremely thin (**inset**) and consists of a endothelial lining *(E)* that rests on a small amount of connective tissue. The tunica media *(TM)* is much thinner than that of the artery; the tunica adventitia *(TA)* is thicker. The tunica media consists largely of smooth muscle. The nuclei of the smooth muscle cells [*SM(N)*] are elongated and readily identified, but the cytoplasmic boundaries cannot be discerned.

The question of distinguishing between an artery and its accompanying vein or veins is usually simplified by their proximity, which enables one to compare histologic features directly, as in this figure.

KEY

AT, adipose tissue
BV, small blood vessels in surrounding connective tissue
E, endothelium
EEM, external elastic membrane
EM, elastic material
E(N), endothelial nuclei
F(N), fibroblast nuclei
IEM, internal elastic membrane
SM(N), smooth muscle nuclei
TA, tunica adventitia
TI, tunica intima
TM, tunica media

PLATE 47

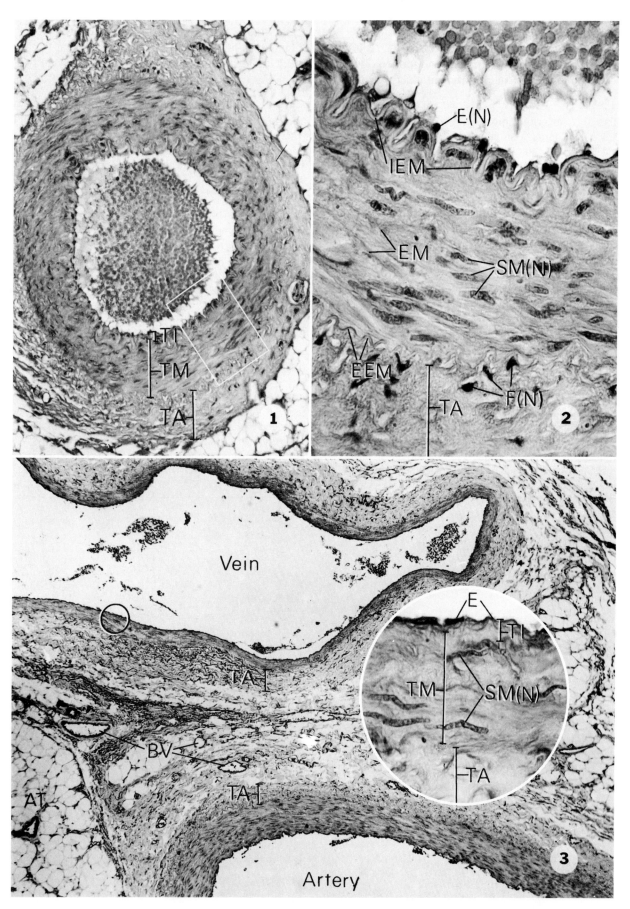

PLATE 48. Arterioles and Lymphatic Vessels

The terminal components of the arterial tree just before a capillary bed or an arterio-venous shunt are the arterioles. Arterioles contain an endothelial lining and smooth muscle in the wall. The muscle component is limited in thickness to one or two cells. There may or may not be an internal elastic membrane, according to the size of the vessel.

FIGURE 1, arteriole, monkey, H&E ×640. A longitudinal section through an arteriole is shown in Figure 1. It branches on the right. The elongated nuclei that line the lumen belong to endothelial cells *(arrows)*. An elastic membrane cannot be seen. The *rectangle* in Figure 1 marks an area comparable with that seen in the electron micrograph in Plate 49. The round nuclei located in the wall of this vessel belong to smooth muscle cells [*SM(N)*] cut in cross section. They should not be confused with cuboidal cells.

FIGURES 2 and 3, arteriole, monkey, H&E ×640. These figures show how, by changing the focus of the optical system, one can obtain information relevant to the shape of the smooth muscle cells. In Figure 2, one sees the elongated nuclei of the endothelial cells *(arrows)* as in Figure 1. Round nuclei are aligned in rows in the wall of the vessel. Four nuclei *(A)* are indicated on the left, and seven *(B)* are indicated on the right. Notice the "shadows" related to the four nuclei on the left.

By changing the focus (Fig. 3), one comes to realize that the round-appearing nuclei are really elongated nuclei that are wrapped around the vessel wall in a circular fashion. Note how the length of the four nuclei in Figure 3 corresponds to the four nuclear "shadows" that are illustrated in Figure 2.

FIGURES 4 and 5, lymphatic vessel, human, H&E ×160 (Fig. 4); ×640 (Fig. 5). *Lymphatic vessels* have extremely thin walls. A lymphatic vessel from the mucosa of the pharynx is shown in Figure 4. It has been cut longitudinally, and two valves *(V)* are included in the section. One of the valves is shown at high magnification in Figure 5. The wall of the lymphatic vessel consists almost exclusively of an endothelial lining. The nuclei *(arrows)* of the endothelial cells appear to be exposed to the lumen. This is because the cytoplasm is so attenuated. At the nuclear poles, the cytoplasm continues as a thin thread. It is not possible to determine where one endothelial cell ends and the next begins. Connective tissue *(CT)* surrounds the lymphatic vessel. Some lymphocytes and precipitated lymph are within the lumen of the vessel. As a general statement, lymphatic vessels possess very large caliber lumina compared with the thickness of the wall (see last paragraph discussing Plate 78, page 486).

KEY

A, smooth muscle cell nuclei at different focus levels
B, smooth muscle cell nuclei at different focus levels
CT, connective tissue
SM(C), smooth muscle cell cytoplasm
SM(N), smooth muscle cell nuclei
V, valves of lymphatic vessel
arrows, endothelial cell nuclei

PLATE 48

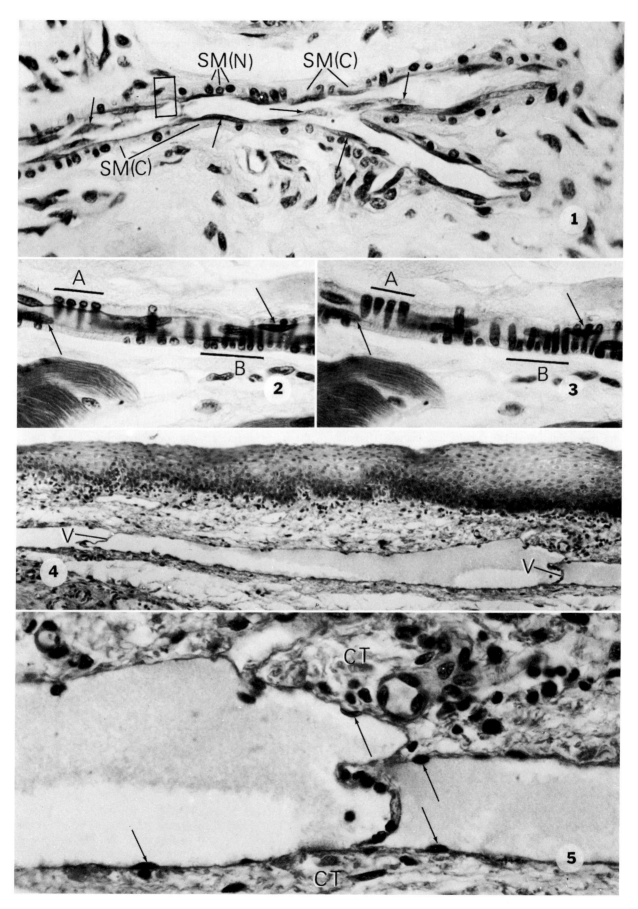

PLATE 49.   Arteriole, Electron Microscopy

Arteriole, electron micrograph ×12,000; inset ×25,000.
The electron micrograph shown here reveals a portion of the wall of a longitudinally sectioned arteriole. The vessel is comparable in size and general structural organization to the arteriole shown in Figure 1 of the preceding plate. For purposes of orientation, the portion of the vessel wall seen in the electron micrograph would correspond to the area indicated by the *rectangle* in Figure 1 of Plate 48.

In comparing the light and electron micrographs, note that with the light microscope the *endothelial* cell boundaries are not delineated, only the nuclei are evident. Also, the cytoplasm of the individual *smooth muscle cells* blends together; only their nuclei, when present in the section, are readily discernible. In contrast, the electron micrograph reveals the individual smooth muscle cells *(SM)* of the vessel wall. Each cell is separated from its neighbor by a definable intercellular space. Evident in the micrograph are portions of two endothelial cells *(End)*, one of which includes part of its nucleus. At the site of apposition, the two endothelial cells are separated by a narrow (~20 nm) intercellular space *(arrows)*.

Between the endothelium and the smooth muscle cells is an internal elastic membrane *(IEM)*. This is typically lacking in the smallest arterioles. The elastic membrane in this vessel is a continuous sheath that is permeated by irregularly shaped openings *(arrowheads)*. Together with the endothelium, it forms the tunica intima *(TI)*. In sectioned material, the openings give the appearance of a discontinuous membrane rather than a true sheath that simply contains fenestrations. The basal lamina *(BL)* of the endothelial and smooth muscle cells are closely applied to the elastic membrane; consequently, other than the elastic material, little extracellular matrix is present in the tunica intima of this vessel.

The tunica media is represented by the single layer of smooth muscle cells. The muscle cells are circumferentially disposed and appear here in cross section; none includes a nucleus. Each muscle cell is surrounded by basal lamina *(BL)*. However, there may be focal sites where neighboring smooth muscle cells come into more intimate apposition to form a nexus or gap junction. At these sites of close membrane apposition, the basal lamina is absent. The cytoplasm of the muscle cell displays aggregates of mitochondria along with occasional profiles of rough endoplasmic reticulum. These organelles tend to be localized along the central axis of the cell at both ends of the nucleus. In addition, numerous cytoplasmic densities *(CD)* are present. They are adherent to the plasma membrane and extend into the interior of the cell to form a branching network. The cytoplasmic densities are regarded as attachment devices for the contractile filaments, analogous to the Z lines in striated muscle.

The tunica adventitia *(TA)* is composed of elastic material *(E)*, numerous collagen fibrils *(C)*, and fibroblasts *(F)*. The elastic material is somewhat more abundant nearest the smooth muscle. If the vessel shown here could be traced back in the direction of the heart, the elastic material would quantitatively increase, ultimately forming a more continuous sheath-like structure, namely, an external elastic membrane. The bulk of the adventitia consists of collagen fibrils, arranged in small bundles, separated by fibroblast processes.

The **inset** shows, at higher magnification, the area within the *circle*. It reveals with somewhat greater clarity the cytoplasmic densities *(CD)* of the smooth muscle cells, the basal lamina *(BL)*, and the collagen fibrils *(C)* and elastic material of the adventitia. A series of pinocytotic vesicles *(PV)* along the plasma membrane of the smooth muscle cell is also evident.

KEY

BL, basal lamina
C, collagen fibrils
CD, cytoplasmic densities
E, elastic material
End, endothelial cell
F, fibroblast
IEM, internal elastic membrane
PV, pinocytotic vesicles
RBC, red blood cell
SM, smooth muscle cell
TA, tunica adventitia
TI, tunica intima
arrows, endothelial cell intercellular space
arrowheads, openings in internal elastic membrane

PLATE 49

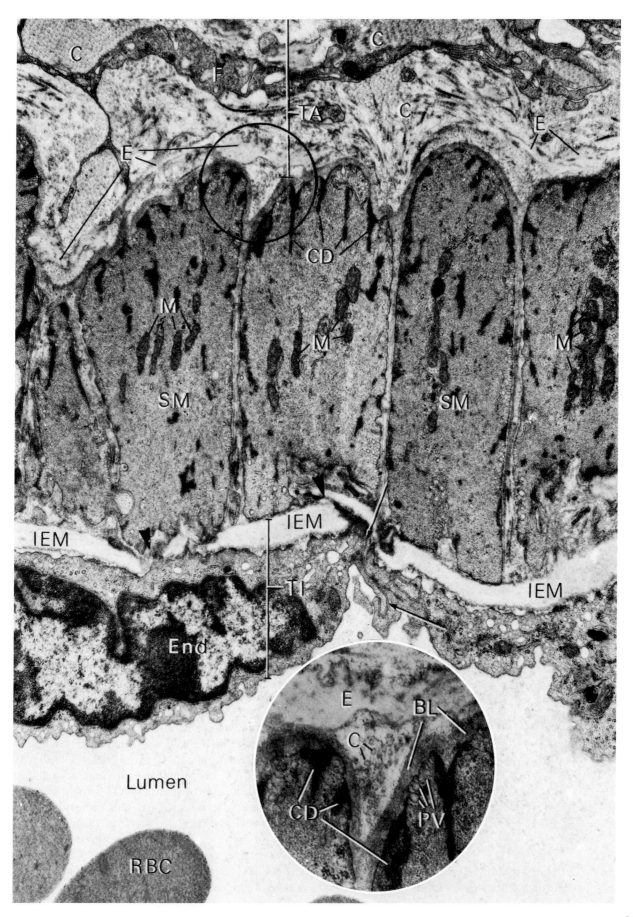

Lymphatic Tissue, Lymphatic Organs, and the Immune System

13

LYMPHATIC TISSUE AND THE IMMUNE RESPONSE

The **lymphatic system** is a specialized form of connective tissue that consists of groups of cells, tissues, and organs that monitor body surfaces and internal fluid compartments and react to the presence of potentially harmful antigenic substances. Included in this system are the **thymus, spleen, lymph nodes, lymphatic nodules,** and **diffuse lymphatic tissue** (Fig 13.1). The several forms of **lymphatic organs and tissue** are often collectively referred to as the **immune system. Lymphatic vessels** (see page 319) connect parts of the system to the blood vascular system.

For over 2000 years, it has been known that people who recover from certain diseases, such as chickenpox, measles, or mumps, are resistant to reinfection with the same disease. Another long-standing observation is that immunity is specific; i.e., an immunity to chickenpox will not prevent infection with measles. It has also been recognized that the immune system sometimes reacts against itself, causing autoimmune diseases such as lupus erythematosus, autoimmune hemolytic anemia, some forms of diabetes mellitus, and autoimmune hypothyroidism.

Lymphocytes Are the Chief Cellular Constituent of Lymphatic Tissue

Lymphocytes and other cells of lymphatic tissue are the key elements in the immune response. Our bodies are constantly exposed to

- Potentially hazardous substances and cells from outside the body (infectious microorganism, toxins, and foreign cells and tissues)

- Changes within the body in our tissues (such as transformation of normal cells to cancerous cells) that give them characteristics that identify them as "nonself"

Our *first line of defense* against external substances and cells is the epithelial covering of the body, i.e. the skin and the epithelial linings of the respiratory, gastrointestinal, and urogenital tracts. Invading substances must cross these epithelial barriers in order to gain access to the body.

The Immune System Provides Resistance to Antigenic and Infectious Materials

Our *second line of defense,* which protects us from invaders that have crossed the epithelial barrier as well as from transformed cells of our own bodies, is lymphatic tissue. This tissue is distributed diffusely throughout the body within the connective tissue that underlies the epithelium and is also organized into the discrete organs of the lymphatic system.

The lymphatic tissue, particularly the thymus and bone marrow, serve as sites where lymphocytes mature and are "processed" so that they become competent to recognize and destroy invading microbes as well as transformed cells within our own bodies. These **immunocompetent cells** have the ability to distinguish between "self" (molecules normally present within an organism) and "nonself" (foreign molecules, i.e., those not normally present) and to provide for the inactivation or destruction of foreign organisms and of substances such as toxins. This protective response of the lymphatic system is known as (acquired) **immunity.** After processing, lymphocytes are transported by the cardiovascular system to sites throughout the body. Some of the immune cells leave the capillaries and move directly among the cells and tissues of the body, especially into the connective tissue that underlies the lining epithelium of the respiratory, gastrointestinal, and urogenital tracts and even into the intercellular spaces of those epithelia.

Supporting cells in the lymphatic organs are organized as loose meshworks. In lymph nodules, lymph nodes, and the spleen, *reticular cells* and the *reticular fibers* that they secrete form meshworks through which blood that contains invading substances passes. Lymphocytes, macrophages, and other cells of the immune system reside in these meshworks as well as in the loose connective tissue of the body. In all of these sites they carry out their mission of surveillance and defense. In the thymus, stellate epithelial cells called *epithelioreticular cells* form the structural meshworks within the tissue. These cells do not secrete or relate to reticular fibers.

Classification of Lymphocytes

Traditionally, Three Groups of Lymphocytes Are Identified on the Basis of Size

Three groups of lymphocytes are often described according to size, i.e., small, medium, and large, measuring approximately 6, 12, and 18 μm in diameter. The range in lymphocyte size is, however, a continuum from about 4 to 18 μm, and after *blastic transformation* (see below), lymphocytes may be up to 30 μm in diameter. Lymphocytes circulating in the blood are mostly of small and medium size, with the vast majority being small. Lymphocytes in immunologically stimulated lymph nodes include the largest cells as well as many small lymphocytes. In understanding the function of the lymphocytes, it is important to realize that most lymphocytes found in blood or lymph represent *recirculating immunocompetent cells*. These are cells that have developed the capacity to recognize and respond to foreign antigen and are in transit from one site of lymphatic tissue to another.

Functionally, Two Types of Lymphocytes Are Identified: T Lymphocytes and B Lymphocytes

The study of the differentiation and function of lymphocytes has established the existence of two classes or categories of cells:

• *T lymphocytes* or *T cells,* involved in cell-mediated immunity
• *B lymphocytes* or *B cells,* involved in humoral immunity and the production of antibodies

Precursors [colony-forming units (CFUs)] give rise to *stem lymphocytes* that will differentiate into the *B lymphocytes* and *T lymphocytes.* In early fetal life, the precursor cells originate in the yolk sac, liver, and spleen. By late fetal life, the CFUs are restricted to the bone marrow and continue to proliferate during postnatal life. In humans, the undifferentiated stem lymphocytes migrate to sites in the bone marrow *(B lymphocytes)* or to the thymus *(T lymphocytes),* where they undergo differentiation that includes the synthesis of the unique internal and membrane proteins essential to the functional activities of the cells (immunocompetence). T lymphocytes, which have a long life span, differentiate into immunocompetent cells in the thymus. *B lymphocytes,* which have variable life spans, also differentiate into immunocompetent cells in the bone marrow. It has been assumed that this occurs in the bone marrow, although recent evidence indicates that the lymphatic tissue of the cecum, appendix, and ileum is also involved.

Primary Lymphatic Organs and Tissues

Thus, in humans and other mammals, the bone marrow and thymus have been identified as *primary* or *central lymphatic organs.* The lymphatic tissue of the distal intestinal tract may now be added to these organs. Lymphocytes undergo their differentiation into immunocompetent cells in these organs. Initially, lymphocytes undergo *antigen-independent proliferation and differentiation* into populations of cells in which individual cells are genetically preprogrammed to recognize a single antigenic determinant out of virtually an infinite number of possible antigens. These immunocompetent cells then enter the blood and lymph and are transported throughout the body where they are dispersed in the connective tissue and penetrate into the epithelia that line mucosal surfaces.

Secondary Lymphatic Organs and Tissues

Immunocompetent lymphocytes, together with plasma cells derived from B lymphocytes and with macrophages, organize around mesenchymal reticular cells and their reticular fibers to form the adult *effector lymphatic tissues and organs,* i.e., lymphatic nodules, lymph nodes, tonsils, and spleen. It is in these *secondary or peripheral lymphatic organs* that T and B lymphocytes undergo *antigen-dependent proliferation and differentiation* into effector lymphocytes and *memory cells.*

Memory cells do not participate in the initial or *primary response* to an antigen; rather, they increase the circulating population of preprogrammed lymphocytes capable of recognizing a particular antigen and responding to a second exposure. This *secondary response* is usually more rapid and more intense than the primary response and is the basis of most immunization programs for common bacterial and viral diseases. Some antigens, such as penicillin and insect venoms, may trigger such violent secondary response as to produce a hypersensitivity reaction or, even, anaphylaxis (see page 196).

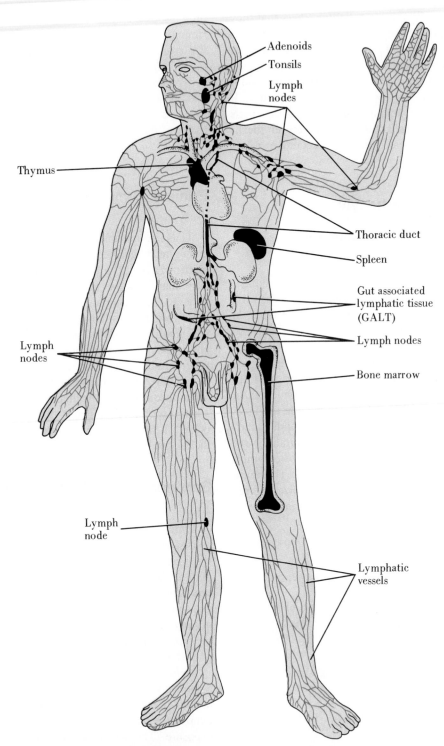

Figure 13.1.   Overview of the structures constituting the lymphatic system. Because lymphatic tissue is the main component of some organs, they are regarded as organs of the lymphatic system (spleen, thymus, lymph nodes). Lymphatic tissue is present as part of other organs, namely, red marrow of bones; as lymphatic nodules of the alimentary canal (tonsils, Peyer's patches) and respiratory system (adenoids, tonsils); and, not shown in the illustration, as diffuse lymphatic tissue of mucous membranes. The lymph nodes are interspersed in the path of lymphatic vessels, and ultimately, the lymphatic vessels empty into the bloodstream by joining the large veins in the root of the neck. The thoracic duct is the largest of the lymphatic vessels. (Based on Jerne NK: *Scientific American* 229:52, 1973.)

In the early 1960s, investigators using chicken embryos demonstrated that the bursa of Fabricius, a mass of lymphatic tissue associated with the cloaca of birds, was one of the anatomic sites of lymphocyte differentiation. The studies showed that when this tissue was destroyed in the chicken embryos (by removing it surgically or by administering high doses of testosterone), the adult chickens lacked the ability to produce antibodies (humoral immunity was impaired). The chickens also demonstrated a marked reduction in the number of lymphocytes found in specific (bursa-dependent areas) regions of the spleen and lymph nodes. The affected lymphocytes were, thus, named B lymphocytes or B cells. The bursa equivalent in mammals (including humans) is believed to be in special microenvironments in the bone marrow, where the B lymphocytes differentiate into immunocompetent cells. However, there is growing evidence that B lymphocytes may also differentiate in gut-associated lymphatic tissue (GALT) in mammals, particularly in the large aggregations of lymphatic tissue in the ileum, cecum, and appendix. Thus, the B may be considered to refer to the bursa of birds or the "bursa equivalent" of mammals.

Investigators studying newborn mice found that removal of the thymus resulted in profound deficiencies in the cell-mediated immune responses (immune responses requiring the presence of cells of the immune system, in contrast to humoral responses involving only circulating antibodies or immunoglobulins). The rejection of transplanted skin from a heterologous donor is an example of cellular immune response. Thymectomized mice demonstrated a marked reduction in the number of lymphocytes found in specific regions of the spleen and the lymph nodes (thymus-dependent areas). The areas of depletion were different from those identified after removal of the bursa of Fabricius in the chicken. The affected lymphocytes were, thus, named T lymphocytes or T cells.

Responses to Antigens

The response of the immune system to antigen progresses along two distinctive pathways:

- *Cell-mediated response,* leading to *cell-mediated immunity*
- *Humoral response,* leading to *antibody-mediated immunity*

The humoral response is mediated by *B lymphocytes,* which produce antibodies that act directly on an invading agent. In some diseases, e.g., tetanus, a nonimmune person can be rendered immune by receiving an injection of antibody purified from the blood of an immune person or animal. The effectiveness of this passive transfer proves that it is the antibody that is responsible for the protection. With other diseases, e.g., smallpox, the passive transfer of antibody is of no value. In these instances, it is necessary to transfer lymphocytes or, more specifically, *T lymphocytes* in order to obtain protection by passive immunity.

The differentiation of the immune system and the origin of immunocompetent lymphocytes presented below are summarized in Figure 13.2.

T and *B lymphocytes* both derive originally from stem lymphocytes in the bone marrow, but they mature by different routes. Lymphocytes engaged in the cell-mediated response derive their immunologic competency in the thymus. For this reason, the response is also called the **thymus-dependent response,** and the effector lymphocytes are designated as T lymphocytes. The sites of maturation of stem lymphocytes into B lymphocytes, as also noted, include the bone marrow and GALT. In birds, the lymphocytes are processed in the bursa of Fabricius, a gut-associated lymphatic organ.

CELLS OF THE LYMPHATIC SYSTEM

B Lymphocytes

B Lymphocytes May Differentiate Into Plasma Cells That Produce Antibodies or Into Memory Cells

A given B lymphocyte reacts only with a single antigen or type of antigenic site to which it is genetically programmed to react. B lymphocytes do not respond when exposed to other antigens. B lymphocytes that have been activated by contact with antigen transform into *immunoblasts (plasmablasts)* that proliferate and then differentiate into

- *Plasma cells,* which synthesize and secrete a specific antibody
- *Memory cells,* which are able to respond more quickly to the next encounter with the same antigen

The specific antibody produced by the plasma cell binds to the stimulating antigen, forming an *antigen-antibody complex.* These complexes are eliminated in a number of ways (Fig. 13.2), including phagocytosis by macrophages and eosinophils. The complexes may also activate a system of plasma proteins, the *complement system,* and cause one of the components, C3, to bind to an antigenic bacterium and act as a ligand for its phagocytosis by macrophages. Complement binding, induced by the antigen-antibody complex, may also cause foreign cells to lyse.

The initial response to an antigen is initiated by only a few or a single B lymphocyte that has been genetically programmed to respond to that specific antigen. Memory cells are only produced after the initial exposure to a specific antigen. Therefore, as noted above, memory cells do not participate in the initial or *primary response* to a specific antigen. However, memory cells are programmed and ready to respond to the same antigen should it appear again. The

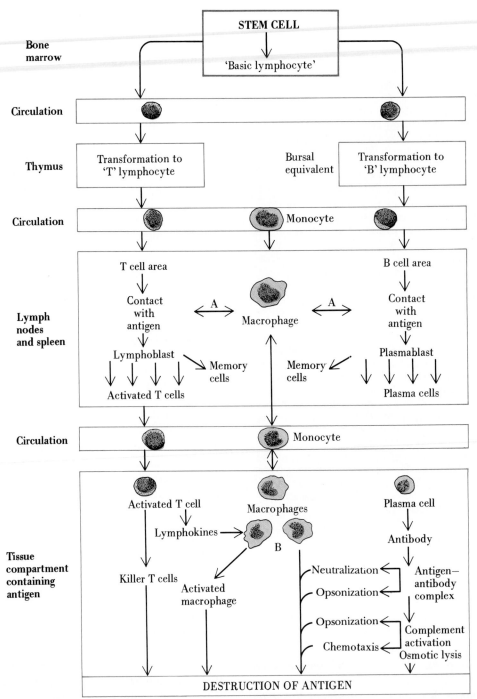

Figure 13.2. Outline of lymphocyte interactions. Mature lymphocytes are designated as either T or B lymphocytes according to whether they are transformed within the thymus or the bursal equivalent in mammals. T and B lymphocytes from the thymus and bursal equivalent populate the spleen, lymph nodes, and lymphatic nodules. On exposure of the lymphatic tissue to antigen, new lymphocytes are generated in these lymphatic organs. The new lymphocytes are activated so that they can react with the specific antigen responsible for their generation. The activated T cells and plasma cells react with the antigen by mechanisms that result in the destruction and removal of the antigen. Reactions involving chiefly T lymphocytes are referred to as constituting the cellular response; reactions involving chiefly B lymphocytes are referred to as constituting the humoral response. In both, macrophages participate with the lymphocytes at two different levels of the chain. They may participate in the initial presentation of antigen to the lymphocyte (A), or they may be involved in the final destruction and disposal of the antigen (B). Memory cells do not participate in the initial response to antigen; they remain in the body, programmed to react at a later time to the same specific antigen in what is designated as the secondary response. The outline depicts those reactions of lymphocytes that are beneficial to the host and that result in the development of immunity. (Modified from Wheater PR, et al: *Functional Histology.* New York, Churchill Livingstone, 1979, p 146.)

response to the same antigen on subsequent exposure is called the *secondary response.* It is more rapid and intense than the primary response because of the presence of a population of specific memory B lymphocytes already programmed to respond to that antigen.

Table 13.1 summarizes the characteristics of various human immunoglobulins (Ig), and Figure 13.3 presents the structure of an antibody molecule in schematic form. Antibodies are produced by B cells and by plasma cells derived from B cells.

HYPERSENSITIVITY

When an individual has been immunologically sensitized by an exposure to an antigen, a subsequent exposure may lead not just to a boosting of the immune response (secondary response) but also to tissue-damaging reactions designated as *hypersensitivity reactions.* Such reactions are observed in sensitized human subjects following insect bites or injections of penicillin. One type of hypersensitivity reaction familiar to many is the allergic reaction. Certain aspects of a hypersensitivity reaction are brought about by the antibody-induced discharge of mast cell granules. These granules contain mediators such as histamine that account for the distressing features of hypersensitivity reactions. Eosinophils are attracted to the site of mast cell degranulation and neutralize the effects of the released mediators. Thus, eosinophils are frequently seen in the connective tissue at allergic or other hypersensitivity reaction sites.

T Lymphocytes

Immunocompetent T lymphocytes that have been activated by interaction with an antigen also transform into lymphoblasts that proliferate and differentiate into several types of effector T lymphocytes and memory cells. Three types of T lymphocytes have been identified:

- *Cytotoxic lymphocytes (CTLs) or killer T cells,* which serve as the primary effector cells in cell-mediated immunity
- *Helper T lymphocytes (T_H cells),* which assist B cells as well as other T cells in their response to antigens
- *Suppressor T lymphocytes (T_S cells),* which suppress the activity of B cells

The primary function of cytotoxic lymphocytes is to screen other cells for signs of viral infection or other signs of abnormality, such as development into cancer cells. The antigen receptors on the killer cells enable them to recognize viral or cancer-related peptides on the surface of cells and to kill the cells by causing them to lyse. A classic target of a CTL is a virus-infected cell that displays viral glycoproteins on its surface.

Helper T cells assist in the stimulation of B lymphocytes to produce antibodies. T_H cells have surface receptors that bind to a surface peptide complex on the membrane of macrophages or B cells that have "processed" an antigen (see page 333). This stimulates the helper T cells to become active, dividing and producing polypeptide hormones called *interleukins* that, in turn, stimulate B cells to divide and produce their antibodies. Few antigenic molecules can stimulate the B cells by themselves. Thus, the major function of the T_H cell is to recognize foreign antigens presented by macrophages and then to secrete *interleukins* that stimulate B cells or other cells that participate in immune reactions, such as CTLs or additional macrophages (see Table 9.5, page 206).

Although all of the functions of suppressor T cells have yet to be elucidated, their existence is now generally accepted. They have been shown to suppress specifically the response to a given antigen, to suppress the immune response generally, to inhibit helper T cells, B cells, and plasma cells directly, and to participate in delayed hypersensitivity reactions (allergic reactions).

The T cells may also function in the regulation of erythroid cell maturation in the bone marrow. The activities of the various types of T lymphocytes are mediated by molecules located on their surface. By employing immunolabeling techniques, it has been possible to identify specific types of T cells and study their function. Some T lymphocytes also form memory cells.

Lymphokines and Interleukins

Lymphokines are soluble substances released by sensitized lymphocytes on contact with a specific antigen. Along with other functions, these substances stimulate the activity of monocytes and macrophages in the cell-mediated immune response. Included among these substances are chemotactic, mitogenic, and migration inhibitory factors, interferon, and lymphotoxin, along with the lymphokines.

The immune system is regulated by hormones in a manner similar to other organ systems. Interleukin-2 was the first hormone of the immune system to be discovered and characterized. Presently, more than 10 interleukins have been identified. However, their functions in the immune response have not been fully elucidated. The most promising current research on therapeutic approaches to autoimmune diseases, acquired immunodeficiency syndrome (AIDS), and organ-transplant rejection is based on the biology of these hormones.

The Number of the Various Types of Lymphocytes in Peripheral Blood Is Related to Disease

Clinical laboratories utilizing immunolabeling techniques can assess the presence of specific classes of lymphocytes in blood samples. This provides an opportunity to assess the immune state of a patient. Elevation or depression of the levels of certain classes of lymphocytes is related to specific diseases. For example, in persons infected

TABLE 13.1. Characteristics of Human Immunoglobulins

ISOTYPE	MOLECULAR WEIGHT	AVERAGE ADULT SERUM LEVEL (mg/ml)	CELLS TO WHICH BOUND VIA Fc REGION	BIOLOGIC PROPERTIES
IgG	150,000	12	Macrophages, neutrophils, eosinophils, and large granular lymphocytes	Activates complement (a group of serum constituents having the capacity to lyse cells and bacteria); crosses placenta, providing the newborn with passive immunity; principal Ig produced during secondary antibody response
IgM	190,000 (950,000)[A]	1	Lymphocytes	Fixes complement; activates macrophages; rheumatoid factor; Ig produced during primary antibody response
IgA	160,000 (385,000)[B]	2	Lymphocytes	Antibody present in body secretions, including tears, colostrum, saliva, and vaginal fluid, and in the secretions of the nasal cavity, bronchi, intestine, and prostate (IgA provides protection against the proliferation of microorganisms in these fluids and aids in the defense against microbes and foreign molecules penetrating the body via the cells lining these cavities)
IgD	175,000	0.03	None	Found mainly on surface of lymphocytes (only traces in serum) and is involved in the differentiation of lymphocytes
IgE	190,000	0.0003	Mast cells and basophils	Stimulates mast cells to release histamine, heparin, leukotrienes (slow-reacting substance of anaphylaxis), and eosinophil chemotactic factor of anaphylaxis (mediates anaphylaxis, allergy)

[A] IgM found in serum as a pentameric molecule.
[B] IgA found in serum as a dimeric molecule.

with the AIDS-causing human immunodeficiency virus (HIV), the number of helper T cells is dramatically reduced. These patients are vulnerable to severe infections that eventually prove fatal. In normal peripheral blood, approximately 20–30% of the total leukocytes are lymphocytes; only 4–10% of the circulating lymphocytes demonstrate immunoglobulins on their surface and are classified as B cells.

Large Lymphocytes

Large Lymphocytes Make Up Only a Small Percentage of Lymphocytes in the Blood

Large lymphocytes, also called *"null cells,"* account for 5–10% of the lymphocytes in peripheral blood (see Plate 25, Figs. 3 and 4, page 211). These cells contain large azurophilic cytoplasmic granules and are nonadherent and nonphagocytic. Two subclasses of large lymphocytes occur:

- *Natural killer (NK) cells,* whose activity does not depend on antigen activation

- A subset of the large lymphocytes that mediate *antibody-dependent cellular cytotoxicity (ADCC)*

NK cells, lacking the surface molecules associated with the activities of T or B lymphocytes, can also cause lysis of target cells. The killing of target cells, usually malignant cell types, is a nonantibody-mediated process. This population of large lymphocytes may play an important role in immune surveillance and the destruction of cells that undergo spontaneous transformation into malignant cells and are, therefore, recognizable as nonself.

ADCC involves binding of an antibody or antibody- and complement-coated *(opsonized)* target cell to an effector cell bearing a receptor for the Fc portion of the antibody (see Fig. 13.3). The binding, through the Fc region, results in the lysis of the target cell.

Antigen-Presenting Cells

Antigen-Presenting Cells Interact with Helper T Cells to Facilitate Immune Responses

The interaction between most antigens and the antibodies on the surface of B cells is insufficient to stimulate B-

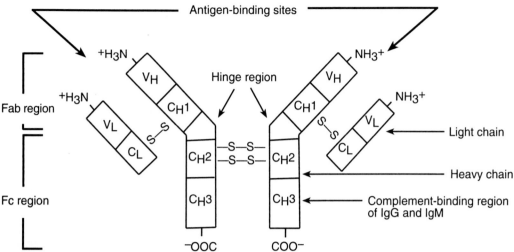

Figure 13.3. Schematic diagram of an antibody molecule. The Y-shaped molecule binds antigens at the two sites indicated where the heavy and light chains are associated with each other. The immunoglobulin isotypes (see Table 13.1) are determined by the type of heavy and light chains present. The four chains (two heavy and two light) making up the molecule are covalently linked by disulfide bonds. Each polypeptide chain is composed of domains of amino acids that are constant (C) or variable (V) in their sequence. The subscripts, H and L, refer to the heavy and light chains. Two regions, Fab and Fc, having unique functions are also indicated. Enzymes can be used to cleave the molecule into two fragments that bind to antigens (Fab) and one fragment that is composed of constant regions of the heavy chains and, in some isotypes, binds complement (Fc). The constant regions of the heavy chain are involved in biologic functions of the immunoglobulin (Ig) molecules. The isotypes demonstrate specific amino acid domains in the three C_H regions of the molecule indicated as C_H1, C_H2, and C_H3. The C_H region at the carboxy terminus functions in the binding of the molecule to Fc receptors of macrophages, lymphocytes, mast cells, basophils, eosinophils, neutrophils, and large granular lymphocytes (see Table 13.1).

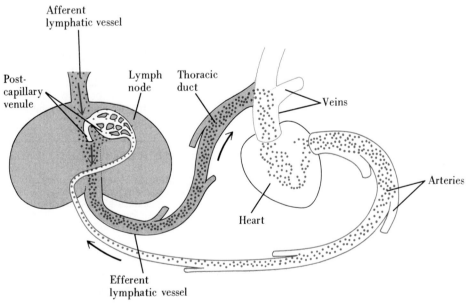

Figure 13.4. Diagram depicting circulation of lymphocytes beginning at a lymph node. Lymphocytes enter lymph nodes by two routes: afferent lymphatic vessels (only one is shown) and through the wall of the postcapillary venules. Some lymphocytes move to the T and B domains of the lymph node; others pass through the substance of the node and leave via an efferent lymphatic vessel. Ultimately, the lymphocytes enter a major lymphatic vessel—in this case the thoracic duct—that opens into the large veins in the root of the neck, whereupon the lymphocytes become components of the blood. The lymphocytes continue to the arterial side of the circulation and, via the arteries, to the lymphatic tissues of the body or to tissues where they participate in immune reactions. From the lymphatic tissues, lymphocytes again return to the lymph nodes to gain entry via the postcapillary venules. The above scheme describes a recirculation of lymphocytes that involves all lymphatic tissue except the thymus. (Based on Gowans JE: *Hospital Practice* 3:34, 1968.)

TABLE 13.2. Characteristics of the Effector Cells of the Immune System[A]

CELL TYPE	FUNCTIONAL SURFACE MOLECULE	CELLULAR FUNCTIONS MEDIATED BY THE SURFACE MOLECULES
T lymphocyte	T3/T-cell-antigen receptor complex (involving T3 receptors and other surface molecules)	Antigen recognition; T-cell activation
	T11	T-cell activation
	T4	Molecule present on helper and some cytotoxic T cells; T4 molecules facilitate antigen recognition; the AIDS virus (HTLV) infects the subset of T cells carrying this surface molecule
	T8	Molecule present on suppressor and cytotoxic T cells that facilitates recognition of antigens via the major histocompatibility complex (MHC) molecules
	Interleukin-2 (IL-2) receptor	Binds IL-2 to T cells
B lymphocyte	Surface immunoglobulins (sIg)[B]	Antigen recognition; cell activation
	IgG Fc receptors	Bind immune complexes
	C3 (complement) receptors	
Large granular lymphocyte	IgG receptors	Bind immune complexes
Monocyte-macrophage	IgG Fc receptors	Bind and phagocytose immune complexes
	C3 (complement) receptors	
	Major histocompatibility complex (MHC) class II antigens	Presentation of antigen to T and B cells
	Chemotactic receptors	Chemotaxis and polarization of cells
Neutrophils	IgG Fc receptors	Bind and phagocytose immune complexes
	C3 (complement) receptors	
	Chemotactic receptors	Chemotaxis and polarization of cells
Eosinophil	IgG Fc receptors	Bind and phagocytose immune complexes
	C3 (complement) receptors	
Basophil-mast cell	IgE Fc receptors	After binding of antigen (allergen)-IgE complexes to receptors, release of granules containing histamine, slow-reacting substance of anaphylaxis, eosinophil chemotactic factor of anaphylaxis, platelet activation factor, neutrophil chemotactic factor, leukotactic activity, heparin, and basophil kallikrein of anaphylaxis
	C3 (complement) receptors	

[A]Modified from Haynes BF, Faver AS: introduction to clinical immunology. In: Braunwald E, et al (eds): *Harrison's Principles of Internal Medicine*, 11th ed. New York, McGraw-Hill, 1987, pp 328–337.
[B]Precursor B cells contain immunoglobulin M in their cytoplasm (cIgM). As they mature in the bone marrow, they express IgM on their surface (sIgM) and no longer express cIgM. With continued maturation, prior to exposure to specific antigens (i.e., antigen-independent maturation), the production of immunoglobulins switches, so that IgD molecules are expressed on the cell surface along with either IgM, IgG, IgA, or IgE. Each B cell expresses Ig molecules of only one heavy and light chain variable and thus are specific for a specific antigen. On contact with that antigen, mature B cells terminally differentiate into antibody-secreting plasma cells or proliferate to produce long-lived memory cells.

cell growth, differentiation, and secretion of soluble antibody. For the lymphocytes to function effectively, antigens are processed and presented to them by ***antigen-presenting cells.*** Although the molecular events involved in this process have not been elucidated fully, it is clear that several cell types are involved, including some B cells, tissue macrophages, perisinusoidal macrophages (Kupffer cells) of the liver, Langerhans' cells in the epidermis, and ***follicular dendritic cells*** found in the germinal center of lymphatic nodules. The follicular dendritic cells, considered to be a subclass of the ***lymphatic dendritic cells*** (see page 339), are pale-staining, nonphagocytic cells with long motile cytoplasmic processes that extend along the reticular meshwork. Most of the antigen-presenting cells phagocytize the "foreign" proteins or toxins, break them down to peptides, and bind the peptides to histocompatibility proteins that are transported to the plasma membrane. Then, helper T cells that have surface receptors for the peptide complex bind to the antigen-presenting cells. This, in turn, stimulates the helper T cells to become active, to divide, and to produce factors called interleukins. These, in turn, stimulate B cells to divide and produce their antibodies.

Table 13.2 presents a brief summary of the characteristics of the effector cells of the immune system and the functions associated with their unique cell surface membrane proteins.

Typically, in a response to a foreign substance, both cellular and humoral immune systems are involved, although one system generally predominates in favor of the other according to the stimulus.

Macrophages and the Immune Response

Macrophages are closely associated with lymphocytes in both types of immune response. Macrophages can

- *Process and present the antigen* to the B cells or helper T cells (A in Fig. 13.2)
- *Destroy (digest) the antigen* (B in Fig. 13.2) after it has been processed by other cells of the immune system

Macrophages Have Important Roles at Several Points in the Immune Response

Normally, the only immune responses that are triggered directly by antigens are those to cells that carry nonself *histocompatibility molecules* on their surface. Histocompatibility molecules (major histocompatibility antigens) are gene products of a "supergene" located on chromosome 6 in humans that is known as the *major histocompatibility gene complex.* The expression of this gene complex produces molecules that insert on cell surfaces and are specific not only for the individual cell that produces them but also for the tissue type and degree of cellular differentiation. In other cases, an effective immune response requires the presence of a cell, other than the lymphocyte, that carries an autologous histocompatibility molecule on its surface (a molecule that is recognized as "self" by the lymphocytes) and presents it to the lymphocyte along with the antigen. It is believed that a macrophage plays this role.

Although the precise mechanism for this *antigen presentation* is unclear, it has been shown that small amounts of antigen bind to the surface of macrophages, that intimate physical contact occurs between macrophages and lymphocytes, and that blockage of macrophages by overloading with inert particulate materials reduces the immune response. In addition, macrophages certainly remove excess antigen, so that the possibility of developing antigen tolerance is reduced. Macrophages also secrete lymphokines that stimulate proliferation and differentiation of lymphocytes.

Some investigators object to this theory. They claim that ordinary macrophages could not discriminate adequately in their phagocytic activity to destroy all but a small amount of the antigen they phagocytize and save it for reinsertion into the plasma membrane. They maintain that it is the *lymphatic dendritic cell* that has all of the properties ascribed to the macrophage in the initiation phase of the immune response. It is still unclear whether these cells represent a distinct population of cells or whether they are merely a particular strain of macrophage, possibly one similar to those found in the lamina propria of the gut, that may originate as the terminal differentiation of the fibroblast-like cell that gives rise to the reticular cells. It does not appear that the dendritic cells are derived from blood-borne monocytes.

Terminal Events in the Immune Response

Macrophages Phagocytose Bacteria and Foreign Cells That Have Been Attacked by Lymphocytes and Lytic Antibodies

Although whether the macrophage plays an important role in *antigen presentation* may be argued, it clearly plays an important role in *antigen disposal* after the immune response has been initiated. Macrophages react even more strongly to cells, bacteria, and materials that have been opsonized (complexed with specific antibody or with antibody and complement components). [Eosinophils and neutrophils may also be stimulated to greater phagocytic activity by opsonization of the material to be phagocytosed.]

Macrophages also play a vital role in sequestration and removal of foreign materials and organisms that either do not provoke an immune response or are ingested but not digested. These include both organic and inorganic particulate materials, such as carbon particles, cellulose, and asbestos, as well as the bacilli of tuberculosis and leprosy and the organisms that cause malaria and other diseases. In these instances, macrophages often fuse to form multinucleate, foreign-body giant cells (Langhans' giant cells) that isolate these pathogens from the body.

LYMPHATIC VESSELS AND THE CIRCULATION OF LYMPHOCYTES

Lymphatic Vessels Are the Route by Which Cells and Large Molecules Pass From the Tissue Spaces Back to the Blood

Lymphatic vessels begin as networks of "blind-ending" capillaries in the loose connective tissue. They are most numerous under the epithelium of skin and mucous membranes. These vessels remove substances and fluid from the extracellular spaces of the connective tissues, thus producing lymph. [The largest amount of lymph originates in the perisinusoidal spaces of the liver (see page 501).] Because the walls of the lymphatic capillaries are more permeable than the walls of blood capillaries, large molecules including foreign substances and cells gain entry more readily into the lymphatic capillaries than into blood capillaries.

As the lymph circulates through the lymphatic vessels, it passes through lymph nodes. Here, foreign substances (antigens) conveyed in the lymph are concentrated by the dendritic cells and presented to the lymphocytes. This leads to the cascade of steps that constitute the immune response.

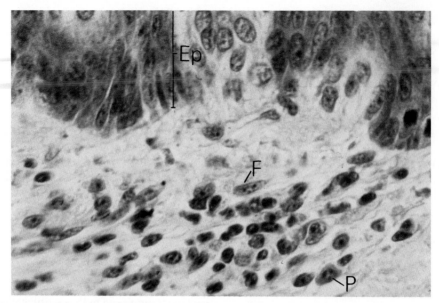

Figure 13.5. Light micrograph of diffuse lymphatic tissue of the tongue. The connective tissue underlying the epithelium *(Ep)* is very cellular. Included in this cell population are some fibroblasts *(F);* the bulk of the cells, however, are lymphocytes and, to a lesser extent, plasma cells *(P).*

Lymphatic vessels ultimately drain the lymph into the bloodstream by joining the venous system at the junctions of the internal jugular and subclavian veins in the neck.

The circulation of lymphocytes through the lymphatic vessels and the bloodstream enables them to move from one part of the lymphatic system to another at different stages in their development and to reach sites within the body where they are needed. An outline of lymphocyte circulation showing a lymph node as a starting point is depicted in Figure 13.4. It shows lymphocytes conveyed in the lymph, entering the node via afferent lymphatic vessels, and lymphocytes conveyed in the blood, entering the node through the wall of postcapillary venules. B and T cells migrate to and populate different regions within the lymph node:

- *B cells* are most numerous in the *medulla* and in the lymphatic *nodules* of the cortex.
- *T cells* are concentrated in the *paracortex* located beneath and around the lymphatic nodules.

Some lymphocytes pass through the substance of the node and leave via the efferent lymphatic vessels. The latter lead ultimately to the right lymphatic duct or, as shown in the illustration, to the thoracic duct. In turn, both of these channels empty into the blood circulation by draining into the large veins in the root of the neck. The lymphocytes are conveyed to and from the various lymphatic tissues via the blood vessels. (The venous component of the blood vascular circulation has not been included in the scheme.) The scheme depicts a recirculation of lymphocytes. Note that all lymphatic tissue except the thymus appears to be in the recirculation route.

Lymphocyte biology is a major subject in immunology and is beyond the scope of this book. The material in this chapter is intended to alert the reader to the realization that the lymphatic system is a dynamic system in which the lymphocytes play a major role in the immune response. Furthermore, lymphocytes are a heterogeneous group of cells that populate the lymphatic organs and tissues and have functions throughout the body. It will be useful in studying the following sections of this chapter to keep in mind the overall functions of the lymphatic system:

- *Concentrate antigens* in certain lymphatic organs
- *Circulate lymphocytes* through these organs so that they can come into contact with antigens
- *Convey products* of the immune response (such as T cells, B cells, plasma cells, and antibodies) to tissues where they are needed
- *Eliminate antigens* from the body

DIFFUSE LYMPHATIC TISSUE AND LYMPHATIC NODULES

Diffuse Lymphatic Tissue and Nodules **Guard the Body From and Respond to Entry of Infectious Organisms and Toxins**

Diffuse Lymphatic Tissue. The alimentary canal, respiratory passages, and genitourinary tract are guarded by accumulations of lymphatic tissue that are not enclosed by a capsule. Lymphocytes and other free cells of this tissue are found in the **lamina propria** (subepithelial tissue) of these tracts. This form of lymphatic tissue is called *diffuse lymphatic tissue* (Fig. 13.5). The cells of the diffuse lymphatic tissue are not static; rather, they are strategically located to intercept and react with antigen and then to travel to regional lymph nodes, where they undergo proliferation and differentiation. Progeny of the cells that have traveled to the regional lymph nodes then return to the lamina propria as effector B and T lymphocytes, as plasma cells, and as memory cells.

The importance of diffuse lymphatic tissue in protecting the body from foreign antigens is emphasized by

- The regular presence of large numbers of plasma cells, especially in the lamina propria of the gastrointestinal tract, a morphologic indication of local antibody secretion
- The presence of large numbers of eosinophils, also frequently observed in the lamina propria of the intestinal and respiratory tracts, an indication of chronic inflammation and hypersensitivity reactions

Lymphatic Nodules. In addition to diffuse lymphatic tissue, localized concentrations of lymphocytes are commonly seen in the walls of the alimentary canal, respiratory passages, and genitourinary tract, as well as in other parts of the body. These concentrations, called ***lymphatic nodules or follicles,*** are sharply defined but are not encapsulated (Fig. 13.6). Generally, the nodules are disposed singly in a random manner. In the alimentary canal, however, some aggregations of nodules are found in specific locations. These include

- ***Appendix*** and ***cecum***
- ***Tonsils,*** which form a ring of lymphatic tissue at the entrance of the oropharynx (see page 424)
- ***Distal small intestine,*** i.e., the ileum ***(Peyer's patches)***

The ***pharyngeal tonsils*** or ***adenoids,*** located in the roof of the pharynx, the ***palatine tonsils*** or, simply, the tonsils, on either side of the pharynx between the faucial pillars, and the ***lingual tonsils,*** in the base of the tongue, all contain aggregates of lymphatic nodules. The intestinal tract also contains numerous isolated nodules as well as aggregations of nodules that are most numerous in the ileum (Fig. 13.7); these are called ***Peyer's patches*** (see page 457). As noted earlier, the diffuse lymphatic tissue and the nodules of the alimentary canal together are referred to as the ***gut-associated lymphatic tissue (GALT).*** All of these nodules are reactive lymphatic tissue and become enlarged during encounters with antigen. Lymphatic nodules also constitute the unit structure in the lymph node (see below).

Lymphatic Nodules Are Oval Concentrations of Lymphocytes Contained in Meshworks of Reticular Cells

A nodule consisting chiefly of small lymphocytes is called a ***primary nodule.*** Many, if not most, nodules are, however, ***secondary nodules*** and have distinctive features:

- A central region, called a ***germinal center*** (see Fig. 13.6) that, in histologic sections, appears to stain less intensely than
- An outer ring of small lymphocytes

The germinal center is a reaction center that develops when a lymphocyte that has recognized an antigen returns

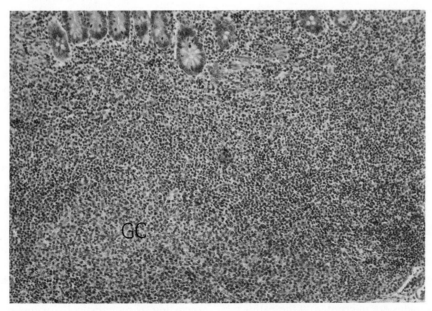

Figure 13.6. Light micrograph of a lymphatic nodule in the lamina propria of the small intestine. The basal portions of some of the intestinal glands are present in the upper part of the micrograph. The remainder of the figure is occupied by the nodule, a compact mass of cells composed mostly of lympho-cytes. A germinal center *(GC)* is evident in the lower left of the nodule. The lymphocytes here are larger than those in Figure 13.5; they have more cytoplasm, and collectively, their nuclei appear as a less compact mass.

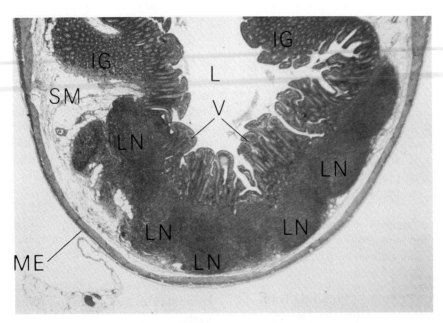

Figure 13.7. Light micrograph showing an aggregation of lymphatic nodules *(LN)* in the wall of the ileum. Such an aggregation is called a Peyer's patch. The nodules originate in the lamina propria located partly in the mucosa and extend into the submucosa *(SM)*. *IG,* intestinal glands; *L,* lumen of ileum; *ME,* muscularis externa; and *V,* villi.

to a primary nodule and undergoes blastic transformation. The lighter staining is due to the fact that the germinal center contains large lymphocytes *(lymphoblasts and plasmablasts)* that have large amounts of dispersed euchromatin in their nuclei rather than the dense heterochromatin of the small lymphocytes. The germinal center is a morphologic indication of lymphatic tissue response to antigen. The presence of a germinal center represents a cascade of events that includes proliferation of lymphocytes, differentiation of plasma cells, and antibody production. Frequently, mitotic figures are observed in the germinal center, a reflection of the proliferation of new lymphocytes at this site. The number of macrophages in the germinal center often increases dramatically following a period of intense response to an antigen. These macrophages phagocytize newly formed lymphocytes that fail to develop correctly.

LYMPH NODES

Lymph Nodes Are Small Encapsulated Organs Located Along the Pathway of Lymphatic Vessels

Lymph nodes are small, bean-shaped, encapsulated lymphatic organs. They range in size from about 1 mm (barely visible with the unaided eye) to about 1–2 cm in their longest dimension. Lymph nodes are interposed in the pathway of lymphatic vessels (Fig. 13.8) and serve as filters through which lymph percolates on its way to the blood. They are widely distributed throughout the body but are concentrated in certain regions such as the axilla, groin, and mesenteries.

Two types of lymphatic vessels serve the nodes:

• *Afferent lymphatic vessels* convey lymph toward the node and enter at various points on the convex surface of the capsule.
• *Efferent lymphatic vessels* convey lymph away from the node and leave at the hilum, a depression on the concave surface of the node that also serves for the entry and exit of blood vessels and nerves.

Note that antigen-transformed lymphocytes, which remain in the lymph node to proliferate and differentiate, are brought to the node primarily by blood vessels.

The supporting elements of the lymph node are

• *Capsule,* composed of dense connective tissue that surrounds the node
• *Trabeculae,* also composed of dense connective tissue, which extend from the capsule into the substance of the node, forming a gross framework
• *Reticular tissue,* composed of reticular cells and reticular fibers that form a fine supporting meshwork throughout the remainder of the organ (Fig. 13.9)

Traditionally, the reticular meshwork of lymphatic tissues and organs (except the thymus) has been described as consisting of reticular cells of mesenchymal origin and reticular fibers and ground substance produced by those cells. The reticular cells appear as stellate or elongated cells with an oval euchromatic nucleus. There is a small amount of acidophilic cytoplasm. These cells can be shown to take up

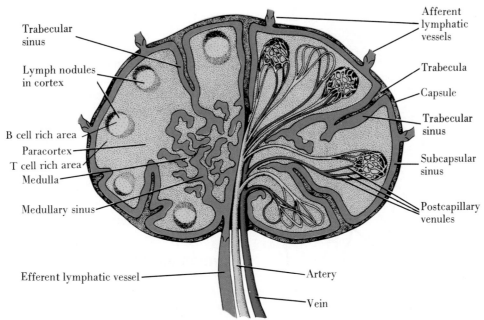

Trabecular
sinus

Lymph nodules
in cortex

B cell rich area
Paracortex
T cell rich area
Medulla

Medullary sinus

Afferent
lymphatic
vessels

Trabecula

Capsule

Trabecular
sinus

Subcapsular
sinus

Postcapillary
venules

Efferent lymphatic vessel

Artery

Vein

Figure 13.8. Schematic diagram of a lymph node. The left side of the figure depicts the general features of a lymph node as seen in a section. The substance of the lymph node is divided into a cortex, including a paracortical region, and a medulla. The cortex is the outermost portion; it contains spherical or oval aggregates of lymphocytes called lymphatic nodules. In an active lymph node, these contain a lighter center called the germinal center. The medulla is the innermost region of the lymph node and extends as far as the hilum of the node. It consists of regions of lymphatic tissue, appearing as irregular cords in section, separated by lymphatic sinuses that, because of their location in the medulla, are referred to as medullary sinuses. The dense population of lymphocytes between the cortex and the medulla constitutes the paracortex. This is the region of the node that contains the postcapillary venules. Surrounding the lymph node is a capsule of dense connective tissue from which trabeculae extend into the substance of the node. Under the capsule and adjacent to the trabeculae are, respectively, the subcapsular (or cortical) sinus and the trabecular lymphatic sinuses. Afferent lymphatic vessels penetrate the capsule and empty into the subcapsular sinus. The subcapsular sinus and trabecular sinuses communicate with the medullary sinuses. The right side of the lymph node also shows an artery and vein and the location of the postcapillary venules of the lymph node. (Based on Bloom W, Fawcett DW: *A Textbook of Histology,* 10th ed. Philadelphia, WB Saunders, 1975, p 473.)

dyes and colloidal materials. Transmission electron microscopy, immunocytochemistry, and autoradiography indicate that there are two populations of cells:

- "Reticular" cells indistinguishable from typical fibroblasts that synthesize and secrete collagen (reticular fibers) and associated ground substance that forms the stroma observed with the light microscope
- "Reticular" cells that have functions characteristic of tissue macrophages (see above, *antigen-presenting cells*)

Processes of the cells with fibroblast function wrap around the bundles of reticular fibers, effectively isolating these structural components from the lymphocytic parenchyma of the lymphatic tissue and organs (Fig. 13.10). The macrophage-like cells (dendritic cells) are splayed along the meshwork formed by the reticular fibers and reticular cell processes, thus increasing the potential surface area for phagocytosis and other cell interactions.

The parenchyma of the lymph node is divided into *cortex* and *medulla* (Fig. 13.11). The *cortex* forms the outer portion of the node except at the hilum. It consists of a dense mass of lymphatic tissue (reticular framework, lymphocytes, macrophages, and plasma cells) and lymphatic sinuses, the lymph channels.

The Lymphocytes in the Outer Part of the Cortex Are Organized Into Nodules

As elsewhere, the lymphatic nodules of the cortex are designated as primary nodules if they consist chiefly of small lymphocytes and as secondary nodules if they possess a germinal center, a region in which new lymphocytes are produced in response to an antigenic stimulus. The portion of the cortex adjacent to the medulla is free of nodules; it is called the *deep cortex,* juxtamedullary cortex, or paracortex. The development of this region is dependent on an adequate supply of T cells. Perinatal thymectomy in animals results in a poorly developed paracortical zone. Because of this observation, the deep cortex is also called the *thymus-dependent cortex.*

The *medulla* is the inner part of the node. It consists of cords of lymphatic tissue separated by lymphatic sinuses called *medullary sinuses.* As described above, a network of reticular cells and fibers traverses the medullary cords and medullary sinuses and serves as the framework of the

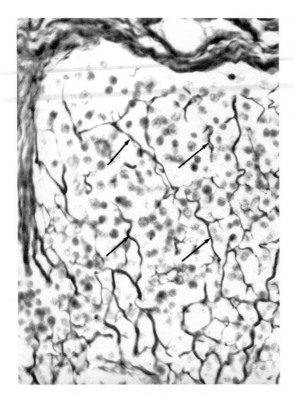

Figure 13.9. Photomicrograph of a lymph node, silver preparation, showing the connective tissue capsule at the top and trabecula extending from it at the left. The reticular fibers *(arrows)* form an irregular anastomosing network.

parenchyma. In addition to reticular cells, the medullary cords contain lymphocytes (mostly B lymphocytes), macrophages, and plasma cells. The medullary sinuses converge toward the region of the hilum, where they drain into efferent lymphatic vessels.

The specific distribution of B and T Lymphocytes may be summarized as follows:

- *B lymphocytes* are most common in the *cortex* and *medullary cords*.
- *T lymphocytes* are most common in the *deep cortex* or *paracortex*.
- Both *B* and *T lymphocytes* are present where the deep and nodular cortex meet.

Lymphatic Sinuses

Just under the capsule of a lymph node there is a sinus interposed between the capsule and the cortical lymphocytes. This is called the **cortical** or **subcapsular sinus**. Afferent lymphatic vessels drain lymph into this sinus. Other lymphatic sinuses extend through the cortex with the trabeculae as **trabecular or peritrabecular sinuses** and drain into medullary sinuses. Lymphocytes and macrophages or their processes readily pass back and forth between the lymphatic sinuses and the parenchyma of the node. The sinuses have a lining of endothelium that is continuous where it is directly adjacent to the connective tissue of the capsule

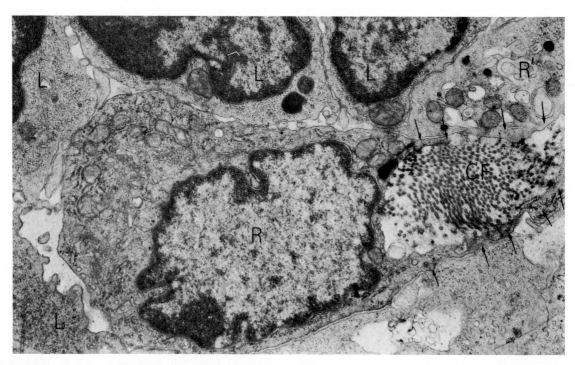

Figure 13.10. Electron micrograph showing a reticular cell *(R)* in association with a bundle of collagen fibrils *(CF)*. With the light microscope and special staining procedures, the bundle of collagen fibrils would be recognized as a reticular fiber. Also present in the micrograph are parts of four lymphocytes *(L)* and the cytoplasm of another reticular cell *(R')*. The collagen fibrils are surrounded by the body and by the processes *(arrows)* of the reticular cells. Thus, the collagen fibrils are not exposed to the lymphocytes.

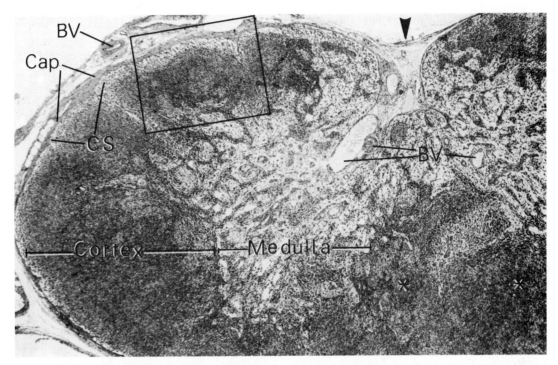

Figure 13.11. Light micrograph of a lymph node. The outermost portion of the lymph node, except at the hilum *(arrowhead)*, is the cortex. It contains dense aggregations of lymphocytes, many organized as lymphatic nodules. The *rectangle* shows a lymphatic nodule with a more lightly stained germinal center. The deep part of the cortex, usually nodule-free *(asterisks)*, is referred to as the paracortex or deep cortex. The innermost portion of the lymph node is the medulla. It extends to the surface of the node at the hilum where blood vessels *(BV)* enter or leave and where efferent lymphatic vessels leave the node. The medulla contains cords of lymphatic tissue and medullary sinuses. Surrounding the lymph node is the capsule *(Cap)* and immediately under this is the cortical sinus *(CS)*. Afferent lymphatic vessels enter the lymph node through the capsule and drain into the cortical sinus. ×20.

or trabeculae but is discontinuous where it faces the lymphatic parenchyma. Even though a macrophage may be in the lymphatic parenchyma, it often sends pseudopods (long cytoplasmic processes) into the sinus through endothelial discontinuities (see Plate 53, page 361). These pseudopods monitor the lymph as it percolates through the sinus.

Lymphatic sinuses are not open spaces, as are blood sinuses. Particularly in the medulla, macrophage processes, along with the reticular fibers surrounded by reticular cell processes, span the lumen of the sinus and form a crisscrossing meshwork that retards the free flow of lymph and enhances the filtration function of the lymph node. Material and cells "trapped" by this mechanical filter are then phagocytosed by the macrophages.

Not only lymph but also lymphocytes constantly circulate through the lymph nodes. Although some lymphocytes enter nodes through afferent lymphatic vessels as components of lymph, more enter the node through the wall of postcapillary venules, located in the deep cortex (see Fig. 13.8 and Plate 51, Fig. 2, page 357). The postcapillary venules are lined by cuboidal or columnar endothelial cells. This unusual endothelium allows lymphocytes to pass through the wall of the vessel but prevents passage of fluid from the vessel to the parenchyma. These cells prevent plasma constituents from reaching the lymphatic parenchyma but allow the lymphocytes to pass through the vessel wall.

Both B and T lymphocytes leave the bloodstream from these postcapillary venules, crossing the endothelium by *diapedesis,* i.e., by migrating between the endothelial cells, in a manner much like a ship passing through a canal lock, and through the basal lamina. The T cells remain in the thymus-dependent cortical zone; the B cells migrate to the nodular cortex. Most lymphocytes leave the lymph node by entering a lymphatic sinus from which they flow to an efferent lymphatic vessel.

Lymph Node Functions

Lymph Nodes Serve as Filters of the Lymph

The phagocytosis of particulate material by phagocytic cells within the lymph nodes can be considered a basic aspect of filtration. The physical obstruction of a lymph node by microorganism and particulate substances conveyed in the lymph and the phagocytosis of the particulate material may lead to concentration of an antigen, thus enhancing its presentation to lymphocytes. As antigens conveyed in the lymph percolate through the sinuses and penetrate the lymph nodules, some of them are trapped on the surface of the follicular dendritic cells. Exposed in this way, the antigens are presented to immunocompetent memory B cells.

Recognition of an antigen by a B cell may necessitate

the involvement of helper T cells to facilitate activation of the B cells. Activated B cells then

- *Migrate to germinal centers*
- *Undergo* a series of *mitotic divisions*
- *Give rise to immature immunoblasts* that proliferate and give rise to plasma cells and memory B cells

The plasma cells then migrate to the medullary cords where they synthesize and release specific antibodies into the lymph flowing through the sinuses. The memory cells may leave the lymph nodes and circulate to various regions through the body. If antigen is encountered, the memory cells proliferate in the manner just described. The presence of memory cells, scattered in various sites throughout the body, results in a more rapid response to an antigen when it is next encountered, i.e., the *secondary* response.

Lymph nodes in which lymphocytes demonstrate response to an antigenic or infectious agent undergo enlargement, reflecting formation of germinal centers and proliferation of lymphocytes. This phenomenon is most often seen in the lymph nodes of the neck in response to nasal or oropharyngeal infection. These enlarged lymph nodes are commonly referred to as "swollen glands." Plasma cells account for 1–3% of the cells in resting lymph nodules. Their number increases dramatically during an immune response, thereby increasing the amount of circulating immunoglobulins.

THYMUS

The thymus is a bilobed organ located in the superior mediastinum anterior to the heart and great vessels. It develops bilaterally from the third (and sometimes also the fourth) branchial (oropharyngeal) pouch. During development, the epithelium invaginates, and the thymic rudiment grows caudally as a tubular prolongation of the endodermal epithelium into the mediastinum of the chest. The advancing tip proliferates and ultimately becomes disconnected from the branchial epithelium.

The Thymus Is Where Stem Lymphocytes Proliferate and Differentiate Into T Lymphocytes

Stem lymphocytes invade the epithelial rudiment and occupy the spaces between the epithelial cells, so that the thymus develops into a lymphoepithelial organ. Although many lymphocytes come to lie between the epithelial cells, the epithelial cells remain joined to one another by desmosomes at the end of long *cytoplasmic* processes. As a consequence, these epithelial cells assume a stellate shape. They form a cytoplasmic reticulum within the parenchyma of the thymus and are designated as *epithelioreticular cells.* The epithelioreticular cells serve as a framework for the thymic lymphocytes; thus, they correspond to the reticular cells and their associated reticular fibers in the other lymphatic tissues and organs. Reticular fibers, however, are *not present* in the thymus.

The essential features of thymic structure illustrated in Figure 13.12 are

- *Cortex,* the outer portion of the parenchyma that contains a high concentration of lymphocytes
- *Medulla,* the inner portion of the parenchyma that contains a lesser number of lymphocytes
- *Capsule,* the external connective tissue that extends trabeculae to the margin of the cortex and medulla

In addition to collagenous fibers and fibroblasts, the connective tissue of the thymus contains variable numbers of plasma cells, granulocytes, lymphocytes, mast cells, fat cells, and macrophages. The capsule and trabeculae also contain blood vessels, efferent *(but not afferent)* lymphatic vessels, and nerves.

The trabeculae establish domains in the thymus called **thymic lobules.** These are not true lobules. They are cortical caps over portions of the highly convoluted but continuous medullary tissue. In some planes of section, the "lobular" arrangement of the cortical cap and medullary tissue superficially resembles a lymphatic nodule with a germinal center. This is often a source of confusion to students. Other morphologic characteristics (described below) allow positive identification of the thymus in histologic sections.

The cortex is extremely basophilic due to the presence of numerous closely packed small lymphocytes with intensely staining nuclei. Some large lymphocytes may be seen close to the capsule. Numerous macrophages are also present for phagocytosis of degenerating (rejected) lymphocytes that were randomly programmed against "self" antigens and, thus, must be destroyed. Macrophages that are heavily laden with lysosomes can be displayed with the periodic acid-Schiff (PAS) reaction. These macrophages have been designated as **PAS cells.**

In contrast, the medulla stains less intensely because, like germinal centers of nodules, it contains mostly large lymphocytes with paler-staining nuclei and quantitatively more cytoplasm than in the small lymphocytes. The epithelioreticular cells of the surrounding meshwork are easily recognized in the medulla. The thymic medulla seen in a histologic section is more heavily infiltrated with lymphocytes than is indicated in the drawing in Figure 13.12.

Thymic or Hassall's Corpuscles Are a Distinctive Feature of the Thymic Medulla

Thymic corpuscles (Fig. 13.13) are isolated masses of closely packed, concentrically arranged epithelioreticular cells. The center of a thymic corpuscle may display evidence of keratinization, a not surprising feature, as the cells are of oropharyngeal origin.

The thymus is fully formed and functional at birth. The characteristic features of thymic structure persist until about

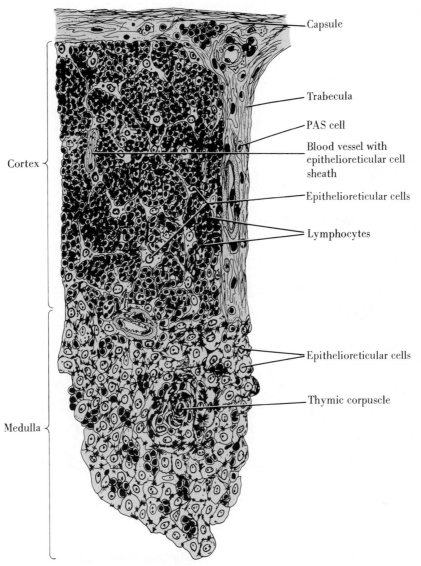

Capsule

Trabecula

PAS cell

Blood vessel with epithelioreticular cell sheath

Epithelioreticular cells

Lymphocytes

Epithelioreticular cells

Thymic corpuscle

Cortex

Medulla

Figure 13.12. Drawing illustrating a portion of a thymic lobule with cortex, medulla, capsule, and trabecula. The cortex contains numerous lymphocytes that are distributed in an apparently random manner between the epithelioreticular cells. The epithelioreticular cells remain joined to each other by means of desmosomes at the ends of long processes. As a consequence, the epithelioreticular cells assume a stellate shape. Fewer lymphocytes are present between the epithelioreticular cells of the medulla. Nevertheless, in an actual thymic section there are more lymphocytes than are depicted in the diagram. Blood vessels within the substance of the thymus are surrounded by epithelioreticular cells or their processes. The concentrically arranged epithelioreticular cells in the medulla constitute a thymic (Hassall's) corpuscle. The capsule and trabecula consist of dense connective tissue. (From Weiss L, Greep RO: *Histology,* 4th ed. New York, McGraw-Hill, 1977, p 505.)

the time of puberty, when lymphocyte processing and proliferation are dramatically reduced and the lymphatic tissue is largely replaced by adipose tissue (involution).

Blood-Thymic Barrier

Blood vessels pass from the trabeculae to enter the substance of the thymus. Typically, the blood vessels enter the medulla from the deeper parts of the trabeculae and carry a sheath of connective tissue along with them. The perivascular connective tissue sheath varies in thickness, being thicker around larger vessels and becoming gradually thin-

ner around smaller vessels. Where it is thick, it contains reticular fibers, fibroblasts, macrophages, plasma cells, and other cells found in loose connective tissue; where it is thin, it may contain only reticular fibers and occasional fibroblasts.

The Blood Vessels of the Thymic Cortex Are Impermeable to Molecules That Pass to the Tissue Spaces in Most Organs

A unique feature of the perivascular connective tissue sheath in the cortex is that it is ensheathed by the epithe-

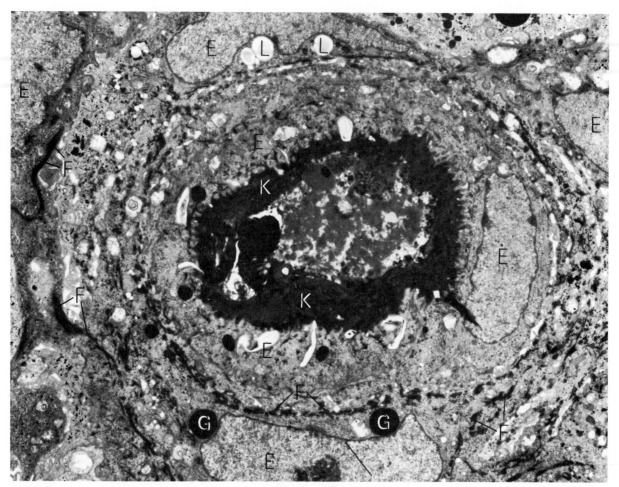

Figure 13.13. Low-power electron micrograph of a thymic (Hassall's) corpuscle. Note the presence of nuclei of concentrically arranged epithelioreticular cells *(E)*, keratohyalin granules *(G)*, bundles of cytoplasmic filaments (tonofilaments) *(F)*, lipid droplets *(L)*, and a fully keratinized epithelioreticular cell *(K)*. (Courtesy of J. G. Rhodin.)

lioreticular cells. Typically, a basal lamina is interposed between the epithelioreticular cells and the perivascular connective tissue. Together, these various layers constitute a **blood-thymic barrier** between the thymic lymphocytes and the lumen of the smallest blood vessels. The components of the barrier, from lumen outward, are

- *Capillary endothelium*
- *Endothelial basal lamina*
- Thin *perivascular connective tissue sheath* containing many macrophages
- *Basal lamina* of the epithelioreticular cell
- *Epithelioreticular cell sheath*

The epithelioreticular cell layer surrounding the vasculature and the endothelium of the capillaries in the cortex are the key functional elements of the blood-thymic barrier. The endothelium has been shown to be highly impermeable to macromolecules and is considered to be the major structural component of the barrier. In addition, because there are no afferent lymphatic vessels to the thymus, it *does not react to lymph-borne antigens*.

Thymic Function

During fetal life, the thymus is populated by functionally immature (stem) lymphocytes that arise in the yolk sac, liver, and spleen. When blood cell formation moves to the bone marrow, the marrow becomes the source of these lymphocytes.

The Thymus Is the Site of the Programming, Differentiation, and Proliferation of T Lymphocytes

Within the thymus there is large-scale proliferation of lymphocytes and large-scale cell death, so that most of the newly formed lymphocytes die within a few days. Nevertheless, the thymus releases large numbers of lymphocytes that are carried by the blood to the lymph nodes, spleen, and other lymphatic tissue where they colonize specific parts of these organs and tissues. The lymphocytes released by the thymus are the T lymphocytes. Under the proper stimulus, T lymphocytes proliferate and participate in the cell-mediated immune response. The T lymphocytes survive for long periods and recirculate through lymphatic tissues.

The transformation of primitive or immature lymphocytes into T lymphocytes is promoted by a thymic humoral factor called **thymosin.** There is evidence that the thymic epithelioreticular cells produce this factor.

When the thymus of newborn mouse is removed, lymph nodes and spleen do not develop normally due to a depletion of T lymphocytes, and as previously described, there is an impairment in the cell-mediated immune response. Thus, in newborn thymectomized mice, tissue grafts from other mice may persist indefinitely, whereas the same type of graft would be rejected by thymus-intact animals. In adult animals, nonthymic lymphatic organs are well stocked with T lymphocytes, and therefore, graft rejection occurs even in thymectomized animals.

SPLEEN

The spleen, which is about the size of a clenched fist, is the largest lymphatic organ. It is located in the upper left quadrant of the abdominal cavity and has a rich blood supply.

The Spleen Filters the Blood and Reacts Immunologically to Blood-Borne Antigens

The spleen has both morphologic and immunologic filtering functions. In addition to large numbers of lymphocytes, it contains specialized vascular spaces or channels, a meshwork of reticular cells and reticular fibers, and a rich supply of macrophages. These contents allow the spleen to monitor the blood immunologically, much as the macrophages of the lymph nodes monitor the lymph.

The substance of the spleen, other than the capsule and trabeculae, consists of splenic pulp. This, in turn, is divided into **white pulp** and **red pulp,** based on color seen in a fresh section. The white pulp appears as circular or elongated whitish-gray areas surrounded by the red pulp.

The spleen is surrounded by a capsule of dense connective tissue from which trabeculae extend into the substance of the organ (Fig. 13.14). The connective tissue of the capsule and trabeculae contains myofibroblasts. Not only are these cells contractile, but they also produce the extracellular connective tissue fibers. In many mammals the spleen has the ability to hold large volumes of red blood cells in reserve. In those species, contraction in the capsule and trabeculae helps discharge stored red blood cells into the systemic circulation. The human spleen normally retains relatively little blood, but it has the capacity for contraction by means of the contractile cells in the capsule and trabeculae.

The hilum, located on the medial surface of the spleen, provides for the passage of the splenic artery and vein, nerves, and lymphatic vessels. The lymphatic vessels originate in the white pulp near the trabeculae and constitute a route for lymphocytes leaving the spleen.

Splenic Pulp

White Pulp Is Rich in Lymphocytes

The white pulp consists of lymphatic tissue, mostly lymphocytes; in hematoxylin-stained sections, the white pulp appears as basophilic areas due to the presence of dense heterochromatin in nuclei of the numerous lymphocytes. Branches of the splenic artery course through the capsule and trabeculae of the spleen and then enter the white pulp. Within the white pulp, the vessel is called the **central artery.** Those lymphocytes aggregated around the central artery constitute the **periarterial lymphatic sheath (PALS).** The PALS has a roughly cylindrical configuration that conforms to the course of the central artery.

In cross sections, the sheath of lymphocytes appears circular and may have the appearance of a nodule. The presence of the central artery, however, distinguishes the PALS from a lymphatic nodule. True lymphatic nodules do occur in the periarterial sheath. They appear as localized expansions of the PALS and tend to displace the central artery, so that it occupies an eccentric rather than a central position (see Plate 55, Fig. 3, page 365).

The nodules are the territory of B lymphocytes; other lymphocytes of the PALS are chiefly T lymphocytes that surround the lymph nodules. Thus, the sheath may be considered to be a thymus-dependent zone similar to the deep cortex of a lymph node. The nodules usually contain germinal centers and, as in other lymphatic tissue, the germinal center is a reaction center that forms in response to antigen exposure. In the human, the germinal centers may become extremely large and visible with the naked eye. The enlarged nodules are called **splenic nodules** or **Malpighian corpuscles** (not to be confused with the renal corpuscles that have the same name).

Red Pulp Contains Large Numbers of Red Blood Cells That It Filters and Degrades

The red pulp has a red appearance in the fresh state as well as in histologic sections because it contains large numbers of red blood cells. Essentially, the red pulp consists of **splenic sinuses** separated by the **splenic cords** (the cords of Billroth). The splenic cords consist of the now-familiar loose meshwork of reticular cells and reticular fibers that contain large numbers of erythrocytes, macrophages, lymphocytes, plasma cells, and granulocytes. Many of the macrophages are engaged in the phagocytosis of damaged red blood cells. The iron from destroyed red blood cells is reutilized in the formation of new red blood cells; the splenic macrophages begin the process of hemoglobin breakdown and iron reclamation. (Megakaryocytes are also present in certain species, such as rodents and the cat, but not in humans except during fetal life.)

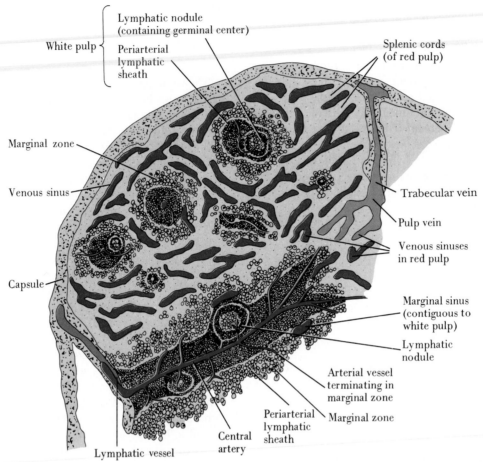

Figure 13.14.   Schematic diagram outlining those features of splenic structure that are evident in a histologic section. The substance of the spleen is divided into white pulp and red pulp. White pulp consists of a cylindrical mass of lymphocytes arranged about a central artery. This mass of lymphocytes constitutes the periarterial lymphatic sheath (PALS). Lymphatic nodules occur along the length of the periarterial sheath. When observed in cross section through part of the sheath that contains a nodule (upper part of figure), the central artery appears eccentrically located with respect to the lymphatic mass. The periarterial lymphatic sheath is surrounded by less densely packed lymphocytes that constitute the marginal zone. The red pulp consists of venous sinuses surrounded by splenic tissue called splenic cords or cords of Billroth. Surrounding the spleen is a capsule. Trabeculae project from the capsule into the substance of the spleen. Both capsule and trabeculae give the appearance of dense connective tissue. The cells in the capsule and trabeculae are myofibroblasts. Blood vessels traverse the capsule and trabeculae before and after passage within the substance of the spleen. Lymphatic vessels begin in the white pulp near the trabeculae. (Based on Weiss L, Tavossoli M: *SEM Hematology* 7:372, 1970.)

The Splenic or Venous Sinuses Are Special Sinusoidal Vessels Lined by Unusually Shaped Endothelial Cells

The cells that line the splenic sinuses, the endothelial cells, are extremely long, with their longitudinal axis parallel to the direction of the vessel (Fig. 13.15). There are few contact points between adjacent cells, thus producing prominent intercellular spaces. This allows blood cells to pass into and out of the sinuses quite readily. Processes of macrophages extend between the endothelial cells and into the lumen of the sinuses to monitor the passing blood for the presence of foreign antigens.

The sinuses do not possess a continuous basal lamina. Strands of basal lamina loop around the outside of the sinus in the same manner that hoops loop around the staves of a barrel. These strands are at right angles to the long axes of the endothelial cells. It is this material that is stained with silver-containing reagents or with the PAS reaction. Neither smooth muscle nor pericytes are found in the wall of splenic sinuses. Reticular cell processes may extend to the basal side of the endothelial cells and are probably associated with the reticular fibers that appear to merge with the perisinusoidal loops of basal lamina. Blood fills both the sinuses and the cords of the red pulp, often to a degree that obscures the underlying structure and makes it difficult, in histologic sections, to distinguish between the cords and the sinuses.

Splenic Circulation

Branches of the splenic artery enter the white pulp from the trabeculae. In the white pulp, the central artery sends

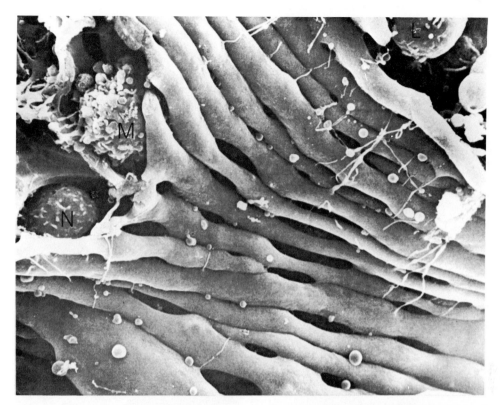

Figure 13.15. **a.** Scanning electron micrograph of the splenic sinus (human), showing the architecture of the sinus wall as seen from the luminal side. Rod-like endothelial cells run in parallel and are intermittently connected with each other by side processes. A nuclear swelling is shown on the bottom left. The tapered ends of a few of the rod cells are seen. The rod cells are provided with a few thread-like microprojections whose significance is unknown. The macrophage *(M)*, neutrophil *(N)*, and lymphocyte *(L)* are outside of the sinus. ×5300. (From Fujita T, et al: *S. E. M. Atlas of Cells and Tissues.* Tokyo, Igaku-Shoin, Ltd, 1981, plate 2.11.)

branches to the white pulp itself and to the sinuses at the perimeter of the white pulp, called *marginal sinuses* (see Fig. 13.14). The central artery continues into the red pulp, where it branches into several relatively straight arterioles called *penicilli (penicillar arterioles)*. The penicilli then continue as arterial capillaries; these may be surrounded by aggregations of macrophages. Arterial capillaries having such arrangements of macrophages are called *sheathed capillaries*.

Disagreement has existed for decades over the pathway taken by blood as it passes through the red pulp of the human spleen to enter the trabecular veins. It is agreed that blood cells do leave the vascular system to populate the white pulp and the red pulp and that they reenter the vascular system in the red pulp. The manner in which this is accomplished has led to two proposed models for circulation:

* *Open circulation model:* In this model, splenic arterioles are presumed to empty directly into the reticular meshwork of the cords rather than connecting to the endothelium-lined splenic sinuses. Blood entering the red pulp in this manner would then percolate through the cords and be exposed to the macrophages of the cords before returning to the circulation by entering a sinus from the extravascular side.

* *Closed circulation model:* In this model, the splenic arterioles would empty directly into the splenic sinuses of the red pulp. To be exposed to the macrophages of the cords, therefore, it would be necessary for blood cells to leave the sinuses first and then reenter them. Although the cells would be extravascular for part of the trip, the system is called "closed" because it describes a continuous vascular channel through the red pulp.

Most experimental and morphologic evidence currently supports the open circulation model. This pathway provides a more efficient exposure of blood to the macrophages of the red pulp. Both transmission and scanning electron micrographs often show blood cells in transit across the endothelium of the sinus, presumably reentering the vascular system from the red pulp cords. The blood collected in the sinuses drains to trabecular veins that converge into larger veins and eventually leaves the spleen by the splenic vein, which, in turn, joins the drainage from the intestine in the hepatic portal vein (see page 496).

Functions of the Spleen

The spleen functions in both the immune and the hematopoietic system.

Immune system functions of the spleen include

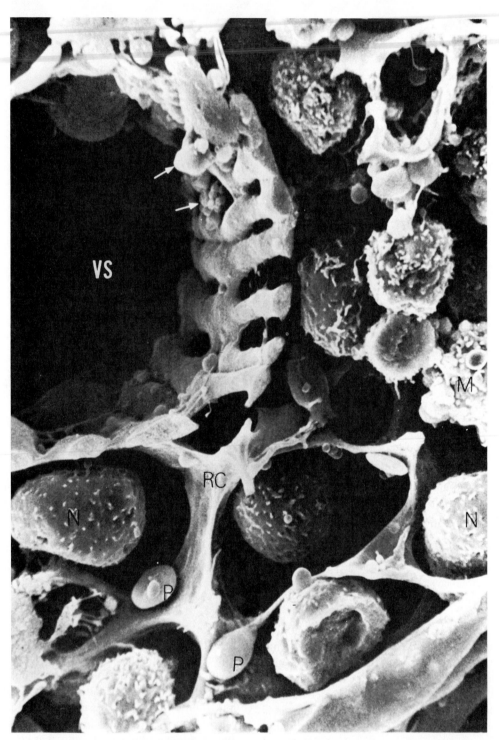

Figure 13.15. **b.** Scanning electron micrograph of the splenic sinus and cord of Billroth (human), showing a cross-sectional view of a venous sinus *(VS)* on the left, revealing the lattice structure of its wall. Rod cells are connected with each other by their side processes. Through the apertures between the rod cells, processes of macrophages *(arrows)* are inserted into the sinus lumen. The cord of Billroth is supported by the wing-like processes of reticular cells *(RC)* whose surface is char- acteristically smooth. The spaces of the reticular cell frame-work contain neutrophils *(N)*, macrophages *(M)*, and blood platelets *(P)*. Red blood cells and many other free cells, which must have filled the spaces in the living state, have been washed away during perfusion for fixation. ×4400. (From Fujita T, et al: *S. E. M. Atlas of Cells and Tissues.* Tokyo, Igaku-Shoin, Ltd, 1981, plate 2.10.)

- Proliferation of lymphocytes
- Production of humoral antibodies
- Removal of macromolecular antigens from the blood

Hematopoietic functions of the spleen include

- Formation of blood cells during fetal life
- Removal and destruction of senile, damaged, and abnormal red blood cells and platelets
- Retrieval of the iron from red cell hemoglobin
- Storage of blood, especially red blood cells, in some species

Proliferation of lymphocytes and differentiation of effector lymphocytes and plasma cells, as well as secretion of humoral antibodies, occur in the white pulp of the spleen. In this regard, the white pulp is the equivalent of other lymphatic organs.

The role of the red pulp is primarily that of **blood filtration,** i.e., removal of particulate material, macromolecular antigens, and aged, abnormal, or damaged blood cells and platelets from the circulating blood. These functions are accomplished by the macrophages embedded in the reticular meshwork of the red pulp. Senescent, damaged, or abnormal red cells are broken down by the lysosomes of the macrophages; the iron of the hemoglobin is retrieved and stored as ferritin or hemosiderin for future recycling. The heme portion of the molecule is broken down to bilirubin, which is transported to the liver via the portal system and there conjugated to glucuronic acid. This is secreted into the bile, to which it gives a characteristic color.

The mechanism by which macrophages recognize old or abnormal blood cells is not yet elucidated. It has been proposed that as red cells age, they become more rigid and are then more easily trapped in the meshes of the red pulp. It has also been suggested that the immune system may respond to changes in the surface of erythrocytes and tag pathologically modified cells with opsonizing antibody. Investigators have recently described changes in the glycosylation of surface proteins in aging erythrocytes that might provide a clue to the mechanism by which they are recognized by macrophages.

Despite this myriad of important functions, the spleen is not essential for human life and can be removed surgically if necessary. This is often done after trauma causes intractable bleeding from the spleen. The removal of aging red blood cells and their destruction then occur in the bone marrow and liver.

PLATE 50. Tonsil

The palatine tonsils (faucial tonsils) are paired, ovoid structures that consist of dense accumulations of lymphatic tissue located in the mucous membrane of the fauces (the junction of oropharynx and oral cavity). The low-magnification (×30) survey micrograph on this page shows the general structural features of part of the human tonsil. The epithelium that forms the surface of the tonsil dips into the underlying connective tissue in numerous places, forming crypts known as tonsillar crypts. One of these crypts is seen in the survey micrograph *(arrows)*. Numerous lymphatic nodules are readily evident in the walls of the crypts.

In addition to the palatine tonsils illustrated here, similar aggregations of lymphatic tissue are present beneath the epithelium of the tongue (lingual tonsils), under the epithelium of the roof of the nasopharynx (pharyngeal tonsils), and in smaller accumulations around the openings of the Eustachian tubes.

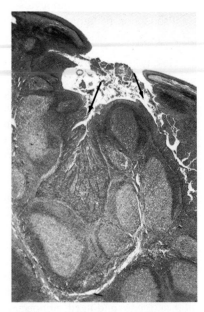

Survey micrograph, tonsil, human, hematoxylin and eosin (H&E) ×30.

FIGURE 1, tonsil, human, H&E ×180. This shows, at a higher magnification, part of the same crypt as in the survey micrograph, as well as the adjacent epithelium *(EP)* and one of the lymphatic nodules *(LN)*. The crypt contains some cellular debris, a frequent occurrence. The lymphatic nodule exhibits a germinal center, the lighter central region of the nodule. The darker-staining peripheral portion of the nodule contains numerous, closely packed small lymphocytes that are intimately related to the epithelium; they have actually become incorporated in the epithelium. Portions of the germinal center have also become incorporated into the epithelium.

FIGURE 2, tonsil, human, H&E ×400; inset ×800. The *rectangular area* in Figure 1 is shown here at higher magnification. The stratified squamous epithelium *(Ep)* is just barely recognized due to the heavy infiltration of lymphocytes. The deeper portion of the epithelium is even more obscured, however. Epithelial cells are present, though difficult to identify, in the germinal center as well as in the periphery of the nodule *(small arrows)*. The **inset** shows the *oval inscribed area* at higher magnification and the epithelial cells *(arrows)* more clearly. In effect, this nodule has literally grown into the epithelium, distorting it and resulting in the disappearance of the well-defined epithelial-connective tissue boundary.

KEY

Ep, epithelium
LN, lymphatic nodule
LP, lamina propria
arrow, survey micrograph, tonsillar crypt

large arrow (Fig. 1), crypt
rectangular area (Fig. 1), shown at higher magnification in Fig. 2

small arrows (Fig. 2), strands of epithelial cells in nodule

PLATE 50

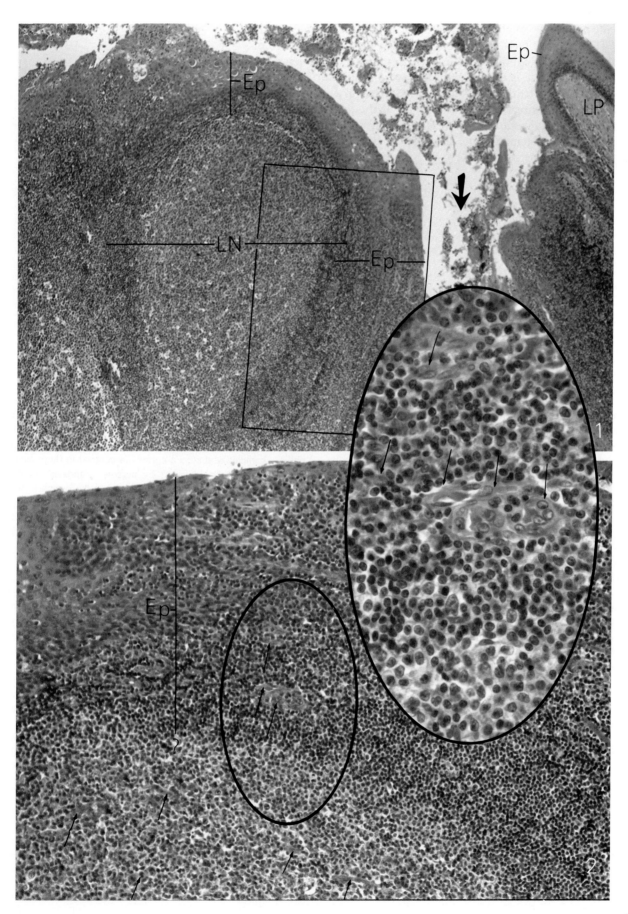

PLATE 51. Lymph Node I

Lymph nodes are small lymphatic organs that are located in the path of the lymph vessels. A low-magnification (×14) micrograph of a section through a human lymph node is shown on this page for orientation. The node is composed of a mass of lymphatic tissue, arranged as a cortex *(C)* that surrounds a less dense area, the medulla *(M)*. The cortex is interrupted at the hilum of the organ *(H)*, where there is a recognizable concavity. It is at this site that blood vessels enter and leave the lymph node; the efferent lymphatic vessels also leave the node at this site.

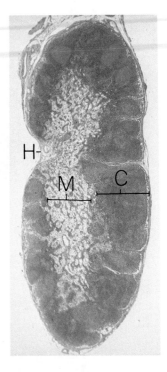

Survey micrograph, lymph node, human, H&E ×14.

FIGURE 1, lymph node, human, H&E ×120. An area from the cortex is shown here at higher magnification. The capsule *(Cap)* is composed of dense connective tissue from which trabeculae *(T)* penetrate into the organ to provide support. Immediately below the capsule is a sinus, the cortical or subcapsular sinus *(CS)*, that receives the lymph from the afferent lymphatic vessels after they penetrate the capsule. The subcapsular sinus is continuous with the trabecular sinuses *(TS)* that course along the trabeculae.

The cortex contains the cortical or lymphatic nodules *(LN)* and a deeper component that lacks the nodules, known as the deep cortex. Whereas the lymph nodules and their lighter-staining germinal centers characterize the outer cortex, a more dense mass of lymphocytes, which impart a distinct basophilia, characterize the deep cortex. In contrast to these areas, the medulla is characterized by narrow strands of anastomosing lymphatic tissue containing numerous lymphocytes, the medullary cords *(MC)*, separated by light-appearing areas known as the medullary sinuses *(MS)*. The medullary sinuses receive lymph from the trabecular sinuses as well as lymph that has filtered through the cortical tissue.

FIGURE 2, lymph node, human, H&E ×400; inset ×640. This higher magnification of a lymphatic nodule from Figure 1 illustrates the germinal center *(GC)* with its population of medium and large lymphocytes and the frequently observed dividing lymphocytes. Germinal centers also contain a number of plasma cells. Dividing lymphocytes are shown at slightly higher magnification in the **inset** *(arrows)*, which corresponds to the area in the *circle* in Figure 2. The **inset** also reveals nuclei of the reticular cells *(RC)* that form the connective tissue stroma throughout the organ. The reticular cell has a large pale-staining nucleus and is usually ovoid. The cytoplasm forms long processes that surround the reticular fibers. In H&E preparations, the reticular fibers and the surrounding reticular cell cytoplasm are difficult to identify. The reticular cells, however, are best seen in the sinuses, where they extend across the lymphatic space and are relatively unobscured by other cells.

A unique vessel, the postcapillary venule *(PCV)*, is found in relation to the lymphatic nodules, particularly in the deep cortex. These vessels have an endothelium composed of tall cells between which lymphocytes migrate from the vessel lumen into the parenchyma. The walls of the postcapillary venules are often infiltrated with migrating lymphocytes, making it difficult to recognize the vessel in some preparations.

KEY

C, cortex
Cap, capsule
CS, cortical or subcapsular sinus
GC, germinal center
H, hilum
LN, lymphatic nodule
M, medulla
MC, medullary cords
MS, medullary sinus
PCV, postcapillary venule
RC, reticular cells
T, trabecula
TS, trabecular sinus
arrows, dividing lymphocytes

PLATE 51

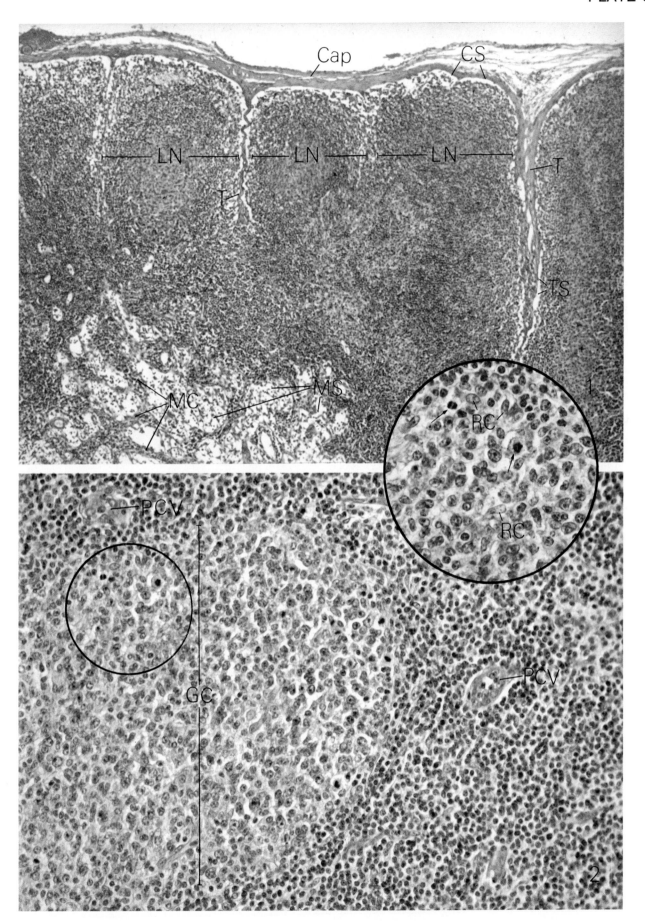

PLATE 52. Lymph Node II

FIGURE 1, lymph node, monkey, H&E ×640; inset ×1300. The nature of the subcapsular (cortical) sinus is revealed at relatively high magnification in this figure. The capsule *(Cap)* is on the left, and a trabecula *(Tr)* extending into the substance of the node is seen at the bottom of the micrograph. The cortical sinus *(CS)* is bounded by endothelium that lines the undersurface of the capsule on one side and by endothelium that covers the lymphatic parenchyma on the opposite side of the sinus. Neither endothelial surface is clearly evident with the light microscope, however, particularly not the endothelial layer adjoining the parenchyma. Extending across the lymphatic sinus are reticular cells *(RC)* and reticular fibers. The reticular cells and their associated fibers, although present throughout the node, are readily identified in the medullary sinuses because here they are not obscured by large numbers of lymphocytes. The nuclei of the reticular cells are usually ovoid and pale staining. The cytoplasm extends into elongate processes that join with those of other reticular cells. The **inset** shows the area within the *circle* at high magnification and reveals the reticular cells with their characteristic processes *(asterisk)*. Note how the cytoplasm of one cell appears to merge with its neighbor, forming a reticular configuration.

FIGURE 3, lymph node, monkey, H&E ×80. This shows, at low magnification, the hilum *(H)* from which connective tissue penetrates into the node as an extension of the capsule. Within this connective tissue are lymphatic vessels *(Ly)* as well as blood vessels. The lymphatic vessels leave the node at the hilum along with a vein. The artery enters the node at the same site. Due to the nature of the section, however, vessels are not seen at the point where they enter and leave the hilum.

FIGURE 2, lymph node, monkey, silver preparation ×500. This figure reveals the distribution of the reticular fibers. They exhibit a blue-black color. Some are present in the capsule *(Cap)* and trabeculae *(Tr)*, mixed with collagen fibers, but the majority of the reticular fibers *(RF)* can be seen forming a network extending across the capsular sinus and into the substance of the lymphatic tissue. Associated with these fibers are the reticular cells that form a cytoplasmic sheath around the fibers. This relationship cannot be visualized with the light microscope but is readily apparent with the electron microscope (see Plate 54, page 363). The medullary sinuses of the node ultimately converge near the hilum and empty into lymphatic vessels that drain the node.

FIGURE 4, lymph node, monkey, H&E ×360. This shows the area in the *rectangle* of Figure 3 at higher magnification. Two of the vessels here are efferent lymphatics; both contain a valve *(V)*. The upper lymphatic vessel exhibits what appears to be an incomplete wall. The openings *(arrows)* are sites in which the medullary sinuses (see area in *rectangle* of Figure 3) are emptying their contents into the lymphatic vessel. Also present are a small artery *(A)* and, at the top of the micrograph (unlabeled), a vein.

KEY

A, artery	**Ly,** lymphatic vessels	**arrows,** openings in which medullary sinuses empty their contents into the lymphatic vessel
Cap, capsule	**M,** macrophage	
CS, cortical or subcapsular sinus	**RC,** reticular cell	
H, hilum	**RF,** reticular fiber	**asterisks,** reticular cells with their characteristic processes
L, lymphocyte	**Tr,** trabecula	
LN, lymphatic nodule	**V,** valve	

PLATE 52

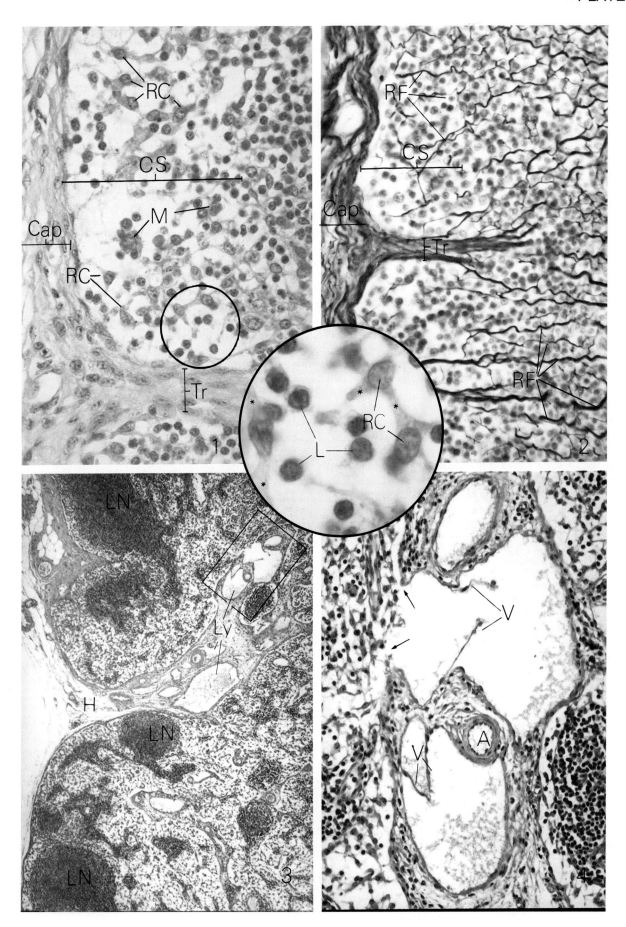

PLATE 53. Lymph Node III, Electron Microscopy

Lymph node, monkey, electron micrograph ×4,300; inset ×16,000. Some of the more significant aspects of the structural organization of the lymph node and its cells are evident in the accompanying electron micrograph. The region of the node shown here corresponds to the light microscopic picture in Plate 52, Figure 1.

The capsule of the lymph node is on the left side of the micrograph. It consists largely of collagen bundles *(C)* and some fibroblasts. The cortical sinus *(CS)*, which lies just below the capsule, can be recognized at the electron microscopic level as a lymphatic channel. It is lined by endothelial cells *(En)* that, in effect, represent a continuation of the lining of the afferent lymphatic vessels that enter the node. The **inset** shows, at higher magnification, portions of two contiguous endothelial cells *(En)* immediately beneath the capsule *(Cap)* that are joined by an intercellular junction *(arrow)*. The connective tissue of the capsule *(Cap)* is to the left of the endothelium, and a portion of a lymphocyte *(L)* within the sinus is seen on the right.

In contrast to the continuous nature of the endothelium that faces the capsule, the portion of the endothelium facing the deep surface of the sinus frequently shows discontinuities. Macrophages *(M)* located within the parenchyma of the node may abut on the sinus wall or may actually project into the sinus through these discontinuities *(curved arrow)*. Here, the endothelium *(En)* shows a gap, and an extension of a macrophage reaches the sinus in the vicinity of the gap. When interposed in this way, the macrophages can be regarded as a component of the sinus wall. However, it is not clear if these macrophages are actually fixed components of the wall or if they are more transient elements. In either case, the macrophage is in a position to monitor and phagocytize substances within the sinus.

A second type of endothelial discontinuity is seen in the lower right of the micrograph *(arrowheads)*. Here, a lymphocyte is in the process of leaving the sinus and entering the parenchyma of the lymph node. The lack of continuity of the endothelium in this instance is clearly transitory, as the endothelium is parted only during the interval that the lymphocyte is moving across the sinus wall.

In addition to the macrophages and the lymphocytes that constitute the bulk of the parenchyma of the node, reticular cells *(RC)* are also a conspicuous cell component when viewed at the electron microscopic level. In identifying these various cell types, the lymphocyte *(L)* is readily recognized by virtue of the dense chromatin (heterochromatin) of its nucleus and relative paucity of cytoplasm. On the other hand, the nuclei of both the macrophage and reticular cell display mostly diffuse chromatin; only a small amount of chromatin is in the condensed form. It is this feature that accounts for the relatively pale staining of the reticular cell and macrophage nuclei as seen with the light microscope. In the electron micrograph, the reticular cell is distinguished from the macrophage by its relative lack of lysosomal granules.

With the light microscope, it is difficult to distinguish macrophages from reticular cells of the parenchyma. The macrophages can be identified, however, if their cytoplasm contains recognizable phagocytosed substances. An additional feature serves to aid in the identification of these cells with the light microscope, namely, macrophages are rarely seen in the cortical sinus. Thus, those cells in the sinus that exhibit lightly stained nuclei can be regarded as reticular cells, particularly if they also exhibit recognizable cytoplasmic processes.

The area within the *rectangle* in the upper right of the micrograph is shown in Plate 54 at higher magnification.

KEY

C, collagen bundles
Cap (inset), capsule
CS, cortical sinus
En, endothelial cells
L, lymphocyte

M, macrophage
RC, reticular cell
RF, reticular fiber
arrow, endothelial cell junction

arrowheads, endothelial discontinuity
curved arrow, macrophage extending into sinus

PLATE 53

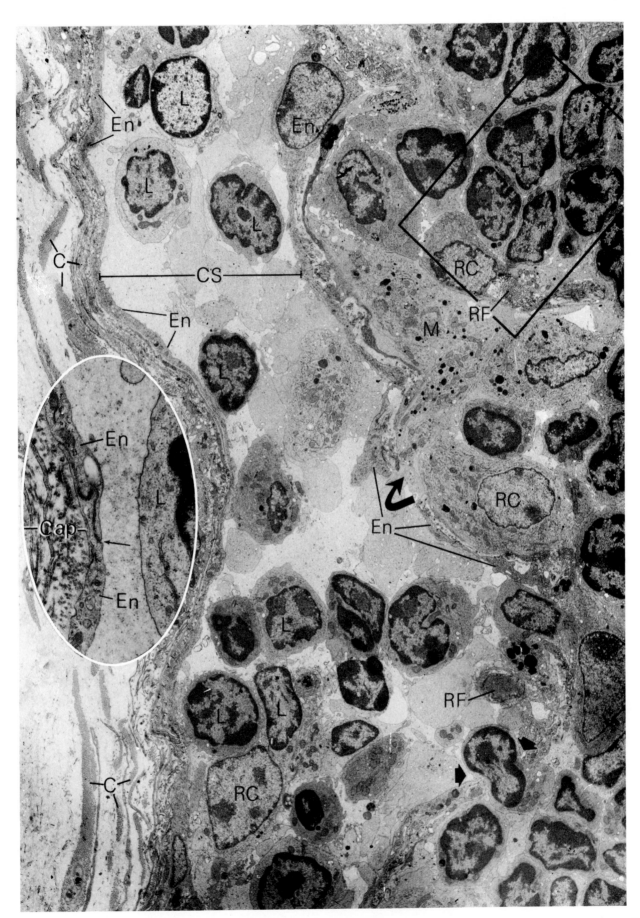

PLATE 54.   Lymph Node IV, Electron Microscopy

Lymph node, monkey, electron micrograph ×18,500.
The electron micrograph shown here illustrates some characterisics of lymphocytes and reticular cells and their relationship to the reticular fibers.

Lymphocytes *(L)* possess large numbers of ribosomes distributed throughout the cytoplasmic matrix; this gives the cytoplasm a stippled appearance. The Golgi area *(GA)* is relatively small and consequently inconspicuous. Mitochondria *(M),* though not numerous in terms of absolute numbers, occupy a relatively substantial portion of the available cytoplasmic volume. Profiles of rough-surfaced endoplasmic reticulum are rare; however, occasional granules are present. In paraffin sections prepared for the light microscope, the cytoplasm of the lymphocyte is inconspicuous, often appearing as nothing more than a light halo around a deeply stained nucleus. In blood smears, where the cells are flattened, however, the cytoplasm is stained pale blue due to the ribosomes.

As already mentioned, the reticular cell can be distinguished from the lymphocyte by the relatively small amount of condensed chromatin in the nucleus. Thus, it is less deeply stained than the lymphocyte nucleus. The cytoplasm of the reticular cell *(RC)* resembles that of the fibroblast, in that it contains moderate numbers of mitochondria *(M),* a relatively extensive Golgi apparatus *(GA),* and profiles of rough-surfaced endoplasmic reticulum. The most distinctive and unique feature of the reticular cell is its relationship to the reticular fibers. Unlike the fibroblast, the reticular cell virtually ensheathes the fiber. Cross sections of the reticular fibers *(RF)* show that it is surrounded by cytoplasmic extension *(arrows)* of the reticular cell. By virtue of this ensheathing, the reticular cell cytoplasm is interposed between the reticular fiber and the lymphocytes. Note that the lymphocytes are tightly packed, with little intercellular space separating the cells. As seen in the illustration, collagen fibrils are conspicuously absent from the space between the lymphocytes.

The reticular fiber of the lymph node consists of a bundle of collagen fibrils that are embedded in and surrounded by a variable amount of matrix. Specific polysaccharides bound to the reticular fibers account for the special silver-staining reaction that distinguishes reticular fibers from collagen fibers.

KEY

GA, Golgi area
L, lymphocytes
M, mitochondria
RC, reticular cell
RF, reticular fibers
arrows, reticular cell process

PLATE 54

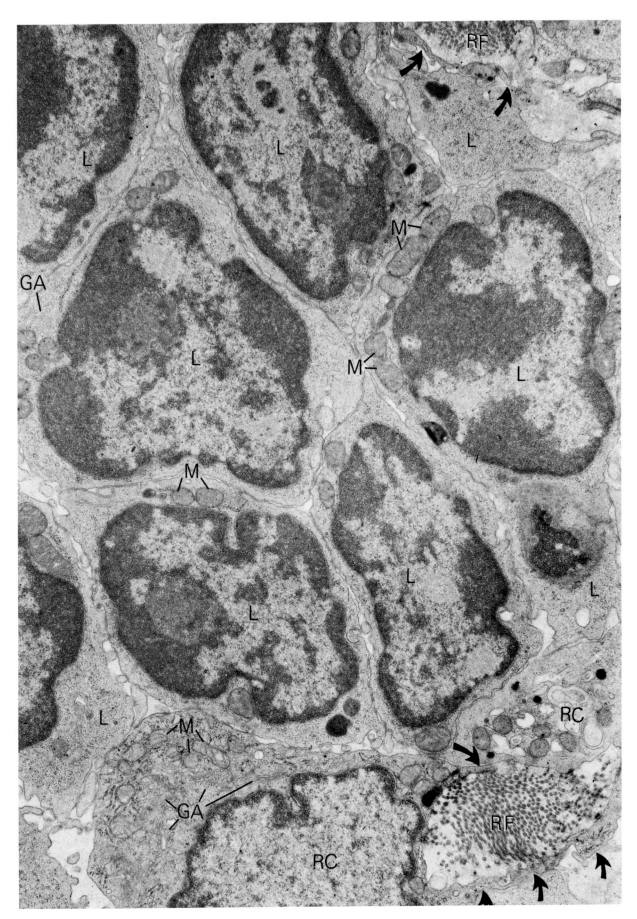

PLATE 55. Spleen I

The spleen is a lymphatic organ surrounded by a capsule and located in the path of the bloodstream (splenic artery and vein).

FIGURE 1, spleen, human, H&E ×65. This low-magnification micrograph of the spleen reveals its two major components, the red pulp *(RP)* and white pulp *(WP)*. Also evident is a portion of the capsule *(Cap)* in the upper right of the figure; in the center, there is a **trabecula** containing a blood vessel, a trabecular vein *(TV)* through which blood leaves the organ. The red pulp constitutes the greater bulk of the splenic tissue. In life, the red pulp has pulp-like texture; it is red due to the natural coloration of the numerous red blood cells present, hence its name.

The white pulp, on the other hand, is so named because its content of lymphocytes appears in life as whitish areas. In tissue sections, however, the nuclei of the closely packed lymphocytes impart an overall blue-staining response. The lymphatic tissue that comprises the white pulp *(WP)* differs from nodules seen elsewhere in that it follows and ensheathes a blood vessel, the central artery. The lymphatic tissue surrounding the artery exhibits periodic expansion, thus forming the nodules. When this occurs, the central artery *(CA)* is displaced peripherally within the nodule.

In those regions where the lymphatic tissue is not in nodular form, it is present as a thin cuff around the central artery and is referred to as the periarterial lymphatic sheath *(PALS)*. If the plane of section does not include the artery, the sheath may appear as a localized and irregular aggregation of lymphocytes *(asterisks)*.

FIGURE 2, spleen, human, H&E ×160. This figure reveals, at a higher magnification, the red pulp and a portion of the trabecular vein from the area enclosed in the *uppermost rectangle* in Figure 1. The red pulp is composed of two elements: venous sinuses *(VS)* and the splenic cords (of Billroth), the tissue that lies between the sinuses. In this specimen, the venous sinuses can be seen to advantage because the red blood cells in the sinuses have lysed and appear as unstained "ghosts;" only the nuclei of the white cells are readily apparent. (This is seen better in Plate 56.) The paler, unstained areas thus represent the sinus lumina.

Near the top of the micrograph, two venous sinuses empty into the trabecular vein *(arrows)*, thus showing the continuity between venous sinuses and the trabecular veins. The wall of the vein is thin, but the trabecula *(T)* containing the vessel gives the appearance of being part of the vessel wall. In humans, as well as other mammals, the capsule and the trabeculae that extend from the capsule contain myofibroblasts. Under conditions of increasing physical stress, contraction of these cells will occur and cause rapid expulsion of blood from the venous sinuses into the trabecular veins and, thus, into the general circulation.

FIGURE 3, spleen, human, H&E ×240. This figure reveals, at higher magnification, the splenic nodule in the *rectangle* in the left portion of Figure 1. Present are a germinal center *(GC)* and a cross section through the thick-walled central artery *(CA)*. As already noted, the central artery is eccentrically placed in the nodule. The marginal zone *(MZ)* is the area that separates white pulp and red pulp *(RP)*. Small arterial vessels and capillaries, branches of the central artery, supply the white pulp, and some pass into the reticular network of the marginal zone, terminating in a funnel-shaped orifice. Venous sinuses are also found in the marginal zone, and occasionally, arterial vessels may open into the sinuses. The details of the vascular supply are, at best, difficult to resolve in typical H&E preparations. The penicillar arterioles, the terminal branches of the central artery, supply the red pulp but are likewise difficult to resolve.

KEY

CA, central artery
Cap, capsule
GC, germinal center
MZ, marginal zone
PALS, periarterial lymphatic sheath
RP, red pulp
T, trabecula
TV, trabecular vein
VS, venous sinus
WP, white pulp
arrows (Fig. 2), venous sinuses emptying into the trabecular vein
asterisks (Fig. 1), lymphocytes of the periarterial lymphatic sheath

PLATE 55

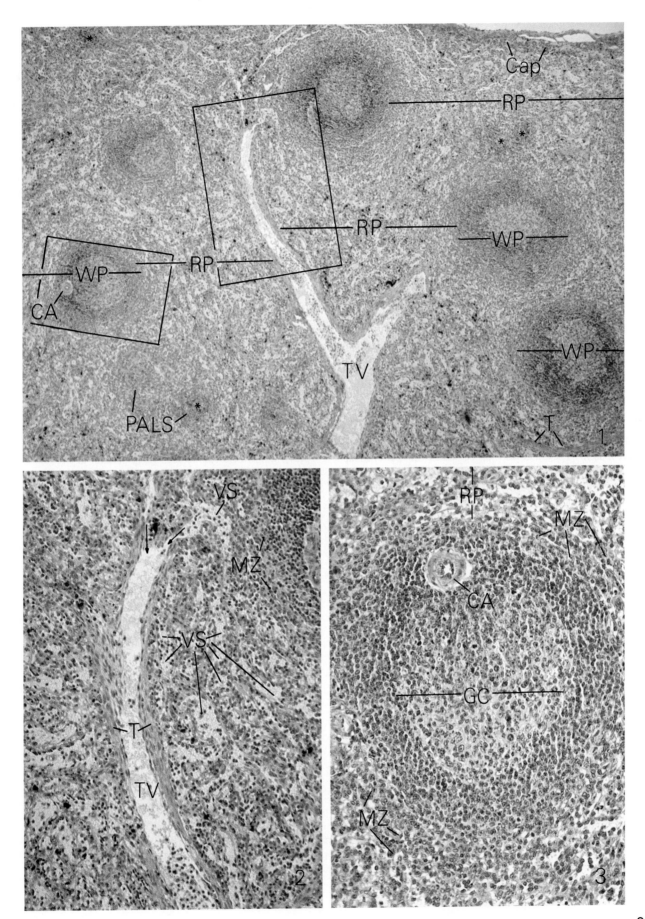

PLATE 56. Spleen II

FIGURE 1, spleen, human, H&E ×360. The red pulp, as noted in the previous plate, has two components: venous sinuses and the splenic cords of Billroth. The venous sinuses *(VS)* can be recognized by their circumscribing endothelial wall. The red cells within the lumen of the vessels are apparent only by virtue of their outline, with the contents of the cells having been lost during the preparation of the tissue (lysed), leaving only a ghost image. The cords are filled with a variety of cell types, among which are numerous lysed red blood cells. These red cells have left the vascular channels; i.e., they are extravascular. Macrophages can be identified in this specimen by the pigment that they have sequestered *(arrows)*, the breakdown product of old red blood cells.

FIGURE 2, spleen, human, H&E ×1200. This figure reveals, at higher magnification, one of the venous sinuses and the surrounding Billroth's cord *(BC)* from the preceding figure. The wall of the sinus consists of elongated rod-like endothelial cells that are oriented parallel to each other in the long axis of the sinus. A narrow but clearly visible intercellular space is usually present between adjacent cells. (The space seen in light microscopic preparations is an exaggeration due to shrinkage during routine preparation.) When a venous sinus is cut in cross section, as in Figure 1, the rod-shaped endothelial lining cells are also cut in cross section, and the cut edges of the adjoining cells are seen in the form of a ring. The narrow intercellular spaces then appear as slits between the cross-sectioned cells. Occasionally, the wall of a sinus is tangentially sectioned, and the cytoplasm of the endothelial cells appears as a series of narrow stripes, as can be seen in the lower left of Figure 1 *(asterisks)*. Each linear component here is a single endothelial cell.

The endothelial cell nuclei *(En)* project into the sinus lumen. In effect, the nuclei form a bleb-like structure that then appears to sit within the lumen of the vessel. Unless carefully examined, they may give the impression that they are nuclei of white blood cells. This is especially true if the white blood cells *(WBC)* within the lumen of the sinus are numerous.

FIGURE 3, spleen, human, silver preparation ×120; inset ×300. The framework of the spleen consists of a capsule, trabeculae that extend from the capsule into the substance of the spleen, and a reticular stroma. The silver-stained reticular stroma is illustrated in this figure. In the white pulp, the germinal centers *(GC)* can be recognized by the circular arrangement and, to some degree, the paucity of the reticular fibers. The central arteries *(CA)* are surrounded by a relative abundance of reticular fibers, hence the dense outline of these vessels. The arrangement of the fibers in the red pulp is more variable in appearance. A special arrangement of blackened fibers is seen in relation to the venous sinus *(VS)* of the red pulp. These fibers often appear as an organized lattice that circumscribes the vessel.

The **inset** in Figure 3 is a higher magnification of the area immediately above it. One of the vessels seen in the **inset** has been sectioned tangentially along its wall, and its circumscribing fibers can be seen lying parallel to one another like the rungs of a ladder *(arrows)*. The vessel above and in very close proximity (with the label *VS* in its lumen) has also been longitudinally sectioned, but the section passes deeper into the vessel; thus, the cut ends of the fibers are seen in cross-sectional profile *(arrowheads)* and give the appearance of a series of dots outlining the wall of the vessel. These fibers are actually composed of basal lamina material. The basal lamina is not a thin sheath in this instance but, rather, forms a cord-like structure that facilitates the passage of cells across the endothelium. The true reticular fibers (composed of collagen fibrils) are darker staining and thicker. They can be seen between the closely apposed vessels.

KEY

BC, Billroth's cord (splenic cord)
CA, central artery
En, endothelial cell nucleus
GC, germinal center
VS, venous sinus

WBC, white blood cells
arrowheads (Fig. 3, inset), silver-positive fibers (basal lamina material) circumscribing the renus sinus endotretium as seen in cross-sectional profile

arrows: Fig. 1, pigment (contained in macrophages); Fig. 3 **(inset),** silver-positive fibers (basal lamina material) circumscribing the venous sinus endothelium
asterisks (Fig. 1), wall of venous sinus seen in tangential section

PLATE 56

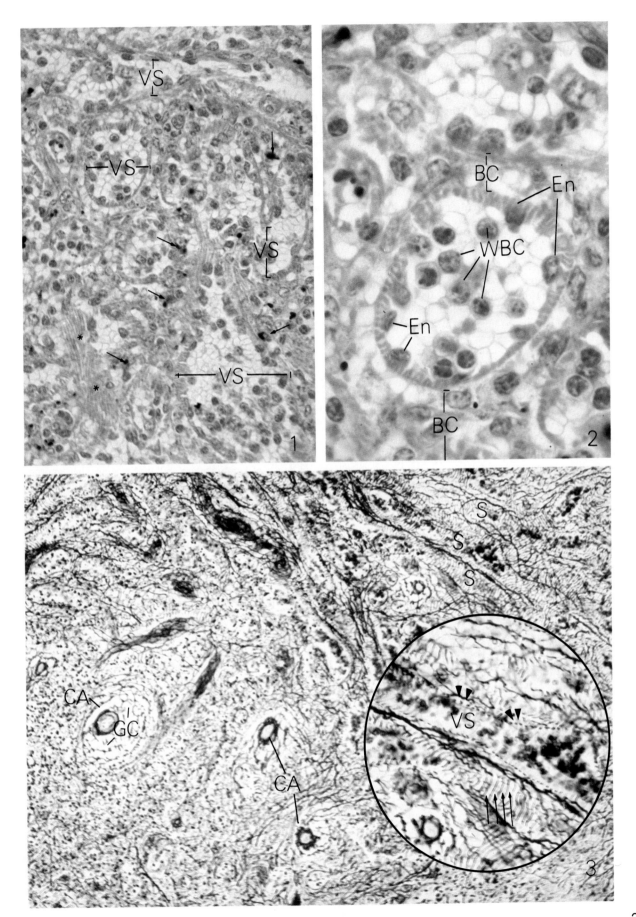

PLATE 57. Thymus

The thymus is a lymphatic organ that exhibits certain unique structural features. The supporting reticular stroma of the thymus arises from endodermal epithelium and produces a cellular reticulum. There are no reticular fibers associated with these cells; instead, the cells, designated epithelioreticular cells, serve as the stroma. Lymphocytes come to lie within the interstices of the cellular reticulum, and these two cellular elements, the lymphocytes and the epithelioreticular cells, comprise the bulk of the organ. The lymphocytes that migrate into the endodermal rudiment during embryonic development derive from the yolk sac and, later, from the red bone marrow. On entering the thymus, the lymphocytes proliferate. Some of these new lymphocytes migrate to other tissues; many of them also die in the thymus.

A connective tissue capsule *(Cap)* surrounds each lobe of the thymus (there are two lobes) and sends trabeculae *(T)* into the substance of the gland to form lobules. The lobules *(L)* are not completely separate units; rather, they interconnect owing to the discontinuous nature of the trabeculae.

FIGURE 1, thymus, human, H&E ×40. Examination of the thymus at low magnification reveals the lobules to be composed of a dark-staining basophilic cortex *(C)* and a lighter-staining and relatively eosinophilic medulla *(M)*. The cortex contains numerous densely packed lymphocytes, whereas the medulla contains fewer lymphocytes and is consequently less densely packed.

FIGURE 2, thymus, human, H&E ×140. It is the relative difference in the lymphocyte population (per unit area) and, in particular, the staining of their nuclei with hematoxylin that creates the difference in appearance between cortex *(C)* and medulla *(M)*. Note that some of the medullary areas bear a resemblance to germinal centers of other lymphatic organs because of the medulla appearing as isolated circular areas (upper left of Fig. 1). The medullary component, however, is actually a continuous branching mass surrounded by cortical tissue. Thus, the "isolated" medullary profiles are actually united with one another, although not within the plane of section. A suggestion of such continuity can be seen on the right in Figure 1, where the medulla appears to extend across several lobules.

The main cellular constituents of the thymus are lymphocytes (thymocytes), with characteristic small, round, dark-staining nuclei, and epithelioreticular supporting cells, with large pale-staining nuclei. Both of the cell types can be distinguished in Figure 3, which provides a high-magnification view of the medulla. Because there are fewer lymphocytes in the medulla, it is the area of choice to examine the epithelioreticular cells. The thymus also contains macrophages; however, they are difficult to distinguish from the epithelioreticular cells.

FIGURE 3, thymus, human, H&E ×600. The medulla usually possesses varying numbers of circular bodies called Hassall's or thymic corpuscles *(HC)*. The corpuscles are large concentric layers of flattened epithelioreticular *(Ep)* cells. They stain readily with eosin and can be distinguished easily with low magnification, as in Figures 1 and 2 *(arrows)*. The center of a corpuscle, particularly a large one, may show evidence of keratinization and appear somewhat amorphous.

The thymus gland remains as a large structure until the time of puberty. At that time, regressive changes occur that result in a significant reduction in the amount of thymic tissue. The young thymus is highly cellular and contains a minimum of adipose tissue. On the other hand, in the older thymus, much adipose tissue is present between the lobules. With continued involution, adipose cells are found even within the thymic tissue itself. Occasional plasma cells may be present in the periphery of the thymic cortex of the involuting thymus gland.

KEY

BV, blood vessels
C, cortex
Cap, capsule
Ep, epithelioreticular cells
HC, Hassall's corpuscles
L, lobule
M, medulla
T, trabeculae
arrowheads, nuclei of epithelioreticular cells of Hassall's corpuscles
arrows (Figs. 1 and 2), Hassall's corpuscles

PLATE 57

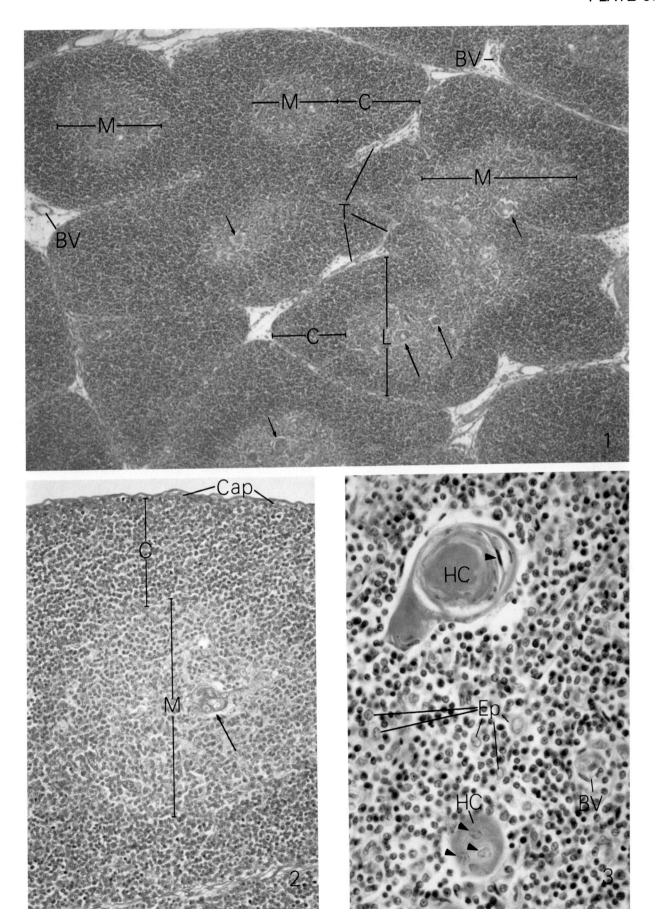

Integumentary System

14

The skin *(integument, cutis)* and its derivatives constitute the integumentary system. It forms the external covering of the body and is the largest organ of the body, constituting 15–20% of its total mass. The skin consists of two main layers:

- *Epidermis,* composed of a keratinized stratified squamous epithelium
- *Dermis,* composed of a dense connective tissue

The *hypodermis,* the subcutaneous connective tissue, is a looser connective tissue than the dermis. It lies deep to the dermis and is the equivalent of the *superficial fascia* described in gross anatomy. The hypodermis contains variable amounts of adipose tissue. In well-nourished individuals and in individuals living in very cold climates, the thickness of the adipose tissue can be considerable.

The epidermal derivatives of the skin include the following organ structures and integumentary products:

- *Hair follicles* and *hair*
- *Sweat (sudoriferous) glands*
- *Sebaceous glands*
- *Nails*
- *Mammary glands*

The integumentary system performs a number of essential functions related to its location on the external surface of the body. These functions include

- *Barrier function* that protects against physical, chemical, and biologic agents in the external environment
- *Homeostatic function* that helps preserve the constancy of the internal environment by regulating body temperature and water loss
- *Sensory function* that brings information about the external environment to the individual and, thus, is both informative and protective
- *"Secretory" function* in converting precursor molecules into vitamin D
- *Excretory function* via the sweat glands

In addition, certain lipid-soluble substances may be absorbed through the skin. Although this is not a function of skin, it is a property that can be taken advantage of in delivery of therapeutic agents.

STRUCTURE OF THICK AND THIN SKIN

The thickness of the skin varies over the surface of the body, from less than 1 μm to more than 5 μm. There are two locations, however, where the skin is obviously different at both gross and histologic levels. The palms of the hands and the soles of the feet, which are subject to the most abrasion, are hairless and have a much thicker epidermal layer than skin in any other location. This hairless skin is referred to as *thick skin.* Elsewhere, the skin possesses a much thinner epidermis and is called *thin skin.* It contains hair follicles in all but a few locations. The terms thick skin and thin skin, as used in histologic description, are misnomers and refer only to the thickness of the epidermal layer. Anatomically, the thickest skin on the body is found on the upper portion of the back where the dermis is exceedingly thick. The epidermis, however, is comparable to that of thin skin found elsewhere on the body. In contrast, in certain other sites such as the eyelid, the skin is extremely thin.

EPIDERMIS

The *epidermis* is composed of stratified squamous epithelium in which four distinct layers can be identified. In the case of thick skin, a fifth layer is observed (Figs. 14.1 and 14.2). Beginning with the deepest layer, these are

- *Stratum basale,* also called *stratum germinativum*
- *Stratum spinosum*
- *Stratum granulosum*
- *Stratum lucidum,* limited to thick skin
- *Stratum corneum*

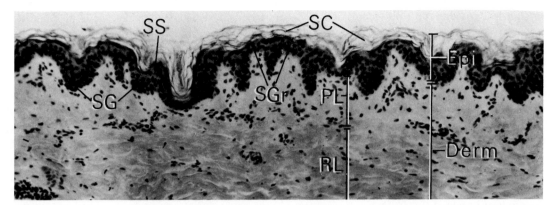

Figure 14.1. Light micrograph showing the layers of thin human skin, the two chief layers of which are epidermis *(Epi)* and dermis *(Derm)*. The epidermis forms the surface; it consists of stratified squamous epithelium that is keratinized. The layers of the epidermis are identified on the basis of location as well as histologic properties. Thus, the deepest layer of cells, adjacent to the dermis, is the stratum germinativum *(SG)*, also called the stratum basale. Adjacent to this is a layer several cells thick, designated as the stratum spinosum *(SS)*. The most superficial layer of nucleated cells is the stratum granulosum *(SGr)*, so designated because of its content of conspicuous cytoplasmic granules, keratohyalin granules, that stain with hematoxylin and give this layer a darker appearance than other layers of the epidermis. The superficial layer of the epidermis is the stratum corneum *(SC)*. It consists of very flat keratinized cells that no longer possess a nucleus. The dermis consists of two layers: the papillary layer *(PL)*, adjacent to the epidermis, and the reticular layer *(RL)*, more deeply positioned. The boundary between these two layers is not conspicuous; the papillary layer is, however, more cellular than the reticular layer. In addition, the collagen fibers of the reticular layer are thick; those of the papillary layer are thin. ×120.

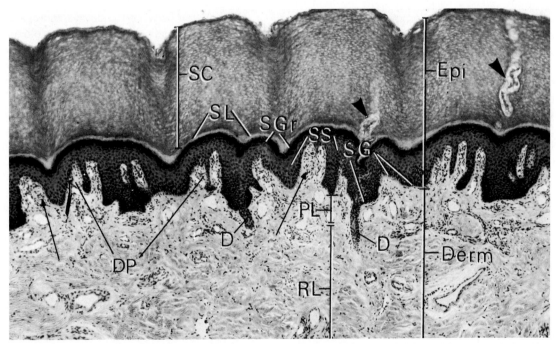

Figure 14.2. Light micrograph showing the layers of thick skin (human). Note the extremely thick stratum corneum *(SC)* and, under this, a thin pale layer, the stratum lucidum *(SL)*. Other layers of the epidermis *(Epi)* are similar to those of thin skin, namely, the stratum basale or germinativum *(SG)*, the stratum spinosum *(SS)*, and the stratum granulosum *(SGr)*. In two locations marked by *arrowheads,* ducts of sweat glands can be seen as they spiral through the epidermis. Only a portion of each duct has been included in the plane of section. The dermis *(Derm)* contains papillae *(DP)* that are more pronounced than those of the thin skin. In several locations, *arrows* point to Meissner's corpuscles. These are sensory receptors and appear as oval bodies within the dermal papillae. Again, notice the greater cellularity of the papillary layer *(PL)* and the fact that collagen fibers of the reticular layer *(RL)* are thicker than those of the papillary layer. In two locations, portions of ducts *(D)* of sweat glands are seen where they enter the epidermis. At the sites where the ducts of the sweat gland enter the epidermis are epidermal downgrowths known as ***interpapillary pegs.*** ×65.

The Stratum Basale Provides for Epidermal Cell Renewal

The *stratum basale* is represented by a single layer of cells that rests on the basal lamina. It contains the *stem cells* from which new cells, the *keratinocytes,* arise by mitotic division. For this reason, the stratum basale is also called the *stratum germinativum.* The cells are small and are cuboidal to low columnar in shape. They have less cytoplasm than the cells in the layer above; consequently, their nuclei are more closely spaced. This, in combination with the basophilic cytoplasm of these cells, imparts a noticeable basophilia to the stratum basale.

As new keratinocytes arise in this layer by mitotic division, they shift into the next layer, thus beginning the process of upward migration. This process terminates when the cell becomes a mature keratinized cell, eventually to be sloughed off at the surface.

The Cells of the Stratum Spinosum Exhibit Numerous Spinous Processes

The *stratum spinosum* is at least several cells thick. The cells are larger than those of the stratum basale. They exhibit numerous cytoplasmic processes or spines, which gives this layer its name. The processes are attached to like processes of adjacent cells by desmosomes. In the light microscope (LM), the site of the desmosome appears as a slight thickening called the *node of Bizzozero.* The processes are usually very conspicuous, in part due to shrinkage of the cells during preparation and the consequent expanded intercellular space that develops between the spines. Because of their appearance, the cells that constitute this layer are often referred to as *prickle cells.* As the cells mature and are moved more superficially, they increase in size and become flattened in a plane parallel to the surface. This is particularly notable in the most superficial spinous cells, where the nuclei also become elongate instead of ovoid, matching the acquired squamous shape of the cells.

The Cells of the Stratum Granulosum Contain Conspicuous Keratohyalin Granules

The stratum granulosum is the most superficial layer of the nonkeratinized portion of the epidermis. This layer varies from one to a few cells thick. The cells contain numerous *keratohyalin granules,* hence the name of the layer. The granules contain cystine-rich and histidine-rich proteins. Keratohyalin granules are variable in size and, because of their intense basophilic staining, are readily seen in routine histologic sections.

The Stratum Corneum Consists of Anucleate Squamous Cells Filled With Keratin

Usually, there is an abrupt transition between the nucleated cells of the stratum granulosum and the very flat-tened, desiccated, anucleate cells of the stratum corneum. The plasma membrane of these cornified keratinized cells is thickened and is coated, at least in the deeper portion of this layer, with a *glycolipid* that forms the major constituent of the *water barrier* in the epidermis.

The stratum corneum is the layer that varies most in thickness, being thickest in thick skin. It is the thickness of this layer that is the principal difference between the epidermis of thick and thin skin. This cornified layer will become even thicker at sites subjected to unusual amounts of friction, as in the formation of calluses on the palm of the hand and on the fingertips.

The *stratum lucidum,* considered a subdivision of the stratum corneum by some histologists, is found only in thick skin. In the LM, it often has a refractile appearance and may stain poorly. This highly refractile layer contains eosinophilic cells in which the process of keratinization is well advanced. The nucleus and cytoplasmic organelles become disrupted and disappear as the cell gradually fills with the intracellular protein *keratin.*

DERMIS

Attachment of Epidermis to Dermis Is Enhanced by an Increased Interface Between the Two Tissues

The junction between the dermis and epidermis as seen with the LM presents an extremely uneven boundary except in the thinnest skin. Sections of skin cut perpendicular to the surface reveal numerous finger-like connective tissue protrusions, *dermal papillae,* that project into the under-surface of the epidermis (Figs. 14.1 and 14.2). The papillae are complemented by what appear to be similar epidermal protrusions, called *epidermal ridges* or *rete ridges,* that seem to project into the dermis. If the plane of section is parallel to the surface of the epidermis and passes at a level to include the dermal papillae, however, the epidermal tissue appears as a continuous sheet of epithelium, containing circular islands of connective tissue within it. The islands are cross sections of true finger-like dermal papillae that project into the epidermis. At sites where there is increased mechanical stress on the skin, the epidermal ridges are much deeper (the epithelium simply being thicker), and the dermal papillae are much longer and more closely spaced. This creates a more extensive interface between the dermis and epidermis. This phenomenon is particularly well demonstrated in histologic sections that show both palmar and dorsal surfaces of the hand, as in a section of a finger.

True *Dermal Ridges* Are Present in Thick Skin in Addition to Dermal Papillae

Dermal ridges tend to have a parallel arrangement, with the dermal papillae located between them. These ridges form a distinctive pattern that is genetically unique for each individual and is reflected in the appearance of epidermal grooves and ridges on the surface of the skin. This is the basis of the science of *dermatoglyphics* or fingerprint and footprint identification.

Where the dermal ridges and papillae are most prominent, in the thick skin of the palmar and plantar surfaces, the basal surface of the epidermis greatly exceeds its free surface. The germinal layer is, thus, spread over a very large area, and assuming a near-constant rate of mitosis in the stratum germinativum, many more cells per unit time would enter the stratum corneum in thick skin than in thin skin. This is thought to account for the greater thickness of the cornified layer in thick skin.

Hemidesmosomes and Other Specializations Strengthen the Attachment of the Epidermis to the Connective Tissue

When studied with the transmission electron microscope (TEM), the basal surface of the basal epidermal cells exhibits a pattern of irregular cytoplasmic protrusions that increase the attachment surface between the epithelial cell and its subjacent basal lamina. A series of specialized attachment sites called *hemidesmosomes* link the basal plasma membrane to the basal lamina. The hemidesmosome is structurally similar to the desmosomal components on other parts of the basal cell membrane except that there is no paired structure linked to it on an adjacent cell. It looks like one-half of a desmosomal junction, hence the name.

The hemidesmosomes attach to the basal lamina by means of fine *anchoring filaments* that extend from the inner leaflet of the plasma membrane to the basal lamina at the site of the hemidesmosome. Beneath the basal lamina at the same site are numerous fibrils called *anchoring fibrils.* The fibrils extend from the basal lamina into the substance of the dermis, where they attach to collagen fibrils, thus enhancing the attachment of the basal lamina to the underlying connective tissue.

The Dermis Is Composed of Two Layers, a Papillary Layer and a Reticular Layer

In examining the full thickness of the dermis at the LM level, one can recognize a division into two structurally distinct layers.

- The *papillary layer,* the more superficial layer, consists of loose connective tissue immediately beneath the epidermis. The collagen fibers located in this part of the dermis are not as thick as those in the deeper portion. Similarly, the elastic fibers here are thread-like and form an irregular network. The papillary layer is relatively thin and includes the substance of the dermal papillae and dermal ridges. It contains blood vessels that serve but do not enter the epidermis. It also contains nerve processes, some of which terminate in the dermis and some of which penetrate the basal lamina to enter the

epithelial compartment. The blood vessels and sensory nerve endings are particularly concentrated and, therefore, particularly apparent in the dermal papillae.
- The *reticular layer* lies deep to the papillary layer; it varies in thickness in different parts of the body but is always considerably thicker and less cellular than the papillary layer. It is characterized by thick, irregular bundles of collagen and by the presence of more coarse elastic fibers. The collagen and elastic fibers are not randomly oriented but form regular lines of tension in the skin, called *Langer's lines.* Skin incisions that are parallel to Langer's lines will heal with the least scarring.

In the skin of the areolae, penis, scrotum, and perineum, smooth muscle cells form a loose plexus in the deepest parts of the reticular layer. This accounts for the puckering of the skin at these sites, particularly in the erectile organs.

Layers of Adipose Tissue, Smooth Muscle, and, in Some Sites, Striated Muscle May Be Found Just Below the Reticular Layer

Deep to the reticular layer is a layer of adipose tissue, the *panniculus adiposus,* that may be quite variable in thickness. Not only is this a major energy storage site, but it also serves as an important insulating layer. It is particularly thick in individuals who live in very cold climates. This layer and its associated loose connective tissue constitute the *hypodermis* or *subcutaneous layer.*

Individual smooth muscle cells or small bundles of smooth muscle cells that originate here form the *arrector pili* muscles that connect the deep part of hair follicles to the more superficial dermis. Contraction of these muscles in humans produces the erection of hairs and puckering of skin called ''goose flesh.'' In animals, the erection of hairs serves both in thermal regulation and in fright reactions.

A thin layer of striated muscle, the *panniculus carnosus,* lies deep to the panniculus adiposus in many animals. Although it is largely vestigial in humans, it remains well defined in the skin of the neck, face, and scalp, where it constitutes the platysma and the muscles of facial expression.

CELLS OF THE EPIDERMIS

Keratinocyte

The keratinocyte is the predominate cell type of the epidermis. On leaving the basal epidermal layer it assumes two essential activities in order to accomplish its functional role:

- Production of keratin, which will ultimately fill the cell
- Creation of an extracellular water barrier

The keratinocytes in the basal layer contain numerous

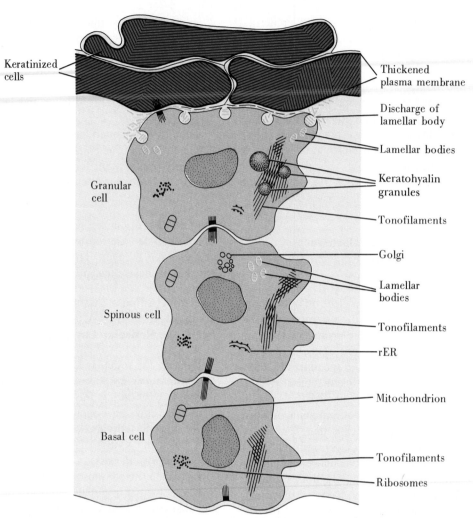

Figure 14.3. Schematic diagram of keratinocytes of the epidermis. The keratinocytes in this figure reflect different stages of the life of the cell as it passes from the basal layer through the spinous and granular layers to the surface keratinized layer. The basal cell begins the synthesis of tonofilaments; these are grouped into bundles and seen with the LM as tonofibrils. The basal cell contains free ribosomes active in the synthesis of tonofilaments. The cell enters the spinous layer where the synthesis of tonofilaments continues. Also in the upper part of the spinous layer, the cells begin the production of keratohyalin granules and glycolipid-containing lamellar bodies. Within the granular layer, lamellar bodies are discharged by the cell; the remainder of the cell cytoplasm contains numerous keratohyalin granules in close association with tonofilaments. The surface cells are keratinized; they contain a thickened plasma membrane and bundles of tonofilaments in a specialized matrix. (From Matoltsy AG, Parrakal PF: In: Zelickson AS (ed): *Ultrastructure of Normal and Abnormal Skin.* Philadelphia, Lea & Febiger, 1967, p 78.)

free ribosomes, scattered 7–9-nm intermediate filaments, a small Golgi complex, mitochondria, and rough endoplasmic reticulum (rER). The cytoplasm of the immature keratinocyte appears basophilic in histologic sections because of the very large number of free ribosomes, most of which are engaged in the synthesis of intermediate filaments. The intermediate filaments, more commonly called *tonofilaments* in the case of the keratinocytes, represent the essential protein in keratin production.

As the cells enter and are moved through the stratum spinosum, the synthesis of tonofilaments continues, and the filaments become grouped into bundles sufficiently thick to be visualized with the LM. These bundles are called *tonofibrils.* The cytoplasm becomes eosinophilic due to the

staining reaction of the tonofibrils that fill more and more of the cytoplasm.

In the upper part of the stratum spinosum (Fig. 14.3), the keratinocytes begin to synthesize *keratohyalin granules* and *lamellar bodies (membrane-coating granules).* The keratohyalin granules are also synthesized by free ribosomes; during their formation, small keratohyalin granules are surrounded by ribosomes (Fig. 14.4).

As the number of granules increases, they become the most distinctive feature of the cells that then constitute the stratum granulosum. A substance contained in the keratohyalin granules combines with the tonofibrils, converting them to keratin. *Keratinization,* i.e., the conversion of granular cells to cornified cells, occurs in 2–6 hours, the

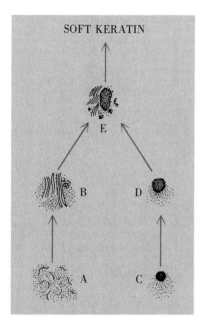

SOFT KERATIN

Figure 14.4. Outline of steps leading to the formation of soft keratin as seen with an electron microscope. Tonofilaments are produced by activity of ribosomes **(A).** The tonofilaments then group as bundles **(B)** that are visible with the LM as tonofibrils. Somewhat later, keratohyalin granules are also produced by the ribosomes **(C** and **D);** at this time the keratohyalin granules are surrounded by a rim of ribosomes. Finally, the tonofilaments (tonofibrils) react with the keratohyalin granules **(E),** which provide a matrix for the fibrils. (From Reith EJ, Rhodin JG: *Fundamentals of Keratinization.* Washington, DC, AAAS, 1962, p 87.)

time it takes for the cells to leave the stratum granulosum and to enter the stratum corneum. The keratin formed in this process is called *soft keratin* in contrast to the *hard keratin* of hair and nails (see below).

The transformation of a granular cell to a cornified cell also involves the breakdown of the nucleus and other organelles and the thickening of the plasma membrane. Finally, there is a regular desquamation of cells from the surface of the stratum corneum. The cells that will desquamate accumulate acid phosphatase, which is thought to participate in the exfoliation of these keratinized cells.

As the keratinocytes in the stratum spinosum begin to produce keratohyalin granules, they also begin to produce the membrane-bounded **lamellar bodies.** The spinous and the granular cells synthesize a glycolipid (Fig. 14.5) that is assembled into the lamellar bodies in the Golgi complex. The content of the granules is then secreted by exocytosis into the intercellular spaces of the upper portion of the stratum granulosum (Fig. 14.6). The glycolipid coating of the membrane, containing acylglucosylceramide, forms the water barrier of the epidermis.

As the cells continue to move toward the free surface, the glycolipid layer is retained, so that it is also present between the stratum granulosum and the stratum corneum and between the deep cells of the cornified layer. Lamellae

may remain as recognizable discs in the intercellular space or may fuse into broad sheets or layers. It has been shown in experiments that animals suffering from essential fatty acid deficiency (EFAD) have an epidermis that is more permeable than normal to water and have membrane-coating granules with fewer lamellae than normal. The destruction of the glycolipid layer over large areas, as in severe burns, can lead to life-threatening loss of fluid from the body.

Melanocyte

Melanocytes Are Pigment-Producing Cells

The epidermal **melanocyte** is a dendritic cell found scattered among the basal cells of the stratum basale (Fig. 14.7). They are called dendritic cells because the rounded cell body resides in the basal layer and extends long processes between the keratinocytes of the stratum spinosum. Neither the processes nor the cell body establishes desmosomal attachments with the neighboring keratinocytes. Hemidesmosomes, however, attach the cell body to the basal lamina. The ratio of melanocyte to keratinocyte or their precursors in the basal layer ranges from 1:4 to 1:10 in different parts of the body; thus, the melanocytes represent a very small portion of the total epidermal cell population. In the LM, the melanocyte is difficult to identify without special staining techniques. With the TEM, however, they can be identified readily by the presence of developing and mature melanin granules in the cytoplasm (Fig. 14.8).

Melanocytes are also present in the dermis in certain regions of the body. They are most numerous in sites where the connective tissue exhibits some degree of pigmentation. The dermal melanocytes are stellate cells with long processes and an elongate nucleus.

Melanocytes Are of Neural Crest Origin

During embryonic life, melanocyte precursor cells migrate from the neural crest and enter the developing epidermis. A specific functional association is then established, the **epidermal-melanin unit,** in which one melanocyte maintains an association with a given number of keratinocytes. As noted earlier, this ratio varies in different parts of the body. The melanocytes maintain the capacity to replicate throughout postnatal life, though at a much slower rate than the keratinocyte, and thus can maintain the appropriate epidermal-melanin unit.

Melanin is produced by the oxidation of **tyrosine** to **3,4-dihydroxyphenylalanine (DOPA)** by **tyrosinase** and the subsequent transformation of DOPA into melanin. These reactions occur initially in membrane-bounded structures, called **premelanosomes,** that are derived from the Golgi complex (Fig. 14.9). The premelanosomes and the early melanosomes, which have a low melanin content, exhibit a finely ordered internal structure in the TEM, reflecting

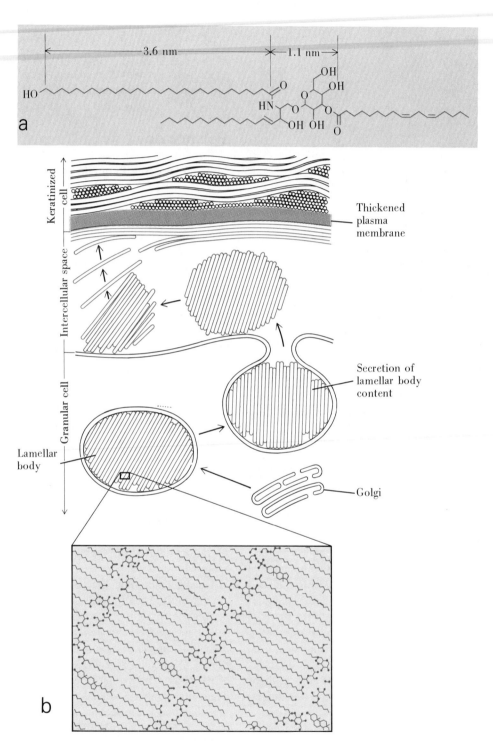

Figure 14.5. Schematic diagram of acylglucosylceramide molecule **(a)** present in lamellar bodies. This molecule, along with other lipid molecules, makes up the lamellae of the lamellar bodies **(b).** The lamellar bodies, produced by an intracellular pathway involving the Golgi complex, are finally discharged by the cell, where they function in the intercellular space as a water barrier. The lamellar arrangement of lipid molecules is depicted in the intercellular space just below the thickened plasma membrane of the keratinized cell. Filaments of the keratinized cell are shown in both longitudinal and cross section. (Based on Wertz P: *Science* 217:1262, 1983, copyright 1983 by the AAAS.)

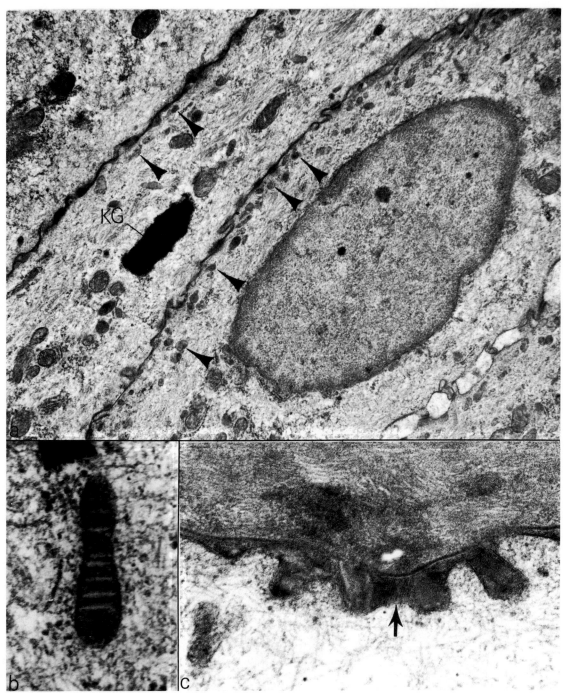

Figure 14.6. Electron micrographs showing keratinocytes with much of their cytoplasm filled with tonofilaments. **a.** One cell exhibits a keratohyalin granule *(KG)*. Near the plasma membrane closest to the surface (upper left), two of the cells display lamellar bodies *(arrowheads)*. **b.** A lamellar body at higher magnification. **c.** Part of a keratinized cell and the underlying keratinocyte. Between the cells is the lamellar material from the lamellar bodies that has been discharged into the intercellular space *(arrow)*. (Courtesy of Dr. A. I. Farbman.)

their content of tyrosinase molecules. As more melanin is produced by oxidation of tyrosine, the internal structure of the premelanosome becomes obscured until the mature melanin granule, the *melanosome,* is formed and then appears as an electron-opaque granule. Premelanosomes are concentrated near the Golgi complex, nearly mature melanosomes are concentrated at the bases of the cell processes,

and mature melanosomes are most commonly found in and at the ends of the processes (Fig. 14.9). The melanosomes are transferred to the keratinocytes by phagocytosis of the tips of the melanocyte processes by the keratinocytes. This process is a type of *cytocrine secretion* because a small amount of cytoplasm surrounding the melanosome is also phagocytosed by the keratinocyte.

SKIN COLOR

The color of an individual's skin is due to a number of factors. The most significant is melanin content. Although the number of melanocytes is essentially the same in all races, there are differences in the nature of the melanin that is produced by the melanocytes. For example, by the lysosomal activity of the keratinocytes, melanin is degraded more rapidly in Caucasian skin than in Negroid skin. In the former, melanosomes are more concentrated in the keratinocytes nearest the basal layer and are relatively sparse in the midregion of the stratum granulosa. In contrast, Negroid epidermis may exhibit melanosomes throughout the epidermis, including the stratum corneum.

In addition, melanin pigment comprises two distinctive forms. One form, *eumelanin,* is a brownish-black pigment. The other form, *pheomelanin,* is a red to yellow pigment. Each is genetically determined. Coloration is most apparent in hair due to the concentration of the melanin pigment granules, but it is also reflected in coloration of the skin.

Exposure to ultraviolet light, particularly the sun's rays, stimulates a more rapid rate of melanin production and, thus, acts as a protection against further radiation effects. Increased pigmentation of the skin may also occur as a result of hormonal imbalance, as, for example, in Addison's disease. Lack of pigmentation occurs in a condition known as albinism. In this instance, premelanosomes are produced by the melanocyte, but because of the absence of tyrosinase, the transformation of tyrosine into 3,4-dihydroxyphenylalanine (DOPA) and the subsequent transformation of DOPA into melanin fail to occur. Thus, there is no pigmentation in the skin or hair of these individuals.

Other normal factors that affect skin coloration include the presence of oxyhemoglobin in the dermal vascular bed, which imparts a red hue, the presence of carotenes, an exogenous orange pigment taken up from foods and concentrated in tissues containing fat, and the presence of certain endogenous pigments. The latter include degradation products of hemoglobin, iron-containing hemosiderin and iron-free bilirubin, all of which impart color to the skin. Hemosiderin is a golden-brown pigment, whereas bilirubin is a yellowish-brown pigment. Bilirubin is normally removed from the bloodstream by the liver and eliminated via the bile. A yellowish skin color due to abnormal accumulations of bilirubin reflects liver dysfunction and is particularly evident in jaundice.

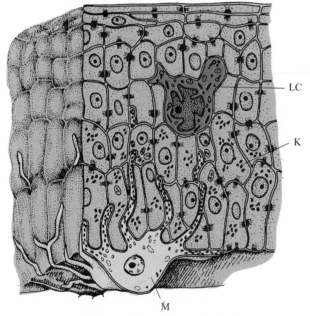

Figure 14.7. Diagram of the epidermis, showing a melanocyte *(M)* interacting with several cells of the stratum germinativum and the stratum spinosum (an epidermal melanin unit). The melanocyte has long dendritic processes that contain accumulated melanosomes and extend between the epidermal cells. The cell higher in the stratum spinosum is a Langerhans cell *(LC),* a dendritic cell often confused with a melanocyte. The Langerhans cell is actually part of the mononuclear phagocytic system that functions as an antigen-presenting cell of the immune system, involved in the initiation of cutaneous hypersensitivity reactions (contact allergic dermatitis). *K,* keratinocyte. (Modified from Weiss L (ed): *Cell and Tissue Biology, A Textbook of Histology,* 6th ed. Baltimore, Urban & Schwarzenberg, 1988, p 548.)

Langerhans Cell

The Langerhans Cell Plays a Role in the Immune Response by Presenting Antigens to T Cells

The Langerhans cell, like the melanocyte, cannot be distinguished with certainty in routine hematoxylin and eosin (H&E)-stained paraffin sections. Like the melanocyte, the Langerhans cell does not form desmosomes with neighboring keratinocytes. They closely resemble, both morphologically and functionally, similar dendritic cells in the lymph nodes, spleen, and thymus. The nucleus stains heavily with hematoxylin, and the cytoplasm is clear. With special techniques, such as gold impregnation, the Langerhans cell is readily seen in the stratum spinosum. It possesses dendritic processes resembling those of the melanocyte. The TEM reveals several distinctive features of the Langerhans cell (Fig. 14.10). Its nucleus is characteristically indented in many places, so that the nuclear profile is very uneven. Also, it possesses characteristic granules that appear as rods, some of which may exhibit a bulbous expansion along their length. A striated band is present at the center of the rod.

In common with macrophages, the Langerhans cell possesses surface Fc, Ia, and C3 receptors. At sites of allergic contact, lymphocytes are seen in close apposition to the Langerhans cell membrane shortly after antigenic challenge. As an antigen-presenting cell, the Langerhans cell is involved in the initiation of cutaneous contact hypersensitivity reactions, i.e., contact allergic dermatitis, and in other cell-mediated immune responses in the skin. Several laboratories have shown that in skin biopsies from individuals with AIDS or AIDS-related complex, Langerhans' cells have the human immunodeficiency virus (HIV) in their cytoplasm. Langerhans' cells appear to be more resistant than

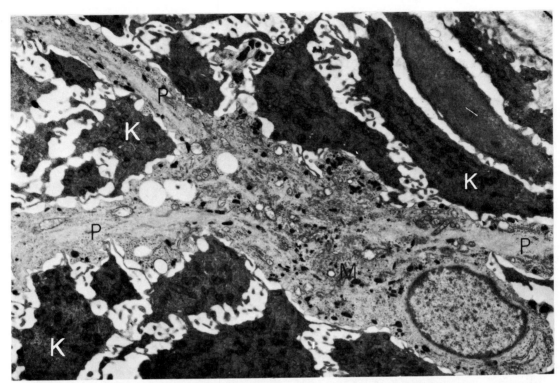

Figure 14.8. Electron micrograph of a melanocyte *(M)* showing melanin granules. Three processes *(P)* can be seen extending between the neighboring keratinocytes *(K).* ×5800. (Courtesy of Dr. B. Munger.)

T cells to the deadly affect of the virus and may, therefore, serve as a reservoir for the virus. The Langerhans cell is most likely derived initially from mesenchyme and is included in the list of cells that constitute the mononuclear phagocytic system.

Merkel Cell

The Merkel Cell Is an Epidermal Cell That Functions in Cutaneous Sensation

Merkel's cells are modified epidermal cells that are located in the stratum basale. They are most abundant in skin where sensory perception is acute, such as the fingertips. Merkel's cells are bound to adjoining keratinocytes by desmosomes and have intermediate (keratin) filaments in their cytoplasm. The nucleus is lobed, and the cytoplasm is somewhat more dense than the cytoplasm of melanocytes and Langerhans' cells. They may have some melanosomes in the cytoplasm, but they are best characterized by the presence of *80-nm dense-cored neurosecretory granules* that resemble those found in the adrenal medulla and the carotid body (Fig. 14.11). Merkel's cells are closely associated with the expanded terminal bulb of an afferent myelinated nerve fiber. The neuron terminal loses its Schwann cell covering and immediately penetrates the basal lamina, where it expands into a disc or plate-like ending that lies in close apposition to the base of the Merkel cell (Fig. 14.12). The combination of the neuron and epidermal cell, called a *Merkel's corpuscle,* is a very sensitive *mechanoreceptor.*

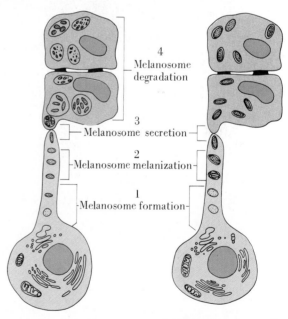

Figure 14.9. Formation of melanin pigment and secretion of pigment granules into keratinocytes. Melanocytes produce melanin within membrane-limited bodies called melanosomes (*1* and *2*). Secretion of melanosomes consists of their passage into neighboring keratinocytes *(3).* In Negroid skin, the melanosomes remain discrete; in Caucasian skin, the melanosomes are degraded *(4)* through the intervention of lysosome-like organelles. (Based on Weiss L, Greep RO: *Histology,* 4th ed. New York, McGraw-Hill, 1977, p 597.)

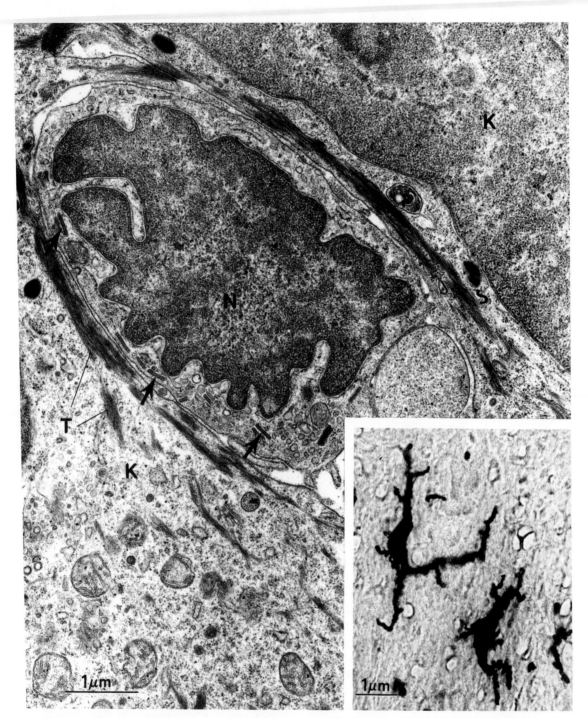

Figure 14.10. Electron micrograph of the Langerhans cell. The nucleus *(N)* is characteristically indented in many places, and the cytoplasm contains distinctive rod-shaped bodies *(arrows)*. Note the presence of tonofilaments *(T)* in adjacent keratino-cytes *(K)* but the absence of these filaments in the Langerhans cell. In the light micrograph **(inset),** the dendritic nature of the Langerhans cell can be seen by application of a special stain. ×19,000; **inset,** ×1,200. (Courtesy of Dr. C. Squier.)

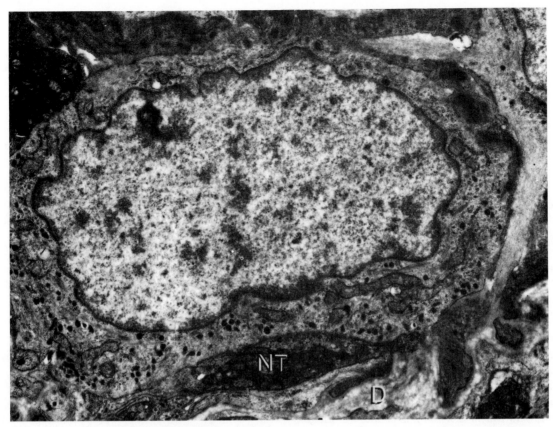

Figure 14.11. Electron micrograph of a Merkel cell. The cell has small granules in the cytoplasm and makes contact with a peripheral terminal *(NT)* of a neuron. The dermis *(D)* is in the lower part of the illustration. ×14,450. (Courtesy of Dr. B. Munger.)

NERVE SUPPLY TO THE SKIN

The skin is endowed with sensory receptors of various types that are peripheral terminals of sensory nerves (Fig. 14.12). It is also well supplied with motor endings to the blood vessels, the arrector pili muscles, and the sudoriferous glands.

The Most Numerous Neuronal Endings Are *Free Nerve Endings* in the Epidermis and the Papillary Dermis

Free nerve endings in the epidermis terminate in the stratum granulosum. The endings are "free" in the sense that they lack a connective tissue or Schwann cell investment. Such neuronal endings subserve multiple sensory modalities including fine touch, heat, and cold, without apparent morphologic distinctions. Networks of free dermal endings surround most hair follicles and attach to their outer root sheath (Fig. 14.13). In this position they are particularly sensitive to hair movement and serve as mechanoreceptors. (This relationship reaches a very sophisticated degree of specialization in the receptors that surround tactile hairs (vibrissae), such as the whiskers of a cat or rodent, in which each vibrissa has a specific representation in the cerebral cortex.)

Other nerve endings in the skin are enclosed in a connective tissue capsule. *Encapsulated nerve endings* include

- *Pacinian corpuscles*
- *Meissner's corpuscles*
- *Ruffini endings*

Pacinian Corpuscles

Pacinian Corpuscles Are Deep Pressure Receptors for Mechanical and Vibratory Pressure

Pacinian corpuscles are large ovoid structures found in the deeper dermis and hypodermis, especially of the fingertips, in connective tissue in general, and in association with joints, periosteum, and internal organs. Pacinian corpuscles are usually of macroscopic dimensions, measuring more than 1 mm in their long axis. They are composed of a myelinated nerve ending surrounded by a capsule structure. The nerve enters the capsule at one pole with its myelin sheath intact. The myelin is retained for one or two nodes and is then lost. The unmyelinated portion of the axon extends toward the opposite pole from which it entered and is covered along its length by a series of tightly packed flattened Schwann cell lamellae that form the **inner core** of the corpuscle. The remainder or bulk of the capsule, the outer core, is formed by a series of concentric lamellae; each lamella is separated from its neighbor by a narrow space containing lymph-like fluid. The appearance of the concentric lamellae as observed in the LM is reminiscent of the cut surface of a hemisected onion. Each lamella is composed of flattened cells that correspond to the endoneurial cells outside of the capsule. In addition to fluid between the lamellae, collagen fibrils are present, though sparse in number, as well as occasional capillaries.

Pacinian corpuscles respond to pressure and vibrations through the displacement of the capsule lamellae. This effectively causes depolarization of the axon.

Meissner's Corpuscles

Meissner's corpuscles (see Fig. 14.12) are touch receptors that are particularly responsive to low-frequency stimuli in the papillary layer of hairless skin, i.e., the lips and the palmar and volar surfaces, particularly those of the fingers and toes. Generally, they are tapered cylinders that measure about 150 μm in their long axis and are oriented perpendicular to the skin surface. Meissner's corpuscles are present at the tip of the dermal papillae just beneath the epidermal basal lamina. In these receptors, one or two unmyelinated endings of myelinated nerve fibers follow spiral paths within the corpuscle. The cellular component consisting of flattened Schwann cells forms several irregular lamellae through which the axons course to the pole of the corpuscle. In H&E-stained slides of sagittal sections, this structure gives an appearance that resembles a loose, twisted skein of wool. It is the Schwann cells that give this impression.

Ruffini Endings

The Ruffini Corpuscle Responds to Mechanical Displacement of Adjacent Collagen Fibers

Ruffini endings are the simplest encapsulated mechanoreceptors. They have an elongated fusiform shape and measure 1–2 μm in length. Structurally, they consist of a thin connective tissue capsule that encloses a fluid-filled space. Collagen fibers from the surrounding connective tissue pass through the capsule. The neural element consists of a single myelinated fiber that enters the capsule, whereupon it loses its myelin sheath and branches to form a dense arborization of fine axonal endings, with each terminating in a small knob-like bulb. The axonal endings are dispersed and intertwined inside the capsule, with the collagen fibers passing through the capsule. The axonal endings respond to displacement of the collagen fibers induced by sustained or continuous mechanical stress.

SKIN APPENDAGES

Skin appendages are derived from downgrowths of epidermal epithelium during development. They include

- **Hair follicles** and their product, **hair**
- **Sebaceous glands** and their product, **sebum**
- **Eccrine sweat glands** and their product, **sweat**
- **Apocrine sweat glands** and their product, **serous secretion**

Both hairs and sweat glands have specific roles in regulation of body temperature. Sebaceous glands secrete an oily material that may have protective functions. Apocrine glands produce a serous secretion that acts as a sex attractant in animals and, possibly, humans. The epithelium of the skin appendages can serve as a source of new epithelial cells for skin wound repair.

HAIR

Hairs Are Composed of Keratinized Cells That Develop From Hair Follicles

Hairs are present over almost the entire body, being absent only from the sides and palmar surfaces of the hands, from the sides and plantar surfaces of the feet, from the lips, and from the region around the urogenital orifices. In some locations, hairs are influenced to a considerable degree by sex hormones; these include, in the male, the thick pigmented facial hairs that begin to grow at puberty and the pubic and axillary hair that develops at puberty in both sexes. In the male, the hairline tends to recede with age, and in both sexes, there is a thinning of the scalp hair with age due to reduction in secretion of estrogen and estrogen-like hormones.

Structure of the Hair Follicle

The hair follicle is responsible for the production and growth of a hair. Coloration of the hair is due to the content and type of melanin (see page 375) that the hair contains. The follicle varies in histologic appearance, depending on whether it is in a growing or a resting phase. The growing follicle shows the most elaborate structure; thus, it is described here.

The growing follicle (see Fig. 14.13) is of nearly uniform diameter except at its base, where it expands to form the **bulb**. The base of the bulb is invaginated by a tuft of vascularized loose connective tissue called, not surprisingly, a **dermal papilla**. The outermost part of the hair follicle is a downgrowth of the epidermis designated the **external (outer) root sheath**. Other cells forming the bulb, including those that surround the connective tissue papilla, are collectively referred to as the matrix, which consists simply of **matrix cells**. Those matrix cells that are immediately adjacent to the dermal papilla represent the germinative layer of the follicle. Scattered melanocytes are present in this germinative layer. They contribute melanosomes to the developing hair cells in a manner analogous to the role they play in the stratum germinativum of the epidermis.

The dividing cells in the germinative layer of the matrix differentiate into the keratin-producing cells of the hair and the *internal root sheath.* The internal root sheath is a multilayered cellular covering that surrounds the deep part of the hair. Both the hair and the internal root sheath have three layers. The hair consists of a *medulla, cortex,* and *cuticle,* and the internal root sheath consists of a *cuticle, Huxley's layer,* and *Henle's layer.* Keratinization of the hair and internal root sheath occurs in a region called the *keratogenous zone* shortly after the cells leave the matrix. By the time the hair emerges from the follicle, it is entirely keratinized as *hard keratin.* The internal root sheath, consisting of *soft keratin,* does not emerge from the follicle with the hair but is broken down at about the level at which sebaceous secretions enter the follicle. The follicle is surrounded by a connective tissue sheath to which the *arrector pili muscle* is attached.

HAIR GROWTH AND HAIR CHARACTERISTICS

Unlike the renewal of the surface epidermis, hair growth is not a continuous process. A period of growth *(anagen)* in which a new hair develops is followed by a brief period in which growth stops *(catagen).* This is followed by a long rest period in which the follicle atrophies *(telogen),* and the hair is eventually lost. In catagen, the germinative zone is reduced to an epithelial strand still attached to a reduced remnant of the dermal papilla. In telogen, the atrophied follicle may contract to one-half or less of its original length. The hair may remain attached to the follicle for several months during this stage and is called a *club hair* because of the shape of its proximal end.

Hairs vary in size from long, coarse *terminal hairs* that may reach a length of a meter or more (scalp hair; beard hair in males) to short, fine *vellus hairs* that may be visible only with the aid of a magnifying lens (vellus hairs of the forehead and anterior surface of the forearm). Terminal hairs are produced by large-diameter, long follicles; vellus hairs are produced by relatively small follicles. Terminal hair follicles may spend up to several *years* in anagen and only a few *months* in telogen. In the balding individual, large terminal follicles gradually convert to small vellus follicles after several growth cycles. The ratio of vellus follicles to terminal follicles increases as baldness becomes more apparent. The "completely bald" scalp is not hairless but is populated by vellus follicles that produce fine hairs and remain in telogen for relatively long periods.

SEBACEOUS GLANDS

Sebaceous Glands Secrete *Sebum* That Coats the Hair and Skin Surface

The sebaceous glands develop as an outgrowth of the external root sheath of the hair follicle, usually producing several glands per follicle (see Fig. 14.13). The oily substance that is produced in the gland, *sebum,* is the product of holocrine secretion. The entire cell produces and becomes filled with the fatty product while it simultaneously undergoes progressive disruption, followed by necrosis, as the product fills the cell. Ultimately, both secretory product and cell debris are discharged from the gland as sebum into the *pilosebaceous canal.* New cells are produced by mitosis of the basal cells at the periphery of the gland, and the cells of the gland remain linked to one another by desmosomes. The basal lamina of these cells is continuous with that of the epidermis and the hair follicle.

The basal cells of the sebaceous gland contain smooth (sER) and rough (rER) endoplasmic reticulum, free ribosomes, mitochondria, glycogen, and a well-developed Golgi complex, but they have few lipid droplets (Fig. 14.14). As the cells move away from the basal layer and begin to produce the lipid secretory product, the amount of sER increases, reflecting the role of the sER in lipid synthesis and secretion. The cells gradually become filled with numerous lipid droplets separated by thin strands of cytoplasm (Fig. 14.14).

FUNCTION OF SEBUM

The function of sebum is not clearly defined. Various investigators have ascribed bacteriostatic, emollient, barrier, and pheromone functions to sebum. Sebum does appear to have a critical role in the development of acne. There is a significant increase in the amount of sebum secreted at puberty in both males and females. Triglycerides contained in sebum are broken down to fatty acids by bacteria on the skin surface, and the free fatty acids liberated may be an irritant in the formation of *acne lesions.*

SWEAT GLANDS

Sweat glands are classified on the basis of their structure and the nature of their secretion. Two types of sweat glands are recognized:

- *Eccrine sweat glands,* distributed over the entire body surface except for the lips and part of the external genitalia
- *Apocrine sweat glands,* limited to the axilla, areola, and nipple of the mammary gland, circumanal region, and the external genitalia

The ceruminous glands of the ear canal and the glands of Moll of the eyelid are also apocrine-type glands.

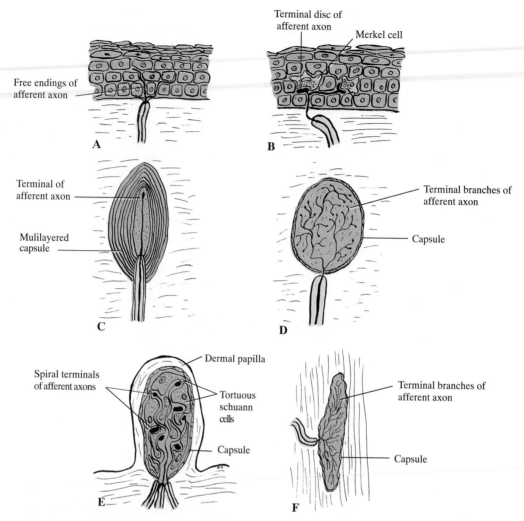

Figure 14.12. Diagram of the sensory receptors in the skin. **A.** Epidermal free ending. **B.** Merkel ending. **C.** Pacinian corpuscle. **D.** Krause end bulb. **E.** Meissner's corpuscle. **F.** Ruffini corpuscle. Note that **C–F** are encapsulated, i.e., surrounded by a capsule of connective tissue.

Eccrine Sweat Glands

Eccrine Sweat Glands Are Simple Coiled Glands That Regulate Body Temperature

The eccrine sweat gland is an independent structure, not associated with the hair follicle, that arises as a downgrowth from the fetal epidermis. It is arranged as a simple coiled tubular structure composed of a secretory segment located deep in the dermis or in the upper part of the hypodermis and a directly continuous duct segment that leads to the epidermal surface.

Secretory and Myoepithelial Cells. Three cell types are present in the secretory segment of the gland: *clear cells* and *dark cells,* both of which are secretory epithelial cells; and *myoepithelial cells,* which are contractile epithelial cells (Fig. 14.15). All of the cells rest on the basal lamina; their arrangement is that of a pseudostratified epithelium.

- *Clear cells* are characterized by abundant glycogen and numerous mitochondria. The glycogen is conspicuous in Figure 14.15*a* by virtue of its amount and intense staining. Membranous organelles include profiles of sER and a relatively small Golgi complex. The plasma membrane is remarkably amplified at the lateral and apical surfaces by extensive cytoplasmic folds. In addition, the basal surface of the cell possesses infoldings, though considerably less complex. The morphology of these cells indicates that they produce the watery component of sweat.
- *Dark cells* are characterized by abundant rER and secretory granules (Fig. 14.15, *a* and *b*). The Golgi complex is relatively large, a feature consistent with the glycoprotein secretion of these cells. The apical cytoplasm contains the mature secretory granules and occupies most of the luminal surface (Fig. 14.15*a*). The clear cells have considerably less cytoplasmic exposure to the lumen; their

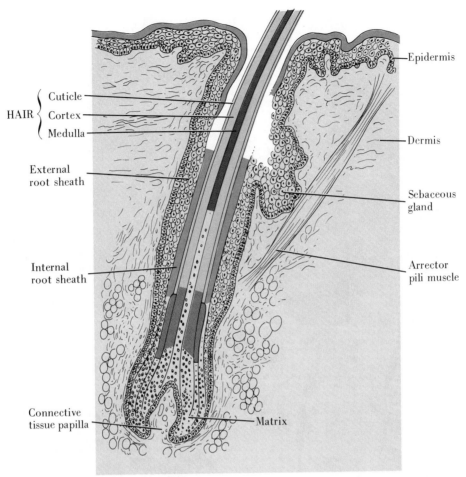

HAIR { Cuticle
       Cortex
       Medulla

External
root sheath

Internal
root sheath

Connective
tissue papilla

Epidermis

Dermis

Sebaceous
gland

Arrector
pili muscle

Matrix

Figure 14.13. Diagram of a hair in a hair follicle, showing the distribution of soft *(medium magenta)* and hard *(pale magenta)* keratin and the keratogenous zone *(dark magenta)* in which the keratin of the hair is produced. (Based on Leblond CP: *Annals of the New York Academy of Sciences* 53:464, 1951.)

secretion is largely via the lateral surfaces of the cell, which are exposed to intercellular canaliculi that allow the watery secretion to reach the lumen where it mixes with the proteinaceous secretion of the dark cells.

- *Myoepithelial cells* are limited to the basal aspect of the tubule. They lie between the secretory cells, with their processes oriented transversally to the tubule. The cytoplasm contains numerous contractile filaments (actin) that stain deeply with eosin, thus making them readily identifiable in routine H&E specimens. Contraction of these cells is responsible for the expression of sweat from the gland.

Duct Cells. The duct of the gland continues from the secretory portion with a similar degree of coiling. In histologic sections, multiple duct profiles may appear among the secretory profiles. As the duct passes upward through the dermis, it takes a gentle spiral course until it reaches the epidermis, where it then continues in a tight spiral to the surface. Where the duct enters the epidermis, however, the duct cells end and the epidermal cells form the wall of the duct. The epithelium of the duct is stratified cuboidal,

consisting of a basal cell layer and a luminal cell layer. The duct cells are smaller and appear darker than the cells of the secretory portion of the gland. Also, the duct has a smaller diameter than the secretory portion. These features can be used to distinguish the duct from the secretory portion in a histologic section.

The basal or peripheral cells of the duct have a rounded or ovoid nucleus and contain a prominent nucleolus. The cytoplasm is filled with mitochondria and ribosomes. The apical or luminal cells are smaller than the basal cells, but their nuclei are similar in appearance. The most conspicuous feature of the luminal cells is a deeply stained, glassy (hyalinized) appearance of the apical cytoplasm. The glassy appearance is due to the presence of large numbers of aggregated tonofilaments in the apical cytoplasm.

The Eccrine Sweat Glands Principally Function in Regulating Body Temperature

The eccrine sweat glands play a major role in temperature regulation through the cooling that results from the evaporation of water from sweat on the body surface. The

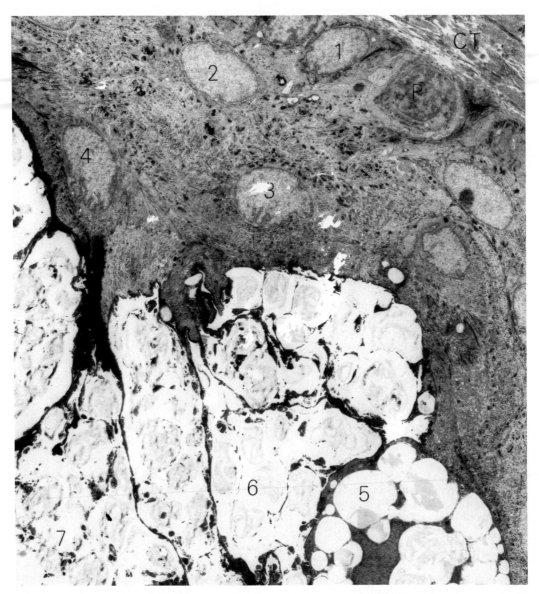

Figure 14.14. Electron micrograph of sebaceous gland. Gland cells *(1)* close to the connective tissue *(CT)* are small and undifferentiated. Among these cells are dividing cells, one of which *(P)* appears to be in early prophase. From this peripheral position the cells move toward the opening of the gland *(2–4)* and produce sebum. The oily product is reflected in the cytoplasm first as small lipid droplets *(5)*, which gradually fuse *(6)* and constitute the secretory product of the gland. The cells perish *(7)* during the secretion. (Courtesy of Dr. B. Munger.)

secretory portion of the glands produces a sweat that is similar in composition to an ultrafiltrate of blood. Resorption of some of the sodium and water in the duct system results in the release of a hypotonic sweat at the skin surface. This hypotonic watery solution is low in protein and contains varying amounts of sodium chloride, urea, uric acid, and ammonia. Thus, the eccrine sweat gland also serves, in part, as an excretory organ. Excessive sweating can lead to loss of other electrolytes, such as potassium and magnesium, and to loss of significant amounts of body water.

Normally, the body loses about 600 mL of water a day through evaporation from the lungs and skin. Under conditions of high ambient temperature, water loss can be increased in a regulated manner by an increased rate of sweating. This ***thermoregulatory sweating*** first occurs on the forehead and scalp, extends to the face and to the rest of the body, and occurs last on the palms and soles. Under conditions of emotional stress, however, the palms, soles, and axillae are the first surfaces to sweat. Whereas control of thermoregulatory sweating is cholinergic, *emotional sweating* may be stimulated by adrenergic portions of the sympathetic division of the autonomic nervous system.

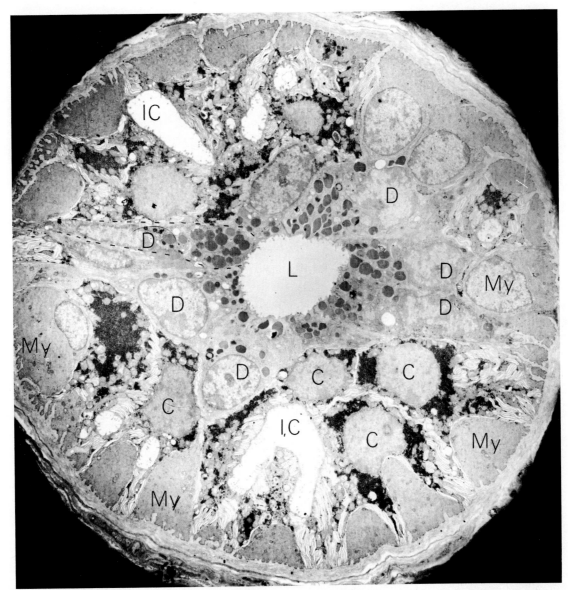

Figure 14.15. a. Electron micrograph of eccrine sweat gland showing myoepithelial cells *(My)* and two distinctive gland cell types, dark cells *(D)* and clear cells *(C)*. The apical portion of the dark cell is broad; it faces the lumen *(L)* of the gland and contains numerous secretory granules. *Dashes* mark the boundary of one dark cell. The clear cell is more removed from the lumen of the gland. Its base rests on the myoepithelial cells or directly on the basal lamina. Most of the free surface of the clear cell faces an intercellular canaliculus *(IC)*. Clear cells contain numerous mitochondria, extensive infoldings of the plasma membrane, and large numbers of glycogen granules. The glycogen appears as the dark material in the electron micrographs. (Courtesy of Dr. J. Terzakis.)

SWEATING AND DISEASE

Although many neural and emotional factors can alter the composition of sweat, altered sweat composition can also be a sign of disease. For example, elevated sodium levels in sweat can serve as a simple indicator of cystic fibrosis. In pronounced uremia, when the kidneys are unable to rid the body of urea, concentrations of urea increase in sweat, and after the water evaporates, crystals may be discerned on the skin, especially on the upper lip. These include urea crystals and are called **urea frost.**

Appocrine Sweat Glands

Apocrine Glands Are Large Lumen Glands Associated With Hair Follicles

Apocrine sweat glands develop from the same downgrowths of epidermis that give rise to the hair follicles. The connection to the follicle is retained, allowing the secretion of the gland to enter the follicle, typically at a level just above the entry of the sebaceous duct, from where it makes its way to the surface.

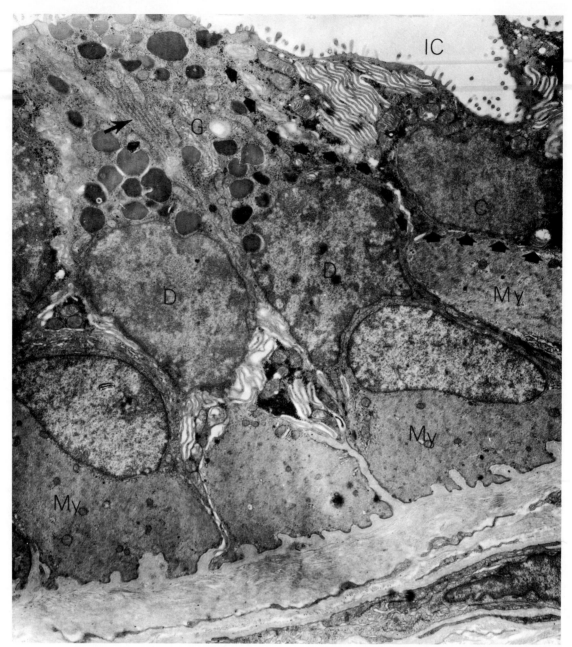

Figure 14.15. b. At higher magnification the dark cells display rER *(arrow)* and a Golgi complex *(G)* in addition to the secretory granules. The clear cells show large amounts of folded membrane, mitochondria, and glycogen. The myoepithelial cells *(My)* contain large numbers of contractile filaments. *Short stubby arrows* (upper right) mark the boundary of the clear cell. (Courtesy of Dr. J. Terzakis.)

Like the eccrine glands, apocrine glands are coiled tubular glands. They are, sometimes, branched. The secretory portion of the gland is deep in the dermis or, more often, in the upper region of the hypodermis.

Secretory and Myoepithelial Cells.   The secretory portion of the apocrine gland differs in several respects from that of the eccrine gland. The most obvious difference, readily noted in the LM, is its very wide lumen (see Plate 60, Fig. 1, page 397). Unlike the eccrine glands, the apocrine glands store their secretory product in the lumen. The secretory portion of the gland is composed of a simple epithelium. Only one cell type is present, and the cytoplasm of the cell is eosinophilic. The apical part of the cell often exhibits a bleb-like protrusion. It was once thought that this part of the cell pinched off and discharged into the lumen as an apocrine secretion, thus the name of the gland. On the basis of TEM studies, it is evident that the secretion is a merocrine type. The apical cytoplasm contains numerous small granules, the secretory component within the cell, that are discharged by exocytosis. Other features of the cell in-

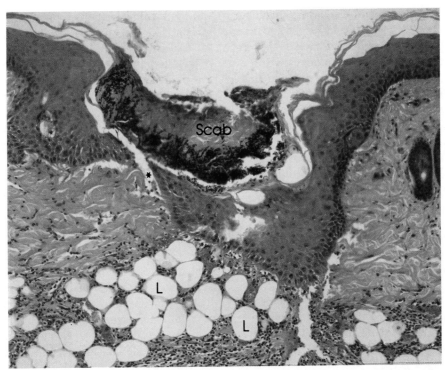

Figure 14.16. Photograph showing a late stage in the epidermal repair of a skin wound. The initial injury was caused by a incision through the full thickness of the skin and partially into the hypodermis, which contains the lipocytes *(L)*. The epidermis has reformed itself beneath the scab. (The *asterisk* marks an artefact where epithelium separated during specimen prep- aration.) The scab, which contains numerous dead neutrophils in its inferior aspect, is nearing the point where it will be released. The dermis at this stage shows little change during the repair process but will ultimately reestablish itself to form a continuous layer. H&E.

clude the presence of numerous lysosomes and lipofuscin pigment granules. The latter represent secondary and tertiary lysosomes. Mitochondria are also numerous. During the refractory phase, after expulsion of the secretion, the Golgi complex becomes enlarged, preparing for a new secretory phase.

Myoepithelial cells are also present in the secretory portion of the gland, situated between the secretory cells and adjacent to the basal lamina. As in the eccrine glands, contraction of the processes of the myoid cell facilitate the expulsion of the secretory product from the gland.

Apocrine Duct. The duct of the apocrine gland is similar to that of the eccrine duct; it has a narrow lumen. However, it continues from the secretory portion of the gland in a relatively straight path to empty into the follicle canal. Because of its straight course, compared with the longer spiral path of the eccrine duct, the chance of viewing both the duct and the secretory portion of the gland in the same histologic section is reduced. Also, in contrast to the eccrine duct, resorption does not take place in the apocrine duct. The secretory product is unaltered in its passage through the duct.

The duct epithelium is stratified cuboidal, usually two but sometimes three cell layers thick. The apical cytoplasm of the luminal cells appears hyalinized. In this they resemble the luminal cells of the eccrine duct. In contrast to the eccrine gland, myoepithelial cells are absent in the duct.

Apocrine Secretions. Apocrine glands produce a secretion that contains protein, carbohydrate, ammonia, lipid, and certain organic compounds that may color the secretion. However, the secretions vary with the anatomic location. In the axilla, the secretion is milky and slightly viscous. When secreted, the fluid is odorless, but through bacterial action on the skin surface it develops an acrid odor.

The apocrine glands become functional only at puberty; as with axillary and pubic hair, development is dependent on sex hormones. In the female, both axillary and areolar apocrine glands undergo morphologic and secretory changes that parallel the menstrual cycle.

In many mammals, similar glands secrete pheromones, chemical signals used in marking territory, in courtship behavior, and in certain maternal and social behavior. It is generally believed that apocrine secretions may function as pheromones in humans.

Innervation of Sweat Glands

Both eccrine and apocrine sweat glands are innervated by the sympathetic portion of the autonomic nervous system. The eccrine sweat glands are stimulated by cholinergic transmitters (usually identified with the parasympathetic component of the autonomic system), whereas the apocrine glands are stimulated by adrenergic transmitters. As described above, the eccrine glands respond differently to heat and to nervous strain. The apocrine glands respond to emotional and sensory stimuli but not to heat.

NAILS

Nails Are Plates of Keratinized Cells Containing Hard Keratin

The slightly arched fingernail or toenail, more properly referred to as the *nail plate,* rests on the *nail bed.* The bed consists of epithelial cells that are continuous with the stratum basale and stratum spinosum of the epidermis (see Plate 63, page 403).

The proximal part of the nail, the *nail root,* is buried in a fold of epidermis and covers the cells of the germinative zone, the *matrix.* The cells of the matrix divide regularly, migrate toward the root of the nail, and there differentiate and produce the keratin of the nail. Nail keratin is a hard keratin, like that of the hair cortex. Unlike soft keratin of the epidermis, it does not desquamate. It consists of densely packed keratin (intermediate) filaments embedded in a matrix of amorphous keratin with a high sulfur content.

The process of hard keratin formation, as with the hair cortex, occurs without the involvement of keratohyalin granules. The constant addition of new cells at the root and their keratinization account for nail growth. As the nail plate grows, it moves over the nail bed.

The crescent-shaped white area near the root of the nail, the *lunula,* derives its color from the thick, opaque layer of partially keratinized matrix cells in this region. When the nail plate becomes fully keratinized, it is more transparent and takes on its coloring from the underlying vascular bed. The edge of the skin fold covering the root of the nail is the *eponychium* or cuticle. This is also composed of hard keratin, and for this reason it does not desquamate. Because of its thinness it tends to break off, or as is the case with many individuals, it is trimmed and pushed back. A thickened epidermal layer, the *hyponychium,* secures the free edge of the nail plate at the fingertip.

SKIN REPAIR

Epidermal Repair Is Effected by Basal Cell Proliferation or, in Extensive Trauma, by Hair Follicle and Sweat Gland Epithelia

An incision or laceration of the skin requires stimulated growth of both the dermis and the epidermis for its repair. Dermal repair involves first, removal of damaged collagen fibers in the wound site, primarily through the effort of macrophage activity, and second, through the proliferation of fibroblasts and subsequent production of new collagen and other extracellular matrix components. By reducing the extent of the repair area through maximal closure of a wound by means of sutures, scar formation is minimized. Surgical incisions are typically made along cleavage lines; the cut tends to parallel the collagen fibers, thus minimizing the need for excess collagen production and the inherent scarring that may occur.

Repair of the epidermis involves the proliferation of the basal keratinocytes in the stratum germinativum in the undamaged site surrounding the wound (Fig. 14.16). Mitotic activity is markedly increased within the first 24 hours.

In a short period of time the wound site is covered by a scab. The proliferating basal cells of the stratum germinativum begin migrating beneath the scab and across the wound surface. The migration rate may be up to 0.5 mm/day, starting within 8–18 hours after wounding. Further proliferation and differentiation occur behind the migration front, leading to restoration of the multilayered epidermis. As the new cells ultimately keratinize and desquamate, the overlying scab is freed with the desquamating cells. This explains why a scab detaches from its periphery inward.

In those cases where the full thickness of the epidermal layer is removed either by trauma or in surgery, the deepest parts of hair follicles and glands that remain as islands of epithelial cells in the dermis will divide and produce cells that migrate over the exposed surface to reestablish a complete epithelial (epidermal) layer. Destruction of all of the epithelial structures of the skin, as in a third-degree burn or full-thickness abrasion, prevents reepithelialization. Such wounds can be healed only by grafting of epidermis to cover the wounded area. In the absence of a graft, the wound would, at best, reepithelialize only slowly and imperfectly by ingrowth of cells from the margins of the wound.

ATLAS PLATES

58–63

PLATE 58. Skin I

The skin or integument consists of two main layers: the *epidermis*, composed of stratified squamous epithelium that is keratinized; and the *dermis*, composed of connective tissue. Under the dermis is a layer of loose connective tissue called the *hypodermis*, which is also generally referred to as the subcutaneous tissue or, by gross anatomists, as the superficial fascia. Typically, the hypodermis contains large amounts of adipose tissue, particularly in the adequately nourished individual. The epidermis gives rise to nails, hairs, sebaceous glands, and sweat glands. On the palms of the hands and the soles of the feet, the epidermis has an outer keratinized layer that is substantially thicker than over other parts of the body. Accordingly, the skin over the palms of the hands and soles of the feet is referred to as *thick skin*, in contrast to the skin over other parts of the body, which is referred to as *thin skin*. There are no hairs in thick skin.

FIGURE 1, skin, human, hematoxylin and eosin (H&E) ×45. In this sample of thick skin, the epidermis *(Ep)* is at the top; the remainder of the field consists of the dermis, in which a large number of sweat glands *(Sw)* can be observed. Although the layers of the epidermis are examined more advantageously at higher magnification (e.g., Fig. 3), it is easy to see, even at this relatively low magnification, that about half of the thickness of the epidermis consists of a distinctive surface layer that stains more lightly than the remainder of the epidermis. This is the keratinized layer. The dome-shaped surface contours represent a cross section through the minute ridges on the surface of thick skin that produce the characteristic fingerprints.

In addition to sweat glands, the dermis displays blood vessels *(BV)* and adipose tissue *(AT)*. The ducts of the sweat glands *(D)* extend from the glands to the epidermis. One of the ducts is shown as it enters the epidermis at the bottom of an epithelial ridge. It will pass through the epidermis in a spiral course to open onto the skin surface.

FIGURE 2, skin, human, H&E ×60. A sample of thin skin is shown here to compare with the thick skin in Figure 1. In addition to sweat glands, thin skin contains hair follicles *(HF)* and their associated sebaceous glands *(SGl)*. Each sebaceous gland opens into a hair follicle. Often, as in this tissue sample, the hair follicles and the glands, both sebaceous and sweat, extend beyond the dermis *(De)* and into the hypodermis. Note the blood vessels *(BV)* and adipose tissue *(AT)* in the hypodermis.

FIGURE 3, skin, human, H&E ×320; inset ×640. The layers of the epidermis of thin skin are shown here at higher magnification. The cell layer that occupies the deepest location is the stratum basale *(SB)*. This is one cell deep. Just above this is a layer several cells in thickness, referred to as the stratum spinosum *(SS)*. It consists of cells that have spinous processes on their surface. These processes meet with spinous processes of neighboring cells and, together, appear as intercellular bridges *(arrows, inset)*. The next layer is the stratum granulosum *(SGr)*, whose cells contain keratohyalin granules *(arrowhead, inset)*. On the surface is the stratum corneum *(SC)*. This consists of keratinized cells, i.e., cells that no longer possess nuclei. The keratinized cells are flat and generally adherent to other cells above and below without evidence of cell boundaries. In thick skin, a fifth layer, the stratum lucidum, is seen between the stratum granulosum and the stratum corneum. The pigment in the cells of the stratum basale is melanin; some of this pigment *(P)* is also present in connective tissue cells of the dermis.

KEY		
AT, adipose tissue	**P,** pigment	**SS,** stratum spinosum
BV, blood vessels	**SB,** stratum basale	**Sw,** sweat gland
D, duct of sweat glands	**SC,** stratum corneum	**arrowhead (inset),** granules in cell of stratum
De, dermis	**SGl,** sebaceous gland	granulosum
Ep, epidermis	**SGr,** stratum granulosum	**arrows (inset),** "intercellular bridges"
HF, hair follicle		

PLATE 58

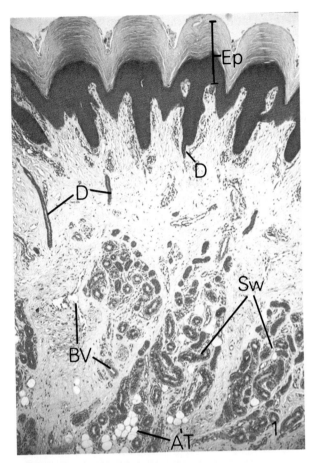

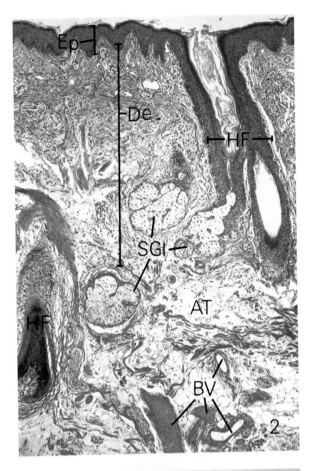

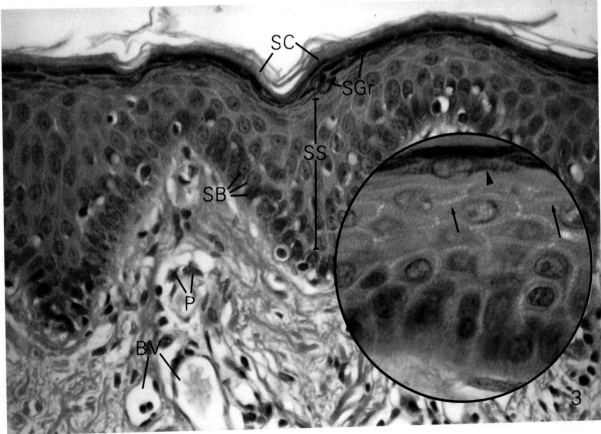

PLATE 59. Skin II

The epidermis contains four distinctive cell types: keratinocytes, melanocytes, Langerhans' cells, and Merkel's cells. Keratinocytes are the most numerous of these cells; they are generated in the stratum basale and move toward the surface. As they do so, they produce the intracellular protein keratin and the special extracellular lipid that serves as a water barrier in the upper reaches of the epidermis. Histologically, the keratinocytes are the cells that show spinous processes in the stratum spinosum. The other three cell types are not readily identified in the H&E-stained paraffin sections. The product of the melanocyte is, however, evident in H&E sections, and this is considered in the first two figures of this plate.

The skin contains pigment, called melanin, that protects the tissue against ultraviolet light. This pigment is chiefly in the epidermis. It is formed by melanocytes that then pass the pigment to the keratinocytes. More pigment is present in Negroid skin than in Caucasian skin; this can be seen by comparing Caucasian skin (Fig. 1) and Negroid skin (Fig. 2). The epidermis and a small amount of the dermis are shown in each figure. Whereas the deep part of the Negroid skin contains considerable pigment, the amount of pigment in Caucasian skin is insufficient to be noticeable at this magnification. Cells for producing the pigment are present in both skin types and *in approximately equal numbers*. The difference is due to more rapid digestion of the pigment by lysosomes of keratinocytes in Caucasian skin. After prolonged exposure to sunlight, pigment would also be produced in sufficient amount to be seen in Caucasian skin.

FIGURE 1, Caucasian skin, human, H&E ×300. In routine H&E-stained paraffin sections of Caucasian skin, such as this sample, the melanocytes are among the cells that appear as small, rounded, clear cells *(CC)* mixed with the other cells of the stratum basale. However, not all clear cells of the epidermis are melanocytes. For example, Langerhans' cells may also appear as clear cells, but they are located more superficially in the stratum spinosum. Merkel's cells may also appear as clear cells, thus making it difficult to identify these three cell types with certainty.

FIGURE 2, Negroid skin, human, H&E ×300. In Negroid skin, most of the pigment is in the basal portion of the epidermis, but it is also present in cells progressing toward the surface and within the nonnucleated cells of the keratinized layer. The *arrows* indicate the melanin pigment in keratinocytes of the stratum spinosum and in the stratum corneum. In Caucasian skin, the melanin is broken down before it leaves the upper part of the stratum spinosum. Thus, pigment is not seen in the upper layers of the epidermis.

FIGURE 3, skin, human, H&E and elastin stain ×200. This figure is included because it shows certain features of the dermis, the connective tissue layer of the skin. The dermis is divided into two layers: the papillary layer *(PL)* of loose connective tissue and the reticular layer *(RL)* of more dense connective tissue. The papillary layer is immediately under the epidermis; it includes the connective tissue papillae that project into the undersurface of the epidermis. The reticular layer is deep to the papillary layer. The boundary between these two layers is not demarcated by any specific structural feature except for the change in the histologic composition of the two layers.

This specimen was stained with H&E and also with a procedure to display elastic fibers *(EF)*. They are relatively thick and conspicuous in the reticular layer (see also **inset**), where they appear as the dark-blue profiles, some of which are elongate, whereas others are short. In the papillary layer, the elastic fibers are thinner and relatively sparse *(arrows)*. The **inset** shows the typical eosinophilic staining of the thick collagenous fibers in the reticular layer. Although the collagenous fibers at the lower magnification of this figure are not as prominent, it is nevertheless possible to note that they are thicker in the reticular layer than in the papillary layer. Finally, as many of the small dark-blue profiles in the reticular layer represent oblique and cross sections through elastic fibers and not nuclei of cells, the papillary layer is evidently more cellular than reticular.

KEY

CC, clear cells
EF, elastic fibers
PL, papillary layer
RL, reticular layer
arrows: Fig. 2, pigment in different layers of epidermis; Fig. 3, delicate elastic fibers

PLATE 59

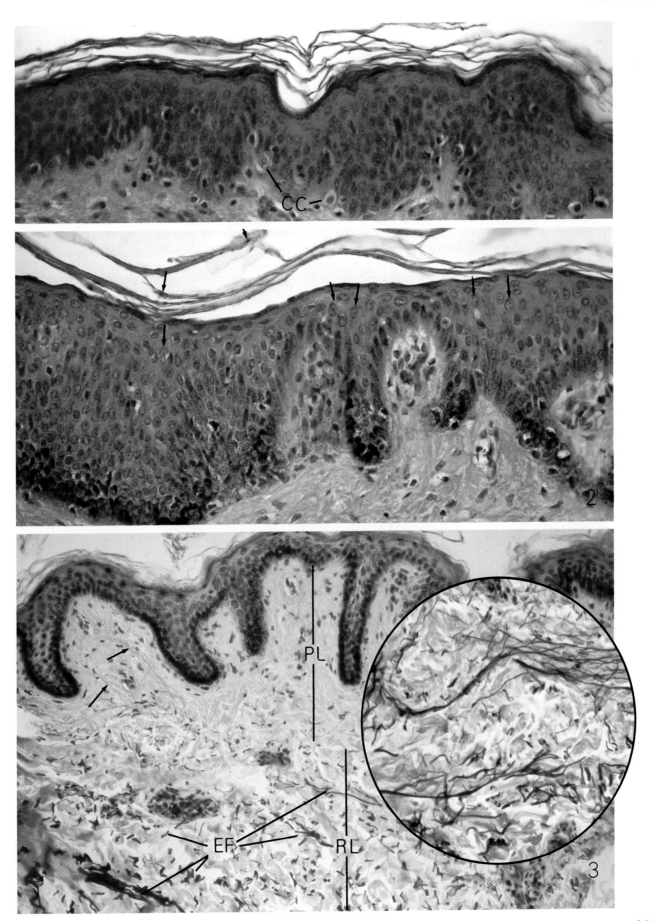

PLATE 60. Eccrine and Apocrine Sweat Glands

Sweat glands are of two types: apocrine and eccrine. Apocrine glands have a limited distribution; in the human they are found in the axilla, anogenital region, and the mammary areola. Apocrine sweat glands are large, tubular structures that are sometimes branched. They empty into the upper portion of the hair follicle and produce a product that becomes odoriferous after being secreted. The apocrine sweat is important in other mammals, serving as a sex attractant and as a marker of territory. Apocrine glands develop at puberty under the influence of sex hormones. They also respond to nerve stimulation but not to heat. In addition to the apocrine glands that are obviously sweat glands, two additional types of glands, namely, the ceruminous glands of the external ear and the glands of Moll in the eyelids, are also classified as apocrine glands.

Eccrine sweat glands in the human are distributed over the entire body surface except for the lips, glans penis, inner surface of the prepuce, clitoris, and labia minora. They serve to regulate body temperature. The eccrine sweat glands are especially numerous in the thick skin of the hands and feet.

FIGURE 1, skin, human, H&E ×120; insets ×1200. This section of adult skin shows both apocrine and eccrine sweat glands. The apocrine sweat glands *(aSG)* are easily identified by virtue of the large lumen of their secretory portion. This histologic feature is in striking contrast to the small lumen displayed by the secretory portion of the eccrine sweat gland *(SG)*. Coincidentally, the apocrine sweat gland is close to a hair follicle *(HF)*. As already mentioned, the apocrine gland opens into the upper portion of a hair follicle. The two *small circular areas* are enlarged in the **circular insets** to show the cell types of the apocrine gland at higher magnification. Note that the *upper small circular area* includes a tangential section through one of the glandular units.

The secretory portion of the apocrine sweat gland consists of a single secretory cell type and myoepithelial cells. These can be seen in the **upper circular inset**. The epithelial cells are either cuboidal or columnar, and if columnar, they typically display granules *(G)* in their apical cytoplasm. The myoepithelial cells are in the basal portion of the epithelial cell layer. Nuclei of myoepithelial cells are elongate and, when cut in cross section, appear as rounded nuclear profiles in the base of the epithelial cell layer *(arrows,* **upper circular inset)**. On the other hand, when seen in different planes of section, the profiles of myoepithelial cell nuclei may appear more elongate, as they are in the **lower circular inset** *(arrows)*. This **inset** also shows the cytoplasmic portion of the myoepithelial cells, cut in cross section *(arrowheads)*, in an adjacent glandular unit.

FIGURE 2, skin, human, H&E ×400; inset ×800. This figure shows eccrine sweat glands at higher magnification. Typically, a section includes profiles of both the secretory portion *(SG)* and the duct portion *(D)* of the gland. The secretory portion of the gland consists of a double layer of cuboidal epithelial cells and, peripherally, along the basal lamina, a conspicuous layer of myoepithelial cells. The duct portion of the gland has a narrower outside diameter than the secretory portion, and the lumen of the duct portion is typically narrower than that of the gland. Occasionally, the duct may be distended *(asterisk)*. The **oval inset** shows where a secretory unit *(SG)* continues into the ductal unit *(D)*. The duct has been cut as it turns, so that in the upper part of the **inset** the duct is seen essentially in cross section, whereas in the middle part of the **inset** it has been cut in a more or less longitudinal plane. Moreover, where the duct has been cut longitudinally, the lumen is not in the plane of section. The duct consists of a double layer of small cuboidal cells and no myoepithelial cells. In addition, there is an acidophilic staining associated with the apical portion of the duct cells that are adjacent to the lumen. This is evident in the duct seen in the **oval inset** and can be contrasted readily with the absence of such staining in the apical region of the secretory cells *(SG)*, also seen in the **oval inset**.

KEY

aSG, apocrine sweat gland
BV, blood vessel
C, capillary
D, duct of eccrine sweat gland
G, granules in apocrine secretory cells
HF, hair follicle
SG, eccrine sweat gland, secretory portion
arrowheads, myoepithelial cells, nuclei
arrows, myoepithelial cells, nuclei
asterisk, lumen of eccrine duct

PLATE 60

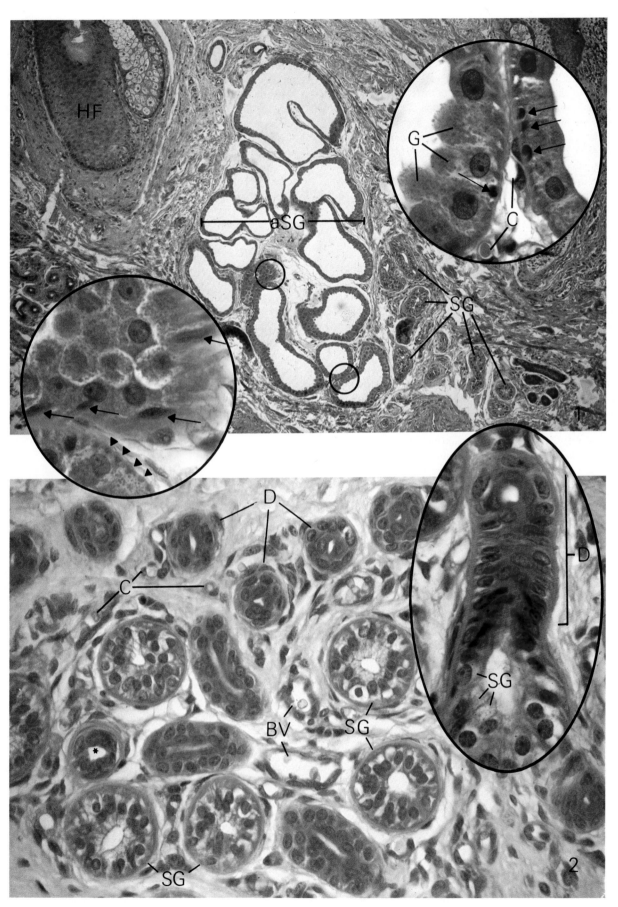

PLATE 61. Sweat and Sebaceous Glands

FIGURE 1, skin, human, H&E ×1000. This section through a sweat gland shows five profiles of the ductal portion *(D)* and two profiles of the secretory portion *(SG)*. The larger secretory segment is through a region either just below or above where a U turn was made; therefore, it shows two luminal profiles. The lumina of both the ductal and secretory units are marked by *asterisks*.

The glandular unit of the eccrine sweat gland contains two epithelial cell types and myoepithelial cells *(M)*. *Arrowheads* show small cross sections of myoepithelial cell cytoplasm; *large arrows* show where more elongate profiles of myoepithelial cytoplasm are evident. The epithelial cells are of two types designated dark cells and clear cells. Unfortunately, the characteristic dark cytoplasmic staining of the dark cells is not evident unless special precautions are taken to preserve the secretory granules in their apical cytoplasm. Nevertheless, note that the dark cells are closer to the lumen, whereas the light cells are closer to the base of the epithelial layer, making contact with either the basal lamina or, more frequently, the myoepithelial cells. In addition, the clear cells are in contact with intercellular canaliculi. Several such intercellular canaliculi are shown in the secretory units *(small arrows)*. This figure also shows that the duct consists of two layers of small cuboidal cells.

FIGURE 2, skin, human, H&E ×160. Sebaceous glands develop from the epithelial cells of the hair follicle and discharge their secretion into the follicle, from where it reaches the skin surface. The sebaceous secretion is rich in lipid, and this is reflected in the cells of the sebaceous gland. A section of a sebaceous gland and its related hair follicle is shown in this figure. At this level, the hair follicle consists of the external root sheath *(RS)* surrounding the hair shaft. The sebaceous gland *(Seb)* appears as a cluster of cells, most of which display a washed-out or finely reticulated cytoplasm. This is because these cells contain numerous lipid droplets and the lipid is lost by dissolution in fat solvents during the routine preparation of the H&E-stained paraffin section. The opening of the sebaceous gland through the external root sheath *(eRS)* and into the hair follicle is shown in the lower right.

FIGURE 3, skin, human, H&E ×320. The same sebaceous gland as in Figure 2 is shown here at higher magnification. *Numbers 1–4* show a series of cells; each is filled with an increasingly greater amount of lipid, and each is progressively closer to the opening of the gland into the hair follicle. The sebaceous secretion includes the entire cell, and therefore, cells need to be replaced constantly in the functional gland. Cells at the periphery of the gland are basal cells *(BC)*. Dividing cells in the basal layer replace those that are lost with the secretion.

KEY

BC, basal cells
CT, connective tissue
D, duct of eccrine sweat gland
eRS, junction between sebaceous gland and external root sheath
M, myoepithelial cell
RS, external root sheath of hair follicle
Seb, sebaceous gland
SG, secretory component of eccrine sweat gland
arrowheads, myoepithelial cell cytoplasm (cross section)
asterisks, lumina of glands
large arrows, myoepithelial cell cytoplasm (longitudinal section)
numbers 1–4 (Fig. 3), see text
small arrows, intercellular canaliculi

PLATE 61

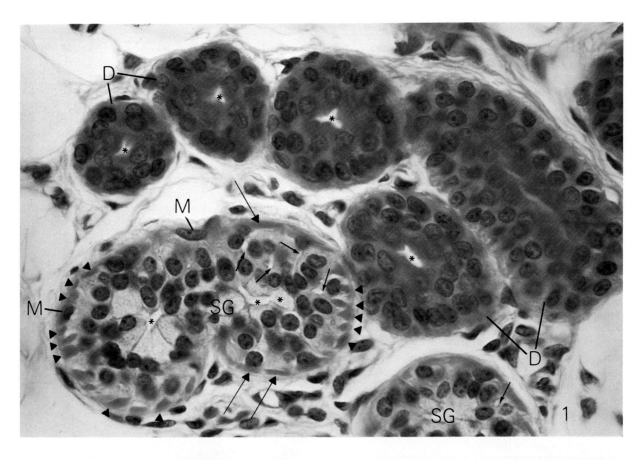

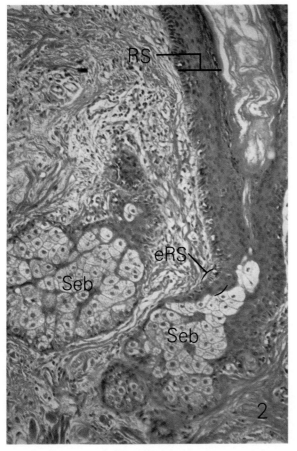

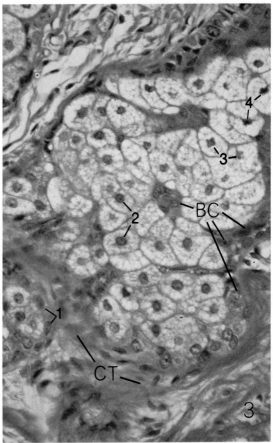

PLATE 62. Integument and Sensory Organs

FIGURE 1, skin, human, H&E ×80. This specimen is a section of thick skin showing the epidermis *(Ep)* and the dermis *(De)* and, under the skin, a portion of the hypodermis *(Hy)*. Note that the thickness of the epidermis is largely due to the thickness of the stratum corneum. Most of this layer is only lightly stained; at the surface, the staining is more intense. Note, also, the thick collagenous fibers in the reticular layer of the dermis and the greater cellularity of the papillary layer of the dermis. Finally, note the presence of some sweat glands in the upper part of the hypodermis. The duct *(D)* of one gland has been labeled.

The main feature of this specimen is that it depicts those sensory receptors that can be recognized in a routine low-power H&E-stained paraffin section. They are the Meissner's corpuscle *(MC)* and the Pacinian corpuscles *(PC)*. Meissner's corpuscles are in the upper part of the dermis, immediately under the epidermis. These corpuscles are small and sometimes difficult to identify at low magnification; however, their location is characteristic. Knowing where they are located is a major step in finding Meissner's corpuscles in a tissue section. Structures suspected of being Meissner's corpuscles should then be examined at higher magnification, which is done in Figure 3.

Pacinian corpuscles are shown in the upper part of the hypodermis. This location is characteristic, although they are often more deeply located. These corpuscles are large, slightly oval structures, and even at low magnification, a layered or lamellated pattern can be discerned.

FIGURE 2, skin, human, H&E ×180. At this higher magnification, the concentric layers or lamellae of the Pacinian corpuscle *(PC)* can be seen to be due to flat cells. These are fibroblast-like cells, and although not evident within the tissue section, these cells are continuous with the endoneurium of the nerve fiber. The space between the cellular lamellae is wide and contains mostly fluid. The neural portion of the Pacinian corpuscle travels longitudinally through the center of the corpuscle. In this specimen, the corpuscles have been cross-sectioned; an *asterisk* has been placed in two of the corpuscles to mark the centrally located nerve fiber. This figure also shows the duct *(D)* of a sweat gland, some nearby blood vessels *(BV)*, and two nerve bundles *(N)*.

FIGURE 3, skin, human, H&E ×550. The two Meissner's corpuscles *(MC)* that were labeled in Figure 1 are shown at higher magnification in this figure. Note the direct proximity of the corpuscle to the undersurface of the epidermis. The section shows the long axis of the corpuscles. A Meissner's corpuscle consists of an axon (sometimes two) taking a zigzag course from one pole of the corpuscle to the other. The nerve fiber terminates at the superficial pole of the corpuscle. Consequently, as seen here, the nerve fibers and supporting cells are oriented approximately at right angles to the long axis of the corpuscle. Meissner's corpuscles are particularly numerous near the tips of the fingers and toes.

KEY

BV, blood vessels
D, ducts of sweat glands
De, dermis
Ep, epidermis
Hy, hypodermis
MC, Meissner's corpuscles
N, nerve bundles
PC, Pacinian corpuscles
asterisks, nerve fiber in center of Pacinian corpuscle

PLATE 62

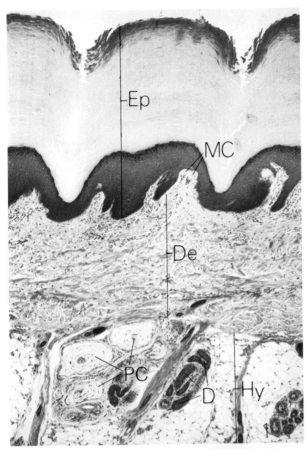

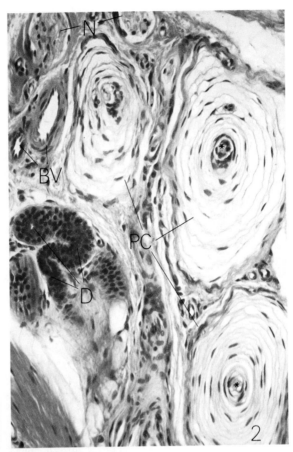

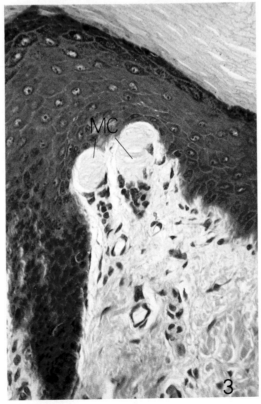

PLATE 63.   Hair Follicle and Nail

FIGURE 1, skin, human, H&E ×300; inset ×440. The growing end of a hair follicle consists of an expanded bulb of epithelial cells that is invaginated by a papilla *(HP)* of connective tissue. The epithelial cells surrounding the papilla at the very tip of the follicle are not yet specialized; they constitute the matrix, the region of the hair follicle where cell division occurs. As the cells leave the matrix, they form cell layers that will become the shaft of the hair and the inner and outer root sheaths of the hair follicle.

The cells that will develop into the shaft of the hair are seen just to the right of the expanded bulb. They constitute the cortex *(C),* medulla *(M),* and cuticle *(asterisks)* of the hair. The cells of the cortex become keratinized. This layer will come to constitute most of the hair shaft as a thick cylinder. The medulla forms the centrally located axis of the hair shaft; it does not always extend through the entire length of the hair and is absent from some hairs. The cuticle consists of overlapping cells that ultimately lose their nuclei and become filled with keratin. The cuticle covers the hair shaft like a layer of overlapping shingles.

The root sheath *(RS)* has two parts: the outer root sheath, which is continuous with the epidermis of the skin, and the inner root sheath, which extends only as far as the level where sebaceous glands enter the hair follicle. The inner root sheath is further divided into three layers: Henle's layer, Huxley's layer, and the cuticle of the inner root sheath. These layers are seen in the growing hair follicle and are shown at higher magnification in the **inset** with *numbers 1–5: 1,* cells of the outer root sheath; *2,* Henle's layer; *3,* Huxley's layer; *4,* cuticle of the inner root sheath; and *5,* future cuticle of the hair.

Many of the cells of the growing hair follicle contain pigment that contributes to the color of the hair. Most of this pigment is inside the cell **(inset);** however, in very dark hair some pigment is also extracellular.

The connective tissue surrounding the hair follicle forms a distinct layer referred to as the sheath or dermal sheath *(DS)* of the hair follicle.

FIGURE 2, skin, human, H&E ×12. A nail is a keratinized plate located on the dorsal aspect of the distal phalanges. A section through a nail plate is shown here. The nail itself *(N)* is difficult to stain. Under the free edge of the nail is a boundary layer, the hyponychium *(Hypon),* that is continuous with the stratum corneum of the adjacent epidermis. The proximal end of the nail is overlapped by skin; here, the junctional region is called the eponychium *(Epon)* and is also continuous with the stratum corneum of the adjacent epidermis. Under the nail is a layer of epithelium, the posterior portion of which is referred to as the nail matrix *(NM).* The cells of the nail matrix function in the growth of the nail. Together, the epithelium under the nail and the underlying dermis *(D)* constitute the nail bed. The posterior portion of the nail, covered by the fold of the skin, is the root of the nail *(NR).*

The relationship of the nail to other structures in the fingertip is also shown in this figure. The bone *(B)* in the specimen represents a distal phalanx. Note that in this bone there is an epiphyseal growth plate *(EP)* at the proximal extremity of the bone but not at the distal extremity. Numerous Pacinian corpuscles *(PC)* are present in the connective tissue of the palmar side of the finger. Also seen to advantage in this section is the stratum lucidum *(SL)* in the epidermis of the thick skin of the fingertip.

KEY

B, bone	**Hypon,** hyponychium	**RS,** root sheath
C, cortex	**M,** medulla	**SL,** stratum lucidum
D, dermis	**N,** nail or nail plate	**asterisks,** cuticle of hair
DS, dermal sheath	**NM,** nail matrix	**numbers: 1,** external root sheath;
EP, epiphyseal plate	**NR,** nail root	**2,** Henle's layer; **3,** Huxley's layer;
Epon, eponychium	**PC,** Pacinian corpuscles	**4,** cuticle of inner root sheath; **5,**
HP, dermal papilla of hair follicle		future cuticle of the hair

PLATE 63

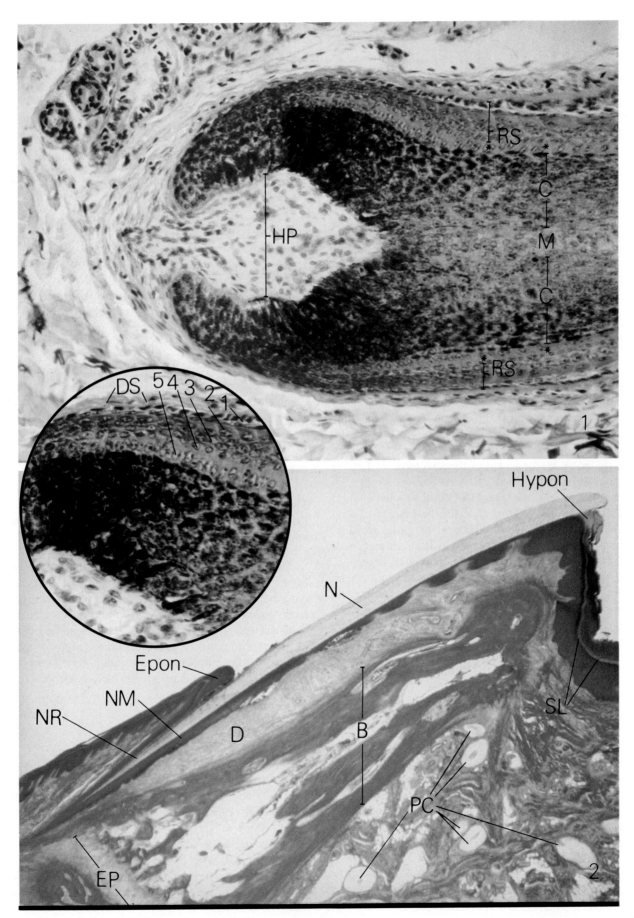

Digestive System I: Oral Cavity and Pharynx

15

The digestive system consists of the *alimentary canal* and its associated organs, namely, the *tongue, teeth, salivary glands, pancreas, liver,* and *gallbladder.*

The Lumen of the Alimentary Canal Is Physically and Functionally *External* to the Body

In passing through the alimentary canal, food is broken down physically and chemically so that the degraded products can be absorbed into the body. The various segments of the alimentary canal are morphologically specialized for particular aspects of digestion and absorption.

After preliminary maceration, moistening, and formation into a bolus by the action of the structures of the oral cavity and the salivary glands, food passes rapidly through the pharynx to the esophagus. (The rapid passage of food through the pharynx keeps it clear for the passage of air.) The food passes more slowly through the gastrointestinal tract, and during its transit through the stomach and small intestine, the major alterations associated with digestion, solubilization, and absorption occur. Absorption occurs chiefly through the wall of the small intestine. Undigested food and other substances within the alimentary canal, such as mucus, bacteria, desquamated cells, and bile pigments, are excreted as the feces.

The Alimentary Mucosa Is the Surface Across Which Most Substances Enter the Body

The alimentary mucosa has numerous functions in its role as an interface between the body and the environment. These include its

- *Barrier function:* The mucosa serves as a barrier to the entry of noxious substances, antigens, and pathogenic organisms.
- *Immunologic function:* Lymphatic tissue in the mucosa serves as a first line of defense of the body by the immune system.
- *Secretory function:* The lining of the alimentary canal *secretes,* at specific sites, digestive enzymes, hydrochloric acid, mucin, and antibodies.

- *Absorptive function:* The epithelium of the mucosa absorbs metabolic substrates, i.e., the breakdown products of digestion, as well as vitamins, water, electrolytes, recyclable materials such as bile components and cholesterol, and other substances essential to the functions of the body.

The digestive system is considered in three chapters that deal, respectively, with the oral cavity and pharynx (I, present chapter), the esophagus and gastrointestinal tract (II, Chapter 16), and the liver, gallbladder, and pancreas (III, Chapter 17).

ORAL CAVITY

The Oral Cavity Consists of the Mouth and Its Contents, i.e., the Tongue, Teeth, Salivary Glands, and Tonsils

The oral cavity is divided into a vestibule and an oral cavity proper. The *vestibule* is that part of the oral cavity lying between the lips and cheeks and the teeth. The *oral cavity proper* lies behind the teeth and is bounded by the hard and soft palates superiorly, the tongue and the floor of the mouth inferiorly, and the entrance to the oropharynx posteriorly. Ducts of the salivary glands empty into the oral cavity. The major salivary glands include the

- *Parotid gland*
- *Submandibular gland*
- *Sublingual gland*

The major salivary glands have relatively long ducts from the secretory portion of the gland to the oral cavity. Minor salivary glands located in the submucosa of the tongue and in the lining of the oral cavity empty directly into the cavity via short ducts.

Lymphatic tissue is organized into a "ring" of immunologic protection at the shared entrance to the digestive and respiratory tracts. This lymphatic tissue, which surrounds the posterior orifice of the oral cavity, the oropharynx, includes the

- Palatine tonsil
- Pharyngeal tonsil
- Lingual tonsil

The Oral Cavity Is Lined by Masticatory Mucosa, Lining Mucosa, and Specialized Mucosa

Masticatory mucosa is found on the gingiva (gums) and the hard palate (Fig. 15.1). The masticatory mucosa has a **keratinized** or **parakeratinized** stratified squamous epithelium (Fig. 15.2). Parakeratinized epithelium is similar to keratinized epithelium except that the cells of the stratum corneum do not lose their nuclei and their cytoplasm does not stain intensely with eosin. The keratinized epithelium of the masticatory mucosa resembles that of the skin but lacks a stratum lucidum. The underlying lamina propria consists of a deep papillary layer of loose connective tissue that contains blood vessels and nerves, some of which send bare axon endings into the epithelium as sensory receptors and some of which end in Meissner's corpuscles. Deep to this is a reticular layer of more dense connective tissue.

As in the skin, the depth and number of papillae contribute to the relative immobility of the masticatory mucosa, thus protecting it from frictional and shearing stress. Except in some places on the hard palate, the mucosa is firmly adherent to the underlying bone, with the reticular layer of the lamina propria blending with the periosteum. Where there is a submucosa underlying the lamina propria on the hard palate (see Fig. 15.1), this contains adipose tissue, anteriorly, and mucous glands, posteriorly, that are continuous with those of the still more posterior soft palate.

In the submucosal regions, thick collagenous bands extend from the mucosa to the bone (Fig. 15.3).

Lining mucosa is found on the lips, cheeks, alveolar mucosal surface, floor of the mouth, inferior surfaces of the tongue, and soft palate. In these sites it covers striated muscle (lips, cheeks, and tongue), bone (alveolar mucosa), and glands (soft palate, cheeks, inferior surface of tongue). The lining mucosa has fewer and shorter papillae so that it can adjust to the movement of its underlying muscles.

Generally, the epithelium is nonkeratinized, although in some places it may be parakeratinized. The epithelium of the vermilion border of the lip is keratinized. The nonkeratinized lining epithelium is thicker than keratinized epithelium (see Plate 71, page 473). It consists of only three layers:

- **Stratum basale**
- **Stratum spinosum**
- **Stratum superficiale,** i.e., the superficial or surface layer

The cells of the mucosal epithelium are similar to those of the epidermis of the skin, including keratinocytes, Langerhans' cells, melanocytes, and Merkel's cells.

The lamina propria contains blood vessels, nerves that send bare axon endings into the basal layers of the epithelium, and encapsulated sensory endings in some papillae. The sharp contrast between the numerous deep papillae of the alveolar mucosa and the shallow papillae in the rest of the lining mucosa allows for a ready identification of the two different regions in a histologic section (see Fig. 15.19).

A distinct submucosa underlies the lining mucosa except on the inferior surface of the tongue. This layer contains

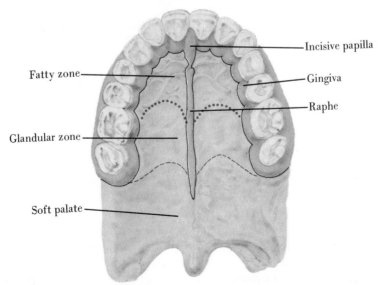

Figure 15.1. Roof of oral cavity proper. The hard palate, containing bone, is bisected into right and left halves by a raphe. Anteriorly, the hard palate contains fatty tissue in the submucosa; posteriorly, there are mucous glands within the submucosa. Neither the raphe nor the gingiva contains a submucosa; instead, the mucosa is attached directly to the bone.

The soft palate has muscle instead of bone in its substance and has glands continuous with those of the hard palate in the submucosa. (Based on Bhaskar SN (ed): *Orban's Oral Histology and Embryology,* 11th ed. St Louis, CV Mosby, 1991, p 284.)

large bands of collagen and elastic fibers that bind the mucosa to the underlying muscle; it also contains the many minor salivary glands of the lips, tongue, and cheeks. Occasionally, sebaceous glands not associated with a hair follicle are found in the submucosa just lateral to the corner of the mouth. They are visible to the eye and are called **Fordyce spots.** The submucosa contains the larger blood vessels, nerves, and lymphatic vessels that supply the subepithelial neurovascular networks in the lamina propria throughout the oral cavity.

Specialized mucosa is restricted to the dorsal surface of the tongue, where it contains *papillae* and *taste buds*.

TONGUE

The *tongue* is a muscular organ projecting into the oral cavity from its inferior surface. The muscles are both extrinsic (having one attachment outside of the tongue) and intrinsic (confined entirely to the tongue without external attachment). The striated muscles of the tongue are arranged in bundles that generally run in three planes, with each arranged at right angles to the other two. This arrangement of muscle fibers allows enormous flexibility and precision in the movements of the tongue that are essential to human speech as well as to its role in digestion and swallowing. This arrangement of muscle is found only in the tongue and allows for easy identification of this tissue as lingual muscle. Variable amounts of adipose tissue are found among the muscle fiber groups.

Grossly, the dorsal surface of the tongue is divided into an anterior two-thirds and a posterior one-third by a V-shaped depression, the **sulcus terminalis** (Fig. 15.4). The apex of the V points posteriorly and is the location of the **foramen cecum,** the remnant of the site from which an evagination of the floor of the embryonic pharynx occurred to form the thyroid gland.

Papillae Cover the Dorsal Surface of the Anterior Portion of the Tongue

Numerous mucosal irregularities and elevations called **papillae** cover the dorsal surface of the tongue anterior to the sulcus terminalis. The papillae and their associated taste buds constitute the **specialized mucosa** of the oral cavity. Four types of papillae are described: *filiform, fungiform, circumvallate,* and *foliate.*

Filiform papillae are the most numerous in humans and the smallest. They are conical, elongated projections of connective tissue that are covered with keratinized stratified squamous epithelium. This epithelium does not contain taste buds. Filiform papillae are distributed over the entire anterior dorsal surface of the tongue, with their tips pointing backward. They appear to form rows that diverge to the left and right from the midline and that parallel the arms of the sulcus terminalis (see Plate 64, Fig. 1, page 427).

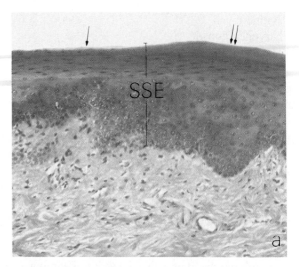

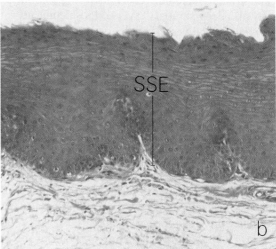

Figure 15.2. Light micrographs showing stratified squamous epithelium *(SSE)* and connective tissue of the mucosa of the hard palate (human). **a.** On the right side, the epithelium is keratinized, and the flattened surface cells *(double arrows)* are devoid of nuclei. On the left side, the flattened surface cells *(single arrow)* display the same staining characteristics as the keratinized cells except that they retain their nuclei; i.e., they are parakeratinized. **b.** Another area from the same specimen of the hard palate. The stratified squamous epithelium is nonkeratinized.

Fungiform papillae, as the name indicates, are mushroom-shaped projections located on the dorsal surface of the tongue. They project above the filiform papillae, among which they are scattered, and are just visible to the unaided eye as small spots (these spots appear light pink in Fig. 15.4). They tend to be more numerous near the tip of the tongue. *Taste buds* are present in the stratified squamous epithelium on the dorsal surface of these papillae.

Circumvallate papillae are the large, dome-shaped structures that reside in the mucosa just anterior to the sulcus terminalis (Fig. 15.4). In humans, 8–12 of these are usually found. Each papilla is surrounded by a moat-like invagination lined with stratified squamous epithelium that

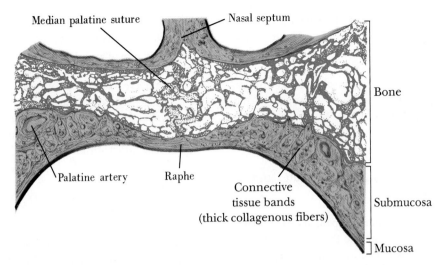

Median palatine suture

Nasal septum

Bone

Palatine artery

Raphe

Connective
tissue bands
(thick collagenous fibers)

Submucosa

Mucosa

Figure 15.3. Frontal section through the hard palate. Connective tissue bands traverse the submucosa and join the mucosa to the periosteum of the bone in the hard palate. Note the absence of a submucosa at the raphe. (Based on Pendleton

EC: *The Journal of the American Dental Association* 21:488, copyright ©1934. Reprinted by permission of ADA Publishing Company, Inc.)

contains numerous taste buds (see Plate 65, Fig. 2, page 429). Ducts of lingual salivary glands (von Ebner's glands) empty their serous secretion into the moats. The secretions presumably flush material from the moat to enable the taste buds to respond rapidly to changing stimuli.

Foliate papillae consist of parallel low ridges separated

by deep mucosal clefts that are aligned at right angles to the long axis of the tongue. They occur on the lateral edge of the tongue. In aged humans, the foliate papillae may not be recognized; in younger individuals, they are easily found on the posterior lateral surface of the tongue and contain many taste buds in the epithelium of the facing walls of

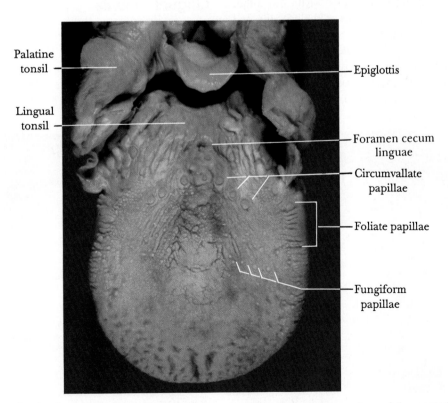

Palatine
tonsil

Lingual
tonsil

Epiglottis

Foramen cecum
linguae

Circumvallate
papillae

Foliate papillae

Fungiform
papillae

Figure 15.4. Photograph of a human tongue. Circumvallate papillae are positioned as a V, separating the anterior two-thirds of the tongue from the posterior third. Fungiform and filiform papillae are on the anterior portion of the dorsal tongue surface; the uneven contour of the posterior tongue surface is due to lingual tonsils. The palatine tonsil is at the junction between the oral cavity and the pharynx. (Specimen courtesy of Dr. G. Von Hagens.)

neighboring papillae (see Plate 65, Fig. 1, page 429). Small serous glands empty into the clefts. In some animals, such as the rabbit, foliate papillae constitute the principal site of aggregation of taste buds.

The dorsal surface of the posterior portion of the tongue exhibits smoother bulges that reflect the presence of the *lingual tonsils* in the lamina propria.

Taste Buds

Taste Buds Are Present on Fungiform, Foliate, and Circumvallate Papillae

In histologic sections, taste buds appear as oval, pale-staining bodies that extend through the thickness of the epithelium (Fig. 15.5). A small opening onto the epithelial surface at the apex of the taste bud is called the *taste pore.*

Three principal cell types are found in taste buds:

- *Neuroepithelial cells*
- *Supporting cells*
- *Basal cells* (Fig. 15.6).

The neuroepithelial cells and supporting cells are mature elongated cells that extend from the basal lamina of the epithelium to the taste pore, through which the tapered apical surface of each cell extends microvilli. The basal cells are located at the periphery of the taste bud, near the basal lamina, and are believed to be stem cells for the two other cell types. The turnover time of neuroepithelial cells and supporting cells is about 10 days.

In addition to the taste buds associated with the papillae, taste buds are also present on the glossopalatine arch, the soft palate, the posterior surface of the epiglottis, and the posterior wall of the pharynx down to the level of the cri-coid cartilage. Nerve fibers are found in the epithelium between taste buds, as networks around taste buds, and within taste buds in association with the neuroepithelial cells. These fibers are from cranial nerves VII, IX, and X.

Taste buds react to only four stimuli: sweet, salty, bitter, and acid. In general, taste buds at the tip of the tongue detect sweet stimuli, those immediately posterolateral to the tip detect salty stimuli, and those on the circumvallate papillae detect bitter stimuli.

INHERITED ABSENCE OF TASTE

The ability to taste, generally or specifically, is genetically determined. At one extreme are those rare individuals, such as wine tasters and tea tasters, who have prodigious taste discrimination and taste memory. At the other extreme are individuals who are totally unable to taste. In one of these rare inherited conditions, *familial dysautonomia*, not only is there a total absence of taste buds, but fungiform papillae are also absent. The disease may be diagnosed easily in the newborn, where the absence of these papillae is particularly clear.

A common test used to identify "tasters" and "nontasters" is to place a drop of a solution containing phenyl-thiocarbamide (PTC) on the tip of the tongue. Tasters report a bitter taste, nontasters are unaware of any taste.

Lingual Tonsils

Lingual tonsils are located in the lamina propria of the root or base of the tongue. They are found posterior to the sulcus terminalis. The lingual tonsils contain lymphatic nodules with germinal centers. These are discussed in Chapter 13.

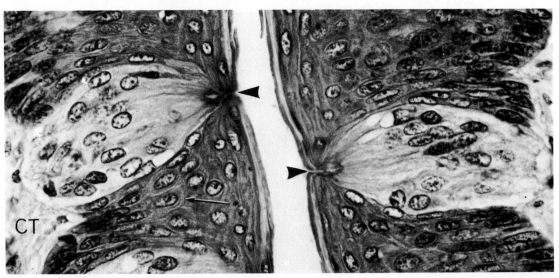

Figure 15.5. Light micrograph of taste buds. The taste buds appear as the light oval structures extending through the full thickness of the epithelium from the connective tissue *(CT)* to the surface. Here, the taste bud opens at the surface by means of a small pore *(arrowheads).* Although three cell types are present in the taste bud, their specific identification in routine paraffin sections is not feasible. Note the intercellular "bridges" between the cells in the stratified squamous epithelium *(arrow).* ×640.

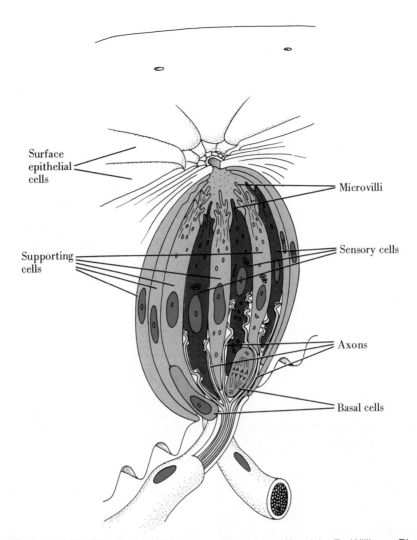

Figure 15.6. Diagram of taste bud showing supporting, sensory, and basal cells. One of the basal cells is in the process of dividing. Nerve fibers terminate about the sensory cells.

(Based on Warwick, R, Williams PL (eds): *Gray's Anatomy,* 35th ed. Edinburgh, Churchill Livingstone, 1973, p 1085.)

Epithelial crypts usually invaginate into the lingual tonsil; the structure of the epithelium may be difficult to distinguish, however, because of the very large number of lymphocytes that normally invade it. Between nodules, the lingual epithelium has the characteristics of lining epithelium. Mucous lingual salivary glands may be seen between lingual tonsils and may extend into the muscle of the tongue root.

Nerve Supply

The Complex Nerve Supply of the Tongue Is Provided by Several Cranial Nerves

General sensation for the anterior two-thirds of the tongue (anterior to the sulcus terminalis) is carried in the trigeminal nerve (cranial nerve V). General sensation for the posterior one-third of the tongue is carried in the glossopharyngeal nerve (cranial nerve IX).

- The musculature of the tongue is innervated by the hypoglossal nerve (cranial nerve XII).
- Taste is carried by the facial nerve (cranial nerve VII) anterior to the sulcus terminalis and by the glossopharyngeal nerve (cranial nerve IX) posterior to the sulcus.

In addition, the tongue has both a sympathetic and parasympathetic innervation for blood vessels and glands. Ganglion cells are often seen within the tongue. These belong to postganglionic parasympathetic neurons and are destined for the minor salivary glands within the tongue. Sympathetic postganglionic neurons have their cell body in the superior cervical ganglion.

TEETH AND SUPPORTING TISSUES

Teeth are a major component of the oral cavity and are essential for the digestive process. Teeth are embedded in and attached to the maxilla and mandible. A child has 10 deciduous teeth in each jaw, consisting, on each side, of

- *A central incisor*
- *A lateral incisor*
- *A canine tooth*
- *Two molar teeth*

Over a period of years, usually beginning at about age 6, these are gradually replaced by 16 permanent teeth in each jaw, consisting, on each side, of

- *A central incisor*
- *A lateral incisor*
- *A canine*
- *Two premolar teeth*
- *Three molar teeth*

Incisors and canines have one root each, premolars usually have two, and molars may have three or four roots. All teeth have the same basic structure, however. This can be illustrated by considering a tooth with one root (Fig. 15.7).

HISTOLOGIC PREPARATION OF TOOTH TISSUES

Because most parts of the tooth are highly mineralized, teeth are prepared for histologic study by methods similar to those used for bone, namely, by means of ground sections and of stained demineralized sections. The ground section is most often used to study an extracted or exfoliated tooth. As in the preparation of bone, the ground section displays mineralized tissue but destroys soft tissue; demineralization removes mineral and retains soft tissue. Demineralized sections have the advantage that they can be used to view a section of a tooth in order to study the relationship of the tooth to the adjacent supporting structures. In routinely demineralized sections of a mature tooth, however, the enamel is dissolved and lost. Therefore, diagrams of a tooth showing features of both enamel and soft tissues are composite diagrams that combine the data derived from both ground and demineralized sections (Fig. 15.7).

The Adult Tooth Consists of Four Distinct Structural Components, the *Enamel* and the *Cementum* on the Outside, the *Dentin* Beneath Them, and the *Pulp* in a Central Pulp Cavity

Enamel covers the crown of the tooth. That part of the crown that is exposed and visible above the gum line is called the **clinical crown;** the **anatomical crown** describes all of the tooth that is covered by enamel, some of which is below the gum line. Enamel varies in thickness over the crown and may be as thick as 2.5 mm on the *cusps* (biting and grinding surfaces) of some teeth. The enamel layer ends at the **neck** or **cervix** of the tooth at the **cementoenamel junction** (Fig. 15.7); the **root** of the tooth is then covered by **cementum,** a bone-like material (see below).

Enamel Is the Hardest Substance in the Body; It Consists of 96–98% *Hydroxyapatite*

The hydroxyapatite (see page 150) of the enamel is arranged in *rods* (Fig. 15.8) or *prisms* that vary in diameter from 4–8 μm. Each enamel rod spans the full thickness of the enamel layer from the dentinoenamel junction to the enamel surface (Fig. 15.9); the spaces between the rods are also filled with hydroxyapatite. Striations observed on enamel rods (contour lines of Retzius) may represent evidence of rhythmic growth of the enamel in the developing tooth. The enamel in a mature tooth is acellular and nonreplaceable.

Although the enamel of an erupted tooth is devoid of cells and cell processes, it is not a static tissue. It is under the influence of substances in saliva, the secretion of the salivary glands, that are essential to its maintenance. The substances in saliva that affect teeth include

- Digestive enzymes
- Antibacterial enzymes
- Antibodies
- Inorganic (mineral) components

Mature enamel contains very little organic material. Despite its hardness, enamel can be damaged by decalcification by acid-producing bacteria acting on food products trapped on the surface of the enamel. This is the basis of the initiation of **dental caries.** Fluoride added to the hydroxyapatite complex hardens the enamel still further, and the widespread use of fluoride in drinking water, tooth pastes, pediatric vitamin supplements, and mouth washes has significantly reduced the incidence of dental caries.

Enamel Formation (Amelogenesis)

Enamel Is Produced by *Ameloblasts* With the Close Cooperation of Other Enamel Organ Cells

The histology of the enamel organ is presented in Plate 70, page 439. The major stages of amelogenesis are the period of matrix production, or the secretory stage, and the period of maturation. In the formation of mineralized tissues of the tooth, dentin is produced first. Then, partially mineralized enamel matrix (see Fig. 15.8) is deposited directly on the surface of the previously formed dentin. The cells producing this partially mineralized organic matrix are referred to as **secretory ameloblasts**. As do osteoblasts in bone, these cells produce an organic proteinaceous matrix by activity of the rough endoplasmic reticulum (rER), Golgi apparatus, and secretory granules. The secretory ameloblasts continue to produce enamel matrix until the full thickness of the future enamel is achieved.

Maturation of the partially mineralized enamel matrix involves the removal of organic material as well as continued influx of calcium and phosphate into the maturing enamel. Cells involved in this second stage of enamel formation are referred to as **maturation ameloblasts.** Maturation ameloblasts differentiate from secretory ameloblasts and function

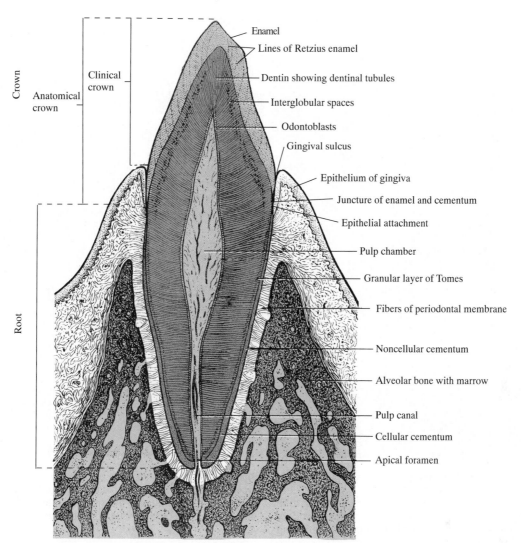

Figure 15.7. Diagram of a section through an incisor tooth and surrounding bony and mucosal structures. The three mineralized components of the tooth are dentin, enamel, and cementum. The central soft core of the tooth is the pulp. The periodontal ligament (membrane) contains bundles of collagenous fibers that bind the tooth to the surrounding alveolar bone. The clinical crown of the tooth is the portion that projects into the oral cavity; the enamel at the tip of the crown shows some abrasion. The anatomical crown is all of the portion of the tooth covered by enamel. (Modified from Copenhaver WM (ed): *Bailey's Textbook of Histology,* 15th ed. Baltimore, Williams & Wilkins, 1964, p 354.)

primarily as a transport epithelium, moving substances into and out of the maturing enamel. Maturation ameloblasts undergo cyclical alterations in their morphology that correspond to cyclical entry of calcium into the enamel.

Secretory ameloblasts are narrow, highly polarized, columnar cells (Fig. 15.10). They are directly adjacent to the developing enamel. At the apical pole of the cell is a process, **Tomes' process,** that is surrounded by the developing enamel. A cluster of mitochondria in the basal extremity of the cell accounts for the eosinophilic staining of this region in hematoxylin and eosin (H&E)-stained paraffin sections. Adjacent to the mitochondria is the nucleus; in the main column of cytoplasm are the rER, Golgi, secretory granules, and other cell elements. Junctional complexes are present at both apical and basal extremities. Contractile filaments joined to these junctional complexes may be involved in moving the secretory ameloblast over the developing enamel. The rod produced by the ameloblast follows in the wake of the cell. Thus, in mature enamel, the direction of the enamel rod is a record of the path taken earlier by the secretory ameloblast.

At their basal poles, the secretory ameloblasts are adjacent to a layer of enamel organ cells called the **stratum intermedium**. The plasma membrane of these cells and that of the basal pole of the ameloblasts is positive for alkaline phosphatase, an enzyme active in calcification. Stellate enamel organ cells are external to the stratum intermedium and are separated from the adjacent blood vessels by a basal lamina.

The histologic feature that marks the cycles of maturation ameloblasts is the presence of a striated or ruffled border (Fig. 15.11). Maturation ameloblasts with a striated border occupy about 70% of a specific cycle, and those that are smooth ended are about 30% of a specific cycle. There

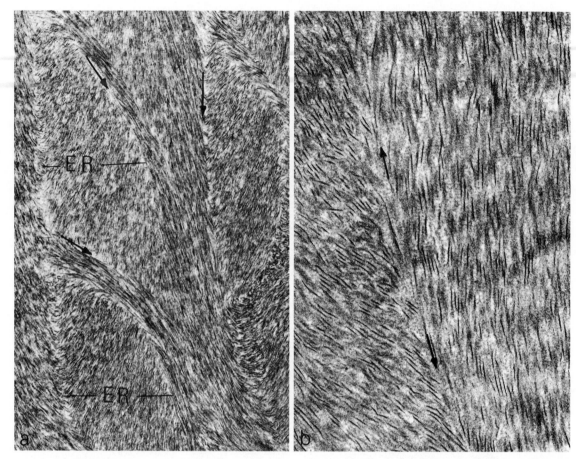

Figure 15.8. Electron micrographs of young enamel. **a.** Enamel rods *(ER)* are cut obliquely. *Arrows* mark the boundaries between adjacent rods. ×14,700. **b.** Parts of two adjacent rods are seen at higher magnification. *Arrows* mark the boundary between the two rods. The dark needle-like objects are young hydroxyapatite crystals; the substance between the hydroxyapatite crystals is the organic matrix of the developing enamel. As the enamel matures, the hydroxyapatite crystals grow, and the bulk of the organic matrix is removed. ×60,000.

is no stratum intermedium in the enamel organ during enamel maturation; stellate *papillary cells* are adjacent to the maturation ameloblasts.

The maturation ameloblasts and the adjacent papillary cells are characterized by the presence of numerous mitochondria. This is indicative of cellular activity that requires large amounts of energy and is a reflection of the fact that the maturation ameloblasts and the adjacent papillary cells function as a transporting epithelium.

The matrix of developing enamel contains three major proteins:

- *Amelogenins*
- *Enamelins*
- *Tuft protein*

Mature enamel contains only enamelins and tuft protein.

Amelogenins are removed during enamel maturation. Tuft protein is located near the dentinoenamel junction. It is present in enamel tufts and accounts for the fact that the enamel tufts are hypomineralized; i.e., they have a higher percentage of organic material than the remainder of the

mature enamel. The maturation of the developing enamel results in the continued mineralization of enamel, so that it becomes the hardest substance in the body. The ameloblasts degenerate after the enamel is fully formed, at about the time of tooth eruption from the gum.

Cementum

Cementum Covers the *Root* of the Tooth

The root is that part of the tooth that fits into its *socket* or *alveolus* in the maxilla or mandible. Cementum is a thin layer of bone-like material that is secreted by *cementocytes,* cells that closely resemble osteocytes. Like bone, cementum has a mineral content of 45–50%. The lacunae and canaliculi in the cementum contain the *cementocytes* and their processes, respectively. They resemble those structures in bone that contain osteocytes and osteocyte processes.

Unlike bone, cementum is avascular. Also, the canaliculi in cementum do not appear to form an interconnecting network. A layer of *cementoblasts* (cells that resemble the osteoblasts of the surface of growing bone) is seen on the outer surface of the cementum, adjacent to the *periodontal ligament.*

Collagen fibers that project out of the matrix of the cementum and embed in the bony matrix of the socket wall form the bulk of the periodontal ligament. These fibers are another example of *Sharpey's fibers* (Fig. 15.12). *Oxytalan fibers* that resemble developing elastic fibers and stain with elastic stains are also a component of the periodontal ligament. This mode of attachment of the tooth in its socket allows slight movement of the tooth to occur naturally and forms the basis of the orthodontic procedures that are used to straighten teeth and reduce malocclusion of the biting and grinding surfaces of the maxillary and mandibular teeth. During such corrective tooth movement, the alveolar bone of the socket is resorbed and resynthesized, but the cementum is not.

Dentin

Dentin Is a Calcified Material That Forms Most of the Tooth Substance

Dentin lies deep to the enamel and cementum. It contains less hydroxyapatite than does enamel, about 70%, but more than is found in bone and cementum. Dentin is secreted by *odontoblasts* that form an epithelial layer over the inner surface of the dentin, i.e., that surface that is in contact with the pulp (Fig. 15.13). Odontoblasts, too, are elongated cylindrical cells that contain a well-developed rER, a large Golgi apparatus, and other organelles associated with the synthesis and secretion of large amounts of protein (Fig. 15.14). The apical surface of the odontoblast is in contact with the forming dentin; junctional complexes between the odontoblasts at that level separate the dentinal compartment from the pulp compartment.

The layer of odontoblasts retreats as the dentin is laid down, leaving odontoblast processes embedded in the dentin in narrow channels called *dentinal tubules* (see Fig. 15.13). The tubules and processes continue to elongate as the dentin continues to thicken by rhythmic growth. The rhythmic growth of dentin produces certain "growth lines" in the dentin (incremental lines of von Ebner and the thicker lines of Owen) that can identify significant developmental times such as birth *(neonatal line)* and may identify when unusual substances such as lead were incorporated into the growing tooth. Study of growth lines has proved useful in forensic medicine.

Predentin is the newly secreted organic matrix, closest to the cell body of the odontoblast, that has yet to be mineralized. An unusual feature of the secretion of collagen and hydroxyapatite by odontoblasts is the presence, in Golgi vesicles, of arrays of a formed filamentous collagen precursor to which granules believed to contain calcium attach. This gives rise to structures called *abacus bodies* (Figs.

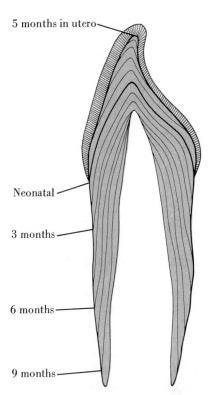

Figure 15.9. Schematic diagram of partially formed tooth. The enamel is drawn to show rods extending from the dentinoenamel junction to the surface of the tooth. Although the full thickness of the enamel is formed, the full thickness of the dentin has not yet been established. The contour lines within the dentin show the extent to which the dentin has developed at a particular time, as labeled in the illustration. Note that the pulp cavity in the center of the tooth becomes smaller as the dentin develops. Contour lines showing increments of enamel development also exist but are not shown in this figure. They are depicted in Figure 15.7. (Based on Schour I, Massler M: *The Journal of the American Dental Association* 23: 1948 copyright ©1936. Reprinted by permission of ADA Publishing Company, Inc.)

15.14 and 15.15). The abacus bodies become more condensed as they mature into secretory granules.

Dentinogenesis

Dentin Is Produced by Odontoblasts

Dentin is the first mineralized component of the tooth to be deposited. During the formation of the very outermost dentin, which is referred to as mantle dentin, it is also formed by subodontoblastic cells that produce small bundles of collagen fibers (von Korff's fibers). The odontoblasts differentiate from cells at the periphery of the dental papilla. The progenitor cells have the appearance of typical mesenchymal cells; i.e., they contain little cytoplasm. During their differentiation into odontoblasts, cytoplasmic volume and organelles characteristic of collagen-producing cells increase. The cells form a layer at the periphery of the dental papilla, and they secrete the organic matrix of dentin, called *predentin,* at their apical pole (the end of the cell away from the dental papilla) (Fig. 15.16). As the thickness of the predentin increases, the odontoblasts move or are displaced centrally (see Fig. 15.9). A wave of mineralization follows the receding odontoblasts; this mineralized product is the dentin. As the cells move centrally, the odontoblastic process becomes increasingly long, with its greatest length being surrounded by the mineralized dentin. In newly formed dentin, the wall of the dentinal tubule is simply the edge of the mineralized dentin. With time, the dentin immediately surrounding the dentinal tubule becomes more highly mineralized; this more mineralized sheath of dentin is referred to as the *peritubular dentin.* The remainder of the dentin is then referred to as the *intertubular dentin.*

Dental Pulp and Pulp Cavity

The Dental Pulp Cavity Is a Connective Tissue Compartment Bounded by the Tooth Dentin

The pulp cavity is the space within a tooth that is occupied by pulp, a loose connective tissue that is richly vascularized and supplied by abundant nerves. The pulp cavity has the general shape of the tooth. The blood vessels and nerves enter the pulp cavity at the tip (apex) of the root, at a site called the *apical foramen.* (The designations apex and apical in this context refer only to the narrowed tip of the root of the tooth rather than to a luminal (apical) surface, as used in describing secretory and absorptive epithelia.)

The blood vessels and nerves extend to the crown of the tooth where they form vascular and neural networks beneath and within the layer of odontoblasts. Some bare nerve fibers also enter the proximal portions of the dentinal tubules and contact odontoblast processes. The odontoblast processes are believed to serve a transducer function in transmitting stimuli from the tooth surface to the nerves in the dental pulp. In teeth with more than one cusp, *pulpal horns* extend into the cusps and contain large numbers of nerve fibers. More of these fibers extend into the dentinal tubules than at other sites. Because dentin continues to be secreted throughout life, the pulp cavity decreases in volume with age.

Alveolar Process and Alveolar Bone

The Alveolar Processes of the Mandible and Maxilla Contain the Sockets or *Alveoli* for the Roots of the Teeth

The *alveolar bone proper,* a thin layer of compact bone, forms the wall of the alveolus (see Fig. 15.7) and is the bone to which the periodontal ligament is attached. The rest of the alveolar process is supporting bone.

The surface of the alveolar bone proper usually shows regions of bone resorption and bone deposition, particularly when a tooth is being moved (Fig. 15.17). Periodontal dis-

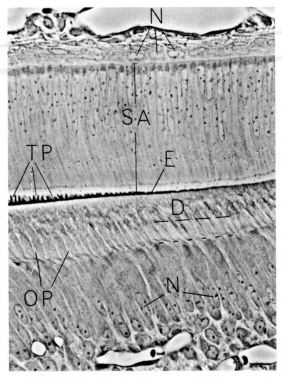

Figure 15.10. Plastic thick section, unstained, viewed with phase contrast optics showing enamel organ cells and odontoblasts as they begin to produce enamel *(E)* and dentin *(D),* respectively. Young enamel is deposited by secretory ameloblasts *(SA)* onto the previously formed dentin. The enamel appears dark in the illustration. On the left, the enamel surface displays a characteristic picket fence pattern due to the sharp contrast between the lightly stained Tomes' processes *(TP)* of the secretory ameloblasts and the darkly stained young enamel product that partly surrounds the cellular processes. The *upper N* marks nuclei of cells constituting the stratum intermedium layer. Other enamel organ cells are not labeled. The *lower N* marks nuclei of odontoblasts in the basal pole of the cell. The apical pole of the odontoblast cell body extends as far as the *short-segment broken line.* At this point, odontoblastic processes *(OP)* continue from the cell body through the predentin (unlabeled) and into the dentin. The *long-segment broken line* marks the boundary between predentin and dentin.

ease usually leads to loss of alveolar bone, as does the absence of functional occlusion of a tooth with its normal opponent.

Periodontal Ligament

The *periodontal ligament* is the fibrous connective tissue joining the tooth to its surrounding bone. The ligament is also called the *periodontal membrane,* but neither term describes its structure and function adequately. The periodontal ligament provides for

- Attachment
- Support
- Bone remodeling (during movement of a tooth)
- Nutrition of adjacent structures

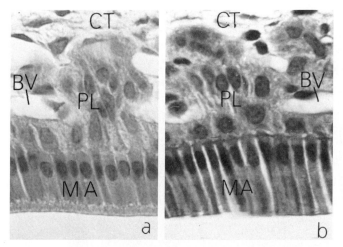

Figure 15.11. Light micrographs of maturation ameloblasts *(MA)* in paraffin sections of demineralized tissue stained with H&E. The maturing enamel has been lost owing to action of the demineralizing solution, and the space below the ameloblasts previously occupied by the enamel appears empty. **a** shows maturation ameloblasts with a striated border, and **b** shows smooth-ended maturation ameloblasts. At the basal pole of the maturation ameloblasts are the cells of the papillary layer *(PL)*. A stratum intermedium is no longer present during the maturation process. *BV*, blood vessels; and *CT*, connective tissue.

- Proprioception
- Tooth eruption

Attachment and support are the most apparent functions.

A histologic section of the periodontal ligament shows it to contain areas of both dense and loose connective tissue. The dense connective tissue contains collagen fibers and fibroblasts that appear elongated parallel to the long axis of the collagen fibers (Fig. 15.17). The fibroblasts are believed to move back and forth, leaving behind a trail of collagen fibers. Periodontal fibroblasts have also been shown to contain internalized collagen fibrils that are digested by

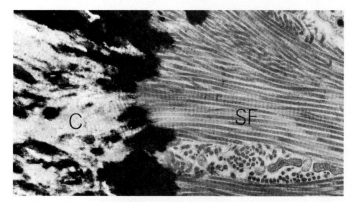

Figure 15.12. Electron micrograph of Sharpey's fibers *(SF)* extending from periodontal ligament (right) into the cementum *(C)*. The Sharpey's fibers consist of collagenous fibrils. Those within the cementum are mineralized; those within the periodontal ligament are not mineralized.

the hydrolytic enzymes of the cytoplasmic lysosomes. These observations indicate that these fibroblasts not only produce collagen fibrils but also resorb collagen fibrils, thereby adjusting continuously to the demands of tooth movement.

The loose connective tissue in the periodontal ligament contains blood vessels and nerve endings in addition to the cells and thin collagenous fibers. The periodontal ligament also contains longitudinally disposed *oxytalan fibers.* They are attached to bone or cementum at each end. Some appear to be associated with the adventitia of blood vessels. As in other connective tissues, oxytalan fibers stain with special elastic stains; ultrastructurally, they resemble developing elastic fibers, with their chief structural component being the microfibril that is characteristic of developing elastic fibers.

Gingiva

The Gingiva Is the Part of the Mucous Membrane Commonly Called the Gums

The gingiva is firmly attached to the teeth and underlying bony tissue. An idealized diagram of the gingiva is presented in Figure 15.18. The *gingival mucosa* is synonymous with the *masticatory mucosa* described above (page 405). The *attachment epithelium* or *junctional epithelium* is firmly adherent to the tooth. Above the attachment of the epithelium to the tooth, the *gingival sulcus,* a shallow crevice, is lined with *crevicular epithelium* that is continuous with the attachment epithelium.

A basal lamina-like material is secreted by the junctional epithelium and adheres firmly to the tooth surface. The cells then attach to this material via hemidesmosomes. The basal lamina and the hemidesmosomes are, together, referred to as the *epithelial attachment.* In young individuals this attachment is to the enamel; in older individuals, where passive tooth eruption and gingival recession expose the roots, the attachment is to the cementum.

The term *periodontium* refers to all the tissues involved in the attachment of a tooth to the jaw. These include the crevicular and junctional epithelium, the cementum, the periodontal ligament, and the alveolar bone.

SALIVARY GLANDS

The Major Salivary Glands Are Paired Glands With Long Ducts

The major salivary glands, as noted earlier, consist of the paired parotid, submandibular, and sublingual glands. The parotid and the submandibular glands are actually located outside the oral cavity; their secretions reach the cavity by ducts. The parotid gland is located subcutaneously, below and in front of the ear, and the submandibular gland is located under the floor of the mouth, close to the mandible. (The submandibular gland is sometimes called the

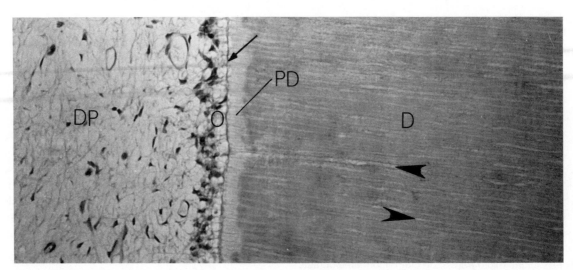

Figure 15.13. Light micrograph of human tooth, decalcified and stained with H&E. On the left is the dental pulp *(DP)*, the soft tissue core of the tooth that resembles embryonic connective tissue, even in the adult tooth. Dentin *(D)* is on the right; two *arrowheads* indicate the dentinal tubules in dentin that contain the odontoblastic processes. The odontoblasts *(O)* are adjacent to the unmineralized dentin called the predentin *(PD)*. At their apical extremities, the odontoblasts form junctional complexes that separate the predentin from the lateral intercellular space of the odontoblasts. This boundary, formed by the junctional complexes of the odontoblasts, appears as a membrane *(arrow)* mostly due to microfilaments within the odontoblasts that are attached to the junctional complexes. ×200.

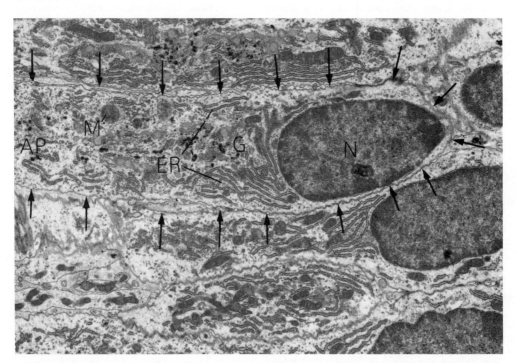

Figure 15.14. Electron micrograph of odontoblasts. The plasma membrane of one odontoblast has been marked with *arrows*. The cell contains a large amount of rough endoplasmic reticulum *(ER)* and a large Golgi apparatus *(G)*. The odontoblastic process is not shown; it would extend from the apical pole *(AP)* of the cell. The black objects in the Golgi region are abacus bodies. The tissue has been treated with pyroantimonate, which forms a black precipitate with calcium. *M,* mitochondria; and *N,* nucleus.

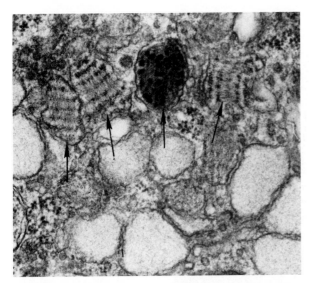

Figure 15.15. Electron micrograph of Golgi region of odontoblast showing numerous large vesicles. Abacus bodies *(arrows)* contain parallel arrays of filaments, and these are studded with granules.

submaxillary gland. This confusion derives from the fact that some British anatomists call the **mandible** the **submaxilla**.) The sublingual gland is located in the floor of the mouth anterior to the submandibular gland.

The minor salivary glands are located in the submucosa of different parts of the oral cavity. They include the **lingual, labial, buccal, molar,** and **palatine glands**.

Each salivary gland arises from the developing oral cavity epithelium. Initially, it takes the form of a solid cord of

cells that enters the mesenchyme (Fig. 15.19). The proliferation of the epithelial cells eventually produces highly branched epithelial cords that have bulbous ends. Degeneration of the innermost cells of the cords and the bulbous ends leads to their canalization. The cords become the ducts, and the bulbous ends become the **secretory acini.**

Secretory Acini Are Organized Into Lobules

The major salivary glands are surrounded by a capsule of moderately dense connective tissue from which septa divide the secretory portions of the gland into lobules and lobes. The septa contain the larger blood vessels and the excretory ducts. The connective tissue associated with the groups of secretory acini blends imperceptibly into the surrounding loose connective tissue. There is no capsule around the minor salivary glands.

Numerous lymphocytes and plasma cells populate the connective tissue surrounding the acini in both the major and minor salivary glands. Their significance in the secretion of salivary antibodies is described below.

Secretory Gland Acini

The acini of salivary glands contain either **serous cells** (protein-secreting), **mucous cells** (mucin-secreting), or both serous and mucous cells. Thus, three types of acini are described:

- **Serous acini**
- **Mucous acini**
- **Mixed acini**

Serous acini are generally spherical; mucous end pieces

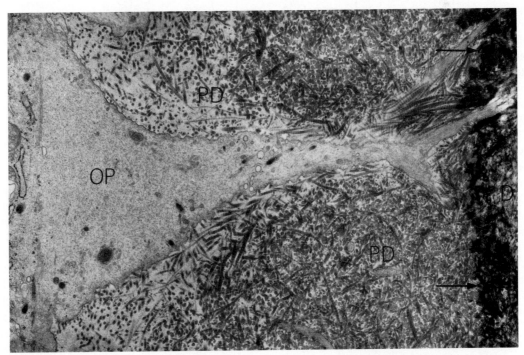

Figure 15.16. Electron micrograph of odontoblastic process *(OP)* of young odontoblast. The process extends through predentin *(PD)* and into dentin *(D)*. Profiles in predentin are collagen fibrils, smaller near the cell body of the odontoblast and larger at the mineralization front *(arrows).*

Bundle bone   Cementum   Fatty tissue

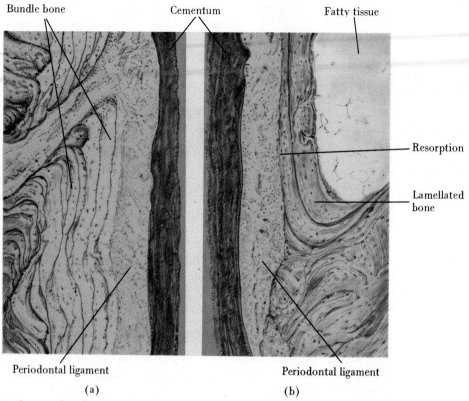

Resorption

Lamellated bone

Periodontal ligament   Periodontal ligament

(a)   (b)

Figure 15.17. Light micrographs of periodontal ligament from two sides of a tooth that is moving to the right. Each micrograph shows cementum, periodontal ligament, and alveolar bone. The other parts of the tooth are not shown. The layered pattern of bone **(a)** is indicative of bone formation; the scalloped edge of the bone **(b)** is indicative of bone resorption. As the tooth moves to the right, bone in the path of the tooth is resorbed, and at the same time, bone is deposited in the wake of the tooth. The cells of the periodontal ligament function to provide constant and adjustable attachment of the tooth during this movement.

are usually more tubular. Nevertheless, the term *acinus*, which is Latin for berry or grape, is used to refer even to the more tubular mucous end pieces.

Mixed Acini. Some mucous acini have a cap of serous cells that secrete into the highly convoluted intercellular space between the mucous cells. Such caps, because of their appearance in histologic sections, are called *serous demilunes* (fr. Fr. for half-moons). The relative frequency of the three types of acini is a prime characteristic by which the major salivary glands may be distinguished.

Serous Cells. Serous cells contain large amounts of rER, free ribosomes, a prominent Golgi apparatus, and numerous secretory granules (Fig. 15.20). As in most protein-secreting cells that store the secretion as zymogen granules, the granules are found in the apical cytoplasm. Most other organelles are in the basal or perinuclear cytoplasm.

In H&E sections, the basal cytoplasm of the serous cell stains with hematoxylin due to the rER and the free ribosomes, whereas the apical region stains with eosin, in large part, due to the presence of the secretory granules.

The base of the serous cell may display infoldings of the plasma membrane and basal-lateral folds in the form of processes that are implicated with similar processes of adjacent cells. The serous cells are joined near their apical surface by junctional complexes. A special feature of the salivary gland acinus is that the lumen may descend between neighboring cells as a narrow, serpentine *canaliculus* extending almost to the basal lamina. In that case, the junctional complex is located at the bottom of the canaliculus.

Mucous Cells. As in other mucus-secreting epithelia, the mucous cells of the mucous salivary acini undergo cycles of activity. During part of the cycle, mucus is synthesized and stored within the cell as mucinogen granules. When the product is discharged, following hormonal or neural stimulation, the cell begins to synthesize mucus again. After discharge of most or all of the mucinogen granules, the cell is difficult to distinguish from an inactive serous cell. However, most mucous cells contain large numbers of mucinogen granules in their apical cytoplasm, and because the mucinogen is lost in H&E-stained paraffin sections, the apical portion of the cell usually has an empty appearance. With the transmission electron microscope (TEM), the rER, mitochondria, and other components are seen chiefly in the basal portion of the cell; this part of the cell also contains the nucleus, which is typically flattened against the base of the cell (Fig. 15.21).

The apical portion of the mucous cell contains numerous mucinogen granules and a large Golgi apparatus in which

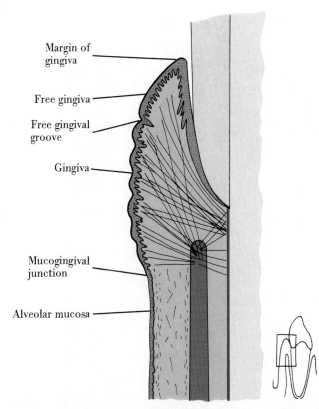

Figure 15.18. Schematic diagram of gingiva. The gingival epithelium is attached to the enamel of the tooth. Here, the junction between epithelium and connective tissue is smooth. Elsewhere, the gingival epithelium is deeply indented by connective tissue papillae, and the junction between the two is irregular. The *black lines* represent collagen fibers from the cementum of the tooth and from the crest of the alveolar bone that extend toward the gingival epithelium. Note the shallow papillae in the lining mucosa (alveolar mucosa) that contrast sharply with those of the gingiva. The schematic diagram of gingiva corresponds to the *rectangular area* of the *small diagram.* (Based on Bhaskar SN (ed): *Orban's Oral Histology and Embryology,* 9th ed. St Louis, CV Mosby, 1980, p 290.)

large amounts of carbohydrate are added to a protein base to synthesize the glycoprotein of the mucin. The mucous cells possess apical junctional complexes, the same as those seen between serous cells. If serous demilunes are present, intercellular canaliculi extend from the lumen, between the mucous cells to the serous cells, and serve as the delivery route for the serous secretions.

Myoepithelial Cells Are Contractile Cells That Embrace the Basal Aspect of the Acinar Secretory Cells

Myoepithelial Cells. Myoepithelial cells are contractile cells with numerous processes. They lie between the basal plasma membrane of the epithelial cells and the basal lamina of the epithelium (Fig. 15.22). Myoepithelial cells also underlie the cells of the proximal portion of the duct system. In both locations, the myoepithelial cells are instrumental in moving secretory products toward the excre-

tory duct. Myoepithelial cells are sometimes difficult to identify in H&E sections. The nucleus of such a cell is often seen as a small, round profile near the basement membrane. The contractile filaments stain with eosin and are often recognized as a thin eosinophilic band in the region where the basement membrane is located.

Salivary Ducts

The lumen of the salivary acinus is continuous with that of a duct system that may have as many as three sequential segments. These are referred to as

- *Intercalated duct*
- *Striated duct*
- *Excretory duct*

There is great variation in the degree of development of the intercalated ducts and striated ducts, depending on the nature of the acinar secretion. Serous glands have well-developed intercalated ducts and striated ducts that modify the serous secretion by both absorption of specific components from the secretion and secretion of additional components to form the final product. Mucous glands, in which the secretion is not modified, have very poorly developed intercalated ducts that may not be recognizable in H&E sections. Moreover, they do not display striated ducts. The excretory duct does not modify the secretion; it simply carries the secretion from the gland to the oral cavity.

Intercalated Ducts Are Located Between a Secretory Acinus and a Larger Duct

Intercalated Ducts. Intercalated ducts are lined by low cuboidal epithelial cells that usually do not have distinctive features to suggest their function other than that of a conduit (see Plate 66, page 431). However, the cells of intercalated ducts possess carbonic anhydrase activity. In ser-

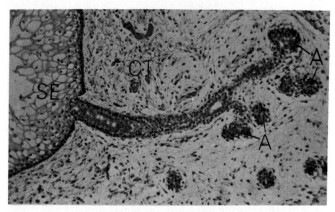

Figure 15.19. Light micrograph of developing salivary gland, H&E section. A cord of cells grows from the surface epithelium *(SE)* into the underlying connective tissue *(CT).* Branching of the cord occurs, and the terminal ends of the branches develop into acini *(A).*

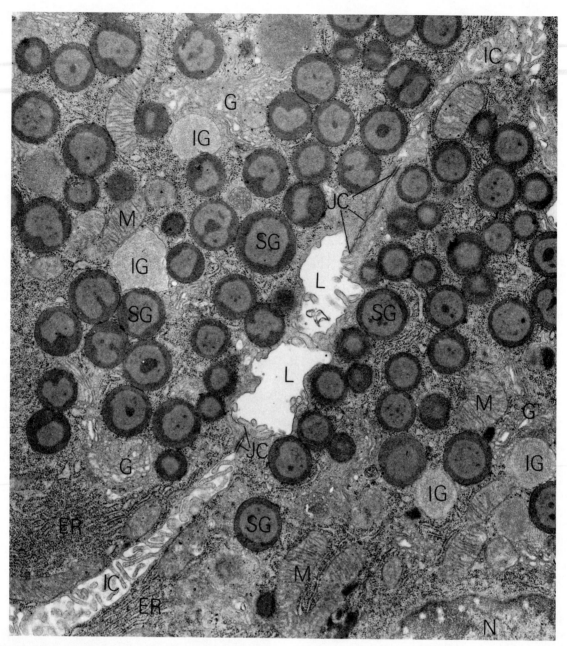

Figure 15.20. Electron micrograph of the apical portion of parotid gland serous cells. The cells are polarized, with their product in the form of secretory granules *(SG)* near the lumen *(L)* of the acinus. The cells display rough endoplasmic reticulum *(ER)* and several Golgi profiles *(G)*. Immature secretory granules *(IG)* are present close to the Golgi apparatus. At the apical pole of the cells are junctional complexes *(JC)*. The intercellular space *(IC)* is dilated, and profiles of sectioned lateral plications are seen. *M,* mitochondria; and *N,* nucleus. ×15,000.

ous-secreting glands and mixed glands, they have been shown to

- *Secrete bicarbonate* ion into the acinar product
- *Absorb chloride* ion from the acinar product

As noted above, intercalated ducts are most prominent in those salivary glands that produce a watery serous secretion. In mucus-secreting salivary glands, the intercalated ducts, when present, are short and difficult to identify.

Striated Duct Cells Have Numerous Infoldings of the Basal Plasma Membrane

Striated Ducts. Striated ducts are lined by a simple cuboidal epithelium that gradually becomes columnar as it approaches the excretory duct. The infoldings of the basal plasma membrane are seen in histologic sections as "striations." Longitudinally oriented, elongated mitochondria are enclosed in the infoldings. Basal infoldings associated with elongated mitochondria are a morphologic specialization al-

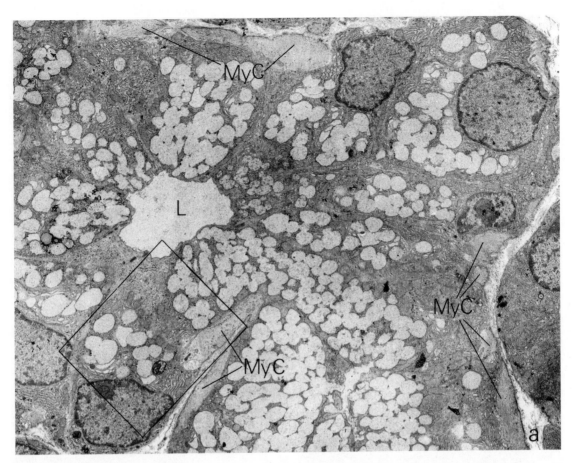

Figure 15.21. a. Low-magnification electron micrograph of a mucous acinus. The mucous cells contain numerous mucinogen granules. Many of the granules have coalesced to form larger irregular masses that will ultimately discharge into the lumen *(L)* of the acinus. Myoepithelial cell processes *(MyC)* are evident at the periphery of the acinus. A portion of one of the secretory cells and part of an underlying myoepithelial cell process *(rectangle)* are shown in **b** at higher magnification. ×5,000.

ways associated with reabsorption of fluid and electrolytes. The striated duct cells also have numerous basal-lateral folds that are implicated with those of adjacent cells. The nucleus typically occupies a central (rather than basal) location in the cell (see Plate 67, Fig. 2, page 433). Striated ducts are the site of

- *Reabsorption of sodium* from the primary secretion
- *Addition of potassium* to the secretion

More sodium is resorbed than potassium is secreted, so the secretion becomes hypotonic. When secretion is very rapid, more sodium and less potassium appear in the final saliva because the reabsorption and secondary secretion systems cannot keep up with the rate of primary secretion. Thus, the saliva may become isotonic to hypertonic.

The diameter of striated ducts often exceeds that of the secretory acinus. Striated ducts are located in the parenchyma of the glands (they are *intralobular ducts*) but may be surrounded by small amounts of connective tissue in which blood vessels and nerves can be seen running in parallel with the duct.

Excretory Ducts Travel in the Interlobular and Interlobar Connective Tissue

Excretory Ducts. Excretory ducts constitute the principal ducts of each of the major glands. They connect, ultimately, with the oral cavity. The epithelium of small excretory ducts is simple cuboidal. It gradually changes to stratified cuboidal or pseudostratified columnar. As the diameter of the duct increases, stratified columnar epithelium is often seen, and as the ducts approach the oral epithelium, stratified squamous epithelium may be found. The parotid duct (Stensen's duct) and the submandibular duct (Wharton's duct) travel in the connective tissue of the face and neck, respectively, for some distance from the gland before penetrating the oral mucosa.

Parotid Gland

The Parotid Glands Are Totally Serous

The paired serous parotid glands are the largest of the major salivary glands. The parotid duct travels from the gland, which is located below and in front of the ear, to

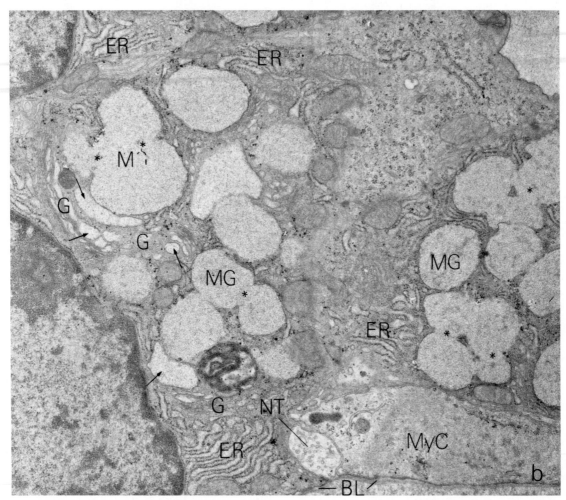

Figure 15.21. b. At this higher magnification, the relationship of the mucinogen granules *(MG)* to the Golgi apparatus *(G)* and rough endoplasmic reticulum *(ER)* is evident. Note that some of the Golgi cisternae are somewhat enlarged *(arrows)* and contain a substance that resembles the mucinogen granules *(MG)*. Also note the nature of the coalescence of the ma- ture mucinogen granules *(asterisks)*. At the lower right, a myoepithelial cell process *(MyC)* can be seen interposed between the surrounding basal lamina *(BL)* and the secretory epithelial cell. A nerve terminal *(NT)* lying in relation to the myoepithelial cell is also evident. ×15,000.

enter the oral cavity opposite the second upper molar tooth. The secretory units in the parotid are *serous* (see Plate 67, page 433) and surround numerous, long, narrow intercalated ducts. Striated ducts are large and conspicuous.

Large amounts of adipose tissue often occur in the parotid gland and may be one of its distinguishing features. The facial nerve (cranial nerve VII) passes through the parotid gland; large cross sections of this nerve, usually found in routine H&E sections of the gland, are useful in identifying the parotid. Mumps, a viral infection of the parotid gland, can damage the facial nerve.

Submandibular Gland

The Submandibular Glands Are Mixed Glands That Are Mostly Serous in Humans

The paired, large, mixed submandibular glands are located under either side of the floor of the mouth, close to the mandible. A duct from each of the two glands runs forward and medially to a papilla located on the floor of the mouth just lateral to the *frenulum* of the tongue. Some mucous acini capped by serous demilunes are generally found among the predominant serous acini (see Plate 66, page 431). Intercalated ducts are less extensive than in the parotid gland.

Sublingual Gland

The Small Sublingual Glands Are Mixed Glands That Are Mostly Mucus Secreting in Humans

The sublingual glands, the smallest of the paired major salivary glands, are located in the floor of the mouth anterior to the submandibular glands. Their multiple small sublingual ducts empty into the submandibular duct as well as directly onto the floor of the mouth. Some of the predominant mucous acini have serous demilunes, but purely

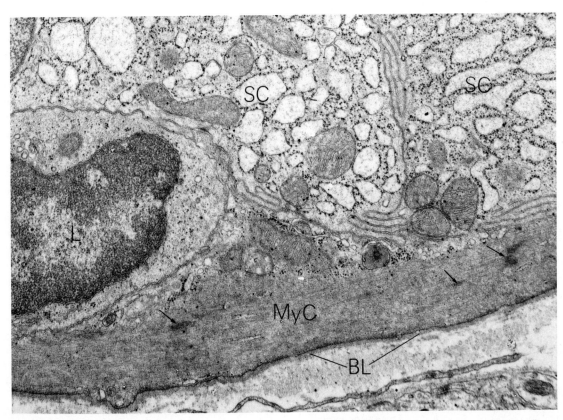

Figure 15.22. Electron micrograph of the basal portion of two secretory cells *(SC)* from a submandibular gland. A myoepithelial cell process *(MyC)* is also present. Again, note the location of the myoepithelial cell on the epithelial side of the basal lamina *(BL)*. The cytoplasm of the myoepithelial cell contains contractile filaments and densities *(arrows)* similar to those seen in smooth muscle cells. The cell on the left with the small nucleus is a lymphocyte *(L)*. Having migrated through the basal lamina, it is also within the epithelial compartment. ×15,000.

serous acini are rarely present (see Plate 68, page 435). Intercalated ducts and striated ducts are difficult to locate or may be absent. The mucous secretory units may be more tubular than purely acinar.

Saliva

Saliva Includes the Combined Secretions of All the Major and Minor Salivary Glands

Most saliva is produced by the salivary glands. A smaller amount derives from the gingival sulcus, tonsillar crypts, and general transudation from the epithelial lining of the oral cavity. One of the unique features of saliva is the large and variable volume produced. The volume (per weight of gland tissue) of saliva exceeds that of other digestive secretions by as much as 40 times. This is undoubtedly related to the fact that saliva has many functions, only some of which are concerned with digestion.

Functions of Saliva. The salivary glands produce about 1200 mL of saliva a day. Saliva has numerous functions relating to metabolic and nonmetabolic activities. These include

* Moistening the oral mucosa
* Moistening dry foods to aid swallowing
* Providing a medium for dissolved and suspended food materials that chemically stimulate taste buds
* Buffering of the contents of the oral cavity through its high concentration of bicarbonate ion
* Digestion of carbohydrates by the digestive enzyme α-amylase that breaks the 1—4 glycoside bonds and continues to act in the esophagus and stomach
* Controlling the bacterial flora of the oral cavity because of the presence of the antibacterial enzyme *lysozyme*

The unique composition of saliva is summarized in Table 15.1.

Saliva Is a Source of Calcium and Phosphate Ions Essential for Normal Tooth Development and Maintenance

Calcium and phosphate in the saliva are essential for posteruptive mineralization of newly erupted teeth and for repair of precarious lesions of the enamel in erupted teeth. In addition, saliva serves several other roles in protecting the teeth. Proteins of the saliva cover the teeth with a protective coat called the *acquired pellicle.* Antibodies and other antibacterial agents serve to retard bacterial action that oth-

TABLE 15.1. Composition of Unstimulated Saliva[A]

	MEAN (mg/mL)
Organic constitutents	
Protein	220.0
Amylase	38.0
Lysozyme	22.0
sIgA	19.0
IgC	1.4
IgM	0.2
Glucose	1.0[B]
Urea	20.0
Uric acid	1.5
Creatinine	0.1
Cholesterol	8.0
cAMP	7.0
Inorganic constituents	
Sodium	15.0
Potassium	80.0
Thiocyanate	
Smokers	9.0
Nonsmokers	2.0
Calcium	5.8
Phosphate	16.8
Chloride	50.0
Fluoride	Traces (according to intake)

[A] Modified from Jenkins GN: *The Physiology and Biochemistry of the Mouth*, 4th ed. Oxford, Blackwell Scientific Publications, 1978.
[B] Higher in patients with uncontrolled hyperglycemia.

erwise would lead to tooth decay. Patients whose salivary glands are irradiated, as in the treatment of salivary gland tumors, fail to produce normal amounts of saliva; these patients typically develop rampant caries.

Immunologic Function of Saliva. Saliva, as noted, contains antibodies, salivary *immunoglobulin A (IgA)*. IgA is synthesized by plasma cells in the connective tissue surrounding the secretory acini of the salivary glands, and both dimeric and monomeric forms are released into the connective tissue matrix (Fig. 15.23a–c). A secretory glycoprotein is synthesized by the salivary gland cells and inserted on the basal plasma membrane where it serves as a receptor for dimeric IgA.

When the dimeric IgA binds to the receptor, the *secretory IgA complex* thus formed is internalized by receptor-mediated endocytosis and carried through the acinar cell to the apical plasma membrane, where it is released into the lumen as secretory IgA (sIgA). This process of synthesis and secretion of IgA is essentially identical with that which occurs in the more distal parts of the gastrointestinal tract where secretory IgA is transported across the absorptive columnar epithelium of the small intestine and colon (see page 462).

Composition of Saliva. Saliva contains chiefly water, proteins and glycoproteins (enzymes and antibodies), and electrolytes. It has a very high potassium concentration about 7 times that of blood, a sodium concentration about one-tenth that of blood, a bicarbonate concentration about 3 times that of blood, and significant amounts of calcium, phosphorus, chloride, thiocyanate, and urea. Lysozyme and α-amylase are the principal enzymes present (see Table 15.1).

Salivation Is Part of a Reflex Arc That Is Normally Stimulated by the Ingestion of Food

Although food ingestion is the most common stimulus for salivation, the sight or smell of food or even thoughts of food can also stimulate salivation. Autonomic stimulation can vary the composition of the saliva. Both sympathetic and parasympathetic nerves end adjacent to salivary acini.

- *Sympathetic stimulation* causes secretion of a *viscous saliva rich in proteins*, i.e., enzymes.
- *Parasympathetic stimulation* causes secretion of a copious, *watery saliva* that serves principally as a lubricant and buffer.

Aldosterone, the adrenal hormone that regulates absorption of sodium and secretion of potassium in the excretory tubules of the kidney (see page 574), also influences the electrolyte composition of saliva. It can greatly increase the reabsorption of sodium and the secretion of potassium in the striated ducts.

PHARYNX

The Pharynx Serves the Respiratory and Digestive Systems as a Common Passage for Air and Food

The pharynx communicates anteriorly with the nasal and oral cavities and with the larynx and continues posteriorly into the esophagus (see Fig. 18.1, page 531). The parts of the pharynx that are subject to abrasion by partially macerated food are lined with a nonkeratinized stratified squamous epithelium that is continuous with that of the oral cavity and the esophagus. Those parts not subject to abrasion are lined with pseudostratified ciliated columnar epithelium that contains goblet cells and that is continuous with that of the nasal cavity and the respiratory tract.

The connective tissue of the pharynx is described as fibroelastic because of the large number of elastic fibers present. External to this layer is the striated skeletal muscle of the pharyngeal constrictor muscles and other pharyngeal muscles.

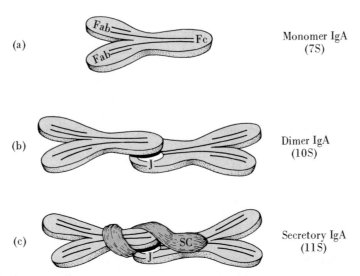

(a)   Monomer IgA (7S)

(b)   Dimer IgA (10S)

(c)   Secretory IgA (11S)

Figure 15.23. Diagram showing the monomer **(a)** and dimer **(b)** of IgA (products of plasma cells), with the J chain *(J)* joining the monomers. The secretory component *(SC),* a product of the epithelial cells, is added to the dimer to form secretory IgA *(sIgA)* **(c).** Fab and Fc indicate parts of basic antibody molecule. (Based on Shaw JH, et al: *Textbook of Oral Biology.* Philadelphia, WB Saunders, 1978, p 765.)

Lymphatic Tissue Surrounds the Pharynx at the Entrance to the Respiratory and Digestive Tracts

Pharyngeal and *palatine tonsils* are located in the sides and roof of the pharynx, respectively, and the *lingual tonsils* (see above) may be said to guard the floor of the pharynx. The palatine tonsils are also called the *faucial tonsils* because they are located in the submucosa of the fauces, the junction between the oral cavity and the pharynx.

- The *palatine tonsils* are the tonsils most commonly subject to chronic inflammation and subsequent tonsillectomy.
- The *pharyngeal tonsils,* also called **adenoids,** are often removed when they become chronically inflamed and enlarged.

The **auditory** or **Eustachian** tube opens into the nasopharynx near the molar teeth, thereby connecting the pharynx and the middle ear. Gingival inflammation from molar tooth eruption or impaction may partially or totally block the opening of the Eustachian tube, causing severe earache.

PLATE 64. Tongue I

The tongue is a muscular organ covered by mucous membrane. The mucous membrane consists of stratified squamous epithelium, keratinized in parts, resting on a loose connective tissue. The undersurface of the tongue is relatively uncomplicated. The mucosa of the dorsal surface, however, is modified to form three types of papillae: filiform, fungiform, and circumvallate. The circumvallate papillae form a V-shaped row that divides the tongue into a body and a root; the dorsal surface of the body, i.e., the portion anterior to the circumvallate papillae, contains filiform and fungiform papillae.

FIGURE 1, tongue, monkey, H&E ×65; inset ×130. This figure shows the dorsal surface of the tongue with the filiform papillae *(Fil P)*. They are the most numerous of the three types of papillae. Structurally, they are bent conical projections of the epithelium, with the point of the projection directed posteriorly. These papillae do not possess taste buds and are composed of stratified squamous keratinized epithelium.

The fungiform papillae are scattered about as isolated, slightly rounded, elevated structures situated among the filiform papillae. A fungiform papilla is shown in the **inset.**

A large connective tissue core (primary connective tissue papilla) forms the center of the fungiform papilla, and smaller connective tissue papillae (secondary connective tissue papillae) project into the base of the surface epithelium *(arrowhead)*. The connective tissue of the papillae is highly vascularized. Because of the deep penetration of connective tissue into the epithelium, combined with a very thin keratinized surface, the fungiform papillae appear as small red dots when the dorsal surface of the tongue is examined by gross inspection.

FIGURE 2, tongue, monkey, H&E ×65. The undersurface of the tongue is shown in this figure. The smooth surface of the stratified squamous epithelium *(Ep)* contrasts with the irregular surface of the dorsum of the tongue. Moreover, the epithelial surface on the underside of the tongue is usually not keratinized. The connective tissue *(CT)* is immediately deep to the epithelium; deeper still is the striated muscle *(M)*.

The numerous connective tissue papillae that project into the base of the epithelium of both the ventral and dorsal surfaces give the epithelial-connective tissue junction an irregular profile. Often, these connective tissue papillae are cut obliquely and then appear as small islands of connective tissue within the epithelial layer (see Fig. 1).

The connective tissue extends as far as the muscle without change in character, and no submucosa is recognized. The muscle *(M)* is striated and is unique in its organization; i.e., the fibers travel in three planes. Therefore, most sections will show bundles of muscle fibers cut longitudinally, at right angles to each other, and in cross section. Nerves *(N)* that innervate the muscle are also frequently observed in the connective tissue septa between the muscle bundles.

The surface of the tongue behind the vallate papillae (the root of the tongue) contains lingual tonsils (not shown). These are similar in structure and appearance to the palatine tonsils illustrated in Plate 50, page 355.

KEY

CT, connective tissue
Ep, epithelium
Fil P, filiform papillae

M, striated muscle bundles
N, nerves

arrowhead (Fig. 1, inset), secondary connective tissue

PLATE 64

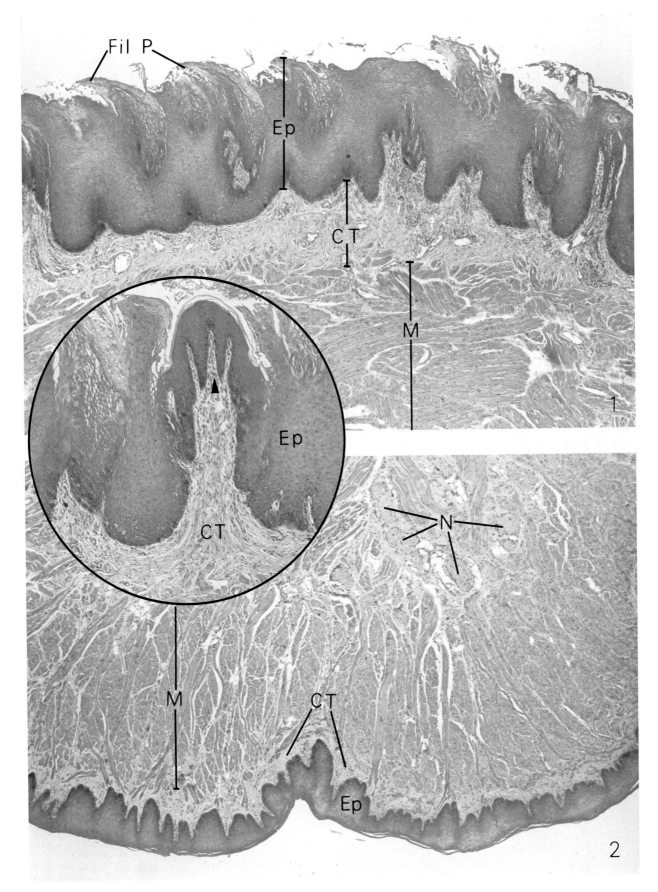

PLATE 65. Tongue II

FIGURE 1, tongue, monkey, H&E ×55. The sides of the tongue contain a series of vertical ridges that bear taste buds. When these ridges are cut at right angles to their long axis, they appear as a row of papillae. These ridges are called *foliate papillae*. Foliate papillae are not always conspicuous in the adult human tongue but are quite evident in the infant tongue. They can immediately be distinguished from fungiform papillae in a section because they appear in rows, whereas fungiform papillae (not illustrated) appear alone. Moreover, numerous taste buds *(TB)* are present on adjacent walls of neighboring foliate papillae. In contrast, fungiform papillae have taste buds on the dorsal surface. The foliate papillae are covered by stratified squamous epithelium that is usually not or is only slightly keratinized. The part of the epithelium *(Ep)* that is on the free surface of the foliate papillae is thick and has a number of secondary connective tissue papillae projecting into its undersurface.

The connective tissue within and under the foliate papillae contains serous-type glands *(Gl)*, called *von Ebner's glands,* that open via ducts *(D)* into the cleft between neighboring papillae. In addition to von Ebner's glands, which are entirely of the serous type, the tongue contains mixed (serous and mucous) glands near the apex and mucous glands in the root (not illustrated).

The dense patches *(arrows)* within the connective tissue consist of accumulations of lymphocytes in the form of diffuse lymphatic tissue. They are typically seen just below the clefts of the papillae.

FIGURE 2, tongue, monkey, H&E ×55; inset ×640. Of the true papillae found on the dorsal surface of the tongue—filiform, fungiform, and circumvallate (vallate)—the circumvallate are the largest. About 7–11 of these form a "V" between the body and root of the tongue. *Circumvallate papillae* are covered by stratified squamous epithelium that may be slightly keratinized. Each circumvallate papilla is surrounded by a trench or cleft. Numerous taste buds *(TB)* are on the lateral walls of the papillae; moreover, the tongue epithelium *(Ep)* facing the papilla within the cleft may contain some taste buds. The dorsal surface of the papilla is rather smooth; however, numerous secondary connective tissue *(CT)* papillae project into the underside of the epithelium. The deep trench surrounding the circumvallate papillae and the presence of taste buds on the sides rather than on the surface are features that distinguish circumvallate from fungiform papillae.

The connective tissue near the circumvallate papillae also contains many serous-type glands *(Gl)*, von Ebner's glands, that open via ducts *(D)* into the bottom of the trench.

The taste buds extend through the full thickness of the stratified squamous epithelium **(inset)** and open at the surface at a small pore *(arrowheads)*. The cells of the taste bud are chiefly spindle shaped and oriented at a right angle to the surface. The nuclei of the cells are elongated and mainly in the basal two-thirds of the bud. At least three cell types are present in the taste bud; one is a special receptor cell, the sensory or neuroepithelial cell. Nerve fibers enter the epithelium and terminate in close contact with the sensory cells of the taste bud, but they cannot be identified in routine H&E preparations. Other cell types in the taste bud include the supporting cells and the basal cells. The latter sometimes exhibit mitotic figures *(asterisk)* and give rise to the other cell types.

KEY

CT, connective tissue	**Gl,** serous (von Ebner's) glands	**arrowheads (inset),** taste bud pore
D, ducts	**M,** striated muscle bundles	**arrows (Fig. 1),** lymphocytes
Ep, epithelium	**TB,** taste buds	**asterisk (inset),** mitotic figure

PLATE 65

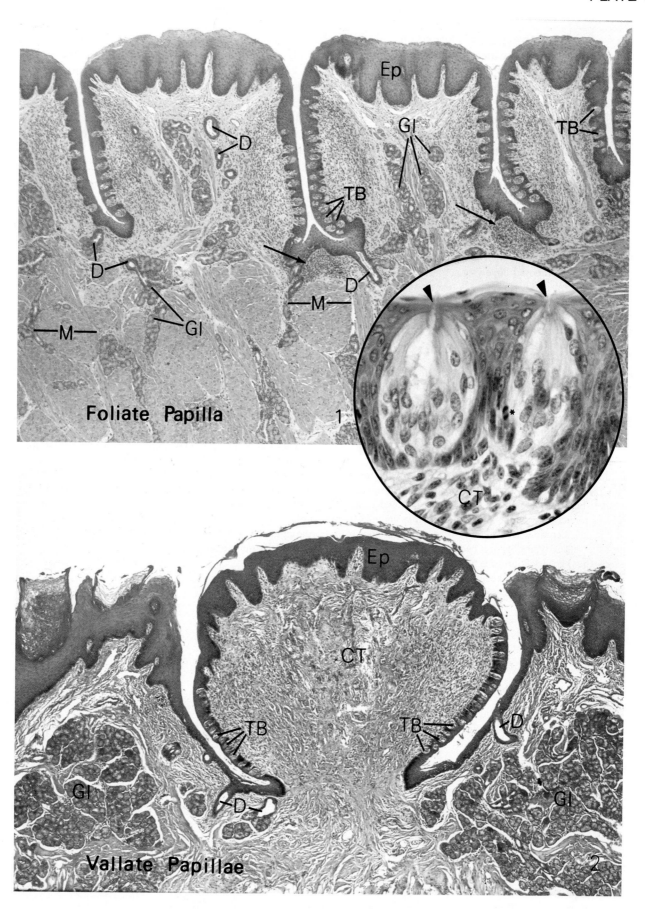

Foliate Papilla 1

Vallate Papillae 2

PLATE 66. Submandibular Gland

The salivary glands are compound (branched) tubuloacinar glands. The secretory unit is the acinus, which is made up of either serous cells (serous acini) or mucous cells (mucous acini). Generally, in H&E preparations, serous cells can readily be distinguished from mucous cells by the deep staining of the cytoplasm of the serous cell in contrast to the empty or washed-out appearance of the mucous cell—a characteristic feature due to loss of the stored mucinogen granules from the cell during tissue preparation. A second distinguishing feature relates to nuclear shape. The nuclei of mucous cells are typically flattened against the base of the cell, whereas nuclei of serous cells are rounded.

FIGURE 1, submandibular gland, human, H&E ×160.

The submandibular glands contain both serous and mucous acini. In humans, the serous components predominate. The *rectangle* reveals a cluster of mucous acini *(MA)*. The mucus-secreting cells of the acini are readily discernible at this low magnification due to their light staining. The remainder of the field is composed largely of serous acini *(SA)*. A few adipose cells *(A)* and various ducts—excretory *(ED)*, striated *(StD)*, and intercalated *(ID)*—are also evident in the field.

The nature of the duct system of the submandibular gland is shown to advantage in this figure. The initial ducts leading from the acinus, the intercalated ducts, are very small. They possess a flattened to cuboidal epithelium and exhibit a distinct lumen. Intercalated ducts in the submandibular gland (and the parotid gland) tend to be relatively long; thus, they are frequently encountered in a section. They merge *(arrows)* to form the larger striated ducts *(StD)*. These ducts have an epithelium of low to tall columnar cells and, at high magnification, show basal striations (see Plate 67).

FIGURE 2, submandibular gland, human H&E ×400.

When examined at higher magnification, as in this figure, the individual mucous cells exhibit distinct cell boundaries. Their nuclei are flattened (except those that are tangentially sectioned). In contrast, the cytoplasm of the serous cells stains deeply, and the nuclei appear ovoid or round.

Serous cells are also found forming a cap known as a serous demilune *(SD)* on the periphery of many of the mucous acini *(MA)*. The cells of the serous demilune secrete via channels between the mucous cells, thereby allowing the secretory product to reach the lumen of the acinus and mix with the mucous secretion. Realize that some acini that appear to be of the serous type *(SA)* and particularly the acini that appear as small spherical profiles may actually be demilunes of mucous acinus that have been cut in a plane that excludes the mucous cells from the section.

Associated with the acinar epithelium are myoepithelial cells. They are located between the basal aspect of the secretory cells and the basal lamina. However, myoepithelial cells are difficult to identify in H&E-stained preparations of salivary gland, and none can be identified with assurance here.

This figure also provides a comparison between an intercalated duct *(ID)* and a small striated duct *(StD)* from the *rectangle* in Figure 1. Outside of the lobule, the striated duct joins the excretory duct *(ED)* (upper left, Fig. 1). The excretory duct is characterized by a wider lumen and a taller columnar epithelium. As the excretory ducts increase in size, the epithelium becomes pseudostratified and, finally, stratified in the main excretory ducts.

KEY

A, adipose cell
ED, excretory duct
ID, intercalated duct
MA, mucous acini
SA, serous acini
SD, serous demilune
StD, striated duct
arrows (Fig. 1), intercalated ducts joining to form a striated duct
asterisks, lumina of mucous acini
rectangle (Fig. 1), cluster of mucous acini

PLATE 66

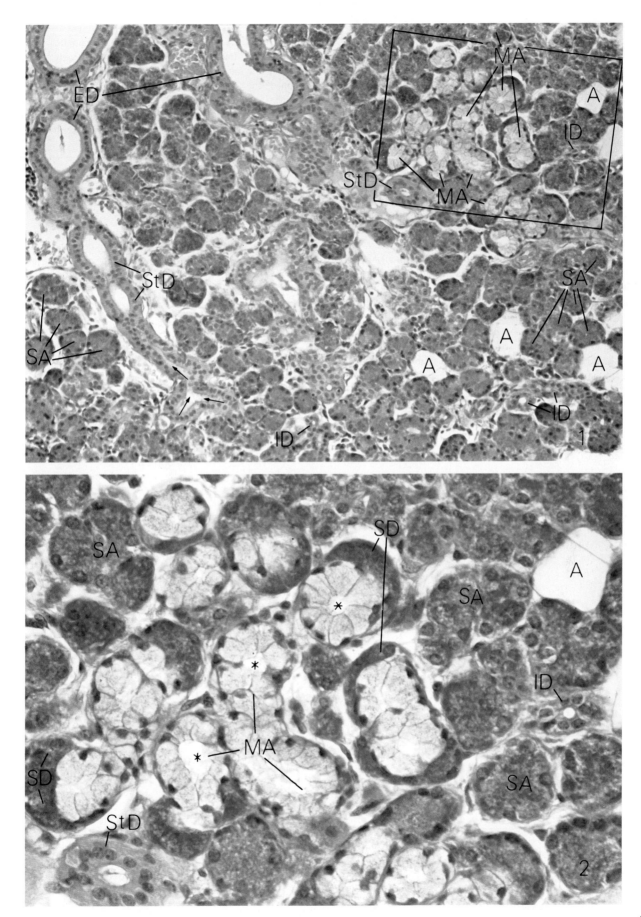

PLATE 67. Parotid Gland

FIGURE 1, parotid gland, human, H&E ×160. The parotid gland in the human is composed entirely of serous acini *(A)* and their ducts. However, numerous adipose cells *(AC)* are usually distributed throughout the gland. Both the serous acini and their duct system in the parotid gland are comparable in structure and arrangement to the same components in the submandibular gland. Within the lobule, the striated ducts *(StD)* are readily observed. They exhibit a simple co-lumnar epithelium. The intercalated ducts are smaller; at the low magnification of this figure, they are difficult to recognize. A few intercalated ducts *(ID)* are indicated. The lower portion of the figure reveals an excretory duct *(ED)* within a connective tissue septum *(CT)*. The epithelium of this excretory duct exhibits two layers of nuclei and is either pseudostratified or, possibly, already true stratified epithelium.

FIGURE 2, parotid gland, monkey, glutaraldehyde-osmium tetroxide fixed, H&E ×640. The serous cells are optimally preserved and reveal their secretory (zymogen) granules. The granules appear as the fine dot-like objects within the cytoplasm. The acinus in the upper right of the figure has been cut in cross section and reveals the acinar lumen *(AL)*. The *small rectangle* drawn in the acinus represents an area comparable to the electron micrograph shown as Figure 15.21. That the acini are not simple spheres but, rather, are irregular elongate structures can be perceived from the large acinar profile to the left of the striated duct *(StD)*. Because of the small size of the acinar lumen and the variability in sectioning an acinus, the lumen is seen infrequently.

A cross-sectional profile of an intercalated duct *(ID)* appears on the left of the micrograph; note its simple cuboidal epithelium. A single flattened nucleus is present at the top of the duct and may represent one of the myoepithelial cells that is associated with the beginning of the duct system as well as with the acini *(A)*. The large duct occupying the center of the micrograph is a striated duct *(StD)*. It is composed of a columnar epithelium. The striations *(S)* that give the duct its name are evident. Also of significance is the presence of plasma cells *(PC)* within the connective tissue surrounding the duct. These cells produce the immunoglobulins taken up and resecreted by the acinar cells, particularly secretory IgA (sIgA).

KEY

A, acinus
AC, adipose cell
AL, acinar lumen
CT, connective tissue
ED, excretory duct
ID, intercalated duct
PC, plasma cells
S, striations of duct cells
StD, striated duct

PLATE 67

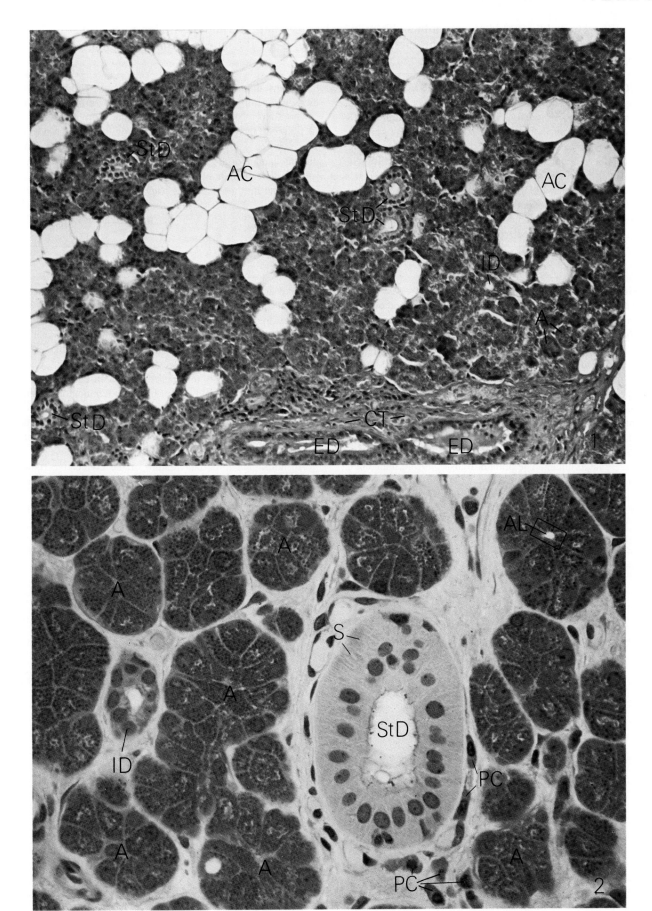

PLATE 68. Sublingual Gland

The sublingual gland resembles the submandibular gland in that it contains both serous and mucous elements. In the sublingual gland, however, the mucous acini predominate.

FIGURE 1, sublingual gland, human, H&E ×160. This figure shows a sublingual gland at low power. The mucous acini *(MA)* are conspicuous due to their light staining. Critical examination of the mucous acini at this relatively low magnification reveals that they are not spherical structures but, rather, elongate or tubular structures with branching outpockets. Thus, the acinus is rather large, and much of it is usually not seen within the plane of a single section.

The serous component of the gland is composed largely of demilunes, but occasional serous acini are present. (As already noted, some of the serous demilunes may be sectioned in a plane that does not include the mucous component of the acinus, thus giving the appearance of a serous acinus.)

The ducts of the sublingual gland that are observed in a section with the greatest frequency are the intralobular ducts. They are the equivalent of the striated duct of the submandibular and parotid glands but lack the extensive basal infoldings and mitochondrial array that creates the striations. One of the intralobular ducts *(InD)* is evident in this figure (upper right). The area within the *rectangle* includes part of this duct and is shown at higher magnification in Figure 2.

FIGURE 2, sublingual gland, human, H&E ×400. Note that through a fortuitous plane of section the lumen of a mucous acinus *(MA)* (upper right) is seen joining an intercalated duct *(ID)*. The juncture between the acinus and the beginning of the intercalated duct is marked by an *arrowhead*. The intercalated duct is composed of a flattened or low columnar epithelium similar to that seen in the other salivary glands. The intercalated ducts of the sublingual gland are extremely short, however, and thus are usually difficult to find. The intercalated duct seen in this micrograph joins with one or more other intercalated ducts to become the intralobular duct *(InD)*, which is identified by its columnar epithelium and relatively large lumen. The point of transition from intercalated to intralobular duct is not recognizable in the micrograph, however, because the duct wall has only been grazed and the shape of the cells cannot be determined.

Examination of the acini at this higher magnification also reveals the serous demilunes *(SD)*. Note how they form a cap-like addition to the mucous end pieces. The cytologic appearance of the mucous cells *(MC)* and serous cells is essentially the same as that described for the submandibular gland. The area selected for this higher magnification also reveals isolated cell clusters that bear some resemblance to serous acini. It is likely, however, that these cells may actually be mucous cells that either have been cut in a plane parallel to their base and do not include the mucinogen-containing portions of the cell or are in a state of activity where, after depletion of their granules, the production of new mucinogen granules is not yet sufficient to give the characteristic "empty" mucous cell appearance.

An additional important feature of the connective tissue stroma is the presence of numerous lymphocytes and plasma cells. Some of the plasma cells are indicated by the *arrows*. The plasma cells are associated with the production of salivary IgA and are also present in the other salivary glands.

KEY

MA, mucous acinus
MC, mucous cells
ID, intercalated duct
InD, intralobular duct
SD, serous demilune
arrowhead, mucous acinus joining intercalated duct
arrows, plasma cells

PLATE 68

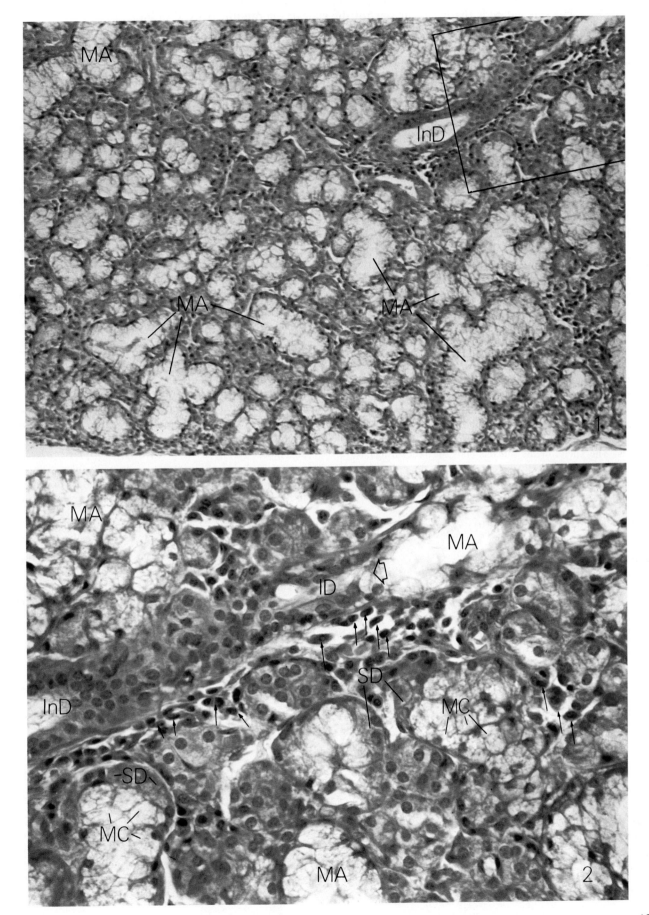

PLATE 69.   Soft Palate

The soft palate is the posterior part of the roof of the mouth. Instead of bone, as in the hard palate, it contains striated muscle between the nasal and oral surfaces. During swallowing, the soft palate separates the nasopharynx from the oropharynx. The oral surface of the soft palate is covered with stratified squamous epithelium. This is also present on the posterior edge and on part of the adjacent "nasal" surface of the soft palate. At some distance from the posterior edge, the stratified squamous epithelium is replaced by pseudostratified ciliated columnar epithelium. At the junction between the two, however, there is a narrow band of stratified columnar epithelium.

Stratified columnar epithelium does not have a wide distribution. It is present where stratified squamous epithelium meets columnar or pseudostratified columnar epithelium as, for example, in large ducts, in the larynx, at the junction of the nasopharynx and oropharynx, on the upper surface of the soft palate, and at the rectoanal junction.

FIGURE 1, soft palate, monkey, H&E ×40.   This figure shows a section through the entire thickness of the soft palate. From top to bottom, the following components can be recognized: the epithelial lining of the nasal surface *(upper Ep)* [a small polyp *(P)* is connected by a stalk to the surface]; the lamina propria *(LP)* of the nasal mucosa; glands *(Gl)*; striated muscle *(StM)*; mucous glands *(MGl)*; lamina propria *(LP)* of the oral mucosa; and epithelial lining of the oral surface *(lower Ep)*.

The muscle of the soft palate is striated. Although striations are not evident at the magnification in this figure, it is possible on the basis of other characteristics (see Plate 72, page 474) to conclude that it is striated and not smooth. Connective tissue is between the muscle bundles.

The oral side of the soft palate contains numerous mucous glands. The nuclei of the mucous cells are pressed against the basal part of the cell, thereby outlining the mucous alveoli.

FIGURE 2, soft palate, monkey, H&E ×160.   The epithelium *(Ep)* lining the nasal surface consists of ciliated pseudostratified columnar cells. Goblet cells *(GC)* are also present in this layer. The epithelium rests on a thick basement membrane *(BM)*. The lamina propria *(LP)* is loose and cellular. It contains an aggregation of lymphocytes *(Lym)* and mixed seromucous glands. Some of the nuclei of the cells that make up these glands are oval in appearance *(arrows)*, whereas others are flattened against the basal part of the cell. The glands may also invade the muscular layer (see Fig. 1).

FIGURE 3, soft palate, monkey, H&E ×160.   The epithelium on the oral surface of the soft palate is stratified squamous. Numerous connective tissue papillae *(asterisks)* project into the undersurface of the epithelium. The dark staining of the deepest part of the epithelium is, in part, due to the cytoplasmic staining of the basal cells. New cells that will migrate to the surface are produced in this layer. As the cells approach the surface, the nuclei become flattened and oriented in a plane parallel to the surface. The presence of nuclei in the surface cells indicates that the epithelium is not keratinized.

The outlining of the mucous acini is seen more clearly in this figure *(arrowheads)*. A duct *(D)* through which these glands empty their secretions onto the surface is also seen in this figure.

KEY		
BM, basement membrane	**Lym,** lymphocytes	**arrows:** Fig. 2, oval nuclei of serous cells; Fig. 3, lymphocytes in epithelial layer
D, duct	**MGl,** mucous glands	
Ep, epithelium	**P,** polyp	
GC, goblet cells	**StM,** striated muscle	**asterisks,** connective tissue papillae
Gl, glands	**arrowheads,** flat nuclei of mucous cells	
LP, lamina propria		

PLATE 69

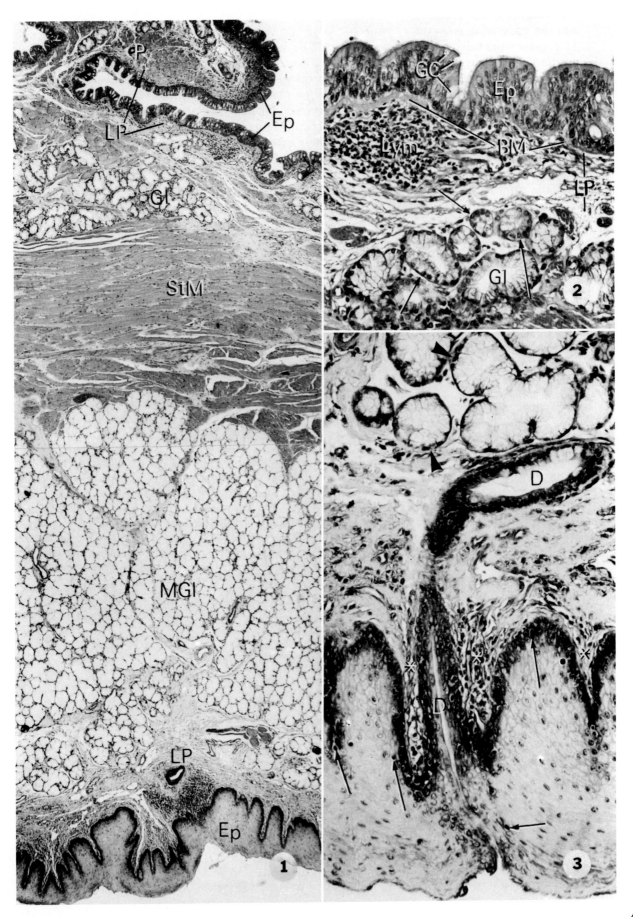

PLATE 70. Developing Tooth

During early fetal development, a plate of epithelium called the dental lamina grows into the underlying embryonic connective tissue (mesenchyme) from the oral epithelium. At regular intervals, where future teeth will be located, the cells of the dental lamina proliferate and become the enamel organs.

In the early stages of enamel formation (amelogenesis), the ameloblasts secrete an organic matrix. Mineralization of this (as with the dentinal matrix) begins almost immediately. However, in teeth with a thin layer of enamel (e.g., the rat), after the enamel reaches its full thickness, it undergoes maturation. Organic material and water are removed, and the enamel continues to mineralize to a greater extent than occurs anywhere else in the body. During maturation, the ameloblasts (see inset, Fig. 3) acquire the characteristics of absorptive or transport cells. The maturation of enamel is a cyclical event marked by the periodic entry of calcium into the maturing enamel.

FIGURE 1, developing teeth, pig, H&E ×16.   The enamel organ (EO) appears as an expanded cell mass that has been invaginated by a connective tissue papilla, the dental papilla (DP). It is attached to the oral epithelium (Ep) by the dental lamina (DL). The junction between the enamel organ and the dental papilla assumes the shape of the future dentinoenamel junction before dentinogenesis or amelogenesis begins. The mesenchyme that surrounds the enamel organ and dental papilla forms a delicate fibrous sac called the dental sac (DS). This sac along with its contents is called the tooth germ (TG).

FIGURE 2, developing teeth, dog, H&E ×40.   This figure shows a tooth germ in which dentinogenesis and amelogenesis have just begun. The parts of the enamel organ are designated the inner enamel epithelium (A) (called ameloblasts once they begin to form enamel), the stratum intermedium (SI), the stellate reticulum (SR), and the outer enamel epithelium (OEE). The dental papilla (DP) will become the future pulp cavity. At the periphery of the dental papilla are the columnar-shaped odontoblasts (O) that produce dentin (D). The enamel (E) is deposited by ameloblasts on the surface of the previously formed dentin.

FIGURE 3, developing teeth, rat, toluidine blue ×65; inset ×160.   This figure shows a tooth, stained with toluidine blue, at a later stage of development. The enamel (E) is unstained; however, the ameloblasts (A), dentin (D), and odontoblasts (O) stain intensely. The most recently formed enamel and dentin are at the bottom of the figure. A serial section of this region, stained with H&E, is examined at higher magnification in Figure 4.

FIGURE 4, developing teeth, rat, H&E ×160; inset ×640.   The sequence of events shown here (and in Fig. 2) is as follows: (1) cells of the enamel organ induce mesenchymal cells of the dental papilla to become odontoblasts; (2) the odontoblasts begin to produce dentin; and (3) when the ameloblasts are confronted with the dentin, they deposit enamel on the outer dentinal surface.

In the formation of dentin, an organic matrix containing collagenous fibers is produced by the odontoblasts. This calcifies to become dentin. The immediate product of the odontoblasts is called predentin (Pd) (inset, Fig. 4). It stains less intensely than the dentin. The odontoblastic process is contained in a dental tubule, and both the process and its tubule extend through the entire thickness of the dentin.

KEY

A, ameloblasts
D, dentin
DL, dental lamina
DP, dental papilla
DS, dental sac

E, enamel
EO, enamel organ
Ep, oral epithelium
O, odontoblasts
OEE, outer enamel epithelium

Pd, predentin
SI, stratum intermedium
SR, stellate reticulum
TG, tooth germ

PLATE 70

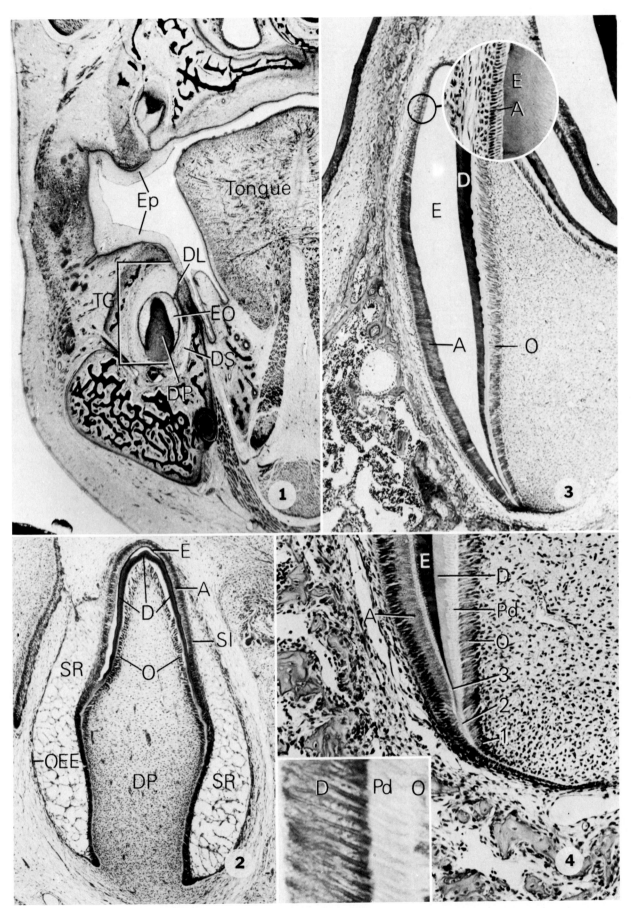

Digestive System II: Esophagus and Gastrointestinal Tract

16

ALIMENTARY CANAL STRUCTURE AND FUNCTIONS

From the esophagus to the rectum, the alimentary canal is a hollow tube of varying diameter. It has the same basic structural organization throughout its length. The wall of the tract is formed by four distinctive layers. From the lumen outward (Fig. 16.1), they are

- *Mucosa,* consisting of a lining epithelium, an underlying connective tissue called the *lamina propria,* and a *muscularis mucosae,* composed of smooth muscle
- *Submucosa,* consisting of dense irregular connective tissue
- *Muscularis externa,* consisting of two layers of muscle
- *Serosa* or *adventitia,* a serous membrane consisting of a simple squamous epithelium, the mesothelium, and a small amount of underlying connective tissue; where the wall is directly attached to adjoining structures, the outer layer is the *adventitia* and is composed of connective tissue

Mucosa

The Mucosa of the Digestive Tract Has Three Principal Functions, a *Barrier* Function, a *Secretory* Function, and an *Absorptive* Function

The epithelium is the barrier that separates the lumen of the digestive tract, which is continuous with the environment, from the body of the organism. It synthesizes and secretes

- *Digestive enzymes* both into the lumen of the alimentary canal and onto the apical plasma membrane of its cells
- *Hormones*
- *Mucus*
- *Antibodies* that it receives from the connective tissue

It selectively absorbs the products of digestion both for its own cells and for transport into the vascular system for distribution to other tissues. The epithelium differs through-

out the alimentary canal, being especially adapted to the specific function of each part of the tube.

The *Lamina Propria* Contains Glands, Vessels That Receive Absorbed Substances, and Elements of the Immune System

In the segments of the digestive tract in which absorption occurs, principally the small and large intestines, the absorbed products of digestion diffuse into the blood and lymphatic vessels of the lamina propria for distribution. Typically, the blood capillaries are of the fenestrated type and receive most of the absorbed metabolites. In addition, in the small intestine, lymphatic capillaries are numerous and receive some absorbed lipids and proteins.

The immunologic barrier consists of

- *Diffuse lymphatic tissue* represented by numerous lymphocytes and plasma cells
- *Lymphatic nodules*
- *Eosinophils* and *macrophages*

Collectively, they function as an integrated system that protects the body against pathogens and other antigens. The diffuse lymphatic tissue and the lymphatic nodules are referred to as *gut-associated lymphatic tissue (GALT).* In the distal small intestine, aggregates of nodules called *Peyer's patches* occupy much of the lamina propria and submucosa on the side of the tube opposite to the attachment of the mesentery. Aggregated lymphatic nodules also occur in the appendix.

The *Muscularis Mucosae* Forms the Boundary Between Mucosa and Submucosa

The *muscularis mucosae,* the deepest portion of the mucosa, consists of smooth muscle cells arranged as an inner circular and an outer longitudinal layer. This muscle can produce movement of the mucosa independent of movement of the entire wall of the digestive tract. It also has a capacity to inhibit invasion of the wall of the intestinal tract by neoplastic cells that arise in the epithelium and invade the lamina propria.

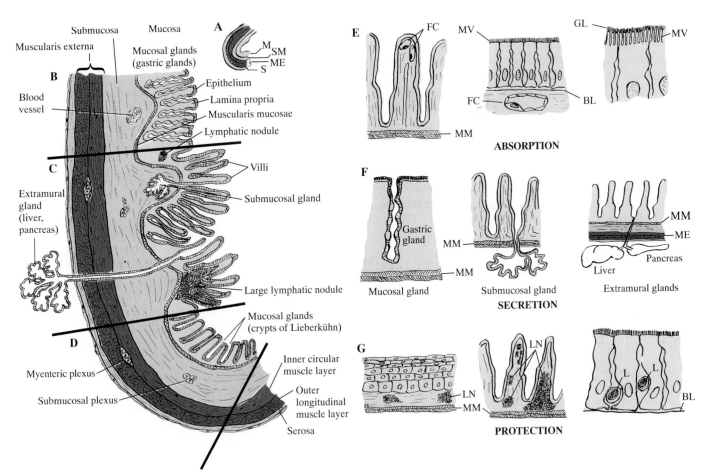

Figure 16.1. **a.** Diagram to show the four layers of the wall of the alimentary canal from the esophagus through the large intestine, namely, the mucosa *(M)*, the submucosa *(SM)*, the muscularis externa *(ME)*, and the serosa *(S)* (or adventitia). **b–d.** This composite diagram shows examples of the stomach **(b),** the small intestine **(c),** and the large intestine (or colon) **(d).** Note that villi, which are characteristic of the small intestine, are not found in any other part of the alimentary canal. Also to be noted are (1) glands in the mucosa, found throughout the tube except sparingly in the esophagus; (2) glands in the submucosa, found in the esophagus and in the proximal part of the small intestine, the duodenum; and (3) extramural glands, which empty only in the duodenum. The **submucosal** (Meissner's) and the **myenteric** (Auerbach's) **plexuses** are nerve plexuses in the submucosa and the muscularis externa, respectively. Large and small **lymphatic nodules** are found in the **lamina propria** throughout the length of the tube. The nerves, bloods vessels, and lymphatic vessels reach the digestive tube via the mesentery or similar sheets of peritoneum (not shown in diagram). Where adventitia is present instead of a serosa, however, vessels and nerves reach the wall of the digestive tube from the adjacent connective tissue. **e–g.** The right-hand side of the figure shows examples of morphologic specialization in the digestive tube and its associated structures related to its major functions. **e.** In areas particularly engaged in ***absorption*** (the small intestine, large in-testine, and gallbladder), there are several morphologic levels at which surface area is increased. Gross submucosal folds (plicae circulares, valves of Kerckring) are indicated in **c. Villi** (mucosal folds) project into the lumen and are covered with absorptive cells whose apical membrane is covered with microvilli *(MV),* i.e., projections from the apical plasma membrane. The microvilli, in turn, are covered with a glycocalyx *(GL),* i.e., glycoproteins that extend from the outer leaflet of the plasma membrane and include many of the terminal digestive enzymes. Note that absorptive fenestrated capillaries *(FC)* immediately underlie the absorptive epithelium. **f.** Portions of the tube engaged in ***secretion,*** namely, the stomach, the proximal duodenum, and the portion of the duodenum that receives the hepatic and pancreatic secretions, are characterized by development of secretory glands that descend into the mucosa **(gastric glands),** into the submucosa [**submucosal glands** (Brunner's glands)], and even through the wall of the alimentary canal to form the **extramural digestive glands, i.e., the liver and pancreas. g.** The ***protective*** function of the alimentary tube is demonstrated by the stratified squamous epithelium of the esophagus, which provides physical protection against abrasion, and by the presence throughout the length of the tube of lymphatic nodules *(LN)* in the lamina propria and of intraepithelial lymphocytes *(L).* These constitute an immunologic barrier that is called the gut-associated lymphatic tissue. *BL,* basal lamina; and *MM,* muscularis mucosae.

Submucosa

The *submucosa* consists of moderately dense, irregular connective tissue. It contains the larger blood vessels that send branches to the mucosa, to the muscularis externa, and to the serosa. The submucosa also contains lymphatic vessels and nerve plexuses. The nerve networks consist of sensory fibers and both parasympathetic and sympathetic fibers of the autonomic nervous system, as well as the motor fibers of the enteric division of the autonomic nervous system that innervate the smooth muscle layers. Interspersed throughout the nerve networks are cell bodies (ganglion cells) of postganglionic parasympathetic neurons and of the enteric neurons. The submucosal network of unmyelinated nerve fibers and ganglion cells constitute the *submucosal plexus (Meissner's plexus).*

Glands occur in the submucosa in certain locations. For example, they are present in the esophagus and the initial portion of the duodenum. The presence of these glands, when observed in a histologic section, often aids in identifying the specific segment or region of the tract.

Muscularis Externa

In most parts of the digestive tract, the *muscularis externa* consists of two concentric and relatively thick layers of smooth muscle. The cells in the inner layer form a tight spiral that is described as a *circularly oriented* layer; those in the outer layer form a very loose spiral that is described as a *longitudinally oriented* layer.

Contractions of the *Muscularis Externa* Mix and Propel the Luminal Contents of the Digestive Tract

Contraction of the inner, circular layer compresses and mixes the contents by constricting the lumen; contraction of the outer, longitudinal layer propels the contents by shortening the tube. The slow rhythmic contraction of these muscle layers under the control of the enteric nervous system produces *peristalsis,* i.e., waves of contraction that move the luminal contents along the intestinal tract.

A few sites along the digestive tube exhibit variation in the nature or organization of the muscularis externa. For example, in the wall of the proximal portion of the esophagus and at the anal sphincter, striated muscle forms the muscularis externa. In the stomach, a third, obliquely oriented layer of the smooth muscle is described internal to the circular layer. Finally, in the large intestine, part of the longitudinal smooth muscle layer is thickened to form three distinct equally spaced longitudinal bands called *teniae coli.* On contraction, the teniae further facilitate the shortening of the tube to move its contents. Between the two muscle layers there is a thin connective tissue layer. In this connective tissue lies the *myenteric plexus (Auerbach's plexus)* of the enteric division of the autonomic nervous system, as well as blood vessels and lymphatic vessels.

The Circular Muscle Layer Forms Sphincters Along the Digestive Tract

At several points along the digestive tract the circular muscle layer is thickened to form sphincters or valves. From the oropharynx distally, these consist of

- *Pharyngoesophageal sphincter,* actually the lowest part of the cricopharyngeus muscle
- *Pyloric sphincter* (gastroduodenal sphincter)
- *Ileocecal valve* (the junction of the small and large intestine)
- *Internal anal sphincter*

Serosa and Adventitia

The *serosa* is a serous membrane consisting of a layer of simple squamous epithelium, the *mesothelium,* and a small amount of underlying connective tissue. It is equivalent to the visceral peritoneum of gross anatomy. The serosa is the most superficial layer of those portions of the digestive tract that are suspended in the peritoneal cavity and, as such, is continuous with the *mesentery* by which they are suspended and with the lining of the abdominal cavity.

Large blood vessels and lymphatic vessels and nerve trunks travel through the *serosa* (from and to the mesentery) to reach the wall of the digestive tract. Large amounts of adipose tissue can develop in the connective tissue of the serosa (and in the mesentery).

The portions of the digestive tract that do not possess a serosa, i.e., the esophagus or the portions of those structures in the abdominal cavity that are fixed to the wall of the cavity—the duodenum, ascending colon, and descending colon, respectively—are attached by a loose connective tissue, the *adventitia.* The adventitia blends with the general connective tissue of adjoining structures.

Secretion

The digestive tube contains numerous glands that provide lubricating mucus, enzymes, water, and other substances that assist digestion (Fig. 16.1). These develop as invaginations of the luminal epithelium to form

- *Mucosal glands* that extend into the lamina propria
- *Submucosal glands* that deliver their secretions to the lumen of mucosal glands or, by ducts that pass through the mucosa, to the luminal surface
- *Extramural glands* that lie outside the digestive tract and deliver their secretions by ducts that pass through the wall of the intestine to the luminal surface

The mucosal glands and submucosal glands are described below in relation to specific regions of the digestive tube. The liver and the pancreas, the extramural digestive glands (covered in Chapter 17), greatly increase the secretory capacity of the digestive system. They deliver their secretions into the duodenum, the first part of the small intestine.

Absorption

Projections of the Mucosa and of the Submucosa Into the Lumen of the Digestive Tract Increase the Surface Available for Absorption

Surface projections are of various sizes and orientation. They consist of the following structural specializations (Fig. 16.1):

- *Rugae* are longitudinally oriented mucosal and submucosal folds in the stomach.
- *Plicae circulares* are circumferentially oriented submucosal folds present along most of the length of the small intestine.
- *Villi* are mucosal projections that cover the entire surface of the small intestine, the principal site of absorption of the products of digestion.
- *Microvilli* are tightly packed microscopic projections of the apical surface of absorptive cells in the intestine.

They further increase the surface available to absorption.

- The *glycocalyx* consists of glycoproteins that project from the apical plasma membrane of the epithelial absorptive cells. It provides additional surface for adsorption and includes enzymes secreted by the absorptive cells that are essential for the final steps of digestion of proteins and sugars.

ESOPHAGUS

The *Esophagus* Is a Muscular Tube That Delivers Food and Liquid From the Oropharynx to the Stomach

In humans, the esophagus (Fig. 16.2) is about 25 cm long and is lined throughout its length with a nonkeratinized stratified squamous epithelium. In many animals, however, the epithelium is keratinized, a reflection of a coarse food diet. In humans, the surface cells may exhibit some keratohyalin granules, but keratinization does not normally occur. The underlying lamina propria is not unique; diffuse lymphatic tissue is scattered throughout, and lymphatic

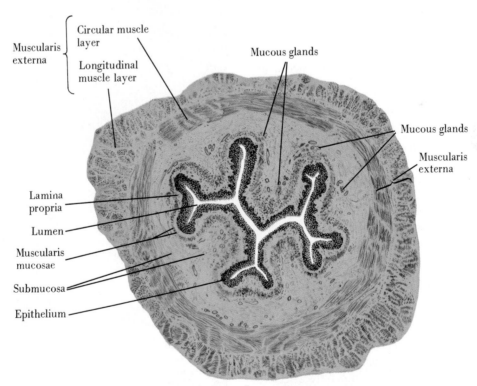

Figure 16.2. Diagram of esophagus in cross section. The esophagus is characteristically collapsed, giving the lumen its branched appearance. The muscularis mucosae is relatively thick, thereby readily marking the extent of the mucosa. Mucous glands are in the submucosa; their ducts, which empty into the lumen of the esophagus, have not been included in the plane of section. Even at this relatively low magnification, it is possible to distinguish the circularly arranged muscle fibers from those that are longitudinally disposed (and, therefore, seen in cross section). The adventitia is not included in the illustration; it is the connective tissue just external to the outer muscle layer. (After Sobotta. In: Bloom W, Fawcett DW: *A Textbook of Histology,* 10th ed. Philadelphia, WB Saunders, 1975, p 640.)

nodules are present, often in proximity to ducts of the esophageal mucous glands (described below). The deep layer of the mucosa, the muscularis mucosae, is composed of longitudinally organized smooth muscle that begins near the level of the cricoid cartilage. It is unusually thick in the proximal portion of the esophagus, presumably functioning as an aid in swallowing.

The *submucosa* along with the muscularis mucosae forms a number of longitudinal folds and creates a highly irregular luminal profile when viewed in cross section. As a bolus of food passes down the esophagus, the folds flatten out, resulting in a localized dilation of the lumen.

The *muscularis externa*, as previously noted, differs from that of the rest of the digestive tract in that the upper one-third is striated muscle, a continuation of the muscle of the oropharynx. Striated muscle and smooth muscle are interwoven in the muscularis externa of the middle third of the esophagus; the muscularis externa of the distal third consists of smooth muscle as in the rest of the digestive tract.

The esophagus is fixed to adjoining structures throughout its length in the thoracic cavity; thus, its outer layer is composed of *adventitia*. After entering the abdominal cavity, the short remainder of the tube is covered by *serosa*.

Glands of the Esophagus

Glands are present in the wall of the esophagus and are of two types. Both are mucus secreting, but their locations differ.

- *Esophageal glands proper* occur in the submucosa and are scattered along the length of the esophagus but are somewhat more concentrated in the upper half. They are small compound tubuloalveolar glands. The excretory duct composed of stratified squamous epithelium is usually conspicuous when present in a section because of its dilated appearance.
- *Esophageal cardiac glands* (so named because of their similarity to the cardiac glands of the stomach) occur in the lamina propria of the mucosa. They are present in the terminal part of the esophagus and frequently, though not consistently, in the beginning portion of the esophagus.

The mucus produced by the esophageal glands proper is slightly acid and serves to lubricate the lumen. Because the secretion is relatively viscous, transient cysts often occur in the ducts. The esophageal cardiac glands produce a neutral mucus. Those glands near the stomach tend to protect the esophagus from regurgitated gastric contents. Under certain conditions, however, they are not fully effective, and excessive reflux results in *pyrosis,* a condition more commonly known as *heartburn.*

Innervation of the Esophagus

The striated musculature in the upper part of the esophagus is innervated by somatic motor neurons of the *vagus*

nerve, cranial nerve X (from the nucleus ambiguus), without synaptic interruption. The smooth muscle of the lower part is innervated by visceral motor neurons of the vagus (from the dorsal motor nucleus) that synapse with postganglionic neurons whose cell bodies are in the wall of the esophagus.

STOMACH

The stomach is an expanded part of the digestive tube that lies under the diaphragm. It receives the bolus of macerated food from the esophagus. Mixing and partial digestion of the food in the stomach by its gastric secretions produces a pulpy fluid mix called *chyme.* The chyme is then passed into the intestine for further digestion and absorption.

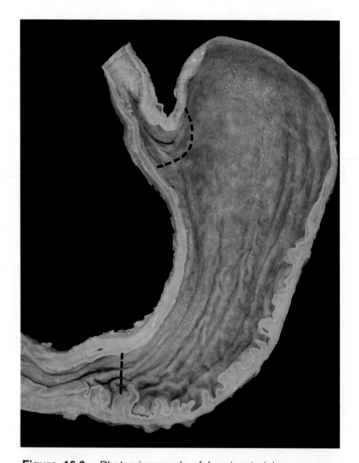

Figure 16.3. Photomicrograph of hemisected human stomach showing the mucosal surface of the posterior wall. Numerous longitudinal folds are evident. These folds or rugae allow the stomach to distend as it fills. The portion of the stomach adjacent to the entrance of the esophagus is the cardiac region in which the cardiac glands are located. A *dashed line* approximates the boundary. A slightly larger region leading toward the pyloric sphincter, the pyloric region, contains the pyloric glands. A *dashed line* approximates its boundary. The remainder of the stomach, the region between the two *dashed lines,* contains the fundic, or gastric, glands. Histologically, this region is designated the fundic region of the stomach.

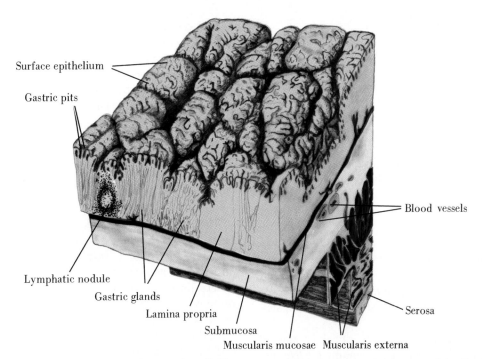

Surface epithelium

Gastric pits

Blood vessels

Lymphatic nodule

Gastric glands

Lamina propria

Submucosa

Muscularis mucosae   Muscularis externa

Serosa

Figure 16.4. Three-dimensional diagram of stomach wall. The elevated areas of the mucosa are referred to as mamillated areas. Tubular depressions from the surface constitute the gastric pits; gastric glands open into the bottom of the pits. Note the lymphatic nodule in the mucosa. (Based on Braus H: *Anatomie der Menschen.* Berlin, Springer, 1924, p 645.)

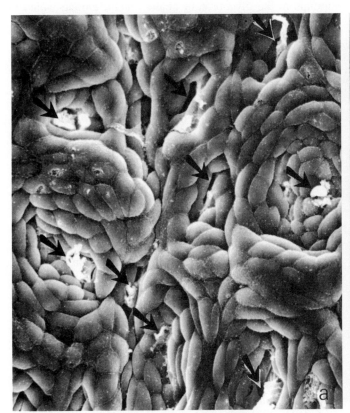

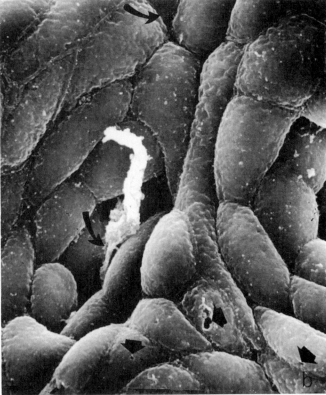

Figure 16.5.   a. Scanning electron micrograph showing the mucosal surface of the stomach. The gastric pits contain secretory material, mostly mucus *(arrows)*. The surface mucus has been washed away to reveal the surface mucous cells. ×1000. **b.** Higher magnification showing the apical surface of the surface mucous cells that line the stomach and the gastric pits. Note the elongate polygonal shape of the cells. The site of the junctional complex between adjoining cells can be seen at some locations *(arrows)*. ×3000.

Structural Organization

The stomach has the same general structural plan throughout, consisting of a mucosa, submucosa, muscularis externa, and a serosa.

Examination of the inner surface of the empty stomach reveals a number of longitudinal folds or ridges called *rugae.* They are prominent in the narrower regions of the stomach but poorly developed in the upper portion (Fig. 16.3). When the stomach is fully distended, the rugae, composed of the mucosa and underlying submucosa, virtually disappear. The rugae do not alter total surface area but, rather, serve as a device to accommodate expansion and filling of the stomach.

A view of the stomach's surface with a hand lens shows that smaller regions of the mucosa are formed by grooves or shallow trenches that divide the stomach surface into bulging irregular areas called *mamillated areas* (Fig. 16.4). In this case the grooves provide some slight increase in surface area for secretion.

At a higher magnification, numerous openings can be observed in the mucosal surface. These are the *gastric pits* or *foveolae.* They can be readily demonstrated with the scanning electron microscope (SEM) (Fig. 16.5, *a* and *b*). The gastric glands empty into the bottom of the gastric pits.

Histologically, the stomach is divided into three distinct parts, with each being designated by the nature of the glands that are present (see Fig. 16.3):

- The *cardia (cardiac region),* the part near the esophageal orifice, contains the *cardiac glands.*
- The *pylorus (pyloric region),* the part proximal to the pyloric sphincter, contains the *pyloric glands.*
- The *fundus (fundic region),* sometimes called the body, the largest part of the stomach, is situated between the cardia and pylorus and contains the *fundic* or *gastric glands.*

Gross anatomists subdivide the body of the stomach into two regions. The fundic region is that part that lies above the level of a horizontal line drawn through the esophageal orifice. The body is that part that lies below this line; the pylorus is simply the distal narrow portion.

Gastric Secretions

The glands of the stomach secrete nearly 2 liters of fluid each day. In addition to water and electrolytes, the gastric secretions include

- *Pepsinogen,* an inactive precursor of the proteolytic enzyme, *pepsin*
- *Hydrochloric acid* (0.16 N HCl), which gives the gastric juice a low pH that promotes acid hydrolysis of substrates and converts pepsinogen to pepsin
- *Intrinsic factor,* a glycoprotein that is essential for the absorption of *vitamin B_{12}* in more distal portions of the digestive tract

In addition, the hormone *gastrin* and other hormones and hormone-like secretions are produced by *enteroendocrine* cells in the gastric epithelium.

The lining of the stomach does not function in an absorptive capacity. However, some water, salts, and lipid-soluble drugs may be absorbed; alcohol and certain drugs, e.g., aspirin, enter the lamina propria by damaging the surface epithelium.

Gastric Mucosa

Surface Mucous Cells Line the Stomach and Gastric Pits

The epithelium that lines the surface and the gastric pits of the stomach is simple columnar. These columnar cells are designated *surface mucous cells.* Each cell possesses a large apical cup of mucinogen granules, thereby creating an epithelial surface that is a glandular sheet of cells (Fig. 16.6 and Plate 74, Fig. 2, page 479). The mucous cup occupies most of the volume of the cell. It typically appears empty in routine hematoxylin and eosin (H&E) sections because the mucinogen is lost in fixation and dehydration. When the mucin is preserved by appropriate fixation, however, the secretion droplets in these cells stain intensely with toluidine blue and with the periodic acid-Schiff (PAS) procedure. The toluidine blue staining reflects the presence of many strongly anionic groups in the glycoprotein of the mucin, among which is bicarbonate ion.

The nucleus and Golgi apparatus of the surface mucous cells are located below the mucous cup. The basal part of the cell contains small amounts of rough endoplasmic reticulum (rER) that may impart a light basophilia to the cytoplasm when observed in well-preserved specimens.

The mucus secretion is described as a *visible mucus* because of its cloudy appearance. It forms a thick viscous, gel-like coat that adheres to the epithelial surface; thus, it provides protection against abrasion from rougher components of the chyme. Additionally, it provides protection to the epithelium from the acid content of the gastric juice by virtue of its high bicarbonate concentration. The bicarbonate that makes the mucus alkaline is secreted by the surface cells but is prevented from mixing rapidly with the contents of the gastric lumen by its containment within the mucus coat.

Fundic Glands of the Gastric Mucosa

Fundic Glands Produce the Digestive Juice of the Stomach

The *fundic glands,* also referred to as *gastric glands,* are present throughout the entire gastric mucosa except for the relatively small regions occupied by the cardiac and pyloric glands. They are simple, branched tubular glands that extend from the bottom of the gastric pits to the muscularis mucosae. Typically, several glands open into a single gastric pit.

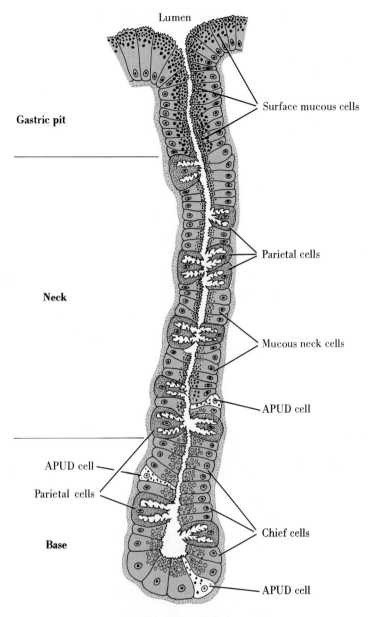

Lumen

Gastric pit

Surface mucous cells

Neck

Parietal cells

Mucous neck cells

APUD cell

APUD cell

Parietal cells

Base

Chief cells

APUD cell

GASTRIC GLAND

Figure 16.6. Diagram of a gastric gland, illustrating the relationship of the gland to the gastric pit. The neck region contains mucous neck cells, parietal cells, and enteroendocrine [amine precursor uptake and decarboxylation (APUD)] cells. Undifferentiated cells (not illustrated) are located in the upper portion of the neck region. The base (or fundus) region contains parietal cells, chief cells, and several different types of enteroendocrine cells. (Based on Ito S, Winchester RJ: The fine structure of the gastric mucosa of the bat. *The Journal of Cell Biology* 16:543, 1963, by copyright permission of The Rockefeller University Press.)

Each gland has a narrow, relatively long **neck segment** and a shorter and wider **base** or **fundic segment.** The base of the gland usually divides into two and, sometimes, three branches that become slightly coiled near the muscularis mucosae.

Fundic Glands Are Composed of Four Functionally Different Cell Types

The cells that constitute the fundic glands are of four functional cell types. Each has a distinctive appearance. In addition, undifferentiated cells that give rise to these cells are also present. Thus, the various cells that can be regarded as constituting the gland are

- *Mucous neck cells*
- *Chief cells*
- *Parietal cells,* also called oxyntic cells
- *Enteroendocrine cells*
- *Undifferentiated cells* present in the upper neck region of the gland that give rise to the mature cells listed

Mucous Neck Cells Are Localized in the Neck Region, Interspersed With Parietal Cells

The *mucous neck cells,* as the name implies, are located in the neck region of the gland. Parietal cells are usually found interspersed between groups of these cells. Compared with the surface mucous cell, the mucous neck cell is much shorter, and the amount of mucinogen in the apical cytoplasm is considerably less. Consequently, these cells do not exhibit a prominent mucous cup. Also, the nucleus tends to be spherical compared with the more prominent, elongate nucleus of the surface mucous cell.

The cell secretes a *soluble mucus* compared with the *insoluble* or *cloudy mucus* produced by the surface mucous cell. Release of the mucinogen granules is effected by vagal stimulation; thus, the secretion from these cells is not present in the resting stomach.

Chief Cells Are Located in the Deepest Part of the Fundic Glands

Chief cells are typical protein-secreting cells (Fig. 16.7). The rER in their basal cytoplasm and the secretory granules in their apical pole account for the basophilia and acidophilia, respectively, of these parts of the cell. The basophilia, in particular, allows for easy identification of these cells in H&E sections. The acidophilia may be weak, however, because the secretory granules are not always adequately preserved. Chief cells secrete *pepsin* in an inactive precursor form designated *pepsinogen* and a weak lipase. On contact with the acid of the gastric juice, the pepsinogen is converted to pepsin, a proteolytic enzyme.

Parietal Cells Secrete HCl and Intrinsic Factor

Parietal (oxyntic) cells are found in the neck of the fundic glands, among the mucous neck cells, and in the deeper parts of the gland. They tend to be most numerous in the upper and middle portions. They are large cells, sometimes binucleate, and appear somewhat triangular in sections, with the apex directed toward the lumen of the gland and the base resting on the basal lamina. The nucleus is spherical, and the cytoplasm stains intensely with eosin and other acid dyes. Their size and distinctive staining characteristic enable the parietal cells to be distinguished easily from other cells in the fundic glands.

When examined with the transmission electron microscope (TEM), parietal cells (Fig. 16.8) are seen to have an extensive *intracellular canalicular system* that communicates with the lumen of the gland. Numerous microvilli project from the surface of the canaliculi, and an elaborate *tubulovesicular membrane system* is present in the cytoplasm adjacent to the canaliculi. Numerous mitochondria with complex cristae and many matrix granules are also evident, indicating that acid secretion requires high levels of energy.

HCl Secretion Is Stimulated by Gastrin

Gastrin, one of the gastrointestinal polypeptide hormones, is the principal effective agent for stimulating the

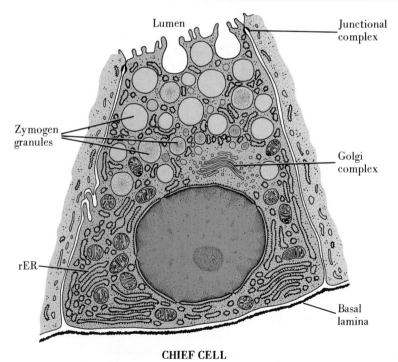

CHIEF CELL

Figure 16.7. Diagram of a chief cell. This cell produces the enzymes of the gastric secretion. The large amount of rER in the basal portion of the cell accounts for the intense basophilic staining seen in this region. Zymogen granules are not always adequately preserved, and thus, the staining in the apical region of the cell is somewhat variable. (Based on Lentz TL: *Cell Fine Structure.* Philadelphia, WB Saunders, 1971, p 165.)

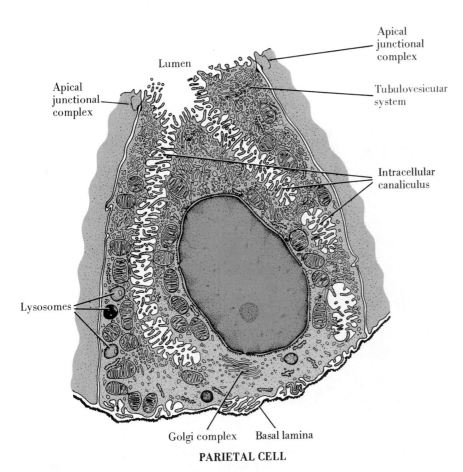

Apical junctional complex

Lumen

Apical junctional complex

Tubulovesicular system

Intracellular canaliculus

Lysosomes

Golgi complex   Basal lamina

PARIETAL CELL

Figure 16.8. Diagram of a parietal cell. The cytoplasm of this cell stains intensely with eosin as a result of the extensive amount of membrane comprising the intracellular canaliculus, tubulovesicular system (tubular endoplasmic reticulum), and mitochondria and of the relatively small number of ribosomes. This cell produces the hydrochloric acid of gastric secretion. (Based on Lentz TL: *Cell Fine Structure*. Philadelphia, WB Saunders, 1971, p 171.)

secretion of HCl. (Histamine and acetylcholine also stimulate HCl secretion.) It is secreted by an enteroendocrine cell (discussed below) within the stomach glands. Receptors for gastrin are present in the parietal cell membrane.

Secretion of HCl occurs across the membranes of the canaliculi and their microvillous extensions, driven by the activity of a Cl⁻-specific ATPase (a chloride pump). In an actively secreting cell, the number of microvilli in the canaliculi increases, and the tubulovesicular system is significantly reduced or disappears. The membranes of the tubulovesicular system are believed to be a reserve that can be inserted into the plasma membrane to increase the surface available for secretion.

In humans, *intrinsic factor* is secreted by the parietal cells (chief cells do so in some other species). Intrinsic factor is a glycoprotein that complexes with vitamin B_{12} in the stomach, a step necessary for subsequent absorption of the vitamin in the ileum.

PERNICIOUS ANEMIA AND ULCER DISEASE

In achlorhydria, a condition characterized by the absence of parietal cells, intrinsic factor is not secreted, thereby leading to **pernicious anemia.** Because the liver has extensive reserve stores of vitamin B_{12}, the disease is often not recognized until long after significant changes in the gastric mucosa take place.

A more common cause of reduced secretion of intrinsic factor and subsequent pernicious anemia is the loss of gastric epithelium due to gastric ulcers. Often, even the healed ulcerated region produces insufficient intrinsic factor. Repeated loss of epithelium and consequent scarring of the gastric mucosa can reduce the amount of functional mucosa significantly.

The use of antiulcer drugs (Zantac and Tagamet), which block attachment of histamine to its receptors in the gastric mucosa, suppress acid production, thereby preventing further mucosal erosion and promoting healing of a previously eroded surface.

Although it has generally been thought that the parietal cells are the direct target of the antiulcer drugs, recent evidence utilizing a combination of in situ hybridization histochemistry and staining with antibodies has unexpectedly revealed that the immunoglobulin A (IgA)-secreting plasma cells and some of the macrophages in the lamina propria displayed a positive reaction for gastrin receptor mRNA, not the parietal cells. These findings indicate that the agents used to treat ulcer disease may act directly on immunocytes (plasma cell and/or macrophage) and then secondarily these cells transmit their effects to the parietal cells to inhibit HCl secretion. The factor that mediates the interaction between the connective tissue cells and the epithelial cells has not been elucidated. These findings relating to the immune system are of particular interest in light of mounting evidence that the majority of common peptic ulcers are actually caused by a chronic infection of the gastric mucosa with the bacterium, **Helicobacterium pylori.**

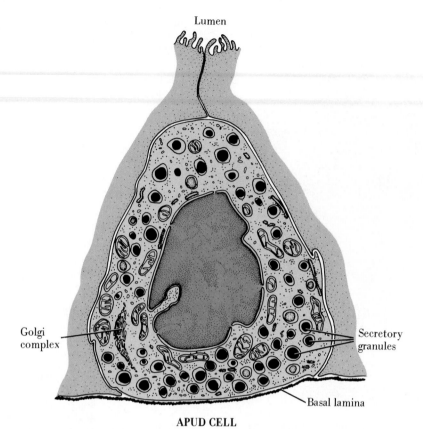

APUD CELL

Figure 16.9. Diagram of an enteroendocrine (APUD) cell. This cell is drawn to show that it does not reach the epithelial surface. The secretory granules are regularly lost during the preparation of paraffin sections, and in the absence of other distinctive stainable organelles, the cell has more or less the appearance of a "clear cell;" i.e., the nucleus appears to be surrounded by a small amount of clear cytoplasm in H&E-stained sections. (Based on Ito S, Winchester RJ: The fine structure of the gastric mucosa of the bat. *The Journal of Cell Biology* 16:574, 1963, by copyright permission of The Rockefeller University Press.)

Enteroendocrine Cells Secrete Their Product Into the Lamina Propria

Enteroendocrine cells may be found at any level of the fundic gland, though they tend to be somewhat more prevalent in the base. They are small cells that rest on the basal lamina and do not always reach the lumen (Fig. 16.9). Some, however, have a thin cytoplasmic extension bearing microvilli that are exposed to the gland lumen. It is thought that these cells sample the contents of the gland lumen and release their hormones based on their sensing response.

Electron micrographs reveal small membrane-bounded secretory granules throughout the cytoplasm; however, the granules are typically lost in H&E preparations, and the cytoplasm appears clear due to the lack of sufficient stainable material. Although these cells are often difficult to identify because of their small size and lack of distinctive staining, the clear cytoplasm of the cell will sometimes stand out in contrast to adjacent chief or parietal cells, thus allowing them to be recognized more easily.

Cardiac Glands of the Gastric Mucosa

The cardiac glands are limited to a narrow region of the stomach (the cardia) surrounding the esophageal orifice. Their secretion, in combination with that of the esophageal cardiac glands, contributes to the gastric juice and also helps protect the esophageal epithelium against gastric reflux. The glands are tubular, somewhat tortuous, and occasionally branched. They are composed mainly of mucus-secreting cells, with occasional interspersed enteroendocrine cells. The mucus-secreting cells are similar in appearance to the cells of the cardiac glands of the esophagus. They have a flattened basal nucleus, and the apical cytoplasm is typically filled with mucin granules. A short duct segment containing columnar cells with elongate nuclei is interposed between the secretory portion of the gland and the shallow pits into which the glands secrete. The duct segment is the site in which the surface mucous cells and the gland cells are produced. The secretory product enters the gastric pits, which are relatively shallow in this part of the stomach.

ENTEROENDOCRINE CELLS ARE COMMON TO THE
EPITHELIUM OF THE DIGESTIVE TRACT

Enteroendocrine cells are present in most of the digestive
tract, including the ducts of the pancreas and liver, and in
the respiratory system, another endodermal derivative that
originates by invagination of the epithelium of the embryonic
foregut. The endocrine islets (of Langerhans) of the pancreas can be considered specialized accumulations of enteroendocrine cells derived from pancreatic buds that also
arise from the embryonic foregut. It has been estimated that
the enteroendocrine cells collectively would constitute the
largest endocrine "organ" in the body. These cells have also
been called **gastroenteropancreatic (GEP) endocrine cells**
and closely resemble neurosecretory cells of the central nervous system that secrete many of the same hormones and
regulatory agents. For that reason, they are also described
as constituting part of a **diffuse neuroendocrine system.**

Some enteroendocrine cells may be classifiable *functionally* as amine precursor uptake and decarboxylation (APUD)
cells because they produce biogenic amines and have

the appropriate enzyme systems. They should not, however,
be confused with the APUD cells that derive from the embryonic neural crest and migrate to other sites in the body.
Enteroendocrine cells differentiate from the progeny of the
same stem cells as do **all** of the other epithelial cells of the
digestive tract. (The fact that two different cells may produce
similar products should not be misinterpreted to imply that
they have the same origin.)

The names given to the enteroendocrine cells in the older
literature were based on their staining with salts of silver and
chromium, i.e., **enterochromaffin cells, argentaffin cells,**
and **argyrophil cells.** Such cells are currently identified and
characterized by immunochemical staining for the more than
20 peptide and polypeptide hormones and hormone-like regulating agents that they secrete (a listing of many of these
agents and their actions is provided in Tables 16.1 and 16.2
and in Fig. 16.18). With the aid of the TEM, at least 17 different types of enteroendocrine cells have been described
on the basis of the size, shape, and density of their secretory granules.

TABLE 16.1. Physiologic Actions of Gastrointestinal Hormones[A]

ACTION	HORMONES[B]			
	GASTRIN	CHOLECYSTOKININ (CCK)	SECRETIN	GASTRIC INHIBITORY PEPTIDE (GIP)
Acid secretion	S			I
Pancreatic bicarbonate ion secretion		S	S	
Pancreatic enzyme secretion		S	S	
Bile bicarbonate ion secretion		S	S	
Gallbladder contraction		S		
Gastric emptying		I		
Insulin release				S
Mucosal growth		S		
Pancreatic growth	S	S	S	

[A]Adapted from Johnson LR (ed): *Gastrointestinal Physiology,* 4th ed. St Louis, CV Mosby, 1991, p 8.
[B]S, stimulates; I, inhibits; blank spaces, not yet tested.

Pyloric Glands of the Gastric Mucosa

Pyloric glands are located in the pyloric antrum (the part
of the stomach between the fundus and the pylorus) and the
pylorus. They are branched, tubular glands that are coiled.
The lumen is relatively wide, and the secretory cells are
very similar in appearance to the surface mucous cells, suggesting a relatively viscous secretion. Enteroendocrine cells
are found interspersed within the gland epithelium along
with occasional parietal cells. The glands empty into deep
gastric pits that occupy about half of the thickness of the
mucosa.

Epithelial Cell Renewal in the Stomach

Surface Mucous Cells Are Renewed Approximately Every 3–5 Days

The relatively short life span of the surface mucous cells,
3–5 days, is accommodated by mitotic activity in the depth
of the pits and in the immediate neck region of the gastric
glands to provide continuous renewal. Most of the newly
produced cells at this site become surface mucous cells.
They migrate upward along the wall of the pit to the lu-

minal surface of the stomach and are ultimately shed into the stomach lumen.

Cells of the Gastric Glands Are Renewed Approximately Once a Year

Other cells from the mucous neck migrate down into the gastric glands to give rise to the parietal cells, chief cells, and enteroendocrine cells that constitute the gland epithelium. These cells have a relatively long life span. They are estimated to live for about a year before they are replaced by new cells migrating downward from the mucous neck.

Lamina Propria and Muscularis Mucosae

The *lamina propria* of the stomach is relatively scant, being restricted to the very limited spaces surrounding the gastric pits and glands. The stroma is composed largely of reticular fibers with associated fibroblasts and smooth muscle cells. Other components consist of cells of the immune system, namely, lymphocytes, plasma cells, macrophages, and some eosinophils. When inflammatory conditions exist, as is often the case, neutrophils may also be prominent. Occasional lymphatic nodules are also present, usually in the vicinity of the muscularis mucosae.

The *muscularis mucosae* is composed of two relatively thin layers, usually arranged as an inner circular and outer longitudinal layer. In some regions a third layer may be present; its orientation tends to be in a circular pattern. Strands of smooth muscle cells extend toward the surface in the lamina propria from the inner layer of the muscularis mucosae. These smooth muscle cells in the lamina propria are thought to play a role in facilitating outflow of the gastric gland secretions.

Gastric Submucosa

The submucosa is composed of a dense connective tissue containing variable amounts of adipose tissue, blood vessels, and nerve fibers and ganglion cells that comprise the *submucosal (Meissner's) plexus*. The latter innervates the vessels of the submucosa and the smooth muscle of the muscularis mucosae.

Gastric Muscularis Externa

The *muscularis externa* of the stomach is traditionally described as consisting of an outer longitudinal layer, a middle circular layer, and an inner oblique layer. This description is somewhat misleading, as distinct layers may be difficult to discern. As with other hollow, spheroid-shaped organs (gallbladder, urinary bladder, and uterus), the smooth muscle of the muscularis externa of the stomach is somewhat more randomly oriented than the description of layers would imply. Moreover, the longitudinal layer is absent from much of the anterior and posterior stomach surfaces, and the circular layer is poorly developed in the periesophageal region. The arrangement of the muscle layers is functionally important, as it relates to its role of mixing the chyme during the digestive process as well as to being able to force the partially digested contents into the small intestine. Groups of ganglion cells and bundles of unmyelinated nerve fibers are present between the muscle layers. Collectively, they represent the myenteric (Auerbach's) plexus, which provides innervation of the muscle layers.

Gastric Serosa

The *serosa* of the stomach is as described previously for the alimentary canal in general. It is continuous with the peritoneum of the abdominal cavity via the omentum. Otherwise, it exhibits no special features.

FUNCTIONS OF GASTRIC MUSCULARIS EXTERNA

Three functions of the stomach depend on its musculature:

- To *receive* large volumes of *ingested food and drink* during a meal
- To *mix* the ingested *food with gastric juices* so that digestion can occur
- To *propel* the gastric *contents into* the small *intestine*

In considering gastric motility, the stomach is divided into an **orad portion** (the anatomical fundus and upper half of the body) and a **caudad portion** (the lower half of the body and the pyloric region). The orad region is said to display relatively little motility; it serves to receive the ingested food by a process termed **receptive relaxation**. This is under the control of neural (vagal) and humoral factors.

The caudad region displays peristaltic contractions that move in a caudad direction. The peristaltic wave moves more rapidly than the stomach contents, and the overtaking peristaltic wave mixes and propels the gastric contents. The propulsion is in both an orad and a caudad direction, but mostly in an orad direction. Because most of the gastric contents are propelled in an orad direction by the overtaking peristaltic wave, only a small amount of gastric contents enters the small intestine with each peristaltic wave.

When the stomach fails to empty properly, the individual complains of nausea, loss of appetite, and fullness. The most common cause of impaired emptying is an obstruction near the gastric outlet, as in gastric cancer and ulcer. Emptying of the stomach is regulated by the vagus (cranial) nerve (X). In some patients, surgical section of the vagus nerve may be necessary to provide relief. In performing a surgical section of the vagus nerve, it may be necessary to modify the gastroduodenal junction surgically in order to facilitate gastric emptying.

Surgical sectioning of the vagus nerve is also used to decrease acid secretion in the treatment of patients with gastric ulcers that do not respond to medical treatment. However, it is important to recognize that most duodenal and gastric ulcers are receptive to histamine H_2-receptor antagonists (such as cimetidine), which may block receptors on parietal cells (see shaded text, page 451) and inhibit acid secretion. Stomal ulcers (in the jejunum) are often resistant to medical therapy. Vagotomy or more extensive gastrectomy is often necessary to decrease acid secretion of the stomach in such cases.

TABLE 16.2. Candidate Hormones[A]

CANDIDATE HORMONE	ACTIONS[B]
VIP (vasoactive intestinal peptide)	↓ Gastric secretion ↑ Insulin release ↑ Intestinal secretion ↑ Pancreatic bicarbonate ion secretion ↑ Glycogenolysis
Pancreatic polypeptide	↓ Pancreatic bicarbonate ion and enzyme secretion
Motilin	↑ Gastric motility ↑ Intestinal motility
Enteroglucagon	↑ Glycogenolysis

[A] Adapted from Johnson LR (ed): *Gastrointestinal Physiology*, 4th ed. St Louis, CV Mosby, 1991, p 9.
[B] ↑, stimulates; ↓ inhibits

SMALL INTESTINE

The small intestine is the longest component of the digestive tract, measuring over 6 meters, and is divided into three anatomic segments:

- *Duodenum* (≈25 cm long)
- *Jejunum* (≈2.5 m long)
- *Ileum* (≈3.5 m long)

Functionally, the small intestine is the principal site for the digestion of food and for absorption of the products of digestion. The chyme from the stomach is received by the duodenum, where enzymes from the pancreas and bile from the liver are also delivered in order to continue the solubilization and digestion process. Enzymes located in the glycocalyx of the microvilli of the **enterocytes,** the **intestinal absorptive cells,** particularly disaccharidases and dipeptidases, contribute to the digestive process by completing the breakdown of most sugars and proteins to monosaccharides and amino acids that are then absorbed. Water and electrolytes that reach the small intestine with the chyme and with the pancreatic and hepatic secretions are also reabsorbed in the small intestine, particularly in the distal portion.

Intestinal Lining

Plicae Circulares, Villi, and Microvilli Increase the Absorptive Surface of the Small Intestine

Amplification of the absorptive surface area of the small intestine is accomplished by tissue and cell specializations of the submucosa and mucosa.

- **Plicae circulares,** also known as the valves of Kerckring, are permanent transverse folds that contain a core of submucosa. Each semilunar fold is circularly arranged and extends about one-half to two-thirds around the circumference of the lumen (Fig. 16.10). The plicae begin to appear about 5–6 cm beyond the pylorus. They are most numerous in the distal part of the duodenum and the beginning of the jejunum and become reduced in size and frequency in the middle of the ileum.
- **Villi** are finger-like and leaf-like projections of the mucosa that extend into the intestinal lumen.
- **Microvilli** of the enterocytes provide the major amplification of the luminal surface. Each cell possesses several thousand closely packed microvilli. They are visible in the light microscope and give the apical region of the cell a striated appearance, the so-called **striated border.** The enterocytes, including their microvilli, are described below.

Mucosa

The villi and intestinal glands (crypts of Lieberkühn) along with the lamina propria and associated GALT and mus-

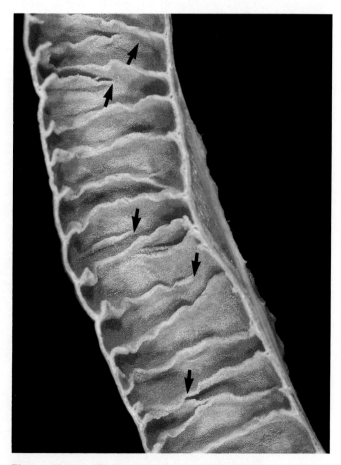

Figure 16.10. Photograph of a longitudinal section of human small intestine showing the mucosal surface. The plicae circulares (valves of Kerckring) appear as a series of transversely oriented ridges that extend partially around the lumen. Consequently, some of the plicae circulares appear to end (or begin) at various sites along the luminal surface *(arrows).* The entire mucosa has a velvety appearance due to the presence of villi.

cularis mucosae constitute the essential features of the small intestinal mucosa.

Villi, as briefly noted, are finger-like and leaf-like projections of the mucosa that extend from the theoretical mucosal surface for 0.5–1.5 mm into the lumen (Figs. 16.1 and 16.11, *a* and *b*). They completely cover the surface of the small intestine, giving it a velvety appearance when viewed with the naked eye. The core of the villus consists of an extension of the lamina propria with a network of fenestrated capillaries located just beneath the epithelial basal lamina. The lamina propria of the villus also contains a central, blind-ending lymphatic capillary, the *lacteal* (Fig. 16.12). Smooth muscle cells derived from the muscularis mucosae extend into the villus and accompany the lacteal. *Myofibroblasts* appear to bridge the diameter of the villus. The presence of these two cell types may account for reports that villi contract and shorten intermittently, an action that may force lymph from the lacteal into the lymphatic vessel network that surrounds the muscularis mucosae.

The *intestinal glands,* or *crypts of Lieberkühn,* are simple tubular structures that extend from the muscularis mucosae through the thickness of the lamina propria, where they open on to the luminal surface of the intestine at the base of the villi (see Fig. 16.11 and Plate 77, page 485). The glands are composed of a simple columnar epithelium

that becomes continuous with the luminal epithelium and the epithelium of the villi.

The *lamina propria,* as in the stomach, surrounds the glands and contains numerous cells of the immune system (lymphocytes, plasma cells, macrophages, and eosinophils), particularly in the villi. The lamina propria also contains numerous nodules of lymphatic tissue that represent a major component of the GALT. The nodules are particularly large and numerous in the ileum, where they are preferentially located on the side of the intestine opposite the mesenteric attachment. These nodular aggregations are given a special name, *aggregated nodules* or *Peyer's patches* (see Plate 79, page 489). In gross specimens, they appear as aggregates of white specks.

The *muscularis mucosae* consists of two thin layers of smooth muscle cells, an inner circular and an outer longitudinal layer. Strands of smooth muscle cells extend from the muscularis mucosae into the lamina propria of the villi.

Cells of the Mucosal Epithelium

The mature cells of the intestinal epithelium are found both in the crypts and on the surface of the villi. They include

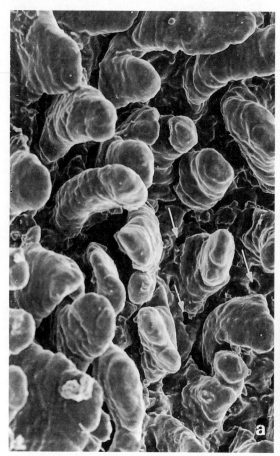
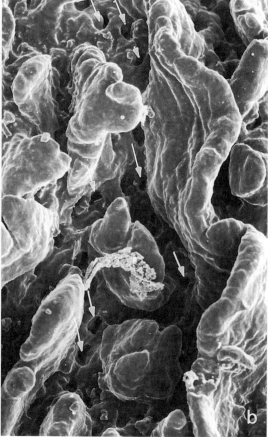

Figure 16.11. Scanning electron micrographs of intestinal villi. In **(a)**, the villi are finger-like. In **(b)**, a prominent leaf-like villus is evident. Between the bases of the villi, openings of the intestinal glands (crypts of Lieberkühn) can be seen in both micrographs *(arrows).*

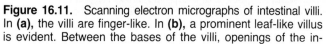

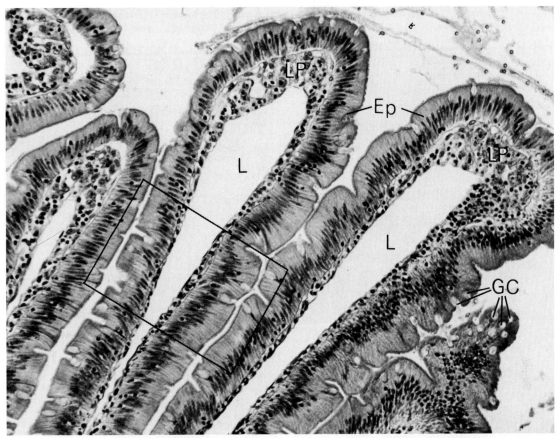

Figure 16.12. Light micrograph of villi. The surface of the villi consists of columnar epithelium *(Ep)*. These are chiefly enterocytes with a striated border. Also evident in the epithelial layer are goblet cells *(GC)*. Under the epithelium is a highly cellular connective tissue called the lamina propria *(LP)*. The center of the villus contains a lymphatic capillary called the lacteal *(L)*. When the lacteals are dilated, as they are in this specimen, they are easily identified. ×160.

- *Enterocytes,* whose primary function is absorption
- *Goblet cells,* unicellular mucin-secreting glands
- *Paneth cells*
- *Enteroendocrine cells*
- *M cells (microfold cells),* a modified enterocyte that covers enlarged lymphatic nodules in the lamina propria

Enterocytes. Enterocytes are specialized for the transport of substances from the lumen of the intestine to the circulatory system. They are tall columnar cells, with a basally positioned nucleus (Figs. 16.12 and 16.13). Microvilli increase the apical surface area as much as 600 times; they are recognized in the light microscope as forming a *striated border* on the luminal surface.

Each microvillus has a core of vertically oriented actin microfilaments that are anchored to the plasma membrane at the tip of the microvillus and that also attach to the plasma membrane of the shaft (Fig. 16.14). The actin microfilaments extend into the apical cytoplasm and insert into the terminal web, a network of horizontally oriented microfilaments that form a layer in the most apical cytoplasm and attach to the intracellular density associated with the zonula adherens. The terminal web contains both actin microfilaments and myosin, and its contractile function may aid in

"closing" the holes left in the epithelial sheet by the exfoliation of aging cells.

Enterocytes are bound to one another and to the goblet, enteroendocrine, and other cells of the epithelium by junctional complexes.

The Junction Establishes a Barrier Between the Lumen and the Intercellular Compartment

Transport mechanisms, "pumps," located in the lateral plasma membrane, especially Na^+-K^+-activated ATPase (the sodium pump enzyme), transiently reduce the cytoplasmic concentration of a substance to be transported across the epithelium so that it can diffuse from lumen, down its concentration gradient, across the apical cell surface. The transport mechanisms also increase the concentrations of specific substances in the intercellular space. These substances then diffuse or flow down their concentration gradients within the intercellular space to cross the epithelial basal lamina and enter the fenestrated capillaries in the lamina propria immediately beneath the epithelium. Those substances that are too large to enter the blood vessels, such as lipoprotein particles, enter the lymphatic lacteal.

The lateral membranes of the enterocytes show elaborate

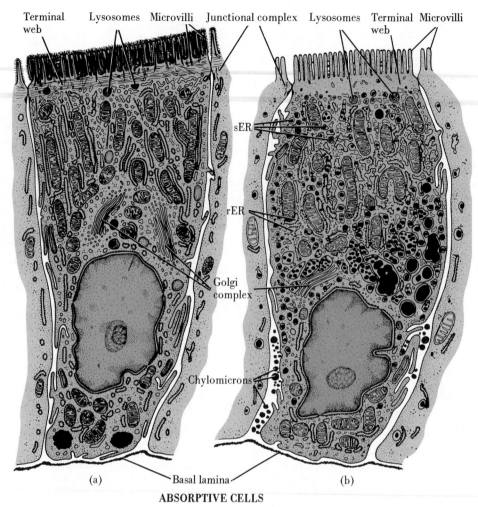

Terminal web · Lysosomes · Microvilli · Junctional complex · Lysosomes · Terminal web · Microvilli

sER

rER

Golgi complex

Chylomicrons

Basal lamina

(a) (b)

ABSORPTIVE CELLS

Figure 16.13. a. Diagram of an enterocyte showing a striated border on its apical (luminal) surface and junctional complexes that seal the lumen of the intestine from the lateral intercellular space. The characteristic complement of organelles is depicted in the diagram. **b.** The cell shows the distribution of lipid during fat absorption as seen with the TEM. Initially, lipid is seen in association with the microvilli of the striated border. The lipid is internalized and seen in vesicles of the smooth endoplasmic reticulum (sER) in the apical portion of the cell. The membrane-bounded lipid can be traced into the center of the cell, where some of the lipid-containing vesicles fuse, and then the lipid is discharged into the lateral intercellular space. The extracellular lipid, recognized as chylomicrons, passes beyond the basal lamina for further transport. (Based on Lentz TL: *Cell Fine Structure.* Philadelphia, WB Saunders, 1971, pp 179 and 181.)

development of flattened processes (plications) that implicate with processes of adjacent cells, thus increasing the amount of plasma membrane containing transport enzymes (see Fig. 4.24). During active absorption, especially of electrolytes, water, and lipids, the *lateral plications* separate, allowing the development of an enlarged intercellular compartment (see Plate 4, page 91). The increased hydrostatic pressure from the accumulated solutes and solvents causes a directional flow through the basal lamina into the lamina propria (see Fig. 4.1).

In addition to the membrane specializations associated with absorption and transport, the cytoplasm of the enterocytes is also specialized for these functions. Elongated mitochondria that provide energy for the transport function of the cells are concentrated in the apical cytoplasm between the terminal web and the nucleus. Tubules and cisternae of the smooth endoplasmic reticulum (sER), which are involved in the absorption of fatty acids and glycerol and in the resynthesis of neutral fat, are found in the apical cytoplasm, beneath the terminal web.

Enterocytes Are Also Secretory Cells, Producing Enzymes Needed for Terminal Digestion and Absorption

The secretory function of the enterocytes, primarily the synthesis of glycoprotein enzymes that will be inserted into the apical plasma membrane, is represented morphologically by vertically aligned stacks of Golgi cisternae in the immediately supranuclear region and by the presence of free ribosomes and rER lateral to the Golgi complex (see Fig. 16.13). Small secretory vesicles containing glycoproteins destined for the cell surface are located in the apical cytoplasm, immediately below the terminal web, and along

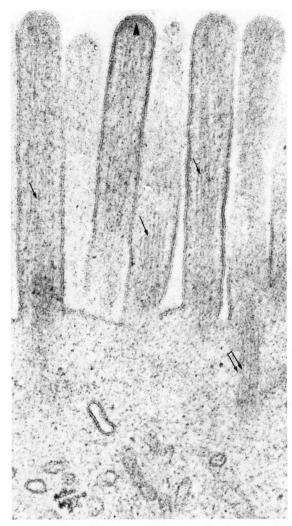

Figure 16.14. Electron micrograph of the microvilli that form the striated border of an enterocyte. The microvilli contain a core of longitudinally disposed microfilaments *(arrows)*. The filaments, composed of actin, are connected to the tip of the microvillus *(arrowhead)* and extend beyond the base of the microvillus *(double arrows)* into the terminal web region of the cell. ×85,000.

the lateral plasma membrane. Histochemical or autoradiographic methods are needed, however, to distinguish these *secretory vesicles* from *endocytic vesicles* or small *primary lysosomes.*

Goblet Cells. Goblet cells are interspersed among the other cells of the intestinal epithelium. Goblet cells increase in number from the proximal to the distal small intestine and are most numerous in the terminal ileum. As in other epithelia, goblet cells produce mucus. Also, as in other epithelia, because water-soluble mucinogen is lost during preparation of routine H&E sections, the part of the cell that normally contains the mucinogen granules appears empty.

Examination with the TEM reveals the presence of a large accumulation of mucinogen granules in the apical cytoplasm that distends the apex of the cell and distorts the shape of neighboring cells (Fig. 16.15a). The characteristic shape

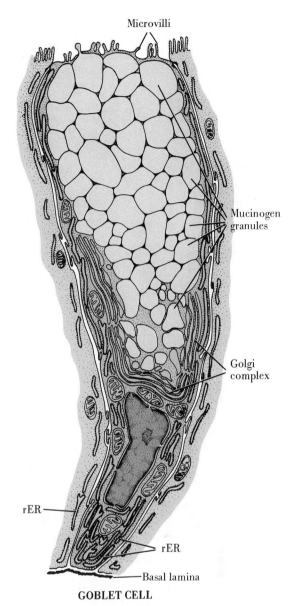

GOBLET CELL

Figure 16.15. **a.** Diagram of a goblet cell. The nucleus is in the basal pole of the cell. The major portion of the cell is filled with mucigen (mucinogen) granules forming the mucous cup that is evident with the light microscope. At the base and lower sides of the mucous cup are flattened saccules of the large Golgi apparatus. Other organelles are distributed throughout the remaining cytoplasm, especially in the perinuclear cytoplasm in the base of the cell. (Based on Neutra M, Leblond CP: *The Journal of Cell Biology* 30:119, 1966, by copyright permission of The Rockefeller University Press.)

of this accumulation of droplets is responsible for the name of the cell. An extensive array of flattened Golgi saccules forms a wide cup around the newly formed mucinogen granules near the basal part of the cell (Fig. 16.15, *a* and *b*). Goblet cells have microvilli that are restricted to a thin rim of cytoplasm (the **theca**) that surrounds the apical-lateral portion of the accumulation of mucinogen granules. Microvilli are more obvious on the immature goblet cells in the deep one-half of the crypt.

The large apical accumulation of mucinogen granules

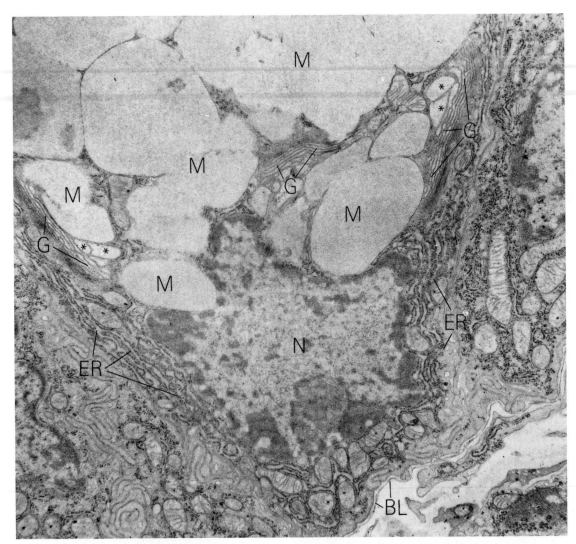

Figure 16.15. b. Electron micrograph of the basal portion of a goblet cell. The cell rests on the basal lamina *(BL)*. The basal portion of the cell contains the nucleus *(N)*, rough endoplasmic reticulum *(ER)*, and mitochondria. Just apical to the nucleus are extensive Golgi profiles *(G)*. As the mucous product accumulates in the Golgi cisternae, they become enlarged *(asterisks)*. The large mucinogen granules *(M)* fill most of the apical portion of the cell and collectively constitute the "mucous cup" seen with the light microscope. ×15,000.

leaves the rest of the cell as a narrow stem forming the basal portion of the cell. This basal portion is intensely basophilic in histologic preparations because it is occupied by the very heterochromatic nucleus, extensive rER, and free ribosomes. Mitochondria are also concentrated in the basal cytoplasm.

Paneth Cells. Paneth cells are found in the bases of the mucosal glands. (They are occasionally found in the normal colon in small numbers; and their number may increase in certain pathologic conditions.) They have a basophilic basal cytoplasm, a supranuclear Golgi complex, and large, intensely acidophilic, refractile apical secretory granules. The granules allow them to be identified easily in routine histologic sections (Fig. 16.16).

The secretory granules contain the antibacterial enzyme lysozyme, other glycoproteins, an arginine-rich protein (probably responsible for the intense acidophilia), and zinc. Lysozyme digests the cell walls of certain groups of bac-

teria. This antibacterial action and the phagocytosis of certain bacteria and protozoa by Paneth cells suggest that Paneth cells have a role in regulating the normal bacterial flora of the small intestine.

Enteroendocrine Cells. Enteroendocrine cells in the small intestine resemble those described in the stomach. They are concentrated in the lower portion of the intestinal crypt but migrate slowly and can be found at all levels of the villus unit (Fig. 16.17). Nearly all of the same hormones and hormone-like secretions identified in this cell type in the stomach can be demonstrated in the enteroendocrine cells of the intestine (Table 16.1). *Cholecystokinin (CCK), secretin,* and *gastric inhibitory peptide (GIP)* are the most active regulators of gastrointestinal physiology that are released in this portion of the gut (Fig. 16.18). These three hormones increase pancreatic and gallbladder activity and inhibit gastric secretory function and motility. Other candidate hormones and hormone-like substances secreted by

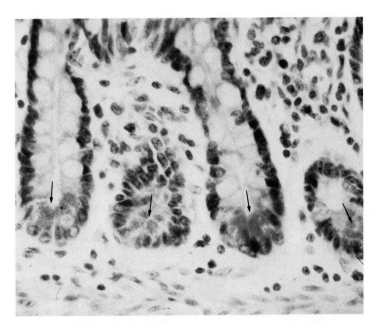

Figure 16.16. Light micrograph of intestinal glands showing Paneth cells. The specimen has been stained with H&E. Paneth cells are typically located in the bottom of the intestinal glands. The cytoplasm contains granules *(arrows)* that stain intensely with eosin.

enteroendocrine cells have similar stimulatory and inhibitory effects on other parts of the digestive tract (Table 16.2).

M Cells (Microfold Cells). The epithelial cells that overlie Peyer's patches and other large lymphatic nodules are different from the surrounding intestinal epithelial cells. They are nearly squamous, have *microfolds* rather than microvilli on their apical surface, and take up macromolecules from the lumen in endocytic vesicles. The vesicles are transported to the basolateral membrane where they discharge their contents into the epithelial intercellular space in the vicinity of lymphocytes that have insinuated themselves into this space. Antigens that reach lymphocytes in this manner stimulate a response in the GALT that is described below.

Intermediate Cells Have Characteristics of Both Immature Absorptive Cells and Goblet Cells

Intermediate Cells. Intermediate cells constitute the majority of the cells in the lower half of the intestinal crypt. These cells are still capable of cell division and usually undergo one or two divisions before they become committed to differentiation into either absorptive or goblet cells. These cells have short, irregular microvilli with long-core filaments extending deep into the apical cytoplasm and numerous macular (desmosomal) junctions with adjacent cells. Small mucin-like secretory droplets form a column in the center of the supranuclear cytoplasm. Intermediate cells that become committed to develop into goblet cells develop a small, rounded collection of secretory droplets just under the apical plasma membrane; those that become committed to develop into absorptive cells lose the secretory droplets and begin to show concentration of mitochondria, rER, and ribosomes in the apical cytoplasm.

Gut-Associated Lymphatic Tissue

As noted above, the lamina propria of the digestive tract is heavily populated with elements of the immune system; approximately one-fourth of the mucosa consists of a loosely organized layer of lymphatic nodules, lymphocytes, macrophages, plasma cells, and eosinophils in the lamina propria. Lymphocytes are also found insinuated between epithelial cells. This gut-associated lymphatic tissue (GALT) serves as an immunologic barrier throughout the length of the gastrointestinal tract. In cooperation with the overlying epithelial cells, particularly the M cells, the lymphatic tissue samples the antigens in the epithelial intercellular spaces. The intraepithelial lymphocytes process antigens and probably migrate to lymphatic nodules in the lamina propria where they undergo blastic transformation (see page 331), leading to antibody secretion by newly differentiated plasma cells.

Most of the plasma cells of the lamina propria of the intestine secrete dimeric IgA rather than the more common IgG; other plasma cells produce IgM and IgE (see, also, Immunologic Function of Saliva, page 423). IgA is transported across the epithelium, linked to a secretory glycoprotein that is synthesized by the enterocytes and inserted in the basal plasma membrane as a receptor for the IgA.

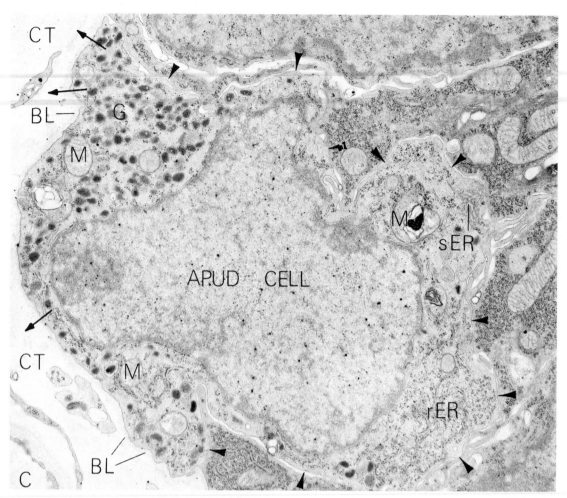

Figure 16.17. Electron micrograph of an enteroendocrine cell of the colon. *Arrowheads* mark the boundary between the enteroendocrine cell and the adjacent epithelial cells. At its base the enteroendocrine cell is adjacent to the basal lamina *(BL)*. This cell does not extend to the epithelial or luminal surface. Numerous secretory granules *(G)* in the base of the cell are secreted in the direction of the *arrows* across the basal lamina and into the connective tissue *(CT)*. C, capillary; *M*, mitochondria; *rER*, rough endoplasmic reticulum; and *sER*, smooth endoplasmic reticulum.

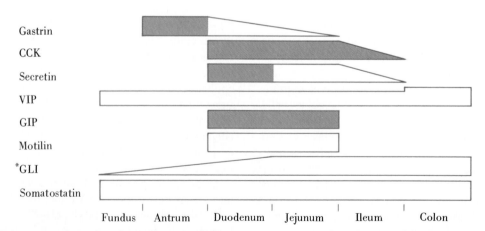

Figure 16.18. Schema to show the distribution of gastrointestinal peptides. The *solid green areas* show where physiologic release of gastrointestinal hormones occurs. *CCK,* cholecystokinin; *GIP,* gastric inhibitory peptide; *GLI,* glucagon-like immunoactivity; and *VIP,* vasoactive intestinal peptide. (Modified from Johnson LR (ed): *Gastrointestinal Physiology,* 4th ed. St Louis, CV Mosby, 1991, p 6.)

The complex of IgA and secretory glycoprotein is taken into the epithelial cell by *endo*cytosis at the basal plasma membrane and is subsequently released from the cell by *exo*cytosis at the apical plasma membrane. In the gut lumen, IgA binds to antigens, toxins, and microorganisms in a process called *immune exclusion* (Fig. 16.23).

IgM is believed to follow a similar secretory pathway and is also found in the lumen of the gut. Some of the IgE binds to the plasma membranes of mast cells in the lamina propria (see page 110), selectively sensitizing them to specific antigens derived from the lumen.

Submucosa

A Distinguishing Characteristic of the Duodenum Is the Presence of Submucosal Glands

The submucosa consists of a dense connective tissue and localized sites that contain aggregates of adipose cells. A conspicuous feature in the duodenum is the presence of submucosal glands (of Brunner).

The branched tubuloalveolar submucosal glands of the duodenum (Brunner's glands; see Plate 77, page 485) have secretory cells with characteristics of both zymogen-secreting and mucus-secreting cells. The secretion of these glands has a pH of 8.1–9.3 and contains neutral and alkaline glycoproteins and bicarbonate ions. This probably serves to protect the proximal small intestine by neutral-izing the acid-containing chyme that is delivered to it and serves to bring the pH of the intestinal contents close to the optimal pH for the pancreatic enzymes that are also delivered to the duodenum.

Muscularis Externa

The *muscularis externa* consists of an inner layer of circularly arranged smooth muscle cells and an outer layer of longitudinally arranged smooth muscle cells. The main components of the myenteric plexus (Auerbach's plexus) are located between these two muscle layers (Fig. 16.19). Two kinds of muscular contraction occur in the small intestine. Local contractions displace intestinal contents both proximally and distally and are designated as *segmentation.* These contractions are primarily of the circular muscle layer. They serve to circulate the chyme locally, mixing it with digestive juices and moving it into contact with the mucosa for absorption. *Peristalsis,* the second type of contraction, largely involves the longitudinal muscle layer and moves the intestinal contents distally.

Serosa

The *serosa* of the parts of the small intestine that are free in the abdominal cavity corresponds to the general description at the beginning of the chapter.

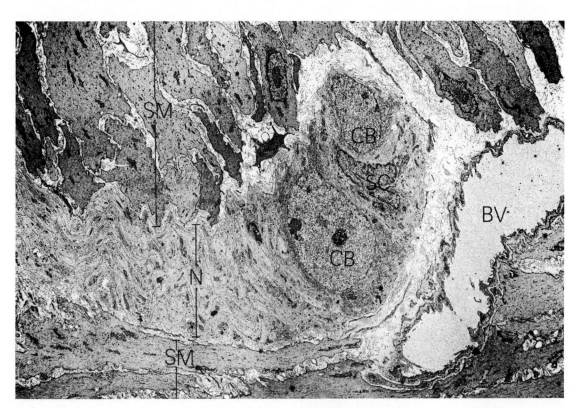

Figure 16.19. Electron micrograph of the myenteric (Auerbach's) plexus in the small intestine. The plexus is located between the two smooth muscle *(SM)* layers of the muscularis externa. It consists of an extensive nerve network *(N).* Neuron cell bodies *(CB)* are also present as part of the network. A Schwann cell *(SC)* is seen in proximity to the neuron cell bodies. *BV,* Blood vessel. ×3800.

GASTROINTESTINAL HORMONES, APUD CELLS, AND PEPTIDES

The mucosa of the gastrointestinal tract produces four principal hormones (see Table 16.1): secretin, gastrin, cholecystokinin (CCK), and gastric inhibitory peptide (GIP). In each case, the hormone is released by the endocrine cells into the lamina propria, where it diffuses into the bloodstream. As it circulates throughout the body, it is bound by receptors on the plasma membrane of target cells. The endocrine cells of the gut are not grouped as clusters in any specific part of the gastrointestinal tract. Rather, they are distributed singly throughout the gastrointestinal epithelium. Figure 16.18 shows the parts of the gastrointestinal tract from which the hormones are released into the blood.

The endocrine cells of the gastrointestinal tract and those of the pancreas are sometimes collectively grouped as the **gastroenteropancreatic (GEP) system.** In addition, some of the endocrine cells of the gastrointestinal tract are part of a group of cells designated as **amine precursor uptake and decarboxylation (APUD) cells** that produce not only gastrointestinal hormones but also paracrine substances. A paracrine substance differs from a hormone in that it diffuses locally to its target cell instead of being carried in the bloodstream to a target cell. A well-known substance that appears to act as a paracrine substance within the gastrointestinal tract and pancreas is **somatostatin.** This inhibits other gastrointestinal and pancreatic islet endocrine cells. APUD cells secrete a variety of regulator substances in tissues and organs including respiratory epithelium, adrenal medulla, islets of Langerhans, thyroid gland (parafollicular cells), and pituitary gland.

In addition to the established gastrointestinal hormones, there are several gastrointestinal peptides whose definite classification as a hormone or paracrine agent has not yet been established; these are designated as candidate or putative hormones. They and their actions are listed in Table 16.2.

Other locally active agents isolated from the gastrointestinal mucosa are neurotransmitters; these are released close to the target cell, usually the smooth muscle of the muscularis mucosae, the muscularis externa, or the tunica media of a blood vessel, from a nerve ending. In addition to acetylcholine (not a peptide), peptides known to be in nerve fibers of the gastrointestinal tract are gastrin, vasoactive intestinal peptide (VIP), and somatostatin. Thus, a particular peptide may be produced by endocrine and paracrine cells and also be localized in nerve fibers.

With the TEM, at least 17 different enteroendocrine cell types have been identified in the epithelium of the gastrointestinal tract. All the cells possess a broad base adjacent to the basal lamina. Some cells extend to the lumen where they display microvilli; others do not reach the lumen. All possess numerous small membrane-limited granules, mostly within the basal cytoplasm (see Fig. 16.17). These granules have been shown to contain an active peptide. The granules discharge their product toward the basal lamina and subjacent connective tissue; the peptide then diffuses locally to the target cell (paracrine) or into the bloodstream and through the blood vessels to the target cells (endocrine). The cells all display relatively little rER and small Golgi profiles.

Histologically, the cells usually appear as clear cells because there is not sufficient RNA to impart cytoplasmic basophilia (as in chief cells), there is not sufficient membrane to impart acidophilia (as in parietal cells), and the small granules are not adequately preserved in H&E paraffin sections. Enteroendocrine cells are difficult to identify in routine H&E sections. In any attempt to do this, one should have a general idea about the frequency of these cells; for gastric mucosa, this is shown in Plate 75, page 481. Granules in some GEP cells can be displayed with silver-staining procedures. These cells were originally designated as **argentaffin** or **argyrophilic cells;** granules in other GEP cells can be displayed with dichromate solutions, and these cells were designated as **enterochromaffin cells.**

In a clinical entity that has been identified as being the result of a tumor of a gastrointestinal endocrine cell, the **Zollinger-Ellison syndrome,** or **gastrinoma,** excessive secretion by gastrin-producing cells of the pylorus (or by pancreatic islet cells) results in excessive secretion of hydrochloric acid by parietal cells. The excess acid cannot be adequately neutralized in the duodenum, thereby leading to duodenal ulcers with complications.

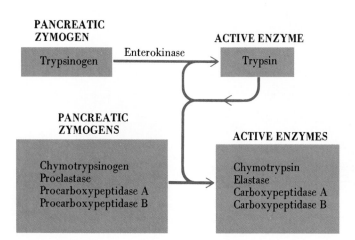

Figure 16.20. Schema to show the events in the activation of the proteolytic enzymes of the pancreas. The chain of events is triggered by enterokinase, which activates trypsinogen. Enterokinase is one of the enzymes of the glycocalyx. In turn, trypsin activates other pancreatic zymogens while at the same time it turns back to continue the activation of the additional trypsinogen. (From Johnson LR (ed): *Gastrointestinal Physiology,* 4th ed. St Louis, CV Mosby, 1991, p 118.)

DIGESTIVE AND ABSORPTIVE FUNCTIONS OF ENTEROCYTES

The plasma membrane of the microvilli of the enterocyte plays a role in digestion as well as absorption. Digestive enzymes are anchored in the plasma membrane, and their functional groups extend outward to become part of the glycocalyx. Note that by this arrangement the end products of digestion are close to the site for their absorption. Included among the enzymes are peptidases and disaccharidases. The plasma membrane of apical microvilli also contains the enzyme *enteropeptidase (enterokinase)*. This is particularly important in the duodenum, where the enzyme converts trypsinogen into trypsin. Trypsin can then continue to convert additional trypsinogen into trypsin, and trypsin converts several other pancreatic zymogens into the active enzyme (Fig. 16.20). A summary of digestion and absorption of the three major foods is outlined in the following paragraphs.

Triglycerides are digested into glycerol, monoglycerides, and long- and short-chain fatty acids. These are emulsified by bile salts and pass into the apical portion of the enterocyte. Here, the glycerol and long-chain fatty acids are resynthesized into triglycerides. The resynthesized triglycerides appear first in apical vesicles of the sER (see Fig. 16.13), then in the Golgi (where they are converted into chylomicrons), and finally in vesicles that discharge the chylomicrons into the intercellular space. The chylomicrons are conveyed away from the intestines via both venous capillaries and the lacteals. Short-chain fatty acids and glycerol leave the intestines exclusively via capillaries that lead to the portal veins and the liver.

The final digestion of carbohydrates is brought about by enzymes bound to the microvilli of the enterocytes (Fig. 16.21). Galactose, glucose, and fructose are conveyed to the liver by the vessels of the hepatic portal system. Some infants and 25–50% of non-Scandinavian adults are unable to tolerate milk and unfermented milk products because of the absence of lactase, the disaccharidase that splits lactose into galactose and glucose. If given milk, they become bloated, due to the gas produced by the bacterial digestion of the unprocessed lactose, and suffer from diarrhea. The condition is alleviated if lactose (milk sugar) is eliminated from the diet.

The digestion and absorption of dietary protein are shown in Figure 16.22. The major end products of protein digestion are amino acids, and these are absorbed by the enterocytes. However, some peptides are also absorbed and are evidently broken down intracellularly. In one disorder of amino acid absorption (Hartnup's disease), free amino acids appear in the blood when the dipeptide is fed to patients but not when the free amino acids are fed. This provides support for the conclusion that the absorption of dipeptides of certain amino acids is by a pathway different from that of the free amino acid.

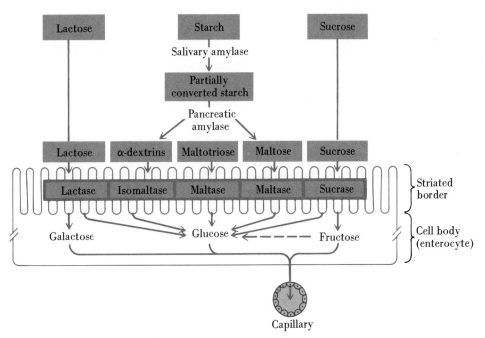

Figure 16.21. Schema to illustrate the digestion and absorption of carbohydrates by an enterocyte. Enzymes superimposed over the striated border are bound to the plasma membranes of the microvilli and act on their substrate in this location. The three absorbed monosaccharides are then passed through the enterocyte and into the underlying capillaries that lead to the portal vein and, via this vein, to the liver. (From Johnson LR (ed): *Gastrointestinal Physiology,* 2nd ed. St Louis, CV Mosby, 1981, fig 12.2.)

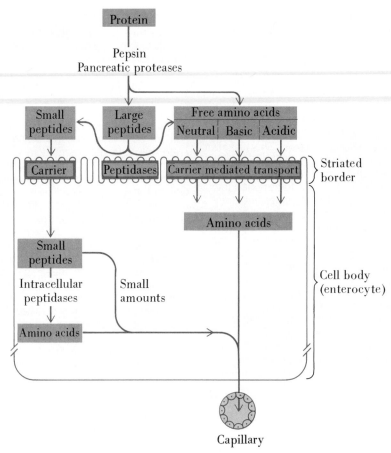

Figure 16.22. Schema to illustrate the digestion and absorption of protein by an enterocyte. Free amino acids are absorbed into the cell; small peptides also enter the cell to be digested by intracellular peptidases; other peptidases are bound to the plasma membrane of the microvilli and act in this location as shown. (From Johnson LR (ed): *Gastrointestinal Physiology,* 4th ed. St Louis, CV Mosby, 1991, fig. 11.10.)

Epithelial Cell Renewal in the Small Intestine

All of the Mature Cells of the Intestinal Epithelium Are Derived From a *Single Stem Cell Population*

Stem cells are localized in the base of the intestinal crypt, and the *zone of cell replication* is usually restricted to the lower one-half of the crypt. A cell destined to be a goblet cell or an absorptive cell usually undergoes two additional divisions after it leaves the pool of stem cells. Epithelial cells migrate from the crypt onto the villus and are shed at the tip of the villus. Autoradiographic studies have shown that the renewal time for absorptive and goblet cells in the human small intestine is 5–6 days (see Fig. 4.32).

Enteroendocrine cells and Paneth cells also derive from the stem cells at the base of the crypt. Enteroendocrine cells appear to go through only one division before differentiating. They migrate with the absorptive and goblet cells but at a slower rate. Paneth cells do not migrate but remain in the bases of the crypts near the stem cells from which they derive. They have a life span of about 4 weeks and are then replaced by differentiation of a nearby "committed" cell in the crypt. Cells that are recognizable as Paneth cells no longer divide.

LARGE INTESTINE

The large intestine is composed of the cecum, ascending colon, transverse colon, descending colon, sigmoid colon, rectum, and anal canal. The four layers characteristic of the alimentary canal are present throughout. There are, however, several distinctive features at the gross level (Fig. 16.24)

- The mucosa has a "smooth" surface; neither plicae circulares nor villi are present.
- The outer longitudinal layer of the muscularis externa exhibits three equally spaced bands.

Mucosa

The mucosa of the large intestine contains numerous straight tubular glands (crypts of Lieberkühn) that extend

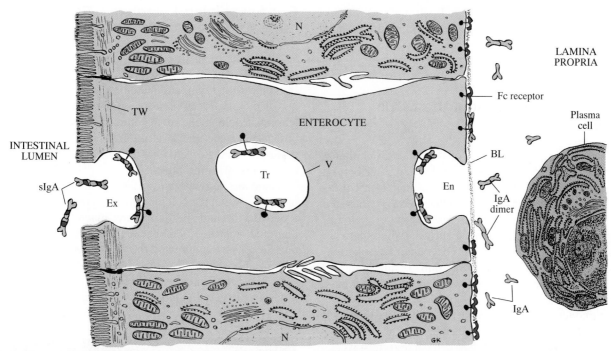

Figure 16.23. Immunoglobulin A (IgA) is secreted by plasma cells into the connective tissue matrix of the lamina propria where it dimerizes and then binds to a transmembrane Fc receptor on the basal plasma membrane of the intestinal cell. The extracellular portion of the membrane receptor will remain with the IgA dimer and will later become the secretory component of the IgA. The IgA-receptor complex enters the cell by endocytosis *(En)* and is carried to the apical surface in membrane-bounded vacuoles *(V)*. This is called transcytosis *(Tr)*. The vacuole fuses with the apical plasma membrane, releasing the IgA-receptor complex as secretory IgA (sIgA), which binds antigen in a process called immune exclusion. The IgA monomers and dimers, the Fc receptors, and the vacuolar transport mechanism are greatly exaggerated in size for clarity. The actual sizes of the vacuoles involved approximate those shown in the adjacent enterocytes. *BL,* basal lamina; *Ex,* exocytosis; *N,* nucleus of enterocyte; and *TW,* terminal web.

through the full thickness of the mucosa (Fig. 16.25*a*). The glands consist of simple columnar epithelium, as does the intestinal surface from which they invaginate. Examination of the luminal surface of the colon at the microscopic level reveals the openings of the crypts, which are arranged in an orderly pattern (Fig. 16.25*b*).

The Principal Functions of the Colon Are Reabsorption of Electrolytes and Water and Elimination of Undigested Food and Waste

The absorptive cells have a morphology essentially identical with that of the enterocytes of the small intestine. The reabsorption of water and electrolytes is accomplished by the same Na^+-K^+-activated ATPase-driven transport system as described above for the small intestine. This is the primary function of the *columnar absorptive cells.*

The elimination of the semisolid to solid waste materials is facilitated by the large amounts of mucus secreted by the numerous goblet cells of the colonic crypts. Goblet cells are more numerous in the large intestine than in the small intestine (Fig. 16.25*a*). They produce mucin that is secreted continuously to lubricate the bowel, facilitating the passage of the increasingly more solid colonic contents.

The Mucosal Epithelium of the Large Intestine Contains the Same Cell Types as the Small Intestine; Paneth Cells Are Normally Absent in the Adult Human

Columnar absorptive cells predominate (4:1) over goblet cells in most of the colon, although this is not always apparent in histologic sections (Fig. 16.25*a*). The ratio decreases, however, approaching 1:1, near the rectum, where the number of goblet cells increases. Although the absorptive cells secrete glycocalyx at a rapid rate (turnover time 16–24 hours in humans), this layer has not been shown to contain digestive enzymes in the colon. As in the small intestine, however, Na^+-K^+-activated ATPase is abundant and is localized in the lateral plasma membranes of the absorptive cells. The intercellular space is often dilated, indicating active transport of fluid.

Goblet cells may mature deep in the crypt, even in the replicative zone (Fig. 16.26). They secrete mucus continuously, even to the point where they reach the luminal surface. Here, the secretion rate exceeds the synthesis rate, and "exhausted" goblet cells appear in the epithelium between the crypts. These cells are tall and thin and have a small number of mucinogen droplets in the central apical cytoplasm. An infrequently observed cell type, the *caveolated "tuft" cell,* has also been described in the colonic epithelium; this cell may, however, be one form of exhausted goblet cell.

Epithelial Cell Renewal in the Large Intestine

As in the small intestine, all of the mucosal epithelial cells of the colon arise from stem cells located at the bottom of the crypt or gland. The lower third of the crypt constitutes the normal replicative zone where newly generated cells undergo 2–3 more divisions as they begin their migration up the crypt to the luminal surface, where they are shed about 5 days after they are generated. The intermediate cell types found in the lower third of the crypt are identical with those seen in the small intestine (see page 461).

The turnover times of the epithelial cells of the colon are similar to those of the small intestine, i.e., about 6 days for the absorptive cells and goblet cells and up to 4 weeks for the enteroendocrine cells. Senile epithelial cells are shed into the lumen at the midpoint between two adjacent crypts.

Lamina Propria

Although the lamina propria of the colon contains the same basic components as in the rest of the digestive tract, there are some additional structural features and greater development of some others. These include

* The *collagen table,* a thick layer of collagen and ground substance just below the free surface
* Elaborate development of the GALT
* A well-developed *pericryptal fibroblast sheath*
* *Absence of lymphatic vessels* in the lamina propria

The *collagen table* is a thick layer of collagen and proteoglycans that lies between the basal lamina of the epithelium and that of the fenestrated absorptive venous capillaries (Fig. 16.27). This layer is as much as 5 μm thick in the normal human colon and can be up to 3 times that thickness in human hyperplastic colonic polyps. The collagen and proteoglycans of this layer are secreted by the mature fibroblasts of the pericryptal sheath that have migrated to this level. Processes of these cells penetrate the layer to remain in intimate apposition to the basal lamina of the epithelium. This specialized portion of the extracellular matrix may, by variations in its degree of supramolecular polymerization, regulate the rate of flow of transported water and electrolytes from the intercellular compartment of the epithelium to the vascular compartment.

Gut-Associated Lymphatic Tissue

The GALT of the lamina propria of the large intestine is continuous with that of the terminal ileum; it is more extensively developed, however, than in most of the small intestine. Large lymphatic nodules distort the regular spacing of the crypts and extend into the submucosa. The extensive development of the immune system in the colon probably reflects the large number and variety of microorganisms and noxious end products of metabolism normally present in the lumen.

There are *no lymphatic vessels* in the core of the lamina propria between the colonic crypts. Lymphatic vessels form a network around the muscularis mucosae, as they do in the small intestine, but no vessels or associated smooth muscle cells extend toward the free surface from that layer. The absence of lymphatic vessels from the lamina propria has great significance in understanding the slow rate of metastasis from certain colon cancers. Cancers that develop in

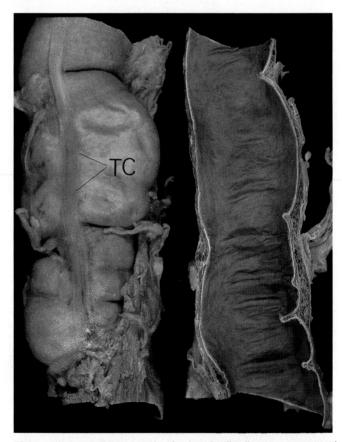

Figure 16.24. Photograph of a longitudinally cut segment of the colon. On the left the outer surface is seen. Note the distinctive smooth muscle band *(TC)* representing one of the three teniae coli that is characteristic of the colon. To the right is the other half of the specimen, showing the characteristic smooth mucosal surface. There are no plicae circulares or villi in the colon. The horizontal creases seen in the specimen are due to contraction of the muscularis externa. Compare the mucosal surface as shown here with that of the small intestine (Fig. 16.9).

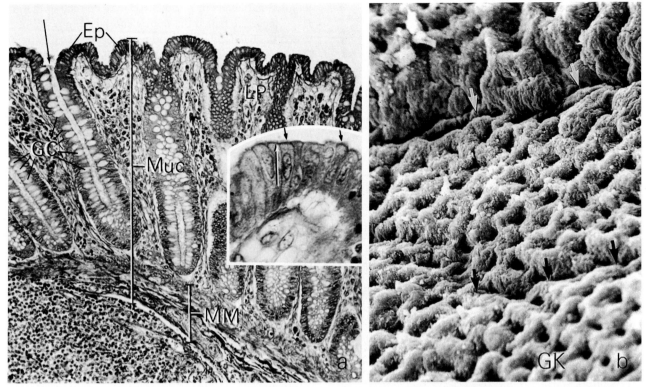

Figure 16.25. **a.** Light micrograph showing the mucosa *(Muc)* and part of the submucosa of the colon. The epithelium of the colonic surface is continuous with the straight, tubular intestinal glands *(arrow)*. A highly cellular lamina propria *(LP)* is under the surface epithelium and around the glands. The **inset** shows the absorptive cells of the colonic surface. These cells possess a small striated border *(arrows)*. Goblet cells *(GC)* are also present on the surface, but they are more numerous in the glands. In the vicinity of the *asterisk,* lymphocytes obscure the muscularis mucosae *(MM)*. **b.** Scanning electron micrograph of normal human colonic mucosal surface. The surface is divided into territories by anastomotic clefts *(arrows)*. Each territory contains 25–100 crypt openings in linear array. ×140. (From Fenoglio CM, Richart RM, Kaye GI: *Gastroenterology* 69:100, 1975.)

large adenomatous colonic polyps may grow extensively within the epithelium and lamina propria before they even have access to the lymphatic vessels at the level of the muscularis mucosae. Lymphatic vessels are found in the submucosa and as a network around the muscularis externa.

Pericryptal Fibroblast Sheath

The pericryptal fibroblasts constitute a population of regularly replicating cells. They have their stem cell zone immediately beneath the base of the crypt, adjacent to the stem cell zone of the epithelium (in both the colon and the small intestine). These cells migrate and differentiate in parallel and in synchrony with the epithelial cells, and they secrete the fine collagen fibers that are identified as the reticular fibers associated with the basement membrane of the crypt. The reticular fibers are arranged in a helical pattern that reflects the helical pathway of migration described for both epithelial cells and pericryptal fibroblasts (Fig. 16.27).

At all levels of the mucosa, the fibroblasts retain some degree of close morphologic apposition to the basal lamina of the epithelium. Near the base of the crypt, this may involve most of the adluminal surface of the fibroblast; under the luminal surface of the colon, the fibroblasts extend cytoplasmic processes through the collagen table to make contact with the basal lamina. Although the ultimate fate of the pericryptal fibroblasts is undetermined, most of these cells, after they reach the level of the luminal surface, take on the morphologic and histochemical characteristics of macrophages, and there is some evidence that the macrophages of the core of the lamina propria in the colon may arise as a terminal differentiation of the pericryptal fibroblasts.

Muscularis Externa

In the colon, as already noted, the outer layer of the muscularis externa is, in part, condensed into prominent

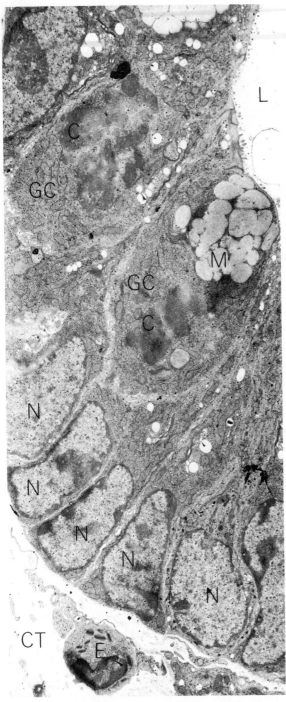

Figure 16.26. Electron micrograph of the intestinal mucosa. This electron micrograph demonstrates that certain cells of the intestine continue to divide even after they have begun to differentiate. Here, two goblet cells *(GC)* are shown in division. One of the goblet cells shows mucinogen granules *(M)* in its apical cytoplasm. The chromosomes *(C)* of the dividing cells are not surrounded by a nuclear membrane. Compare with the nuclei *(N)* of nondividing intestinal epithelium. The lumen of the gland *(L)* is on the right. *CT,* connective tissue; and *E,* eosinophil. ×5000.

longitudinal bands of muscle that may be seen at the gross level; these are called the ***teniae coli*** (see Fig. 16.24). Between the bands, the longitudinal layer forms an extremely thin sheet. In the rectum, the outer longitudinal layer of smooth muscle is a uniformly thick layer, as in the small intestine.

Bundles of muscle from the teniae coli penetrate the inner, circular layer of muscle at irregular intervals along the length and circumference of the colon. These apparent discontinuities in the muscularis externa allow segments of the colon to contract independently, leading to the formation of ***saccules (haustra)*** in the colon wall.

The muscularis externa of the large intestine produces two major types of contraction: segmentation and peristalsis. The segmenting type of contraction is local and does not result in the propulsion of contents. The peristaltic contractions result in mass movements distally of colonic contents. The mass peristaltic movements do not occur frequently; in a healthy person, they usually occur once a day in order to empty the distal colon.

Submucosa and Serosa

The ***submucosa*** corresponds to the general description already given. Where the large intestine is directly in contact with other structures (as on much of its posterior surface), its outer layer is an adventitia; elsewhere, the outer layer is a typical serosa.

Cecum and Appendix

The cecum forms a blind pouch just distal to the ileocecal valve; the appendix is a thin, finger-like extension of this pouch. The histology of the cecum closely resembles that of the rest of the colon; the appendix differs from it in having a complete layer of longitudinal muscle in the muscularis externa (Fig. 16.28). The most conspicuous feature of the appendix is the large number of lymphatic nodules that fuse and extend into the submucosa. In many adults, the normal structure of the appendix is lost, and the appendage is filled with fibrous scar tissue.

Rectum and Anus

The rectum is the ***dilated*** distal portion of the alimentary canal. Its upper part is distinguished from the rest of the colon by the presence of folds called ***transverse rectal folds.*** The most distal portion of the alimentary canal is the anal canal. It extends from the anorectal junction to the anus. The upper part of the anal canal has longitudinal folds called

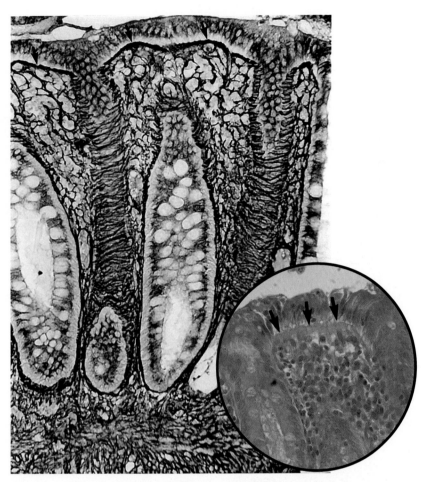

Figure 16.27. Photomicrograph of the mucosa of the colon, stained for reticular fibers. The fibers are arranged circumferentially around the crypts in what appears to be a spiral configuration. This is particularly evident where the section grazes the crypt wall. Note the thickening and condensation of the reticular fibers under the surface epithelial cells at the lumen *(arrows)*. This represents the collagen table. Laidlow (silver) stain. ×340. **Inset.** Photomicrograph of normal human colon stained with hematoxylin-phloxine-safran. In this specimen, the collagen is stained yellow. The thick collagen table *(arrows)* beneath the absorptive epithelial surface cells is particularly prominent.

anal columns (Fig. 16.29). Depressions between the anal columns are called *anal sinuses.*

The mucosa of the rectum is similar to that of the rest of the distal colon, having straight, tubular intestinal glands with many goblet cells.

Anal Canal

In the anal canal, *anal glands* extend into the submucosa and even into the muscularis externa. These are branched, straight tubular glands that secrete mucus onto the anal surface through ducts lined with stratified columnar epithelium. The distal portion of the anal canal is lined with stratified squamous epithelium that is then continuous with that of the skin of the perineum. Stratified columnar epithelium may be found between the simple columnar epithelium of the upper portion of the anal canal and the stratified squamous epithelium of the lower portion of the anal canal.

Large apocrine glands, the *circumanal glands,* are found in the skin surrounding the anal orifice. In some animals, the secretion of these glands acts as a sex attractant. Hair follicles and sebaceous glands are also found at this site.

The submucosa of the anal columns contains the terminal ramifications of the superior rectal artery and the rectal venous plexus. Enlargements of these submucosal veins constitute *internal hemorrhoids.* There are no teniae coli at the level of the rectum; the longitudinal layer of the muscularis externa forms a complete sheet. The muscularis mucosae disappears at about the level of the rectoanal margin, but at the same level, the circular layer of the muscularis externa thickens to form the *internal anal sphincter.* The external anal sphincter is formed by the striated muscles of the perineum.

IMMUNE FUNCTIONS OF THE ALIMENTARY CANAL

Immunologists have shown that the gut-associated lymphatic tissue (GALT) not only responds to antigenic stimuli, but that it functions in a monitoring capacity. This function has been partially clarified for the lymphatic nodules of the intestinal tract. The epithelium covering the nodules contains a special cell, the **M cell,** with distinctive surface *microfolds* or with thick microvilli. (These two surface configurations may reflect different functional variations of the cell surface.) The cells are readily identified with the scanning electron microscope because the thick microvilli and microfolds contrast sharply with the thinner microvilli that constitute the striated border of the adjacent enterocytes.

It has been shown with horseradish peroxidase (an enzyme used as an experimental marker) that the M cells are able to pinocytose protein from the intestinal lumen, transport the pinocytotic vesicles through the cell, and discharge the protein by exocytosis into deep recesses of the adjacent extracellular space (Fig. 16.29). Lymphocytes within the deeply recessed extracellular space sample the luminal protein, including antigens, and thus have the opportunity to stimulate development of specific antibodies against the antigens. The destination of these exposed lymphocytes has not yet been totally determined. Some remain within the local lymphatic tissue, but others may be destined for other sites in the body, such as salivary glands and mammary glands. Remember that in the salivary gland, cells of the immune system (plasma cells) secrete IgA, which the glandular epithelium then converts into secretory IgA (sIgA). Certain experimental observations suggest that antigen contact for the production of IgA by these plasma cells occurs in the lymphatic nodules of the intestines.

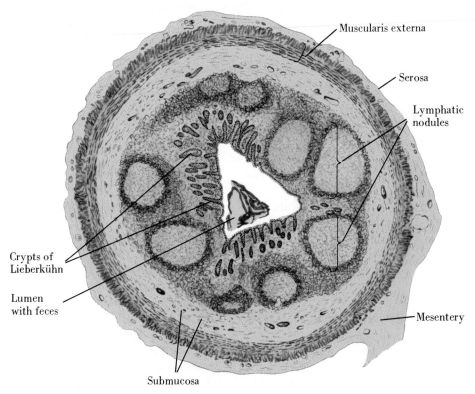

Figure 16.28. Drawing of a cross section through the appendix. The appendix displays the same four layers as those of the large intestine except that the diameter of the appendix is much less. Typically, lymphatic nodules are seen around the entire appendix, often extending into the submucosa. (After Sobotta. In: Bloom W, Fawcett DW: *A Textbook of Histology,* 10th ed. Philadelphia, WB Saunders, 1975, 674.)

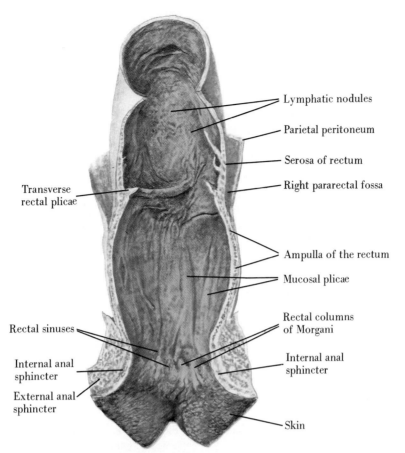

Figure 16.29. Drawing of the rectum and anorectal junction. The rectum is the terminal portion of the large intestine. The permanent plicae are transversely arranged. Characteristic mucosa of the large intestine extends as far as the rectal sinuses. Below the rectal sinuses, the epithelium is in transition to that of the skin, being first stratified columnar (or cuboidal) and then stratified squamous. (Based on Braus H: *Anatomie der Menschen.* Berlin, Springer, 1924.)

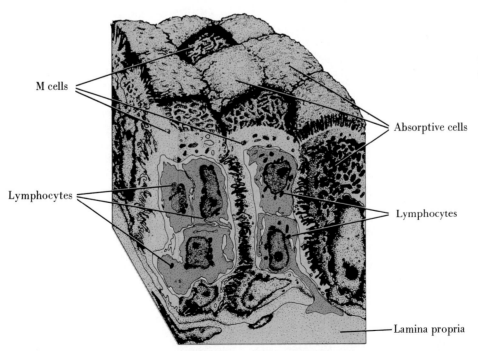

Figure 16.30. Diagram showing cells that cover a lymphatic nodule of the intestine. Some of these cells are typical of absorptive cells. Other cells display large blunt microvilli or blunt microfolds (M cells). The M cells have deep recesses that contain lymphocytes. The M cells are considered to monitor intestinal contents and present antigen to the lymphocytes. (Based on Owen RC, Nemanic P (eds): *Scanning Electron Microscopy.* O'Hare, IL, SEM Inc AMF, 1978.)

PLATE 71. Lip, A Mucocutaneous Junction

Survey micrograph, lip, human, H&E ×8. A sagittal section through the lip is shown in this low-power orientation photomicrograph. It reveals the skin of the face, the red margin of the lip, and the transition to the oral mucosa of the mouth. The *numbered rectangles* indicate representative areas of each of these sites; these are shown at higher magnifications in Figures 1, 3, and 5, respectively, on the adjacent plate. In examining the low-power orientation micrograph, note the change in thickness of the epithelium from the exterior or facial portion of the lip (the vertical surface on the right) to the interior surface of the oral cavity (the surface beginning with *rectangle 5* and continuing down the left surface of the lip).

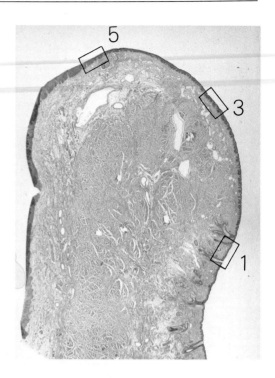

FIGURES 1, 3, 5, lip, human, H&E ×120. The epithelium *(Ep)* of the face (Fig. 1) is relatively thin and has the general features of thin skin found in other sites. Associated with it are hair follicles *(HF)* and sebaceous glands *(SGl)*.

FIGURE 3. The epithelium of the red margin of the lip is much thicker than that of the face. The stratum granulosum is still present (see Fig. 4); thus, the epithelium is keratinized. The principal feature that accounts for the coloration of the red margin in life is the deep penetration of the connective tissue papillae into the epithelium *(arrowheads)*. Note how thin the epithelium is where it overlies the papillae. The thinness of the epithelium at these sites in combination with the extensive vascularity of the underlying connective tissue, particularly the extensive venous vessels *(BV)*, allows the color of the blood to show through the epithelium. The deep connective tissue papillae are more numerous than is suggested by the micrograph, where only two are apparent; the several other more shallow-appearing papillae have been cut in a plane that does not reveal their depth.

FIGURE 5. The transition from the keratinized red margin to the fairly thick stratified squamous parakeratinized epithelium of the oral mucosa is evident in this figure. Note how the stratum granulosum suddenly ends. This is more clearly shown at higher magnification in Figure 6.

FIGURES 2, 4, 6, lip, human, H&E ×380. The *circled area* in Figure 1 is shown at higher magnification here. The reddish brown material in the basal cells is the pigment melanin *(M)*, and the dark blue near the surface is the stratum granulosum *(SG)* with its deep-blue-stained keratohyalin granules.

FIGURE 4. The sensitivity of the red margin to stimuli such as light touch is due to the presence of an increased number of sensory receptors. In fact, each of the two deep papillae contains a Meissner's corpuscle, one of which *(MC)* is more clearly seen in this figure.

FIGURE 6. Beyond the site where the stratum granulosum cells disappear, nuclei are seen in the superficial cells up to the surface *(arrows)*. The epithelium is also much thicker at this point and remains so throughout the oral cavity.

KEY

BV, venous blood vessels
Ep, epithelium
HF, hair follicle
M, melanin pigment

MC, Meissner's corpuscle
SG, stratum granulosum
SGl, sebaceous gland

arrowheads, connective tissue papillae
arrows, nuclei of superficial cells up to surface

PLATE 71

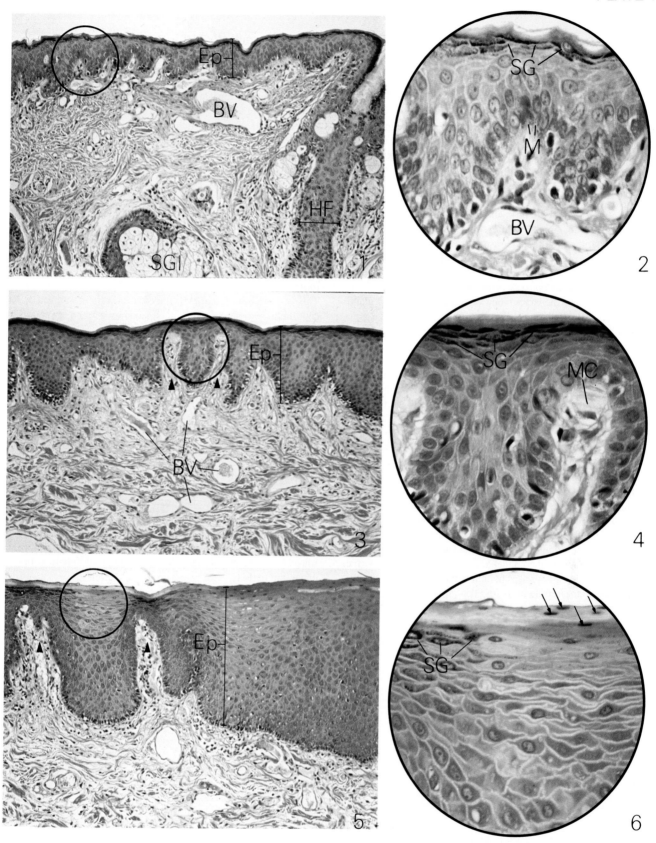

PLATE 72. Esophagus

The esophagus is a muscular tube that conveys food and other substances from the pharynx to the stomach.

FIGURE 1, esophagus, monkey, H&E ×60; inset ×400. A cross section of the wall of the esophagus is shown here. The mucosa *(Muc)* consists of stratified squamous epithelium *(Ep)*, a lamina propria *(LP)*, and muscularis mucosae *(MM)*. The boundary between the epithelium and lamina propria is distinct, although uneven, as a result of the presence of numerous deep connective tissue papillae. The basal layer of the epithelium stains intensely, appearing as a dark band that is relatively conspicuous at low magnification. This is, in part, due to the cytoplasmic basophilia of the basal cells. That the basal cells are small results in a high nuclear-cytoplasmic ratio, which further intensifies the hematoxylin staining of this layer.

The submucosa consists of irregular dense connective tissue that contains the larger blood vessels and nerves. No glands are seen in the submucosa in this figure, but they are regularly present throughout this layer and are likely to be included in a section of the wall. Whereas the boundary between the epithelium and lamina propria is striking, the boundary between the mucosa *(Muc)* and submucosa *(SubM)* is less well marked, though it is readily discernible.

The muscularis externa *(ME)* shown here is composed largely of smooth muscle, but it also contains areas of striated muscle. Although the striations are not evident at this low magnification, the more densely stained eosinophilic areas *(asterisks)* prove to be striated muscle when observed at higher magnification. Reference to the **inset,** which is from an area in the lower half of the figure, substantiates this identification.

The **inset** shows circularly oriented striated and smooth muscle. The striated muscle stains more intensely with eosin, but of greater significance are the distribution and number of nuclei. In the midarea of the **inset,** numerous elongated and uniformly oriented nuclei are present; this is smooth muscle *(SM)*. Above and below, few elongated nuclei are present; moreover, they are largely at the periphery of the bundles. This is striated muscle *(StM);* the cross-striations are just perceptible in some areas. The specimen shown here is from the middle of the esophagus, where both smooth and striated muscle are present. The muscularis externa of the distal third of the esophagus would contain only smooth muscle, whereas that of the proximal third would consist of striated muscle.

External to the muscularis externa is the adventitia *(Adv)* consisting of dense connective tissue.

FIGURE 2, esophagus, monkey, H&E ×300. As in other stratified squamous epithelia, new cells are produced in the basal layer, from which they move to the surface. During this migration, the shape and orientation of the cells change. This change in cell shape and orientation is also reflected in the appearance of the nuclei. In the deeper layers, the nuclei are spherical; in the more superficial layers, the nuclei are elongated and oriented parallel to the surface. That nuclei can be seen throughout the epithelial layer, particularly the surface cells, indicates that the epithelium is not keratinized. In some instances, the epithelium of the upper regions of the esophagus may be parakeratinized or, more rarely, keratinized.

As shown in this figure, the lamina propria *(LP)* is a very cellular, loose connective tissue containing many lymphocytes *(Lym)*, small blood vessels, and lymphatic vessels *(LV)*. The deepest part of the mucosa is the muscularis mucosae *(MM)*. That layer of smooth muscle defines the boundary between mucosa and submucosa. The nuclei of the smooth muscle cells of the muscularis mucosae appear spherical because the cells have been cut in cross section.

KEY

Adv, adventitia
Ep, stratified squamous epithelium
L, longitudinal layer of muscularis externa
LP, lamina propria
LV, lymphatic vessel
Lym, lymphocytes
ME, muscularis externa
MM, muscularis mucosae
Muc, mucosa
SM, smooth muscle
StM, striated muscle
SubM, submucosa
arrows (Fig. 2), lymphocytes in epithelium
asterisks (Fig. 1), areas containing striated muscle in the muscularis externa

PLATE 72

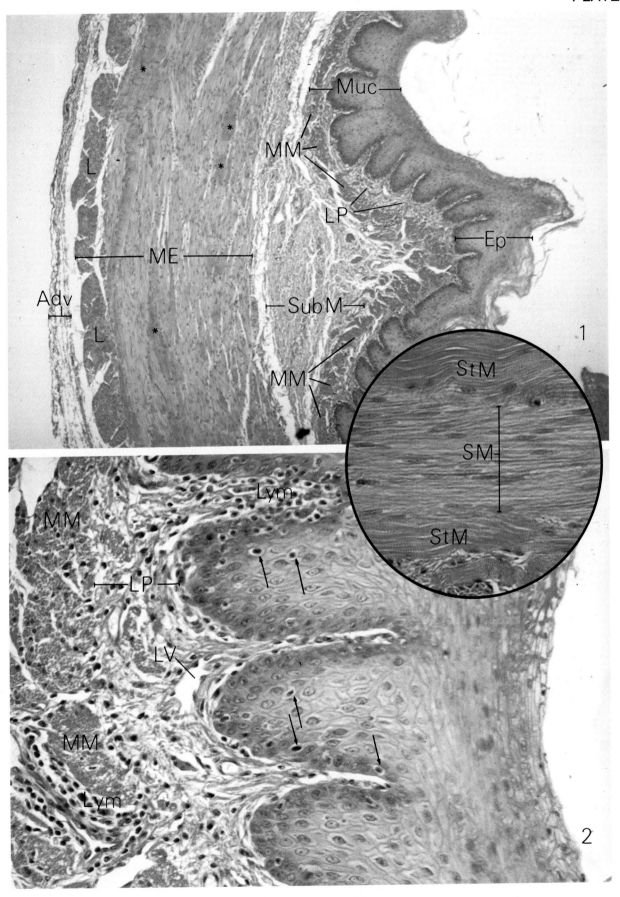

PLATE 73. Esophagus and Stomach, Cardiac Region

FIGURE 1, esophagogastric junction, H&E ×100. The junction between the esophagus and stomach is shown here. The esophagus is on the right and the cardiac region of the stomach on the left. The *large rectangle* marks a representative area of the cardiac mucosa seen at higher magnification in Figure 2; the *smaller rectangle* shows part of the junction examined at higher magnification in Figure 3.

As noted in Plate 72, the esophagus is lined by stratified squamous epithelium *(Ep)* that is indented on its undersurface by deep connective tissue papillae. When these are sectioned obliquely (as five of them have been), they appear as islands of connective tissue within the thick epithelium. Under the epithelium are the lamina propria and the muscularis mucosae *(MM)*. At the junction between the esophagus and the stomach (see also Fig. 3), the stratified squamous epithelium of the esophagus ends abruptly, and the simple columnar epithelium of the stomach surface begins.

The surface of the stomach contains numerous and relatively deep depressions called gastric pits *(P)* or foveolae that are formed by epithelium similar to and continuous with that of the surface. Glands *(Gl)* open into the bottom of the pits; they are cardiac glands. The entire gastric mucosa contains glands. There are three types of gastric glands: cardiac, fundic, and pyloric. Cardiac glands are in the immediate vicinity of the opening of the esophagus, pyloric glands are in the funnel-shaped portion of the stomach that leads to the duodenum, and fundic glands are throughout the remainder of the stomach.

FIGURE 2, esophagogastric junction, H&E ×260. The cardiac glands and pits seen in Figure 1 are surrounded by a very cellular lamina propria. At this higher magnification, it can be seen that many cells of the lamina propria are lymphocytes and other cells of the immune system. Large numbers of lymphocytes *(L)* may be localized between the smooth muscle cells of the muscularis mucosae *(MM)*, and, thus, the muscularis mucosae in these locations appears to be disrupted.

The cardiac glands *(GL)* are limited to a narrow region around the cardiac orifice. They are not sharply delineated from the fundic region of the stomach that contains parietal and chief cells. Thus, at the boundary, occasional parietal cells are seen in the cardiac glands.

In certain animals (e.g., ruminants and pigs), the anatomy and histology of the stomach are different. In these, at least one part of the stomach is lined with stratified squamous epithelium.

FIGURE 3, esophagogastric junction, H&E ×440. The columnar cells of the stomach surface and gastric pits *(P)* produce mucus. Each surface and pit cell contains a mucous cup in its apical cytoplasm, thereby forming a glandular sheet of cells named surface mucous cells *(MSC)*. The content of the mucous cup is usually lost during the preparation of the tissue, and, thus, the apical cup portion of the cells appears empty in routine H&E paraffin sections such as the ones shown in this plate.

FIGURE 4, esophagogastric junction, H&E ×440. The epithelium of the cardiac glands *(Gl)* also consists of mucous cells *(MGC)*. As seen in the photomicrograph, the nucleus of the gland cell is typically flattened; one side is adjacent to the base of the cell, while the other side is adjacent to the pale-staining cytoplasm. Again, mucus is lost during processing of the tissue, and this accounts for the pale-staining appearance of the cytoplasm. Although the cardiac glands are mostly unbranched, some branching is occasionally seen. The glands empty their secretions via ducts *(D)* into the bottom of the gastric pits. The cells forming the ducts are columnar, and the cytoplasm stains well with eosin. This makes it easy to distinguish the duct cells from mucous gland cells. Among the cells forming the duct portion of the gland are those that undergo mitotic division to replace both surface mucous and gland cells. Cardiac glands also contain enteroendocrine cells, but they are difficult to identify in routine H&E paraffin sections.

KEY

D, ducts of cardiac glands
Ep, epithelium
Gl (Fig. 1 and 4), cardiac glands
GL (Fig. 2), cardiac glands
L, lymphocytes
LP, lamina propria
MGC, mucous gland cells
MM, muscularis mucosae
MSC, surface mucous cells
P, gastric pits
arrows, intraepithelial lymphocytes

PLATE 73

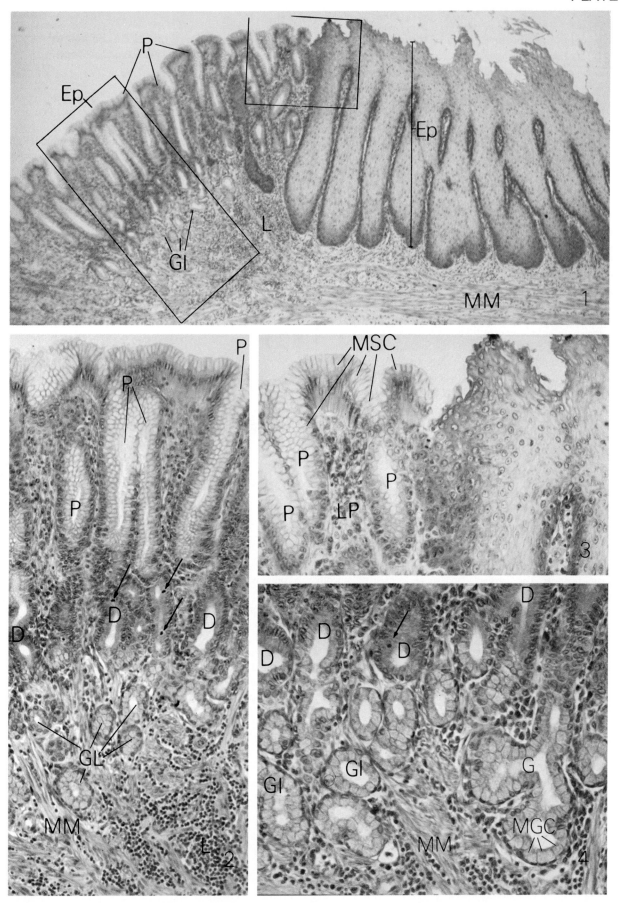

PLATE 74. Stomach I

The major portion of the stomach mucosa contains glands referred to as fundic glands; the portion of the stomach with such glands in the mucosa is referred to as the fundic stomach.

FIGURE 1, stomach, H&E.   As with other parts of the gastrointestinal tract, the wall of the stomach consists of four layers: a mucosa *(Muc)*, a submucosa *(SubM)*, a muscularis externa *(ME)*, and a serosa. The mucosa is the innermost layer and reveals three distinctive regions *(arrows)*. The most superficial region contains the gastric pits; the middle region contains the necks of the glands, which tend to stain with eosin; and the deepest part of the mucosa stains most heavily with hematoxylin. The cells of these regions and their staining characteristics are considered in Figure 1 of Plate 75. The cell types of the deep (hematoxylin-staining) portion of the fundic mucosa are also considered in Figure 3 of this plate.

The inner surface of the empty stomach is thrown into long folds referred to as rugae. One such cross-sectioned fold is shown here. It consists of mucosa and submucosa *(asterisks)*. The rugae are not permanent folds; they disappear when the stomach wall is stretched, as in the distended stomach. Also evident are mamillated areas *(M)*, which are slight elevations of the mucosa that resemble cobblestones. The mamillated areas consist only of mucosa without submucosa.

The submucosa and muscularis externa stain predominantly with eosin; the muscularis externa appears darker. The smooth muscle of the muscularis externa gives an appearance of being homogeneous and uniformly solid. In contrast, the submucosa, being connective tissue, may contain areas with adipocytes and contains numerous profiles of blood vessels *(BV)*. The serosa is so thin that it is not evident as a discrete layer at this low magnification.

FIGURE 2, stomach, H&E.   This figure and Figure 3 show the junction between the cardiac and fundic regions of the stomach. This junction can be identified histologically on the basis of the structure of the mucosa. The gastric pits *(P)*, some of which are seen opening at the surface *(arrows)*, are similar in both regions, but the glands are different. The boundary between cardiac glands *(CG)* and fundic glands *(FG)* is marked by the *dashed line* in each figure.

The full thickness of the gastric mucosa is shown here, as indicated by the presence of the muscularis mucosae *(MM)* deep to the fundic glands. The muscularis mucosae under the cardiac glands is obscured by a large infiltration of lymphocytes forming a lymphatic nodule *(LN)*.

FIGURE 3, stomach, H&E.   This figure provides a comparison between the cardiac and fundic glands at higher magnification. The cardiac glands *(CG)* consist of mucous gland cells arranged as a simple columnar epithelium; the nucleus is in the most basal part of the cell and is somewhat flattened. The cytoplasm appears as a faint network of lightly stained material. The lumina *(L)* of the cardiac glands are relatively wide. On the other hand, the fundic glands *(FG)* (left of the *dashed line*) are small, and a lumen is readily seen only in certain fortuitously sectioned glands. As a consequence, most of the glands appear to be cords of cells.

Because this is a deep region of the fundic mucosa, most of the cells are chief cells. The basal portion of the chief cell contains the nucleus and extensive ergastoplasm, thus, its basophilia. The apical cytoplasm, normally occupied by secretory granules that were lost during the preparation of the tissue, stains poorly. Interspersed among the chief cells are parietal cells *(P)*. These cells typically have a round nucleus that is surrounded by eosinophilic cytoplasm. Among the cells of the lamina propria are some with pale elongate nuclei. These are smooth muscle cells *(SM)* that extend into the lamina propria from the muscularis mucosae.

KEY

BV, blood vessels
CG, cardiac glands
FG, fundic glands
L, lumen
LN, lymphatic nodule
M, mamillated areas
ME, muscularis externa

MM, muscularis mucosae
Muc, mucosa
P: Fig. 2, gastric pits; Fig. 3, parietal cells
SM, smooth muscle cells
SubM, submucosa

arrows: Fig. 1, three differently stained regions of fundic mucosa; Fig. 2, opening of gastric pits
asterisks, submucosa in ruga
dashed line, boundary between cardiac and fundic glands

PLATE 74

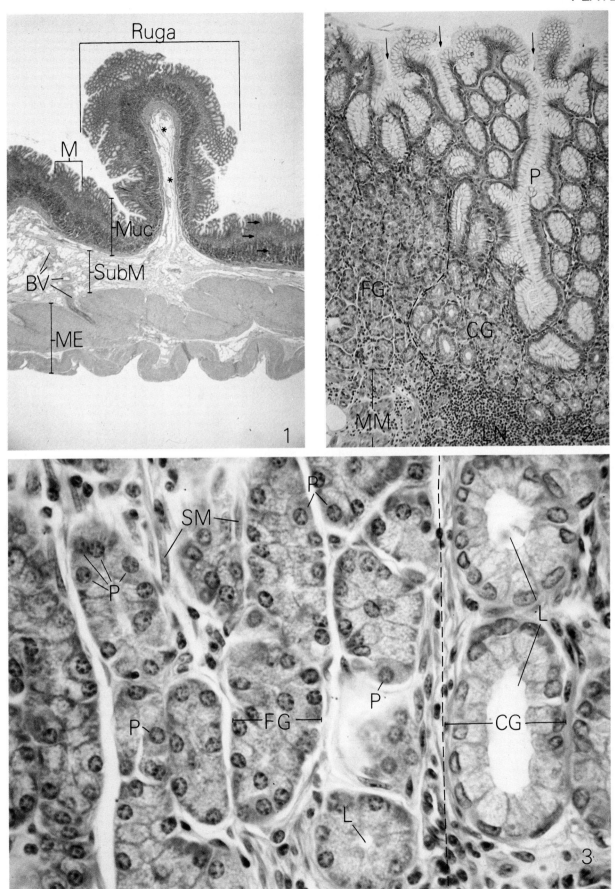

PLATE 75. Stomach II

FIGURE 1, stomach, monkey, H&E ×320. This figure shows an area of the fundic mucosa that includes the bottom of the gastric pits and the neck and deeper part of the fundic glands. It includes the areas marked by the *arrows* in Figure 1 of Plate 74. The surface mucous cells *(MSC)* of the gastric pits are readily identified because the mucous cup in the apical pole of each cell has an empty, washed-out appearance. Just below the gastric pits are the necks *(N)* of the fundic glands in which one can identify mucous neck cells *(MNC)* and parietal cells *(PC)*. The mucous neck cells produce a mucous secretion that is different from that produced by the surface mucous cells. As seen here, the mucous neck cells display a cytoplasm that is lightly stained; there are no cytoplasmic areas that stain intensely, nor is there a characteristic local absence of staining as in the mucous cup of the surface mucous cells. The mucous neck cells are also the stem cells that divide to give rise to the surface mucous cells and the gland cells.

Parietal cells are distinctive primarily because of the pronounced eosinophilic staining of their cytoplasm. Their nucleus is round, like that of the chief cell, but tends to be located closer to the basal lamina of the epithelium than to the lumen of the gland because of the pear-like shape of the parietal cell.

This figure also reveals the significant characteristics of chief cells *(CC)*, namely, the round nucleus in a basal location; the ergastoplasm, deeply stained with hematoxylin (particularly evident in some of the chief cells where the nucleus has not been included in the plane of the section); and the apical, slightly eosinophilic cytoplasm (normally occupied by the secretory granules).

FIGURE 2, stomach, monkey, H&E ×320. This figure shows the bottom of the stomach mucosa, the submucosa *(SubM)*, and part of the muscularis externa *(ME)*. The muscularis mucosae *(MM)* is the deepest part of the mucosa. It consists of smooth muscle cells arranged in at least two layers. As seen in the photomicrograph, the smooth muscle cells immediately adjacent to the submucosa have been sectioned longitudinally and display elongate nuclear profiles. Just above this layer, the smooth muscle cells have been cut in cross section and display rounded nuclear profiles.

The submucosa consists of connective tissue of moderate density. Present in the submucosa are adipocytes *(A)*, blood vessels *(BV)*, and a group of ganglion cells *(GC)*. These particular cells belong to the submucosal plexus [Meissner's plexus *(MP)*]. The **inset** shows some of the ganglion cells *(GC)* at higher magnification. These are the large cell bodies of the enteric neurons. Each cell body is surrounded by satellite cells intimately apposed to the neuron cell body. The *arrowheads* point to the nuclei of the satellite cells.

FIGURE 3, stomach, silver stain ×160. Enteroendocrine cells constitute a class of cells that can be displayed with special histochemical or silver-staining methods but that are not readily evident in H&E sections. The distribution of cells demonstrable with special silver-staining procedures is shown here *(arrows)*. Because of the staining procedure, these cells are properly designated as argentaffin cells. The surface mucous cells *(MSC)* in the section mark the bottom of the gastric pits and establish the fact that the necks of the fundic glands are represented in the section. The argentaffin cells appear black in this specimen. The relatively low magnification permits the viewer to assess the frequency of distribution of these cells.

FIGURE 4, stomach, silver stain ×640. At higher magnification, the argentaffin cells *(arrows)* are almost totally blackened by the silver staining, although a faint nucleus can be seen in some cells. The silver stains the secretory product lost during the preparation of routine sections, and, accordingly, in H&E-stained paraffin sections the argentaffin cell appears as a clear cell. The special silver staining in this figure and in Figure 3 shows that many of the argentaffin cells tend to be near the basal lamina and away from the lumen of the gland.

KEY

A, adipocytes
BV, blood vessels
CC, chief cells
GC, ganglion cells
ME, muscularis externa

MM, muscularis mucosae
MNC, mucous neck cells
MP, Meissner's plexus
MSC, surface mucous cells
N, neck of fundic glands

PC, parietal cells
SubM, submucosa
arrows, argentaffin cells
arrowheads, nuclei of satellite cells

PLATE 75

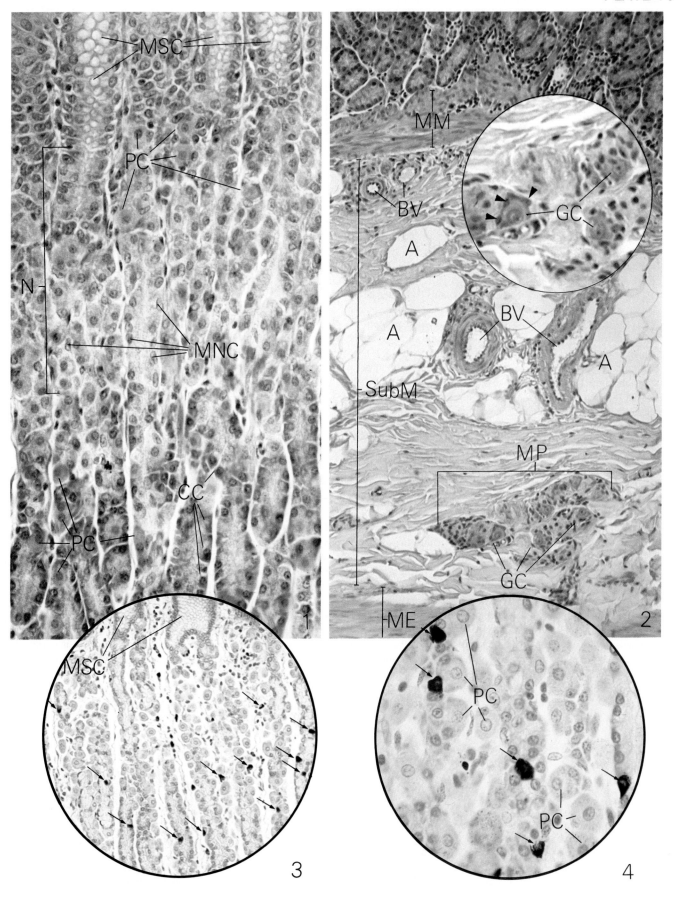

PLATE 76. Gastroduodenal Junction

FIGURE 1, stomach-duodenum, monkey, H&E ×40. The junction between the stomach and the duodenum is shown here. Most of the mucosa shown in the micrograph belongs to the stomach; it is the pyloric mucosa *(PMuc)*. The pyloric sphincter *(PS)* appears as a thickened region of the smooth muscle below the pyloric mucosa. On the far right is the duodenal mucosa, the first part of the intestinal mucosa *(IMuc)*. The area marked by the *rectangle* is shown at higher magnification in Figure 2. It provides a comparison of the two mucosal regions and also shows the submucosal glands (Brunner's glands).

The gastric mucosa and intestinal mucosa exhibit different histologic characteristics. There are also distinctive features in the submucosa of the duodenum and in the muscularis externa of the stomach. These are evident in the low-magnification panoramic view afforded in this figure and are considered first.

The submucosa of the duodenum contains submucosal (Brunner's) glands. These are below the muscularis mucosae; therefore, this structure serves as a useful landmark in identifying the glands. In the stomach, the muscularis mucosae is readily identified as narrow bands of muscular tissue *(MM)*. It can be followed toward the right into the duodenum but is then interrupted in the region between the two *asterisks*.

This figure also shows the thickened region of the gastric muscularis externa where the stomach ends. This is the pyloric sphincter *(PS)*. Its thickness, mostly due to the amplification of the circular layer of smooth muscle of the muscularis externa, can be appreciated by comparison with the muscularis externa in the duodenum *(ME)*.

FIGURE 3, stomach-duodenum, monkey ×640. The *rectangular area* in Figure 2 is considered at higher magnification here. It shows how the epithelium of the stomach differs from that of the intestine. In both cases, the epithelium is simple columnar, and the underlying lamina propria *(LP)* is highly cellular due to the presence of large numbers of lymphocytes. The boundary between gastric and duodenal epithelium is marked by the *arrow*. On the stomach side of the *arrow*, the epithelium consists of surface mucous cells *(MSC)*. The surface cells contain an apical cup of mucous material that typically appears empty in an H&E-stained paraffin section. In contrast, the absorptive cells *(AC)* of the intestine do not possess mucus in their cytoplasm. Although goblet cells are found in the intestinal epithelium and are scattered among the absorptive cells, they do not form a complete mucous sheet. The intestinal absorptive cells also possess a striated border, which is shown in Plate 78, page 487.

FIGURE 2, stomach-duodenum, monkey ×120.
Examination of this region at higher magnification reveals that in addition to intestinal glands *(IGl)* within the mucosa, there are glands within the duodenal submucosa. These are submucosal (Brunner's) glands *(BGl)*. Some of the glandular elements *(arrows)* can be seen to pass from the submucosa to the mucosa, thereby interrupting the muscularis mucosae *(MM)*. The submucosal glands empty their secretions into the duodenal lumen by means of ducts *(D)*. In contrast, the pyloric glands *(PGl)* are relatively straight for most of their length but are coiled in the deepest part of the mucosa and are sometimes branched. They are restricted to the mucosa and empty into deep gastric pits. The boundary between the pits and glands is, however, hard to ascertain in H&E sections.

With respect to the mucosal aspects of gastroduodenal histology, it has already been mentioned that the glands of the stomach empty into gastric pits. These are depressions; accordingly, when the pits are sectioned in a plane that is oblique or at right angles to the long axis of the pit, as in this figure, the pits can be recognized as being depressions because they are surrounded by lamina propria. In contrast, the inner surface of the **small intestine has villi (V).** These are projections into the lumen of slightly varying height. When the villus is cross-sectioned or obliquely sectioned, it is surrounded by space of the lumen, as is one of the villi shown here. In addition, the villi have lamina propria *(LP)* in their core.

KEY

AC, absorptive cells
BGl, Brunner's glands
D, ducts
IGl, intestinal glands
IMuc, intestinal mucosa
LP, lamina propria
ME, muscularis externa

MM, muscularis mucosae
MSC, surface mucous cells
PGl, pyloric glands
PMuc, pyloric mucosa
PS, pyloric sphincter
V, villi

arrows: Fig. 2, Brunner's gland element that passes from the submucosa to the mucosa; Fig. 3, boundary between gastric and duodenal epithelium
asterisks, interruption in muscularis mucosae

PLATE 76

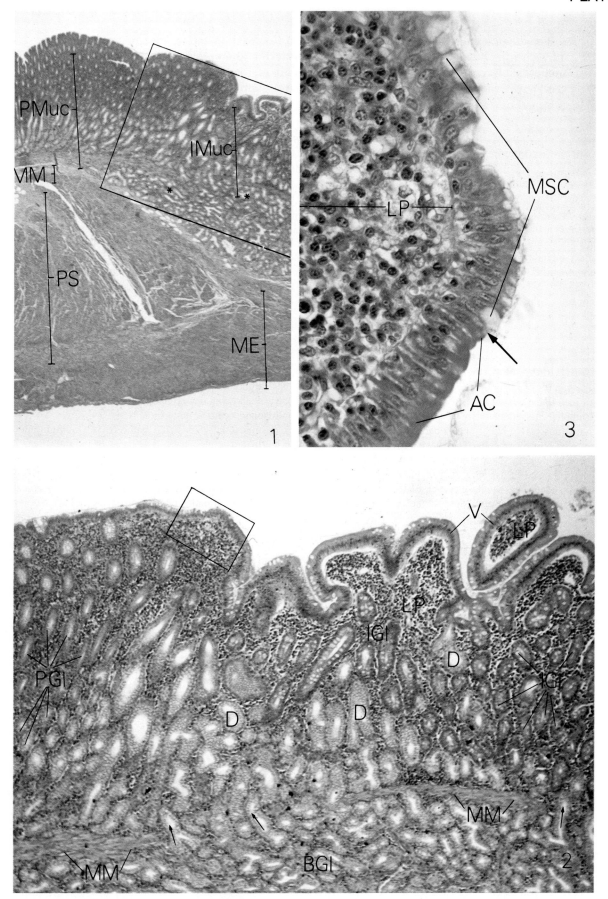

PLATE 77.   Duodenum

The duodenum is the first and shortest part of the small intestine, measuring about 10–12 inches in humans. It is adherent to the posterior abdominal wall and is, therefore, immobile. It receives the partially digested bolus of food from the stomach, as well as secretions from the stomach, pancreas, liver, and gallbladder. As already noted, it contains submucosal (Brunner's) glands.

FIGURE 1, duodenum, monkey, H&E ×120. This figure shows a segment of the duodenal wall. As in the stomach, the layers of the wall, in order from the lumen, are the mucosa *(Muc)*, the submucosa *(SubM)*, the muscularis externa *(ME)*, and the serosa *(S)*. Both longitudinal *(L)* and circular *(C)* layers of the muscularis externa can be distinguished. Although plicae circulares are found in the wall of the small intestine, including the duodenum, none is included in this photomicrograph.

A distinctive feature of the intestinal mucosa is the presence of finger-like and leaf-like projections into the intestinal lumen, called villi. Most of the villi *(V)* shown here display profiles that correspond to their description as finger-like.

One villus, however, displays the form of a leaf-like villus *(asterisk)*. The *dashed line* marks the boundary between the villi and the intestinal glands (also called crypts of Lieberkühn). The latter extend as far as the muscularis mucosae *(MM)*.

Under the mucosa is the submucosa, containing the Brunner's glands *(BGl)*. These are branched tubular or branched tubuloalveolar glands whose secretory components, shown at higher magnification in Figure 2, consist of columnar epithelium. A duct *(D)* through which the glands open into the lumen of the duodenum is shown here and, at higher magnification, in Figure 2, where it is marked by an *arrow*.

FIGURE 2, duodenum, monkey, H&E ×240. The histologic features of the duodenal mucosa are shown at higher magnification here. Two kinds of cells can be recognized in the epithelial layer that forms the surface of the villus: enterocytes (absorptive cells) and goblet cells *(GC)*. Most of the cells are absorptive cells. They have a striated border that will be seen at higher magnification in Plate 78; their elongate nuclei are located in the basal half of the cell. Goblet cells are readily identified by the presence of the apical mucous cup, which appears empty. Most of the dark round nuclei also seen in the epithelial layer covering the villi belong to lymphocytes.

The lamina propria *(LP)* makes up the core of the villus. It contains large numbers of round cells whose individual identity cannot be ascertained at this magnification. Note, however, that these are mostly lymphocytes (and other cells of the immune system), which accounts for the designation of the lamina propria as diffuse lymphatic tissue. The lamina propria surrounding the intestinal glands *(IGl)* similarly consists largely of lymphocytes and related cells. The lamina propria also contains components of loose connective tissue and isolated smooth muscle cells.

The intestinal glands *(IGl)* are relatively straight and tend to be dilated at their base. The bases of the intestinal crypts contain the stem cells from which all of the other cells of the intestinal epithelium arise. They also contain Paneth cells. These cells possess eosinophilic granules in their apical cytoplasm. The granules contain lysozyme, a bacteriolytic enzyme thought to play a role in regulating intestinal microbial flora. The main cell type in the intestinal crypt is a relatively undifferentiated columnar cell. These cells are shorter than the enterocytes of the villus surface; they usually undergo two mitoses before they differentiate into absorptive cells or goblet cells. Also present in the intestinal crypts are some mature goblet cells and enteroendocrine cells.

KEY

BGl, Brunner's glands
C, circular (inner) layer of muscularis externa
D, duct of Brunner's gland
GC, goblet cells
IGl, intestinal glands (crypts)
L, longitudinal (outer) layer of muscularis externa

LP, lamina propria
ME, muscularis externa
MM, muscularis mucosae
Muc, mucosa
S, serosa
SubM, submucosa

V, villi
arrow, duct of Brunner's gland
asterisk, leaf-like villus
dashed line (Fig. 1), boundary between base of villi and intestinal glands

PLATE 77

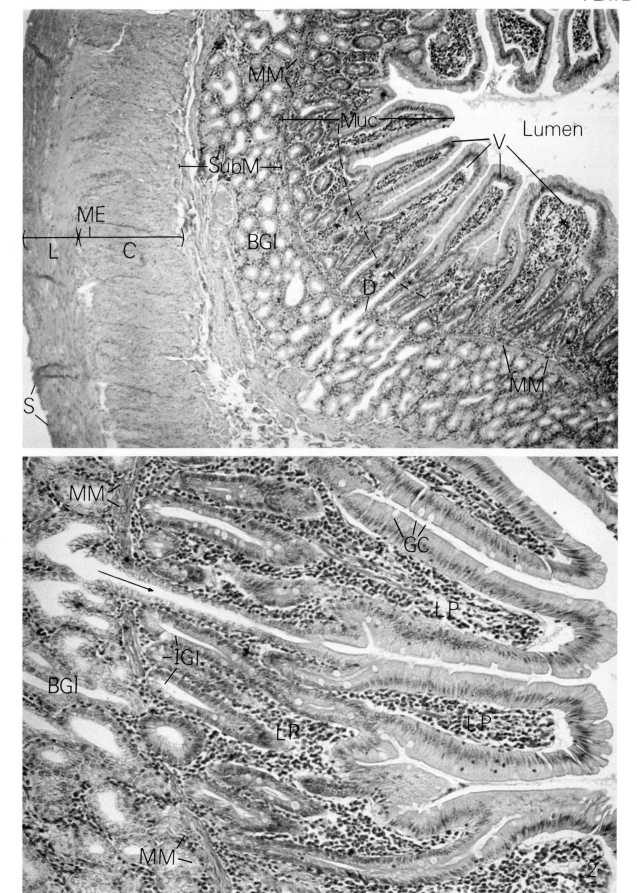

PLATE 78. Jejunum

FIGURE 1, jejunum, monkey, H&E ×22. This is a longitudinal section of the jejunum showing the permanent circular folds of the small intestine, the plicae circulares *(PC)*. These folds or ridges are mostly arranged with their long axis at roughly right angles to the longitudinal axis of the intestine; therefore, the plicae circulares shown here are cut in cross section. The plicae circulares consist of mucosa *(Muc)* as well as submucosa *(SubM)*. The broad band of tissue external to the submucosa is the muscularis externa *(ME)* and is not included in the plicae. (The serosa cannot be distinguished at this magnification.)

Most of the villi *(V)* in this specimen have been cut longitudinally, thereby revealing their full length as well as the fact that some are slightly shorter than others. The shortening is considered to be due to the contraction of smooth muscle cells in the villi. Also seen here are the lacteals *(L)*, which in most of the villi are dilated. Lacteals are lymphatic capillaries that begin in the villi and carry certain absorbed dietary lipids and proteins from the villi to the larger lymphatic vessels of the submucosa.

FIGURE 2, jejunum, monkey, H&E ×60. Part of the plica marked by the *bracket* in Figure 1 is shown at higher magnification. Note the muscularis mucosae *(MM)*, the intestinal glands *(Gl)*, and the villi *(V)*. The boundary between the glands and villi is marked by the *dashed line*. Some of the glands are cut longitudinally, some are cut in cross section; most of the villi have been cut longitudinally. In conceptualizing the mucosal structure of the small intestine, it is important to recognize that the glands are epithelial depressions that project into the wall of the intestine, whereas the villi are projections that extend into the lumen. The glands are surrounded by cells of the lamina propria; the villi are surrounded by space of the intestinal lumen. The lamina propria with its lacteal occupies a central position in the villus; the lumen occupies the central position of the gland. Also note that the lumen of the gland tends to be dilated at its base. Studies of enzymatically isolated preparations of mucosa show that the bases of the glands are often divided into two to three fingerlike extensions resting on the muscularis mucosae.

FIGURE 3, jejunum, monkey, H&E ×500. This figure shows the epithelium from portions of two adjacent villi at higher magnification. The epithelium consists chiefly of enterocytes. These are columnar absorptive cells that typically exhibit a striated border *(SB)* at their apical surface. The dark band at the base of the striated border is due to the terminal web of the cell, a layer of actin filaments that extends across the apex of the cell to which the actin filaments of the cores of the microvilli of the bush border attach. The nuclei of the enterocytes have essentially the same shape, orientation, and staining characteristics. Even if the cytoplasmic boundaries were not evident, the nuclei would be an indication of the columnar shape and orientation of the cells. The enterocytes rest on a basal lamina not evident in H&E-stained paraffin sections. The eosinophilic band *(arrows)* at the base of the cell layer, where one would expect a basement membrane, actually consists of flat lateral cytoplasmic processes from the enterocytes (see Plate 4). These processes partially delimit the basal-lateral intercellular spaces *(asterisks)* that are dilated, as can be seen here, during active transport of absorbed substrates.

The epithelial cells with an expanded apical cytoplasm in the form of a cup are goblet cells *(GC)*. In this specimen, the nucleus of almost every goblet cell is just at the base of the cup, and a thin cytoplasmic strand (not always evident) extends to the level of the basement membrane. The scattered round nuclei within the epithelium belong to lymphocytes *(Ly)*.

The lamina propria *(LP)* and the lacteal *(L)* are located beneath the intestinal epithelium. The cells forming the lacteal are simple squamous epithelium (endothelium). Two nuclei of these cells *(EC)* appear to be exposed to the lumen of the lacteal; another elongate nucleus slightly removed from the lumen belongs to a smooth muscle cell *(M)* accompanying the lacteals.

KEY

EC, endothelial cell	**ME,** muscularis externa	**arrows,** basal processes of enterocytes
GC, goblet cell	**MM,** muscularis mucosae	
Gl, intestinal glands (crypts)	**Muc,** mucosa	**asterisks,** basal-lateral intercellular spaces
L, lacteal	**PC,** plicae circulares	
LP, lamina propria	**SB,** striated border	**dashed line,** boundary between villi and intestinal glands
Ly, lymphocytes	**SubM,** submucosa	
M, smooth muscle cell	**V,** villi	

PLATE 78

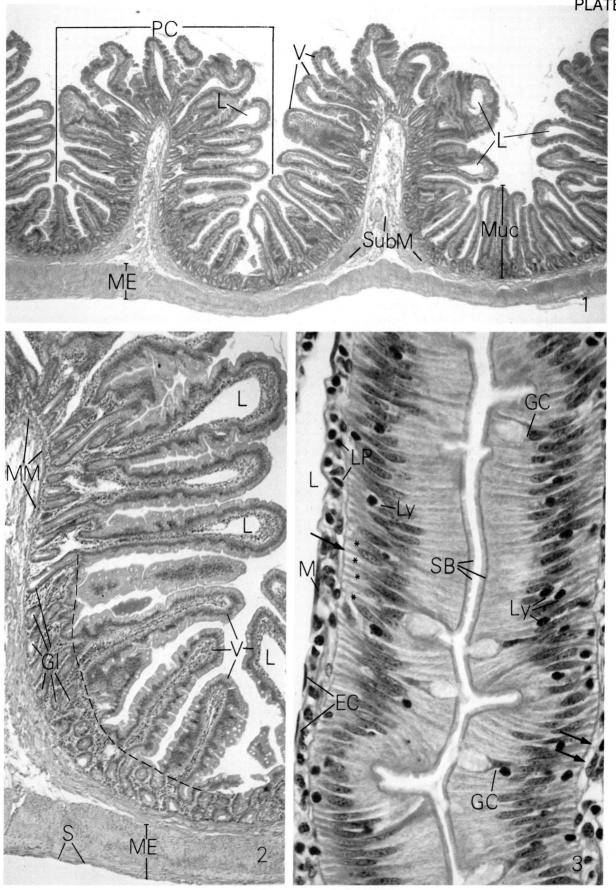

PLATE 79. Ileum

The ileum exhibits essentially the same histologic features as those seen in the jejunum. The differences are chiefly in the degree to which certain features are present. For example, the villi occur frequently in the form of leaf-like structures, and lymphatic nodes are present in greater frequency, forming Peyer's patches.

FIGURE 1, ileum, monkey, H&E ×20. For purposes of orientation, the submucosa *(SM)* and muscularis externa *(ME)* have been marked in the cross section through the ileum shown here. Just internal to the submucosa is the mucosa; external to the muscularis externa is the serosa. The mucosa reveals several longitudinally sectioned villi *(V)* that have been labeled and other unlabeled villi that can be identified easily on the basis of their appearance as islands of tissue completely surrounded by the space of the lumen. They are, of course, not islands because this appearance is due to the plane of section that slices completely through some of the villi obliquely or in cross section, thereby isolating them from their base. Below the villi are the intestinal glands, many of which are obliquely or transversely sectioned and can be readily identified, as was done in the preceding plates, because they are totally surrounded by lamina propria.

There are about 8–10 projections of tissue into the intestinal lumen that are substantially larger than the villi. These are the plicae circulares. As already noted, plicae generally have circular orientation, but they may travel in a longitudinal direction for short distances and may branch. In addition, even if all the plicae are arranged in a circular manner, if the section is somewhat oblique, the plicae will be cut at an angle, as appears to be the case with several plicae in this figure. One of the distinctive features of the small intestine is the presence of single and aggregated lymph nodules in the intestinal wall. Isolated nodules of lymphatic tissue are common in the proximal end of the intestinal canal. As one proceeds distally through the intestines, however, the lymph nodules occur in increasingly larger numbers. In the ileum, large aggregates of lymph nodules are regularly seen; they are referred to as Peyer's patches. Several lymphatic nodules *(LN)* forming a Peyer's patch are shown in this figure. The nodules are partly within the mucosa of the ileum and extend into the submucosa. Although not evident in the figure, the nodules are characteristically located opposite to where the mesentery connects to the intestinal tube.

FIGURE 2, ileum, monkey, H&E ×40. Sometimes, even in a cross section through the intestine, a plica displays a cross-sectional profile such as that shown here. Note, again, that the submucosa *(SM)* constitutes the core of the plica. Although many of the villi in this figure present profiles *(V)* that would be expected if the villus were a finger-like projection, others clearly do not. In particular, one villus (marked with three *asterisks*) shows the broad profile of a longitudinally sectioned leaf-like villus. If this same villus were cut at a right angle to the plane shown here, it would appear as a finger-like villus.

FIGURE 3, ileum, monkey, H&E ×100; inset ×200. Part of a lymphatic nodule and part of the overlying epithelium are shown here at higher magnification. The lymphocytes and related cells are so numerous that they virtually obscure the muscularis mucosae. Their location, however, can be estimated as being near the presumptive label *(MM??)*, inasmuch as the muscularis mucosae is ordinarily adjacent to the base of the intestinal glands *(Gl)*. Moreover, on examination of this area at higher magnification **(inset)**, groups of smooth muscle cells *(MM)* can be seen separated by numerous lymphocytes close to the intestinal glands *(Gl)*. Clearly, the lymphocytes of the nodule are on both sides of the muscularis mucosae and, thus, within both the mucosa and the submucosa.

In places, the lymph nodule is covered by the intestinal epithelium. Whereas the nature of the epithelium cannot be appreciated fully with the light microscope, electron micrographs (both scanning and transmission) have shown that among the epithelial cells are special cells, designated M cells, that sample the intestinal content (for antigen) and present this antigen to the lymphocytes in the epithelial layer.

KEY

GI, intestinal glands
LN, lymphatic nodules
ME, muscularis externa
MM, muscularis mucosae
MM??, presumptive location of muscularis mucosae
SM, submucosa
V, villi
asterisks, leaf-like villus

PLATE 79

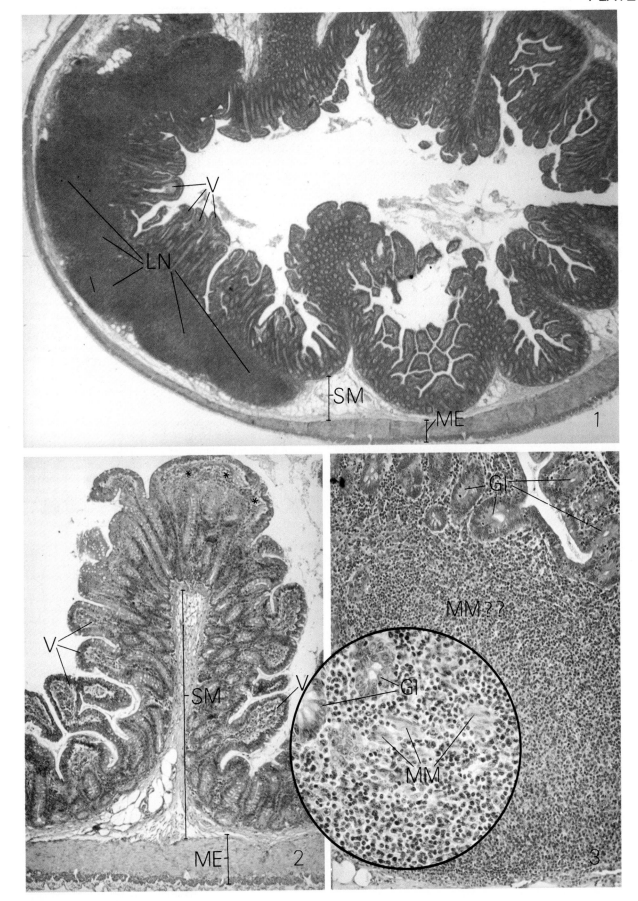

PLATE 80. Colon

FIGURE 1, colon, monkey, H&E ×30. A cross section through the large intestine is shown at low magnification. It shows the four layers that make up the wall of the colon: the mucosa *(Muc)*, the submucosa *(SubM)*, the muscularis externa *(ME)*, and the serosa *(S)*. Although these layers are the same as those in the small intestine, several differences should be noted. The large intestine has no villi, nor does it have plicae circulares. On the other hand, the muscularis externa is arranged in a distinctive manner, and this is evident in the photomicrograph. The longitudinal layer *[ME(l)]* is substan-

tially thinner than the circular layer *[ME(c)]* except in three locations where the longitudinal layer of smooth muscle is present as a thick band. One of these thick bands, called a tenia coli *(TC)*, is shown in this figure. Because the colon is cross-sectioned, the tenia coli is also cross-sectioned. The three teniae coli extend along the length of the large intestine as far as, but not into, the rectum.

The submucosa consists of a rather dense irregular connective tissue. It contains the larger blood vessels *(BV)* and areas of adipose tissue (see *A*, Fig. 2).

FIGURE 2, colon, monkey, H&E ×140. The mucosa, shown at higher magnification, contains straight, unbranched, tubular glands (crypts of Lieberkühn) that extend to the muscularis mucosae *(MM)*. The *arrows* identify the openings of some of the glands at the intestinal surface. Generally, the lumen of the glands is narrow except in the deep-

est part of the gland, where it is often slightly dilated *(asterisks,* Fig. 3). Between the glands *(Gl)* is a lamina propria *(LP)* that contains considerable numbers of lymphocytes and other cells of the immune system. Two *rectangles* mark areas of the mucosa that are examined at higher magnification in Figures 3 and 4.

FIGURE 3, colon, monkey, H&E ×525. This figure reveals the muscularis mucosae *(MM)* and the cells in the lamina propria *(LP)*, many of which can be recognized as lymphocytes and plasma cells. The smooth muscle cells of the muscularis mucosae are arranged in two layers. Note that the smooth muscle cells marked by the *arrowheads* show rounded nuclei; however, other smooth muscle cells appear as more or less rounded eosinophilic areas. These smooth muscle cells have been cut in cross section. Just above these cross-sectioned smooth muscle cells are others that have been cut longitudinally; they display elongate nuclei and elongate strands of eosinophilic cytoplasm.

FIGURE 4, colon, monkey, H&E ×525. The cells that line the surface of the colon and the glands are principally absorptive cells *(AC)* and goblet cells *(GC)*. The absorptive cells have a thin striated border that is readily evident where the *arrows* show the opening of the glands. Interspersed among the absorptive cells are the goblet cells *(GC)*. As the absorptive cells are followed into the glands, they become fewer in number, whereas the goblet cells increase in number. Other cells in the gland are enteroendocrine cells, not easily identified in routine H&E-stained paraffin sections, and, in the deep part of the gland, undifferentiated cells of the replicative zone, derived from the stem cells in the base of the crypt. The undifferentiated cells are readily identified if they are undergoing division by virtue of the mitotic figures *(M)* that they display (see Fig. 3).

Paneth cells are not usually seen in the crypts of the colon, although they are described as sometimes being present, especially in pathologic specimens.

KEY

A, adipose tissue
AC, absorptive cells
BV, blood vessels
GC, goblet cells
Gl, intestinal glands
LP, lamina propria
M, mitotic figures

ME, muscularis externa
ME(c), circular layer of muscularis externa
ME(l), longitudinal layer of muscularis externa
MM, muscularis mucosae
Muc, mucosa

S, serosa
SubM, submucosa
TC, tenia coli
arrowheads, smooth muscle cells showing rounded nuclei
arrows, opening of intestinal glands
asterisks, lumen of intestinal glands

PLATE 80

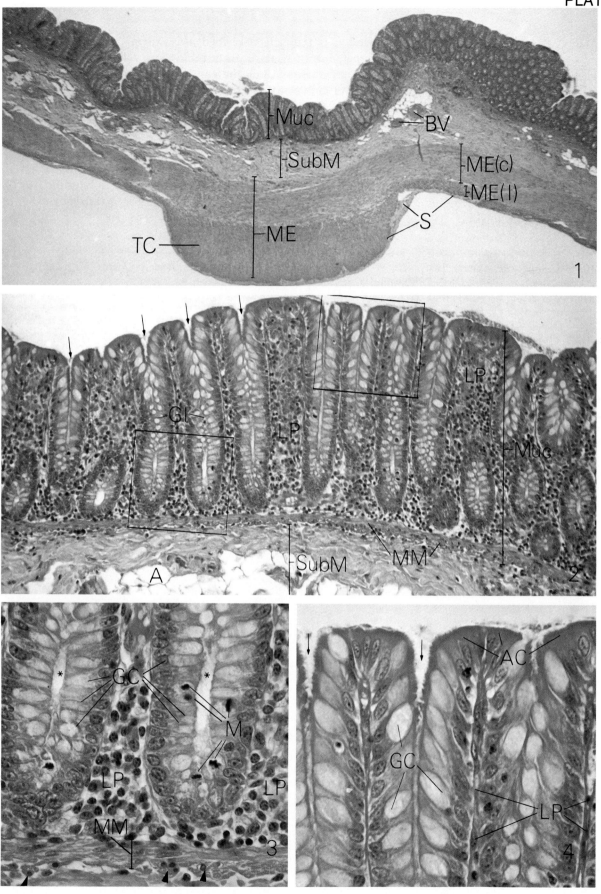

PLATE 81. Appendix

The appendix, vermiform appendix, is typically described as a worm- or finger-like structure (fr. L. *vermis*, worm; *forma*, form). It arises from the cecum, forming a blind-ending tube ranging from $2\frac{1}{2}$ cm to as much as 13 cm in length, with an average length of approximately 8 cm. In infants and children it is longer than in adults and contains numerous lymphatic nodules. Its wall is structured much like the small intestine; however, villi are not present, nor are there plicae circulares. Its mucosa, on the other hand, is similar to that of the colon. Although the appendix is often described as a vestigial organ, the abundant lymphatic tissue that it contains during early life suggests that it is functionally a lymphatic organ having an immunologic role. Recent evidence suggests that it is a principal site for the differentiation of immunocompetent B lymphocytes. In later life, the amount of lymphatic tissue within the organ regresses; thus, there is a consequent reduction in size.

FIGURE 1, appendix, human, H&E ×25. Cross section of an appendix from a preadolescent, showing the various structures composing its wall. The lumen *(L)*, mucosa *(Muc)*, submucosa *(Subm)*, muscularis externa *(ME)*, and serosa *(S)* are identified.

FIGURE 2, appendix, human, H&E ×80. This micrograph is a higher magnification of the *boxed area* in Figure 1. It reveals the straight tubular glands *(Gl)* that extend to the muscularis mucosae. Below is the submucosa *(Subm)* in which the lymphatic nodules *(LN)* and considerable diffuse lymphatic tissue are present. Note the distinct germinal centers *(GC)* of the nodules and the cap region *(Cap)* that faces the lumen. The more superficial part of the submucosa blends and merges with the mucosal lamina propria due to the numerous lymphocytes in these two sites. The deeper part of the submucosa is relatively devoid of lymphocyte infiltration and contains the large blood vessels *(BV)* and nerves. The muscularis externa *(ME)* is composed of a relatively thick circular layer and a much thinner outer longitudinal layer. The serosa *(S)* is only partially included in this micrograph.

Inset, appendix, human, H&E ×200. Higher magnification of the *circled area* in Figure 2. Note that the epithelium of the glands in the appendix is similar to that of the large intestine. Most of the epithelial cells contain mucin; thus, the light appearance of the apical cytoplasm. The lamina propria, as noted, is heavily infiltrated with lymphocytes, and the muscularis mucosae at the base of the glands is difficult to recognize.

KEY

BV, blood vessel
Cap, cap of lymphatic nodule
GC, germinal center
Gl, gland
L, lumen
LN, lymphatic nodule
ME, muscularis externa
Muc, mucosa
S, serosa
Subm, submucosa

PLATE 81

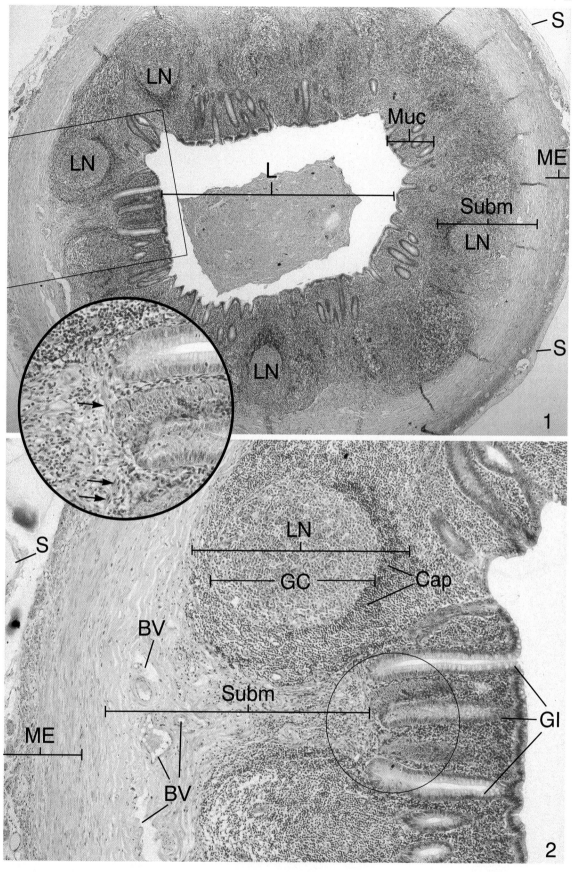

S

LN

LN

Muc

L

ME

Subm

LN

LN

S

1

S

LN

GC

Cap

BV

Subm

ME

GI

BV

2

PLATE 82. Anorectal Junction

At the anorectal junction, there is a transition from the simple columnar epithelium of the intestinal mucosa to the keratinized stratified squamous epithelium of the skin. Between these two distinctly different epithelia there is a narrow region where the epithelium is first stratified columnar (or cuboidal) and then stratified squamous. In addition, the circularly arranged smooth muscle of the intestinal canal becomes thickened and serves as an internal anal sphincter.

FIGURE 1, anorectal junction, H&E ×40. A view of the anorectal junction is shown here at low magnification. The mucosa characteristic of the large intestine is seen on the upper left of the micrograph. This region is the upper part of the anal canal, and the intestinal glands are the same as those present in the colon. The muscularis mucosa *(MM)* is readily identified as the narrow band of tissue under the glands. Both the intestinal glands and the muscularis mucosae terminate within the *left rectangular area* of the field, and here, at the *diamond*, there is the first major change in the epithelium. This area is examined at higher magnification in Figure 2. The *right rectangular area* includes the stratified squamous epithelium *(StS)* of the skin and is examined at higher magnification in Figure 3.

Between the two *diamonds* in the *rectangular areas* shown here is epithelium of the lower part of the anal canal. Under this epithelium, there is a lymphatic nodule that has a well-formed germinal center. Isolated lymphatic nodules under mucous membranes should not be construed to have fixed locations. Rather, they may or may not be present according to local demands.

Also, at this low magnification, note the internal anal sphincter muscle *(IAS)*, i.e., the thickened, most distal portion of the circular layer of smooth muscle of the muscularis externa. Under the skin on the right is the external anal sphincter muscle *(EAS)*. It is composed of striated muscle fibers, which are seen in cross section.

FIGURE 2, anorectal junction, H&E ×160; inset ×300. The junction between the simple columnar *(SC)* and the stratified *(St)* epithelium is marked with the *diamond*. The simple columnar epithelium of the upper part of the anal canal contains numerous goblet cells, and as in the mucosa of the colon, this epithelium is continuous with the epithelium of the intestinal glands *(IG)*. These glands continue to about the same point as the muscularis mucosae *(MM)*. Characteristically, the lamina propria contains large numbers of lymphocytes *(Lym)*, which is particularly so in the region marked. A higher magnification of the stratified columnar epithelium *(StCol)* and stratified cuboidal epithelium *(StC)* found in the transition zone is shown in the **inset.**

FIGURE 3, anorectal junction, H&E ×160. The final change in epithelial type that occurs at the anorectal junction is shown here. On the right is the stratified squamous epithelium of skin [*StS(k)*]. The keratinized nature of the surface is readily apparent. On the other hand, the stratified squamous epithelium *(StS)* below the level of the *diamond* is not keratinized, and nucleated cells can be seen all the way to the surface. Again, numerous lymphocytes *(Lym)* are in the underlying connective tissue and many have migrated into the epithelium in the nonkeratinized area.

KEY

EAS, external anal sphincter
IAS, internal anal sphincter
IG, intestinal glands
LN, lymphatic nodules
Lym, lymphocytes
MM, muscularis mucosae

SC, simple columnar epithelium
St, stratified epithelium
StC, stratified cuboidal epithelium
StCol, stratified columnar epithelium
StS, stratified squamous epithelium

StS(k), stratified squamous epithelium (keratinized)
arrow, termination of muscularis mucosae
diamonds, junctions between epithelial types

PLATE 82

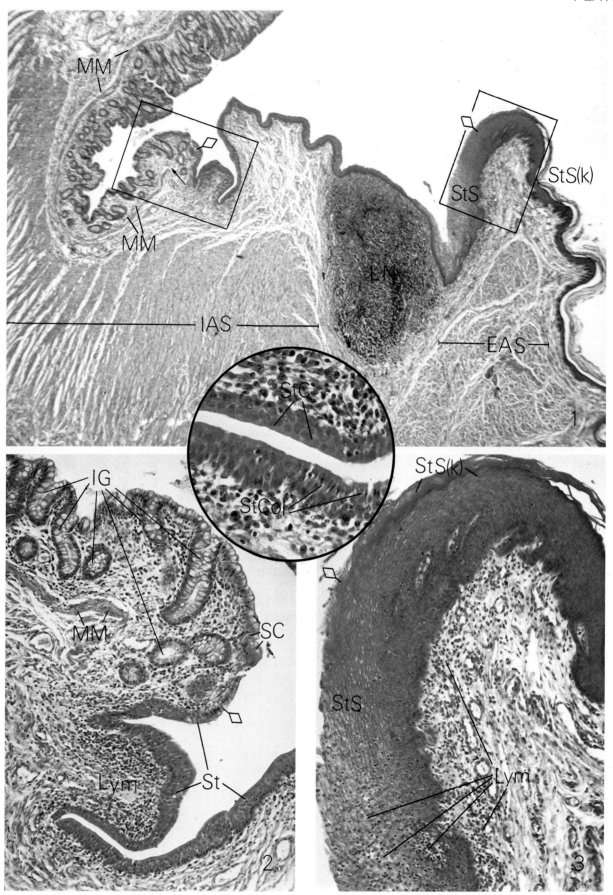

Digestive System III: Liver, Gallbladder, and Pancreas

17

LIVER

The liver is the largest mass of glandular tissue in the body and is also the largest internal organ. It is unique among the organs because it receives its major blood supply from the *hepatic portal vein,* which carries venous blood from the digestive tube, pancreas, and spleen. Thus, the liver stands directly in the pathway of blood vessels that convey substances absorbed from the digestive tube. Whereas this gives the liver the first chance to receive metabolic substrates and nutrients, it also makes the liver the first organ exposed to toxic substances that have been absorbed. The liver normally degrades or *conjugates* toxic substances to render them harmless, but it can be overwhelmed by such substances and damaged.

The Liver Has Both Exocrine and Endocrine Functions

The liver is an organ engaged in numerous metabolic conversions involving substrates brought to it from the digestive tube, pancreas, and spleen. Some of the products of these metabolic conversions are carried in the exocrine secretion of the liver, called *bile.* Bile (Table 17.1) contains conjugated and degraded waste products that are delivered back to the intestine for disposal, as well as substances that bind to metabolites in the intestine to aid in absorption. Bile is carried from the parenchyma of the liver by *bile ducts* that fuse to form the *hepatic duct.* The *cystic duct* then carries the bile into the *gallbladder* where it is concentrated before being returned, via the cystic duct, to the *common bile duct,* which delivers bile from the liver and gallbladder to the duodenum (see Fig. 17.11).

The endocrine secretions of the liver are released directly into the blood that supplies the liver parenchyma. These secretions include substances synthesized by the liver cells, i.e.,

- *Albumin*
- The protein portion of the several varieties of *lipoproteins*

- *Nonimmune α- and β-globulins*
- *Prothrombin*
- Numerous glycoproteins, including *fibronectin*

Glucose, released by hydrolysis of stored glycogen in the liver cells, is also secreted directly into the blood, as is *triiodothyronine* (T_3), the more active deiodination product of the thyroid hormone *thyroxine* (T_4) (see page 605). Other important metabolic products that are included in the endocrine secretions of the liver include modified secretions from other organs and end products of carbohydrate metabolism.

Some of the metabolic and secretory functions of liver cells are summarized in Table 17.2.

Blood Supply to the Liver

To appreciate the myriad functions of the liver introduced above, it is necessary, first, to understand its unique blood supply and how that blood is distributed to bathe the epithelial cells of the liver, the *hepatocytes.*

The Liver Receives Blood That Initially Supplied the Small Intestine, Pancreas, and Spleen

The hepatic portal vein carries about 75% of the blood supply to the liver. It brings to the liver blood from the major abdominal organs that is largely depleted of oxygen. The portal blood carried to the liver contains

- Nutrients and noxious materials absorbed in the intestine
- Blood cells and breakdown products of blood cells from the spleen
- Endocrine secretions of the pancreas

The *hepatic artery,* a branch of the celiac trunk, carries oxygenated blood to the liver. It provides the remaining 25% of the blood supply to the liver. Blood from the two sources is mixed as it perfuses the hepatocytes of the liver parenchyma, however, so that the liver cells are never exposed to the fully oxygenated blood.

Within the liver, the distributing branches of the portal vein and hepatic artery, which supply the *sinusoidal cap-*

496

TABLE 17.1. The Composition of Bile

COMPONENT	FUNCTION
Water	Solute in which other components are carried
Cholesterol and phospholipids (i.e., lecithin)	Metabolic substrates for other cells in the body; precursors of membrane components and steroids; largely reabsorbed in the gut and recycled
Bile salts (also called bile acids); glyco-cholic and taurocholic acid	Emulsifying agents that aid in the digestion and absorption of lipids from the gut and help to keep the cholesterol and phospholipids of the bile in solution, largely recycled, going back and forth between the liver and gut
Bile pigments, principally the glucuronide of the bilirubin produced in the spleen by the breakdown of hemoglobin	Detoxify bilirubin and carry it to the gut for disposal
Electrolytes: Na^+, Cl^-, HCO_3^-, K^+, Ca^{2+}, Mg^{2+}	Establish and maintain bile as an isotonic fluid; also largely reabsorbed in the gut

TABLE 17.2. Major Functions of Hepatocytes

FUNCTION	MAIN ORGANELLE
Protein synthesis and secretion (albumin, prothrombin, fibrinogen)	rER, Golgi
Bile formation and secretion (recycling of many bile constituents to and from intestine)	sER
Metabolism of lipid-soluble drugs (including detoxification) and steroids (including cholesterol synthesis)	sER
Lipoprotein synthesis and secretion	rER, sER, Golgi
Carbohydrate metabolism	sER, cytosol (also rER in the newborn?)
Urea formation from ammonium ion (urea cycle)	Mitochondria, cytosol?

ANATOMIC RELATIONSHIPS OF THE LIVER

The liver is located in the upper right quadrant of the abdominal cavity and is divided into four lobes. These are evident on the surface and are important in gross anatomy because of their relationships to other abdominal organs. Surrounding the liver is a capsule of fibrous connective tissue (Glisson's capsule) and a serous covering (visceral peritoneum) outside the capsule, except where the liver is directly adherent to the abdominal wall or the other organs.

The major vessels that bring blood to the liver, i.e., the portal vein and the hepatic artery, enter the liver at a hilum or **porta hepatis,** the same site at which the common bile duct, carrying the bile secreted by the liver, and the lymphatic vessels leave the liver.

The liver develops in the embryo as an evagination of the wall of the foregut. The original stalk of the evagination becomes the common bile duct. This duct receives the exocrine secretions of the liver, which it then delivers to the duodenum.

illaries *(sinusoids)* that bathe the hepatocytes, and the draining branches of the bile duct system, which lead to the common hepatic duct, course together in a relationship termed the **portal triad.** Although a convenient term, it is a misnomer because one or more vessels of the lymphatic drainage system of the liver always travel with the vein, artery, and bile duct.

The sinusoids are in intimate contact with the hepatocytes and provide for the exchange of substances between the blood and the liver cells. The sinusoids lead to a venous network through which blood leaves the liver. The largest of these veins, the **hepatic veins,** empty into the inferior vena cava.

Structural Organization of the Liver

As introduced above, the structural components of the liver include

- Hepatocytes, organized as plates of cells
- Connective tissue stroma
- Blood vessels, nerves, lymphatic vessels, and bile ducts that travel in the stroma
- Sinusoidal capillaries (sinusoids) between the plates of hepatocytes

With this as background, it is now possible to consider

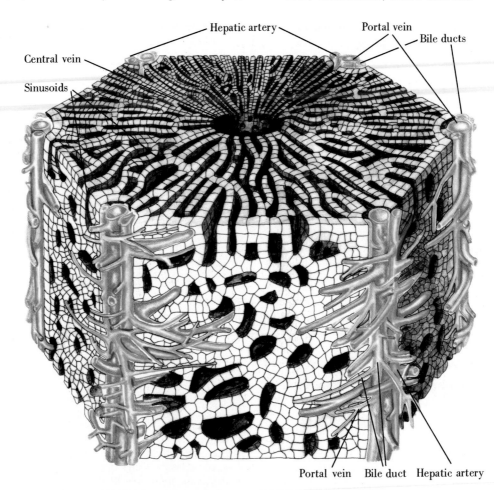

Figure 17.1. A liver lobule schematically diagramed as a six-sided polyhedral prism with portal triads (hepatic artery, portal vein, and bile duct) at each of the corners, i.e., the "classic" lobule. The vessels of the portal triads send distributing branches along the sides of the lobule, and these branches open into the sinusoids. The long axis of the lobule is traversed by the central vein, and this vessel receives blood from the sinusoids. Interconnecting sheets of hepatocytes are disposed in a radial pattern from the central vein to the perimeter of the lobule. (Based on Weiss L (ed): *Cell and Tissue Biology, A Textbook of Histology,* 6th ed. Baltimore, Urban & Schwarzenberg, 1988, p 687.)

several ways of describing the organization of these structural elements in order to understand the major functional relationships of the liver.

Liver Lobules

There are three ways of describing the structure of the liver in terms of a functional unit: the *"classic" lobule,* the *portal lobule,* and the *liver acinus.* The classic lobule is the traditional description of the organization of the liver parenchyma and one that is relatively easy to visualize. It is based on the distribution of the branches of the portal vein and hepatic artery within the organ and the pathway that blood from them follows as it ultimately perfuses the liver cells.

The Classic Hepatic Lobule Is a Roughly Hexagonal Block of Tissue

The classic lobule (Fig. 17.1) is regarded as consisting of stacks of *anastomosing plates* of hepatic cells, 1–2

cells thick, separated by the anastomosing system of *sinusoids* that perfuse the cells with the mixed portal and arterial blood. It measures about 2.0×0.7 mm. At the center of the lobule is a relatively large venule, the *terminal hepatic venule (central vein),* into which the sinusoids drain. The plates of cells radiate from the central vein to the periphery of the lobule, as do the sinusoids. At the angles of the hexagon are the *portal areas (portal canals),* loose stromal connective tissue characterized by the presence of the portal triads. This connective tissue is, ultimately, continuous with the fibrous capsule of the liver. The portal canal is bordered by the outermost hepatocytes of the lobule. At the edges of the portal canal, between the connective tissue stroma and the hepatocytes, is a small space called the *space of Mall* (see Fig. 17.9*b*). This is thought to be one of the sites where lymph originates in the liver.

In some species, e.g., the pig (Fig. 17.2), the classic lobule is easily recognized because the portal areas are con-

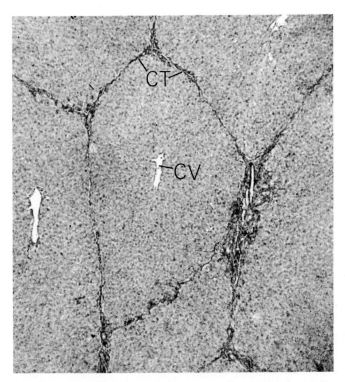

Figure 17.2. Light micrograph of pig liver lobules in cross section, showing the central vein *(CV)* and connective tissue *(CT)* surrounding the lobules. Some interlobular blood vessels can be seen in the connective tissue. At this relatively low magnification, the substance of the lobule appears as a uniform array of hepatocytes because their arrangement as sheets separated by sinusoids is difficult to discern.

nected by relatively thick layers of connective tissue. In humans, however, there is normally very little interlobular connective tissue, and it is necessary, when examining histologic sections of liver, to draw imaginary lines between portal areas surrounding a central vein in order to get some sense of the size of the classic lobule (see Plate 83, Fig. 1, page 521).

The *Portal Lobule* Emphasizes the Exocrine Functions of the Liver

The major exocrine function of the liver is bile secretion. Thus, the morphologic axis of the **portal lobule** is the interlobular bile duct of the portal triad of the "classic" lobule. Its outer margins are imaginary lines drawn between the three central veins that are closest to that portal triad (Fig. 17.3). This defines a roughly triangular block of tissue that includes those portions of three classic lobules that secrete the bile that drains into its axial bile duct. This concept allows description of hepatic parenchymal structure in terms comparable to those used for other exocrine glands.

The *Liver Acinus* Provides the Best Correlation Among Blood Perfusion, Metabolic Activity, and Liver Pathology

The liver acinus, variously described as diamond shaped or lozenge shaped, is the smallest functional unit in the hepatic parenchyma. The *short axis* of the acinus is defined by the terminal branches of the portal triad that lie along the border between two "classic" lobules. The *long axis* is a line drawn between the two central veins closest to the short axis (Figs. 17.3 and 17.4).

This concept allows description of the exocrine secretory function of the liver in terms comparable to those derived form the portal lobule. More importantly, it allows description and interpretation of patterns of degeneration, regeneration, and specific toxic effects in the liver parenchyma relative to the degree or quality of vascular perfusion of the hepatic cells.

The hepatocytes in each liver acinus are described as being arranged in three concentric elliptical zones surrounding the short axis. Thus,

- Zone 1 is closest to the axis.
- Zone 3 is farthest from the axis and closest to the terminal hepatic vein (Fig. 17.4).
- Zone 2 lies between zones 1 and 3 but has no sharp boundaries.

The cells in zone 1 are the first to receive both nutrients and toxins in the blood and are the first to show morphologic changes following bile duct occlusion (bile stasis). These cells are also the last to die, if circulation is impaired, and the first to regenerate. The cells in zone 3, on the other hand, are the first to show ischemic necrosis (centrilobular necrosis) in situations of reduced perfusion and the first to show fat accumulation. They are the last to respond to toxic substances and to bile stasis. Normal variations in enzyme activity, the number and size of cytoplasmic organelles, and the size of cytoplasmic glycogen deposits are also seen between zones 1 and 3. The cells in zone 2 have functional and morphologic characteristics and responses intermediate to (between) those of zones 1 and 3.

Having presented three ways of describing the basic morphologic unit of the liver parenchyma, it is now necessary to examine the cells and tissues that make up that unit.

Blood Vessels of the Parenchyma

The blood vessels that occupy the portal canals are called **interlobular vessels.** Only the interlobular vessels that form the smallest portal triads send blood into the sinusoids. The larger interlobular vessels branch into distributing vessels that are located at the periphery of the lobule. These dis-

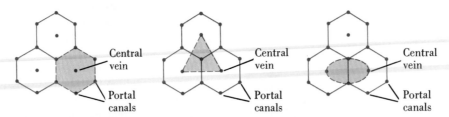

Figure 17.3. Comparison of the different interpretations of liver lobules (shown in blue). The classic lobule **(left)** has the central vein at the center of the lobule and the portal canals at the peripheral angles of the lobule. The portal lobule **(center)** has a portal canal at the center of the lobule and central veins at the peripheral angles of the lobule. The liver acinus **(right)** has distributing vessels at the equator and central veins at each pole. (Based on Weiss L: *Histology,* 5th ed. New York, Elsevier, 1983, p 713.)

tributing vessels send inlet vessels to the sinusoids (Fig. 17.1). In the sinusoids, the blood flows centripetally toward the central vein. The central vein courses through the central axis of the classic liver lobule, becoming larger as it progresses through the lobule and empties into a ***sublobular vein.*** Several sublobular veins converge to form larger ***hepatic veins*** that empty into the inferior vena cava.

The ***portal vein*** and its branches within the liver have a structure typical of veins in general. The lumen is much larger than that of the artery associated with it. The ***hepatic artery*** has a structure typical of other arteries, i.e., a thick muscular wall. In addition to providing arterial blood directly to the sinusoids, it provides arterial blood to the connective tissue and other structures in the larger portal ca-

nals. Capillaries in these larger portal canals return the blood to the interlobular veins before those veins empty into the sinusoid.

The ***central vein*** is a thin-walled vessel receiving blood from the hepatic sinusoids. The endothelial lining of the central vein is surrounded by small amounts of spirally arranged connective tissue fibers. The central vein, so named because of its central position in the classic lobule, is actually the terminal venule of the system of hepatic veins and, thus, is more properly called the ***terminal hepatic venule.*** The sublobular vein, the vessel that receives blood from the terminal hepatic venules, has a distinct layer of connective tissue fibers, both collagenous and elastic, just external to the endothelium. The sublobular veins as well as

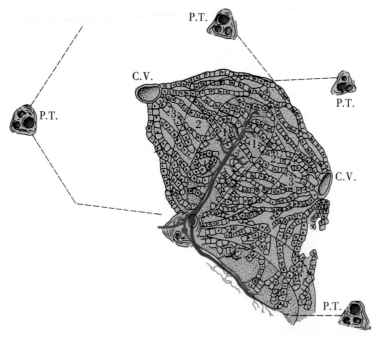

Figure 17.4. The liver acinus is a functional interpretation of liver organization. It consists of adjacent sectors of neighboring hexagonal fields of classic lobules (see Fig. 17.3) partially separated by distributing blood vessels. The zones marked *1, 2,* and *3* are supplied with blood that is most oxygenated and richest in nutrients in *zone 1* and least so in *zone 3*. The central veins *(C.V.)* in this interpretation are at the edges of the acinus instead of in the center, as in the classical lobule. The vessels of the portal space, namely, branches of the portal vein and hepatic artery that, along with the smallest bile ducts, make up the portal triad *(P.T.)*, are shown at some corners of the hexagon that outlines the cross-sectioned profile of the classic lobule. (Based on Rappaport AM, et al: *Anatomical Record* 119:11, 1954.)

the hepatic veins into which they drain travel alone. Being solitary vessels, they can readily be distinguished in a histologic section from the portal veins that are members of a triad. There are no valves in hepatic veins.

Sinusoids

Hepatic Sinusoids Are Lined With a Thin Discontinuous Endothelium

The discontinuous sinusoidal endothelium has a discontinuous basal lamina that is absent over large areas. The discontinuity of the endothelium is evident in two ways:

- *Large fenestrae*, without diaphragms, are present in the endothelial cells.
- *Large gaps* are present between neighboring endothelial cells.

Hepatic sinusoids differ from other sinusoids in that a second cell type, the ***stellate sinusoidal macrophage*** or ***Kupffer cell*** (Fig. 17.5), is a regular part of the vessel lining.

Kupffer Cells Belong to the Mononuclear Phagocytic System

Like other members of the mononuclear phagocytic system, Kupffer cells are derived from monocytes. The scan-

ning electron microscope and the transmission electron microscope (TEM) clearly show that the Kupffer cells form part of the lining of the sinusoid, although they had earlier been described as lying on the luminal surface of the endothelial cells. This older histologic description probably derived from the fact that processes of the Kupffer cells occasionally overlap endothelial processes on the luminal side. Kupffer cells do not form junctions with neighboring endothelial cells.

Processes of Kupffer cells often seem to span the sinusoidal lumen and may even partially occlude it. The presence of red cell fragments and iron in the form of ferritin in the cytoplasm of Kupffer cells suggests that they may be involved in the final breakdown of some damaged or senile red blood cells that reach the liver from the spleen. This function is greatly increased after splenectomy and is then essential for red blood cell disposal.

Perisinusoidal Space (Space of Disse)

The Perisinusoidal Space Is the Site of Exchange of Materials Between Blood and Liver Cells

The *perisinusoidal space* lies between the basal surfaces of the hepatocytes and the basal surfaces of the endothelial cells and Kupffer cells that line the sinusoids. Irregular microvillous processes project into this space from the basal plasma membrane of the hepatocytes (Fig. 17.6).

The basal microvillous processes of the hepatocytes in-

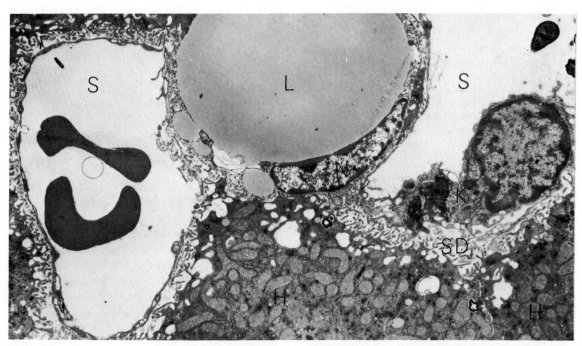

Figure 17.5. Electron micrograph showing two sinusoids *(S)*, one of which displays a sinusoidal macrophage or Kupffer cell *(K)*. The other sinusoid is lined by thin cytoplasmic sheets that belong to endothelial cells. Surrounding each sinusoid is the perisinusoidal space of Disse *(SD)*, which contains numerous hepatocyte *(H)* microvilli. Also seen in the space of Disse is a cell (Ito cell) with a large lipid droplet. This is a lipocyte *(L)*. Its nucleus *(N)* is shaped to conform to the curve of the lipid droplet. ×6600.

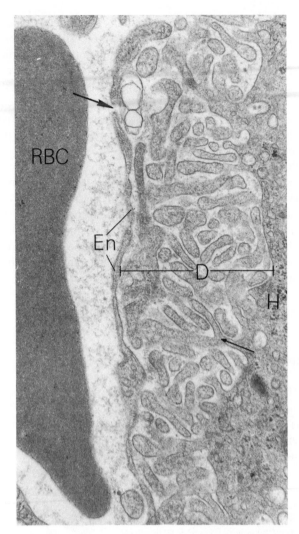

Figure 17.6. Electron micrograph showing the perisinusoidal space of Disse *(D)* between hepatocyte *(H)* and sinusoid. A gap *(large arrow)* separates the endothelial cells *(En)* that line the sinusoid. Such gaps allow for easy passage of small substances between the sinusoid and space of Disse. Numerous microvilli extend from the hepatocytes into the space of Disse. These are long and frequently branch *(small arrow)*. A red blood cell (RBC) is within the sinusoid. ×18,000.

crease the surface area available for exchange of materials between hepatocytes and plasma by as much as 6 times. Because of the large gaps in the endothelial layer and the absence of a continuous basal lamina, there is no significant barrier between the blood plasma in the sinusoid and the hepatocyte plasma membrane that forms the parenchymal border of the perisinusoidal space. Proteins and lipoproteins synthesized by the hepatocyte (see Table 17.2) are transferred into the blood in the perisinusoidal space. This is the pathway for the endocrine secretions of the liver.

A third cell type, the *lipocyte* or *adipose* cell (commonly called an Ito cell), is found in the perisinusoidal space. These cells have been shown to be the primary storage site for vitamin A; the vitamin is transported from the liver to the retina, where it is used in the synthesis of the visual pig-

ments. For many years and in many countries, fish liver oils (e.g., cod liver oil) have been medically and economically important nutritional sources of vitamin A.

When depleted of lipid, these cells resemble fibroblasts; many investigators believe that they secrete the fine type III collagen fibers *(reticular fibers)* that can be found in the space of Disse and that constitute the only stroma of the parenchymal portion of the lobule. This fine perisinusoidal reticular stroma is continuous with the connective tissue of the portal space and the connective tissue surrounding the central vein. An increase in the amount of perisinusoidal stroma is an early sign of hepatic response to toxins and can, with continued insult, lead to fibrosis.

In the fetal liver, the space between blood vessels and hepatocytes contains islands of blood-forming cells. In cases of chronic anemia in the adult, blood-forming cells may appear again in the perisinusoidal space.

Lymphatic Pathway

Hepatic Lymph Originates in the Perisinusoidal Space

Plasma that remains in the perisinusoidal space drains to the periportal connective tissue where a small space, the *space of Mall* (see Fig. 17.9*b*), is described between the stroma of the portal canal and the outermost hepatocytes. From this collecting site, the fluid then enters lymphatic capillaries that travel with the other components of the portal triad.

The lymph moves, in progressively larger vessels, in the same direction as the bile, i.e., from the level of the hepatocytes toward the portal canals and, eventually, to the hilum of the liver. About 80% of the hepatic lymph follows this pathway and drains into the thoracic duct, forming the major portion of the thoracic duct lymph.

Hepatocytes

Hepatocytes Make Up the Anastomosing Cell Plates of the Liver Lobule

Hepatocytes are large polygonal cells measuring between 20 and 30 μm in each dimension. They constitute about 80% of the cell population of the liver.

Nuclei of hepatocytes are large and spherical and occupy the center of the cell. Many cells in the adult liver are binucleate; most cells in the adult liver are tetraploid (i.e., they contain the 4*n* amount of DNA). Heterochromatin is present as scattered clumps in the nucleoplasm and as a distinct band under the nuclear envelope. Two or more well-developed nucleoli are present in each nucleus.

Hepatocytes are relatively long lived for cells associated with the digestive system; their average life span is about 5 months. In addition, liver cells are capable of considerable regeneration when liver substance is lost to hepatotoxic processes, disease, or surgery.

The hepatocyte cytoplasm is generally acidophilic. Specific cytoplasmic components may be identified by routine and special staining procedures. These include

- Basophilic regions that represent rough endoplasmic reticulum (rER) and free ribosomes.
- Numerous mitochondria; as many as 800–1000 mitochondria per cell can be demonstrated by vital staining or enzyme histochemistry.
- Large deposits of glycogen can be stained by means of the periodic acid-Schiff (PAS) procedure.
- Lipid droplets of various sizes can be seen after appropriate fixation and Sudan staining.

- Several small Golgi complexes can be seen in each cell after specific staining.

In routinely prepared histologic sections, irregular spaces and round spaces are seen that represent dissolved glycogen and lipid, respectively. Lipid droplets or the spaces left when they were dissolved increase in hepatocytes after injection or ingestion of certain hepatotoxins, including ethanol.

As noted above, the liver cell is polyhedral in shape; for convenience, it is described as having six surfaces, although there may be more. A schematic section of a cuboidal hepatocyte is shown in Figure 17.7. Two of its surfaces appear facing the perisinusoidal space. Two surfaces

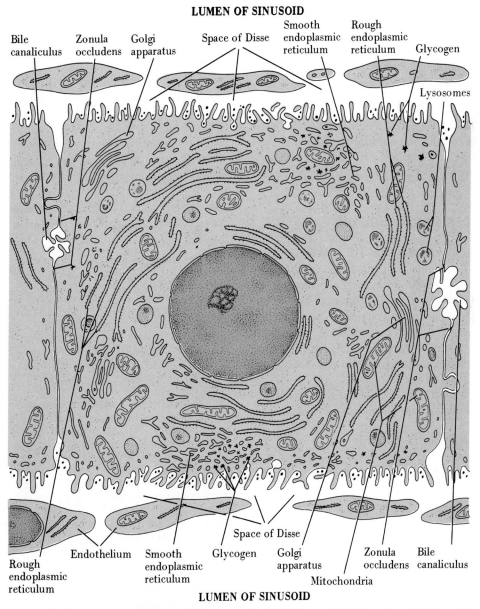

Figure 17.7. Schematic diagram of a hepatocyte showing representative cytoplasmic constituents. Two sides of the cell are shown facing sinusoids; two sides of the cell are shown facing bile canaliculi. Assuming that the cell is cuboidal in shape, the two additional sides of the cell, not shown, would also be facing bile canaliculi.

show the plasma membrane facing its neighbor and facing a bile canaliculus. The remaining two surfaces, parallel to the plane of the page, one above and one below, also face neighboring cells and bile canaliculi. The surfaces that face the perisinusoidal space correspond to the basal surface of other epithelial cells; the surfaces that face neighboring cells and the bile canaliculus correspond to the lateral and apical surfaces, respectively, of other epithelial cells.

Hepatocytes Are Rich in Peroxisomes

Hepatocytes have as many as 200–300 *peroxisomes* per cell. They are relatively large, varying in diameter from 0.2–1.0 μm (see Fig. 17.10*a*). Peroxisomes are involved in the breakdown of hydrogen peroxide produced in many of the general cytoplasmic metabolic activities. In addition, peroxisomes have specific oxidative functions in

- Gluconeogenesis
- Metabolism of purines
- Metabolism of alcohol
- Metabolism of lipids

In fact, about one-half of the ethanol that one might drink is converted to acetaldehyde by enzymes contained in liver peroxisomes. In humans, *catalase* and D-amino acid oxidase, as well as *alcohol dehydrogenase,* are found in peroxisomes.

Smooth Endoplasmic Reticulum

The smooth endoplasmic reticulum (sER) in hepatocytes may be extensive but varies with metabolic activity (see Fig. 17.10). The sER contains enzymes involved in degradation and conjugation of toxins and drugs as well as enzymes responsible for synthesizing cholesterol and the lipid portion of lipoproteins. Under conditions of hepatocyte challenge by drugs, toxins, or metabolic stimulants, the sER may become the predominant organelle in the cell.

Certain Drugs and Hormones Stimulate Increased Activity in the Smooth Endoplasmic Reticulum

In addition to stimulating sER activity, certain drugs and hormones induce synthesis of new sER membranes and their associated enzymes. The sER hypertrophies after the administration of

- Phenobarbital
- Ethanol
- Anabolic steroids and progesterone
- Certain cancer chemotherapeutic agents

Stimulation of the sER by one drug (e.g., ethanol) enhances its ability to detoxify other drugs, certain carcinogens, and some pesticides. On the other hand, metabolism by the sER actually can make some toxic compounds, such as carbon tetrachloride (CCl_4) and 3,4-benzpyrene, more damaging to hepatocytes.

Golgi Apparatus

Examination of hepatocytes with the TEM shows the Golgi complex to be much more elaborate than would have been expected from examining routine histologic preparations. Heavy-metal preparations (Golgi stains) of thick sections of liver give an indication of the extent of the Golgi network.

Transmission Electron Microscopy Demonstrates as Many as 50 Golgi Units in Each Hepatocyte

Each of the Golgi units consists of three to five closely stacked cisternae, many large and small vesicles, and associated lysosomes. These "units" are actually branches of the tortuous Golgi complex seen in heavy-metal preparations. Elements of the Golgi complex concentrated near the bile canaliculus are believed to be associated with the "exocrine" secretion of bile. Golgi cisternae and vesicles near the sinusoidal surfaces of the cell, however, contain electron-dense granules 25–80 nm in diameter that are believed to be very-low-density lipoproteins (VLDL) and other lipoprotein precursors that are subsequently released into the circulation as part of the "endocrine" secretory function of the hepatocytes. Similar dense globules are seen in dilated portions of the sER and, occasionally, in the dilated ends of rER cisternae where they are synthesized.

LIPOPROTEINS

Lipoproteins are multicomponent complexes of proteins and lipids that are involved in the transport of cholesterol and triglycerides in the blood. Cholesterol and triglycerides do not circulate free in the plasma because lipids, on their own, would be unable to remain in suspension. The association of the protein with the lipid-containing core makes the complex sufficiently hydrophilic to be suspended in the plasma.

Five classes of lipoproteins, from largest and least dense to smallest and most dense, have been defined by their characteristic density, molecular weight, size, and chemical composition: chylomicrons; very-low-density lipoproteins (VLDL); intermediate-density lipoproteins (IDL); low-density lipoproteins (LDL); and high-density lipoproteins (HDL). High levels of LDL are directly correlated with increased risk of developing cardiovascular disease; high levels of HDL or low levels of LDL have been associated with decreased risk. The lipoproteins serve a variety of functions in cellular membranes and in the transport and metabolism of lipids. Precursors of the lipoproteins are produced in hepatocytes. The lipid component is produced in the sER; the protein component, in the rER. The lipoprotein complexes pass to the Golgi where secretory vesicles containing electron-dense lipoprotein particles bud off and then are released into the plasma at the cell surface bordering the perisinusoidal space.

Lysosomes Concentrated Near the Bile Canaliculus Correspond to the Peribiliary Dense Bodies Seen in Histologic Sections

Hepatocyte lysosomes are so heterogeneous that they may be identified positively, even at the TEM level, only by histochemical means. They have varied contents including

- Pigment granules (lipofuscin)
- Partially digested cytoplasmic organelles
- Myelin figures

Hepatocyte lysosomes may also be a normal storage site for iron (as a ferritin complex) and a site of iron accumulation in certain storage diseases. Lysosomes increase in a number of pathologic conditions ranging from simple obstructive bile stasis to viral hepatitis and anemia. It is noteworthy, however, that over a very wide range of normal liver function, specifically bile secretion rate, there are no statistically significant morphologic changes in the Golgi complex and lysosomes of the peribiliary cytoplasm.

Biliary Tree

The system of conduits of increasing diameter that bile flows through from the hepatocytes to the gallbladder as well as the intestine is called the biliary tree. The smallest branches of this system are the canaliculi into which the hepatocytes secrete the bile.

The Bile Canaliculus Is a Small Canal Formed by Grooves in Neighboring Cells

The *canaliculus* contains short, irregular microvilli from the hepatocyte. It is sealed by zonulae occludentes, which prevent its contents from escaping into the adjacent intercellular space. The bile canaliculi form a ring about the hepatocyte (Fig. 17.8) and constitute a network that drains into small bile ducts, the *canals of Hering* (Fig. 17.9); these, in turn, drain into the bile ducts of the portal canals. Thus, *liver cells are organized for easy exchange of substances with the blood and for the delivery of bile to the duodenum through a system of canaliculi and ducts.*

Bile Canaliculi Are Formed by Apposed Grooves in the Surface of Adjacent Hepatocytes

In three dimensions, bile canaliculi may form a complete loop around four sides of the idealized six-sided hepatocytes (Fig. 17.8). They range in diameter from 0.5 to 1.5 μm and are isolated from the rest of the intercellular compartment by junctional complexes consisting of tight junctions, zonulae adherentes, gap junctions, and desmosomes. Microvillous processes of the two adjacent hepatocytes extend into the canalicular lumen. Adenosine triphosphatase

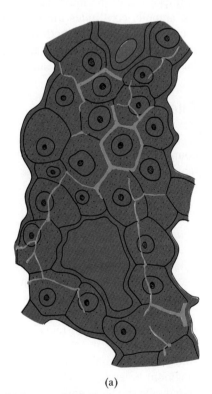

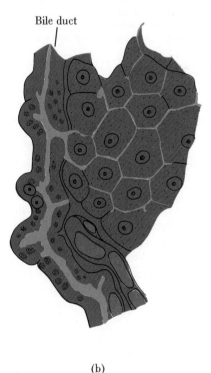

(a)   (b)

Figure 17.8. Network of bile canaliculi demonstrated by intravenous injection of indigo carmine. Some bile canaliculi are clearly seen to form a band (green) about the hepatocyte in **a** and **b.** In **b,** bile canaliculi are seen draining into a bile duct at the periphery of the lobule. (Special preparation fixed in potassium chloride-formol; frozen section mounted in glycerin). (Based on Elias H: *American Journal of Anatomy* 85:379, 1949.)

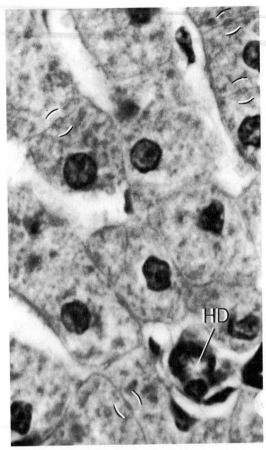

Figure 17.9. a. Light micrograph of liver cells and a small bile duct *(HD)*. Because this duct is still surrounded by hepatocytes, it is called an intralobular canal or canal (ductule) of Hering. The *parentheses* mark cross-sectioned bile canaliculi. ×1240.

(ATPase) and other alkaline phosphatases can be localized on the plasma membranes of the canaliculi, suggesting that bile secretion into this space is an active process.

Bile Flow in the Canaliculi Is *Centrifugal*

The flow of bile is in a direction opposite to the flow of blood, i.e., from the region of the central vein toward the portal canal. Near the portal canal, but still within the lobule, bile canaliculi join to form small **ductules,** the *canals of Hering* (Fig. 17.9*a*), that are lined with cuboidal cells that are not hepatocytes. The ductule epithelium is subtended by a complete basal lamina, as is the rest of the distal biliary tree.

Intrahepatic Bile Ducts

The ductules, which have a diameter of about 1.5 μm, carry the bile through the boundary of the lobule to the *interlobular bile ducts* that form part of the portal triad (Fig. 17.9*b*). These ducts range from 15 to 40 μm in diameter

and are lined by an epithelium that is cuboidal near the lobules and gradually becomes columnar as the ducts near the porta hepatis. The columnar cells have well-developed microvilli, as do those of the extrahepatic bile ducts and the gallbladder. As the bile ducts get larger, they gradually acquire a dense connective tissue investment containing numerous elastic fibers. Smooth muscle cells appear in this connective tissue as the ducts near the hilum. Interlobular ducts join to form the right and left *lobar ducts* that, in turn, join at the hilum to form the *common hepatic duct* (Fig. 17.11).

Extrahepatic Bile Ducts

Extrahepatic Bile Ducts Carry the Bile to the Gallbladder and Intestine

The *common hepatic duct* is about 3 cm long and is lined with tall columnar epithelial cells that closely resemble those of the gallbladder as described below. All of the layers of the alimentary canal (see page 441) are represented in the duct, except for a muscularis mucosae. The *cystic duct* connects the common hepatic duct to the gallbladder and carries bile both *into* and *out of* the *gallbladder*. Distal to the junction with the cystic duct, the fused duct is called the *common bile duct* and extends for about 7 cm to the wall of the duodenum at the *ampulla of Vater*. A thickening of the muscularis externa of the duodenum at the ampulla constitutes the *sphincter of Oddi,* which surrounds the openings of both the common bile duct and the *pancreatic duct* (see below) and acts as a valve to regulate the flow of bile and pancreatic juice into the duodenum.

Bile

The composition of bile and the functions of most of its components are indicated in Table 17.1. As noted in the table, many components of the bile are recycled via the portal circulation.

- About 90% of the *bile salts,* a component of bile, is reabsorbed by the gut and transported back to the liver in the portal blood. The bile salts are then reabsorbed and resecreted by the hepatocytes. Lost bile salts are replaced by new synthesis in the hepatocytes.
- *Cholesterol* and *lecithin,* as well as most of the *electrolytes* and *water* delivered to the gut with the bile, are also reabsorbed and recycled.

Bilirubin glucuronide, the detoxified end product of hemoglobin breakdown, is not recycled. It is ultimately excreted with the feces and gives it its color. Failure to absorb the bilirubin or failure to conjugate it or to secrete the glucuronide can produce *jaundice.*

The adult human liver secretes, on average, about 1 liter

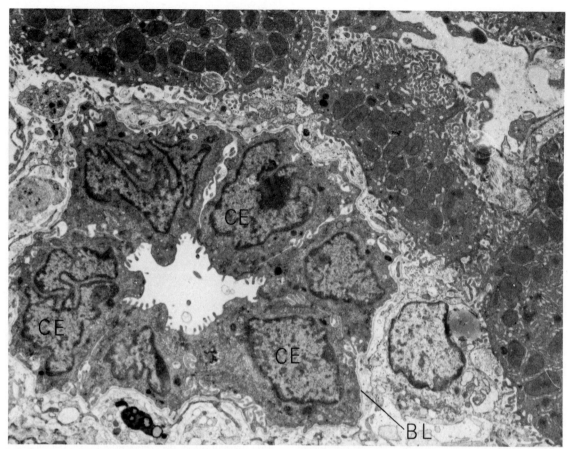

Figure 17.9. **b.** Electron micrograph showing the first portion of a bile duct, the ductule or canal of Hering. The ductule collects bile from the canaliculi. It is close to the hepatocytes, but the actual connection between bile canaliculi and the canal of Hering is not evident in the plane of section. The ductule is composed of cuboidal epithelium *(CE)* with a complete basal lamina *(BL)*. The narrow space in the upper left quadrant of the micrograph, into which microvillous processes of hepatocytes project, is the space of Mall, not the space of Disse. ×6000.

of bile a day. Bile flow from the liver is increased by hormones such as secretin, cholecystokinin (CCK), and gastrin released by the enteroendocrine cells during digestion. The rate of blood flow to the liver and the concentration of bile salts in the blood also exert regulatory effects on the flow. Bile that leaves the liver via the common hepatic duct flows through the cystic duct to the gallbladder. The gallbladder stores and concentrates the bile up to 10 times (see below). Following hormonal stimulation, the gallbladder contracts and delivers the bile to the duodenum via the common bile duct.

Nerves of the Liver

The liver receives nerves from both sympathetic and parasympathetic divisions of the autonomic nervous system. The nerves enter the liver at the porta hepatis and ramify through the liver in the portal canals along with the members of the portal triad. Sympathetic fibers are believed to innervate blood vessels; parasympathetic fibers are assumed to innervate the large ducts (those that contain smooth muscle in their walls) and possibly blood vessels.

Cell bodies of parasympathetic neurons are often seen near the porta hepatis.

GALLBLADDER

The gallbladder is a pear-shaped organ (Fig. 17.11); it is a distensible sac with a volume of about 50 mL in humans. It is attached to the posteroinferior surface of the liver. The gallbladder is a secondary derivative of the embryonic foregut, arising as an evagination of the primitive bile duct that connects the embryonic liver to the developing intestine.

The Gallbladder Concentrates and Stores Bile

The gallbladder is a blind pouch that leads, via a neck, to the cystic duct. Through this duct it receives dilute bile from the hepatic duct. After stimulation by hormones secreted by the enteroendocrine cells of the small intestine in response to the presence of fat in the proximal duodenum, contractions of the smooth muscle of the gallbladder result

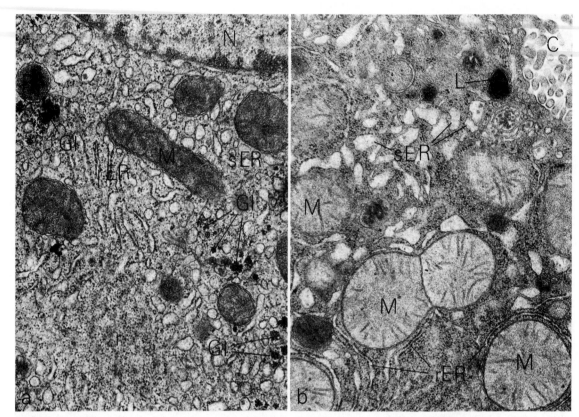

Figure 17.10. Electron micrographs. **a** shows typical cytoplasmic constituents near the nucleus *(N)* of a hepatocyte. These include a peroxisome *(P)*, mitochondria *(M)*, glycogen *(Gl)*, smooth endoplasmic reticulum *(sER)*, and rough endoplasmic reticulum *(rER)*. In the lower left, the membranes of the rER have been cut in a tangential plane showing the ribosomes *(r)* on the cytoplasmic face of the membrane. **b** shows a region of cytoplasm near a canaliculus *(C)*. It includes a lysosome *(L)*, mitochondria *(M)*, and endoplasmic reticulum, both sER and rER. Note the numerous microvilli in the canaliculus. ×18,000.

in discharge of concentrated bile into the common bile duct through which it is carried to the duodenum.

Mucosa

The empty or partially filled gallbladder has numerous deep mucosal folds (Fig. 17.12). The mucosal surface consists of a simple columnar epithelium. The tall epithelial cells exhibit the following features

- Numerous, well-developed *apical microvilli*
- *Apical junctional complexes* that join adjacent cells and form a barrier between the lumen and the intercellular compartment
- Localized *concentrations of mitochondria* in the apical and basal cytoplasm
- Complex *lateral plications* (Fig. 17.13)

In these characteristics, as well as in the localization of Na⁺-K⁺-activated ATPase on the lateral plasma membrane (see Fig. 1.3, page 7) and the presence of secretory vesicles filled with glycoproteins in the apical cytoplasm, these cells closely resemble the absorptive cells of the intestine (see page 457).

The lamina propria of the mucosa is particularly rich in fenestrated capillaries and small venules, but there are *no lymphatic vessels* in this layer. The lamina propria is also very cellular, containing large numbers of lymphocytes and plasma cells. The characteristics of the lamina propria resemble the situation in the colon, another organ specialized for the absorption of electrolytes and water.

Mucin-secreting glands are sometimes seen in the lamina propria in normal human gallbladders, especially near the neck of the organ, but are more commonly found in inflamed gallbladders. Cells that appear identical with enteroendocrine cells of the intestine are also found in these glands.

Muscularis Externa, Adventitia, and Serosa

External to the lamina propria is a muscularis externa that has numerous collagen and elastic fibers among the bundles of smooth muscle cells. Despite its origin from a foregut-derived tube, the gallbladder does not have a muscularis mucosae or a submucosa. The smooth muscle bundles are somewhat randomly oriented, unlike the layered

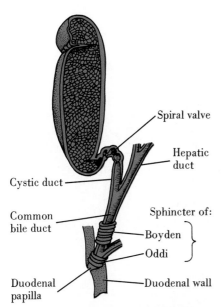

Figure 17.11. Schematic diagram of gallbladder and its ducts. The gallbladder is a blind pouch joined to a single cystic duct. Thickenings in this duct are called the spiral valve. The cystic duct joins with the hepatic duct, and together they form a common bile duct that leads to the duodenum. At the entry to the duodenum, the common bile duct is joined by the pancreatic duct, and together they enter the duodenum at the duodenal papilla. Sphincters guard the common bile duct (Boyden) and the common opening of this and the pancreatic duct (Oddi). (Based on Grant JCB: *A Method of Anatomy,* 10th ed. Baltimore, Williams & Wilkins, 1980, p 165.)

organization of the intestine. Contraction of the smooth muscle reduces the volume of the bladder, forcing its contents out through the cystic duct.

External to the muscularis externa is a thick layer of dense connective tissue (Fig. 17.12). This layer contains large blood vessels, an extensive lymphatic network, and the autonomic nerves that innervate the muscularis externa and the blood vessels (cell bodies of parasympathetic neurons are found in the wall of the cystic duct). The connective tissue is also rich in elastic fibers and adipose tissue. Where the gallbladder is attached to the liver surface, this layer is referred to as the **adventitia.** The unattached surface is covered by a serosa or visceral peritoneum consisting of a layer of mesothelium and a thin layer of loose connective tissue.

In addition, deep diverticula of the mucosa, called Rokitansky-Aschoff sinuses, sometimes extend through the muscularis externa (see Plate 86, Fig. 4). They are thought to presage pathologic changes. Bacteria may accumulate in these sinuses, causing chronic inflammation.

Concentration of Bile Requires the Coupled Transport of Salt and Water

The epithelial cells actively transport both Na^+ and Cl^- (and HCO_3^-) from the cytoplasm into the intercellular compartment of the epithelium. Transport ATPase is lo-

cated in the lateral plasma membranes of the epithelial cells. This transport mechanism is essentially identical with that described in Chapter 16 for the enterocytes of the small intestine and the absorptive cells of the colon.

MECHANISM OF FLUID TRANSPORT IN THE GALLBLADDER

The gallbladder actively transports Na^+, Cl^-, and HCO_3^- across the lateral plasma membrane into the intercellular (paracellular) compartment. The increased concentration of electrolytes in the intercellular space creates an osmotic gradient between the intercellular space and the cytoplasm and between the intercellular space and the lumen. Water moves from the cytoplasm and from the lumen into the intercellular space because of the osmotic gradient; i.e., it moves down its concentration gradient (Fig. 17.13*b*). Despite the ability of the intercellular space to distend below the apical junctional complex by loosening of the implicated lateral margins, often to a degree visible with the LM, it is nevertheless of limited distensibility. The movement of electrolytes and water into the space creates a hydrostatic pressure that forces a nearly isotonic fluid out of the intercellular compartment into the subepithelial connective tissue (the lamina propria). The fluid that enters the lamina propria quickly passes into the numerous fenestrated capillaries and the venules that closely underlie the epithelium. Studies of fluid transport in the gallbladder first demonstrated the essential role of the intercellular compartment in explaining the morphologic basis of transepithelial transport of an isotonic fluid from the lumen to the vasculature.

In some individuals, there are ducts, the **ducts of Luschka,** located in the connective tissue between the liver and the gallbladder, near the neck of the gallbladder. These connect with the cystic duct, not with the lumen of the gallbladder. They are histologically similar to the intrahepatic bile ducts and may be remnants of aberrant embryonic bile ducts.

PANCREAS

The Pancreas Is an Exocrine and Endocrine Gland

Unlike the liver, in which the exocrine and endocrine functions reside in the same cell, the pancreas restricts the functions to two structurally distinct components in the gland.

- The *exocrine component* is a serous gland that synthesizes and secretes, into the duodenum, enzymes that are essential for digestion in the intestine.
- The *endocrine component* synthesizes and secretes, into the blood, **insulin** and **glucagon,** hormones that regulate glucose, lipid, and protein metabolism in the whole body.

The exocrine pancreas is a continuum throughout the organ

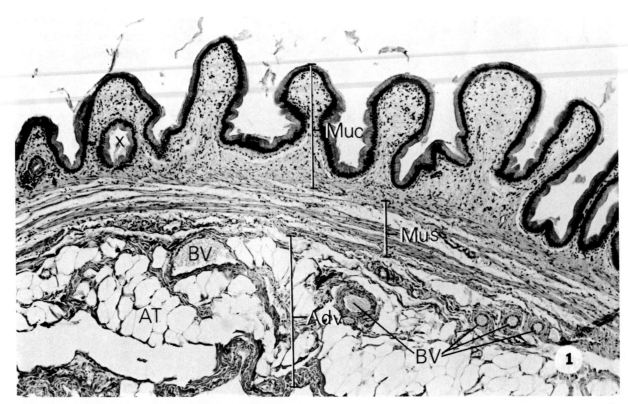

Figure 17.12. Light micrograph of gallbladder. The mucosa (*Muc*) consists of a lining of columnar epithelial cells and a lamina propria of loose connective tissue with many fenestrated capillaries and venules. Under this is a thin muscular layer (*Mus*), and external to the muscle is an adventitia (*Adv*) containing adipose tissue (*AT*) and blood vessels (*BV*). The portion of the gallbladder not attached to the liver will show a typical serosa instead of an adventitia. ×75.

within which the endocrine pancreas called *islets of Langerhans* is dispersed as distinct cell masses.

ANATOMIC RELATIONSHIPS OF THE PANCREAS

The pancreas is an elongate gland with a head, body, and tail. The **head** is an expanded portion that lies in the C-shaped curve of the duodenum (Fig. 17.14). It is joined to the duodenum by connective tissue. The centrally located **body** of the pancreas crosses the midline of the human body, and the **tail** extends toward the hilum of the spleen. The **pancreatic duct (duct of Wirsung)** extends through the length of the gland and empties into the duodenum at the **ampulla of Vater** (through which the common bile duct from the liver and gallbladder also enters the duodenum). In some individuals, there is also an accessory pancreatic duct, a vestige of the fact that the pancreas forms from two embryonic primordia that evaginate from the foregut.

A thin layer of loose connective tissue forms a capsule for the gland. From this capsule, septa extend into the gland, dividing it into ill-defined lobules. Within the lobules, a stroma of loose connective tissue surrounds the parenchymal units. Between the lobules, larger amounts of connective tissue surround the larger ducts, blood vessels, and nerve fibers. Moreover, in the connective tissue surrounding the pancreatic duct, there are small mucous glands that empty into the duct.

Exocrine Pancreas

The exocrine pancreas is a serous gland that closely resembles the parotid gland, with which it can be confused. The secretory units are acinar or tubuloacinar in shape and are formed by a simple epithelium of pyramidal serous cells (Fig. 17.15). The cells have a narrow free (luminal) surface and a broad basal surface. Periacinar connective tissue is minimal.

The serous secretory cells of the acinus produce the digestive enzyme precursors secreted by the pancreas. Pancreatic acini are unique among glandular acini, in that the initial duct that leads from the acinus, the intercalated duct, actually begins within the acinus (Fig. 17.15). The duct cells located inside the acinus are referred to as *centroacinar cells.*

The acinar cells are characterized by a distinct basophilia in the subnuclear cytoplasm and by the presence of acidophilic *zymogen granules* in the apical cytoplasm (Fig. 17.15). Zymogen granules are more numerous in the pancreas of fasting animals. The squamous centroacinar cells lack both ergastoplasm and secretory granules; thus, they stain very lightly with eosin. This weak staining is an aid to their identification in routine histologic sections.

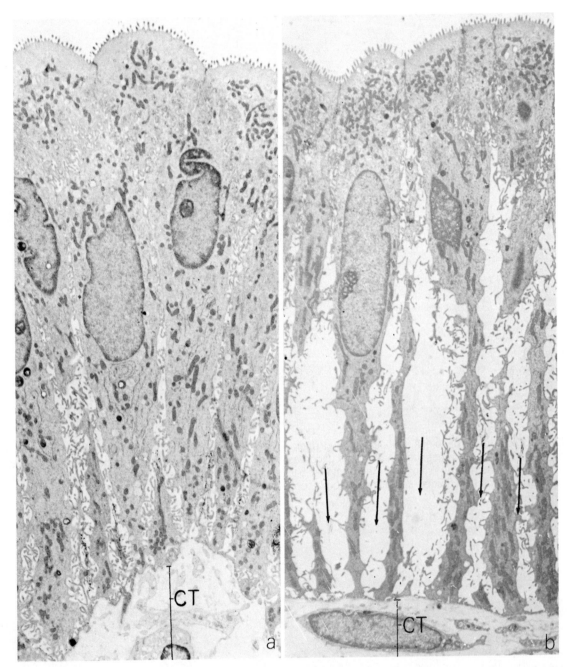

Figure 17.13. Electron micrographs of gallbladder epithelium. **a.** The tall columnar cells display features typical of absorptive cells, with microvilli on their apical surface, an apical junctional complex separating the lumen of the gallbladder from the lateral intercellular space, and apical concentrations of mitochondria. **b.** During active fluid transport, salt is pumped from the cytoplasm into the intercellular space, and water follows the salt. Both salt and water then diffuse into the cell from the lumen. This process continues so that the intercellular space becomes greatly distended *(arrows)*. Fluid moves from the engorged intercellular space across the basal lamina into the underlying connective tissue *(CT)* and then into blood vessels. The increase in size of the lateral intercellular space during active fluid transport is sufficient to be evident with the LM.

Zymogen Granules Contain a Variety of Digestive Enzymes in an Inactive Form

Pancreatic enzymes are capable of digesting most food substances. The inactive enzymes or proenzymes contained in pancreatic zymogen granules are listed below along with the specific substances they digest when activated.

- *Trypsinogen, pepsinogen,* and *procarboxypeptidase* digest proteins.
- *Amylase* digests carbohydrates.
- *Lipase* digests lipids.
- *Deoxyribonuclease and ribonuclease* digest nucleic acids.

The pancreatic digestive enzymes are activated only af-

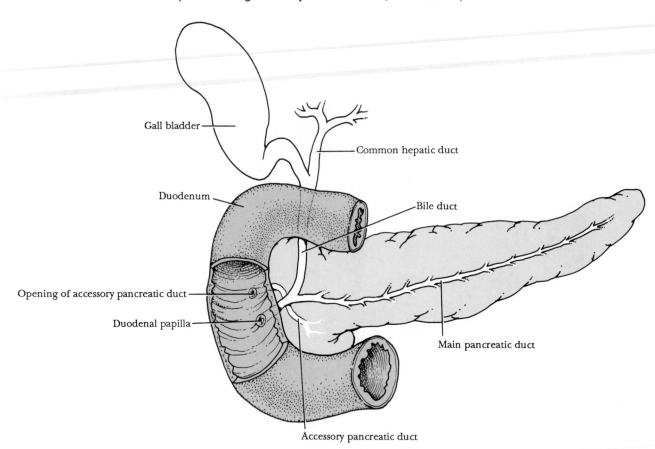

Figure 17.14. Diagram of pancreas, duodenum, and ducts. The main pancreatic duct traverses the length of the pancreas and enters the duodenum after joining with the common bile duct. An accessory pancreatic duct is sometimes also present, as shown. The site of duct entry is typically marked by a papilla on the inner surface of the duodenum. (Based on Grant JCB: *A Method of Anatomy,* 10th ed. Baltimore, Williams & Wilkins, 1980, p 173.)

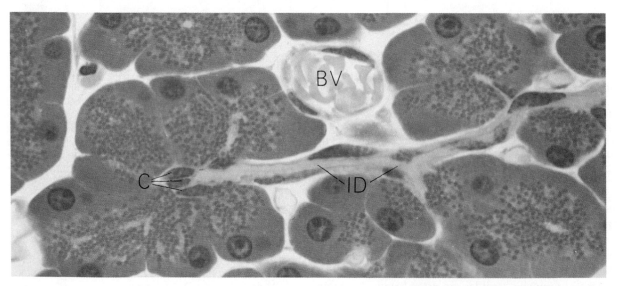

Figure 17.15. Plastic section (light micrograph) of a pancreatic acinus and the intercalated duct *(ID)* leading from it. The duct can be seen beginning within the acinus. The cells forming the duct within the acinus are known as centroacinar cells *(C)*. The acidophilic zymogen granules are clearly seen in the apical cytoplasm. *BV,* blood vessel.

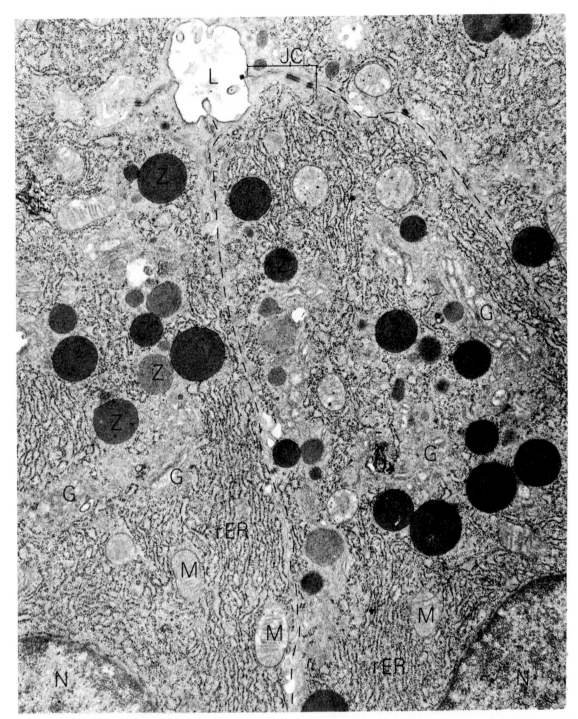

Figure 17.16. Electron micrograph of the apical cytoplasm of several pancreatic acinar cells. (One of the cells is outlined by the *broken line*.) Nuclei *(N)* of adjoining cells are evident at the bottom left and right of the micrograph. The apical cytoplasm contains rER, some mitochondria *(M)*, the zymogen se-cretory granules *(Z)*, and profiles of Golgi apparatus *(G)*. At the apices of the cells, a lumen *(L)* is present into which the zymogen granules are discharged. A junctional complex *(JC)* is also evident near the lumen. ×20,000.

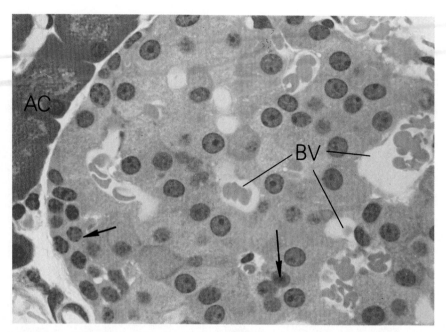

Figure 17.17.   Light micrograph of islet of Langerhans. Identification of specific cell types without special stains is difficult. At best, one can identify small cells *(arrows)* at the periphery of the cell mass, i.e., in proximity to the adjacent connective tissue, that are probably A cells. *AC,* acinar cells; and *BV,* blood vessels.

ter they reach the lumen of the small intestine. Initially, the proteolytic activity of enzymes *(enterokinases)* in the glycocalyx of the microvilli of the intestinal absorptive cells converts trypsinogen to **trypsin,** a potent proteolytic enzyme. Trypsin then catalyzes the conversion of the other inactive enzymes as well as the digestion of proteins in the chyme.

The cytoplasmic basophilia of the pancreatic acinar cells when observed in the TEM appears as an extensive array of rER and free ribosomes. This correlates with the high level of protein synthetic activity of the acinar cells (Fig. 17.16). A well-developed Golgi complex is present in the supranuclear zone and is involved in concentration and "packaging" of the secretory products. Mitochondria are small and, although found throughout the cell, are concentrated among the rER cisternae. Acinar cells are joined to one another by junctional complexes at their apical poles, thus forming an isolated lumen into which small microvilli extend from the apical surfaces of the acinar cells and into which the zymogen granules are released by exocytosis.

Duct System

The centroacinar cells (Fig. 17.15) are the beginning of the duct system of the exocrine pancreas. They have a centrally placed nucleus and attenuated cytoplasm, forming a squamous cell.

Centroacinar Cells Are *Intercalated Duct Cells* Located in the Acinus

Centroacinar cells are continuous with the cells of the short **intercalated duct** that lies outside the acinus. The

TABLE 17.3. Principal Cell Types in Pancreatic Islets

CELL TYPE	%	CYTOPLASMIC STAINING WITH MALLORY-AZAN	PRODUCT	GRANULES (TEM)
A	15–20	Red	Glucagon	About 250 nm; dense, eccentric core surrounded by light substance
B	60–70	Brownish orange	Insulin	About 300 nm; many with dense, crystalline (angular) core surrounded by light substance
D	5–10	Blue	Somatostatin	About 325 nm; homogeneous matrix

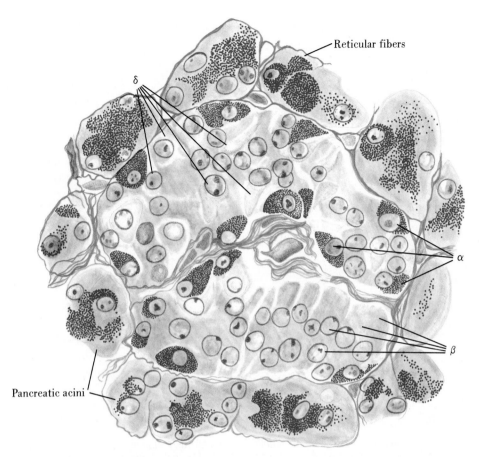

Reticular fibers

δ

α

β

Pancreatic acini

Figure 17.18. Diagram of islet of Langerhans, Mallory-Azan stain. A cells (α) display red cytoplasmic staining; B cells (β) (comprising most of the islet cells) display brownish-orange staining (see Table 17.3) but are indicated in this figure as pale gray-green staining; and D cells (δ) show a blue cytoplasm.

structural unit of the acinus and centroacinar cells resembles a balloon (the acinus) into which a drinking straw (the intercalated duct) has been pushed. The intercalated ducts are short and drain to *intralobular collecting ducts. There are no striated (secretory) ducts in the pancreas.*

The complex, branching network of intralobular ducts drains to the larger *interlobular ducts,* which are lined with a low columnar epithelium in which enteroendocrine cells and occasional goblet cells may be found. The interlobular ducts, in turn, drain directly into the *main pancreatic duct,* which runs the length of the gland parallel to its long axis, giving this portion of the duct system a herringbone-like appearance (see Fig. 17.14). A second large duct, the *ductus choledochus (accessory pancreatic duct)* arises in the head of the pancreas.

The Intercalated Ducts Add Bicarbonate and Water to the Exocrine Secretion

The pancreas secretes about 1 liter of fluid per day, about equal to the initial volume of the hepatic bile secretion. Whereas the bile is concentrated in the gallbladder, the entire volume of the pancreatic secretion is delivered to the duodenum. While the acini secrete a small volume of pro-tein-rich fluid, the intercalated duct cells secrete a large volume of fluid rich in sodium and bicarbonate (HCO_3^-). The bicarbonate serves to neutralize the acidity of the chyme that enters the duodenum from the stomach and to establish the optimum pH for the activity of the major pancreatic enzymes.

Hormonal Control of Exocrine Secretion

Two hormones secreted by the enteroendocrine cells of the duodenum, *secretin and CCK,* also called *pancreozymin,* are the principal regulators of the exocrine pancreas (see Tables 16.1 and 16.2). The entry of the acidic chyme into the duodenum stimulates the release of these hormones into the blood.

- *Secretin* is a polypeptide hormone (27 amino acid residues) that stimulates the duct cells to secrete a large volume of fluid with a high HCO_3^- concentration but little or no enzyme content.
- *CCK* is a polypeptide hormone (33 amino acid residues) that causes the acinar cells to secrete their proenzymes.

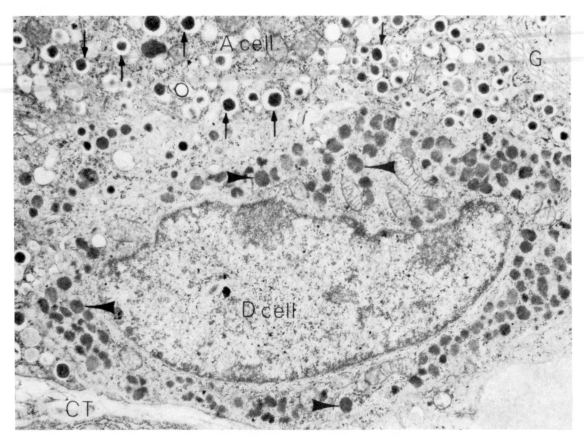

Figure 17.19. Electron micrograph of pancreatic islet cells. The cell in the upper part of the illustration is an A cell. It contains characteristic granules *(arrows)* showing a dense spherical core surrounded by clear area and then a membrane. The A cell also displays a characteristically well-developed Golgi *(G).* The cell in the bottom of the illustration is a D cell. It contains numerous membrane-bounded granules of moderately low density *(arrowheads).* CT, connective tissue. ×15,000.

TABLE 17.4. Minor Cell Types in Pancreatic Islets

CELL TYPE	SECRETION	LOCATION (in Addition to Islet)	ACTIONS
PP cell (F cell)[A]	Pancreatic polypeptide		Stimulates gastric chief cells, inhibits bile secretion and intestinal motility, inhibits pancreatic enzymes and HCO_3^- secretion
D-1 cell	Vasoactive intestinal peptide (VIP)	Also in exocrine acini and duct epithelium[B]	Similar to those of glucagon (hyperglycemic and glycogenolytic); also affects secretory activity and motility in gut; stimulates pancreatic exocrine secretion
EC cell[A]	Secretin, motilin, substance P	Also in exocrine acini and duct epithelium[B]	Secretin—acts locally to stimulate HCO_3^- secretion in pancreatic fluid and pancreatic enzyme secretion; motilin—increases gastric and intestinal motility; substance P—???

[A] PP, protein polypeptide; and EC, enterochromaffin cell.
[B] This localization further emphasizes the ontogeny of the pancreas from the embryonic intestine.

TABLE 17.5. Characteristics of Pancreatic Hormones

HORMONE	MW	STRUCTURE
Insulin	5700–6000	Two protein chains linked by disulfide bridges: α chain, 21 amino acids; β chain, 30 amino acids
Glucagon	3500	Linear polypeptide: 29 amino acids
Somatostatin	1638	Cyclic polypeptide: 14 amino acids
VIP	3300	Linear polypeptide: 28 amino acids
Pancreatic polypeptide	4200	Linear polypeptide

The coordinated action of the two hormones produces the secretion into the duodenum of a large volume of enzyme-rich, alkaline fluid. In addition to hormonal influences, the pancreas also receives autonomic innervation. Sympathetic nerve fibers are involved in regulation of pancreatic blood flow. Parasympathetic fibers stimulate activity of acinar as well as centroacinar cells. Cell bodies of neurons occasionally seen in the pancreas belong to parasympathetic postganglionic neurons.

Endocrine Pancreas

The Endocrine Pancreas Is a Diffuse Organ That Secretes Hormones That Regulate Blood Glucose Levels

The *islets of Langerhans,* the endocrine component of the pancreas, are scattered throughout the organ. The islets constitute about 1–2% of the volume of the pancreas but are most numerous in the tail. Individual islets may contain only a few cells or may contain many hundreds of cells. The polygonal cells are arranged in short, irregular cords that are profusely invested with a network of fenestrated capillaries. The definitive endocrine cells of the islets develop between 9 and 12 weeks of gestation.

In hematoxylin and eosin (H&E)-stained sections, the islets of Langerhans appear as clusters of pale-staining cells surrounded by more intensely staining pancreatic acini. It is not practical to try to identify the several cell types found in the islets in routinely prepared specimens (Fig. 17.17). After Zenker-formol fixation and staining by the Mallory-Azan method, however, it is possible to identify three principal cell types designated A, B, and D cells (Tables 17.3 and Fig. 17.18). With this method, the A cells stain red,

the B cells stain brownish-orange, and the D cells stain blue. About 5% of the cells appear to be unstained after this procedure. TEM allows identification of the principal cell types by the size and density of their secretory granules.

Islet Cells, Other Than the B Cells, Have a Counterpart in the Enteroendocrine Cells of the Gastrointestinal Mucosa

Three principal and three minor islet cell types have been identified by using a combination of the TEM and immunocytochemistry (Tables 17.3 and 17.4). Each cell type can be correlated with a specific hormone, and each has a specific location in the islet.

Principal Cell Types of the Islet

The *B cells* constitute about 70% of the total islet cells in humans and are generally located in its central portion. They secrete *insulin* (Table 17.3). B cells contain numerous secretory granules of about 300-nm diameter with a dense polyhedral core and a pale matrix. The polyhedral core is believed to be crystallized insulin.

The *A cells* constitute about 15–20% of the human islet population and are generally located peripherally in the islets. They secrete *glucagon* (Table 17.3). A cells contain secretory granules of about 250-nm diameter that are more uniform in size and more densely packed in the cytoplasm than the granules of the B cells. The granule is the site of stored glucagon (Fig. 17.19).

The *D cells* constitute about 5–10% of the total pancreatic endocrine tissue and are also located peripherally in the islets. D cells secrete *somatostatin,* which is contained in secretory granules that are larger than those of the A and B cells (300–350 nm) and contain material of low to medium electron density (Fig. 17.19).

The minor islet cells constitute about 5% of the islet tissue and may be equivalent to the pale cells seen after Mallory-Azan staining. Their characteristics and functions are summarized in Table 17.4.

There is evidence that some cells may secrete more than one hormone. Immunocytochemical staining has localized several hormones in addition to glucagon in the cytoplasm of the A cell. These include *gastric inhibitory peptide (GIP), CCK,* and *adrenocorticotropic hormone (ACTH)–endorphin.* Although there is no clear morphologic evidence for the presence of G cells (gastrin cells) in the islets, *gastrin* may also be secreted by one or more of the islet cells. Certain pancreatic islet cell tumors secrete large amounts of gastrin, thereby producing excessive acid secretion in the stomach (Zollinger-Ellison syndrome).

Functions of Pancreatic Hormones

All of the hormones secreted by the endocrine pancreas regulate metabolic functions either systemically, regionally (in the gastrointestinal tract), or locally (in the islet itself).

Insulin, the Major Hormone Secreted by the Islet Tissue, Lowers Blood Glucose

Insulin is the most abundant endocrine secretion. Its principal effects are on the liver, skeletal muscle, and adipose tissue. Insulin stimulates

- *Uptake of glucose* from the circulation
- *Utilization and storage of glucose* by all cells
- *Phosphorylation of glucose* in the cells
- *Synthesis of glycogen* from the phosphorylated glucose

Absence or inadequate amounts of insulin lead to elevated blood glucose levels and the presence of glucose in the urine, a condition known as *diabetes mellitus.*

In addition to its effects on glucose metabolism, insulin stimulates glycerol synthesis in adipose cells and inhibits lipase activity in these cells. Circulating insulin also increases the amount of amino acids taken up by cells (this may involve a cotransport with glucose) and inhibits protein catabolism. Insulin appears to be essential for normal cell growth and function, particularly as demonstrated in tissue culture systems.

Glucagon, Secreted in Amounts Second Only to Insulin, Raises Blood Glucose

The actions of *glucagon* are essentially reciprocal to those of insulin. It stimulates release of glucose into the bloodstream, and stimulates gluconeogenesis (synthesis of glucose from metabolites of amino acids) and glycogenolysis (breakdown of glycogen) in the liver. Glucagon also stimulates proteolysis to promote gluconeogenesis, mobilizes fats from adipose cells, and stimulates hepatic lipase.

Somatostatin is secreted by the D cells of the islets. It is identical with the hormone secreted by the hypothalamus that regulates somatotropin (growth hormone) release from the anterior pituitary gland (see page 603). The precise role of somatostatin in the islets is unclear, but it has been shown to inhibit both insulin and glucagon secretion.

The molecular characteristics of the major and some minor islet hormones are summarized in Table 17.5.

REGULATION OF ISLET ACTIVITY

A blood glucose level *above* the normal 70 mg/100 mL (70 mg/dL) stimulates release of insulin from B cells, leading to uptake and storage of glucose by liver and muscle. The resultant reduction in blood sugar stops insulin secretion. Some amino acids also stimulate insulin secretion, either alone or in concert with elevated blood glucose. Increased blood fatty acid levels will also stimulate insulin release, as will circulating *gastrin, CCK, and secretin.* CCK and *glucagon,* released in the islet by the A cells, act as paracrine secretions to stimulate B-cell secretion of insulin.

Blood glucose levels *below* 70 mg/100 mL (70 mg/dL) stimulate release of glucagon; blood glucose levels significantly *above* 70 mg/100 mL inhibit glucagon secretion. Glucagon is also released in response to low levels of fatty acids in the blood. Insulin inhibits release of glucagon by A cells, but because of the cascading circulation in the islet (see below), this is effected by a hormonal action of insulin carried in the general circulation.

The islets have both sympathetic and parasympathetic innervation. About 10% of the islet cells have nerve endings directly on their plasma membrane. There are well-developed gap junctions between islet cells. Ionic events triggered by synaptic transmitters at the nerve endings are carried from cell to cell across these junctions. Autonomic nerves may have direct effects on hormone secretion by A and B cells.

Parasympathetic (cholinergic) stimulation increases secretion of both insulin and glucagon; sympathetic (adrenergic) stimulation increases glucagon release but inhibits insulin release. This may contribute to the availability of circulating glucose in stress reactions.

INSULIN SYNTHESIS: AN EXAMPLE OF POSTTRANSLATIONAL PROCESSING

Insulin is a small protein consisting of two polypeptide chains joined by disulfide bridges. Its biosynthesis presents a clear example of the importance of posttranslational processing in the achievement of the final, active structure of a protein (see page 28).

Insulin is originally synthesized as a single polypeptide chain with a molecular weight of about 12,000, called *preproinsulin*; this is reduced to a polypeptide with a molecular weight of about 9,000, called *proinsulin,* as the molecule is inserted into the cisternae of the rER. Proinsulin is a single polypeptide chain of 81–86 amino acids that has the approximate shape of the *letter G.* Two disulfide bonds connect the bar of the G to the top loop.

During packaging and storage of the proinsulin in the Golgi complex, a cathepsin-like enzyme cleaves most of the side of the loop, leaving the bar of the G as an *A chain* of 21 amino acids cross-linked by the disulfide bridges to the top of the loop, which becomes the *B chain* of 30 amino acids. The 35 amino acid peptide removed from the loop is called a *C peptide* (connecting peptide). It is stored in the secretory vesicles and released with the insulin in equimolar amounts. No function has been identified for the C peptide.

The Blood Supply of the Pancreas Provides a Cascading Perfusion of the Islets and Acini

Several arterioles enter the periphery of the islets and branch into fenestrated capillaries. In humans, the capillaries first perfuse the A and D cells peripherally before the blood reaches the B cells centrally. Larger vessels that travel in septa that penetrate the central portion of the islet are also accompanied by A and D cells, so that blood reaching the B cells has *always* first perfused the A and D cells.

Large *efferent capillaries* leave the islet and branch into the capillary networks that surround the acini of the exocrine pancreas. This cascading flow resembles the portal systems of other endocrine glands (pituitary, adrenal). Secretions of the islet cells have regulatory effects on the acinar cells:

- Insulin, vasoactive intestinal peptide (VIP), and CCK stimulate exocrine secretion.
- Glucagon, pancreatic polypeptide (PP), and somatostatin inhibit exocrine secretion.

PLATE 83. Liver I

The liver consists of large numbers of functional units called lobules. The classic lobule is traditionally described as roughly cylindrical with a venous channel, the central vein that courses through its long axis. Irregular interconnecting sheets or plate-like arrangements of hepatic cells radiate outward from the central vein and constitute the parenchyma of the lobule. Sinusoids separate the sheets of hepatic cells and empty into the central veins. In the human, the lobules are poorly delineated from their neighbors, and it is often difficult to determine where one lobule ends and the next begins.

FIGURE 1, liver, human, H&E ×65; inset ×65. At the low magnification shown here, large numbers of hepatic cells appear to be uniformly disposed throughout the specimen. The hepatic cells are arranged in plates one cell thick, but when sectioned, they appear as interconnecting cords one or more cells thick according to the plane of section. The sinusoids appear as light areas between the cords of cells; they are more clearly shown in Figure 2 *(asterisks)*.

Also present in this figure is a portal canal. It is a connective tissue septum that carries the branches of the hepatic artery *(HA)* and portal vein *(PV)*, bile ducts *(BD)*, and lymphatic vessels and nerves. The artery and vein, along with the bile duct, are collectively referred to as a portal triad.

The hepatic artery and the portal vein are easy to identify because they are found in relation to one another within the surrounding connective tissue of the portal canal. The vein is typically thin walled; the artery is smaller in diameter and has a thicker wall. The bile ducts are composed of a simple cuboidal or columnar epithelium, depending on the size of the duct. Multiple profiles of the blood vessels and bile ducts may be evident in the canal due to either branching or their passage out of the plane of section and then back in again.

The vessel through which blood leaves the liver is the hepatic vein. It is readily identified because it travels alone **(inset)** and is surrounded by an appreciable amount of connective tissue *(CT)*. If more than one profile of a vein is present within this connective tissue, but no arteries or bile ducts are present, the second vessel will also be a hepatic vein. Such is the case in the **inset,** where a profile of a small hepatic vein is seen just above the larger hepatic vein *(HV)*.

FIGURE 2, liver, human, H&E ×160. The central veins *(CV)* are the most distal radicals of the hepatic vein, and like the hepatic vein, they also travel alone. Their distinguishing features are the sinusoids that penetrate the wall of the vein and the paucity of surrounding connective tissue. These characteristics are shown to advantage in Plate 84.

It is best to examine low-magnification views of the liver to define the boundaries of a lobule. A lobule is best identified when it is cut in cross section. The central vein then appears as a circular profile, and the hepatic cells appear as cords radiating from the central vein. Such a lobule is outlined by the *dotted lines* in Figure 1.

The limits of the lobule are defined, in part, by the portal canal. In other directions, the plates of the lobule do not appear to have a limit; i.e., they have become contiguous with plates of an adjacent lobule. One can estimate the dimensions of the lobule, however, by approximating a circle with the central vein as its center and incorporating those plates that exhibit a radial arrangement up to the point where a portal canal is present. If the lobule has been cross-sectioned, the radial limit is set by the location of one or more of the portal canals as indicated by the bile ducts *(BD)* in this figure.

KEY

BD, bile duct
CT, connective tissue
CV, central vein
HA, hepatic artery
HV, hepatic vein
L, lymphatic nodule
PV, portal vein
asterisks (Fig. 2), blood sinusoids
dotted line (Fig. 1), approximates the limits of a lobule

PLATE 83

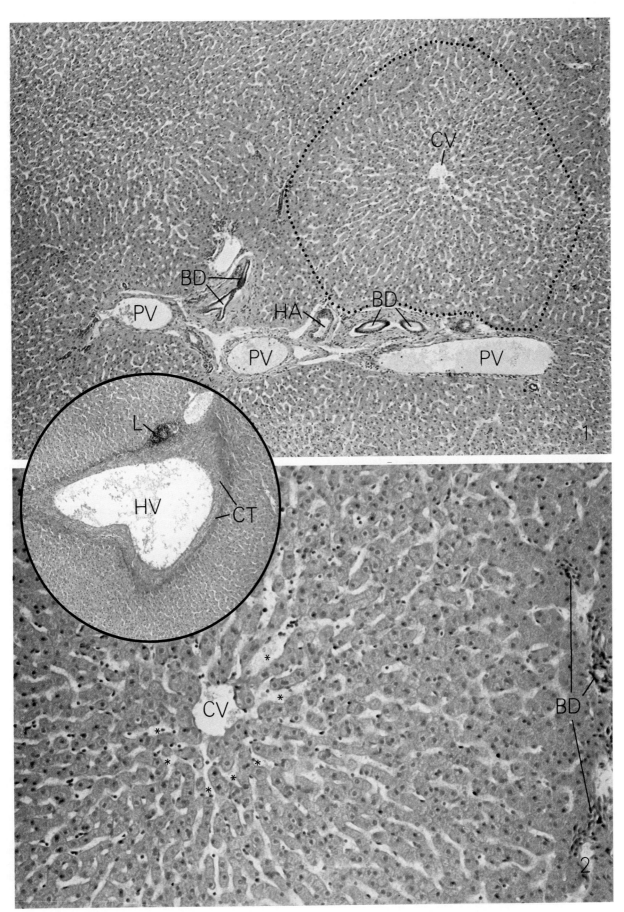

PLATE 84.   Liver II

FIGURE 1, liver, human, H&E ×500; inset ×800. The central vein and surrounding hepatocytes from Figure 2 of Plate 83 are shown here at higher magnification. The cytoplasm of the hepatocytes in this specimen exhibits a foamy appearance due to extraction of glycogen and lipid during tissue preparation. The boundaries between individual hepatocytes are discernible in some locations but not between those cells where the knife has cut across the boundary in an oblique plane. Frequently, when cell boundaries are observed at still higher magnification **(inset)**, a very small circular or oval profile is observed midway along the boundary. These profiles represent the bile canaliculi *(BC)*.

The cells that line the sinusoids *(S)* show little, if any, cytoplasmic detail in routine preparations. Perisinusoidal macrophages [Kupffer cells *(KC)*] are generally recognized by their ovoid nuclei and the projection of the cell into the lumen. The endothelial cell, in contrast, is a squamous cell that has a smaller, attenuated or elongated nucleus. Some nuclei of this description are evident in the micrograph.

The termination of two of the sinusoids and their union with the central vein *(CV)* is indicated by the *curved arrows*. Note that the wall of the vein is strengthened by connective tissue, mostly collagen, that appears as the homogeneous eosin-stained material *(asterisks)*. Fibroblasts *(F)* within this connective tissue can be identified and distinguished from the endothelial cell *(En)* lining of the vein.

FIGURE 2, liver, rat, glutaraldehyde-osmium fixation, toluidine blue ×900. This figure shows a plastic-embedded liver specimen fixed by the method normally used for transmission electron microscopy. In contrast to the H&E-stained preparation, this specimen demonstrates to advantage the cytologic detail of the hepatocytes and the sinusoids *(S)*. The hepatocytes are deeply colored with toluidine blue. Note that the cytoplasm exhibits irregular magenta masses *(arrows)*. This is glycogen that has been retained by the fixation procedure and metachromatically stained by the toluidine blue. (Retention of the glycogen is due to the glutaraldehyde, the initial fixative employed in preserving the specimen.) Also evident are lipid droplets *(L)* of varying size that have been preserved and stained black by the osmium used as the secondary fixative. The quantities of lipid and glycogen are variable and, under normal conditions, reflect dietary intake. Careful examination of the hepatocyte cytoplasm also reveals small, punctate, dark-blue bodies contrasted against the lighter-blue background of the cell. These are the mitochondria. Another feature of this specimen is the clear representation of the bile canaliculi *(BC)* between the liver cells. They appear as empty circular profiles, when cross-sectioned, and as elongate channels (lower right), when longitudinally sectioned.

Examination of the sinusoidal lining cells reveals two distinct cell types. The Kupffer cell *(KC)* is the more prominent cell. These cells exhibit a large nucleus and a substantial amount of cytoplasm. They tend to protrude into the lumen and sometimes give the appearance of occluding the vascular channel. Though a Kupffer cell may span the lumen, it actually does not block the channel. The surface of the Kupffer cell exhibits a very irregular or jagged contour due to the numerous processes that provide the cell with an extensive surface area. The endothelial cell *(En)* has a smaller nucleus, attenuated cytoplasm, and a smooth surface contour. [A third cell type, the less frequently observed perisinusoidal lipocyte (Ito cell), is not seen in this micrograph. This cell would appear as a light cell containing numerous lipid droplets. The lipid droplets contain stored vitamin A.]

KEY		
BC, bile canaliculus	**KC,** Kupffer cell	**asterisks,** connective tissue of central vein
CV, central vein	**L,** lipid droplet	
En, endothelial cell	**S,** sinusoid	**curved arrows,** opening of sinusoid into central vein
F, fibroblast	**arrows (Fig. 2),** glycogen	

PLATE 84

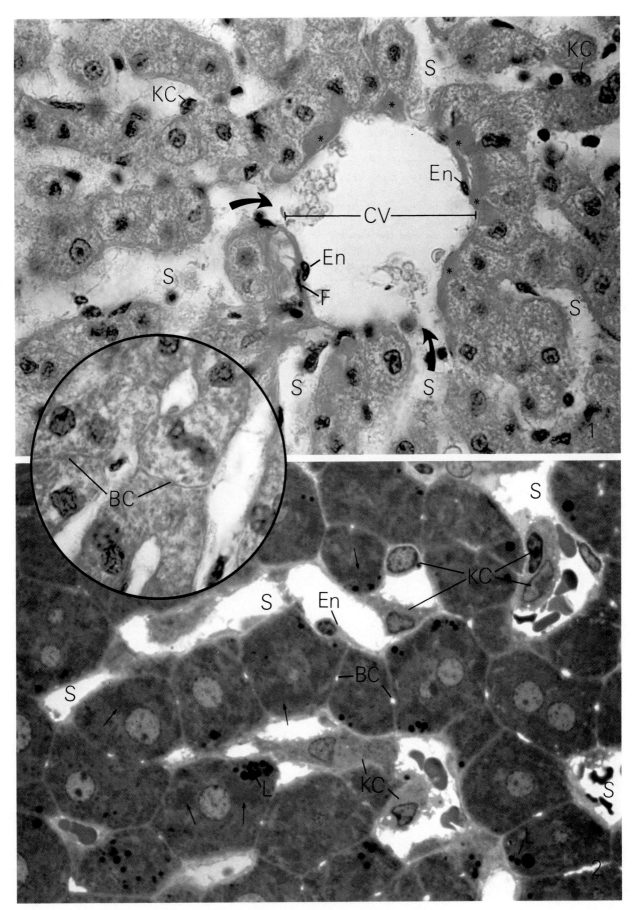

PLATE 85. Liver III, Electron Microscopy

Liver, mouse, electron micrograph ×5100; inset ×6000. A more detailed analysis of liver structural organization is provided by this electron micrograph; it should be compared with the plastic section, Figure 2, in Plate 84. Shown in the electron micrograph are portions of two liver cords that join one another in the upper left of the micrograph. A sinusoid *(S)* is seen between the two cords, but it turns out of the plane of section where the cords join. The nucleus of one of the hepatocytes is included in the section. This nucleus (center) displays the same characteristic, sparse heterochromatin distribution as is seen in the hepatocyte nuclei in the plastic section.

The cytoplasm displays numerous patches of glycogen particle aggregates *(G)*. They correspond to the pink (metachromatic) stained areas in the toluidine blue specimen in Plate 84. Also relatively conspicuous are numerous ovoid mitochondria and profiles of rER *(ER)*. A few small lipid droplets *(L)* are also present.

At this low magnification, the perisinusoidal space [space of Disse *(D)*] can be recognized as a narrow space containing small cytoplasmic processes or microvilli. The space of Disse is separated from the lumen of the sinusoid *(S)* by a thin endothelium, which, at higher magnifications, shows gaps of various sizes; i.e., one can detect open pathways between the space of Disse and the lumen. The Kupffer cells *(KC)* can be seen forming a portion of the sinusoid wall. They seemingly substitute in places for the endothelial cells, but the bulk of the cell lies within the sinusoid lumen. The **inset** shows a Kupffer cell with its nucleus. Note the presence of secondary lysosomes. They appear as irregular, electron-dense bodies within the cytoplasm. Also, note the numerous microvilli that project from the hepatocytes into the space of Disse.

The last feature of note is the bile canaliculi *(BC)* seen on the left side of the micrograph. The boundaries between adjoining cells can just be made out at this low magnification, and the canaliculus is seen where the two adjoining membranes part to form this small canal.

KEY

BC, bile canaliculus
D, space of Disse
ER, rough endoplasmic reticulum (rER)
G, Golgi apparatus
KC, Kupffer cell
L, lipid droplet
S, sinusoid

PLATE 85

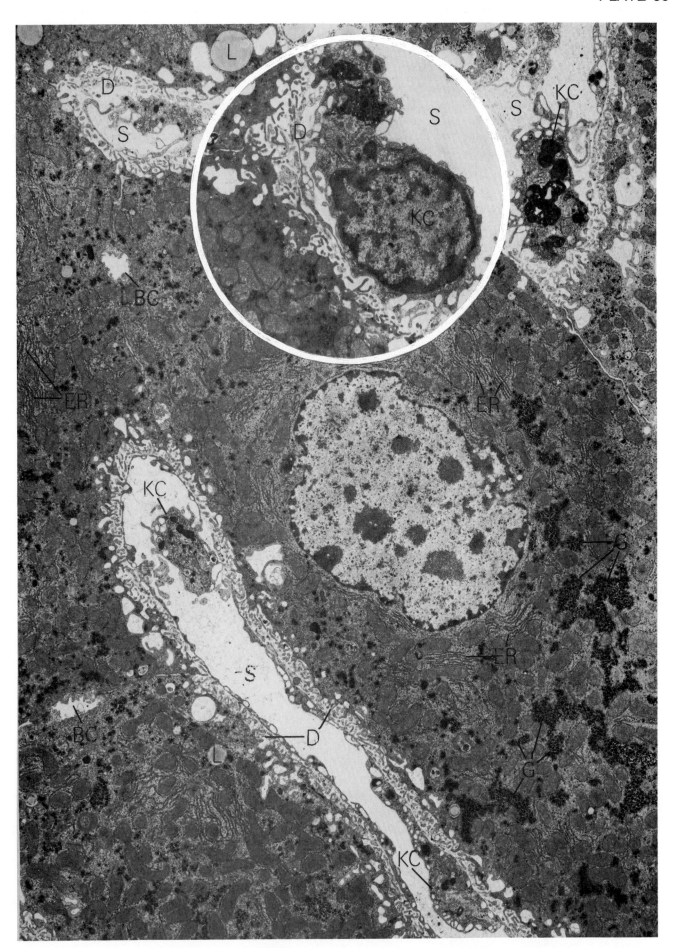

PLATE 86. Gallbladder

FIGURE 1, gallbladder, H&E ×45. The gallbladder is a hollow, pear-shaped organ that concentrates and stores the bile. The full thickness of its wall is shown here. It is composed of a mucosa *(Muc)*, muscularis *(Mus)*, and adventitia *(Adv)* and, on its free surface (not shown), a serosa. The mucosa is considered at higher magnification in Figure 2. The muscularis consists of interlacing bundles of smooth muscle *(SM)*. The adventitia *(Adv)* consists of irregular, dense connective tissue through which the larger blood vessels *(BV)* travel and, more peripherally, of varying amounts of adipose tissue *(AT)*.

The mucosa is thrown into numerous folds that are particularly pronounced when the muscularis is highly contracted. This is the usual histologic appearance of the gallbladder unless, of course, steps are taken to fix and preserve it in a distended state. Occasionally, the section cuts through a recess in a fold, and the recess may then resemble a gland *(arrows)*. The mucosa, however, does not possess glands except in the neck region, where some mucous glands are present (see Fig. 4).

FIGURE 2, gallbladder, human, H&E ×325. The mucosa consists of a tall simple columnar absorptive epithelium *(Ep)* resting on a lamina propria of loose irregular connective tissue *(CT)*. The epithelium has characteristics that distinguish it from the absorptive epithelium of other organs such as the intestines. Only one cell type, tall columnar cells, is present in the epithelial layer (see Fig. 3). The nuclei are in the basal portion of the cell. The cells possess a thin apical striated border. However, this is not always evident in routine H&E-stained sections. The cytoplasm stains rather uniformly with eosin. This is related to its absorptive function and is in contrast to the staining of cells that are engaged in the production of protein. Lastly, with respect to its absorptive function, the epithelial cells frequently exhibit distended intercellular spaces at their basal aspect (see Fig. 3, *arrows)*. This is a feature associated with the transport of fluid across the epithelium and, as previously noted, commonly seen in intestinal absorptive cells.

FIGURE 3, gallbladder, human, H&E ×550. The lamina propria underlying the epithelium is usually relatively cellular. In this specimen, in addition to the presence of lymphocytes *(L)*, a relatively common finding, there is also a large number of plasma cells *(PC)* present within the lamina propria. (The high concentration of plasma cells suggests a chronic inflammation.) Another feature of note in the lamina propria is the presence of several glands and gland-like profiles *(Gl)* other than those seen in the mucosa and already noted. These are readily apparent in Figure 1. Two of these structures, marked by *asterisks* in Figure 1, are shown at higher magnification in Figure 4.

FIGURE 4, gallbladder, human, H&E ×550. The smaller of the two gland-like structures is comprised of mucous cells *(MC)* and represents a section through a mucous gland. This specimen was taken from a site near the neck of the gallbladder where mucous glands are often present. Note the characteristic flattened nuclei at the base of the cell and the lightly stained appearance of the cytoplasm, features characteristic of mucin-secreting cells. In contrast, the epithelium of the large gland-like profile that is only partially included in the micrograph has rounded or ovoid nuclei. This epithelial-lined structure is not a true gland but represents an invagination of the mucous membrane that extends into and often through the thickness of the muscularis. These invaginations are known as Rokitansky-Aschoff sinuses. Their role or significance, if any, is unknown. (Some authorities contend that they result from disease, but they are also found in small numbers in gallbladders that appear normal in all other respects.)

KEY

Adv, adventitia
AT, adipose tissue
BV, blood vessel
CT, connective tissue, lamina propria
Ep, epithelium
Gl, gland or gland-like structure
L, lymphocytes
MC, mucous cells
Muc, mucosa
Mus, muscularis mucosae
PC, plasma cells
SM, smooth muscle
arrows: Fig. 1, recess in luminal surface; Fig. 3, intercellular spaces
asterisks (Fig. 1), gland or gland-like structure

PLATE 86

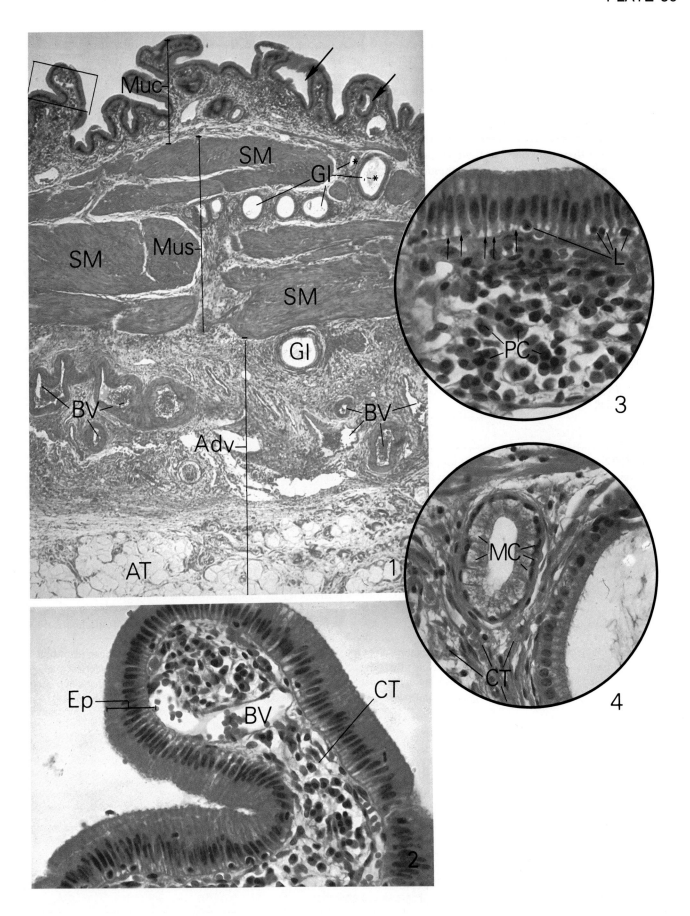

PLATE 87. Pancreas

The pancreas is an elongated gland with a head nestled in the C-shaped bend of the duodenum, a body, and a tail extending across the back of the abdomen. It is a mixed gland containing both an exocrine component and an endocrine component. The exocrine component is a compound tubuloacinar gland with a branching network of ducts that convey the exocrine secretions to the duodenum. The endocrine component is composed of the islets of Langerhans. The islet cells discharge their secretion (hormones) into the connective tissue from which the hormones diffuse to local blood vessels. The hormones are then conveyed to their respective target tissues. Other secretions, referred to as paracrine secretions or parahormones, are also produced by the islets. Paracrine secretions act locally by diffusing to their target cells. Paracrine secretions of the A and D cells help to regulate the activity of the B cells.

FIGURE 1, pancreas, H&E. The pancreas is surrounded by a delicate capsule of moderately dense connective tissue. Septa from the capsule divide the pancreas into lobules, one of which is shown here, bounded by connective tissue *(CT)*. Larger blood vessels *(BV)* travel in the connective tissue septa; nerves also travel in the septa, but they are seen infrequently. Within the lobule are the numerous acini of the exocrine component, an intralobular duct *(InD)*, intercalated ducts (not readily evident at this low magnification), and islets of Langerhans *(IL)*. Also within the lobule are the small blood vessels and the connective tissue serving as a stroma for the parenchymal elements of the gland.

This figure shows an islet of Langerhans *(IL)* among the far more numerous acini. (Islets are most numerous in the tail of the pancreas and least numerous in the head). Cells within the islets are arranged as irregular cords. In routine preparations, it is not possible to identify the various cell types within the islets. Note, however, that B cells are the most numerous; these produce insulin. The next most numerous are A cells; these produce glucagon. The **inset** also shows numerous capillaries *(arrows)*. The labels *A* and *B* are not intended to identify specific cells but rather to show those parts of the islets where A and B cells are found in greatest number.

FIGURE 2, pancreas, H&E. Acini of the pancreas consist of serous cells. In sections, the acini present circular and irregular profiles. The lumen of the acinus is small, and only in fortuitous sections through an acinus is the lumen included *(asterisks)*. The nucleus is characteristically in the base of the acinar cell. There is a region of intense basophilia adjacent to the nucleus. This is the ergastoplasm *(Er)*, and it reflects the presence of rER that is active in the synthesis of pancreatic enzymes. Some acini reveal a centrally positioned cell with cytoplasm that shows no special staining characteristics in H&E-stained paraffin sections. These are centroacinar cells *(CC)*. They are the beginning of the intercalated ducts.

This figure demonstrates particularly well the morphology and relationships of the intercalated ducts. Note, first, the cross-sectioned intralobular duct *(InD)* consisting of cuboidal epithelium. (There are no striated ducts in the pancreas.)

Leading to the intralobular duct is an intercalated duct *(ID)*, which is seen in cross section at the furthest distance from the intralobular duct and then, in longitudinal section, in the center of the illustration as it travels toward the intralobular duct. The lumen is evident where the intercalated duct is seen in cross section but is not evident where it is seen in longitudinal section. This is because the plane of section cuts chiefly through the cells rather than the lumen. As a consequence, this figure provides a good view of the nuclei of the duct cells. They are elongate, with their long axis oriented in the direction of the duct. In addition, they display a staining pattern similar to that of centroacinar cells and different from that of nuclei of the parenchymal cells.

Once the cells of the intercalated duct have been identified in one part of the section, their staining characteristics and location can be used to identify the intercalated ducts in other parts of the lobule, several of which are marked *(ID)*.

KEY		
A, region with most A cells	**CT,** connective tissue	**InD,** intralobular duct
B, region with most B cells	**Er,** ergastoplasm	**arrows,** capillaries
BV, blood vessels	**ID,** intercalated ducts	**asterisks,** lumen of acini
CC, centroacinar cells	**IL,** islets of Langerhans	

PLATE 87

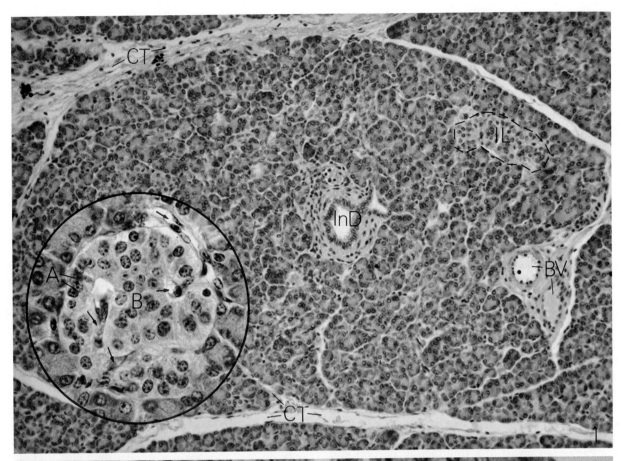

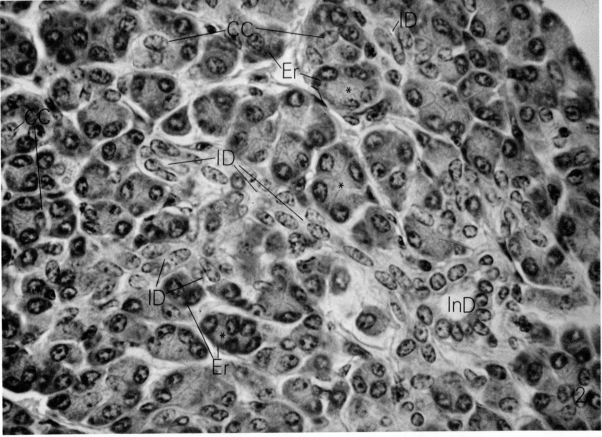

Respiratory System

18

The respiratory system consists of the paired lungs and a series of air passages that lead to and from the lungs. As the air passages continue within the lung, they branch into increasingly smaller tubes until the very smallest air spaces, called *alveoli,* are reached (Fig. 18.1). Three principal functions are performed by this system, namely, *air conduction, air filtration,* and *gas exchange (respiration).* The latter occurs in the alveoli. In addition, air passing through the *larynx* is used to produce speech, and air passing over the *olfactory mucosa* in the *nasal cavities* carries the stimuli for the *sense of smell.*

The Air Passages Consist of a Conducting Portion and a Respiratory Portion

The *conducting portion* of the respiratory system consists of those air passages that lead to the sites of respiration within the lung where gas exchange takes place. The conducting passages include those located outside as well as within the lungs.

The passages external to the lungs consist of

- *Nasal cavities* (and, during forced breathing, the *mouth*)
- *Nasopharynx* and *oropharynx*
- *Larynx*
- *Trachea*
- *Paired primary bronchi*

Within the lungs are the *internal bronchi,* which undergo extensive branching to give rise to the distributing *bronchioles.* They represent the terminal part of the conducting passages. Collectively, the internal bronchi and the bronchioles constitute the *bronchial tree.*

The *respiratory portion* is that portion of the respiratory tract in which *gas exchange* occurs. It sequentially includes

- *Respiratory bronchioles*
- *Alveolar ducts*
- *Alveolar sacs*
- *Alveoli*

Blood vessels enter the lung with the bronchi. The ar-

teries branch into smaller vessels as they follow the bronchial tree into the substance of the lung. Capillaries come into intimate contact with the terminal respiratory units, the alveoli. This intimate relationship between the alveolar air spaces and the pulmonary capillaries is the structural basis for gas exchange within the lung parenchyma.

Air passing through the respiratory passages must be conditioned before reaching the terminal respiratory units. *Conditioning* of the air occurs in the conducting portion of the system and consists of *warming, moistening,* and *removal of particulate materials.* Mucous and serous secretions play a major role in the conditioning process. Not only do they moisten the air, but they also trap particles that were not trapped by special short thick hairs, *vibrissae,* in the nasal cavities. Mucus, augmented by secretions of serous glands, also prevents the dehydration of the underlying epithelium by the moving air. It covers almost the entire luminal surface of the conducting passages and is constantly produced by goblet cells and mucus-secreting glands in the walls of the passages. The mucus and other secretions are moved toward the pharynx by means of coordinated sweeping movements of cilia and are then normally swallowed.

NASAL CAVITIES

The nasal cavities are paired chambers separated by a bony and cartilaginous septum (Fig. 18.2). Each chamber is divided into three regions:

- *Vestibule* (nostril)
- *Respiratory segment*
- *Olfactory segment*

Vestibule of the Nasal Cavity

The *vestibule* communicates anteriorly with the external environment. It is lined with stratified squamous epithelium, a continuation of the skin of the face, and contains the hairs that filter out large particulate matter before it is

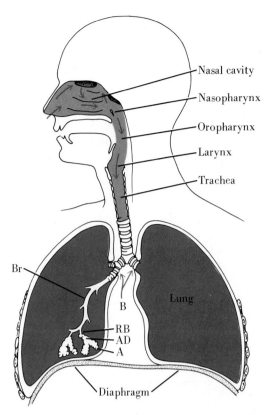

Figure 18.1. Diagram of respiratory passages. The nasal cavities, nasopharynx, oropharynx, larynx, trachea, bronchi *(B)*, and bronchioles *(Br)* are the conducting portion of the respiratory passages. Gas exchange occurs between the blood and air spaces of the respiratory bronchioles *(RB)*, alveolar ducts *(AD)*, and terminal alveoli *(A)*. (After Grant JCB: *A Method of Anatomy,* 10th ed. Baltimore, Williams & Wilkins, 1980, p 51.)

carried in the airstream to the rest of the cavity. Sebaceous glands are also present, and their secretions assist in the entrapment of particulate matter. Posteriorly, where the vestibule ends, the stratified squamous epithelium becomes thinner and undergoes a transition to the pseudostratified epithelium that characterizes the respiratory segment. At this site the sebaceous glands end.

Respiratory Segment of the Nasal Cavity

The respiratory segment constitutes most of the volume of the nasal cavities. It is lined by a ciliated, pseudostratified columnar epithelium. The underlying lamina propria is attached to the periosteum of the adjacent bone.

The medial wall of the respiratory segment, the *nasal septum,* is smooth, but the lateral walls are thrown into folds by the presence of three shelf-like, bony projections called *turbinates* or *conchae*. The turbinates play a dual role. They increase surface area as well as cause turbulence in airflow to allow more efficient conditioning of inspired air.

The ciliated, pseudostratified columnar epithelium of the respiratory segment is composed of five cell types:

- *Ciliated cells*
- *Goblet cells*
- *Brush cells,* a general name for those cells in the respiratory tract that bear short, blunt microvilli
- *Small granule cells,* cells that resemble the basal cell but contain secretory granules
- *Basal cells,* stem cells from which the other cell types arise

The epithelium of the respiratory segment of the nasal cavity is essentially the same as the epithelium covering (lining) most of the parts that follow in the conducting system. Because the respiratory epithelium of the trachea is usually studied and examined in preference to that of the nasal cavity, the above cell types are discussed in the section on the trachea.

The Mucosa of the Respiratory Segment Warms, Moistens, and Filters Inspired Air

The lamina propria of the respiratory segment has a rich, vascular network that includes a complex set of capillary loops. The arrangement of the vessels allows the inhaled air to be warmed by blood flowing through the part of the loop closest to the surface. The capillaries that reside near the surface are arranged in rows; the blood flows perpendicular to the airflow, much as one would find in a mechanical heat exchange system. These same vessels may become extensively engorged and leaky during allergic reactions or viral infections such as the common cold. The lamina propria then becomes distended with fluid, resulting in marked swelling of the mucous membrane with a consequent restriction of the air passage. This makes breathing difficult. The lamina propria also contains mucous glands, many with serous demilunes. Their secretion supplements that of the goblet cells in the respiratory epithelium.

The turbinates, by increasing surface area, provide efficiency in warming the inspired air. Inspired air is also more efficiently filtered by *turbulent precipitation.* The airstream is broken into eddies by the turbinates. Particulate matter suspended in the airstream is thrown out of the stream and adheres to the mucus-covered wall of the nasal cavity. Particles trapped in this layer of mucus are transported to the pharynx by means of coordinated sweeping movements of cilia and are then swallowed.

Olfactory Segment of the Nasal Cavity

Part of the dome of each nasal cavity and, to a variable extent, the contiguous lateral and medial nasal walls form the *olfactory segment* and are lined with *olfactory mucosa*. When observed in life it can be distinguished by a slight yellowish-brown color due to the presence of pigment in the *olfactory epithelium* and the associated *olfactory glands*. In humans the total surface area of the *olfactory mucosa* is only a few square centimeters, whereas in animals with acute

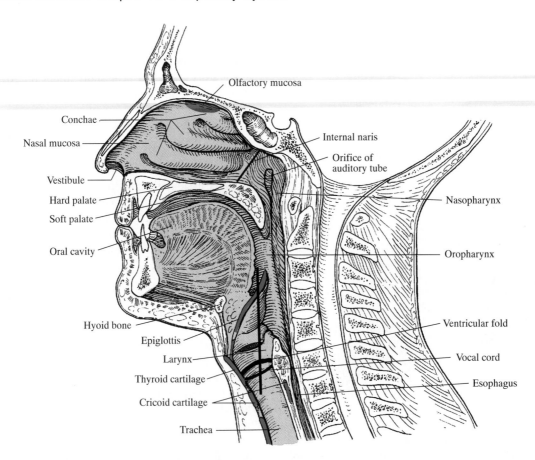

Figure 18.2.   Diagram of sagittal section of head, showing the relationship of the pharynx to the respiratory and digestive systems. The pharynx, with its three parts labeled, is located posteriorly. It serves both systems. The *unlabeled vertical line* drawn through the larynx corresponds to the cutting plane of the histologic section shown in Figure 18.5. Note that the upper part of the section includes the part of the tongue that contains the lingual tonsils. The plane also obviously transects the epiglottis and laryngeal folds; lateral to the laryngeal folds is the thyroid cartilage (open in back), and below the folds is the ring-like cricoid cartilage.

sense of smell the total surface area of the olfactory mucosa is considerably more extensive.

The olfactory epithelium, like the epithelium of the respiratory segment, is also pseudostratified, but it contains very different cell types. Also, it lacks goblet cells (Fig. 18.3). The olfactory epithelium is composed of the following cell types:

- *Olfactory cells, bipolar neurons* that span the thickness of the epithelium
- *Supporting* or *sustentacular cells,* columnar cells that provide mechanical and metabolic support to the olfactory cells
- *Basal cells,* stem cells from which new olfactory cells and supporting cells differentiate
- *Brush cells,* the same cell type that occurs in the respiratory epithelium

Olfactory Cells Are Bipolar Neurons That Possess an Apical Projection Bearing Cilia

The apical (luminal) pole of each olfactory neuron is a dendritic process that projects above the epithelial surface

as a knob-like structure called the *olfactory vesicle.* A number of cilia with typical basal bodies arise from the olfactory vesicle and extend radially in a plane parallel to the epithelial surface (Fig. 18.3). The cilia are regarded as being nonmotile, though some believe they may have limited motility. Their plasma membrane is the site of olfactory receptors. The basal pole of the cell gives rise to an axonal process that leaves the epithelial compartment to enter the connective tissue, where it joins with axons from other olfactory cells to give rise to the *olfactory nerve (cranial nerve I).* Autoradiographic studies have shown that olfactory cells have a normal life span of about 1 month. If injured, they are quickly replaced. Olfactory cells (and some neurons of the enteric division of the autonomic nervous system) appear to be the only neurons that are replaced during postnatal life.

Supporting Cells Provide Mechanical and Metabolic Support for the Olfactory Cells

Supporting cells are the most numerous cells in the olfactory epithelium. The nuclei of these tall columnar cells

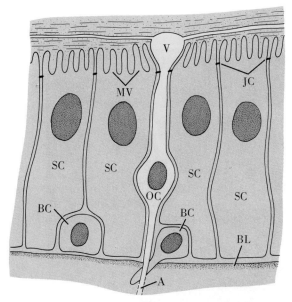

Figure 18.3. Diagram of major cell types of the olfactory mucosa. These are sustentacular cells *(SC)*, olfactory cells *(OC)*, and basal cells *(BC)*. The olfactory cell is the receptor cell; it has an expansion, the olfactory vesicle *(V)*, from which long nonmotile cilia extend, and it sends an axon *(A)* into the connective tissue that joins with axons of other olfactory cells to form the olfactory nerves. The basal cell extends beyond the basal lamina *(BL)* to enclose the first part of the olfactory axon. Occasional brush cells (not illustrated) are also found in the olfactory mucosa. *JC*, junctional complex; and *MV*, microvilli.

occupy a more apical position in the epithelium than do those of the other cell types, thus aiding in their identification in light microscopic specimens. They have numerous microvilli on their apical surface, and mitochondria are abundant. Numerous profiles of smooth-surfaced endoplasmic reticulum (sER) and, to a more limited extent, rough-surfaced endoplasmic reticulum (rER) are observed in the cytoplasm. They also possess lipofuscin granules. Adhering junctions are present between these cells and the olfactory cells, but gap and tight junctions are absent. The supporting cells function in a manner comparable with glial cells, providing both metabolic and physical support to the olfactory cells.

Brush Cells Are Specialized for Transduction of General Sensation

The olfactory epithelium also contains cells present in much smaller numbers, called **brush cells.** These cells are present in the epithelium of the other parts of the conducting air passages, as previously noted. They are columnar cells that in the electron microscope exhibit large, blunt microvilli at their apical surface, a feature that gives them their name. The basal surface of the brush cell is in synaptic contact with nerve fibers that penetrate the basal lamina. The nerve fibers are terminal branches of the **trigeminal nerve (cranial nerve V)** that function in general sensation

rather than olfaction. Brush cells appear to be involved in transduction of general sensory stimulation of the mucosa.

Basal Cells Are Progenitors of the Other Mature Cell Types

Basal cells are small rounded cells located close to the basal lamina. Their nuclei are frequently invaginated and lie at a level below those of the olfactory cell nuclei. The cytoplasm contains few organelles, a feature consistent with their role as a reserve or stem cell. They proliferate and differentiate into supporting cells. Also, a feature consistent with their differentiation into supporting cells is the observation of processes in some basal cells that partially ensheathe the first portion of the olfactory cell axon. They thus maintain a relationship to the olfactory cell even in this undifferentiated state.

Lamina Propria. The lamina propria of the olfactory mucosa is directly contiguous with the periosteum of the underlying bone. This connective tissue contains numerous blood and lymphatic vessels, unmyelinated olfactory nerves, myelinated nerves, and olfactory glands (Bowman's glands).

The **olfactory glands,** a characteristic feature of the mucosa, are branched tubuloalveolar serous glands that deliver their secretions via ducts onto the olfactory surface (Fig. 18.4). They secrete a proteinaceous material. Lipofuscin granules are prevalent in the gland cells, and in combination with the lipofuscin granules in the supporting cells of the olfactory epithelium, they give the mucosa its natural yellow-brown coloration. Short ducts leading from the glands, composed of cuboidal cells, are present within the lamina propria. As the ducts pass through the basal lamina into the olfactory epithelium, the duct cells become squamous and are then difficult to discern in the light microscope.

The serous secretion of the olfactory glands serves as a trap and solvent for odoriferous substances. Constant flow from the glands rids the mucosa of remnants of detected odoriferous substances so that new scents can be continuously detected as they arise.

The feature that allows one to identify the olfactory region of the nasal mucosa in a histologic preparation is the presence of the olfactory nerves in combination with the olfactory glands in the lamina propria. The nerves are particularly conspicuous due to the relatively large diameter of the individual unmyelinated fibers that they contain (Fig. 18.4).

Sinuses

Paranasal Sinuses Are Air-Filled Spaces in the Bones of the Walls of the Nasal Cavity

The paranasal sinuses are pockets in the wall of the nasal bones that are lined by respiratory epithelium. The sinuses are named for the bone in which they are found, i.e., the

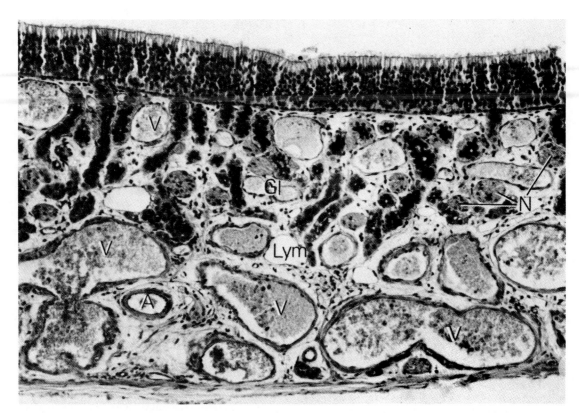

Figure 18.4. Photomicrograph of olfactory mucosa including the olfactory epithelium and the underlying connective tissue that extends as far as the bone (not shown). This micrograph shows numerous blood vessels [artery *(A)* and veins *(V)*], lymphatic vessels *(Lym)*, nerves *(N)*, and Bowman's glands *(Gl)*. ×160.

ethmoid, frontal, sphenoid, and maxillary bones. The sinuses communicate with the nasal cavities via narrow openings onto the respiratory mucosa. The mucosal surface of the sinuses is a thin, ciliated, pseudostratified columnar epithelium with numerous goblet cells. Mucus produced in the sinuses is swept into the nasal cavities by coordinated ciliary movements. The sinuses are often subject to acute infection following viral infection of the upper respiratory tract. Severe cases may require physical drainage.

PHARYNX

As described in detail in Chapter 15, the pharynx connects the nasal and oral cavities to the larynx and esophagus. It serves as a passageway for air and food and provides a resonating chamber for speech. The pharynx is located posterior to the nasal and oral cavities and is divided regionally into the **nasopharynx** and **oropharynx,** respectively (see Fig. 18.2). The **auditory (Eustachian) tubes** connect the nasopharynx to each middle ear. Diffuse lymphatic tissue and lymphatic nodules are found in the wall of the nasopharynx. The concentration of such nodules in the posterior wall is called the **pharyngeal tonsil.**

LARYNX

The passageway for air between the oropharynx and trachea is the **larynx** (see Fig. 18.2). It is a complex tubular segment of the respiratory system that is formed by irregularly shaped plates of hyaline and elastic cartilage. In addition to serving as a conduit for air, the larynx serves as the organ for speech (phonation).

Vocal Folds Control the Flow of Air Through the Larynx and Vibrate to Produce Sound

The **vocal folds,** also referred to as **vocal cords,** are two folds of mucosa that project into the lumen of the larynx (Fig. 18.5). They are oriented in an anteroposterior direction and define the lateral boundaries of the opening of the larynx, the **glottis.** A supporting ligament and skeletal muscle, the **vocalis muscle,** is contained within each vocal fold. Ligaments and the **intrinsic skeletal muscles** join the adjacent cartilaginous plates and are responsible for generating tension in the vocal folds and for opening and closing the glottis. The **extrinsic laryngeal muscles** insert on cartilages of the larynx but originate in extralaryngeal structures and move the larynx during swallowing **(deglutition).**

Expelled air passing through the glottis can be induced to cause the vocal folds to vibrate. The vibrations are al-

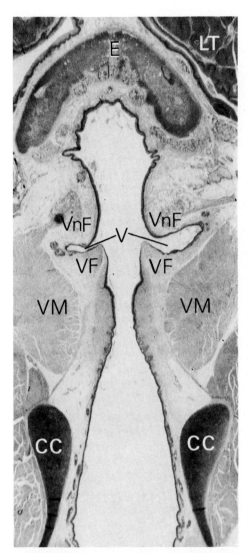

Figure 18.5. Photomicrograph of larynx sectioned in a plane marked by the *line* in Figure 18.2. The roof of the larynx contains the epiglottis *(E)*. Above this is a small space of the oral cavity, and then, above this is part of the tongue. The posterior portion of the tongue contains lingual tonsils *(LT)*. The objects of main interest within the larynx are the vocal folds *(VF)*, seen in cross section, above which are the ventricles *(V)* and, above these, the ventricular folds *(VnF)*. The vocalis muscle *(VM)* is under the vocal folds. *CC*, cricoid cartilage.

tered by modulating the tension on the vocal folds and by changing the degree of glottal opening. This alteration of the vibrations produces sounds of different *pitch*.

The Ventricular Folds Located Above the Vocal Folds Are the "False Vocal Cords"

Above the vocal folds is an elongated recess in the larynx called the ***ventricle***. Immediately above the ventricle is another pair of mucosal folds, the ***ventricular folds*** or ***false vocal cords*** (Fig. 18.5). These do not have the intrinsic muscular investment of the true vocal cords and,

therefore, do not modulate in phonation. They and the ventricle are, however, important in creating sound *resonance*.

Stratified Squamous and Ciliated, Pseudostratified Columnar Epithelium Line the Larynx

The luminal surface of the vocal cords is covered with stratified squamous epithelium, as is most of the epiglottis. This serves to protect the mucosa from abrasion caused by the rapidly moving airstream. The rest of the larynx is lined with the ciliated, pseudostratified columnar epithelium that characterizes the respiratory tract (see Plate 89, page 551). The connective tissue of the larynx contains mixed mucoserous glands that secrete through ducts onto the laryngeal surface.

METAPLASIA

In human respiratory mucosa, changes may occur from the ciliated pseudostratified epithelium to stratified squamous. This is a normal occurrence on the rounded more exposed portions of the turbinates, on the vocal folds, and in certain other regions. Changes in the character of the respiratory epithelium may, however, occur in other ciliated epithelial sites when the pattern of airflow is altered or when forceful airflow occurs, such as in chronic coughing. Typically, in chronic bronchitis and in bronchiectasis the respiratory epithelium changes in certain regions to a stratified squamous form. The altered epithelium is more resistant to physical stress or insult, but it is less effective functionally. In the case of smokers, a similar epithelial change occurs. Initially, the ciliated cells begin to lose synchrony of ciliary beating due to noxious elements in smoke. This results in impaired removal of mucus. To compensate, the individual begins to cough, thereby facilitating the expulsion of accumulated mucus in the airway, particularly in the trachea. With time, there is a reduction in the number of ciliated cells due to chronic coughing. This further impairs the normal epithelium and results in a squamous replacement epithelium at affected sites in the airway.

Epithelial alterations of this kind are referred to as ***metaplasia***, i.e., a change from one type of fully differentiated adult cell to a different type of adult cell. A given mature cell does not change to another type of mature cell; rather, it is replaced by basal cell proliferation to give rise to the new differentiated cell type. Such cellular changes are considered to be controlled and adaptive.

TRACHEA

The ***trachea*** is a short tube about 2.5 cm in diameter and about 10 cm long. It serves as a conduit for air; additionally, its wall assists in conditioning inspired air. The trachea extends from the larynx to about the middle of the thorax, where it divides into the two ***primary bronchi (extrapulmonary bronchi)***.

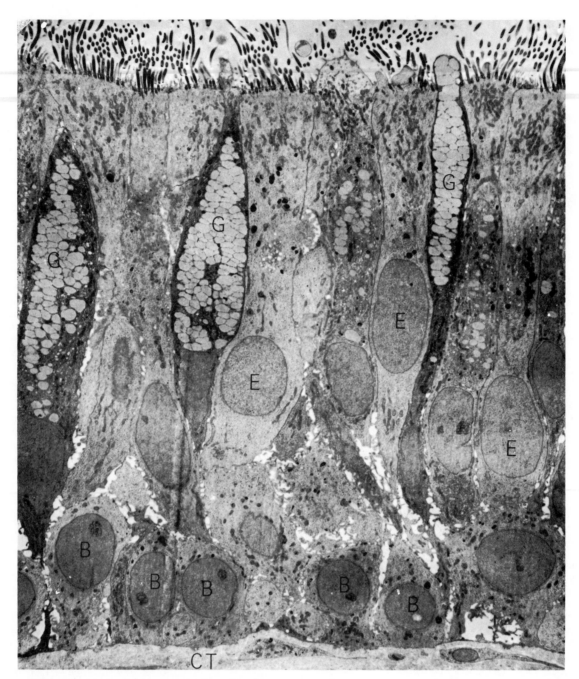

Figure 18.6. Electron micrograph of human trachea. The three main cell types of this respiratory epithelium are ciliated epithelial cells *(E)* extending to the surface, where they possess cilia; goblet cells *(G),* with mucinogen granules; and basal cells *(B),* which are confined to the basal portion of the epithelial layer near the connective tissue *(CT).* ×1,800. (Courtesy of J. Rhodin.)

The wall of the trachea consists of four definable layers:

- *Mucosa,* composed of ciliated, pseudostratified epithelium and an elastic fiber-rich lamina propria
- *Submucosa,* composed of a slightly more dense connective tissue than the lamina propria
- *Cartilaginous layer,* composed of C-shaped hyaline cartilages

- *Adventitia,* which binds the trachea to adjacent structures

A unique feature of the trachea is the presence of the C-shaped hyaline cartilages that are stacked on one another to form a supporting structure (see Fig. 7.8). The cartilages, which might be described as a skeletal framework, prevent collapse of the tracheal lumen, particularly during

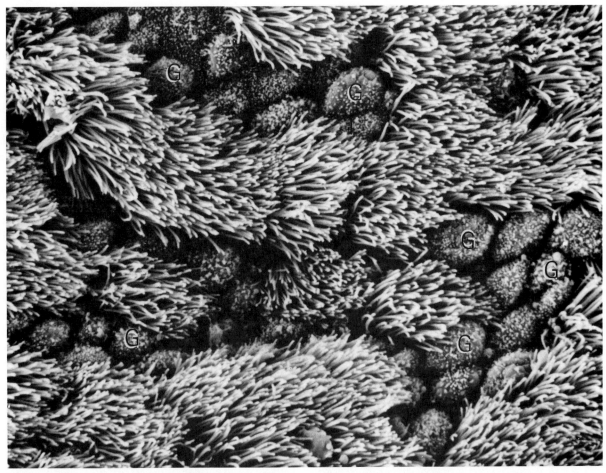

Figure 18.7. Scanning electron micrograph of the luminal surface of a bronchus. The nonciliated cells are the goblet cells *(G)*. Their surface is characterized by small blunt microvilli that give a stippled appearance to the cell at this low magnification. The cilia of the many ciliated cells occupy the remainder of the micrograph. Note how all are "synchronously" arrayed, i.e., uniformly leaning in the same direction, appearing just as they were when fixed at a specific moment during their wave-like movement.

expiration. Fibroelastic tissue and smooth muscle, the *trachealis muscle,* bridge the gap between the free ends of the C-shaped cartilages at the posterior border of the trachea, adjacent to the esophagus.

Tracheal Epithelium Is Similar to Respiratory Epithelium in Other Parts of the Conducting Airway

Ciliated columnar cells, mucous (goblet) cells, and basal cells are the principal cell types in the tracheal epithelium (Figs. 18.6 and 18.7). Brush cells are also present but in small numbers, as are the small granule cells.

- *Ciliated cells,* the most numerous of the cell types, extend through the full thickness of the epithelium. Cilia appear in histologic sections as short hair-like projections from the apical surface. Immediately below the cilia is a dark line formed by the aggregated ciliary basal

bodies. The cilia provide a coordinated sweeping motion of the mucous coat from the furthest reaches of the air passages toward the pharynx. In effect, the ciliated cells provide a "ciliary escalator" that serves as an important protective mechanism for removing small inhaled particles from the lungs.

- *Mucous cells* are similar in appearance to the intestinal goblet cells and, thus, are often referred to by the same name. They are interspersed among the ciliated cells and also extend through the full thickness of the epithelium. They are readily seen with the light microscope after accumulating mucinogen granules in their cytoplasm. Although the granules are typically washed out in hematoxylin and eosin (H&E) preparations, the identity of the cell is made apparent by the remaining clear area in the apical cytoplasm and the lack of cilia at the apical surface.

- *Brush cells* have the same general features as those

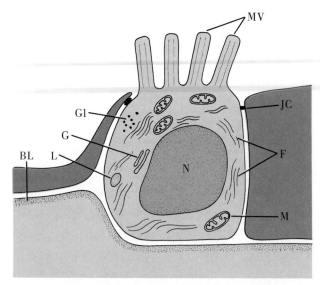

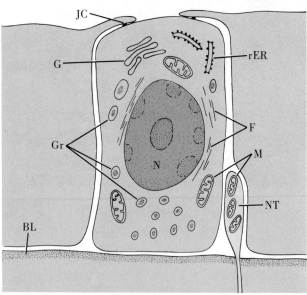

Figure 18.8. **Top.** Diagram of brush cell between pulmonary type I and II cells in a lung alveolus. Large blunt microvilli *(MV)* are distinctive features of the brush cell. The cytoplasm typically shows a Golgi complex *(G)*, lysosomes *(L)*, filaments *(F)*, mitochondria *(M)*, and glycogen *(Gl)*. *BL,* basal lamina; *JC,* junctional complex; and *N,* nucleus. **Bottom.** Diagram of dense-core granule cell between two Clara cells, as in a terminal or respiratory bronchiole. The cell contains small granules *(Gr)*, most of which are basal to the nucleus *(N)*. In addition to the granules, the most conspicuous organelles of the cell are filaments *(F)*, rough-surfaced endoplasmic reticulum *(rER)*, a Golgi complex *(G)*, and mitochondria *(M)*. A nerve terminal *(NT)* is adjacent to the cell. *BL,* basal lamina; and *JC,* junctional complex.

described in the respiratory epithelium of the nasal cavity (Fig. 18.8a). They are columnar cells that bear microvilli. The basal surface of the cells is in synaptic contact with an afferent nerve ending (epitheliodendritic synapse). Thus, the brush cell is regarded as a receptor cell.

- *Small granule cells* are a representation in respiratory epithelium of the general class of enteroendocrine cells of the gut and gut derivatives (Fig. 18.8b). Their presence is explained by the fact that the respiratory tract and lungs develop in the embryo as an evagination from the primitive foregut. The small granule cells usually occur singly in the trachea, dispersed sparsely among the other cell types. They are difficult to distinguish from basal cells in the light microscope without special techniques such as silver staining in which there is a reaction with the granules. The nucleus is located near the basement membrane; the cytoplasm is somewhat more extensive than that of the smaller basal cells. In the transmission electron microscope (TEM), a thin, tapering cytoplasmic process is sometimes observed extending to the lumen. Also, with the TEM, the cytoplasm exhibits numerous, membrane-bounded, dense-core granules. In one type of small granule cell the secretion is a catecholamine. A second cell type produces a polypeptide hormone. Some but not all small granule cells appear to be innervated. The function of the small granule cell is not well understood. Some cells have been found in groups in association with nerve fibers, forming what is described as neuroepithelial bodies that are thought to function in reflexes regulating the airway or vascular caliber.
- *Basal cells* serve as a reserve population by maintaining individual cell replacement in the epithelium. The basal cells tend to be prominent because their nuclei form a row in close proximity to the basal lamina. Although the small granule cell nuclei reside at this same general level within the epithelium, they are relatively sparse in number. Thus, most of the nuclei near the basement membrane are those of basal cells.

Basement Membrane and Lamina Propria

A Thick "Basement Membrane" Is Characteristic of Tracheal Epithelium

Beneath the tracheal epithelium there is a distinctive layer typically referred to as a "basement membrane." It usually appears as a glassy or homogeneous, light-staining layer approximately 25–40 µm in thickness (see Fig. 4.2). Electron microscopy reveals it to consist of densely packed collagenous fibers that lie immediately under the epithelial basal lamina. Structurally, it can be regarded as an unusually thick and dense reticular lamina and, as such, is part of the lamina propria. In smokers, particularly those who experience chronic coughing, this layer may be considerably thicker, a response to irritation of the mucosa.

The lamina propria, excluding that part just designated as basement membrane, appears as a typical loose connective tissue. It is very cellular, containing numerous lymphocytes, many of which infiltrate the epithelium. Plasma cells, mast cells, eosinophils, and fibroblasts are the other

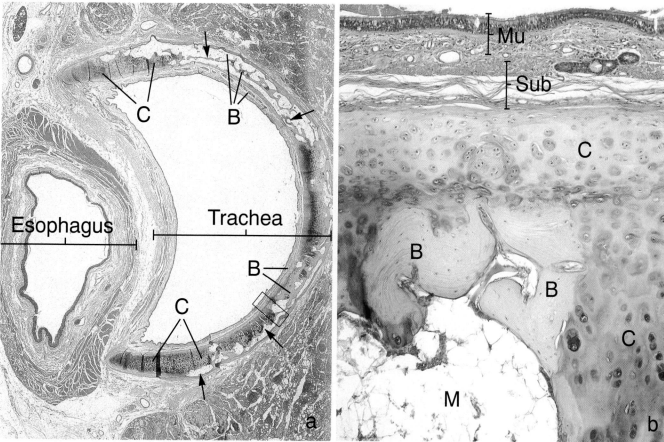

Figure 18.9. **a.** Photomicrograph of a section through the esophagus and trachea of a 66-year-old individual. The C-shaped tracheal cartilage ring has transformed, in part, to bone. The darker-staining material represents cartilage *(C)*, whereas most of the lighter-staining material has been replaced by bone tissue *(B)*. The very light areas *(arrows)* are marrow spaces in the bony portion of the tracheal ring. H&E, ×3.25. **b.** Photomicrograph of the *boxed area* in **a.** At the top of the photomicrograph are the tracheal mucosa *(Mu)* and submucosa *(Sub)*. Below is the tracheal ring. The tracheal ring cartilage *(C)* that is still intact is indicated. In this particular region, however, more than half of the cartilage tissue has been replaced by bone tissue *(B)* or marrow *(M)*. The bone tissue exhibits typical lamellae and osteocytes. The cartilage tissue, in contrast, exhibits nests of chondrocytes and a more amorphous-appearing intercellular matrix. The staining difference in the cartilage is a reflection of loss of sulfate groups in the outer portions of the cartilage matrix. H&E, ×100.

cell types readily observed in this layer. Lymphatic tissue, in both diffuse and nodular forms, has a constant presence in the lamina propria and submucosa of the tracheal wall. It is also present in other parts of the respiratory system concerned primarily with conduction of air. This lymphatic tissue is the developmental and functional equivalent of the *gut-associated lymphatic tissue (GALT)*.

The Boundary Between Mucosa and Submucosa Is Defined by an Elastic Membrane

Interspersed among the collagenous fibers are numerous elastic fibers. Where the lamina propria ends, the elastic material is more extensive, and in specimens stained for these fibers, a distinct band of elastic material is present. This band or *elastic membrane* marks the boundary between the lamina propria and submucosa. In H&E preparations, however, the boundary is not obvious.

The submucosa is unlike that of most other organs where this connective tissue typically has a dense character. In the trachea the submucosa is a relatively loose connective tissue similar in appearance to the lamina propria, thus making it difficult to determine where it begins. Diffuse lymphatic tissue and lymphatic nodules characteristically extend into this layer from the lamina propria. The submucosa contains the larger distributing vessels and lymphatics of the tracheal wall.

Submucosal glands composed of mucus-secreting acini with serous demilunes are also present in the submucosa. Their ducts, consisting of a simple cuboidal epithelium, extend through the lamina propria to deliver the product, largely glycoproteins, on the epithelial surface. The glands are especially numerous in the cartilage-free gap on the posterior portion of the trachea. Some penetrate the muscle layer at this site and, thus, also lie in the adventitia. The submucosal layer ends where its connective tissue fibers blend with the perichondrium of the cartilage layer.

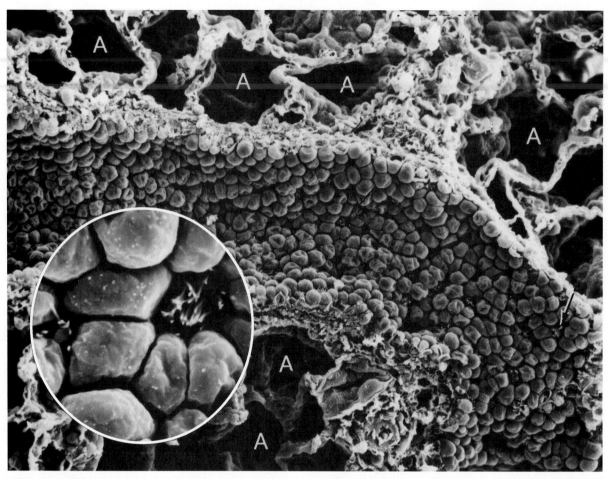

Figure 18.10. Scanning electron micrograph of a terminal bronchiole and surrounding alveoli *(A)*. The bronchiole has been broken open in a longitudinal plane and shows the apical surface of the lining Clara cells. In various areas, isolated ciliated cells are present; the cilia *(arrow)* are barely perceptible at this magnification. The **inset** shows some of the Clara cells at a higher magnification, with the cilia of a ciliated cell clearly visible. Note the relatively few cilia present on these small cells.

The Tracheal Cartilages and Trachealis Muscle Separate Submucosa From Adventitia

The tracheal cartilages, about 16–20 in number in the human, represent the next layer of the tracheal wall. As noted, the cartilages are C-shaped. They sometimes anastomose with adjacent cartilages, but their arrangement is such that they provide flexibility to the tracheal pipe and at the same time maintain patency of the lumen. With age, the hyaline cartilage may be partially replaced by bone tissue (Fig. 18.9), thus losing much of its flexibility.

The *adventitia,* the outer layer, lies peripheral to the cartilage rings and trachealis muscle. It binds the trachea to adjacent structures in the neck and mediastinum and contains the largest blood vessels and nerves that supply the tracheal wall, as well as the larger lymphatics that drain the wall.

BRONCHI

The trachea divides into two branches forming the *primary or extrapulmonary bronchi*. Anatomically, these divisions are more frequently described simply as *right and left bronchi,* terms that are more useful in view of the physical difference between the two. The right bronchus is wider and significantly shorter than the left. On entering the lungs the bronchi become the *intrapulmonary bronchi,* which branch immediately to give rise to the *lobar bronchi (secondary bronchi).*

The left lung is divided into two lobes, whereas the right lung is divided into three lobes. Thus, the right bronchus divides into three lobar bronchial branches, and the left, into two lobar bronchial branches, with each branch supplying one lobe. The left lung is further divided into eight *bronchopulmonary segments,* and the right lung, into ten such segments. Thus, in the right lung the lobar bronchi

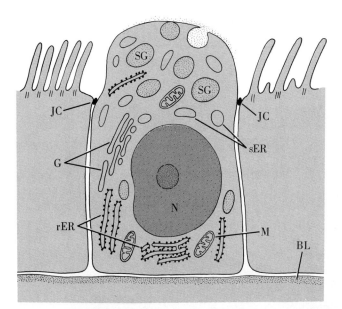

Figure 18.11. Diagram of a Clara cell between bronchiolar epithelial cells. The nucleus *(N)* is in a basal location. Rough-surfaced endoplasmic reticulum *(rER)*, a Golgi complex *(G)*, and mitochondria *(M)* are chiefly in basal and paranuclear locations. Smooth-surfaced endoplasmic reticulum *(sER)* and secretory granules *(SG)* are chiefly in the apical cytoplasm. One of the secretory granules is shown discharging its contents onto the surface of the cell. *BL,* basal lamina; and *JC,* junctional complex.

divide to give rise to ten *segmental bronchi (tertiary bronchi);* the lobar bronchi of the left lung give rise to eight segmental bronchi. A segmental bronchus and the lung parenchyma that it supplies constitute a bronchopulmonary segment. The significance of the bronchopulmonary segment in human lung becomes apparent when considering the need for surgical resection, which may be required in certain disease states. The segments, each with its own blood supply and connective tissue septa, are convenient subunits that facilitate surgical resection.

Bronchial Structure

The bronchi initially have the same general histologic structure as the trachea. At the point where the bronchi enter the lungs to become intrapulmonary bronchi, the structure of the bronchial wall changes. The cartilage rings are replaced by cartilage plates of irregular shape. The plates are distributed in a linear array around the entire circumference of the wall, giving the bronchi a circular or cylindrical shape in contrast to the ovoid shape with a flattened posterior wall of the trachea. As the bronchi become reduced in size, due to branching, the cartilage plates become smaller and fewer in number. They ultimately disappear at the point where the airway reaches a diameter of about 1 mm, whereupon it is designated as a bronchiole.

Bronchi Can Be Identified by Their Cartilage Plates and a Circular Layer of Smooth Muscle

The second change observed in the wall of the intrapulmonary bronchus is the addition of smooth muscle to form a complete circumferential layer. The smooth muscle becomes an increasingly conspicuous layer as the amount of cartilage diminishes. Initially, the smooth muscle is in the form of interlacing bundles forming a continuous layer. In the smaller bronchi, the smooth muscle may appear discontinuous.

Because the smooth muscle forms a separate layer, namely, a *muscularis,* the wall of the bronchus can be regarded as having five layers. These layers can be described as follows:

- *Mucosa* is composed of a pseudostratified epithelium having the same cellular composition as the trachea. The height of the cells decreases as the bronchi become reduced in diameter. In H&E specimens the ''basement membrane'' is conspicuous in the primary bronchi but quickly diminishes in thickness and disappears as a discrete structure. The lamina propria is similar to that of the trachea but is reduced in amount in proportion to the diameter of the bronchi.
- *Muscularis* is a continuous layer of smooth muscle in the larger bronchi. It is more attenuated and loosely organized in smaller bronchi where it may appear discontinuous because of its spiral course. Contraction of the muscle maintains the appropriate diameter of the airway.
- *Submucosa* remains as a relatively loose connective tissue. Glands are present as well as adipose tissue in the larger bronchi.
- *Cartilage layer* consists of discontinuous cartilage plates that become reduced in size as the bronchial diameter diminishes.
- *Adventitia* is moderately dense connective tissue that is continuous with that of adjacent structures, such as pulmonary artery and lung parenchyma.

BRONCHIOLES

The bronchopulmonary segments are further subdivided into *pulmonary lobules;* each lobule is supplied by a *bronchiole.* Delicate connective tissue septa that partially separate adjacent lobules may be represented on the surface of the lung as faintly outlined polygonal areas. *Pulmonary acini* are smaller units of structure that make up the lobules. Each acinus consists of a *terminal bronchiole* and the *respiratory bronchioles* and *alveoli* aerated by the terminal bronchiole (Fig. 18.10). The smallest functional unit of pulmonary structure is, thus, the *respiratory bronchiolar unit.* It consists of a single respiratory bronchiole and the alveoli that it supplies.

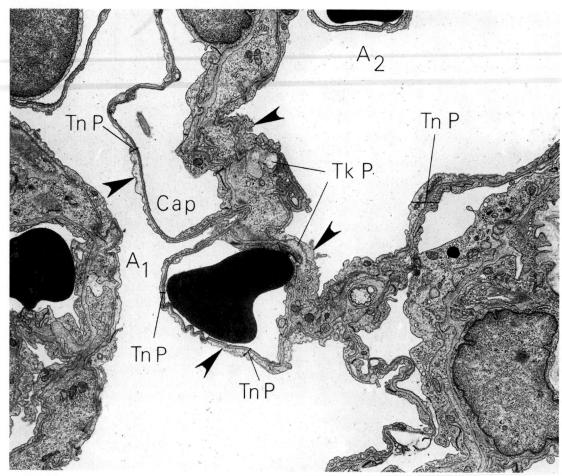

Figure 18.12. Electron micrograph showing two alveolar spaces, A_1 and A_2, and the intervening septal wall (marked by the *facing arrowheads*). The septal wall contains capillaries *(Cap)*, some of which contain red blood cells. The septal wall displays thin portions *(Tn P)* and thick portions *(Tk P)*. These can be seen in the higher magnification shown in Figure 18.15.

Bronchiolar Structure

Bronchioles are air-conducting ducts that measure 1 mm or less in diameter. The larger bronchioles represent branches of the segmental bronchi. These ducts branch repeatedly, giving rise to the smaller **terminal bronchioles** that also branch. They finally give rise to the **respiratory bronchioles.**

Cartilage and Glands Are Not Present in Bronchioles

The larger diameter bronchioles initially have a ciliated, pseudostratified columnar epithelium that gradually transforms to a simple ciliated columnar epithelium as the duct narrows. Goblet cells are still present in the largest bronchioles but are not found in the terminal bronchioles that follow. An exception is in smokers and others exposed to irritants in the air. There are no subepithelial glands in bronchioles. Cartilage plates, characteristic of the bronchi, are absent in bronchioles. Instead, a relatively thick layer of smooth muscle is present in the wall of all bronchioles.

Small bronchioles have a simple cuboidal epithelium. The smallest conducting bronchioles, the **terminal bronchioles,** are lined with a simple cuboidal epithelium in which **Clara cells** (see below) are found among the ciliated cells. The Clara cells increase in number as the ciliated cells decrease along the length of the bronchiole. Occasional brush cells and dense-core granule cells are also present (Figs. 18.10 and 18.11). A small amount of connective tissue underlies the epithelium, and a circumferential layer of smooth muscle underlies the connective tissue in the conducting portions.

Clara cells are nonciliated cells that have a characteristic rounded or dome-shaped apical surface projection. They display TEM characteristics of protein-secreting cells (Fig. 18.11). They have a well-developed basal rER, a lateral or supranuclear Golgi complex, secretory granules that stain for protein, and numerous cisternae of sER in the apical cytoplasm. Clara cells secrete a surface-active agent, a lipoprotein. The functional role of this agent is to prevent luminal adhesion should the wall of the airway fold on itself, particularly during expiration.

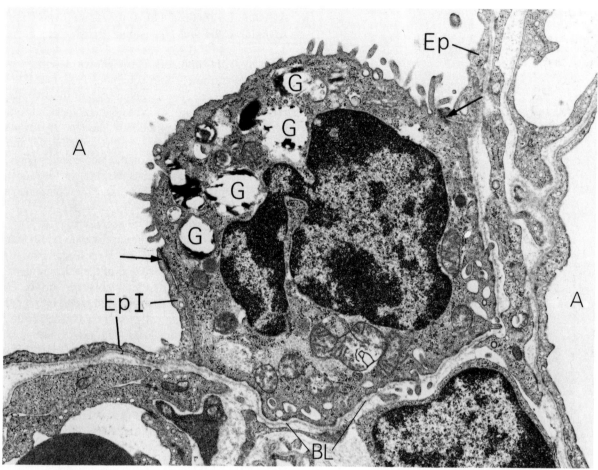

Figure 18.13. Electron micrograph of a type II alveolar cell. The cell has a dome-shaped apical surface with a number of short microvilli present at its periphery and a relatively smooth-contoured apical center. The lateral cell margins are overlain to a variable degree by the type I alveolar cells *(Ep I)* that are joined to the type II cell by occluding junctions *(arrows)*. Both cell types rest on the basal lamina *(BL)*. The granules *(G)* in this specimen are largely dissolved, but their lamellar character is shown to advantage in Figure 18.14. *A,* alveolar air space.

Respiratory Bronchioles Are the First Part of the Bronchial Tree That Allows Gas Exchange to Occur

Respiratory bronchioles constitute a transitional zone in the respiratory system concerned with both air conduction and gas exchange between air and blood. They have a narrow diameter and are lined by a cuboidal epithelium. The epithelium of the initial segments of the respiratory bronchioles contains both ciliated cells and Clara cells (Fig. 18.11). Distally, the Clara cells predominate. Occasional brush cells and dense-core granule cells are also found along the length of the respiratory bronchiole. Scattered, thin-walled outpocketings, *alveoli,* extend from the lumen of the respiratory bronchioles (see Fig. 18.10). It is at these sites where air may leave and enter the bronchiole to allow gas exchange.

CYSTIC FIBROSIS

Cystic fibrosis is a chronic obstructive pulmonary disease of children and young adults. It is an autosomal recessive disorder that affects the viscosity of the secretion of the exocrine glands. Almost all exocrine glands secrete abnormally viscid mucus that obstructs the glands and their excurrent ducts.

The course of the disease is largely determined by the degree of pulmonary involvement. The lungs are normal at birth. The pulmonary lesion is probably initiated by obstruction of the bronchioles by the unusually thick mucous secretions. This blocks the airways and leads to thickening of the walls of the bronchioles and to other degenerative changes. Because fluids remain trapped in the lungs, individuals with this disease often suffer from respiratory tract infections.

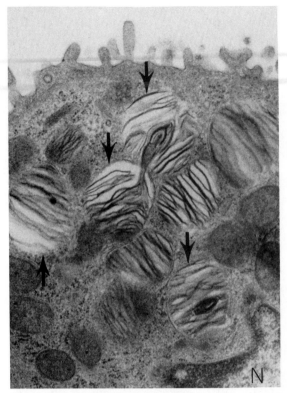

Figure 18.14. Higher magnification electron micrograph showing the typical lamellar pattern of the secretory granules of the type II pneumocytes. The granules are composed of the precursors of pulmonary surfactant. (Courtesy of A. Mercuri.)

ALVEOLI

Alveoli Are the Site of Gas Exchange

Alveoli are the terminal air spaces of the respiratory system and are the actual site of gas exchange between the air and the blood. About 100 million alveoli are found in each lung. Each alveolus is a thin-walled polyhedral chamber approximately 0.2 mm in diameter. At some point, each alveolus is confluent with a respiratory bronchiole, by means of an alveolar duct, and an alveolar sac.

- *Alveolar ducts* are elongate airways that have almost no walls, only alveoli, as their peripheral boundary with rings of smooth muscle in the knob-like interalveolar septa (see below).
- *Alveolar sacs* are spaces surrounded by clusters of alveoli. The surrounding alveoli open into these spaces.

Alveolar sacs usually occur at the termination of an alveolar duct but may occur anywhere along its length. Alveoli are surrounded and separated from one another by a thin connective tissue layer that contains numerous blood capillaries. The tissue between adjacent alveolar air spaces is called the **alveolar septum** (Fig. 18.12).

Alveolar Epithelium Is Composed of Type I and II Alveolar Cells and Occasional Brush Cells

Type I alveolar cells, also known as *type I pneumocytes,* are extremely thin squamous cells that line most of the surface of the alveoli, about 95% of the alveolar surface area. These cells are joined to one another and to the other cells of the alveolar epithelium, the *type II alveolar cells,* also called *type II pneumocytes* or *septal cells,* and the occasional **brush cells,** by zonulae occludentes (Fig. 18.13). These tight junctions enable the cells to form an effective barrier between the air space and the components of the septal wall.

Type II alveolar cells are secretory cells. They are cuboidal cells interspersed among the type I cells but tend to concentrate at septal junctions. Type II cells are as numerous as type I cells, but because of their different shape they cover only about 5% of the alveolar air surface. The type II cells, like the Clara cells, tend to bulge into the air space (Fig. 18.13). Their apical cytoplasm is filled with granules that are resolved in the TEM (Fig. 18.14) as stacks of parallel membrane lamellae *(lamellar bodies).* The lamellae are rich in phospholipids, among which is the surface active agent **surfactant.** The lamellar bodies are released into the alveolar space by exocytosis, and the surfactant forms a monomolecular layer over the alveolar epithelium, thus reducing the surface tension at the air-epithelium interface. Without adequate secretions of surfactant, the alveoli would collapse on exhalation. This occurs in premature infants whose lungs have not developed sufficiently to produce surfactant (respiratory distress syndrome).

Brush cells are also present in the alveolar wall, but they are extremely few in number. They may serve as receptors that monitor air quality in the lung.

The Alveolar Septum Is the Site of the Air-Blood Barrier

The components of the alveolar septum are

- *Alveolar epithelial cells*
- *Basal lamina* of the alveolar epithelium
- *Basal lamina* of the capillary endothelium
- *Endothelial cells* of the rich capillary network
- Other connective tissue elements, including fibroblasts, macrophages, collagen fibers, and elastic fibers (Figs. 18.12, 18.13, and 18.15)

Most of the basal surface of the alveolar epithelium is in intimate association with the capillaries of the septum. Any one capillary may be shared by two or more alveoli.

The **air-blood barrier** refers to the cells and cell products across which gases must diffuse between the alveolar compartment and capillary compartment. The thinnest air-blood barrier consists of a monomolecular layer of surfactant, a

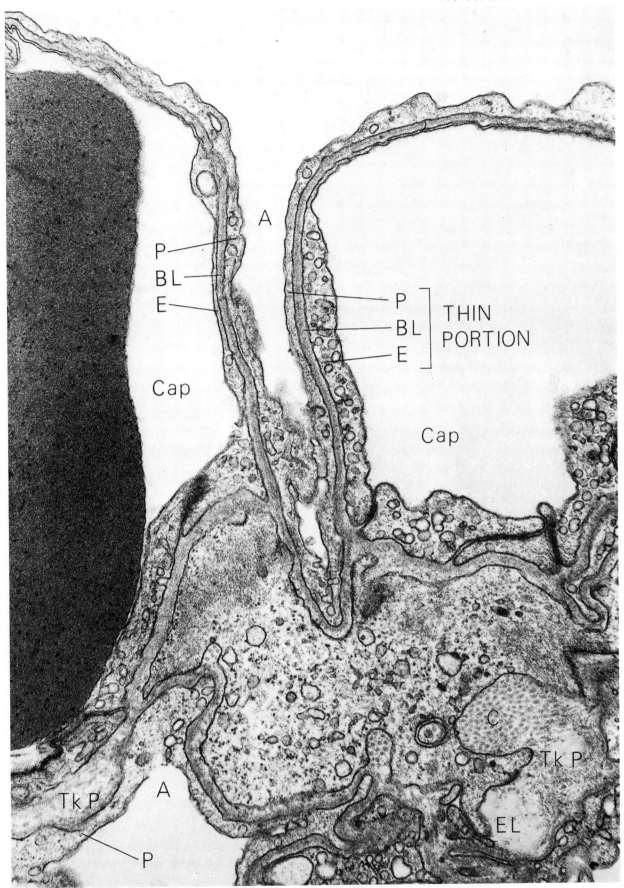

Figure 18.15. Electron micrograph of part of septal wall showing the alveolar capillary complex. The thin portion consists of a pneumonocyte type I cell *(P)*, capillary endothelium *(E)*, and the fused basal lamina *(BL)* shared by both cells. In the thick portion *(Tk P)*, the pneumonocyte type I cell rests on a basal lamina; under this is connective tissue in which collagen fibrils *(C)* and elastic fibers *(EL)* are evident. *A*, alveolar air space; and *Cap*, capillary. ×33,000.

type I epithelial cell and its basal lamina, and a capillary endothelial cell and its basal lamina. Often, these two basal laminae are fused (Fig. 18.15). Connective tissue cells and fibers that may be present between the two basal laminae widen the air-blood barrier. These two arrangements produce a **thin portion** and a **thick portion** of the barrier (Figs. 18.12 and 18.15). It is believed that most gas exchange occurs across the thin portion of the barrier. The thick portion is believed to be a site in which tissue fluid can accumulate and, even, cross into the alveolus. Lymphatic vessels in the connective tissue of the terminal bronchioles drain fluid that accumulates in the thick portion of the septum.

EMPHYSEMA

Emphysema is a condition of the lung characterized by permanent enlargement of the air spaces distal to the terminal bronchiole. This is caused by chronic obstruction of airflow, most often because of narrowing of the bronchioles, and is accompanied by destruction of the alveolar wall. Thus, significant area for gas exchange is lost in this disease. The disease is common. It is seen in about half of all autopsies and is easily recognized. Pathologists identify several types of emphysema. The severity of the disease is clinically more important, however, than the recognition of the specific type. Emphysema is often caused by chronic inhalations of foreign particulate material such as coal dust, textile fibers, and construction dust. The most common cause, however, is cigarette smoking.

The destruction of the alveolar wall may be associated with excess lysis of elastin and other structural proteins in the alveolar septa. Elastase and other proteases are derived from lung neutrophils, macrophages, and monocytes. A specific genetic disease, α_1-antitrypsin deficiency, causes a particularly severe emphysema in both heterozygous and homozygous individuals. It is usually fatal in homozygotes if untreated, but its severity can be reduced by supplying the enzyme inhibitor exogenously.

Alveolar Macrophages Remove Inhaled Particulate Matter From the Air Spaces and Red Blood Cells From the Septum

Alveolar macrophages are unusual in that they function both in the connective tissue of the septum and in the air space of the alveolus. In the air spaces, they scavenge the surface to remove inhaled particulate matter, e.g., dust and pollen, thus giving them one of their alternate names, **dust cells**. Alveolar macrophages also phagocytize red blood cells that may enter the alveoli in heart failure. Some engorged macrophages pass up the bronchial tree in the mucus and are disposed of by swallowing or expectoration when they reach the pharynx. Other macrophages return to or remain in the septal connective tissue, where, filled with accumulated phagocytized material, they may stay for much of an individual's life. Thus, the lungs of a smoker at autopsy will usually show many alveolar and septal macrophages filled with carbon particles. Alveolar macrophages also phagocytose infectious organisms such as tubercle bacilli, which can be recognized in the cells in appropriately stained specimens. These bacilli are not digested by the macrophages, however, and other infections or conditions that damage alveolar macrophages can lead to release of the tubercle bacillus and recurrent tuberculosis.

Collateral Air Circulation Through Alveolar Pores Allows Air to Pass Between Alveoli

Scanning electron microscopic studies of alveolar structure show openings in the interalveolar septa that allow circulation of air from one alveolus to another. These **alveolar pores (of Kohn)** can be of great significance in some pathologic conditions in which obstructive lung disease blocks the normal pathway of air to the alveoli. The alveoli distal to the blockage may continue to be aerated, via the pores, from an adjacent lobule or acinus.

BLOOD SUPPLY

The Lung Has both a *Pulmonary Circulation* and a *Bronchial Circulation*

The **pulmonary circulation** supplies the capillaries of the alveolar septum and is derived from the pulmonary artery that leaves the right ventricle of the heart. The branches of the pulmonary artery travel with those of the bronchi and bronchioles and carry blood down to the capillary level at the alveoli. This blood is oxygenated and collected by pulmonary venous capillaries that join to form venules. They ultimately form the four pulmonary veins that return blood to the left atrium of the heart. The pulmonary venous system is located at a distance from the respiratory passages at the periphery of the bronchopulmonary segments.

The **bronchial circulation,** via bronchial arteries that branch from the aorta, supplies all of the lung tissue other than the alveoli, e.g., the walls of the bronchi and bronchioles and the connective tissue of the lung other than that of the alveolar septum. The finest branches of the bronchial arterial tree also open into the pulmonary capillaries. Therefore, the bronchial and pulmonary circulations anastomose at about the level of the junction between the conducting and respiratory passages. Bronchial veins drain only the connective tissue of the hilar region of the lungs. Most of the blood reaching the lungs via the bronchial arteries leaves the lungs via the pulmonary veins.

LYMPHATIC VESSELS

There is also a dual lymphatic drainage of the lungs that parallels the dual blood supply. One set of lymphatic vessels drains the parenchyma of the lung and follows the air passages to the hilum. Lymph nodes are found along the route of the larger lymphatic vessels. A second set of lymphatic vessels drains the surface of the lung and travels in the connective tissue of the *visceral pleura,* a serous membrane consisting of a surface mesothelium and the underlying connective tissue.

NERVES

Most of the nerves that serve the lung are not visible at the level of the light microscope. They are components of the sympathetic and parasympathetic divisions of the autonomic nervous system and mediate reflexes that modify the dimensions of the air passages (and blood vessels) by contraction of the smooth muscle of their walls.

PLATE 88. Olfactory Mucosa

The olfactory mucosa is located in the roof and part of the walls of the nasal cavity. Its epithelium is pseudo-stratified as in the nonsensory epithelium, but it is thicker and is modified to serve as the receptor for smell. Three cell types are present: basal cells, supporting (sustentacular) cells, and olfactory receptor cells. A brush cell is also present in smaller numbers in the olfactory epithelium, but it is not recognizable in routine hematoxylin and eosin (H&E) preparations.

The receptor cell is a bipolar neuron that has an apical (dendritic) process with a knob-like terminal expansion, the olfactory vesicle. Nonmotile cilia that serve as receptors extend from the vesicle and lie in the secretions on the epithelial surface. The basal portion of the cell tapers into an axonal process that enters the lamina propria and joins axons from other receptor cells. After a short distance in the lamina propria, the axons are ensheathed by Schwann cells. The ensuing nerve has a unique appearance, the large cuboidal Schwann cells being the prominent feature of the nerve.

The supporting cell has more extensive cytoplasm and apical microvilli. It attaches to the receptor cells by adhering junctions and provides metabolic support of the olfactory cells.

The basal cell is small and confined to the basal region of the epithelium. It is able to divide and differentiate into supporting cells.

The lamina propria contains tubuloalveolar Bowman's glands in addition to olfactory nerves and is rich in blood and lymphatic vessels. The glands produce a watery serous secretion that reaches the olfactory surface via ducts. The continual washing effect allows renewal of olfactory sensation, as well as a moist surface to trap odorant substances.

FIGURE 1, olfactory mucosa, human, Azan ×75. This low-magnification orientation micrograph shows part of the wall of the nasal cavity. The olfactory mucosa (OM) and adjacent ethmoid bone (EB) are indicated. The olfactory mucosa is directly attached to the bone tissue; no submucosa is present. In this specimen, however, the mucosa is separated from the bone tissue due to shrinkage, a frequently encountered artefact. The olfactory epithelium (OEp) is pseudostratified, like respiratory epithelium; however, it is typically thicker. Note the respiratory epithelium (REp) included in the lower right of the micrograph. The feature that is most useful in identifying olfactory mucosa is the presence of numerous large, unmyelinated nerves (N) and extensive olfactory (Bowman's) glands (BG) in the connective tissue of the mucosa. Note that the adjacent respiratory epithelium lacks the nerves and exhibits a relative paucity of glands.

FIGURE 2, olfactory mucosa, human, Azan. At this higher magnification, it is possible to distinguish in a general way the three principal cell types of the olfactory epithelium on the basis of nuclear location and appearance, as well as by certain cytoplasmic characteristics. For example, the nuclei of the supporting cells (SC) are relatively dense and are located closest to the epithelial surface. They are arranged in an almost discrete, single layer. The supporting cell has a cylindrical shape and extends from the basement membrane through the full thickness of the epithelium. Immediately beneath this layer are the cell bodies of the olfactory receptor cells (OC). They lie at different levels within the thickness of the epithelium. Careful examination of the nuclei of these bipolar neuronal cells reveals that they contain more euchromatin than the nuclei of the supporting cells and often exhibit several nucleoli. In this preparation, the nucleoli appear as small round red bodies. In some cases, particularly when there is shrinkage, the thin tapering dendritic process that extends to the olfactory surface may be observed. Similarly, an axonal process may sometimes be observed extending basally. The basal cells (BC), the least numerous of the principal cell types, are characterized by their small round nuclei and scant cytoplasm. They are irregularly spaced and lie in proximity to the basement membrane.

The lamina propria contains numerous blood vessels (C, V), lymphatics, olfactory nerves (N), and olfactory (Bowman's) glands (BG). The Bowman's glands are branched tubuloalveolar structures. They exhibit a very small lumen (arrows). The duct elements extend from the secretory portion of the gland beginning in close proximity to the overlying epithelium (arrowhead) and pass directly through the epithelium to deliver their secretions at the surface. The ducts are very short, making it difficult to identify them. The very thin axonal processes (AP) of the olfactory cells are sometimes evident within the lamina propria prior to being ensheathed by Schwann cells to form the prominent olfactory nerves. The nuclei present within the olfactory nerves represent Schwann cell nuclei (ScC).

KEY		
A, artery	**ES,** ethmoid sinus	**SC,** supporting cell nuclei
AP, axonal process	**N,** olfactory nerves	**ScC,** Schwann cell nuclei
BC, basal cells	**OC,** olfactory cells	**V,** vein
BG, Bowman's glands	**OEp,** olfactory epithelium	**arrows,** lumina of Bowman's glands
C, capillary	**OM,** olfactory mucosa	**arrowhead,** duct of a Bowman gland
EB, ethmoid bone	**REp,** respiratory epithelium	entering epithelium

PLATE 88

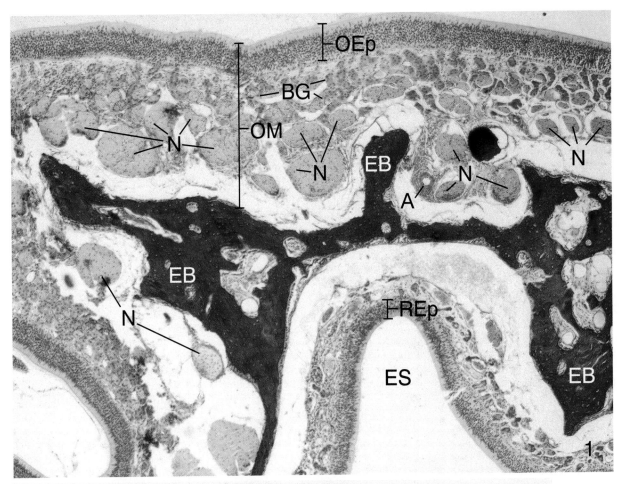

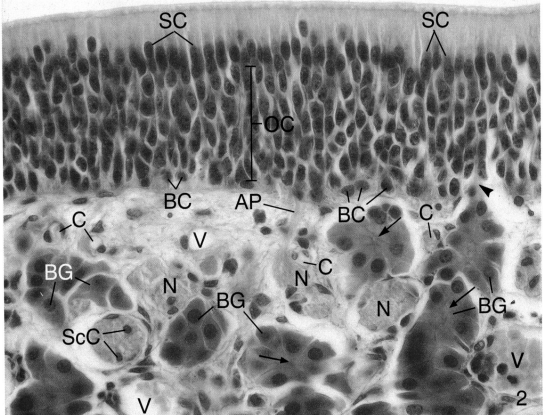

PLATE 89. Larynx

The larynx is the part of the respiratory passage that functions in the production of sound. It consists of a cartilaginous framework, to which muscles are attached, and a mucosal surface that varies in character in different regions. The muscles move certain cartilages with respect to others; in doing so, they bring about a greater or lesser opening of the glottis and a greater or lesser tension on the vocal folds (cords). In this way, vibrations of different wavelengths are generated by the passing air, and sound is produced.

FIGURE 1, larynx, monkey, H&E ×15. The vocal folds are ridge-like structures that are oriented in an anteroposterior (ventral-dorsal) direction. In frontal sections, the vocal folds *(VF)* are cross-sectioned, giving the appearance seen here. The two vocal folds and the space between them constitute the glottis. Just above each vocal fold is an elongated recess called the ventricle *(V)*, and above the ventricle is another ridge called the ventricular fold *(VnF)* or, sometimes, the false vocal fold. Below and lateral to the vocal folds are the vocalis muscles *(VM)*. Within the vocal fold is a considerable amount of elastic material, although it is usually not evident in routine H&E preparations. This elastic material is part of the vocal ligament. It lies in an anteroposterior direction within the substance of the vocal fold and plays an important role in phonation.

FIGURE 2, larynx, monkey, H&E ×160. The surfaces of a vocal fold and the facing ventricular fold within *rectangle 2* in Figure 1 are turned 90° clockwise and shown at higher magnification in this figure. Medially, both are lined by stratified squamous epithelium *(SSE)*. Here, the contact between surfaces is considerable. Laterally, the surfaces consist of stratified columnar epithelium *(SCE)*. The contact between these surfaces is less wearing. Small glands *(Gl)* are in the lamina propria of the laryngeal mucosa.

FIGURE 3, larynx, monkey, H&E ×160. *Rectangle 3* in Figure 1 is shown at higher magnification in this figure. It shows the junction between the stratified squamous epithelium *(SSE)*, with its flat surface cells, and the stratified columnar epithelium *(SCE)*, with its columnar surface cells. The lamina propria consists of loose connective tissue in which glands *(Gl)* are present.

FIGURE 4, larynx, monkey, H&E ×160. Just below the portion of the larynx shown in Figure 1, the epithelium changes again, giving way, below, to the ciliated pseudostratified columnar epithelium *(PSE)* shown here. Note the cylinders of cytoplasm that clearly indicate the columnar nature of the surface cells. In the upper part of the figure, the epithelium is stratified columnar; in the lower part of the figure, it is pseudostratified columnar. This distinction is difficult to make from the examination of a single sample such as that shown here, and other information is needed to make the assessment. The additional information is the presence of cilia on the pseudostratified columnar epithelium; this epithelium is typically ciliated. Although not evident in the photomicrographs, note that stratified columnar epithelium has a very limited distribution, usually occurring between stratified squamous epithelium and some other epithelial types (e.g., pseudostratified columnar here or simple columnar at the anorectal junction). The lamina propria is a loose cellular connective tissue, and it also shows some glands *(Gl)*.

KEY

Gl, glands
PSE, pseudostratified columnar epithelium
SCE, stratified columnar epithelium
SSE, stratified squamous epithelium
V, ventricles
VF, vocal folds
VM, vocalis muscles
VnF, ventricular folds

PLATE 89

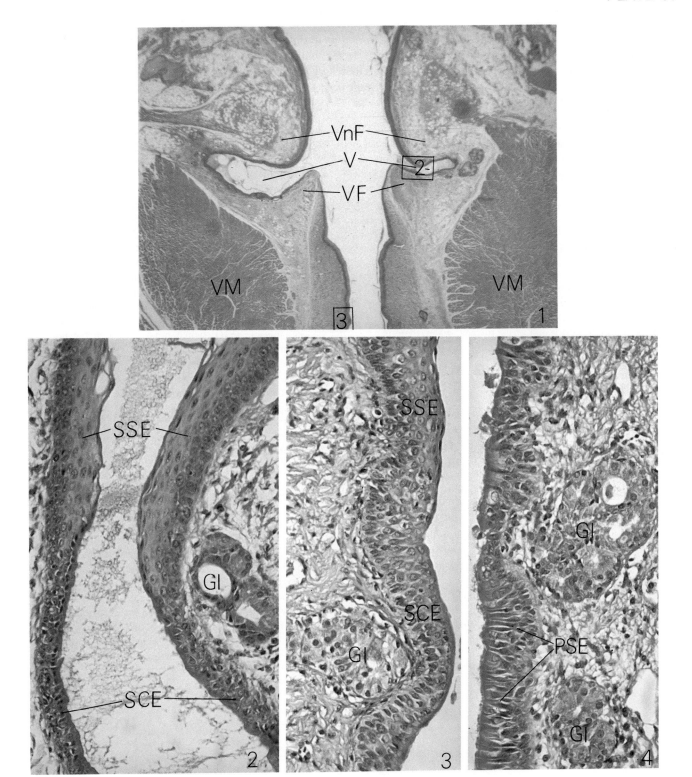

PLATE 90.   Trachea and Bronchus

The trachea extends from the larynx to about the middle of the thorax, where it divides into two bronchi. Its primary function is to serve as a conduit for air. The lumen of the trachea is held open by a series of C-shaped hyaline cartilages that form the structural framework of the wall. Posteriorly, cartilage is lacking, but smooth muscle and fibroelastic tissue are present.

FIGURE 1, trachea, dog, H&E ×65.   The wall of the trachea consists of the following layers: from the inside (luminal surface) there is a *mucosa (Muc)*, a *submucosa (Submuc)*, a *cartilaginous layer (Cart)*, and an *adventitia (Adv)*. The *rectangle* outlines the area shown at higher magnification in Figure 2.

FIGURE 2, trachea, dog, H&E ×160.   The mucosa consists of ciliated pseudostratified columnar epithelium *(Ep)* resting on a highly elastic lamina propria *(LP)*. A division between the mucosa and submucosa is not evident in H&E sections, but the boundary *(double-headed arrow)* is marked by the presence of an elastic layer that is revealed with special elastic tissue stains. Seromucous glands *(Gl)* and their ducts *(Duct)* are present in the submucosa. Glands are also present in the posterior part of the trachea, where there is no cartilage; here, they often extend through the muscle layer into the adventitia.

FIGURE 4, bronchus, dog, H&E ×40.   The trachea divides into two bronchi, one of which goes into each lung. The bronchi branch several times, decrease somewhat in diameter, and undergo certain structural changes (Fig. 4). The large C-shaped cartilages are now replaced by smaller plates *(Cart)* that collectively surround the bronchus. The connective tissue of the bronchus contains a large number of elasticfibers. The discrete elastic layer is, however, replaced by smooth muscle *(SM)*, which now appears at the boundary between the mucosa and submucosa. The mucosa remains essentially the same except for the presence of smooth muscle. The description of ciliated pseudostratified columnar epithelium given above also applies to the epithelium of the bronchi.

FIGURE 3, trachea, monkey, H&E ×640.   Three major cell types are evident in the tracheal epithelium: basal cells, ciliated columnar cells, and goblet cells. Brush cells and dense-core granule cells are also present, but they are not apparent in typical H&E preparations. The dense-core granule cells (argyrophilic cells) are demonstrable with special silver stains. The basal cells, located at the base of the epithelial layer, can be recognized by their spherical, densely staining nuclei *(N Bas)*, which are close to the basement membrane. These cells contain little cytoplasm.

The ciliated columnar cells extend from the basement membrane to the surface. The nuclei of these cells *(N Col)* are generally oval and tend to be located in the midregion of the cell. Moreover, they are somewhat larger and paler staining than the basal cell nuclei. At their free surface they contain numerous cilia that, together, give the surface a brush-like appearance. At the base of the cilia one sees a dense line. This is due to the linear aggregation of structures referred to as basal bodies located at the proximal end of each cilium.

Interspersed between the ciliated cells are mucus-secreting goblet cells *(GC)*. They appear empty because the mucus is lost during tissue preparation. Characteristically, the flattened nuclei are at the base of the mucous cup *(arrows)*.

Although basement membranes are not ordinarily seen in H&E preparations, a structure identified as such is regularly seen under the epithelium in the human trachea. Conspicuous because of its thickness, it is composed of closely packed collagen fibrils that appear as a layer beneath the epithelium; thus, it is not a true basement membrane structure.

KEY

Adv, adventitia
Cart, cartilaginous layer
Duct, duct of seromucous gland
Ep, epithelium
GC, goblet cells
Gl, glands

LP, lamina propria
Muc, mucosa
N Bas, nuclei of basal cells
N Col, nuclei of columnar cells
SM, smooth muscle

Submuc, submucosa
arrows (Fig. 3), nuclei of goblet cells
double-headed arrow (Fig. 2), approximate boundary between mucosa and submucosa

PLATE 90

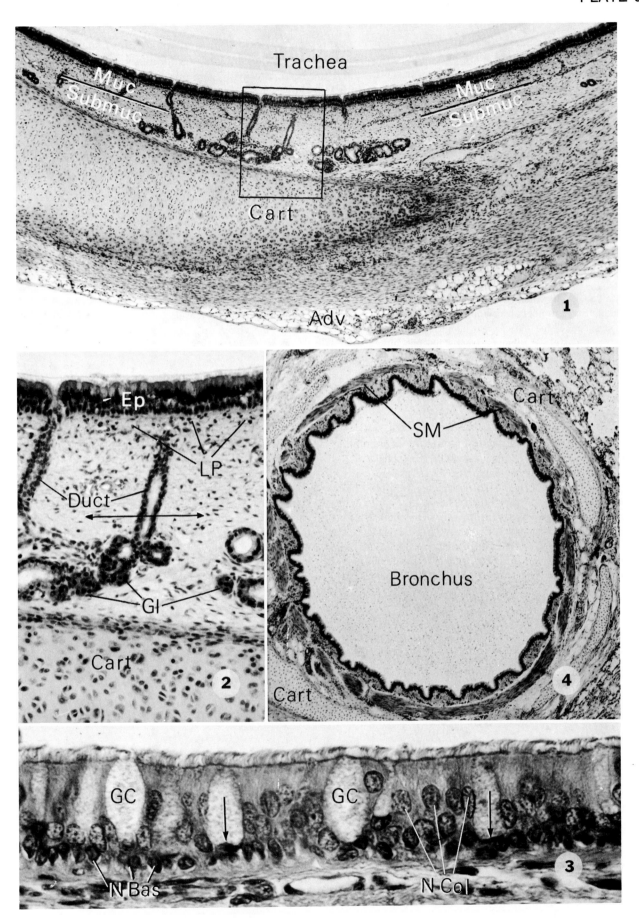

PLATE 91. Bronchiole and End Respiratory Passages

A primary bronchus enters each lung and then, within the lung, divides into smaller secondary and tertiary bronchi. As the bronchi become smaller, components of the wall are lost or changed in amount. Ultimately, the respiratory passage has distinctly different features from those of the bronchus, and it is termed a bronchiole. Chief among the changes in the formation of a bronchiole is the reduction and, finally, disappearance of cartilage. Among the other changes that occur are disappearance of submucosal glands; reduction in the number and, finally, disappearance of goblet cells; change from pseudostratified columnar epithelium to ciliated columnar epithelium, with some columnar cells that are nonciliated; and smooth muscle occupation of a larger proportion of the bronchiolar wall.

FIGURE 1, bronchiole, H&E. A typical bronchiole is shown here. Characteristically, blood vessels *(BV)* are adjacent to the bronchiole. The main features of the bronchiolar wall that are evident in the figure are bundles of smooth muscle *(SM)* and the lining epithelium (shown at higher magnification in Plate 92). Higher magnification would reveal the epithelium to be ciliated. The connective tissue is minimal and, at this low magnification, not conspicuous. Nevertheless, it is present and separates the muscle into bundles (i.e., the muscle layer is not a single continuous layer). The connective tissue contains collagenous and some elastic fibers. Glands are not present in the wall of the bronchiole. Surrounding the bronchiole, comprising most of the lung substance, are the air spaces or alveoli of the lung.

FIGURE 3, alveoli, H&E. The most distal component of the respiratory passage is the alveolus. Groups of alveoli clustered together and sharing a common opening are referred to as an alveolar sac *(AS)*. Alveoli that form a tube are referred to as alveolar ducts *(AD)*.

The outer surface of lung tissue is the serosa *(S)*; it consists of a lining of mesothelial cells resting on a small amount of connective tissue. This is the layer that gross anatomists refer to as the visceral pleura.

FIGURE 2, bronchiole and respiratory bronchioles, H&E. In this figure, a short length of a bronchiole *(B)* is shown longitudinally sectioned as it branches into two respiratory bronchioles *(RB)*. The last portion of a bronchiole that leads into respiratory bronchioles is called a terminal bronchiole. It is not engaged in exchange of air with the blood; the respiratory bronchiole does engage in air exchange. *Arrows* mark the place where the terminal bronchiole ends. Not uncommonly, as shown here, cartilage *(C)* is found in the bronchiolar wall where branching occurs. Blood vessels *(BV)* and a nodule of lymphocytes *(L)* are adjacent to the bronchiole.

The respiratory bronchiole has a wall that is composed of two components: one consists of recesses that have a wall similar to that of the alveoli and, thus, is capable of gas exchange; the other has a wall formed by small cuboidal cells that appear to rest on a small bundle of eosinophilic material. This is smooth muscle surrounded by a thin investment of connective tissue. Both of these components are shown at higher magnification in Plate 92.

KEY		
AD, alveolar ducts	**C,** cartilage	**S,** serosa
AS, alveolar sacs	**L,** nodule of lymphocytes	**SM,** smooth muscle
B, bronchiole	**RB,** respiratory bronchiole	**arrows,** end of terminal bronchiole
BV, blood vessels		

PLATE 91

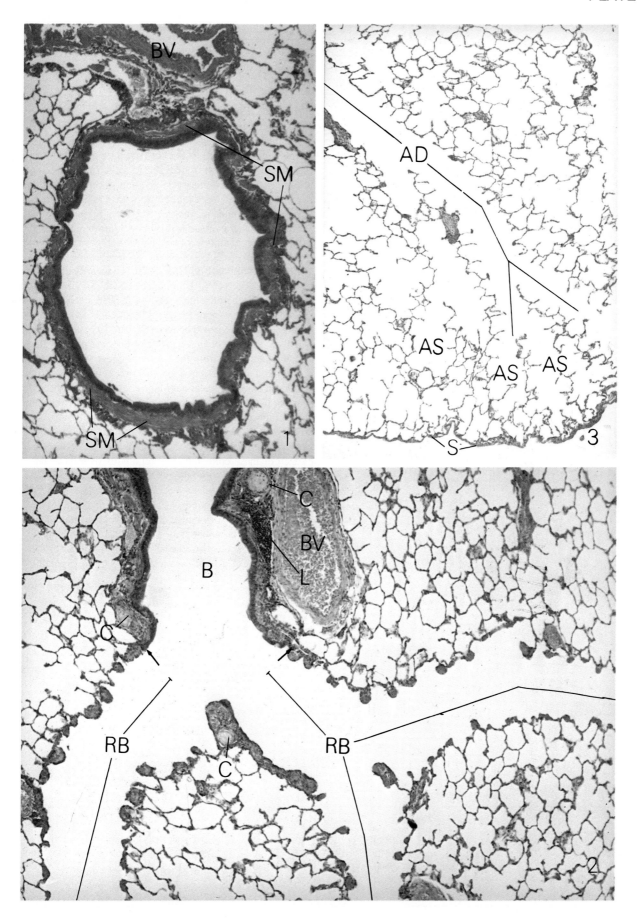

FIGURE 1, terminal bronchiole, H&E. The histologic features of the terminal bronchiolar wall are shown here. Ciliated epithelium extends from the top of the figure to the *diamond*. This is ciliated pseudostratified columnar epithelium. Some basal cells are still present, therefore, the designation as pseudostratified columnar. Elsewhere, the epithelium might be ciliated simple columnar, and just before it becomes a respiratory bronchiole, the epithelium may include cuboidal or low columnar nonciliated cells. These nonciliated cells are Clara cells (*CC, beyond the diamond*). Clara cells produce a surface-active agent that is instrumental in expansion of the lungs. The smooth muscle *(SM)* in the bronchiolar wall is organized in bundles; other cells under the epithelium and around the smooth muscle belong to the connective tissue.

FIGURE 3, respiratory bronchiole, H&E. The respiratory bronchiole shown in Figure 3 is slightly more distal than the area seen in Figure 2. Structurally, it shows essentially the same features as those seen in Figure 2 except that there are fewer Clara cells and the smooth muscle is somewhat thinner.

FIGURE 2, respiratory bronchiole, H&E. The wall of a respiratory bronchiole is shown here and in Figure 3. The alveoli *(A)* are terminal air spaces on the left in each of the two figures. The lumen of the respiratory bronchiole is on the right. Characteristically, the wall of the respiratory bronchiole consists of alternating thick and thin regions. The thick regions are similar to the wall of the bronchiole except that cuboidal Clara cells instead of columnar epithelium form the surface. Thus, as seen here, Clara cells *(CC)* are the surface-lining cells of the thick regions, and smooth muscle bundles *(SM)* are under the Clara cells, with a small amount of intervening connective tissue. The thin regions have a wall similar to the alveolar wall; this is considered below.

FIGURE 4, alveolus, H&E. The alveolar wall is shown in Figure 4. The central component of the wall is the capillary *(C)* and, in certain locations, associated connective tissue. On each side, where it faces the alveolus *(A)*, a flat, squamous cell is interposed between the capillary and the air spaces. This is a pneumocyte type I cell. In some places, the type I cell is separated from the capillary endothelial cell by a single basal lamina shared by the two cells. This is the thin portion of the alveolar-capillary complex, readily seen in the upper part of the figure *(arrows)*. Gas exchange occurs through the thin portion of the alveolar-capillary complex. Elsewhere, connective tissue is interposed between the pneumocyte type I cell and the endothelial cell of the capillary; each of these epithelial cells retains its own basal lamina.

A second cell type, the pneumocyte type II cell or the septal cell *(SC)*, also lines the alveolar air space. This cell typically displays a rounded (rather than flattened) shape, and the nucleus is surrounded by a noticeable amount of cytoplasm, some of which may appear clear. The septal cell produces a surface-active agent, different from that of the Clara cell, that also acts in permitting the lung to expand.

KEY

A, alveolus
C, capillary
CC, Clara cells
PsEp, pseudostratified squamous epithelium

SC, septal cell
SM, smooth muscle
arrows (Fig. 4), thin portion of alveolar-capillary complex

diamond, junction between pseudostratified columnar epithelium and Clara cells

PLATE 92

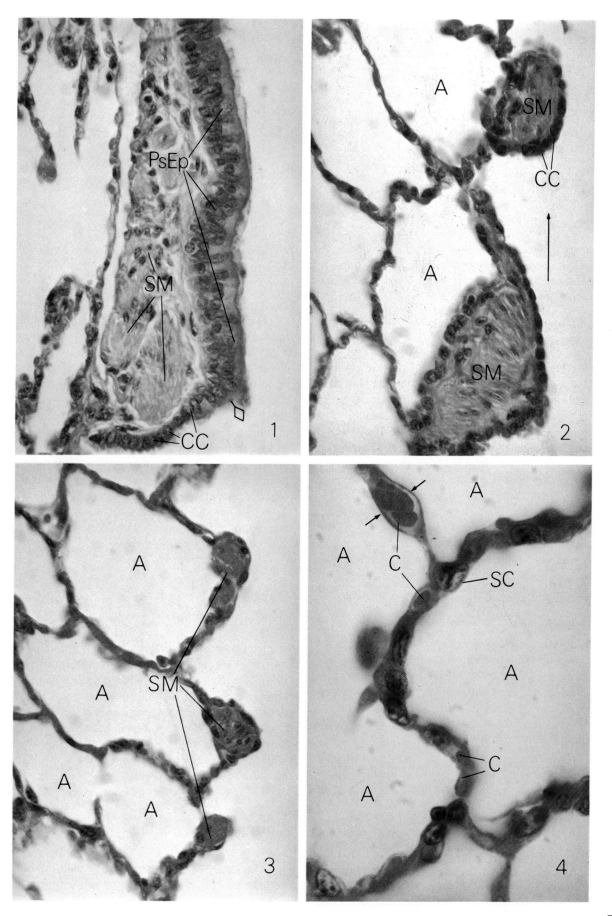

19

Urinary System

The urinary system consists of the paired **kidneys,** the paired **ureters,** which lead from the kidneys to the **bladder,** and the **urethra,** which leads from the bladder to the exterior of the body.

Kidneys Conserve Body Fluid and Electrolytes and Remove Metabolic Waste

Like the lungs and liver, the kidneys retrieve essential materials and dispose of wastes. They conserve water, essential electrolytes, and metabolites, and they remove certain waste products of metabolism from the body.

The kidneys are highly vascular organs. They receive approximately 25% of the cardiac output. The kidneys produce **urine,** initially an *ultra*filtrate of the blood, that is then modified by selective resorption and specific secretion by the cells of the kidney. The final urine is conveyed by the ureters to the urinary bladder, where it is stored until discharged at the body surface via the urethra.

The final urine contains water and electrolytes as well as waste products, such as urea, uric acid, and creatinine, and breakdown products of various substances.

Kidneys Also Function as Endocrine Organs

The endocrine activities of the kidneys include

- Synthesis and secretion of **erythropoietin,** a growth factor regulating red blood cell formation (see page 203)
- Synthesis and secretion of **renin,** a hormone involved in control of blood pressure and blood volume (see page 570)
- Hydroxylation of **vitamin D,** a steroid prohormone, to produce its active form

---

VITAMIN D

Despite its name, vitamin D is actually a steroid prohormone. It is converted to the highly active 1,25-(OH)$_2$ vitamin D by successive metabolic steps that take place first in the liver and then in the kidney. This hormone plays an essential role in calcium balance. It is noteworthy that patients on prolonged renal dialysis, unless treated, often suffer severe disturbance of calcium homeostasis.

KIDNEY STRUCTURE

The kidneys are large, reddish, bean-shaped organs located on either side of the spinal column in the retroperitoneal tissue of the posterior abdominal cavity. Each kidney measures approximately 10 cm long × 6.5 cm wide (from concave to convex border) × 3 cm thick. On the upper pole of each kidney, embedded within the renal fascia and a thick protective layer of perirenal adipose tissue, lies an *adrenal gland.* The medial border of the kidney is concave and contains a deep vertical fissure, called the **hilum,** through which the renal vessels and nerves pass and through which the expanded, funnel-shaped origin of the ureter, called the **renal pelvis,** leaves. A section through the kidney shows the relationship of these structures as they lie just within the hilum of the kidney in a space called the **renal sinus** (Fig. 19.1). Although not shown in the illustration, the space between and around these structures is filled largely with loose connective tissue and adipose tissue.

Capsule

The kidney surface is covered by a thin but tough connective tissue capsule. The capsule consists of an outer layer of fibroblasts and collagen fibers and an inner layer of myofibroblasts (Fig. 19.2). The contractility of the myofibroblasts may aid in resisting the volume and pressure variations that can accompany variations in kidney function. The capsule passes inward at the hilum, where it forms the connective tissue covering of the sinus and becomes continuous with the connective tissue forming the walls of the calyces and renal pelvis (Fig. 19.1).

Cortex and Medulla

Examination with the naked eye of the cut face of a fresh, hemisected kidney reveals that its substance can be divided into two distinct regions (see Plate 93, page 585):

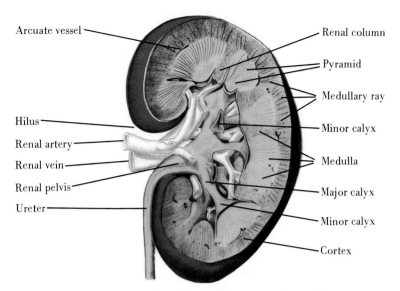

Figure 19.1. Diagram of a kidney seen from behind. Part of the kidney has been removed to show the internal structure.

(Based on Braus H: *Anatomie der Menschen*. Berlin, Springer, 1924.)

- *Cortex,* the outer reddish brown-colored part
- *Medulla,* the much lighter-colored inner part

The color seen in the cut surface of the unfixed kidney reflects the distribution of blood in the organ. Approximately 90–95% of the blood passing through the kidney is in the cortex; 5–10% is in the medulla.

The Cortex Is Characterized by *Renal Corpuscles* and Their Tubules

The cortex consists of *renal corpuscles,* along with the convoluted and straight tubules of the *nephron, the collecting tubules,* and an extensive vascular supply. The nephron is the basic functional unit of the kidney and is described later. The renal corpuscles are spherical structures, barely visible with the naked eye. They comprise the beginning segment of the nephron and contain a unique capillary network called a *glomerulus.*

Examination of a section cut through the cortex at an angle perpendicular to the surface of the kidney reveals a series of vertical striations that appear to emanate from the medulla. These are the *medullary rays* (of Ferrein). The name reflects their appearance, as the striations seem to radiate from the medulla.

The Medullary Ray Is an Aggregation of Straight Tubules and Straight Collecting Tubules

Each medullary ray contains *straight collecting tubules* and straight tubule components of the nephrons. Each nephron and its *collecting tubule* (which connects to a collecting duct) form a functional unit of the kidney, the *uriniferous tubule.* There are 400–500 medullary rays projecting into the cortex from the medulla. The regions between medullary rays contain the convoluted tubules of the neph-

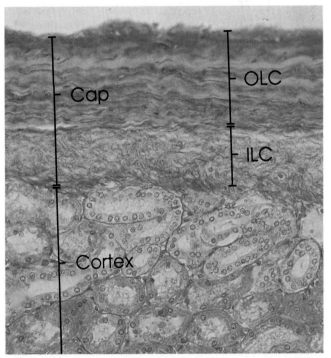

Figure 19.2. Light micrograph of human kidney, showing the capsule *(Cap)* and underlying cortex. The outer layer of the capsule *(OLC)* is composed of dense connective tissue. The fibroblasts in this part of the capsule are relatively few in number; their nuclei appear as narrow, elongate, red-staining profiles against a blue background representing the stained collagen fibers. The inner layer of the capsule *(ILC)* consists of large numbers of myofibroblasts whose nuclei appear as round and elongate, red-staining profiles, depending on their orientation within the section. Note that the collagen fibers in this layer are relatively sparse. Mallory-Azan.

rons and the renal corpuscles. These areas are referred to as *cortical labyrinths.*

The Medulla Is Characterized by Straight Tubules, Collecting Ducts, and a Special Capillary Network

The straight tubular segments of the nephrons and the collecting ducts continue from the cortex into the medulla. They are accompanied by a capillary network, the *vasa recta,* that runs in parallel with the various tubules. These vessels represent the vascular part of the *countercurrent exchange* mechanism that determines the ultimate concentration of the urine.

The tubules in the medulla, because of their arrangement and because of differences in length, collectively form a number of conical structures called *pyramids.* Usually 8–12 but as many as 18 pyramids may occur in the human kidney. The bases of the pyramids face the cortex and the apices face the renal sinus. Each pyramid is divided into an *outer medulla* or *outer zone* (adjacent to the cortex) and an *inner medulla* or *inner zone.* The outer zone is further divided into an inner and an outer stripe. The zonation and the stripes are readily recognized in a sagittal section through the pyramid of a fresh specimen. They are a reflection of the location of distinct segments of the nephron at specific levels within the pyramid (Fig. 19.3).

The Renal Columns Represent Cortical Tissue Contained Within the Medulla

The caps of cortical tissue that lie over the pyramids are sufficiently extensive that they extend peripherally around the lateral portion of the pyramid, forming the *renal columns* (of Bertin).

Although the renal columns contain the same components as the rest of the cortical tissue, they are regarded as part of the medulla. In effect, the amount of cortical tissue is sufficiently extensive that it ''spills'' over the side of the pyramid much as a large scoop of ice cream will extend beyond and overlap the sides of a cone.

The apical portion of each pyramid, which is known as the *papilla,* projects into a *minor calyx,* a cup-shaped structure that represents an extension of the renal pelvis. The tip of the papilla, also known as the *area cribrosa,* is perforated by the openings of the collecting ducts (Fig. 19.4). The minor calyces are branches of the two or three *major calyces* that, in turn, are major divisions of the renal pelvis (see Fig. 19.1).

Kidney Lobes and Lobules

The Number of Lobes in a Kidney Equals the Number of Medullary Pyramids

Each medullary pyramid and the associated cortical tissue at its base and sides (one-half of each adjacent renal column) constitutes a *lobe* of the kidney.

The lobar organization of the kidney is conspicuous in the developing fetal kidney. Each lobe is reflected as a convexity on the outer surface of the organ, but these convexities usually disappear after birth. The surface convexities that are typical of the fetal kidney may persist, however, until the teen-age years and, in some cases, into adulthood. Each human kidney contains 8–18 lobes. Kidneys of some animals possess only one pyramid (Fig. 19.5); these kidneys are classified as unilobar, in contrast to the multilobar kidney of the human.

The Lobule Consists of a Collecting Duct and All the Nephrons That It Drains

The lobes of the kidney are further subdivided into *lobules* consisting of a central medullary ray and the surrounding cortical material (Fig. 19.5). Although the center or axis of a lobule is readily identified, the boundaries between adjacent lobules are not obviously demarcated from one another by connective tissue septa. The concept of the lobule has an important physiologic basis; the medullary ray containing the collecting duct for a group of nephrons that drain into that duct constitutes the renal secretory unit. It is the equivalent of a glandular secretory unit or lobule.

Nephron

The Nephron Is the Functional Unit of the Kidney

The nephron is the fundamental structural and functional unit of the kidney (Fig. 19.3). In the human there are about 2 million nephrons in each kidney. They are responsible for the production of urine and correspond to the secretory part of other glands. It is the collecting tubule that is responsible for the final concentration of the urine. Thus, the collecting tubules are analogous to the ducts of those exocrine glands that are responsible for modifying the concentration of the secretory product. Unlike the typical exocrine gland where the secretory and duct portions arise from a single epithelial outgrowth, the nephrons and their collecting tubules arise from separate primordia and only later become connected.

The *renal corpuscle* represents the beginning of the nephron. It consists of the *glomerulus,* a tuft of capillaries composed of 10–20 capillary loops, surrounded by a double-layered epithelial cup, the *renal* or *Bowman's capsule.* Bowman's capsule is the initial portion of the nephron where blood flowing through the glomerular capillaries undergoes a filtration process to produce the initial urine filtrate.

The glomerular capillaries are supplied by an *afferent arteriole* and are drained by an *efferent arteriole* that then branches, forming a new capillary network to supply the kidney tubules. This is then an arterial portal system. Where the afferent and efferent arterioles penetrate and exit from the parietal layer of Bowman's capsule is called the *vascular pole.* Opposite this site is the *urinary pole* of the

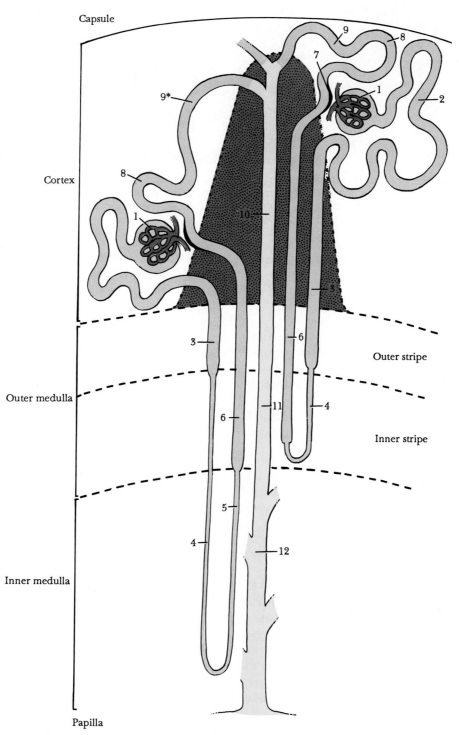

Figure 19.3. Schematic diagram of a long-looped *(left side)* and a short-looped nephron *(right side)* together with the associated collecting duct system. The relative position of the cortex, medulla, papilla, and capsule are indicated. The cone-shaped *gray area* in the cortex represents a medullary ray. *1,* renal corpuscle including the glomerulus (tuft of capillaries) and Bowman's capsule; *2,* proximal convoluted tubule; *3,* proximal straight tubule; *4,* descending thin limb; *5,* ascending thin limb; *6,* thick ascending limb (distal straight tubule); *7,* macula densa located in the final portion of the thick ascending limb; *8,* distal convoluted tubule; *9,* connecting tubule; *9*,* collecting tubule that forms an arch (arched collecting tubule); *10,* cortical collecting duct; *11,* outer medullary collecting duct; and *12,* inner medullary collecting duct. (Modified from Kriz W, Bankir L: A standard nomenclature for structures of the kidney. Used with permission from *Kidney International* 33:1–7, 1988.)

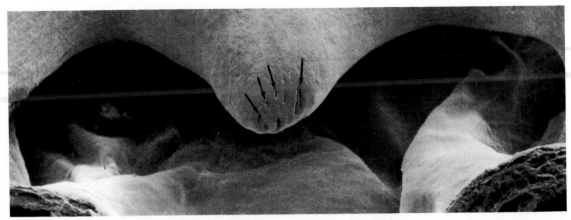

Figure 19.4. Scanning electron micrograph of renal papilla and calyx, showing a conical structure, the apex of the renal papilla, projecting into a space, the renal calyx. The apex of the papilla contains openings *(arrows)* of the ducts of Bellini. These ducts deliver urine from the pyramids to the calyx. The surface of the apex of the papilla containing the openings is designated the area cribrosa. (Courtesy of C. C. Tisher.)

renal corpuscle, where the proximal convoluted tubule begins (Fig. 19.6).

Continuing from Bowman's capsule, the remaining segments of the nephron, namely, the tubular parts, are

- *Proximal thick segment,* consisting of the *proximal convoluted tubule (pars convoluta)* and the *proximal straight tubule (pars recta)*
- *Thin segment,* which constitutes the thin limb of the loop of Henle
- *Distal thick segment,* consisting of the *distal straight segment (pars recta)* and the *distal convoluted tubule (pars convoluta)*

The distal convoluted tubule connects to the collecting tubule, often through a *connecting tubule,* thus forming the *uriniferous tubule,* i.e., the nephron plus collecting tubule (see Fig. 19.3).

Proximal Segment

The proximal thick segment of the nephron begins as the *proximal convoluted tubule* at Bowman's capsule; it makes a short turn toward the cortex and then returns to its site of origin where it follows a very tortuous or convoluted course. It then enters a medullary ray and continues as the descending proximal straight tubule into the pyramid. Next, the *thin segment* descends farther toward the apex of the pyramid, but at some point before reaching the apex, it makes a hairpin turn and returns toward the cortex.

Distal Segment

The distal thick segment ascends through the pyramid and medullary ray as the ascending distal straight tubule to the vicinity of its renal corpuscle of origin. The distal tubule then leaves the medullary ray and makes contact with the vascular pole of its parent renal corpuscle. At this point, the epithelial cells of the tubule adjacent to the afferent arteriole of the glomerulus are modified to form the *macula densa.* The distal tubule then leaves the region of the corpuscle and becomes the *distal convoluted tubule.* The distal convoluted tubule is less tortuous than the proximal convoluted tubule; thus, in a section showing the cortical labyrinth, there are fewer distal tubule profiles than proximal tubule profiles. At its termination, the distal convoluted tubule empties into either an *arched collecting tubule* or a shorter tubule simply called a *connecting tubule* (see Fig. 19.3). Both, in turn, lead to a straight collecting tubule that lies in the medullary ray.

Loop of Henle

The Loop of Henle Is the Entire U-Shaped Portion of a Nephron

The descending limb of the proximal thick segment, the thin segment and its hairpin turn, and the ascending limb of the distal thick segment are collectively called the *loop of Henle.* In some nephrons, the thin segment is extremely short, and the hairpin turn may be made by the distal thick segment.

Types of Nephrons

Several types of nephrons are identified, based on where their renal corpuscles are located in the cortex (see Fig. 19.3):

- *Cortical* or *subcapsular nephrons* have their renal corpuscles located in the outer part of the cortex. They have short loops of Henle, extending only into the outer region of the pyramid. They are typical of the nephrons

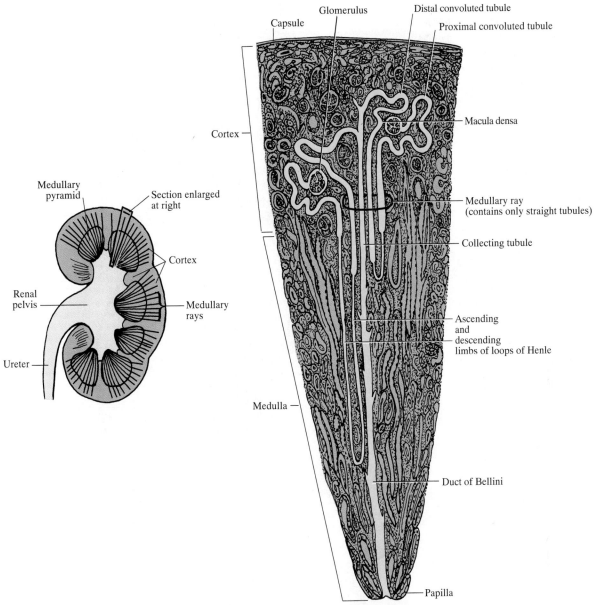

Figure 19.5. Diagrams of adult human kidney showing, on the *left,* a hemisection for orientation and, on the *right,* an enlarged portion emphasizing the relationship of two nephrons and their collecting tubules and ducts (yellow) to the cortex and medulla. The upper nephron, a midcortical nephron, extends only a short distance into the medulla and possesses a short thin segment in the loop of Henle. The lower nephron, a juxtamedullary nephron, has a long loop of Henle that extends deep into the medulla. Both drain into the collecting tubules and duct that form the core of a medullary ray.

described above, wherein the hairpin turn occurs in the distal thick segment.

- *Juxtamedullary nephrons* have their renal corpuscles in proximity to the base of a medullary pyramid. They have long loops of Henle and long thin segments that extend well into the inner region of the pyramid. This is an essential structural feature of the urine concentrating mechanism, which is described later.
- *Intermediate nephrons* have their renal corpuscles in the

midregion of the cortex. Their loops of Henle are of intermediate length.

The straight collecting tubules empty into larger ducts in the medullary ray, the *cortical collecting ducts,* which, in turn, continue into the medulla or pyramid. These ducts travel to the apex of the pyramid, where they join to form larger collecting ducts, called *ducts of Bellini,* that open into the calyx (see Fig. 19.4). The area on the papilla that

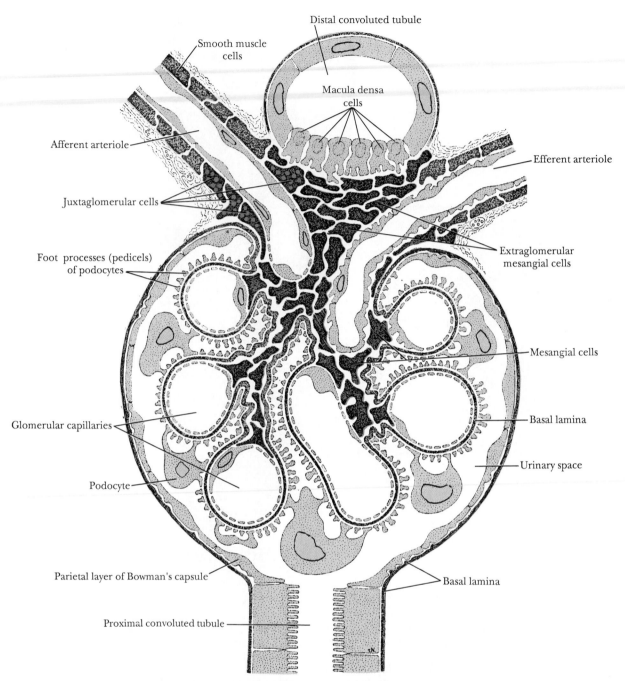

Figure 19.6. Schematic diagram of a renal glomerulus and the structures associated at the vascular pole *(top)* and urinary pole *(bottom)* (not drawn to scale). Mesangial cells are associated with the capillary endothelium and the glomerular basement membrane. The macula densa cells of the distal tubule are shown intimately associated with the juxtaglomerular cells of the afferent arteriole and the extraglomerular mesangial cells. (Modified from Kriz W, Sakai T: Morphological aspects of glomerular function. In: *Nephrology: Proceedings of the Tenth International Congress of Nephrology.* London, Bailliere-Tindall, 1987.)

contains the openings of these collecting ducts is called the **area cribrosa.**

In summary, the gross appearance of the kidney parenchyma reflects the structure of the nephron. The renal corpuscle and the proximal and the distal convoluted tubules are all located in and make up the substance of the **cortical** **labyrinths.** The portions of the straight segments of the proximal and distal tubules (the ascending and descending portions of the loop of Henle) in the cortex are located in and make up the major portion of the **medullary rays.** The thin limb of the loop of Henle is always located in the medulla. Thus, the arrangement of the nephrons (and the collecting tubules and ducts) accounts for the characteristic appearance of the cut surface of the kidney, as can be seen in Figure 19.2.

Renal (Malpighian) Corpuscle

The Renal Corpuscle Contains the Filtration Apparatus of the Kidney

The renal corpuscle consists of the glomerular capillary tuft and the surrounding visceral and parietal epithelial lay-

ers of Bowman's capsule (Figs. 19.6 and 19.7). The filtration apparatus, enclosed by the parietal layer of Bowman's capsule, consists of three components:

- Endothelium of the glomerular capillaries
- Visceral layer of Bowman's capsule
- Basal lamina lying between these two cellular elements

The filtration apparatus may thus be described as a *semipermeable barrier* having two discontinuous cellular layers applied to either side of a continuous extracellular layer, the basal lamina.

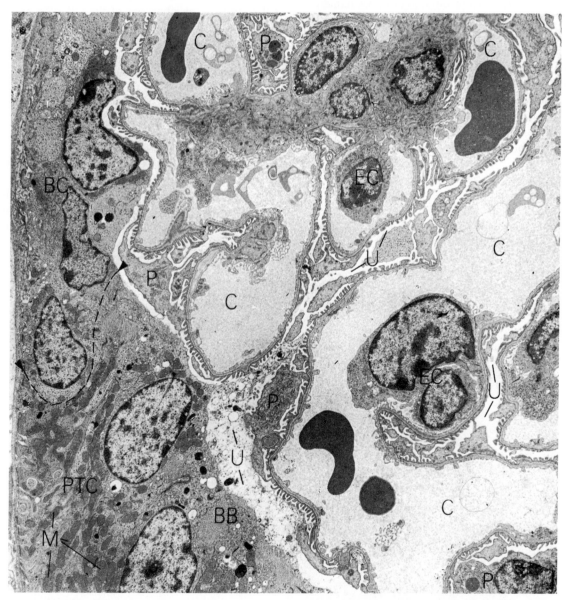

Figure 19.7. Transmission electron micrograph of a glomerulus in the region of the urinary pole. The nuclear and perinuclear regions of the endothelial cells *(EC)* that line the glomerular capillaries *(C)* bulge into the vascular lumen. On the outer surface of the capillaries are the processes of the podocytes *(P)*. External to the podocytes is the urinary space *(U)*. Bowman's capsule *(BC)* is shown on the left; it is continuous at the *broken line* (marked by *arrowheads*) with the proximal tubule cells *(PTC)* of the tubule. Note the numerous mitochondria *(M)* in the base of these cells and the brush border *(BB)* at the apex, projecting into the urinary space. The nuclei of three adjacent mesangial cells can be seen in the upper right corner of the micrograph. ×4700.

The endothelium of the glomerular capillaries has numerous fenestrations (Fig. 19.8). These fenestrations are larger (70–90 nm in diameter), more numerous, and more irregular in outline than fenestrations in other capillaries. Moreover, the diaphragm that spans the fenestrations in other capillaries is absent in the glomerular capillaries.

Podocytes Constitute the Visceral Layer of Bowman's Capsule

The *podocytes,* the cells of the inner or visceral layer of Bowman's capsule, extend processes around the glomerular capillaries (Fig. 19.9). Each process, in turn, has numerous secondary processes called *pedicels* or *foot processes.* The foot processes interdigitate with foot processes of neighboring podocytes, a feature that can be clearly demonstrated with the scanning electron microscope (SEM) (Figs. 19.10, *a* and *b,* and 19.11). The elongated spaces between the interdigitating foot processes, called *filtration slits,* are about 25 nm wide and allow the filtrate from the blood to enter the Bowman's space. The foot processes contain numerous *microfilaments* (actin) that are thought to have a role in regulating the size and patency of the filtration slits. An additional factor that may influence the passage of substances through the filtration slits is the presence of a thin membrane similar to the diaphragm of capillary fenestrations. This membrane, the *filtration slit membrane,* spans the slits (Fig. 19.11, *inset*).

The thick (300–350 nm) basal lamina is the joint product of the endothelium and the podocytes. It is the principal component of the filtration barrier. Because of its thickness, it is prominent in histologic sections stained with the periodic acid-Schiff (PAS) procedure and is, therefore, usually called the *glomerular basement membrane (GBM).*

The Glomerular Basement Membrane Acts as a *Physical Barrier* and an *Ion-Selective Filter*

The GBM contains type IV collagen, sialoglycoproteins, and other noncollagenous glycoproteins (e.g., laminin), as well as proteoglycans and glycosaminoglycans, particularly heparan sulfate (Fig. 19.12). The components tend to localize in particular portions of the GBM:

- The *lamina rara interna,* adjacent to the capillary endothelium
- The *lamina rara externa,* adjacent to the podocyte processes
- The *lamina densa,* the fused portion of the basal laminae, sandwiched between the laminae rarae

The *laminae rarae* are particularly rich in polyanions, such as heparan sulfate, that impede specifically the passage of positively charged molecules. Type IV collagen is concentrated in the *lamina densa,* which is organized into a feltwork that acts as a physical filter. The sialoglycoproteins are involved in the attachment of the endothelial cells and podocytes to the GBM.

The GBM restricts the movement of particles, usually

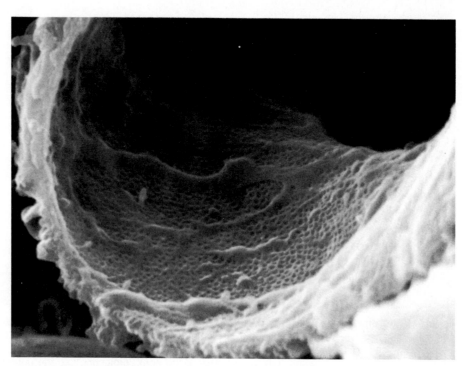

Figure 19.8. Scanning electron micrograph of the interior surface of a glomerular capillary. The wall of the capillary shows horizontal ridges formed by the cytoplasm of the endothelial cell. Elsewhere, fenestrations are seen as numerous dark oval and circular profiles. (Courtesy of C. C. Tisher.)

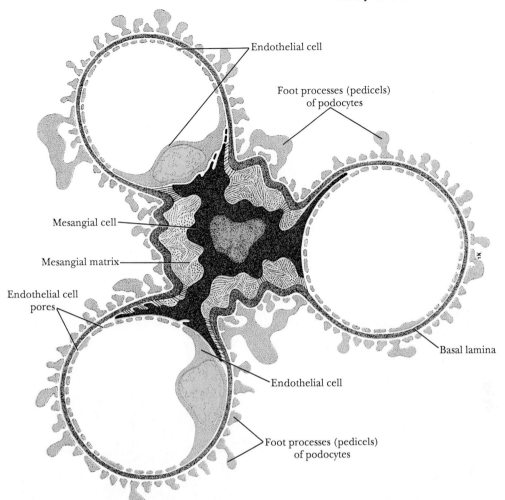

Endothelial cell

Foot processes (pedicels)
of podocytes

Mesangial cell

Mesangial matrix

Endothelial cell
pores

Basal lamina

Endothelial cell

Foot processes (pedicels)
of podocytes

Figure 19.9. Schematic diagram showing the relationship between the intraglomerular mesangial cells and the glomerular capillaries. The mesangial cell and its surrounding matrix are enclosed by the basal lamina of the glomerular capillaries. Note that the mesangial cells are in the same compartment as the endothelium and that they can be intimately associated with the basal lamina as well as with the endothelial cells. (Modified from Sakai T, Kriz W: *Anatomy and Embryology* 176:373–386, 1987.)

proteins, larger than approximately 70,000 Daltons, e.g., albumin or hemoglobin. The fact that albumin, though not a usual constituent, may sometimes be found in urine emphasizes that the size of albumin is close to the effective pore size of the filtration barrier. Despite the ability of the filtration barrier to restrict protein, several grams of protein do pass through the barrier each day. This protein is reabsorbed by endocytosis in the proximal convoluted tubule. In contrast, the presence of significant amounts of albumin or hemoglobin in the urine (***albuminuria*** or ***hematuria***) indicates physical or functional damage to the GBM. The polyanionic glycosaminoglycans of the laminae rarae restrict the movement of cationic particles and molecules across the GBM, even those that are smaller than 70,000 Daltons.

The narrow slit pores formed by the pedicels and the filtration slit membranes also act as physical barriers to bulk flow and free diffusion. The glycoproteins of the filtration slit membrane and of the glycocalyx of the pedicels probably act in a manner similar to that of the glycosaminoglycans of the laminae rarae of the GBM. Lastly, the fenestrae

of the capillary endothelium restrict the movement of blood cells and other formed elements of the blood from the capillaries. In addition to the structural barriers, the flow rate and the pressure of the blood in the glomerular capillaries also have an effect on the filtration function of the renal corpuscle.

URINALYSIS

Urinalysis is an important part of the examination of patients who are thought to be suffering from renal disease. Part of this analysis includes the determination of the amount of protein excreted in the urine. The excretion of excessive amounts of protein, i.e., ***proteinuria*** (albuminuria), is an important diagnostic sign of renal disease. Normally, less than 150 mg of protein is excreted in the urine each day. Although excessive excretion of protein is almost always an indication of renal disease, extreme exercise, such as jogging, or severe dehydration may produce increased proteinuria in individuals without renal disease.

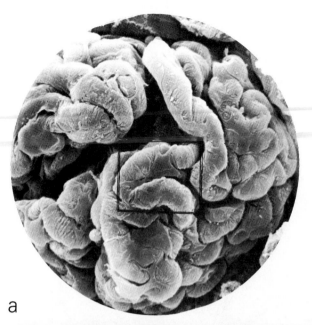

a

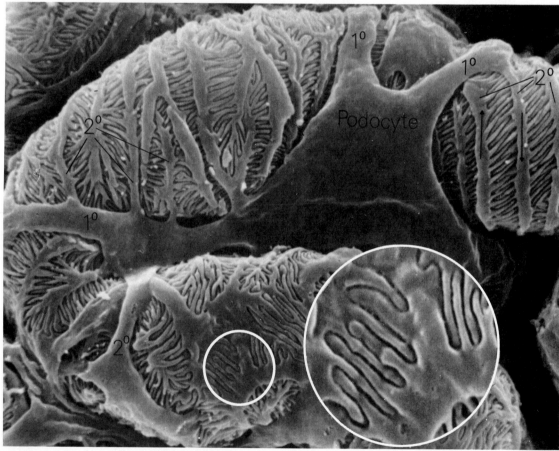

b

Figure 19.10. **a.** Scanning electron micrograph of a glomerulus at low magnification. The parietal layer of Bowman's capsule has been removed, revealing the tortuous course of the glomerular capillaries covered by podocytes within the renal corpuscle. ×700. **b.** A higher magnification of the area in the *rectangle* in **a,** showing the epithelial podocytes (visceral layer of Bowman's capsule) covering the capillary. Note the podocyte and its processes embracing the capillary wall. The primary processes *(1°)* of the podocyte give rise to secondary processes *(2°)*, and these, in turn, give rise to the pedicels. The space between the interdigitating pedicels creates the slit pores. The area in the **inset** (enlarged from the area indicated by the *white circle*) reveals the slit pores at higher magnification. An interesting feature is that alternating pedicels belong to the secondary process of one cell; the intervening pedicels belong to the process of another cell. For example, the *two arrows on the right* of the micrograph are aligned on secondary processes; the *arrow pointing down* is on a process of the podocyte visible from the perspective shown, whereas the process with the *arrow pointing up* is from another podocyte that is not visible from the perspective shown here. Note how each secondary process provides pedicels that then interdigitate with the opposing pedicel of the other cell's secondary process. ×4000; **inset,** ×6000.

568

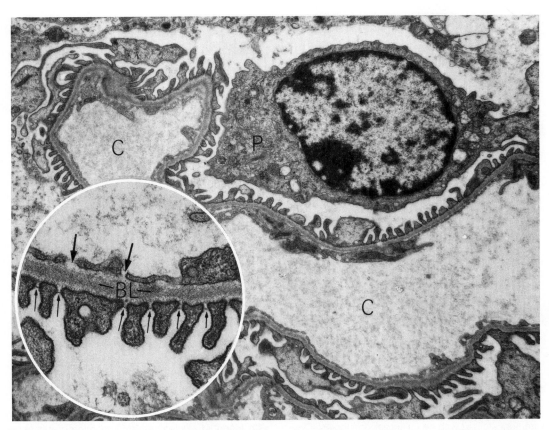

Figure 19.11. Transmission electron micrograph of glomerular capillary *(C)* and adjacent podocyte *(P)*. The pedicels of the podocytes rest on the basal lamina surrounding the capillary endothelium, and together, the three components—the capillary endothelium, basal lamina, and podocytes—form a filtration apparatus. These are seen at higher magnification in the **inset.** *Large arrows* point to the fenestrations in the capillary; external to these is the basal lamina *(BL),* and external to this are the pedicels of the podocytes. Note the slit membrane *(small arrows)* spanning the gap between adjacent pedicels.

The outer layer of Bowman's capsule, called the ***parietal layer,*** is a simple squamous epithelium. At the ***urinary pole*** of the renal corpuscle, it is continuous with the cuboidal epithelium of the proximal convoluted tubule (see Figs. 19.6 and 19.7).

The space between the visceral and parietal layers of Bowman's capsule is called the ***urinary*** or ***Bowman's space*** (see Fig. 19.7). It is the receptacle for the plasma filtrate produced by the filtration apparatus of the renal corpuscle. At the urinary pole of the renal corpuscle, the urinary space is continuous with the lumen of the proximal convoluted tubule.

Mesangium

The renal corpuscle contains an additional group of cells called ***mesangial cells.*** These cells and their extracellular matrix constitute the ***mesangium.*** It is most obvious at the vascular stalk of the glomerulus and at the interstices of adjoining glomerular capillaries. Mesangial cells are positioned much the same as pericytes, in that they are enclosed by the basal lamina of the glomerular capillaries (see Fig.

19.9). The mesangial cells are not entirely confined to the renal corpuscle; some are located outside of the corpuscle along the vascular pole where they are also designated as ***lacis cells*** and form part of what is called the ***juxtaglomerular apparatus*** (see Fig. 19.6).

Although all of the functions of mesangial cells are not yet fully understood, the following functions have been demonstrated:

- Mesangial cells are phagocytic; they can remove trapped residues and aggregated proteins from the GBM, thus keeping the glomerular filter free of debris.
- Mesangial cells and their matrix provide structural support for the podocytes where the epithelial basement membrane is absent or incomplete.

The cleaning of the GBM is believed to be the primary function of the mesangial cells. Clinically, it has been observed that mesangial cells proliferate in certain kidney diseases in which abnormal amounts of protein and protein complexes are trapped in the basement membrane. Mesangial cells are contractile. Thus, they may also play a role in regulating glomerular blood flow.

Embryologically, mesangial cells and the juxtaglome-

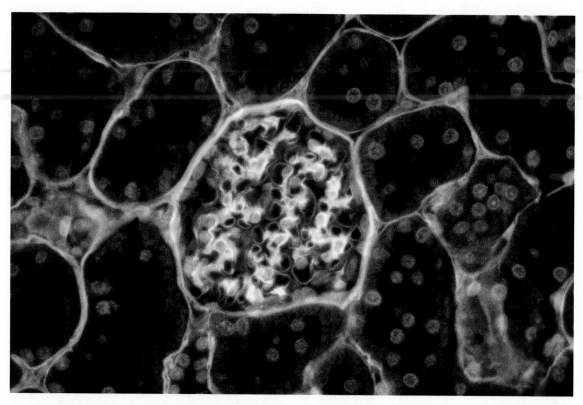

Figure 19.12. A triple-exposure micrograph of a normal adult rat glomerulus immunostained with two different antibodies. One antibody recognizes specific extracellular components, namely, **basement membrane heparan sulfate proteoglycan** (BM-HSPG, rhodamine label). The other antibody recognizes basement membrane **chondroitin sulfate proteoglycan** (BM-CSPG, fluorescein label). Because it is a triple-exposure micrograph, a yellow color occurs where the two fluorescent labels exactly codistribute. The blue fluorescence is nuclear counterstaining with Hoechst nuclear stain. The micrograph shows that compartmentalization occurs with respect to glomerular proteoglycan populations. The glomerular capillary basement membrane is composed exclusively of BM-HSPG, whereas the mesangial matrix (yellow) contains both BM-HSPG and BM-CSPG. Bowman's capsule appears to be strongly stained by only BM-CSPG antibodies. (Courtesy of Dr. K. J. McCarthy.)

rular cells are derived from smooth muscle cell precursors. Although mesangial cells are clearly phagocytic, they are unusual in the sense that they are not derived from the usual precursor cells of the mononuclear phagocytic system, the blood-borne monocytes.

Juxtaglomerular Apparatus

The Juxtaglomerular Apparatus Includes the Macula Densa, the Juxtaglomerular Cells, and the Extraglomerular Mesangial Cells

Lying directly adjacent to the afferent and efferent arterioles and adjacent to some extraglomerular mesangial cells at the vascular pole of the renal corpuscle is the terminal portion of the distal thick segment of the nephron. It contains, as part of its wall, cells that collectively are referred to as the *macula densa.* When viewed with the light microscope, the cells of the macula densa are distinctive, in that they are narrower and usually taller than other distal tubule cells. The nuclei of these cells appear crowded, even to the extent that they appear partially superimposed over one another—thus, the name macula densa.

In this same region, the smooth muscle cells of the adjacent afferent arteriole (and, sometimes, the efferent arteriole) are modified. They contain secretory granules, and their nuclei are spherical, as opposed to the typical elongate smooth muscle cell nucleus. These modified smooth muscle cells, referred to as *juxtaglomerular cells* (see Fig. 19.6), require special stains to reveal the granules in the light microscope.

The Juxtaglomerular Apparatus Regulates Blood Pressure

The granules of the juxtaglomerular cells contain an aspartyl peptidase, called *renin,* that is synthesized, stored, and released into the blood from the modified smooth muscle cells. In the blood, renin catalyzes the hydrolysis of circulating *angiotensinogen* to produce the decapeptide *angiotensin I.* Then,

• Angiotensin I is converted to the active octapeptide *angiotensin II* by an enzyme in the lung. Angiotensin II is the active agent in blood pressure regulation and functions as follows.

- Angiotensin II stimulates the release of the hormone *aldosterone* from the *zona glomerulosa of the adrenal gland* (see page 613).
- Aldosterone, in turn, increases distal tubular resorption of sodium and concomitant resorption of water, thereby raising blood volume and pressure.
- Angiotensin II is also a potent vasoconstrictor that has a regulatory role in the control of renal and systemic vascular resistance.

The juxtaglomerular apparatus functions both as an endocrine organ that helps to regulate blood composition and volume and as a sensor of blood composition and volume. Decreased blood volume or decreased sodium concentration in the blood are believed to be stimuli for the release of renin by the juxtaglomerular cells. In vitro experiments on microperfused juxtaglomerular apparatus have demonstrated that a decrease in NaCl concentration stimulates renin secretion. The cells of the macula densa monitor the NaCl concentration in the afferent arteriole and regulate the release of renin by the juxtaglomerular cells in a paracrine manner. An increase in blood volume sufficient to cause stretching of the juxtaglomerular cells in the afferent arteriole may be the stimulus that closes the feedback loop and stops secretion of renin.

RENIN-ANGIOTENSIN SYSTEM AND HYPERTENSION

Although cardiologists and nephrologists for years have believed that chronic essential hypertension, the most common form of hypertension, was somehow related to an abnormality in the renin-angiotensin system, 24-hour urine renin levels in such patients were usually normal. It was not until a factor in the venom of a South American snake was shown to be a potent inhibitor of the angiotensin conversion enzyme (ACE) in the lung that investigators had both a clue to the cause of chronic essential hypertension and a new series of drugs with which to treat this common disease.

The "lesion" in chronic essential hypertension is now believed to be excessive production of angiotensin II in the lung. The development of the so-called ACE inhibitors, captopril, enalapril, and related derivatives of the original snake venom factor, has had truly revolutionary effects in the treatment of chronic essential hypertension, while avoiding many of the debilitating and often dangerous side effects of the diuretics and β blockers that were previously the most commonly used drugs for control of this condition.

KIDNEY TUBULE FUNCTION

As the glomerular filtrate passes through the uriniferous and collecting tubules of the kidney, it undergoes changes that involve both active and passive absorption, as well as secretion.

- Certain substances within the filtrate are reabsorbed, some partially, e.g., water, sodium, and bicarbonate, and some completely, e.g., glucose.
- Other substances, e.g., creatinine and organic acids and bases, are added to the filtrate, i.e., the primary urine, by secretory activity of the tubule cells.

Thus, the volume of the filtrate is reduced substantially, and the urine is made hypertonic. The long loops of Henle and the collecting tubules that pass parallel to similarly arranged blood vessels, the *vasa recta,* serve as the basis for the *countercurrent multiplier mechanism* that is instrumental in concentrating the urine and, thereby, making it hypertonic.

Proximal Thick Segment

The Proximal Thick Segment Is the Initial and Major Site of Reabsorption

The *proximal convoluted tubule* receives the primary filtrate from the urinary space of Bowman's capsule. The cuboidal cells of the tubule have the elaborate surface specializations associated with cells engaged in absorption and fluid transport. They exhibit the following features:

- A *brush border,* composed of numerous, relatively long microvilli (Fig. 19.13)
- A *terminal bar apparatus,* consisting of a narrow tight junction and a zonula adherens that seal off the intercellular space from the lumen of the tubule
- Large, flattened processes, *plicae* or folds, on the lateral surfaces of the cells, which alternate with similar processes of adjacent cells (Fig. 19.13)
- Extensive *interdigitation of basal processes* of adjacent cells (Figs. 19.14 and 19.15)
- *Basal striations,* consisting of elongate mitochondria concentrated in the basal processes and oriented normal to the basal surface (Fig. 19.14)

In well-fixed histologic preparations, the basal striations and the apical brush border help to distinguish the cells of the proximal convoluted tubule from those of the other tubules.

At the very base of the cell, in the interdigitating processes, bundles of 6-nm microfilaments are present (see *arrows,* Figs. 19.14 and 19.15). It has been suggested that these actin filaments play a role in regulating the movement of fluid from the basolateral extracellular space across the tubule basal lamina toward the adjacent peritubular capillary.

The Proximal Convoluted Tubule Reabsorbs 80% of the Primary Filtrate

Water and Electrolyte Reabsorption. The proximal convoluted tubule reabsorbs about 150 liters of fluid per day. As in the intestinal and gallbladder epithelia, this re-

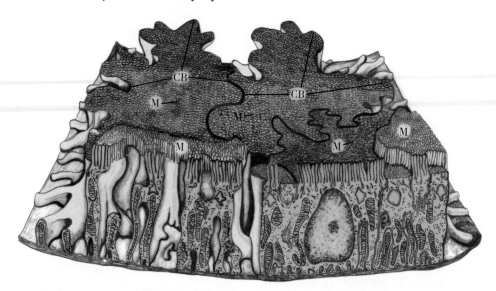

Figure 19.13.   Diagram showing both sectioned faces and three-dimensional aspects of proximal convoluted tubule cells. The basolateral interdigitations are numerous; some of the interdigitating processes extend the full height of the cell. The processes are long in the basal region and create an elaborate extracellular compartment adjacent to the basal lamina (see Fig. 19.15). Apically, the microvilli *(M)* constitute a brush border. In some locations, the microvilli have been omitted, thereby revealing the convoluted character of the apical cell boundary *(CB)*. (Based on Bulger R: *American Journal of Anatomy* 116:253, 1965.)

sorption of fluid is driven by active transport of Na^+ into the lateral intercellular space. The pump enzyme, ***Na⁺-K⁺-activated ATPase,*** is localized in the plasma membrane of the lateral folds. The active transport of Na^+ is followed by passive diffusion of Cl^- to maintain electrochemical neutrality. The accumulation of NaCl in the lateral intercellular spaces creates an osmotic gradient that draws water from the lumen into the intercellular compartment. This compartment distends as the amount of fluid in it increases; the lateral folds separate to allow this distension.

The hydrostatic pressure head that then builds up in the distended intercellular compartment, presumably aided by contractile activity of the actin filaments in the base of the tubule cells, drives an essentially isosmotic fluid through the basement membrane of the tubule into the renal connective tissue. Here, the fluid is reabsorbed into the vessels of the ***peritubular capillary network.***

The Proximal Tubule Reabsorb Amino Acids, Sugars, and Polypeptides

Amino Acid, Sugar, and Protein Reabsorption.   As in the intestine, the microvilli of the proximal tubule cell are covered with a well-developed glycocalyx that contains several ATPases, peptidases, and high concentrations of disaccharidases. In addition to amino acids and monosaccharides, the primary filtrate also contains small peptides and disaccharides. The latter adsorb on the glycocalyx for further digestion before internalization of the resulting amino acids and monosaccharides (including glucose). Also, as in the gut, amino acid and glucose resorption are dependent on active Na^+ transport.

Proteins and Large Peptides Are Reabsorbed by Endocytosis in the Proximal Tubule

There are deep tubular invaginations between the microvilli of the proximal tubule cells. Proteins in the filtrate, on reaching the tubule lumen, bind to the glycocalyx that covers the plasma membrane of the invaginations. Then endocytic vesicles containing the bound protein bud from the invaginations and fuse in the apical cytoplasm to form large protein-containing vacuoles (Fig. 19.14). These vacuoles concentrate the protein in their lumen before fusing with primary lysosomes. The proteins are degraded by the acid hydrolases of the lysosomes, and the amino acids produced are recycled into the circulation via the intercellular compartment and the interstitial connective tissue.

Also, the pH of the primary filtrate is modified in the proximal convoluted tubule by the reabsorption of bicarbonate and by the specific secretion into the lumen of exogenous organic acids and organic bases derived from the peritubular capillary circulation.

Proximal Straight Segment

The cells of the straight segment of the proximal tubule, i.e., the thick descending limb of the loop of Henle, are not as specialized for absorption as are those of the convoluted segment. They are shorter, with a less well-developed brush border and with fewer and less complex lateral and basal-lateral processes. The mitochondria are smaller than those of the cells of the convoluted segment and are randomly distributed in the cytoplasm. There are fewer apical invaginations and endocytic vesicles, as well as fewer lysosomes.

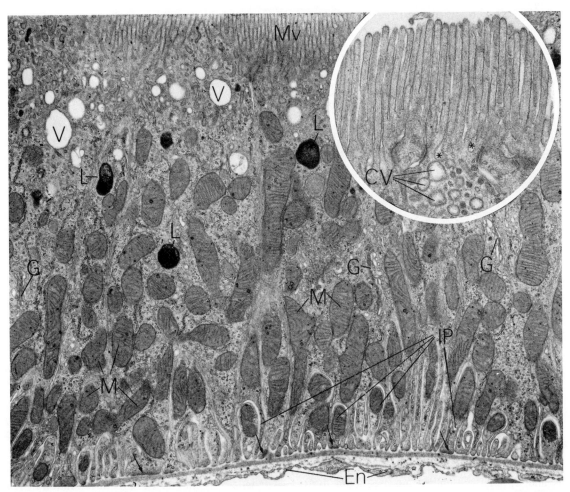

Figure 19.14. Electron micrograph of a proximal tubule cell. The apical surface of the cell shows numerous microvilli *(Mv)* that collectively are recognized as the brush border in the light microscope. Numerous vesicles *(V)* are evident in the apical cytoplasm. These form by fusion of smaller vesicles *(CV,* **inset**) that pinch off from the plasma membrane at the base of the microvilli *(asterisks,* **inset**). Also present in the apical region and midregion of the cell are lysosomes *(L)* and Golgi profiles *(G).* The nucleus has not been included in the plane of section. Many longitudinally oriented mitochondria *(M)* are seen within the interdigitating processes *(IP)* directly adjacent to the infolded plasma membrane. The mitochondria are responsible for the appearance of the basal striations seen in the light microscope, particularly if the extracellular space is enlarged. In the base of the foot processes there is a dense material *(arrows)* that represents bundles of cross-sectioned microfilaments (these are the same filaments as seen in longitudinal section in Fig. 19.15). The electron micrograph also reveals a small amount of connective tissue and the fenestrated endothelium *(En)* of an adjacent peritubular capillary. ×15,000.

Thin Segment

As noted earlier, the length of the thin segment of a nephron varies with its location in the cortex. Juxtaglomerular nephrons have the longest thin segment; cortical nephrons have the shortest. Furthermore, the type of cell that constitutes the thin segment shows variation. In the light microscope it is possible to detect at least two kinds of thin segment tubules, one with an epithelium more squamous than that of the other. Examination of the thin segments of the various nephrons by electron microscopy reveals further differences, namely, the existence of four types of epithelial cells (Fig. 19.16).

- *Type I* epithelium is found in the thin segment of the loop of Henle of short-looped nephrons. It consists of a thin, simple epithelium. The cells have almost no interdigitations with neighboring cells and have few organelles.
- *Type II* epithelium, found in the thin descending limb of long-looped nephrons, consists of taller epithelium. These cells possess abundant organelles and have many small, blunt microvilli. The extent of lateral interdigitation with neighboring cells shows species variation.
- *Type III* epithelium, found in the thin descending limb in the inner medulla, consists of a thinner epithelium. The cells have simpler structure and have fewer microvilli than cells of the type II epithelium. Lateral interdigitations are absent.
- *Type IV* epithelium, found at the bend of long-looped

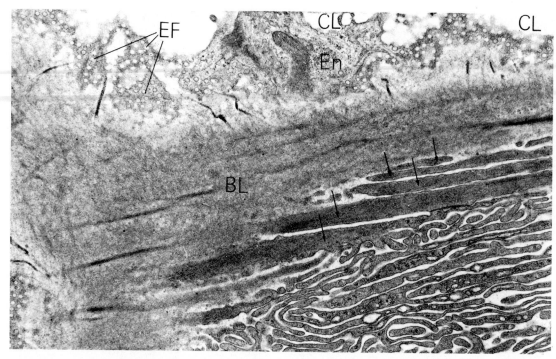

Figure 19.15. Electron micrograph of a section that is almost tangential to the base of a proximal convoluted tubule cell and the subjacent basal lamina and capillary. In the upper part of the micrograph is the capillary lumen *(CL)* bounded by the capillary endothelium *(En)*. Characteristically, the endothelium possesses numerous fenestrations *(EF)*, and in this plane of section, the fenestrations are seen in face view, displaying cir-cular profiles. The basal lamina *(BL)* appears as a broad band of homogeneous material. Below that (lower right) are the in-terdigitating basal processes of the proximal tubule cells. The long, straight processes contain longitudinally oriented micro-filaments *(arrows)*. In this plane of section, the basal extra-cellular space appears as a maze between the cellular pro-cesses. ×15,000.

nephrons and through the entire thin ascending limb, consists of a low, flattened epithelium without micro-villi. The cells possess few organelles.

The specific functional roles of the four cell types in the thin segment are not yet clear, although this segment is part of the countercurrent exchange system that functions in concentrating the urine. Morphologic differences, such as microvilli, mitochondria, and degree of cellular interdigi-tation, probably reflect specific active or passive roles in this process.

Permeability of the Thin Segment. The descending portion of the thin segment is **permeable,** permitting free passage or **equilibration** of salt and water between the lu-men of the nephron and the peritubular connective tissue. Because the interstitial fluid in the medulla is hypertonic (read about the countercurrent multiplier system under His-tophysiology of the Kidney), water diffuses out of, and salt diffuses into, the nephron at this site.

The hypertonicity of the interstitium is directly related to the transport activity of the cells of the ascending portion of the thin segment of the loop of Henle, which actively pump Cl^- into the intercellular compartment from which it diffuses to the interstitium. As in most pump systems, a counter ion, in this case Na^+, follows passively in order to maintain electrochemical neutrality. Further, the ascending portion of the thin segment is largely **impermeable** to water,

so that at this site, as the salt concentration increases in the interstitium, the interstitium becomes hypertonic and the fluid in the lumen of the nephron becomes hypotonic.

Distal Thick Segment

The *thick, straight, ascending segment of the distal tu-bule,* as previously noted, is the third part of the loop of Henle and includes both medullary and cortical portions, with the latter in the medullary rays. The straight segment of the distal tubule, like the ascending thin segment, trans-ports ions from the tubular lumen to the interstitium. The large, cuboidal cells of the distal tubule have extensive basal-lateral plications and numerous large mitochondria associ-ated with these basal folds (Fig. 19.17). They have con-siderably fewer and less well-developed microvilli than proximal tubule cells (compare Figs. 19.14 and 19.17).

In routine histologic preparations, the cells stain lightly with eosin, and the lateral margins of the cells are indis-tinct. The nucleus is located in the apical portion of the cell and sometimes, especially in the straight segment, causes the cell to bulge into the lumen.

The Distal *Convoluted* Tubule Exchanges Na^+ for K^+ Under Aldosterone Regulation

The distal *convoluted* tubule, located in the cortical lab-yrinth, is only about one-third as long (~5 mm) as the

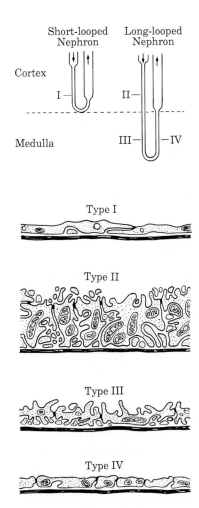

Type I

Type II

Type III

Type IV

Figure 19.16. Schematic diagrams of a short-looped nephron *(top, left side)*, a long-looped nephron *(top, right side)*, and four regions of the epithelium of the thin limb of the loop of Henle. *Roman numerals (I–IV)* identify the various segments of the epithelium and the region where they are found in the thin limb of the loop. The diagrams of the epithelium do not include nuclear regions of the epithelial cells. See text for further explanation. (Modified from Madsen KM, Tisher CC: Physiologic anatomy of the kidney. *Kidney Hormones* 3:45–100, 1986.)

proximal convoluted tubule. This short segment is responsible for

- *Reabsorption of Na$^+$* and *secretion of K$^+$* in order to conserve Na$^+$
- Continued *reabsorption of bicarbonate ion,* with concomitant secretion of hydrogen ion, leading to further acidification of the urine
- *Conversion of ammonia to ammonium ion* that then can enter the urea cycle in order to avoid the toxic effects of ammonia

Aldosterone, secreted by the adrenal gland and released under stimulation by angiotensin II, increases the reabsorption of Na$^+$ and secretion of K$^+$. This has the effect of increasing blood volume and blood pressure in response to increased blood Na$^+$ concentration. Angiotensin conversion

enzyme inhibitors thus regulate blood pressure by secondarily inhibiting aldosterone secretion.

Antidiuretic hormone (ADH), a neurosecretion from the *hypothalamus* that is released by the *posterior pituitary gland* (see page 600), can act on the terminal portion of the distal convoluted tubule to increase the permeability of the tubule to water, thereby producing a more concentrated urine. Increase in plasma osmolality or decrease in blood volume stimulates release of ADH, as does nicotine. The latter effect was the basis for one of the common clinical tests of posterior pituitary function. The action of this hormone is more significant in the collecting tubules and collecting ducts (see below).

Collecting Tubules and Collecting Ducts

The collecting tubules begin in the cortical labyrinth, as either *connecting tubules* or *arched collecting tubules,* and proceed to the medullary ray where they continue as *straight collecting tubules.* Straight collecting tubules, in turn, merge in the medullary ray to form *cortical collecting ducts.* These collecting ducts continue into the pyramids where they continue to merge, ultimately forming large ducts (up to 200 μm), the *papillary ducts* (ducts of Bellini).

Both the collecting tubules and ducts are composed of a simple epithelium. The arched and cortical collecting tubules have flattened cells, somewhat squamous to cuboid in shape. The medullary collecting ducts have cuboidal cells, with a transition to columnar cells as the ducts increase in size. The collecting tubules and ducts are readily distinguished from proximal and distal tubules by virtue of the cell boundaries that can be seen in the light microscope.

Cytologically, two distinct types of cells are present in the collecting system:

- *Light cells,* also called *collecting duct or CD cells,* are the principal cells of the system. They are pale-staining cells with basal infoldings, true infoldings rather than processes that implicate with those of adjacent cells. They possess a single cilium and have relatively few short microvilli (Fig. 19.18). They contain small, spherical mitochondria.
- *Dark cells,* also called *intercalated (IC) cells,* occur in considerably smaller numbers. They have many mitochondria, and their cytoplasm appears more dense. Microplicae, cytoplasmic folds, are present on their apical surface, as well as microvilli. The microplicae are readily observed in the SEM but may be mistaken for microvilli with the transmission electron microscope (TEM) (Fig. 19.18). They do not show basal infoldings but have basally located interdigitations with neighboring cells. Numerous vesicles are present in the apical cytoplasm.

The cells of the collecting ducts gradually become taller as the ducts pass from the outer to the inner medulla and become columnar in the region of the renal papilla. The dark cells gradually decrease in number until none are present in the ducts as they approach the papilla.

HORMONAL REGULATION OF COLLECTING DUCT FUNCTION

As noted above, the water permeability of the epithelium of the collecting ducts is regulated by **antidiuretic hormone (ADH)**, released from the posterior pituitary. In the absence of ADH, a copious, dilute urine is produced. This condition is called **diabetes insipidus.** Increased secretion of ADH can produce an extremely hypertonic urine, thereby conserving water in the body. Excess consumption of water can inhibit ADH release, thereby promoting the production of a large volume of hypotonic urine. Inadequate consumption of water or loss of water as a result of sweating, vomiting, or diarrhea stimulates release of ADH. This leads to an increase in the permeability of the epithelium of the distal and collecting tubules and promotes the production of a small volume of hypertonic urine.

INTERSTITIAL CELLS

The connective tissue of the kidney parenchyma, called **interstitial tissue,** surrounds the components of the nephrons, the ducts, and the blood and lymphatic vessels. This tissue increases considerably in amount from the cortex (where it constitutes about 7% of the volume) to the inner region of the medulla and papilla (where it may constitute more than 20% of the volume).

In the cortex, two types of interstitial cells are recognized: cells that resemble fibroblasts, found between basement membrane of the tubules and the adjacent peritubular capillaries, and occasional macrophages.

In their intimate relationship with the base of the tubular epithelial cells, the fibroblasts resemble the subepithelial fibroblasts of the intestine (see page 467), another transporting tissue. These cells synthesize and secrete the collagen and glycosaminoglycans of the extracellular matrix of the interstitium.

In the medulla, the principal interstitial cells resemble myofibroblasts. They are oriented normal to the long axes of the tubular structures and may have a role in compressing these structures. The cells contain prominent bundles of actin filaments, abundant rough endoplasmic reticulum (rER), a well-developed Golgi complex, and lysosomes. Prominent lipid droplets in the cytoplasm appear to increase and decrease in relationship to the diuretic state. Some experimental evidence suggests that these cells may secrete a hormone-like material that reduces blood pressure, but this has been neither isolated nor characterized. In addition, it has been reported that prostaglandins and prostacyclin are synthesized in the interstitium.

HISTOPHYSIOLOGY OF THE KIDNEY

The Countercurrent Multiplier System Creates Hypertonic Urine

The ability to excrete a hypertonic urine depends on a combination of three morphologic specializations:

- *Loop of Henle*
- *Vasa recta,* which form a loop paralleling the loop of Henle
- Arrangement of the collecting ducts in the medulla

A Standing Gradient of Ion Concentration Produces a Hypertonic Urine

The loop of Henle is the structure that allows the creation and maintenance in the medullary interstitium of a gradient of ion concentration that increases from the corticomedullary junction to the renal papilla. As noted previously, the descending limb of the loop of Henle is freely permeable to Na^+, Cl^-, and water, whereas the ascending limb of the loop of Henle is impermeable to water. Further, the ascending limb actively transports Cl^- from the lumen to the interstitium; Na^+ follows passively to maintain electrochemical neutrality.

Because water cannot leave the ascending limb, the interstitium becomes hypertonic relative to the luminal contents. Although some of the Cl^- and Na^+ of the interstitium diffuse back into the nephron at the descending limb, the ions are transported out again in the ascending limb. This produces the **countercurrent multiplier** effect. Thus, the concentration of NaCl in the interstitium gradually increases down the length of the loop of Henle and, consequently, through the thickness of the medulla from the corticomedullary junction to the papilla.

Collecting Ducts and Vasa Recta Are Countercurrent Exchangers

To explain the countercurrent exchange mechanism, it is necessary to return briefly to a description of the renal circulation and to resume the description of this system at the point at which the efferent arteriole leaves the renal corpuscle.

Vasa Recta

The efferent arterioles of the renal corpuscles of most of the cortex branch to form the capillary network that surrounds the tubular portions of the nephron in the cortex, the **peritubular capillary network.** The efferent arterioles of the juxtamedullary renal corpuscles form several unbranched arterioles that descend into the medullary pyramid. These **arteriolae rectae** make a hairpin turn deep in the medullary pyramid and ascend as the **venulae rectae.** Together, the descending arterioles and the ascending ven-

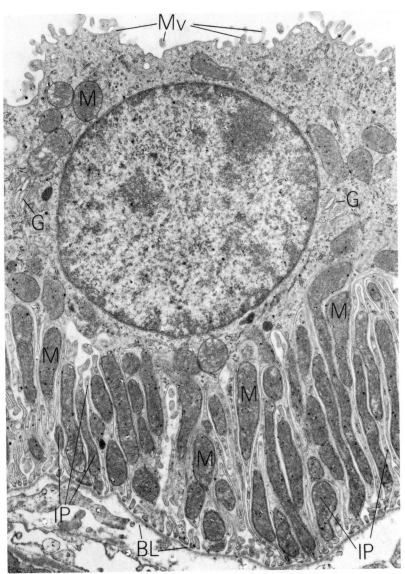

Figure 19.17. Electron micrograph of a distal convoluted tubule cell cut in longitudinal section. The apical surface of the cell displays some microvilli *(MV)*, but they are not sufficiently long or numerous to give the appearance of a brush border (compare with Fig. 19.14). The nucleus and Golgi profiles *(G)* are in the upper portion of the cell. Mitochondria *(M)* are chiefly in the basal region of the cell within the interdigitating processes *(IP)*. As in the proximal tubule cell, the mitochondria account for the appearance of basal striations in the light microscope. Beneath the distal tubule cell is a basal lamina *(BL)*. ×12,000.

ules are called the *vasa recta.* The arteriolae rectae form capillary plexuses, lined by fenestrated endothelium, that supply the tubular structures at the various levels of the medullary pyramid.

Countercurrent Exchange Occurs Between the Collecting System and the Vasa Recta

Because the ascending limb of the loop of Henle has a high level of transport activity and because it is impermeable to water, the modified filtrate that ultimately reaches the distal convoluted tubule is *hypotonic.* When ADH is present, the distal convoluted tubules, the collecting tubules, and the collecting ducts are highly permeable to water. Therefore, within the cortex, in which the interstitium is isotonic with blood, the modified filtrate equilibrates to isotonicity in the distal convoluted tubule, partly by loss of water to the interstitium and partly by addition of ions other than Na^+ and Cl^- to the filtrate. In the medulla, increasing amounts of water leave the filtrate as the collecting ducts pass through the increasingly hypertonic interstitium on their course to the papillae.

As noted above, the vasa recta also form loops in the medulla that parallel the loop of Henle. Because of this arrangement, the vessels can provide circulation to the medulla without disturbing the osmotic gradient that is established by the active chloride pump in the epithelium of the ascending limb of the loop of Henle.

The vasa recta form a countercurrent exchange system in the following manner: Both the arterial and venous sides of the loop are thin-walled vessels that form plexuses of fenestrated capillaries at all levels in the medulla. As the arterial vessels descend through the medulla, the blood loses water to the interstitium and gains salt from the interstitium so that at the tip of the loop, deep in the medulla, the blood is essentially in equilibrium with the hypertonic interstitial fluid.

As the venous vessels ascend toward the corticomedullary junction, the process is reversed; i.e., the hypertonic blood loses salt to the interstitium and gains water from the interstitium. This passive countercurrent exchange of water and salt between the blood and the interstitium occurs **without expenditure of energy** by the endothelial cells. The energy that drives this system is the same energy that drives the multiplier system, namely, the active transport of Cl^- by the water-impermeable ascending limb of the loop of Henle.

BLOOD SUPPLY

Specific aspects of the blood supply of the kidney have been described in relation to specific functions, i.e., glomerular filtration, control of blood pressure, and countercurrent exchange. It remains, however, to provide an overall description of the blood supply of the kidney.

Each kidney receives a large branch from the abdominal aorta, called the **renal artery.** The artery branches within the renal sinus and sends **interlobar** branches into the substance of the kidney (Fig. 19.19). The interlobar arteries travel between the pyramids as far as the cortex and then turn to follow an arched course along the base of the pyramid between the medulla and the cortex. Thus, this artery is designated as an **arcuate artery.**

Interlobular arteries branch from the arcuate arteries and ascend through the cortex toward the capsule. Although the boundaries between lobules are not distinct, the interlobular arteries, when included in the section, are located at some midpoint between adjacent medullary rays, traveling in the cortical labyrinth. As they traverse the cortex toward the capsule, the interlobular arteries give off branches, the **afferent arterioles,** with one to each glomerulus. A single afferent arteriole may spring directly from the interlobular artery, or a common stem from the interlobular artery may branch to form several afferent arterioles. (The common stem, having left the interlobular location to enter the lobule, is properly called an **intralobular artery**). Some interlobular arteries terminate near the periphery of the cortex, whereas others enter the kidney capsule to provide its arterial supply.

Afferent arterioles give rise to the glomerular tuft of capillaries. The glomerular capillaries reunite to form an **ef-**

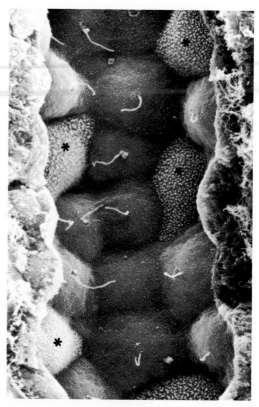

Figure 19.18. Scanning electron micrograph of a collecting tubule showing dark cells *(asterisks),* with numerous short lamellipodia or microridges on their surface, and light cells, each with a single cilium on its free surface along with small microvilli. [Note that the terms "light" and "dark" refer to the staining character of sectioned cells. Here, the density differences reflect charge characteristics of the coated surface of the specimen.] (Courtesy of C. C. Tisher.)

ferent arteriole that, in turn, gives rise to a second network of capillaries, the **peritubular capillaries.** The arrangement of these capillaries differs according to whether they spring from cortical or juxtamedullary glomeruli.

* *Efferent arterioles from cortical glomeruli* lead into a peritubular capillary network that surrounds the local uriniferous tubules (see *G1* and *G2,* Fig. 19.19).
* *Efferent arterioles from juxtamedullary glomeruli* descend into the medulla alongside the loop of Henle; they break up into smaller vessels that continue toward the apex of the pyramid but make hairpin turns at various levels to return again as straight vessels toward the base of the pyramid (see *G3* and *G4,* Fig. 19.19). Thus, the efferent arterioles of the juxtamedullary glomeruli give rise to these **vasa recta** and the peritubular capillary networks derived from them, which are described above in the explanation of the countercurrent exchange system.

Generally, venous flow in the kidney follows a reverse course to arterial flow, with the veins running in parallel with the corresponding arteries (Fig. 19.20). Thus,

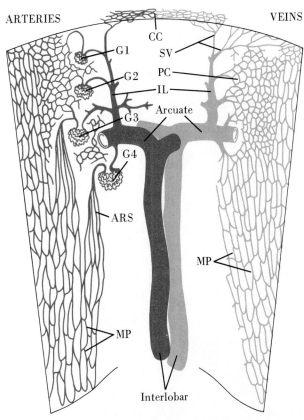

ARTERIES   VEINS

CC
G1
SV
G2
PC
IL
G3
Arcuate
G4

ARS

MP

MP

Interlobar

Figure 19.19. Schematic diagram of the renal blood supply. Renal arteries give rise to interlobar arteries that branch into arcuate arteries at the border between medulla and cortex. Interlobular arteries *(IL)* branch from the arcuate arteries and travel toward the renal capsule, giving off afferent arterioles to the glomeruli *(G)*. Glomeruli in the outer part of the cortex *(G1, G2)* send efferent arterioles to the peritubular capillaries *(PC)* that surround the tubules in the cortex; glomeruli near the medulla *(G3, G4)*, the juxtamedullary glomeruli, send efferent arterioles almost entirely into the medullary plexus *(MP)* of capillaries via the arteriolae rectae spuriae *(ARS)*. Blood returns from the capillaries via veins that enter the interlobular (or arcuate) veins. Stellate veins near the capsule drain both the capsular *(CC)* and the peritubular capillaries. (Based on Morrison DM: *American Journal of Anatomy* 37:75, 1926.)

- Peritubular cortical capillaries drain to interlobular veins, which, in turn, drain to arcuate veins, interlobar veins, and the renal vein.
- The medullary vascular network drains to arcuate veins and so forth.
- Peritubular capillaries near the kidney surface and capillaries of the capsule drain to stellate veins (so called because of the pattern of their distribution when viewed from the kidney surface), which drain to interlobular veins, and so forth.

LYMPHATIC VESSELS

The kidneys contain two major networks of lymphatic vessels. These are not usually visible in routine histologic

sections but can be demonstrated by experimental methods. One lymphatic network is located in the outer regions of the cortex and drains to larger lymphatic vessels in the capsule. The other network is located more deeply in the substance of the kidney and drains to large lymphatic vessels in the renal sinus. There are numerous anastomoses between the two lymphatic networks.

NERVE SUPPLY

The fibers that form the renal plexus are mostly derived from the sympathetic division of the autonomic nervous system. They cause contraction of vascular smooth muscle and consequent vasoconstriction.

- *Constriction of the afferent arterioles* to the glomeruli reduces the filtration rate and decreases the production of urine.
- *Constriction of the efferent arterioles* from the glomeruli increases the filtration rate and increases the production of urine.
- Loss of sympathetic innervation leads to an increased urinary output.

It is evident, however, that the *extrinsic nerve supply is not necessary for normal renal function*. The nerve fibers to the kidney are cut during renal transplantation and transplanted kidneys subsequently function normally.

EXCRETORY PASSAGES

The urine that is excreted at the **area cribrosa** flows sequentially

- To the *minor calyx* of that papilla
- To a *major calyx*
- To the *renal pelvis*
- Through the *ureter* to the *urinary bladder,* where it is stored
- Through the *urethra,* where it is voided

All of these excretory passages except the urethra have the same general structure, namely, a mucosa, a muscularis, and an adventitia (or, in some regions, a serosa).

Transitional Epithelium

Transitional Epithelium Lines All of the Excretory Passages

Transitional epithelium (Fig. 19.20) is essentially impermeable to salts and water. The ability of transitional ep-

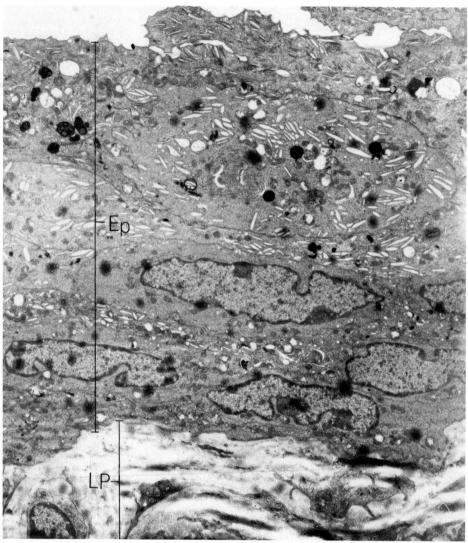

Figure 19.20.   Transmission electron micrograph of epithelial cells of the urinary bladder. The mucous membrane of the urinary bladder consists of transitional epithelium *(Ep)* with an underlying lamina propria *(LP).* The surface cells of transitional epithelium are large; the plasma membrane facing the lumen of the bladder possesses unique areas, designated plaques, seen at higher magnification in Figure 19.21. ×5000.

ithelium to become thinner and flatter allows distensibility of the lining of all these excretory passages. The structure of the surface cells of transitional epithelium is uniquely adapted to accommodate the distensibility of the epithelium.

In routine histologic sections, the surface cells appear as rounded cells that bulge into the lumen of the passages. The apical surface of the cell is very irregular, with deep clefts penetrating into the apical cytoplasm. When examined with the TEM, modified areas of plasma membrane called *plaques* (Fig. 19.21) are seen on the luminal surface of the cells. These plaques appear to be more rigid and thicker (up to 12 nm) than the rest of the apical plasma membrane. Fine filaments can be seen stretching from the inner surface of the plaques into the apical cytoplasm.

- In the *undistended* urinary bladder, the plaques appear to fold inward into the apical cytoplasm where they appear in sections as *fusiform vesicles* because their continuity with the apical surface is not evident (Fig. 19.21).
- In the *distended* urinary bladder, the clefts and the fusiform vesicles (plaques) are reinserted into the cell surface (Fig. 19.22) as the mucosa unfolds and the transitional epithelium flattens.

Connective Tissue and Muscle

A dense collagenous lamina propria underlies the transitional epithelium throughout the excretory passages. There is neither a muscularis mucosae nor a submucosal layer in their walls. In the tubular portions (ureters and urethra), there are usually two layers of smooth muscle beneath the lamina propria:

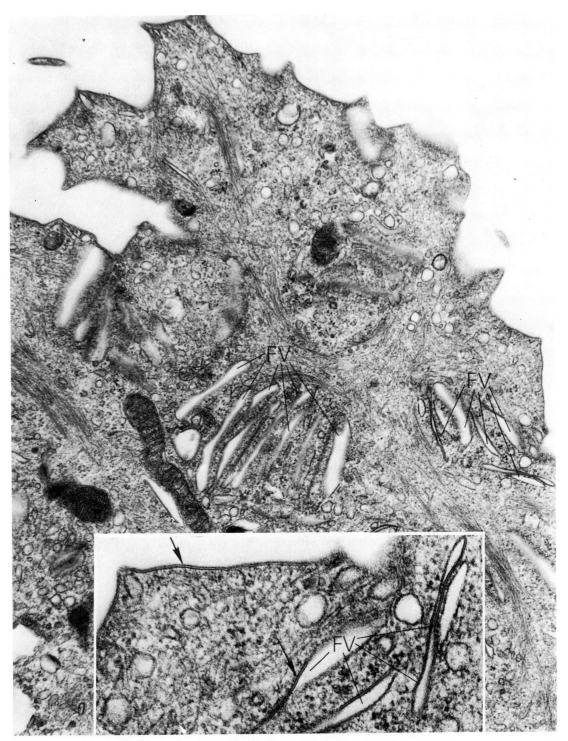

Figure 19.21. Transmission electron micrograph of the apical region of a transitional epithelial cell. The cytoplasm displays small vesicles, filaments, and mitochondria, but the most distinctive feature of the cell is its fusiform-shaped vesicles *(FV)*. At higher magnifications **(inset)**, the membrane forming the vesicles is seen to be similar to the plasma membrane of the cell surface *(arrows)*. Both of these are thickened and give the impression of possessing a degree of rigidity greater than that of plasma membrane in other locations. The thickened plasma membrane represents a sectioned view of a surface plaque. The fusiform vesicles are formed by the infolding of the plaques in the relaxed urinary bladder. ×27,000; **inset,** ×60,000.

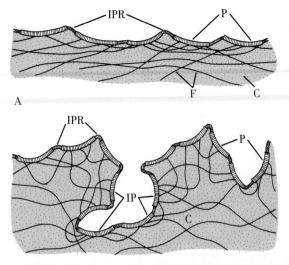

Figure 19.22. Diagrams of luminal surface of transitional epithelial cells in distended **(upper drawing)** and relaxed **(lower drawing)** bladder. The plasma membrane is thickened in regions to form plaques *(P)*. The interplaque regions *(IPR)* consist of membrane that is not thickened. In the relaxed bladder, the plaques are invaginated into the cell, and although they retain their continuity with the surface, the invaginated plaques *(IP)* typically appear as isolated fusiform vesicles in electron micrographs. Filaments *(F)* attached to the undersurface of the plaques may prevent undue stretching in the distended bladder. (Modified from Staehelin LA, et al: *The Journal of Cell Biology* 53:73, 1972, by permission of The Rockefeller University Press.)

- The inner layer is arranged in a loose spiral described as a *longitudinal layer.*
- The outer layer is arranged in a tight spiral described as a *circular layer.*

Note that this arrangement of the smooth muscle is opposite to that of the muscularis externa of the intestinal tract.

The smooth muscle of the urinary passages is mixed with connective tissue, so that it forms parallel bundles rather than pure muscular sheets. Peristaltic contractions of the smooth muscle move the urine from the minor calyces through the ureter to the bladder.

The smooth muscle of the bladder wall is less regularly arranged than that of the tubular portions of the excretory passages, and thus, there is more random mixing of muscle and collagen bundles. Contraction of the smooth muscle of the bladder muscle compresses the whole viscus and forces the urine into the urethra.

URETERS

The ureters conduct urine from the renal pelvis to the bladder and follow an oblique path through the wall of the bladder. As the bladder distends with urine, the openings of the ureters are compressed, reducing the possibility of reflux of urine into the ureters. Contraction of the smooth muscle of the bladder wall also compresses the openings of

the ureters into the bladder. This is important in protecting the kidney from the spread of infection from the bladder and urethra, frequent sites of chronic infection, particularly in the female.

In the terminal portion of the ureters, a thick outer layer of longitudinal muscle is described in addition to the two listed above, particularly in the portion of the ureter that passes through the bladder wall. Old descriptions of the bladder indicate that this continues into the wall of the bladder to form a principal component of the bladder wall. The smooth muscle of the bladder is not, however, that clearly separated into layers (see above).

URINARY BLADDER

The bladder is a distensible reservoir for urine located in the pelvic region of the abdominopelvic cavity; its size and shape change as it fills. It contains three openings, two for the ureters and one for the urethra. The smooth muscle of the bladder wall forms an **internal sphincter,** a ring-like arrangement of muscle around the opening of the urethra.

The triangular region defined by these three openings, the **trigone,** is relatively smooth and constant in thickness, whereas the rest of the bladder wall is thick and folded when the bladder is empty and thin and smooth when the bladder is distended. These differences reflect the embryologic origins of the trigone and the rest of the bladder wall, with the trigone deriving from the embryonic mesonephric ducts and the major portion of the wall originating from the cloaca.

The bladder is innervated by both the sympathetic and parasympathetic divisions of the autonomic nervous system.

- *Sympathetic fibers* form a plexus in the adventitia of the bladder wall. These fibers probably innervate blood vessels in the wall.
- *Parasympathetic fibers* end in ganglia in the muscle bundles and the adventitia and are the efferent fibers of the **micturition reflex.**
- *Sensory fibers* from the bladder to the sacral portion of the spinal cord are the afferent fibers of the micturition reflex.

URETHRA

In the male, the urethra is about 20 cm long and serves as the terminal duct of both the urinary and genital systems. It has three distinct segments:

- *Prostatic urethra* extends for 3–4 cm from the neck of the bladder through the prostate gland (see page 662).

- *Membranous urethra* extends for about 1 cm from the apex of the prostate gland through the body wall.
- *Penile urethra* extends for about 15 cm through the length of the penis to open on the body surface at the *glans penis.*

The *prostatic* urethra is lined with transitional epithelium. The ejaculatory ducts of the genital system (see page 658) enter the posterior wall of this segment, and many small prostatic ducts also empty into this segment. The *membranous* urethra passes through the pelvic and urogenital diaphragms of the body wall to the bulb of the *corpus cavernosum* of the penis.

The skeletal muscles of the pelvic and urogenital diaphragms that surround the membranous urethra form the *external (voluntary) sphincter of the urethra.* Transitional epithelium ends in the membranous urethra. This segment is usually described as lined with a stratified or pseudostratified columnar epithelium that resembles the epithelium of the genital duct system more than it resembles the epithelium of the more proximal portions of the urinary duct system.

The *penile urethra* is surrounded by the *corpus spongiosum* as it passes through the length of the penis. It is lined with pseudostratified columnar epithelium except at its distal end, where it is lined with stratified squamous epithelium continuous with that of the skin of the penis. Ducts of the bulbourethral glands and of the mucus-secreting glands of Littré empty into the penile urethra.

In the female, the urethra is short, measuring 3–5 cm in length from the bladder to the vestibule of the vagina, where it normally terminates just below the clitoris. The mucosa is traditionally described as having longitudinal folds. As in the male urethra, the lining is initially transitional epithelium, a continuation of the bladder epithelium, but this changes to stratified squamous epithelium before its termination. Some investigators have reported the presence of stratified columnar and pseudostratified columnar epithelium in the midportion of the female urethra.

Numerous small glands, the *paraurethral* and *periurethral glands,* which are homologous to the prostate gland in the male, open into the urethra. They produce an alkaline secretion. The lamina propria is a highly vascularized layer of connective tissue that resembles the corpus spongiosum in the male. Where the urethra penetrates the urogenital diaphragm, the striated muscle of this structure forms the external (voluntary) urethral sphincter.

PLATE 93. Kidney I

The kidney is a flattened, bean-shaped structure with a hilum, an indented region, on its medial border. Blood vessels, nerves, and lymphatic vessels enter or leave the kidney through the hilum; in addition, the funnel-shaped pelvis of the ureter leaves the kidney at the hilum.

FIGURE 1, kidney, human, fresh specimen ×3. A section through the hilum is shown here. The hilar region of the kidney is below, and the convex lateral border is above. The outer part of the kidney (except at the hilum) has a reddish-brown appearance; this is the cortex. It is easily distinguished from the inner portion, the medulla, which is further divided into an outer portion *(OM)*, identified here by the presence of straight blood vessels, the vasa recta *(VR)*, and an inner portion *(IM)*, which has a light appearance. The medulla consists of pyramidal structures, the pyramids, which have their base facing the cortex and their apex in the form of a papilla *(P)* facing the hilar region of the kidney. The pyramids are separated, sometimes only partially in this figure, by cortical material that is designated the renal columns *(RC)*. Note, also, that the two pyramids depicted in the illustration share the same papilla. Most of the pyramid belonging to the other papilla, on the left, has not been included in the plane of the section. The papillae are free tips of the pyramids that project into the first of a series of large collecting vessels, the minor calyces *(MC);* the inner surface of the calyx is white. Minor calyces drain into major calyces, and in turn, these open into the pelvis, which funnels into the ureter.

An interesting feature in this specimen is that the blood has been retained in many of the vessels, thereby allowing for visualization of several renal vessels in their geographic location. Among the vessels that can be identified in the cut face of the kidney shown here are the interlobular vessels *(IV)* within the cortex; the arcuate veins *(AV)* at the base of the pyramids; and, in the medulla, the vessels going to and from the capillary network of the pyramid. The latter vessels, both arterioles and venules, are relatively straight and are designated collectively as the vasa recta *(VR)*.

FIGURE 2, kidney, human, hematoxylin and eosin (H&E) ×20. A histologic section including the cortex and part of the medulla is shown here. Located at the boundary between the two (partly marked by the *dashed line*) are numerous profiles of arcuate arteries *(AA)* and arcuate veins *(AV)*. The most distinctive feature of the renal cortex, regardless of the plane of section is the presence of the renal corpuscles *(RC)*. These are spherical structures composed of a glomerulus (glomerular vascular tuft) surrounded by the visceral and parietal epithelium of Bowman's capsule. Also seen in the cortex are groups of tubules that are more or less straight and disposed in a radial direction from the base of the medulla *(arrows);* these are the medullary rays. In contrast, the medulla presents profiles of tubular structures that are arranged as gentle curves in the outer part of the medulla, turning slightly to become straight in the inner part of the medulla. The disposition of the tubules (and blood vessels) gives the cut face of the pyramid a slightly striated appearance that is also evident in the gross specimen (Fig. 1).

KEY

AA, arcuate arteries
AV, arcuate veins
IM, inner medulla
IV, interlobular vessels
MC, minor calyx

OM, outer medulla
P, papilla
RC: Fig. 1, renal column; Fig. 2, renal corpuscles

VR, vasa recta
arrows, medullary rays
dashed line (Fig. 2), boundary between cortex and medulla

PLATE 93

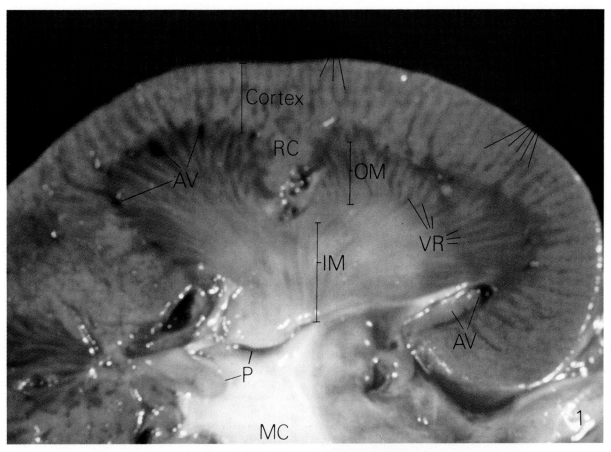

Cortex

RC

AV

OM

VR

IM

AV

P

MC

1

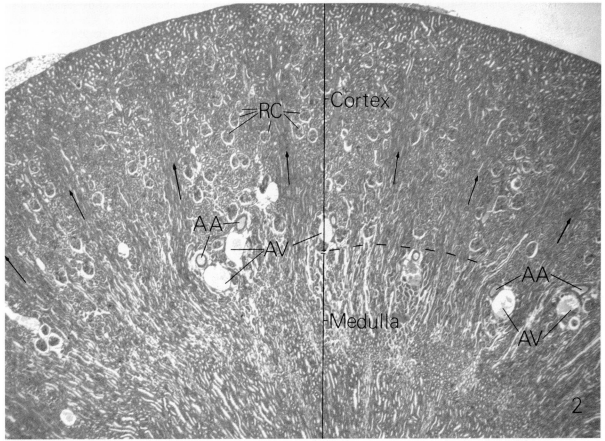

RC

Cortex

AA

AV

AA

AV

Medulla

2

PLATE 94. Kidney II

The nephron is the functional unit of the kidney. It is made up of the following parts: the renal corpuscle (consisting of a glomerulus and Bowman's capsule) and the renal tubule, which itself consists of three major segments: the proximal thick segment (proximal convoluted tubule and the descending limb of Henle's loop); the thin segment; and the distal thick segment (ascending limb of Henle's loop, macula densa, and distal convoluted tubule). Nephrons empty into collecting ducts that drain into progressively slightly larger ducts that ultimately pass from the cortex into the pyramid, where they open at the papilla into a calyx. The collecting ducts opening at the papilla are called ducts of Bellini.

FIGURE 1, kidney, human, H&E ×60. The renal cortex can be divided into regions referred to as the cortical labyrinth *(CL)* and the medullary rays *(MR)*. The cortical labyrinth contains the renal corpuscles *(RC)*, which appear as relatively large spherical structures. Surrounding each renal corpuscle are the proximal and distal convoluted tubules. They are also part of the cortical labyrinth. The convoluted tubules, particularly the proximal, because of their tortuosity, present a variety of profiles, most of which are oval or circular; others, more elongate, are in the shape of a J, a C, or even an S. The medullary rays are composed of groups of straight tubules oriented in the same direction and appear to radiate from the base of the pyramid. When the medullary rays are cut longitudinally, as they are in this figure, the tubules present elongated profiles. The medullary rays contain proximal thick segments (descending limb of Henle's loop), distal thick segments (ascending limbs of Henle's loop), and collecting tubules.

FIGURE 2, kidney, human, H&E ×120. This figure presents another profile of the renal cortex, at a somewhat higher magnification, cut in a plane at a right angle to the section in Figure 1. The peripheral part of the micrograph shows the cortical labyrinth in which the tubules display chiefly round and oval profiles but also some that are more elongate and curved. The appearance is the same as the cortical labyrinth areas of Figure 1. A renal corpuscle *(RC)* is also present in the cortical labyrinth. In contrast, the profiles presented by the tubules of the medullary ray in this figure are quite different from those seen in Figure 1. All of the tubules bounded by the *dashed line* belong to the medullary ray *(MR)*, and all are cut in cross section.

A general survey of the tubules within the medullary ray reveals that several distinct types can be recognized on the basis of the size of the tubule, shape of the lumen, and size of the tubule cells. These features as well as those of the cortical labyrinth are considered in Plate 95.

KEY		
CL, cortical labyrinth **MR,** medullary ray	**RC,** renal corpuscle	**dashed line,** approximate boundary of the medullary ray

PLATE 94

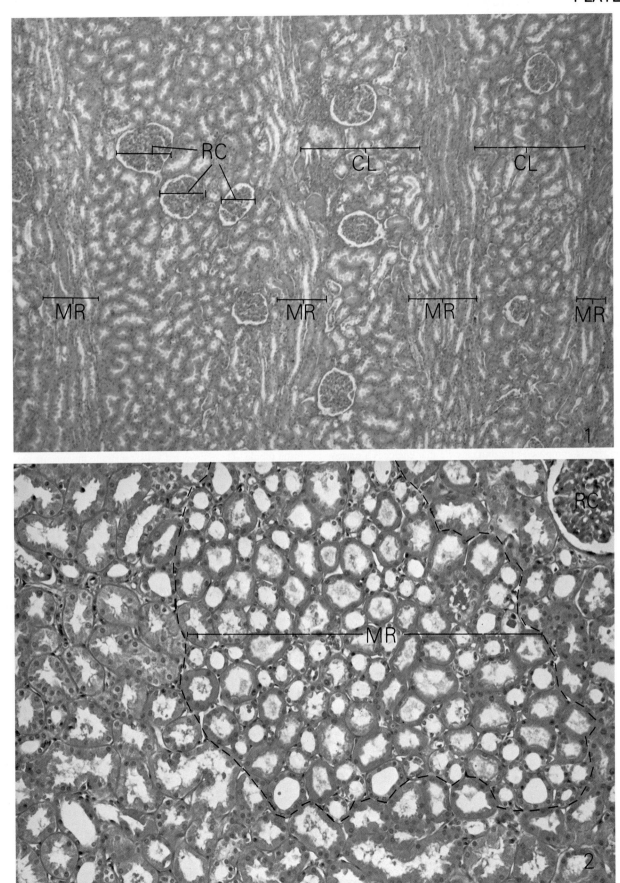

PLATE 95.   Kidney III

Proximal and distal convoluted tubules display features that allow for their identification in H&E-stained paraffin sections. The proximal convoluted tubule is more than twice as long and more tortuous than the distal convoluted tubule; thus, the majority of the tubular profiles in the cortical labyrinth will be proximal.

FIGURE 1, kidney, human, H&E ×240.   In this figure, an area of cortical labyrinth, there are six distal convoluted *(DC)* tubule profiles. The proximal tubules (unlabeled) have a slightly larger outside diameter than do the distal tubules. The proximal tubules have a brush border, whereas the distal tubules have a cleaner, sharper luminal surface. The lumen of the proximal tubules is often star shaped; this is not the case with distal tubules. Typically, fewer nuclei appear in a cross section of a proximal tubule than in an equivalent segment of a distal tubule.

Most of the above points can also be utilized in distinguishing the straight portions of the proximal and distal thick segments in the medullary rays. There are, however, certain differences. The medullary rays consist of tubules that are straight and parallel. Thus, instead of the occasional U, J, or S shapes seen in the cortical labyrinth, the proximal and distal thick segments within the medullary rays all display essentially the same profiles, be they rounded or elongate.

FIGURE 2, kidney, human, H&E ×240.   In this figure, all of the tubular profiles are rounded except for a proximal convoluted tubule *(PC)* included in the lower right corner of the figure (it belongs to the adjacent cortical labyrinth). Secondly, the number of proximal *(P)* and distal *(D)* tubular profiles are about equal in the medullary ray, as is shown by the labeling of each tubule in this figure. Note that, in contrast to the distal tubules, the proximal tubules display a brush border and have a larger outside diameter, with many displaying a star-shaped lumen. The medullary ray also contains collecting tubules *(CT)*. They are considered in Plate 96.

FIGURES 3 and 4, kidney, human, H&E ×360.   The renal corpuscle appears as a spherical structure whose periphery is composed of a thin capsule that encloses a narrow clear-appearing space, the urinary space *(asterisks),* and a capillary tuft or glomerulus that appears as a large cellular mass. The capsule of the renal corpuscle, known as Bowman's capsule, actually has two parts: a parietal layer, which is marked *(BC),* and a visceral layer. The parietal layer consists of simple squamous epithelial cells. The visceral layer consists of cells, called podocytes *(Pod),* that lie on the outer surface of the glomerular capillary. Except where they clearly line the urinary space, as the labeled cells do in Figure 3, podocytes may be difficult to distinguish from the capillary endothelial cells. To complicate matters, the mesangial cells are also a component of the glomerulus. In general, nuclei of podocytes are larger and stain less intensely than the endothelial and mesangial cells.

A distal *(DC)* and two proximal *(PC)* convoluted tubules are marked in Figure 3. The cells of the distal tubule are more crowded on one side, as is also the case in the adjacent distal tubule. These crowded cells constitute the macula densa *(MD)* of the distal thick segment. The macula densa is adjacent to the afferent arteriole.

In Figure 4, both the vascular pole and the urinary pole of the renal corpuscle are evident. The vascular pole is characterized by the presence of arterioles *(A),* one of which is entering or leaving *(double-headed arrow)* the corpuscle. The afferent arteriole possesses modified smooth muscle cells with granules, the juxtaglomerular cells (not evident in Fig. 4). At the urinary pole, the parietal layer of Bowman's capsule is continuous with the beginning of the proximal convoluted tubule *(PC).* Here, the urinary space of the renal corpuscle continues into the lumen of the proximal tubule, and the lining cells change from simple squamous to simple cuboidal or low columnar with a brush border.

KEY

A, arteriole
BC, Bowman's capsule (parietal layer)
CT, collecting tubule
D, distal thick segment (straight portion)

DC, distal convoluted tubule
MD, macula densa
P, proximal thick segment (straight portion)
PC, proximal convoluted tubule

Pod, podocyte (visceral layer of Bowman's capsule)
asterisks, urinary space
double-headed arrow (Fig. 4), blood vessel at vascular pole of renal corpuscle

PLATE 95

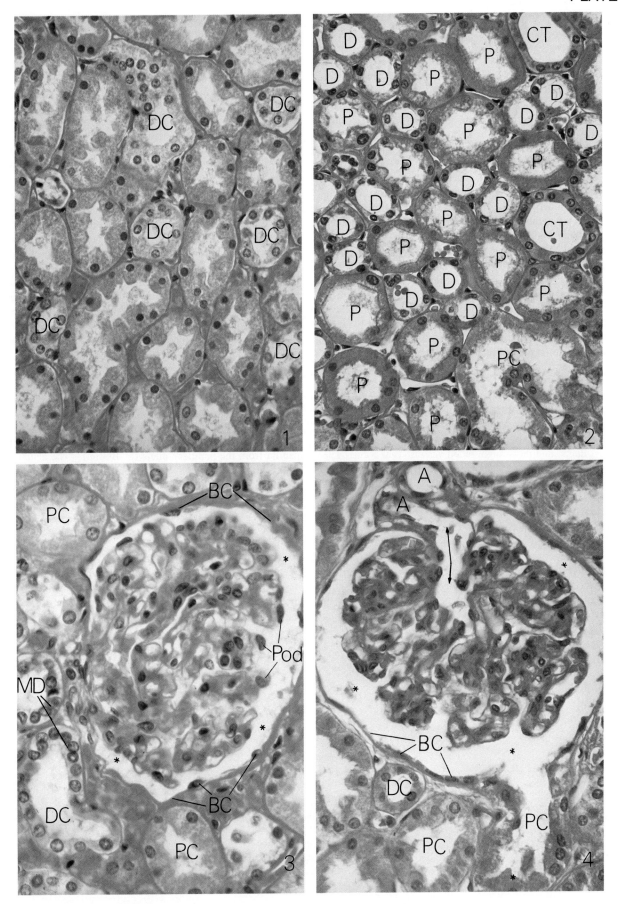

PLATE 96. Kidney IV

FIGURE 1, kidney, human, H&E ×240. A section through the outer portion of the medulla is shown in this figure. This region contains proximal and distal thick segments, thin segments, and collecting tubules. All of the tubules are parallel, and all are cut in cross section; thus, they present circular profiles. The proximal *(P)* thick segments display typical star-shaped lumina and a brush border (or the fragmented apical cell surface from which the brush border has been partially broken). These tubules have outside diameters that are generally larger than those of the distal tubules *(D)*. As mentioned previously and as shown here, the distal tubules display a larger number of nuclei than do comparable segments of proximal tubule cells. Note, also, that the lumen of the distal tubule is more rounded and the apical surface of the cells is sharper. The collecting tubules *(CT)* have outer diameters that are about the same as those of the proximal tubules and larger than those of distal tubules. The cells forming the collecting tubules are cuboidal and smaller than those of proximal tubules; thus, they also display a relatively larger number of nuclei than comparable segments of proximal tubule cells. Count them! Finally, boundaries between the cells

that constitute the collecting tubules are usually evident *(asterisks);* this serves as one of the most dependable features for the identification of collecting tubules.

The thin segments *(T)* have the thinnest walls of all renal tubules seen in the medulla. They are formed by a low cuboidal or simple squamous epithelium, as seen here, and the lumina are relatively large. Occasionally, a section includes the region of transition from a thick to a thin segment and can be recognized even in a cross section through the tubule. One such junction is evident in this figure (the tubule with *two arrows* in the lumen). On one side, the tubule cell *(left-pointing arrow)* is characteristic of the proximal segment; it possesses a distinctive brush border. The other side of the tubule *(right-pointing arrow)* is composed of low cuboidal cells that resemble the cells forming the thin segments. In addition to the renal and collecting tubules, there are many other small tubular structures in this figure. Thin-walled and lined by endothelium, they are small blood vessels. These vessels (along with the loops of Henle and collecting tubules) play an important role in the countercurrent mechanism that concentrates urine in the pyramids.

FIGURE 2, kidney, human, H&E ×20. This figure shows a renal pyramid at low magnification. The pyramid is a conical structure composed principally of medullary straight tubules, ducts, and the straight blood vessels (vasa recta). The *dashed line* at the left of the micrograph is placed at the junction between cortex and medulla; thus, it marks the base of the pyramid. Note the arcuate vessels *(AV)* that lie at the boundary of cortex and medulla. They define the boundary line. The few renal corpuscles *(RC),* upper left, belong to the medulla. They are referred to as juxtamedullary corpuscles.

The pyramid is somewhat distorted in this specimen, as evidenced by regions of longitudinally sectioned tubules, lower left, and cross-sectioned and obliquely sectioned tubules in other regions. In effect, part of the pyramid was bent, thus the change in the plane of section of the tubules.

The apical portion of the pyramid, known as the renal papilla, is lodged in a cup- or funnel-like structure referred to as the calyx. It collects the urine that leaves the tip of the papilla from the papillary ducts (of Bellini). (The actual tip of the papilla is not seen within the plane of section, nor are the openings of the ducts at this low magnification.) The surface of the papilla that faces the lumen of the calyx is simple columnar or cuboidal epithelium *(SCEp).* (In places, this epithelium has separated from the surface of the papilla and appears as a thin strand of tissue.) The calyx is lined by transitional epithelium *(TEp).* Although not evident in the low magnification shown here, the boundary between the columnar epithelium covering the papilla and the transitional epithelium covering the inner surface of the calyx is marked by the *diamonds.*

KEY

AV, arcuate vessels	**TEp,** transitional epithelium	**left-pointing arrow (Fig. 1),** proximal tubule cell
CT, collecting tubules	**arrowhead,** location of apex of pyramid	**right-pointing arrow (Fig. 1),** thin segment cell
D, distal thick segment	**asterisks,** boundaries between cells of collecting tubule	
P, proximal thick segment	**diamonds,** boundary between transitional and columnar epithelium	
RC, renal corpuscle		
SCEp, simple columnar epithelium		
T, thin segment		

PLATE 96

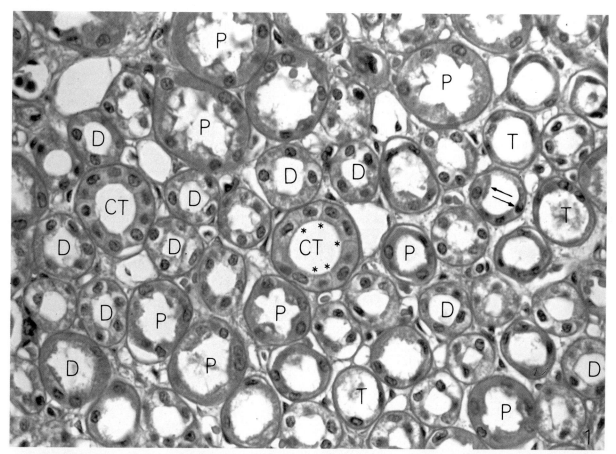

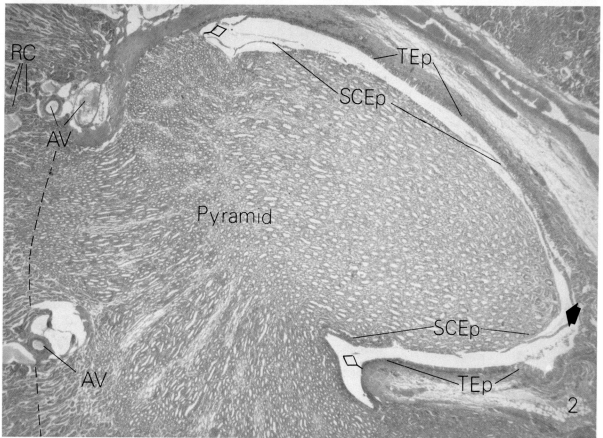

PLATE 97.   Ureter

The ureters are paired tubular structures that convey urine from the kidneys to the urinary bladder. They not only serve as a route to the bladder but also contribute to the flow of urine by means of their regular peristaltic activity.

FIGURE 1, ureter, monkey, H&E ×35.   As shown in this low-power orientation micrograph, the wall of the ureter consists of a mucosa *(Muc)*, a muscularis *(Mus)*, and an adventitia *(Adv)*. Note that the ureters are located behind the peritoneum of the abdominal cavity in their course to the bladder. Thus, a serosa *(Ser)* may be found covering a portion of the circumference of the tube. Also, due to contraction of smooth muscle of the muscularis, the luminal surface is characteristically folded, thus creating a star-shaped lumen.

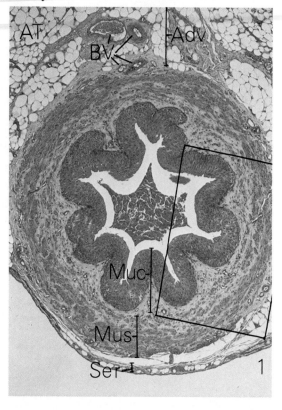

FIGURE 2, ureter, monkey, H&E ×160.   The wall of the ureter is examined at higher magnification in this figure. One can immediately recognize the thick epithelial lining, which appears distinct and sharply delineated from the remainder of the wall. This is the transitional epithelium *(Ep)*. The remainder of the wall is made up of connective tissue *(CT)* and smooth muscle. The latter can be recognized as the darker-staining layer. The section also shows some adipose tissue *(AT)*, a component of the adventitia.

The transitional epithelium and its supporting connective tissue constitute the mucosa *(Muc)*. A distinct submucosa is not present, although the term is sometimes applied to the connective tissue that is closest to the muscle.

The muscularis *(Mus)* is arranged as an inner longitudinal layer *[SM(l)]*, a middle circular layer *[SM(c)]*, and an outer longitudinal layer *[SM(l)]*. However, the outer longitudinal layer is present only at the lower end of the ureter. In a cross section through the ureter, the inner and outer smooth muscle layers are cut in cross section, whereas the circular middle layer of the muscle cells is cut longitudinally. This is as they appear in this figure.

FIGURE 3, ureter, monkey, H&E ×400.   This figure shows the inner longitudinal smooth muscle layer *[SM(l)]* at higher magnification. Note that the nuclei appear as round profiles, indicating that the muscle cells have been cross-sectioned.

This figure also shows the transitional epithelium to advantage. The surface cells are characteristically the largest, and some are binucleate *(arrow)*. The basal cells are the smallest, and typically, the nuclei appear crowded due to the minimal cytoplasm of each cell. The intermediate cells appear to consist of several layers and are composed of cells larger in size than the basal cells but smaller than the surface cells.

KEY

Adv, adventitia
AT, adipose tissue
BV, blood vessels
CT, connective tissue
Ep, transitional epithelium

Muc, mucosa
Mus, muscularis
Ser, serosa
SM(c), circular layer of smooth muscle

SM(l), longitudinal layer of smooth muscle
arrow (Fig. 3), binucleate surface cell

PLATE 97

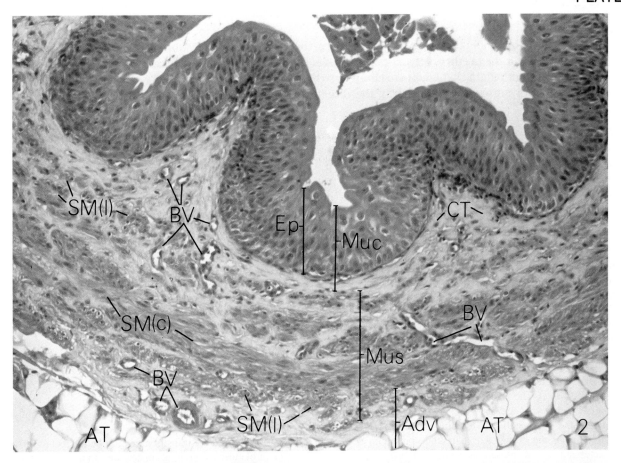

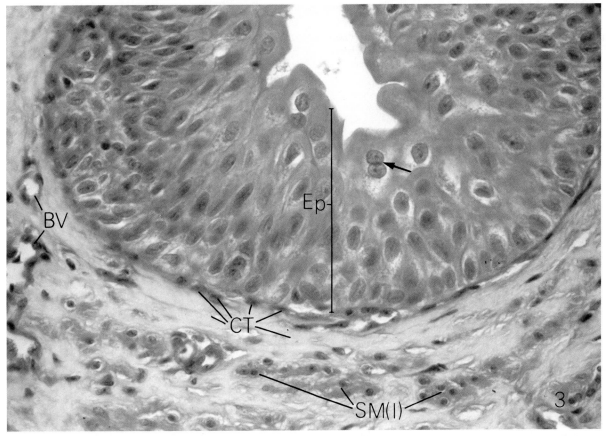

PLATE 98. Urinary Bladder

The urinary bladder receives urine from the two ureters and stores it until it is discharged via the urethra. Its structure reflects these functions. It possesses a lining of transitional epithelium that adapts to changes in bladder volume, and the wall contains bundles of smooth muscle that function in the discharge of urine.

FIGURE 1, urinary bladder, H&E ×65. The full thickness of the urinary bladder is illustrated here. It shows the mucosa *(Muc)*, the muscularis *(Mus)*, and the serosa *(S)*. The mucosa consists of transitional epithelium *(Ep)* and its supporting connective tissue *(CT)*. A distinct submucosa is not present, although, as with the ureter, the connective tissue closest to the muscle is sometimes referred to as a submucosa. The muscularis consists of smooth muscle that, like the muscularis of the ureter, is arranged in three layers: an inner longitudinal [*SM(L)*], a middle circular [*SM(C)*], and an outer longitudinal [*SM(L)*]. The smooth muscle in this preparation stains more intensely than the connective tissue. On the basis of organization, the bundles of smooth muscle cells can be recognized because they are surrounded by connective tissue. This relationship is especially evident when the smooth mus-

cle is cut obliquely or in cross section. When the smooth muscle is cut longitudinally, the relationship is less evident, but then the elongated profiles of the smooth muscle cell nuclei serve as a diagnostic feature. Another extremely useful criterion for distinguishing smooth muscle from connective tissue in this figure is that the number of nuclei in a given area of smooth muscle *(white circle)* is greater than the number of nuclei in a comparable area of connective tissue *(black circle)*.

A serosa is present on the upper surface of the bladder; it consists of a layer of simple squamous epithelium (mesothelium) that rests on a small amount of supporting connective tissue. Elsewhere, the outer layer of the wall consists of a fibrous adventitia.

FIGURES 2 and 3, urinary bladder, H&E ×160 (Fig. 2); ×640 (Fig. 3). The *rectangles* in Figure 1 and in Figure 2 indicate areas that are shown at higher magnification in Figures 2 and 3, respectively, to demonstrate the transitional epithelium. In the contracted state, the epithelium *(Ep)* is characterized by the presence of dome-shaped cells at the free surface and large numbers of pear-shaped cells immediately under the surface cells. The cells at the surface are large and sometimes have two nuclei *(arrows)*. The deeper cells, on the other hand, are smaller. Because of the absence

of connective tissue papillae, the epithelial-connective tissue junction is rather even. An aggregation of lymphocytes *(Lym)* is immediately under the epithelial surface. This is not an unusual observation.

The thickness of the transitional epithelium depends on the degree of bladder (or ureteral) distension. In the empty ureter or bladder, it appears to be about five cells deep. When the bladder is distended, however, it appears to have a thickness of only three cells: a basal layer, an intermediate cell layer, and a surface cell layer.

KEY

CT, connective tissue	**Mus,** muscularis	**SM(L),** longitudinal layer of
Ep, epithelium	**S,** serosa	smooth muscle
Lym, lymphocytes	**SM(C),** circular layer of smooth	**arrows,** binucleate cells
Muc, mucosa	muscle	

PLATE 98

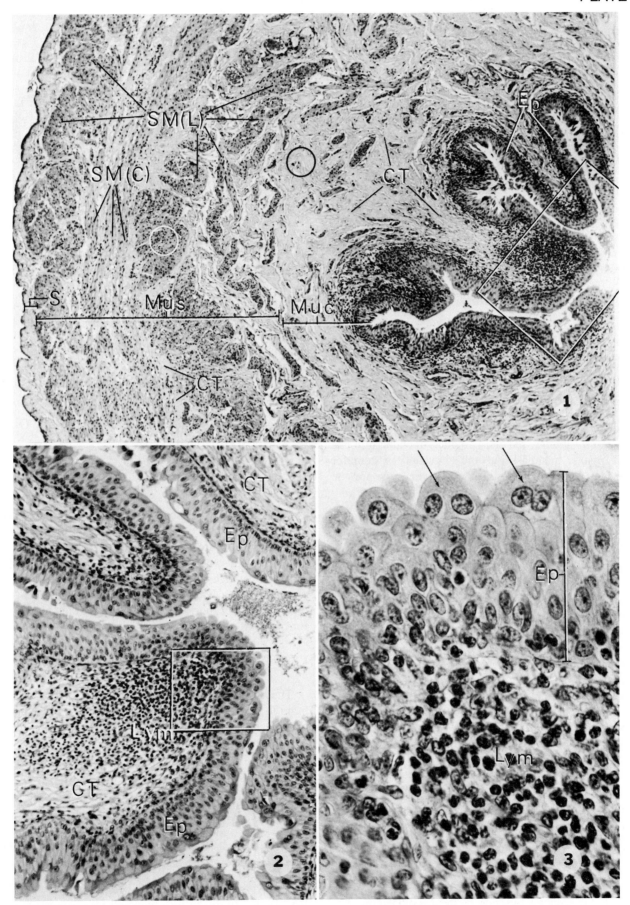

Endocrine Organs

20

Communication between cells is necessary to maintain homeostasis and coordinate growth and development. The primary function of two major organ systems, the *nervous system* and the *endocrine system,* is intercellular communication.

- The *nervous system* communicates through the transmission of neural impulses along nerve cell processes and release of neurotransmitters in the immediate vicinity of the target cell.
- The *endocrine system* communicates through the release of *hormones,* secretory products of endocrine cells and organs, that pass into the circulatory system for transport to target cells that possess *receptors* for the hormone.

The endocrine system produces a slower and more prolonged response than the nervous system. The release of hormones also induces a more generalized response as the hormones reach target cells in widely separated organs or tissues.

Functionally, these two systems are closely interrelated and may overlap in function. Both systems may act simultaneously on the same target cells and tissues, and some nerve cells secrete hormones. The *hypothalamus,* a part of the brain, coordinates most endocrine functions of the body and serves as one of the major controlling centers of the autonomic nervous system.

Endocrine Hormones Include Three Classes of Compounds

Cells of the endocrine system release over 50 hormones that are chemically divided into three classes of compounds:

- *Steroids,* cholesterol-derived compounds, are synthesized and secreted by cells of the ovaries, testes, and adrenal cortex.
- *Small peptides, proteins, and glycoproteins* are synthesized and secreted by cells of the hypothalamus, hy-

pophysis (pituitary), thyroid, parathyroid, pancreas, and scattered endocrine cells (the enteroendocrine cells) of the gastrointestinal tract and lungs.
- *Amino acid analogues and derivatives,* including the *catecholamines* (norepinephrine and epinephrine), are synthesized and secreted by many neurons as well as cells of the adrenal medulla. Also included in this group of compounds is *thyroxine,* an *iodinated amino acid* that is synthesized and secreted by cells of the thyroid gland.

Hormone-Secreting Cells Are Present in Many Organs to Regulate Their Activity

In other chapters, the endocrine function of cells within the gonads, liver, kidney, and gastrointestinal system are discussed. The cells of the gastroenteropancreatic (GEP) system (see page 453) constitute the largest collection of endocrine cells in the body. In addition to their endocrine function, cells of the GEP exercise *paracrine* control of the activity of adjacent epithelial cells by diffusion of peptide secretions through the extracellular spaces. This chapter deals primarily with a description of the discrete endocrine glands that release their hormones for delivery to the bloodstream for transport to target cells and organs.

HYPOPHYSIS (PITUITARY GLAND)

The *hypophysis* and the hypothalamus, the portion of the brain to which the hypophysis is attached, are morphologically and functionally linked in the endocrine and neuroendocrine control of other endocrine glands. Because they play central roles in a number of regulatory feedback systems, they are often called the "master organs" of the endocrine system.

Gross Structure and Development

The Hypophysis Is Composed of Glandular Epithelial Tissue and Neural (Secretory) Tissue

The hypophysis is a pea-sized, compound endocrine gland. It is located in the base of the skull in a depression of the sphenoid bone, called the *sella turcica*. A short stalk, the *infundibulum*, attaches the pituitary to the hypothalamus. The hypophysis weighs 0.5 g in normal males and 1.5 g in multiparous females.

The hypophysis has two functional components:

- *Adenohypophysis* (anterior pituitary), the glandular epithelial tissue
- *Neurohypophysis* (posterior pituitary), the neural secretory tissue

These two portions are of different embryologic origin. The adenohypophysis is derived from an evagination of the ectoderm of the oropharynx toward the brain (Rathke's pouch). The neurohypophysis is derived from a downgrowth (the future infundibulum) of neuroectoderm of the floor of the third ventricle (diencephalon) of the developing brain (Fig. 20.1).

The adenohypophysis consists of three derivatives of Rathke's pouch:

- *Pars distalis,* which comprises the bulk of the adenohypophysis and arises from the thickened anterior wall of the pouch
- *Pars intermedia,* a thin remnant of the posterior wall that abuts against the infundibulum
- *Pars tuberalis,* which develops from the thickened lateral walls of the pouch and forms a collar or sheath around the pars intermedia

The embryonic infundibulum gives rise to the neurohypophysis. The neurohypophysis consists of

- *Pars nervosa,* which contains the neurosecretory nerve endings
- *Infundibulum,* continuous with the **median eminence,** which contains the axons of the neurosecretory nerves

Blood Supply

A knowledge of the unusual blood supply of the hypophysis is important in understanding how it functions. Its supply is derived from two sets of vessels (Fig. 20.2):

- *Superior hypophyseal arteries* supply the pars tuberalis, median eminence, and infundibular stem. These vessels arise from the internal carotid arteries and posterior communicating artery of the circle of Willis.
- *Inferior hypophyseal arteries* primarily supply the pars nervosa. These vessels arise solely from the internal carotid arteries. An important functional observation is that *most of the anterior lobe of the hypophysis has no direct arterial supply.*

Hypophyseal Portal System

The arteries that supply the pars tuberalis, median eminence, and infundibular stem give rise to fenestrated capillaries (the *primary capillary plexus*). These capillaries drain into portal veins, called the **hypophyseal portal veins,** that run along the pars tuberalis and give rise to a second fenestrated sinusoidal capillary network (the *secondary capillary plexus*). This system of vessels carries neuroendocrine secretions of hypothalamic nerves from their sites of

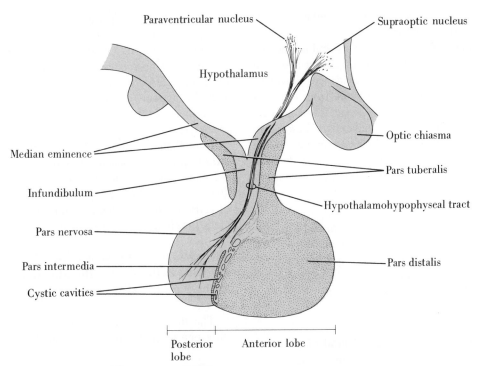

Figure 20.1. Drawing of a section through the human pituitary and related regions of the hypothalamus. The adenohypophysis consists of the pars distalis, pars tuberalis, and pars intermedia; the neurohypophysis consists of the infundibulum and pars nervosa. (Based on Netter FH: *CIBA Collection of Medical Illustrations.*)

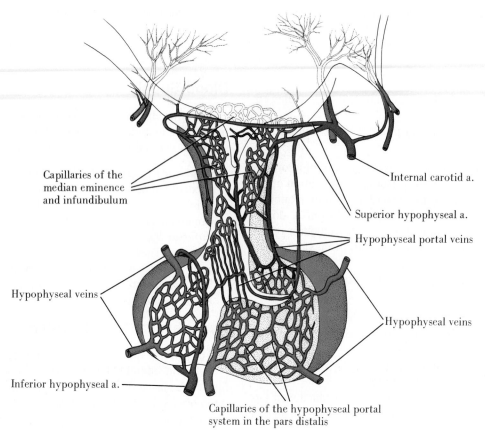

Capillaries of the
median eminence
and infundibulum

Internal carotid a.

Superior hypophyseal a.

Hypophyseal portal veins

Hypophyseal veins

Hypophyseal veins

Inferior hypophyseal a.

Capillaries of the hypophyseal portal
system in the pars distalis

Figure 20.2. Diagram of the blood supply to the pituitary. The hypophyseal portal veins are indicated. They begin in the capillary beds of the median eminence and infundibulum and end in the capillaries of the pars distalis. (Based on Netter FH: *CIBA Collection of Medical Illustrations.*)

release in the median eminence and infundibular stem directly to the cells in the pars distalis.

Most of the blood from the hypophysis drains into the cavernous sinus at the base of the diencephalon and then into the systemic circulation. There is evidence, however, that blood can flow via short portal veins from the pars distalis to the pars nervosa and that blood from the pars nervosa may flow toward the hypothalamus. These short pathways provide a route by which the hormones of the adenohypophysis could provide feedback directly to the brain without making the full circuit of the systemic circulation.

Nerve Supply

The nerves that enter the infundibular stem and pars nervosa from the hypothalamic nuclei are components of the neurohypophysis (see below). The nerves that enter the adenohypophysis are postganglionic fibers of the autonomic nervous system and have vasomotor function.

Adenohypophysis

The Adenohypophysis Is the Master Gland of the Endocrine System, Regulating Other Endocrine Glands

Most of the adenohypophysis has the typical organization of endocrine tissue. The cells are organized in clumps and cords that are separated by fenestrated sinusoidal capillaries of relatively large diameter. These cells respond to signals from the hypothalamus and synthesize and secrete a number of hormones, called *tropic hormones,* that regulate the activity of cells in other endocrine glands and tissues throughout the body (Fig. 20.3). The general nature and effects of these tropic hormones are summarized in Table 20.1.

Pars Distalis.   Early descriptions of the cells within the *pars distalis* were based solely on the staining properties of secretory granules within the cells. Using mixtures of acidic and basic dyes (Fig. 20.4), histologists identified three types of cells according to their staining reaction, viz., *basophils* (10%), *acidophils,* (40%), and *chromophobes* (50%).

Histochemical, Physiologic, and Immunocytochemical Methods Better Define the Functions of the Cell Types in the Pars Distalis

The three methods used to define the functions of the different cell types of the pars distalis are

- *Histochemistry:* The use of histochemical stains for specific chemical groups, such as the periodic acid-Schiff (PAS) reaction for carbohydrates of glycoproteins, trichrome stains (Mallory's, Cleveland-Wolfe, etc.), and other empirically derived combinations of stains (e.g., aldehyde-fuchsin), enables investigators to characterize the cells further. Acidophils and basophils have been subdivided into smaller groups that more closely correlate staining properties with function, as is summarized in Table 20.2.

- **Histophysiologic studies:** The cells in Table 20.2 are characterized as acidophils and basophils on the basis of their staining characteristics. The identification of the role of the cells, however, was made by combining information on staining properties with changes in the number, size, and staining intensity of the cells as physiologic manipulations were made on the target organs of the pituitary hormones. Pathologic conditions were also correlated with the absence or overgrowth of specific hypophyseal cells. The physiologic and pathologic observations have led to the recognition that many of the cells originally identified as chromophobes are actually transiently degranulated forms of secretory cells.
- **Electron microscopy and immunocytochemistry:** Ultrastructurally, the cells of the adenohypophysis have relatively distinctive characteristics based on comparison of cell size and shape, degree of development of cytoplasmic organelles, and secretory granule size, density, and distribution (Table 20.3).

All known hormones of the adenohypophysis are small proteins or glycoproteins. This important fact has led to definitive identification of specific cell types by immunocytochemistry. These studies have shown that in at least two cases a single cell type produces more than one hormone: The *adrenocorticolipotropes* (the most common basophils) produce both adrenocorticotropic hormone (ACTH) and lipotropic hormone (LPH), and *gonadotropes* (small basophils) produce both luteinizing hormone (LH) and follicle-stimulating hormone (FSH). The large basophils are *thyrotropes* that produce thyroid-stimulating hormone (TSH). Among the acidophils, the most common are the small *somatotropes* that produce somatotropin, a growth hormone (GH). *Lactotropes* (mammotropes) are variable and scattered acidophils that produce prolactin (PR) or lactogenic hormone (LTH) and undergo hypertrophy during lactation.

Pars Intermedia. In humans, the *pars intermedia* surrounds a series of small cystic cavities that represent the residual lumen of Rathke's pouch. The endocrine cells of the pars intermedia surround the colloid-filled cysts. The nature of this colloid is yet to be determined. The pars intermedia contains basophilic and chromophobic cells (Fig. 20.5). Frequently, basophilic cells and cysts extend into the pars nervosa.

The function of the cells of the pars intermedia in the human remains unclear. From studies of other species, however, it is known that basophils have scattered granules in their cytoplasm that contain either α or β endorphin (a morphine-related compound). In frogs, the basophils produce melanocyte-stimulating hormone (MSH) that stimulates pigment production in melanocytes and pigment dis-

persion in melanophores. In humans, MSH is not a distinct, functional hormone but is a byproduct of LPH posttranslational processing. Because MSH is found in the human pars intermedia in small amounts, the basophils of the pars intermedia are assumed to be adrenocorticolipotropes.

Pars Tuberalis. The *pars tuberalis* is a highly vascular region containing the veins of the hypophyseal portal system. The endocrine cells are arranged in short clusters or cords in association with the blood vessels. Nests of squamous cells and small follicles lined with cuboidal cells are scattered in this region. Some functional gonadotropes are present in this region.

HORMONAL REGULATING FACTORS

The release of hormones from the adenohypophysis is regulated by the hypothalamus through the release of *hypothalamic regulating factors* (hormones) into the hypophyseal portal veins. These hypothalamic regulating factors can stimulate secretion *(releasing factors)* or inhibit it *(inhibitory factors).* The regulating factors are produced in the cells of the hypothalamus in response to circulating levels of hormones. Thus, the cells of the adenohypophysis can be selectively inhibited or stimulated. A simple negative feedback system controls the synthesis and discharge of the releasing factors. Consider the production of thyroid hormones (Fig. 20.3). If blood levels of thyroid hormones are high, thyrotropin-releasing factor (TRF) is not produced or released. If blood levels of thyroid hormones are low, the hypothalamus discharges TRF into the hypophyseal portal vein. This stimulates specific cells within the adenohypophysis to produce TSH or thyrotropin, which, in turn, stimulates the thyroid to produce and release more thyroid hormone. As the thyroid hormone level rises, the negative feedback system stops the hypothalamus from discharging TRF. Most of the tropic hormones produced by the adenohypophysis are regulated by releasing factors. Prolactin production is regulated by an inhibitory factor; i.e., prolactin secretion is tonically inhibited by the release of prolactin-inhibiting factor (PIF) by the hypothalamus.

Neurohypophysis

The Neurohypophysis Is a Nerve Tract Whose Terminals Store and Release Secretory Product From the Hypothalamus

The neurohypophysis consists of the *pars nervosa* and the *infundibulum* that connects it to the hypothalamus. The *pars nervosa,* the neural lobe of the pituitary, contains nonmyelinated axons and nerve endings of approximately 100,000 *neurosecretory neurons* whose cell bodies lie in the *supraoptic* and *paraventricular nuclei* of the hypothalamus. These neurons are unique in two respects. First, they do not terminate on other neurons or target cells but end in close proximity to the fenestrated capillary network of the pars nervosa. Second, they contain *secretory granules* in all parts of the cells, i.e., the cell body, axon, and axon terminal. These granules may be specifically stained

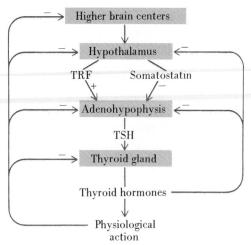

Figure 20.3. Hypothalamic-adenohypophyseal-thyroid interaction. Production of thyroid hormones is regulated through a negative feedback system. Both the thyroid hormones and the physiologic actions that they induce, such as an increase in the metabolic rate, can feed back on the system and inhibit further release of thyroid hormones. Such inhibition may occur at the level of the thyroid gland, adenohypophysis, hypothalamus, or higher brain centers. The system is activated in response to low thyroid hormone levels or in response to metabolic needs. *TRF,* thyrotropin-releasing factor; and *TSH,* thyroid-stimulating hormone.

with the aldehyde-fuchsin, aldehyde-thionine, and chromhematoxylin methods, by specific procedures for the disulfide groups of cystine, and most specifically by immunochemical reactions. Due to their intense secretory activity, the neurons have very well developed Nissl bodies and, in this respect, resemble ventral horn and ganglion cells.

The neurohypophysis is *not an endocrine gland.* Rather, it is a *storage site for neurosecretions* of the neurons of the *supraoptic* and *paraventricular nuclei* of the hypothalamus. The nonmyelinated axons convey neurosecretory products to the pars nervosa. Other neurons from hypothalamic nuclei, which are described later, also release their secretory products in close proximity to the fenestrated capillary network of the infundibulum, the first capillary bed of the hypophyseal portal system.

Electron Microscopy Reveals Three Morphologically Distinct Neurosecretory Granules in the Nerve Endings of the Pars Nervosa

Three sizes of membrane-bounded granules are present in the pars nervosa:

* Neurosecretory granules with diameters ranging between 10 and 30 nm accumulate in the axon terminals. They also form accumulations that dilate portions of the axon near the terminals (Fig. 20.6). These dilations, called **Herring bodies,** are visible with the light microscope (LM) (Fig. 20.7).
* The nerve terminals also contain 30-nm vesicles that

contain acetylcholine. These granules may play a specific role in the release of the neurosecretory granules.
* Larger, 50–80-nm vesicles that resemble the dense core granules of the adrenal medulla (see page 619) and adrenergic nerve endings are present in the same terminal as the other membrane-bounded granules.

The membrane-bounded neurosecretory granules that aggregate to form the Herring bodies contain either *oxytocin* or *vasopressin (antidiuretic hormone) (ADH)* (Table 20.4). These two compounds are octapeptides that differ in only two amino acids. In addition to one of the two hormones, each granule contains ATP and a **neurophysin,** a specific hormone-binding protein that is bound to the hormone by noncovalent bonds. Oxytocin and vasopressin are synthesized as a part of a large molecule that includes the hormone and its specific neurophysin. The large molecule splits into hormone and neurophysin as it travels from the perikaryon to the axon terminal. Immunocytochemical staining demonstrates that the two hormones are secreted by different cells in the hypothalamic nuclei.

Antidiuretic Hormone Controls Blood Pressure by Altering the Permeability of Kidney Collecting Tubules

ADH derived its original name, vasopressin, from the fact that in large nonphysiologic doses it increases blood pressure by promoting the contraction of smooth muscle in small arteries and arterioles. The primary physiologic effect of ADH is to increase the permeability of the distal portions of the nephron, i.e., the distal convoluted tubule and collecting ducts. This causes rapid resorption of water across the tubular epithelium. In the absence or reduced production of ADH, most commonly due to hypothalamic and neurohypophyseal lesions, large volumes of dilute urine are produced. Persons with this condition, called **diabetes insipidus,** produce up to 20 liters of urine per day and have extreme thirst.

Plasma osmolality and blood volume are monitored by specialized receptors of the cardiovascular system (e.g., carotid bodies and juxtaglomerular apparatus). A rise in osmolality or a drop in volume causes ADH to be released. Additionally, the cell bodies of the hypothalamic secretory neurons may also serve as osmoreceptors, initiating ADH release. Pain, trauma, emotional stress, and drugs, such as nicotine, also stimulate release of ADH. A standard clinical test in the differential diagnosis of **diabetes** is nicotine-induced release of ADH.

Oxytocin Promotes Contraction of Smooth Muscle of the Uterus and Myoepithelial Cells of the Breast

Oxytocin is a more potent promoter of smooth muscle contraction than is ADH. Its primary effects include promotion of contraction of

TABLE 20.1. Tropic Hormones of the Adenohypophysis

HORMONE	NATURE	MW	FUNCTIONS
Somatotropin (growth hormone, GH)	Straight-chain protein (191 aa)	21,700	Stimulates kidney and liver to synthesize and secrete *somatomedin,* which stimulates the growth of long bones
Prolactin (PR) (lactogenic hormone, LTH)	Straight-chain protein (198 aa)	22,500	Promotes mammary gland development; initiates and maintains milk secretion
Adrenocorticotropic hormone (ACTH)	Small polypeptide (39 aa)	4,500	Maintains structure and stimulates secretion of glucocorticoids and gonadocorticoids by the zona fasciculata and zona reticularis of the adrenal cortex
Lipotropins (LPH)	Small polypeptides (β 90 aa and α 55 aa)		No known function in humans; broken down to melanocyte-stimulating hormone (β-MSH) and β endorphin
Follicle-stimulating hormone (FSH)	2-chain glycoprotein[A] (α 90 aa)	25,000	Stimulates follicular development in the ovary and spermatogenesis in the testis
Luteinizing hormone (LH); also known as interstitial cell-stimulating hormone (ICSH)	2-chain glycoprotein[A] (α 90 aa; β 116 aa)	30,000	Regulates final maturation of ovarian follicle, ovulation, and corpus luteum formation; stimulates steroid secretion by follicle and corpus luteum; in males, it is essential for maintenance of and androgen secretion by the interstitial (Leydig) cells of the testis
Thyrotropin (TSH)	2-chain glycoprotein[A] (α 90 aa; β 112 aa)	26,600	Stimulates growth of thyroid epithelial cells and release of thyroid hormones to the blood

[A]The α chains of FSH, LH, and TSH are now known to be identical; the β chains are specific for each hormone.

- Uterine smooth muscle during copulation and parturition
- Myoepithelial cells of the secretory alveoli and alveolar ducts of the breast

Oxytocin secretion is triggered by neural stimuli that reach the hypothalamus. This initiates a neurohumoral reflex that resembles a simple sensorimotor reflex. In the uterus, the neurohumoral reflex is initiated by distension of the vagina and cervix. In the breast, the reflex is initiated by nursing (suckling). Contraction of the myoepithelial cells that surround the base of the alveolar secretory cells and the cells of the larger ducts causes milk to be released and pass through the ducts that open onto the nipple, i.e., milk ejection (see page 713).

The Pituicyte Is the Only Cell Specific to the Neurohypophysis

In addition to the numerous axons and terminals of the hypothalamic neurosecretory neurons, the neurohypophysis contains fibroblasts, mast cells, and *pituicytes* associated with the fenestrated capillaries. The *pituicyte* is the only cell type that is specific to the neurohypophysis. These cells are irregular in shape, with many branches, and resemble glial cells. Their nuclei are round or oval, and pigment granules are present in the cytoplasm. Like astroglia, they often have processes that terminate in the perivascular space. Because of their many processes and relationships to the blood, the pituicyte may serve a role similar to the astrocyte in the rest of the CNS (see page 269).

The Hypothalamus Regulates Hypophyseal Function

The hypothalamus is the site of production of a number of neurosecretory proteins. In addition to oxytocin and ADH, the hypothalamic neurons secrete proteins that promote and inhibit the secretion and release of adenohypophyseal hormones (Table 20.5). These other hypothalamic peptides also accumulate in nerve endings near the median eminence and infundibular stalk and are released into the first capillary bed of the hypophyseal portal system for transport to the pars distalis.

A Feedback System Regulates Endocrine Function at Two Levels: Hormone Production in the Hypophysis and Tropic Hormone Production in the Hypothalamus

The circulating level of a specific secretory product of a target organ, a hormone or its metabolite, may act directly

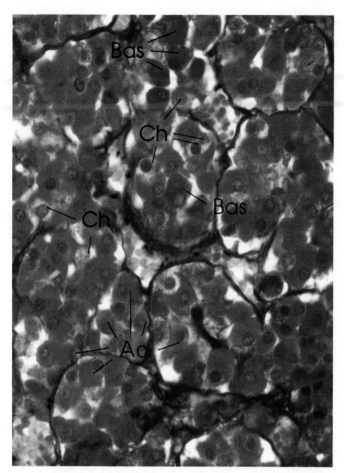

Figure 20.4. Photomicrograph of human pars distalis. The cords of cells are surrounded by a thin layer of connective tissue. The capillaries (sinusoids) are seen in close association with the parenchyma. In the region shown here, the acidophils *(Ac)* are the most numerous cell type present. Their cytoplasm stains cherry red. The basophils *(Bas)* stain blue. The chromophobes *(Ch)*, though few in number in this particular region, are virtually unstained. The collagen stains blue, and the erythrocytes stain yellow. Stain, brilliant crystal scarlet, aniline blue, and Martius yellow.

on the cells of the adenohypophysis or on the cells of the hypothalamus to regulate the secretion of specific tropic hormones (see Fig. 20.3). The two levels of feedback allow exquisite sensitivity in the control of secretory function. The hormone, itself, normally regulates the secretory activity of the cells in the hypothalamus and hypophysis that regulate its secretion.

In addition, information from most physiologic and psychologic stimuli that reach the brain also reaches the hypothalamus. The hypothalamic-hypophyseal feedback loop then provides a regulatory path whereby general information from the central nervous system contributes to the regulation of the adenohypophysis and, consequently, to the regulation of the entire endocrine system. The secretion of hypothalamic regulatory peptides is the primary mechanism by which changes in emotional state are translated into changes in the physiologic homeostatic state.

PINEAL GLAND

The pineal gland (pineal body) is now described as an endocrine or neuroendocrine gland, but its functions in humans are not clearly defined. It develops from the neuroectoderm of the posterior portion of the roof of the diencephalon and remains attached to the brain by a short stalk. In humans, it is a flattened, cone-shaped structure that measures 5–8 mm high and 3–5 mm in diameter and weighs between 100 and 200 mg (Fig. 20.8).

The Human Pineal Gland Relates Light Intensity and Duration to Endocrine Activity

In many animals, extracts of pineal glands contain numerous neurotransmitters and neuroendocrine regulatory peptides including norepinephrine, dopamine, serotonin, histamine, melatonin, somatostatin, and TRF. Melatonin functions in regulating reproductive function in mammals by inhibiting the steroidogenic activity of the gonads (Table 20.6). In humans, pineal activity, as indicated by changes in the plasma level of melatonin, rises during darkness and falls during light. Clinically, tumors that destroy the pineal gland are associated with precocious (early-onset) puberty.

From animal studies, it is well known that information on changes in the length of day comes to the pineal gland from photoreceptors in the retina. Pineal gland function then influences seasonal sexual activity. Recent studies in humans suggest that the pineal gland has a role in adjusting to sudden changes in day length, such as those experienced by travelers who suffer from *jet lag,* and in regulating emotional responses to reduced day length during winter in temperate and subarctic zones (seasonal affective disorder, SAD).

The Pineal Gland Contains Two Basic Types of Parenchymal Cells: Pinealocytes and Interstitial (Glial) Cells

Pinealocytes are the most common parenchymal cell in the pineal gland. They are arranged in clumps or cords within the lobules formed by connective tissue septa that extend into the gland from the pia mater that covers its surface. These cells have a large, deeply infolded nucleus with one or more prominent nucleoli and contain lipid droplets within their cytoplasm. When examined with the transmission electron microscope (TEM), pinealocytes show typical cytoplasmic organelles along with numerous, dense-cored, membrane-bounded granules in their elaborate, elongated cytoplasmic processes. The processes also contain numerous parallel bundles of microtubules. The expanded, club-like endings of the processes are associated with the blood capillaries. This feature is strongly suggestive of neuroendocrine activity.

The *interstitial (glial) cells* comprise about 5% of the cells in the gland. They have staining and ultrastructural features that closely resemble those of astrocytes and are reminiscent of the pituicytes of the neurohypophysis.

TABLE 20.2. Staining of Adenohypophyseal Cell Types

CELL TYPE	GENERAL STAINING	SPECIFIC STAINING	PRODUCT
Somatotropes	Acidophils	Orange G	Somatotropin (STH; growth hormone, GH)
Mammotropes	Acidophils	Orange G Erythrosin Carmine	Luteotropic hormone (LTH)
Adrenocortico-lipotropes	Basophils	Periodic acid-Schiff (PAS)	Adrenocorticotropic hormone (ACTH); lipotropin (LPH)
Gonadotropes	Basophils	PAS and aldehyde-fuchsin	Follicle-stimulating hormone (FSH) and luteinizing hormone (LH; interstitial cell-stimulating hormone, ICSH)
Thyrotropes	Basophils	PAS (weak) and aldehyde-fuchsin (intense)	Thyrotropic hormone (TSH)

In addition to the two cell types, the human pineal gland is characterized by the presence of calcified concretions, called **corpora arenacea** or **brain sand** (Fig. 20.9). These concretions appear to derive from precipitation of calcium phosphates and carbonates on carrier proteins that are released into the cytoplasm when the pineal secretions are released by exocytosis. The concretions are recognizable in childhood and increase in number with age. Because they are opaque to x-rays, they serve as convenient markers in radiographic and computed tomography scanning studies.

THYROID GLAND

The Thyroid Is a Bilobed Endocrine Gland Located in the Neck, Anterolateral to the Larynx and Upper Trachea

The two large lobes of the thyroid gland (each ≈5 cm in the superior-inferior dimension and 20–30 g in weight) lie on either side of the larynx and upper trachea. The lobes are connected by a thin band of thyroid tissue, the **isthmus**, that crosses anterior to the upper part of the trachea. A **pyramidal lobe** may extend upward from the isthmus. A thin connective tissue capsule surrounds the gland. It sends trabeculae into the parenchyma to partially outline irregular lobes and lobules. Secretory follicles constitute the functional units of the gland.

Thyroid Gland Function Is Essential to Normal Growth and Development

The thyroid gland produces three hormones, each of which is essential to normal metabolism and homeostasis:

- **Thyroxine (tetraiodothyronine) (T_4)** and **triiodothyronine (T_3)** regulate cell and tissue metabolism.
- **Calcitonin** regulates blood calcium levels.

Follicular Cells

The Follicle Is the Structural Unit of the Thyroid Gland

A **follicle** is a roughly spheroidal cyst-like compartment with a wall formed by a simple squamous or cuboidal epithelium, the **follicular epithelium**. Hundreds of thousands of follicles that vary in diameter from about 0.2 to 1.0 mm constitute nearly the entire mass of the human thyroid. The lumina of the follicles are filled with a gel-like mass called **colloid** (Fig. 20.10). The apical surfaces of the follicular epithelial cells are in contact with the colloid, and the basal surfaces rest on a typical basal lamina.

Two basic cell types are present in the follicles: **principal** or **follicular cells** and **parafollicular** or **C cells.** They have different embryologic origins:

- **Follicular cells,** the cells that secrete T_4 and T_3, arise from a downward growth of endoderm in the midline of the floor of the pharyngeal portion of the foregut, near the base of the tongue.
- **Parafollicular cells,** the cells that secrete calcitonin, arise from neural crest cells that migrate into the developing thyroid gland.

The follicles are surrounded by an extensive network of fenestrated capillaries derived from the superior and inferior thyroid arteries. Blind-ending lymphatic capillaries are present in the interfollicular connective tissue and may also provide a second route for conveying the hormones from the gland.

The synthesis, storage, and secretion of the thyroid hormones involve a number of functional events that can be correlated with the structure of the follicular epithelial cells (Fig. 20.11).

The nuclei of follicular epithelial cells are spherical and contain one or more prominent nucleoli. With the LM, a supranuclear Golgi complex, lipid droplets, and PAS-positive droplets can be identified in the basophilic cytoplasm. Ultrastructural studies of the active cuboidal or columnar cells reveal the presence of organelles commonly associated with both secretory and absorptive cells. This is shown schematically in Figure 20.12. The organelles include typical junctional complexes at the apical end of the lateral plasma membrane, short microvilli on the apical surface of the cells, numerous profiles of rough-surfaced endoplasmic reticulum (rER) in the basal region, a well-developed supranuclear Golgi complex, numerous small vesicles in the apical cytoplasm that are morphologically similar to vesicles associated with the Golgi complex, abundant lysosomes and multivesicular bodies, and membrane-limited vesicles, identified as *colloidal resorption droplets*, in the apical region.

Colloid Contains *Thyroglobulin*, the Inactive Storage Form of the Thyroid Hormones

The colloid stains with both basic and acidic dyes and is strongly PAS-positive. Its principal component is a large iodinated glycoprotein called *thyroglobulin*. It also contains several enzymes and other glycoproteins. The protein portion of thyroglobulin is synthesized in the rER of the follicular epithelial cells and glycosylated there and in the Golgi complexes before it is secreted by exocytosis into the lumen of the follicle. Thyroglobulin is not a hormone. It is an inactive storage form of the thyroid hormones. Active thyroid hormones are liberated from the thyroglobulin and

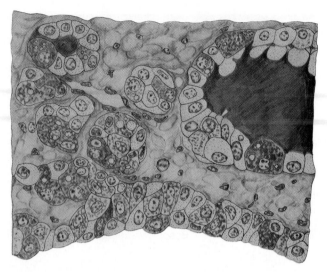

Figure 20.5. Drawing of a section through the pars intermedia of an adult human pituitary gland. Cords of basophilic (darkly staining) and chromophobic (lightly staining) cells grow into the neural lobe. Vesicles filled with colloid (black) are present within some of the cords of cells. (Based on Kelley RO: *Bailey's Textbook of Histology,* 17th ed. Baltimore, Williams & Wilkins, 1978, fig. 21.7.)

released into the fenestrated blood capillaries that surround the follicles only after further cellular processing. The thyroid is unique among endocrine glands because it stores large amounts of its secretory product extracellularly.

Thyroglobulin Is Iodinated in the Colloid at the Microvillar Surface of the Follicular Cells

The follicular epithelial cells actively transport iodide from the blood into their cytoplasm, establishing a concentration that is 30–40 times the serum level. The iodide is oxidized to iodine by thyroperoxidase in the cytoplasm. It is then

TABLE 20.3. Electron Microscopic Characteristics of Adenohypophyseal Cells

CELL TYPE	SIZE/SHAPE	GRANULE SIZE/ CHARACTERISTICS	OTHER CYTOPLASMIC CHARACTERISTICS
Somatotropes	Small/round	Dense—350 nm, closely packed	
Mammotropes	Variable	Inactive—200 nm, sparse Active—dense, pleiomorphic, 600 nm, sparse	Lysosomes increase after lactation
Adrenocorticolipotropes	Round/oval	100–300 nm	Lipid droplets, 6–8-nm filaments
Gonadotropes			
FSH	Large/round	Dense, 200 nm	Distended rER vesicles
LH	Small/round	Dense, 250 nm	Minimal rER
Thyrotropes	Large/ polygonal	Dense, <150 nm	

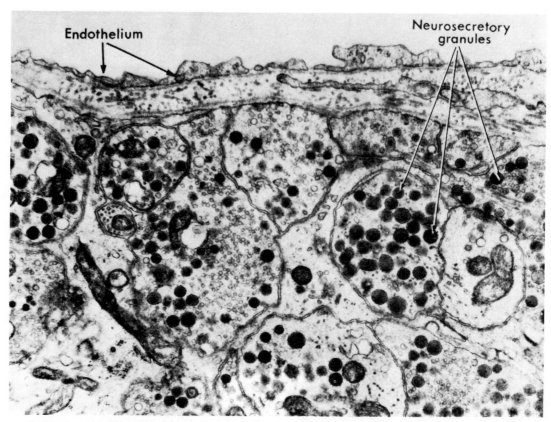

Figure 20.6. Electron micrograph of rat neurohypophysis. Neurosecretory granules and small vesicles are present in the terminal portions of axonal processes of the fibers of the hy- pothalamohypophyseal tract. Capillaries with fenestrated en- dothelium are present in close proximity to the nerve endings. ×22,000. (Courtesy of P. Orkland and S. L. Palay.)

released into the follicular lumen where iodination of some tyrosine residues of the thyroglobulin occurs near the microvilli of the apical cell surface.

The Synthesis, Storage, and Release of Thyroid Hormones Are Controlled by Thyroid-Stimulating Hormone From the Adenohypophysis

Under the influence of TSH, thyroid follicular epithelial cells increase in size and activity. The cells become more columnar in shape, and both the iodide pump and the extracellular iodination of thyroglobulin are stimulated. In addition, thyroglobulin synthesis, endocytosis, and lysosomal breakdown increase, resulting in the release of large amounts of the thyroid hormones.

In response to TSH, the follicular cells take up the thyroglobulin from the colloid by the process of receptor-mediated endocytosis. The **colloidal resorption droplets** are endocytic vacuoles and are larger than the secretory vesicles. They can be seen in the apical cytoplasm with the LM. Primary lysosomes fuse with the colloidal resorption droplets and hydrolyze the thyroglobulin into its constituent amino acids and carbohydrates. If the levels of TSH remain high, the amount of colloid in the follicle is reduced because it is synthesized, secreted, iodinated, and resorbed too rapidly to accumulate.

The **thyroid hormones** are formed by the coupling of two iodinated tyrosine residues to produce **thyroxine (tetraiodothyronine, T_4)** and **triiodothyronine (T_3)**. These active thyroid hormones (in a T_4:T_3 ratio of 20:1) cross the basal plasma membrane and enter blood and lymphatic capillaries. Most of the released hormones are immediately bound to specific plasma proteins, leaving only small amounts of free circulating hormones that are metabolically active. T_3 is the more active thyroid hormone, and most of the circulating T_3 is formed in the liver by deiodination of T_4. The free hormone also functions in the feedback system that regulates the secretory activity of the thyroid.

SUMMARY FEEDBACK CONTROL OF THYROID HORMONE SYNTHESIS

The release of the thyroid hormones T_3 and T_4 is regulated by a simple feedback system. The secretion of thyroid hormones is controlled by the release of thyroid-simulating hormone (TSH) or thyrotropin from the adenohypophysis into the bloodstream. The TSH stimulates the principal cells of the thyroid to release T_3 and T_4. Low levels of free T_3 and T_4 initiate the release of thyrotropin-releasing factor (TRF) from the hypothalamus. In turn, TRF stimulates thyrotropic cells in the adenohypophysis to secrete TSH. High serum levels of free T_3 and T_4 inhibit the synthesis and release of TSH. Somatostatin, released from the hypothalamus, functions as an antagonist to TRF, inhibiting TSH release (see Fig. 20.3).

Thyroid Hormones Play an Essential Role in Normal Fetal Development and the Regulation of Metabolism

In humans, the fetal thyroid gland begins to function during the tenth week of gestation and its secretions are essential to normal growth and development (Table 20.7). Thyroid hormone deficiency during fetal development results in irreversible damage to the central nervous system, including reduced numbers of neurons, defective myelination, and mental retardation, as well as generalized stunted body growth, a constellation of symptoms called *cretinism.*

Thyroid hormones stimulate carbohydrate, lipid, and protein metabolism. T_3 and T_4 bind to the inner mitochondrial membranes of cells in responsive (target) tissues (e.g., liver) but not in nonresponsive tissues (e.g., spleen). Recent studies have shown that the primary effect of thyroid hormones is to modulate the activity of the sodium and other ion pumps of the plasma membrane and, thereby, to regulate the entry of metabolites into cells.

ABNORMAL THYROID FUNCTION

A *goiter* is an enlarged thyroid gland and may be indicative of either hypothyroidism or hyperthyroidism. Congenital hypothyroidism in infants and children leads to cretinism. In adults, hypothyroidism can be caused by insufficient dietary iodine (iodine-deficiency goiter, endemic goiter) or by one of several inherited autoimmune diseases, such as Hashimoto's thyroiditis. The low levels of circulating thyroid hormone stimulate release of excessive amounts of TSH that cause hypertrophy of the thyroid through synthesis of more thyroglobulin. Adult hypothyroidism is called myxedema and is characterized by mental and physical sluggishness and edema of the connective tissue.

In hyperthyroidism (toxic goiter, Graves' disease), thyroid cells are stimulated, as shown by an increase in number and size. However, there is little colloid. Thyroid hormones secreted at abnormally high rates cause an increase in metabolic processes. Often, toxic amounts of hormone are produced (thyrotoxicosis). Levels of TSH are usually normal in hyperthyroidism. In some cases, an abnormal immunoglobulin called long-acting thyroid stimulator (LATS) appears to bind to the TSH receptors on the follicular cells and leads to continuous stimulation of the cells.

Parafollicular Cells

Parafollicular Cells Are Present Within the Follicular Epithelium or Are Scattered in the Connective Tissue

The *parafollicular cells (C cells, calcitonin cells)* are the second type of endocrine cell found in the thyroid. They are pale-staining cells that occur as solitary cells or small clusters of cells in the wall of the follicle or in the interfollicular space (Fig. 20.12). In the follicles, they are located near the basal lamina and do not extend to the follicular lumen to contact the colloid. In this site they are

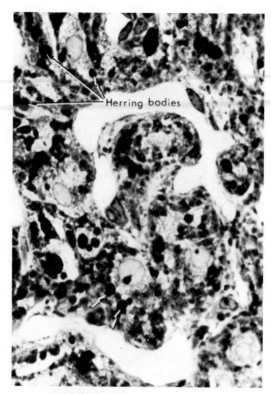

Figure 20.7. Photomicrograph of rat neurohypophysis. Note the dark rounded masses called Herring bodies that are present in nerve endings adjacent to the capillaries. ×950. (Courtesy of P. Orkland and S. L. Palay.)

partially surrounded by follicle cell cytoplasm, but a portion of the parafollicular cell rests directly on the basal lamina. Human parafollicular cells are difficult to identify with light microscopy. The most characteristic feature of these cells seen with the TEM is the presence of numerous, small (0.1–0.5 μm in diameter), membrane-bounded secretory granules.

Parafollicular Cells Produce Calcitonin, a Hormone That Lowers Blood Calcium Levels

Calcitonin (thyrocalcitonin) is a physiologic antagonist to parathyroid hormone (PTH) (see below). These two hormones act in concert to maintain the normal concentration of calcium in the serum and the extracellular fluids. Calcitonin lowers blood calcium levels by suppressing bone resorption and increasing the rate of osteoid calcification. Secretion of calcitonin is regulated directly by blood calcium levels. High levels of calcium stimulate secretion; low levels inhibit it. Secretion of calcitonin is unaffected by the hypothalamus and pituitary gland. Although calcitonin is used to treat patients with hypercalcemia, no clinical disease has been associated with its deficiency or, even, its absence after total thyroidectomy.

PARATHYROID GLANDS

The parathyroid glands are small endocrine glands closely associated with the thyroid. They are ovoid, a few milli-

TABLE 20.4. Hormones of the Neurohypophysis

HORMONE[A]	SOURCE	FUNCTION
Oxytocin	Cell bodies of neurons located in the supraoptic and paraventricular nuclei of the hypothalamus[B]	Stimulates activity of the contractile cells around the ducts of the mammary glands to eject milk from the glands; stimulates contraction of smooth muscle cells in the pregnant uterus
Antidiuretic hormone (ADH) or vasopressin	Cell bodies of neurons located in the supraoptic and paraventricular nuclei of the hypothalamus[B]	Decreases urine volume by causing the kidneys to remove water from newly formed urine; decreases the rate of perspiration in response to dehydration; causes rise in blood pressure by stimulating contractions of smooth muscle cells in the wall of arterioles

[A]Oxytocin and ADH are peptide hormones.
[B]Immunocytochemical studies indicate that oxytocin and ADH are produced by separate sets of neurons within the supraoptic and paraventricular nuclei of the hypothalamus. Biochemical studies have demonstrated that the supraoptic nucleus contains equal amounts of both hormones, whereas the paraventricular nucleus contains more oxytocin than ADH, but less than the amount found in the supraoptic nucleus.

meters in diameter, and arranged in two pairs, to comprise the **superior** and **inferior parathyroid glands.** They are usually located in the connective tissue on the posterior surface of the thyroid. However, the number and location may vary. In some individuals (estimates on the frequency vary from 2% to 10%), additional glands are associated with the thymus.

Development and Structure

Embryologically, the inferior parathyroid glands (and the thymus) derive from the third branchial pouch; the superior glands, from the fourth branchial pouch. Normally, the inferior parathyroids separate from the thymus and come to lie below the superior parathyroids. Failure of these structures to separate results in the atypical association of the parathyroids with the thymus in the adult.

Structurally, each parathyroid gland is surrounded by a thin connective tissue capsule that separates it from the thyroid. Septa extend from the capsule into the gland to divide it into poorly defined lobules and to separate the densely packed cords of cells. The connective tissue is more evident in the adult as the number of fat cells increases with age, ultimately reaching as much as 60–70% of the glandular mass.

The glands receive their blood supply from the inferior thyroid arteries or from anastomoses between the superior and inferior thyroid arteries. Typical of endocrine glands, rich networks of fenestrated blood capillaries and lymphatic capillaries surround the parenchyma of the parathyroids.

Principal (Chief) Cells and Oxyphil Cells Constitute the Epithelial Cells of the Parathyroid Gland

• **Principal cells,** the more numerous of the parenchymal cells of the parathyroid (Fig. 20.13), are responsible for the secretion of PTH. They are small, polygonal cells, with a diameter of 7–10 μm and a centrally located nucleus. The pale-staining, slightly acidophilic cytoplasm contains lipofuscin granules, large accumulations of glycogen, and lipid droplets. Small, dense, membrane-limited granules seen with the TEM or after using special stains with the LM are thought to be the storage form of PTH.

• **Oxyphil cells** constitute a minor portion of the parenchymal cells and are not known to have a secretory role. They are more rounded and considerably larger than the principal cells and have a distinctly acidophilic cytoplasm. They are found singly or in clusters and increase in number with age. Mitochondria almost fill the cytoplasm and are responsible for the strong acidophilia of these cells. No secretory granules are present, and little if any rER is present. Cytoplasmic inclusion bodies consist of occasional lysosomes, lipid droplets, and glycogen distributed among the mitochondria.

Function

The parathyroids function in the regulation of blood ion levels of calcium and phosphate. Parathyroid hormone is essential for life. Therefore, care must be taken during thyroidectomy to leave some functioning parathyroid tissue. If the glands are totally removed, death will ensue because muscles, including the laryngeal and other respiratory muscles, go into tetanic contraction as the blood calcium level falls.

Parathyroid Hormone Regulates Calcium and Phosphate Levels in the Blood

The parathyroids produce **parathyroid hormone (PTH),** also known as **parathormone** (Table 20.8). Release of this

TABLE 20.5. Hypothalamic Regulatory Peptides

PEPTIDE NAME	CHARACTERIZATION	COMMENTS
Growth hormone-releasing factor (GRF)	?	
Growth hormone-inhibiting factor (GIF)	14-amino acid peptide	
Prolactin-releasing factor (PRF)	A tripeptide?	May be identical to thyrotropin-releasing factor (TRF)
Prolactin-inhibiting factor	?	
Corticotropin-releasing factor (CRF)	41-amino acid polypeptide	
Gonadotropin-releasing factor (GnRF)	A decapeptide	Stimulates release of both FSH and LH
Thyrotropin-releasing factor (TRF)	A modified tripeptide	

hormone causes the level of calcium in the blood to increase. Simultaneously, it reduces the concentration of phosphate. Secretion of PTH is regulated by the serum calcium level through a simple feedback system. Low levels of serum calcium stimulate secretion of PTH; high levels of serum calcium inhibit its secretion.

PTH functions at several sites:

- *Bone resorption* is *stimulated* by PTH. The hormone probably has a direct effect on osteoclasts (osteoclastic osteolysis) and on osteocytes (osteocytic osteolysis). During osteolysis, calcium and phosphate are both released from calcified bone matrix into the extracellular fluid.
- *Kidney excretion of calcium* is *reduced* by PTH stimulation of tubular resorption, thus conserving calcium. *Phosphate excretion,* however, is *increased* by PTH stimulation, thus decreasing phosphate concentration in the blood and extracellular fluids.
- *Intestinal absorption of calcium* is *increased* under the influence of PTH. Vitamin D, however, has a greater effect than PTH on intestinal absorption of calcium.

Parathyroid Hormone and Calcitonin Have Reciprocal Effects in the Regulation of Blood Calcium Levels

Although PTH raises blood calcium levels, the peak increase following its release is not reached for several hours. PTH appears to have a rather slow, long-term homeostatic action. PTH secretion, itself, is regulated by blood calcium levels. The level of PTH goes up as blood calcium levels go down; the level of PTH goes down as blood calcium levels go up.

Calcitonin, however, rapidly lowers blood calcium lev-

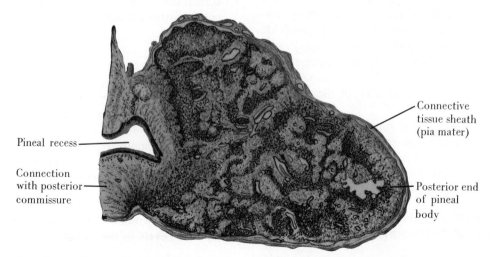

Pineal recess

Connection with posterior commissure

Connective tissue sheath (pia mater)

Posterior end of pineal body

Figure 20.8. Drawing of a median section through the pineal gland of a newborn child. The blood vessels are empty. ×25.

(After Schaffer: In: Bloom W, Fawcett DW: *A Textbook of Histology,* 10th ed. Philadelphia, WB Saunders, 1975, p 557.)

TABLE 20.6. Hormones of the Pineal Gland

HORMONE[A]	SOURCE	FUNCTION
Melatonin	Pinealocytes	Function obscure in humans; in other mammals, slows steroid secretion by the ovaries; may function in regulating endocrine activity of the gonads, particularly as related to the menstrual cycle

[A]Melatonin is an indolamine.

els and has its peak effect in about 1 hour. Calcitonin has a rapid, acute homeostatic action.

ADRENAL GLANDS

The **adrenal (suprarenal) glands** secrete both steroid hormones and catecholamines. They have a flattened triangular shape and are embedded in the perirenal fat at the superior poles of the kidneys.

The glands are covered with a thick connective tissue capsule from which trabeculae extend into the parenchyma, carrying blood vessels and nerves. The secretory parenchymal tissue is organized in **cortical** and **medullary** regions:

• The **cortex** is the steroid-secreting portion. It lies beneath the capsule and constitutes nearly 90% of the gland by weight.

• The **medulla** is the catecholamine-secreting portion. It lies deep to the cortex and forms the center of the gland.

Parenchymal Cells of the Cortex and Medulla Are of Different Embryologic Origin

Embryologically, the cortical cells originate from mesodermal mesenchyme, whereas the medulla originates from neural crest cells that migrate into the developing gland. Although embryologically distinct, the two portions of the adrenal are functionally related (see below). The parenchymal cells of the adrenal cortex are controlled, in part, by the adenohypophysis and function in regulating metabolism and maintaining normal electrolyte balance (Table 20.9).

Blood Supply

The adrenal glands are supplied with blood by the superior, middle, and inferior adrenal arteries. These vessels

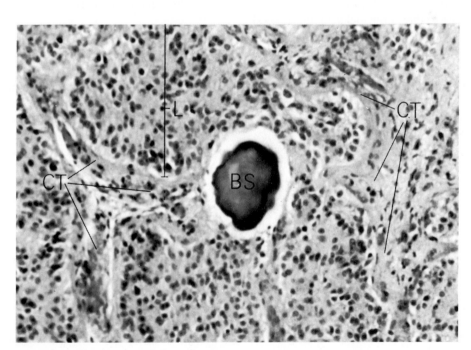

Figure 20.9. Photomicrograph of human pineal gland. A characteristic concretion called brain sand *(BS)* or *corpora arenacea* can be seen. Lobules *(L)* of the gland are surrounded by connective tissue *(CT)*. ×250.

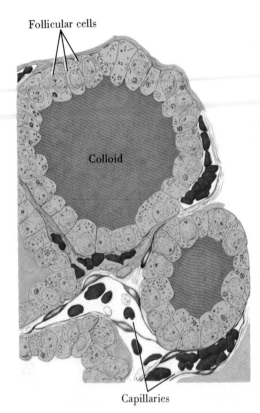

Follicular cells

Colloid

Capillaries

Figure 20.10. Drawing of a section through follicles of a human thyroid gland. Follicles consist of a single layer of epithelial cells surrounding a central mass of colloidal material. (Based on Bensley RR: In: Bloom WA, Fawcett DW: *A Textbook of Histology,* 10th ed. Philadelphia, WB Saunders, 1975, p 528.)

branch before entering the capsule to produce many small arteries that penetrate the capsule. In the capsule, the arteries branch to give rise to three principal patterns of blood distribution (Figs. 20.14 and 20.15). The vessels form a system that consists of

- *Capsular capillaries* that supply the capsule
- *Fenestrated cortical sinusoidal capillaries* that supply the cortex and then drain into the fenestrated *medullary capillary sinusoids*
- *Medullary arterioles* that traverse the cortex traveling within the trabeculae and bring arterial blood to the medullary capillary sinusoids

The medulla thus has a dual blood supply: arterial blood from the medullary arterioles and "venous" blood from the cortical sinusoidal capillaries that have already supplied the cortex. The venules that arise from the cortical and medullary sinusoids drain to the small medullary veins that join to form the large medullary vein (adrenal vein). It then drains to the inferior vena cava. In humans, the medullary vein and its tributaries are unusual in that they have a tunica media containing conspicuous, longitudinally oriented bundles of smooth muscle cells.

Lymphatic vessels are present in the capsule and the con-

nective tissue around the larger blood vessels in the gland. No lymphatic vessels are present in association with the parenchyma of the gland.

Adrenal Medullary Parenchymal Cells Are Innervated by Preganglionic Sympathetic Neurons

Numerous myelinated, preganglionic sympathetic nerve fibers pass directly to the parenchymal cells of the medulla. When nerve impulses carried by the sympathetic fibers reach the catecholamine-secreting medullary cells, they release their secretory products. Therefore, the medullary cells are considered to be equivalent to postganglionic neurons. However, they lack axonal processes. Thus, they resemble typical endocrine secretory cells. Their secretory product enters the bloodstream via the fenestrated capillaries, as is typical of other endocrine and neurosecretory glands. Ganglion cells are also present in the medulla. They innervate the smooth muscle of the medullary veins.

Zonation of the Adrenal Cortex

The adrenal cortex is divided into three zones on the basis of the arrangement of its parenchymal cells (see Figs. 20.14 and 20.15). The zones are designated

- *Zona glomerulosa,* the narrow outer zone that constitutes 15% of the cortical volume
- *Zona fasciculata,* the thick middle zone that constitutes nearly 80% of the cortical volume
- *Zona reticularis,* the inner zone that constitutes only 5–7% of the cortical volume but is thicker than the glomerulosa due to its more central location

Zona Glomerulosa. The cells of the zona glomerulosa are arranged in closely packed ovoid clusters and curved columns that are continuous with the cellular cords in the zona fasciculata. They are relatively small columnar or pyramidal cells whose spherical nuclei appear closely packed and stain densely. In the human, some areas of the cortex may lack a recognizable zona glomerulosa. A rich network of fenestrated sinusoidal capillaries surrounds each cell cluster. The cells have abundant smooth-surfaced endoplasmic reticulum (sER), multiple Golgi complexes, large mitochondria with shelf-like cristae, free ribosomes, and some rER. Lipid droplets are sparse.

The Zona Glomerulosa Secretes Aldosterone That Functions in the Control of Blood Pressure

The cells of the zona glomerulosa secrete *mineralocorticoids,* compounds that function in the regulation of sodium and potassium homeostasis and water balance. The principal secretion, *aldosterone,* acts on the distal tubules and collecting tubules of the nephron in the

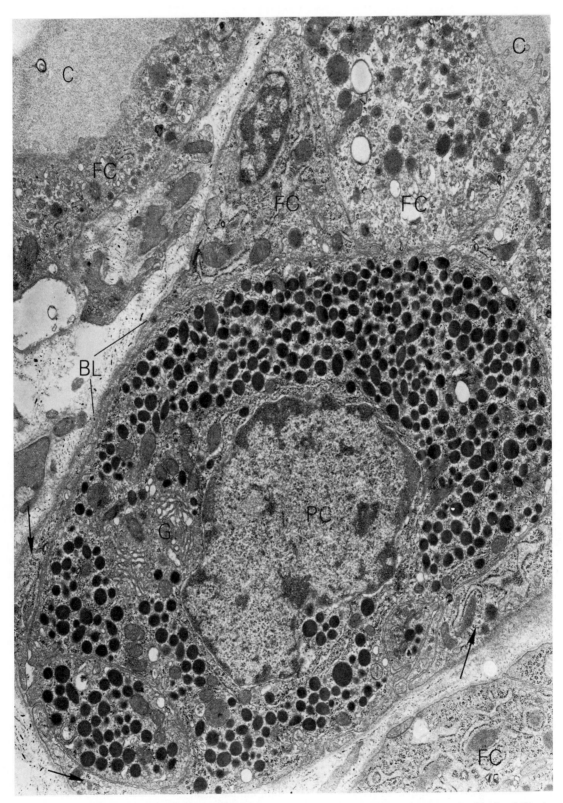

Figure 20.11. Electron micrograph of a parafollicular cell. Cytoplasmic processes of follicular cells *(arrows)* partially surround the parafollicular cell *(PC)*, which contains numerous electron-dense granules and a prominent Golgi complex *(G)*. Basal lamina *(BL)* is associated with the follicular cells *(FC)*. The central mass of colloidal material (C) in two adjacent follicles can be seen in the upper portion of the micrograph. ×12,000 (Courtesy of E. Nunez.)

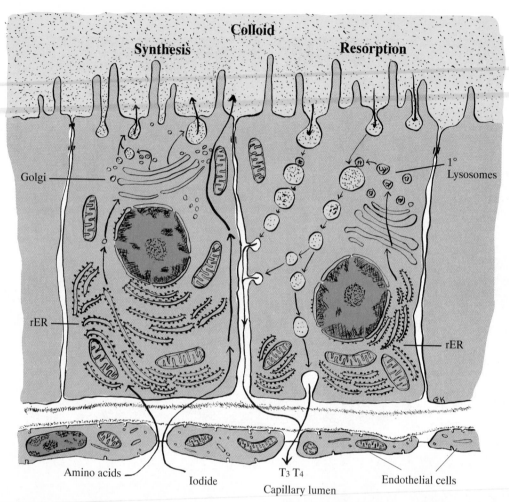

Figure 20.12. Diagram illustrating structural-functional relationships in thyroid follicular cells. *Arrows* indicate the general metabolic pathways. The cell under *Synthesis* illustrates the pathways of synthesis, glycosylation, secretion, and iodination of the thyroglobulin that is stored in the colloid. Iodide is absorbed at the basal surfaceof the cell, oxidized in the apical portion of the cell, and secreted into the colloid, where it iodinates tyrosine residues in the thyroglobulin. The cell under *Resorption* illustrates the pathways of colloid resorption by endocytosis and digestion by lysosomal enzymes that liberate iodinated tyrosine dimers [triiodothyronine and tetraiodothyronine (thyroxine)] from the thyroglobulin. These thyroid hormones are released into the extracellular space at the lateral and basal cell surfaces and diffuse into the underlying capillary.

TABLE 20.7. Hormones of the Thyroid Gland

HORMONE[A]	SOURCE	FUNCTION
Tetraiodothyronine (T_4) or thyroxine Triiodothyronine (T_3)	Principal cells	Calorigenic effect—regulates tissue metabolism (increases rate of carbohydrate utilization, protein synthesis and degradation, and fat synthesis and degradation); influences body and tissue growth and development of the nervous system in the fetus and young child[B]; increases absorption of carbohydrates from the intestine
Thyrocalcitonin	Parafollicular cells	Lowers blood calcium level by inhibiting bone resorption and stimulating absorption of calcium by the bones

[A]T_3 and T_4 are iodinated tyrosine derivatives (T_3 acts more rapidly and is more potent): thryrocalcitonin is a peptide hormone.
[B]Deficiency of T_3 and T_4 during development results in fewer and smaller neurons, defective myelination, and mental retardation.

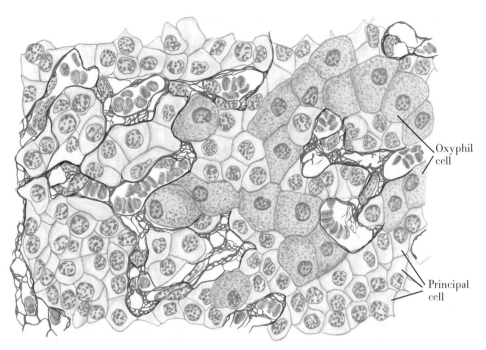

Figure 20.13. Drawing of cells within the human parathyroid gland. Principal cells are small and often vacuolated. The oxyphilic cells are much larger and contain fine granules. (Modified from Bloom W, Fawcett DW: *A Textbook of Histology,* 10th ed. Philadelphia, WB Saunders, 1975, p 536.)

kidney, on the gastric mucosa, and on the salivary and sweat glands to stimulate resorption of sodium at all of these sites, as well as to stimulate excretion of potassium by the kidney.

The Renin-Angiotensin System Provides Feedback Control of the Function of the Zona Glomerulosa

The zona glomerulosa is under feedback control of the *renin-angiotensin* system (see page 570). The juxtaglomerular cells in the kidney release renin in response to a fall in blood pressure or a low blood sodium level. Circulating renin catalyzes the conversion of circulating *an-giotensinogen* to *angiotensin I,* which, in turn, is converted by an enzyme in the lung to *angiotensin II*. Angiotensin II then stimulates the cells of the zona glomerulosa to secrete aldosterone. As the blood pressure, sodium concentration, and blood volume then rise in response to aldosterone, release of renin from the juxtaglomerular cells is inhibited. Drugs that have been designed as inhibitors of the angiotensin conversion enzyme of the lung are very effective in the treatment of chronic essential hypertension.

Zona Fasciculata. The cells of the zona fasciculata are large and polyhedral. They are arranged in long straight cords, one or two cells thick, that are separated by the si-

TABLE 20.8. Hormones of the Parathyroid Glands

HORMONE[A]	SOURCE	FUNCTION
Parathyroid hormone (PTH) or parathormone	Principal or chief cells[B]	Increases blood calcium level in three ways: (1) promotes calcium release from bone (increases relative number of osteoclasts); (2) stimulates calcium resorption by tubular cells of kidney while inhibiting phosphate resorption; (3) causes formation of 1,25-dihydroxycholecalciferol in the kidneys (hormone that promotes absorption of calcium by the intestinal epithelial cells)

[A]PTH is a peptide hormone.
[B]Some evidence suggests that oxyphilic cells, which first appear in the parathyroid gland at about 4–7 years of age and increase in number after puberty, may also produce PTH.

TABLE 20.9. Hormones of the Adrenal Glands

HORMONE[A]	SOURCE	FUNCTION
ADRENAL CORTEX		
Mineralocorticoids (95% of mineralocorticoid activity in aldosterone)	Parenchymal cells of the zona glomerulosa	Aid in controlling electrolyte homeostasis (act on distal tubule cells of kidney to increase sodium resorption and decrease potassium resorption); function in maintaining the osmotic balance in the urine and in preventing serum acidosis
Glucocorticoids (hydrocortisone, corticosterone, and cortisone; 95% of glucocorticoid activity in hydrocortisone)	Parenchymal cells of the zona fasciculata (and to a lesser extent of the zona reticularis)	Promote normal metabolism, in particular, affect carbohydrate metabolism (increase rate of amino acid transport to liver, promote removal of protein from skeletal muscle and its transport to the liver, reduce rate of glucose metabolism by cells and stimulate glycogen synthesis by liver, stimulate mobilization of fats from storage deposits for energy utilization); provide resistance to stress; suppress inflammatory response and some allergic reactions
Gonadocorticoids (sex steroids)	Parenchymal cells of the zona reticularis (and to a lesser extent of the zona fasciculata)	Amount usually so small that it is insignificant (for specific functions, see chapters on male and female reproductive systems)
ADRENAL MEDULLA		
Norepinephrine and epinephrine (in human, 80% epinephrine)	Chromaffin cells	Sympathomimetic (produce effects similar to those induced by the sympathetic division of the autonomic nervous system)[B]: increase heart rate, increase blood pressure, reduce blood flow to viscera and skin; stimulate conversion of glycogen to glucose; increase sweating; induce dilation of bronchioles; increase rate of respiration; decrease digestion; decrease enzyme production by digestive system glands; decrease urine production

[A]Mineralocorticoids, glucocorticoids, and gonadocorticoids are steroid hormones (cholesterol derivatives); epinephrine and norepinephrine are catecholamines (amino acid derivatives).
[B]The catecholamines influence the activity of glandular epithelium, cardiac muscle, or smooth muscle located in the walls of blood vessels or viscera.

nusoidal capillaries. The cells of the zona fasciculata have a lightly staining spherical nucleus. Binucleate cells are common in this zone. The generally acidophilic cytoplasm contains numerous lipid droplets but usually appears vacuolated in routine histologic sections because of the extraction of the lipid during dehydration. The lipid droplets contain neutral fats, fatty acids, cholesterol, and phospholipids that are precursors for the steroid hormones secreted by these cells. In the TEM, the cells have the characteristics of steroid-secreting cells, i.e., a highly developed sER (more so than cells of the zona glomerulosa) and mitochondria with tubular cristae. They also have a well-developed Golgi complex and numerous profiles of rER that may give a slight basophilia to some parts of the cytoplasm (Fig. 20.16).

The Principal Secretion of the Zona Fasciculata Is Glucocorticoids That Regulate Glucose and Fatty Acid Metabolism

The zona fasciculata secretes *glucocorticoids,* so called because of their role in regulating *gluconeogenesis (glucose synthesis)* and *glycogenesis (glycogen polymerization).* The most important of the glucocorticoids secreted by the zona fasciculata is *hydrocortisone (cortisol).* This compound acts on many different cells and tissues to increase the metabolic availability of glucose and fatty acids, both of which are immediate sources of energy. Within this broad function, glucocorticoids may have different, even opposite effects in different tissues, e.g.:

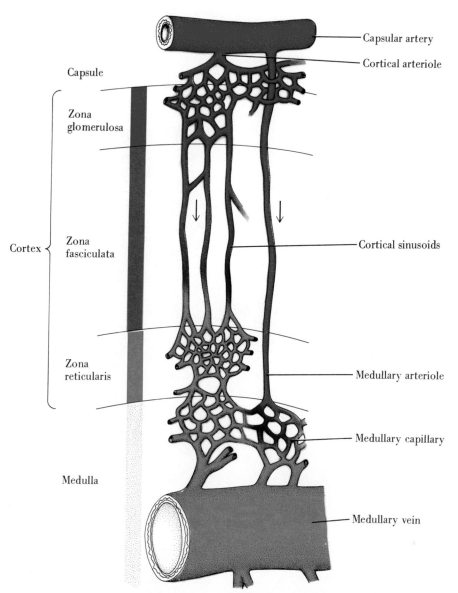

Capsular artery

Cortical arteriole

Capsule

Zona
glomerulosa

Cortex

Zona
fasciculata

Cortical sinusoids

Zona
reticularis

Medullary arteriole

Medullary capillary

Medulla

Medullary vein

Figure 20.14. Diagram illustrating the blood supply to the human adrenal gland. The region of the capsule, the zones within the cortex, and the medulla are indicated. (Modified from Warwick R, Williams PL (eds): *Gray's Anatomy,* 35th ed. Edinburgh, Churchill Livingstone, 1973.)

- In the liver, glucocorticoids stimulate conversion of amino acids to glucose, stimulate the polymerization of glucose into glycogen, and promote the uptake of amino acids and fatty acids.
- In adipose tissue, the glucocorticoids stimulate the breakdown of lipids to glycerol and free fatty acids.
- In other tissues, they reduce the rate of glucose utilization and promote the oxidation of fatty acids.
- In cells such as fibroblasts, they inhibit protein synthesis and even promote protein catabolism by cells in order to provide amino acids for conversion to glucose in the liver.

Glucocorticoids depress the immune response and the inflammatory response and, as a result of the latter, inhibit wound healing. They depress the inflammatory response by inhibiting macrophage recruitment and migration. They also stimulate destruction of lymphocytes in lymph nodes and inhibit mitosis by transformed lymphoblasts. Note, also, that the cells of the zona fasciculata secrete small amounts of gonadocorticoids, principally androgens.

The Corticotropin-Releasing Factor-Adrenocorticotropic Hormone System Provides Feedback Control of the Function of the Zona Fasciculata

The zona fasciculata is under feedback control of the *hypothalamic-hypophyseal corticotropin-releasing factor*

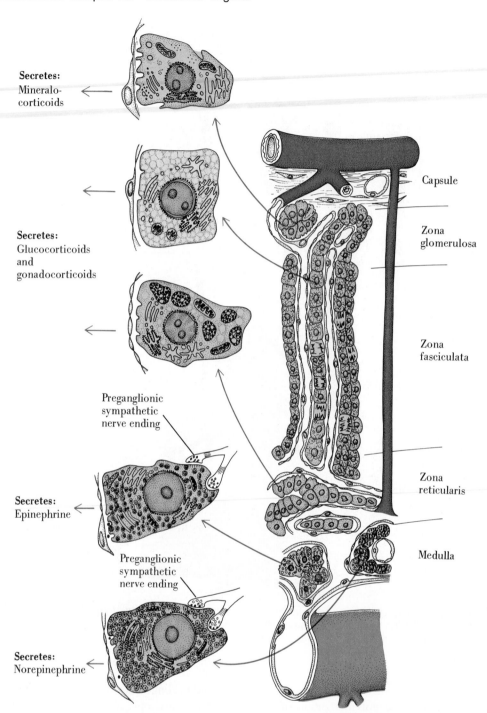

Secretes:
Mineralo-
corticoids

Secretes:
Glucocorticoids
and
gonadocorticoids

Preganglionic
sympathetic
nerve ending

Secretes:
Epinephrine

Preganglionic
sympathetic
nerve ending

Secretes:
Norepinephrine

Capsule

Zona
glomerulosa

Zona
fasciculata

Zona
reticularis

Medulla

Figure 20.15.   Diagram illustrating the organization of the cells within the adrenal gland and their relationship to the blood vessels. Refer to Figure 20.14 for identification of the blood vessels. The ultrastructural features of the basic cell types and a brief description of their function are included. (Modified from Warwick R, Williams PL (eds): *Gray's Anatomy,* 35th ed. Edinburgh, Churchill Livingstone, 1973.)

(CRF)-adrenocorticotropic hormone (ACTH) system. Cells of the fasciculata atrophy after hypophysectomy. Not only is ACTH necessary for cell growth and maintenance, but it also stimulates steroid synthesis and increases blood flow through the adrenal gland. Exogenous ACTH maintains the structure and function of the zona fasciculata after hypophysectomy. In intact animals, administration of ACTH causes hypertrophy of the zona fasciculata.

Circulating glucocorticoids may act directly on the hypophysis but, most commonly, exert their feedback control on neurons in the *arcuate nucleus* of the hypothalamus. This causes CRF to be released into the hypothalamic-hypophyseal portal circulation. There is also evidence that circulating glucocorticoids and the physiologic effects that they produce stimulate higher brain centers that, in turn, cause the hypothalamic neurons to release CRF (Fig. 20.17).

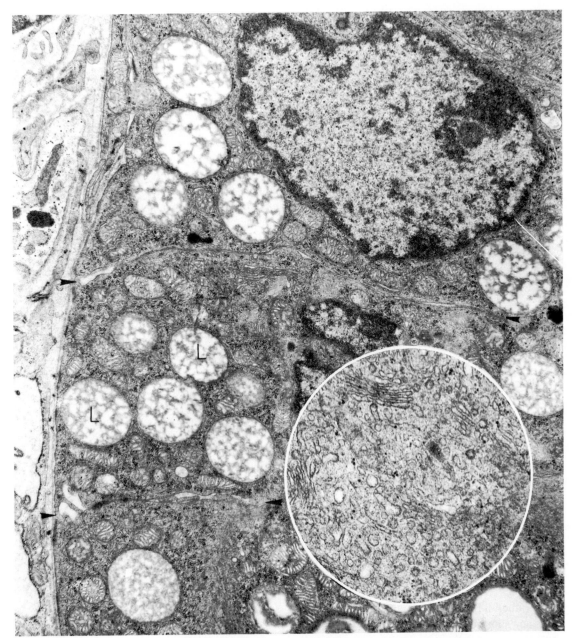

Figure 20.16. Electron micrograph of portions of several adrenal cortical cells from the outer part of the zona fasciculata. The boundary between adjacent cells of the cord is indicated by the *arrowheads*. Lipid droplets *(L)* are numerous (the lipid has been partially extracted), as are the mitochondria. A higher magnification **(inset)** of an area in the cell at the top of the micrograph reveals the extensive sER that is characteristic of steroid-secreting cells. A portion of the Golgi complex is also evident. ×15,000; **inset,** ×40,000.

The Zona Reticularis Produces Glucocorticoids and Androgens

Zona Reticularis. The cells of the zona reticularis are noticeably smaller than those of the zona fasciculata, and their nuclei are more deeply stained. They are arranged in anastomosing cords, separated by fenestrated capillaries. The cells have relatively few lipid droplets. Both light and dark cells are seen. In the dark cells, abundant large lipofuscin pigment granules and deeply staining nuclei are evident. Because the cells in this zone are small, due to less cytoplasm than the cells in the zona fasciculata, the nuclei appear closely packed. They exhibit the features of steroid-secreting cells, namely, a well-developed sER and numerous elongated mitochondria with tubular cristae, but they have little rER.

The Principal Secretions of the Zona Reticularis Are Weak Androgens

The principal secretion of the cells in the zona reticularis consists of weak androgens, mostly *dehydroepiandroster-*

one (DHA). The cells also secrete some glucocorticoids, in much smaller amounts than those of the zona fasciculata. Here, too, the principal glucocorticoid secreted is *hydrocortisone.*

The zona reticularis is also under feedback control of the CRF-ACTH system and atrophies after hypophysectomy. Exogenous ACTH maintains the structure and function of the zona reticularis after hypophysectomy.

CHOLESTEROL

Cholesterol is the basic precursor of corticosteroid hormones. These hormones are synthesized from cholesterol by removal of part of the side chain and modifications at specific sites on the remainder of the molecule. The enzymes catalyzing these modifications are located in different zones of the cortex as well as in different cytoplasmic sites within the cells. A precursor molecule may move from the sER to a mitochondrion and back again several times before the definitive molecular structure of a given corticosteroid is obtained.

Low-density lipoproteins (LDLs) carried in the blood are the primary source of the cholesterol used in these synthetic processes. Under conditions of acute or prolonged ACTH stimulation, the lipid stores in the adrenal cortical cells will be used for corticosteroid synthesis.

Adrenal Medulla

Adrenal Medullary Cells Are Modified Postganglionic Neuronal Cells That Have a Secretory Function

The central portion of the adrenal gland, the *medulla,* is composed of a parenchyma of large, pale-staining epithelioid cells, called *chromaffin cells,* connective tissue, numerous sinusoidal blood capillaries, and nerves. The parenchymal cells are, in effect, modified neurons (see shaded text). They are epithelioid in character and are organized in ovoid clusters and short interconnecting cords. The blood capillaries are arranged in intimate relation to the parenchyma. They originate either from the cortical capillaries or, as branches, from the cortical arterioles.

Ultrastructurally, the parenchymal cells are characterized by numerous membrane-bounded secretory granules with diameters of 100–300 nm, profiles of rER, and a well-developed Golgi complex. The secretory material in the vesicles can be stained specifically to demonstrate histochemically that the catecholamines epinephrine and norepinephrine secreted by the medullary cells are produced by different cell types. Similarly, the TEM reveals two populations of cells distinguished by the nature of the membrane-bounded granules (Fig. 20.18).

- One population of cells contains only large *dense core granules.* These cells secrete norepinephrine.

- The other population of cells contains granules that are smaller, more homogeneous, and less dense. These cells secrete epinephrine.

The exocytosis of these secretory granules is triggered by release of acetylcholine by the preganglionic sympathetic axons that synapse with each adrenal medullary cell.

Epinephrine and norepinephrine account for less than 20% of the contents of the medullary secretory granules. The granules also contain large amounts of soluble proteins, called *chromogranins,* that appear to impart the density to the granule contents. These proteins, along with ATP and Ca^{2+}, may help to bind the low-molecular-weight catecholamines and are released with the hormones during exocytosis. The catecholamines, synthesized in the cytosol, are transported into the granules through the action of a magnesium-activated ATPase in the membrane of the granule. Drugs such as *reserpine,* which cause depletion of catecholamines from the granules, may act by inhibiting the transport mechanism.

CHROMAFFIN CELLS

Chromaffin cells (named because they react with chromate salts) of the adrenal medulla are a part of the APUD system of cells. The chromaffin reaction is thought to involve oxidation and polymerization of the catecholamines contained within the secretory granules of the cells. Classically, chromaffin cells have been defined as being derived from neuroectoderm, innervated by preganglionic sympathetic nerve fibers, and capable of synthesizing and secreting catecholamines. Chromaffin cells are found in the adrenal medulla, in paravertebral and prevertebral sympathetic ganglia, and in various other locations. Those scattered groups of chromaffin cells located among or near the components of the autonomic nervous system are called *paraganglia.*

The exocytosis of these secretory granules is triggered by release of acetylcholine by the preganglionic sympathetic axons that synapse with each adrenal medullary cell.

Glucocorticoids Secreted in the Cortex Induce the Conversion of Norepinephrine to Epinephrine in Medullary Cells

Glucocorticoids produced in the adrenal cortex reach the medulla directly through the continuity of the cortical and medullary sinusoidal capillaries. They induce the enzyme that catalyzes the methylation of norepinephrine to produce epinephrine. The nature of the blood flow correlates with regional differences in distribution of norepinephrine- and epinephrine-containing medullary cells. The epinephrine-containing cells are more numerous in areas of the medulla supplied with blood that has passed through the cortical si-

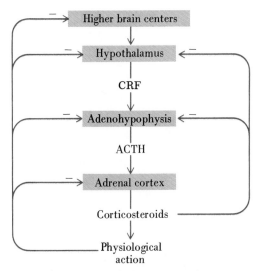

Figure 20.17. Diagram illustrating the neuroendocrine control of the adrenal cortex. Both the corticosteroids, themselves, and the physiologic effects that they induce can inhibit further release of corticosteroids through negative feedback. As is indicated, inhibition may occur at a number of levels. The system is activated in response to metabolic needs (stress).

nusoids and, thus, contains secreted glucocorticoids. This arrangement, which allows the glucocorticoids to reach the medulla directly, can be considered a portal system. The norepinephrine-containing cells are more numerous in those regions of the medulla that are supplied by capillaries de-

rived from the cortical arterioles. Thus, the distribution of norepinephrine- and epinephrine-containing cells within the medulla is determined by its dual blood supply.

The Catecholamines, in Concert with the Glucocorticoids, Prepare the Body for the "Fight-or-Flight" Response

The sudden release of catecholamines establishes conditions for maximum utilization of energy and, thus, maximum physical effort. Both epinephrine and norepinephrine stimulate glycogenolysis (releasing glucose into the bloodstream) and mobilization of free fatty acids from adipose tissue. The release of catecholamines also causes a rise in blood pressure, dilation of the coronary blood vessels, vasodilation of vessels supplying skeletal muscle, vasoconstriction of vessels conveying blood to the skin and gut, an increase in heart rate and output, and an increase in the rate and depth of breathing.

Fetal Adrenal Gland

The Fetal Adrenal Consists of an Outer Narrow Permanent Cortex and an Inner Thick Fetal Zone

The fetal adrenal, once fully established, is unusual in terms of its organization and its large size relative to other

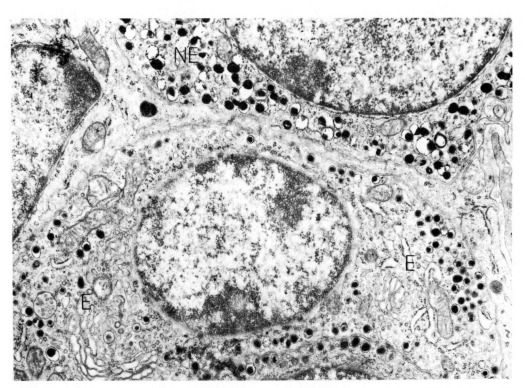

Figure 20.18. Electron micrograph of secretory cells in the mouse adrenal medulla. Two types of medullary cells are present. The norepinephrine-secreting cells *(NE)* contain granules with very dense cores; the epinephrine-secreting cells *(E)* contain less intensely staining granules. ×15,000.

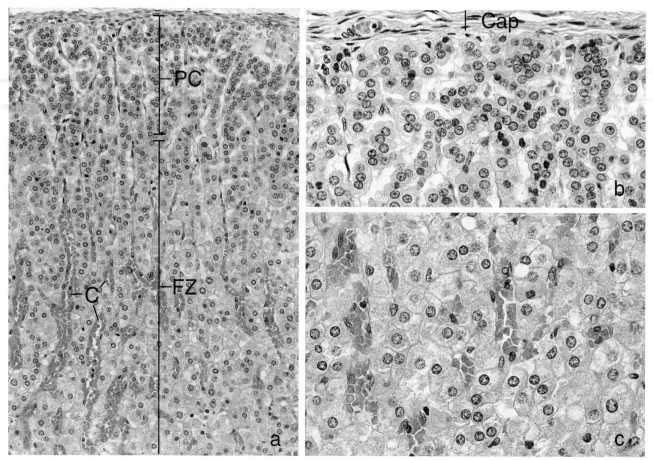

Figure 20.19. **a.** Low-power micrograph of the fetal adrenal gland. The permanent cortex *(PC)* is indicated in the upper portion of the micrograph. Below is the fetal zone *(FZ)* in which the cells are arranged in anastomosing linear cords. Some of the capillaries *(C)* are engorged with red blood cells, thereby making them more apparent. ×100. **b.** Higher power micrograph showing the capsule *(Cap)* and the underlying permanent cortex. The cells are arranged in arched groups that extend into short cords. Note the close proximity of the nuclei and the small amount of cytoplasm. ×200. **c.** This micrograph shows the cells of the fetal zone at the same magnification as in **b.** Note the slightly larger size of the nuclei and the considerable amount of cytoplasm in each of these cells of the fetal zone. Also note the eosinophilia of the cytoplasm compared with the more basophilic cytoplasm of the cells of the permanent cortex. ×200. (Original specimen courtesy of Dr. William H. Donnelly.)

developing organs. The gland arises from mesothelial cells located between the root of the mesentery and the developing gonad. The mesothelial cells penetrate the underlying mesenchyme and give rise to a large eosinophilic cell mass that will become the functional fetal adrenal. Later, a secondary wave of cells from the mesothelium enters the mesenchyme and surrounds the primary cell mass. By the fourth fetal month, the adrenal reaches its maximum mass in terms of body weight and is only slightly smaller than the adjacent kidney. At term, the adrenals are equivalent in size and weight to those of the adult and produce 100–200 mg of steroid compounds per day, about twice that of the adult adrenals.

The histologic appearance of the fetal adrenal gland superficially resembles the adrenal gland of the adult. During late fetal life, the major portion of the gland consists of cords of large eosinophilic cells that make up approximately 80% of its mass. This portion of the gland, referred to as the *fetal zone,* arose from the initial mesothelial cell migration. The remainder of the gland is made up of the peripheral layer of small cells with scanty cytoplasm. This portion, referred to as the *permanent cortex,* arose from the secondary mesothelial cell migration. The narrow permanent cortex, when fully established in the embryo, appears similar to the adult zona glomerulosa. The cells are arranged in arched groups that extend into short cords. They, in turn, become continuous with the cords of the underlying fetal zone (Fig. 20.19). In H&E preparations, the cytoplasm of the cells in the permanent cortex is basophilic; in combination with the closely packed nuclei, this gives this part of the gland a blue appearance, in contrast to the eosinophilic staining of the fetal zone.

With the TEM, the cells of the permanent cortex exhibit small mitochondria with shelf-like cristae, abundant ribosomes, and small Golgi profiles. The cells of the fetal zone, in contrast, are considerably larger and are arranged in irregular cords of varying width. With the TEM, these cells exhibit spherical mitochondria with tubular cristae, small lipid droplets, an extensive sER, which accounts for the eosinophilia of the cytoplasm, and multiple Golgi profiles. Collectively, these are features characteristic of steroid-secreting cells.

The fetal adrenal lacks a definitive medulla. Chromaffin cells are present but are scattered among the cells of the fetal zone and are difficult to recognize in H&E preparations. The chromaffin cells originate from the neural crest and invade the fetal zone at the time of its formation. They remain in this location in small, scattered cell clusters during fetal life.

The blood supply to both the permanent cortex and the fetal zone is through sinusoidal capillaries that course between the cords and join to form larger venous channels in the center of the gland. Unlike the postnatal adrenal, arterioles are absent in the parenchyma of the fetal adrenal gland.

Functionally, the fetal adrenal is under the control of the CRF-ACTH feedback system through the fetal pituitary (see page 615). It interacts with the placenta to function as a steroid-secreting organ because it lacks certain enzymes necessary for steroid synthesis that are present in the placenta. Similarly, the placenta lacks certain enzymes necessary for steroid synthesis that are present in the fetal adrenal. Thus, the fetal adrenal is part of a fetal-placental unit. Precursor molecules are transported back and forth between the two organs to enable synthesis of glucocorticoids, aldosterone, androgens, and estrogens.

At birth, the fetal zone undergoes a rapid involution, reducing the gland within the first postnatal month to about a quarter of its size. The permanent cortex undergoes growth and maturation to form the characteristic zonation of the adult cortex. With the involution and disappearance of the fetal zone cells, the chromaffin cells aggregate to form the medulla.

PLATE 99. Pituitary Gland I

The pituitary gland or hypophysis cerebri is located in a small bony fossa in the floor of the cranial cavity. It is connected by a stalk to the base of the brain. Although it is joined to the brain, only part of the pituitary gland develops from the neural ectoderm; this is referred to as the neurohypophysis. The larger part of the pituitary gland develops from the oral ectoderm; this part is called the adenohypophysis. The adenohypophysis develops as a diverticulum of the buccal epithelium, called Rathke's pouch. In the fully developed gland, the lumen of Rathke's pouch may be retained as a vestigial cleft.

Both the adenohypophysis and the neurohypophysis are further subdivided as follows:

Adenohypophysis
       Pars distalis (anterior lobe)
       Pars tuberalis
       Pars intermedia

Neurohypophysis (posterior lobe)
       Pars nervosa
       Infundibulum (infundibulum stem and median eminence of tuber cinereum)

Pituitary, monkey, hematoxylin and eosin (H&E) ×40.
The parts of the pituitary are shown in a sagittal section of the gland in this figure. The neurohypophysis is marked by the *broken lines*. The pars nervosa is the expanded portion that is continuous with the infundibulum *(I)*. The pars tuberalis *(PT)* is located around the infundibular stem. The pars intermedia *(PI)* is between the pars distalis and the pars nervosa. It borders a small cleft *(C)* that constitutes the remains of the lumen of Rathke's pouch. The pars distalis is the largest part of the pituitary gland. It contains a variety of cell types that are not uniformly distributed. This accounts for differences in staining (light and dark areas) that are seen throughout the pars distalis.

The parts of the pituitary gland can be identified largely on the basis of their location and relation to each other. For example, the pars nervosa can be identified readily if it is continuous with a stem or stalk of essentially the same kind of material. The pars intermedia is in an intermediate location and in relation to the vestigial cleft; the cleft may not be evident, however, and the pars intermedia may be more extensive (in this specimen it continues along the surface of the gland). On considering the cell types at higher magnification (Plate 100), one comes to realize that these also serve as a major indication of the part of the gland that is being examined.

The blood supply to the pars distalis of the pituitary gland is unique and requires special mention, in that it involves two sets of vessels. Capillaries at the outer layer of the pars distalis receive blood from arteries in the usual manner; most of the capillary plexuses receive blood via the *hypophyseal portal system*. The latter originates in capillaries located in the median eminence and infundibulum (see Fig. 20.2, page 598). They then drain into a venous network that flows to the pars distalis, where they empty into a second capillary network. This system serves as a route whereby releasing factors (hormones) from the hypothalamus are conveyed to the pars distalis. There is a specific releasing factor for each of the anterior pituitary hormones. The releasing factors cause the release or discharge of the specific pituitary hormones, and in this way the hypothalamus regulates the secretory activity of the pars distalis.

KEY

C, vestigial cleft of Rathke's pouch   **PI,** pars intermedia   **PT,** pars tuberalis
I, infundibulum

PLATE 99

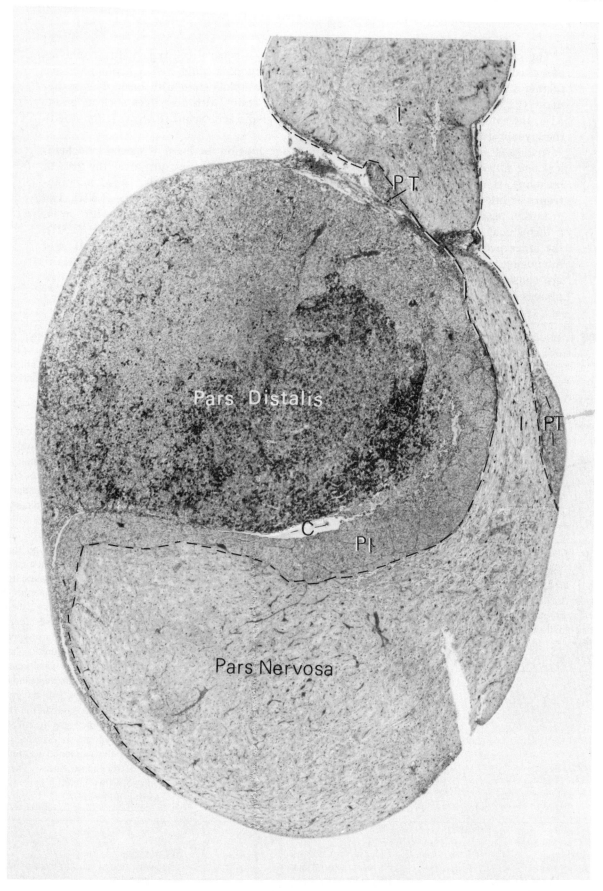

PLATE 100. Pituitary Gland II

The parenchyma of the pars distalis consists of two general cell types: chromophobes and chromophils. Chromophobes stain poorly; chromophils stain well. Chromophils are further subdivided into acidophils and basophils. Basophils stain with basic dyes or hematoxylin, whereas the cytoplasm of the acidophil stains with acid dyes such as eosin. Also, the cytoplasm of basophils stains with the periodic acid-Schiff (PAS) reaction due to the glycoprotein in the secretory granules.

Acidophils can be further subdivided into two groups on the basis of special cytochemical and ultrastructural features. One group, called somatotropes, produces the growth hormone, somatotropic hormone (STH); the other group of acidophils, called mammotropes or luteotropes, produces the lactogenic hormone, luteotropic hormone (LTH). The groups of basophils can also be distinguished with the electron microscope and with special cytochemical procedures. One group produces the thyroid-stimulating hormone (TSH); the other produces the gonadotropic hormones, follicle-stimulating hormone (FSH) and luteinizing hormone (LH). Chromophobes are also a heterogeneous group of cells. Many are considered to be depleted acidophils or basophils; however, one group of chromophobes is considered to produce the adrenocorticotropic hormone (ACTH).

FIGURE 1, pituitary, cat, H&E ×640. A region of the pars distalis that shows a large number of basophils is illustrated in this figure. The field also contains acidophils, chromophobes, and stromal elements. The basophils (B) can be distinguished from acidophils (A) because the basophils are slightly larger and the cytoplasm of the acidophils stains with eosin. Both of these cell types can be distinguished from the chromophobes (C), which contain only a small amount of poorly staining cytoplasm. The parenchymal components of the pars distalis are arranged as cords of cells. These are separated by a delicate connective tissue stroma that contains capillaries. The elongated nuclei (arrows) belong either to cells of the connective tissue stroma or to the endothelial cells.

FIGURE 2, pituitary, cat, H&E ×640. A region of pars distalis in which acidophils predominate is shown in this figure. Eosinophilic cytoplasm can be seen in each cell. In contrast, the nuclei of chromophobes (C) are surrounded by a small amount of poorly staining cytoplasm.

FIGURE 5, pituitary, cat, H&E ×400. The neurohypophysis, seen here, contains cells called pituicytes and nonmyelinated nerve fibers from the supraoptic and paraventricular nuclei of the hypothalamus. The pituicytes are comparable with neuroglial cells of the central nervous system. The nuclei of the cells are round or oval; the cytoplasm extends from the nuclear region of the cell as long processes. In H&E preparations, the cytoplasm of the pituicytes cannot be distinguished from the nonmyelinated nerve fibers. The hormones of the neurohypophysis, oxytocin and antidiuretic hormone (ADH) (also called vasopressin because of its action on vascular smooth muscle), are formed in the hypothalamic nuclei and pass via the fibers of the hypothalamohypophyseal tract to the neurohypophysis, where they are stored in the expanded terminal portions of the nerve fibers. The stored neurosecretory material appears as the Herring bodies (HB).

FIGURE 3, pituitary, cat, H&E ×400. The pars tuberalis, seen here, surrounds the infundibular stem. It consists of small acidophil and basophil cells. Frequently, these are arranged as small vesicles (V) that contain colloid. The function of the colloid is not known.

FIGURE 4, pituitary, cat, H&E ×400. The pars intermedia (PI), seen in this figure, varies in size in different mammals. It is relatively small in the human. It consists of cords of cells that resemble basophils, except that they are smaller. They sometimes form colloid-filled vesicles. Cells from the pars intermedia are occasionally seen in the pars nervosa (PN). The function of the pars intermedia in humans is not clear. Studies with frogs indicate that a hormone from the intermedia, called the melanocyte-stimulating hormone (MSH), brings about a darkening of the skin.

KEY		
A, acidophils	**HB,** Herring bodies	**V,** vesicles
B, basophils	**PI,** pars intermedia	**arrows,** nuclei of stromal or vascular cells
BV, blood vessel	**PN,** pars nervosa	
C, chromophobes		

PLATE 100

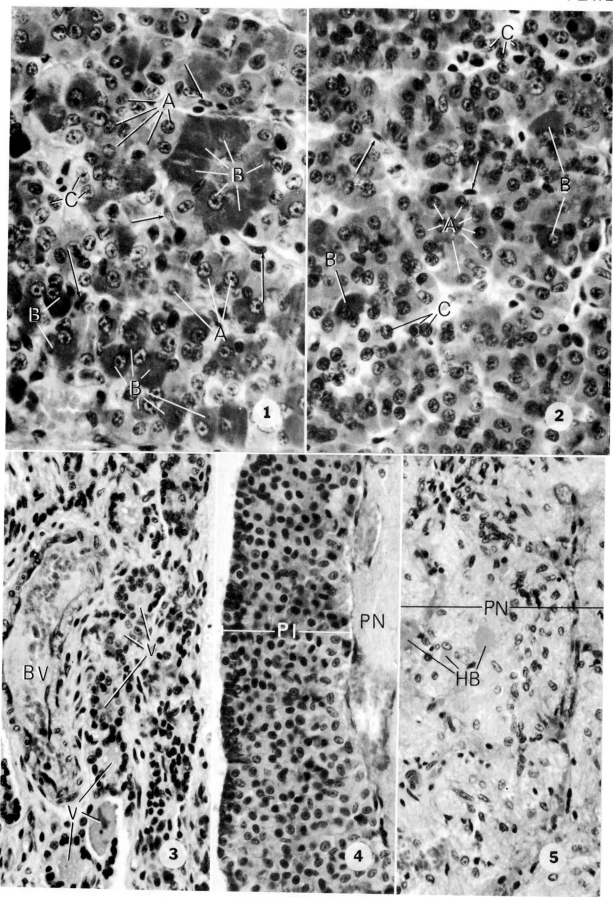

PLATE 101. Pineal Gland

The *pineal gland (pineal body, epiphysis cerebri)* is located in the brain above the superior colliculi. It develops from neuroectoderm but, in the adult, bears little resemblance to nerve tissue.

Two cell types have been described within the pineal gland: parenchymal cells and glial cells. The full extent of these cells cannot be appreciated without the application of special methods. These would show that the glial cells and the parenchymal cells have processes and that the processes of the parenchymal cells are expanded at their periphery. The parenchymal cells are more numerous. In an H&E preparation, the nuclei of the parenchymal cells are pale staining and somewhat vesicular. The nuclei of the glial cells, on the other hand, are smaller and stain more intensely.

Although the physiology of the pineal gland is not well understood, the secretions of the gland evidently have an antigonadal effect. For example, hypogenitalism has been reported in pineal tumors that consist chiefly of parenchymal cells, whereas sexual precocity is associated with nonparenchymal tumors (presumably in these the parenchymal cells have been destroyed). In addition, numerous experiments with laboratory animals indicate that the pineal gland has a neuroendocrine function whereby the pineal gland serves as an intermediary that relates endocrine function (particularly gonadal function) to cycles of light and dark. The external photic stimuli reach the pineal gland via optical pathways that connect with the superior cervical ganglion. In turn, the superior cervical ganglion sends postganglionic nerve fibers to the pineal gland. The extent to which these findings with laboratory animals apply to humans is not yet clear.

FIGURE 1, pineal gland, human, H&E ×80. The pineal gland is surrounded by a capsule *(Cap)* except at its stalk. The capsule is formed by the *pia mater.* Trabeculae extend from the capsule into the substance of the gland and divide it into lobules. The lobules *(L)* appear as the indistinct groups of cells surrounded by connective tissue *(CT)*. The adult pineal body contains calcareous deposits *(BS)* that are regularly found in histologic sections. They are called *brain sand* or *corpora arenacea.* When viewed with higher magnification, they can be seen to possess a lamellated structure.

FIGURE 2, pineal gland, human, H&E ×185. In this figure, two nuclear types can be seen. The more numerous nuclei are the larger ones; they stain less intensely and are somewhat vesiculated; they belong to parenchymal cells *(PC)*. The less numerous nuclei are the smaller ones; they stain more intensely and belong to glial cells *(GC)*.

KEY		
BS, brain sand	**CT**, connective tissue	**L**, lobules
Cap, capsule	**GC**, nuclei of glial cells	**PC**, nuclei of parenchymal cells

PLATE 101

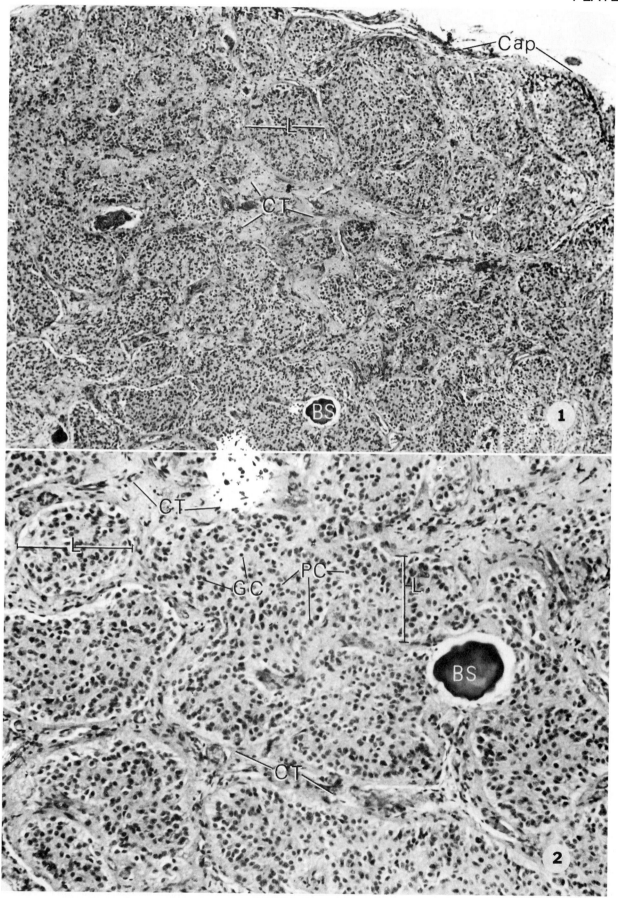

PLATE 102. Parathyroid and Thyroid Glands

The parathyroid glands are usually four in number. Each is surrounded by a capsule and lies on or is partially embedded in the thyroid gland. Connective tissue trabeculae extend from the capsule into the substance of the gland.

The parathyroid glands elaborate a hormone that influences calcium and bone metabolism. Injection of parathyroid hormone into laboratory animals results in the release of calcium from bone by the action of osteocytes (osteocytic osteolysis) and osteoclasts (osteoclasia). Removal of parathyroid glands results in a rapid drop in blood calcium levels.

The thyroid gland is located in the neck in close relation to the upper part of the trachea and the lower part of the larynx. It consists of two lateral lobes that are joined by a narrow isthmus. The follicle, which consists of a single layer of cuboidal or low columnar epithelium surrounding a colloid-filled space, is the functional unit of the thyroid gland. A rich capillary network is present in the connective tissue that separates the follicles. The connective tissue also contains lymphatic capillaries.

FIGURE 1, parathyroid gland, human, H&E ×320. As seen here, the larger blood vessels are associated with the trabeculae *(BV)* and, occasionally, with adipose cells *(A)*. The parenchyma of the parathyroid glands appears as cords or sheets of cells separated by capillaries and delicate connective tissue septa.

Two parenchymal cell types can be distinguished in routine H&E sections: chief cells (principal cells) and oxyphil cells. The chief cells *(CC)* are more numerous. They contain a spherical nucleus surrounded by a small amount of cytoplasm. Oxyphil cells *(OC)* are less numerous. They are conspicuously larger than chief cells but have a slightly smaller and more intensely staining nucleus. Their cytoplasm stains with eosin, and the boundaries between the cells are usually well marked. Moreover, the oxyphils are arranged in groups of variable size that appear scattered about in a much larger field of chief cells. Even with low magnification it is often possible to identify clusters of oxyphil cells because a unit area contains fewer nuclei than a comparable unit area of chief cells, as is clearly evident in this figure. Oxyphil cells appear during the end of the first decade of life and become more numerous around puberty. A further increase may be seen in older individuals.

In addition to the chief and oxyphil cells, which are easy to identify, there may be other cells intermediate between these two and more difficult to identify. The significance of these intermediate cell types is not clear at present. Observations with the electron microscope verify the presence of cells that appear to be transitional between chief and oxyphil cells. This finding tends to support the concept that chief and oxyphil cells represent two functional variations of the same cell.

FIGURE 2, thyroid gland, human, H&E ×200. A histologic section of the thyroid gland is shown here. The follicles *(F)* vary somewhat in size and shape and appear closely packed. The homogeneous mass in the center of each follicle is the colloid. The thyroid cells appear to form a ring around the colloid. Although the individual cells are difficult to distinguish at this magnification, the nuclei of the cells serve as an indication of their location and arrangement.

Large groups of cells are seen in association with some follicles. Where the nuclei are of the same size and staining characteristics, one can conclude that in these sites, the section includes the wall of the follicle *(arrows)* in a tangential manner without including the lumen.

KEY

A, adipose cells	**CT,** connective tissue	**arrows,** tangential section of follicle
BV, blood vessels	**F,** follicles	wall
CC, chief cells	**OC,** oxyphil cells	**asterisks,** shrinkage artifact

PLATE 102

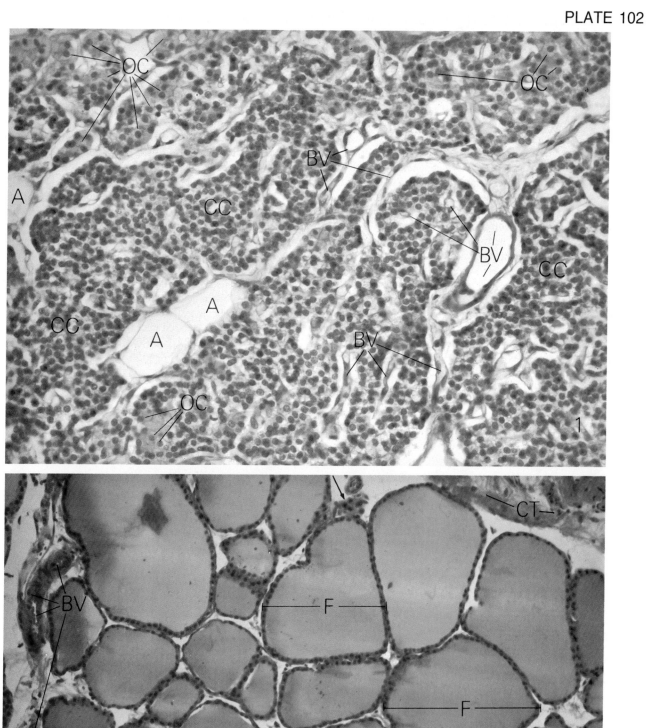

PLATE 103. Thyroid Follicle Cells, Light and Electron Microscopy

Thyroid gland, electron micrograph ×1600; inset, H&E ×480. The **inset** shows parts of three thyroid follicles. The colloid is generally homogeneous in each, although different follicles show different degrees of staining. In one, the colloid has separated from the cells *(asterisk);* this is an artefactual separation. The cuboidal follicular cells are the principal secretory cell type of the thyroid gland. They synthesize thyroglobulin and secrete it into the follicle. Later, the cells remove the colloid from the follicle by endocytosis, degrade the thyroglobulin of the colloid, and discharge the products into the underlying blood vessels.

A second secretory cell type is also found in the thyroid gland, namely, the parafollicular cell, also called the C cell. These cells may be present singly or in small groups. They produce calcitonin. The cell with the large amount of cytoplasm at the junction of the three follicles **(inset)** may be a parafollicular cell. In many places, adjacent follicles are extremely close to each other, separated only by a small amount of connective tissue in which there are capillaries *(arrows)* and sometimes nerves (see below). The electron micrograph shows portions of two adjacent follicles from a region roughly equivalent to the one marked by the two *arrows.*

The most conspicuous organelles of the thyroid follicular cells are numerous profiles of rough-surfaced endoplasmic reticulum, Golgi profiles, and mitochondria. Less obvious are the small microvilli on their apical surface, lysosomes, small vesicles, and—when endocytosing colloid—large apical pseudopods extending into the colloid. Because such apical pseudopods are not seen within the colloid in this specimen, these cells are not likely to be engaged in removal of colloid. The main point of the electron micrograph is to show the minimal space between follicles. At its narrowest point, the space contains a bundle of nonmyelinated nerve fibers *(NF)* and a thin cellular process of a fibroblast. Also to be noted in the electron micrograph are the capillaries in proximity to the follicle cells in the upper and lower part of the micrograph. The fenestrated capillary endothelium *(En)* is extremely thin; the electron micrograph shows very little perinuclear cytoplasm. There are red blood cells *(RBC)* within the capillaries.

KEY

En, capillary endothelium
NF, nerve fibers
RBC, red blood cells

arrows (inset), perifollicular connective tissue with blood vessels

asterisk, artefactual separation of colloid from follicular cells

PLATE 103

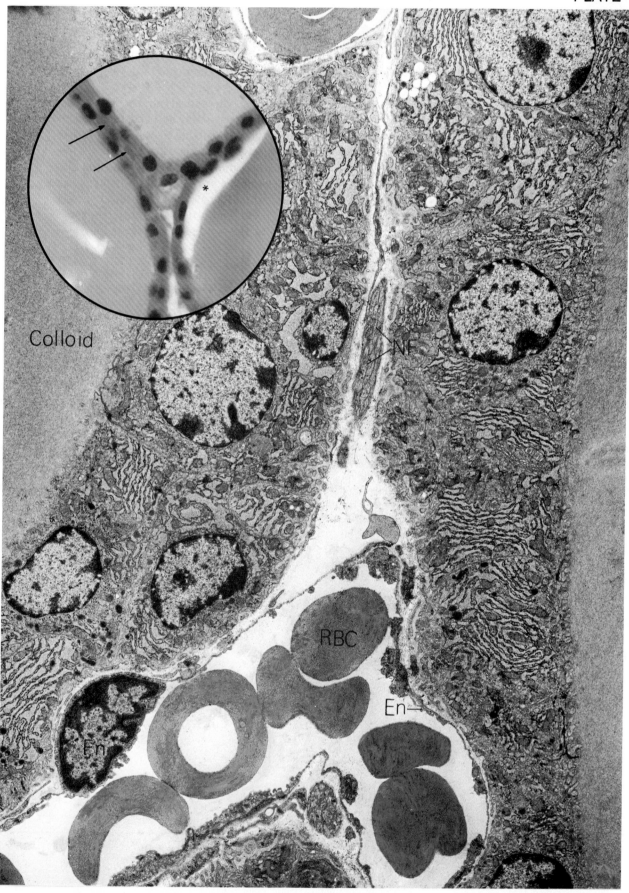

Colloid

NF

RBC

En

En

PLATE 104.   Adrenal Gland I

There are two adrenal glands, with one situated at the upper pole of each kidney. An adrenal gland is a composite of two distinct structural and functional components: the cortex and the medulla. The cortex develops from mesoderm; the medulla develops from neuroectoderm.

The cortex is divided into three parts according to the type and arrangement of cells. These are designated as the zona glomerulosa, the zona fasciculata, and the zona reticularis. The zones of the adrenal cortex not only are morphologically distinct but also reflect a functional specialization. The zona glomerulosa secretes the mineralocorticoids (aldosterone and deoxycorticosterone). On the other hand, the zona fasciculata secretes the glucocorticoids (cortisol, cortisone, and corticosterone), and the zona reticularis is active in the production of adrenal androgens. The zona fasciculata has also been found to secrete adrenal androgens. There is yet another functional distinction in that the inner two zones of the adrenal cortex are regulated by ACTH, whereas the zona glomerulosa is not.

FIGURE 1, adrenal gland, monkey, H&E ×30.   This low-magnification micrograph of a section through the entire thickness of an adrenal gland readily shows several significant histologic features. The outer part of the gland, the cortex, has a distinctly different appearance, in both structural organization and staining characteristics, from the inner portion, the medulla. Very large blood vessels *(V)* are typically found in the medulla. These are veins that drain both the cortex and the medulla. A capsule *(Cap)* surrounds the gland, and from it delicate trabeculae extend into the substance of the gland (see, also, Fig. 2).

FIGURE 2, adrenal gland, monkey, H&E ×400.   The zona glomerulosa *(ZG)* is located at the outer part of the cortex, immediately under the capsule. The parenchyma of this zone consists of small cells that appear as arching cords or as oval groups. The nuclei of the parenchymal cells are spherical, and the cells possess a small amount of lightly staining cytoplasm. Because of the small amount of cytoplasm, the nuclei in this zone appear relatively crowded. Between the cords of cells are elongated nuclei *(arrows;* see, also, Fig. 3) that belong either to cells of the delicate connective tissue stroma or to the endothelial cells of the capillaries that course between the cell cords.

The zona fasciculata consists of radially oriented cords and sheets of cells, usually two cells in width. It can be divided into two parts, an outer and an inner, based on the appearance of the cells in routine H&E preparations. The outer part of the zona fasciculata *(ZF)* is shown where it begins just beneath the zona glomerulosa in this figure. A deeper portion of the zona fasciculata is shown in Figure 3.

FIGURE 3, adrenal gland, monkey, H&E ×400.   The nuclei of the cells of the zona fasciculata are about the same size or slightly larger than those of the zona glomerulosa; however, there is more cytoplasm, and consequently, the nuclei are more distant from one another than those of the zona glomerulosa. Occasionally, binucleate cells *(asterisk)* are seen in the zona fasciculata. These may be difficult to recognize because the cell boundaries are not always conspicuous. The cells of the outer part of the zona fasciculata contain a considerably greater amount of lipid than the cells in the other parts of the cortex. During the preparation of routine H&E specimens, the lipid is lost, and the cytoplasm then has a noticeably foamy or spongy appearance.

KEY		
Cap, capsule	**ZG,** zona glomerulosa	**asterisk,** binucleate cell
V, vein of medulla	**arrows,** nuclei of endothelial cells	
ZF, zona fasciculata	or of connective tissue cells	

PLATE 104

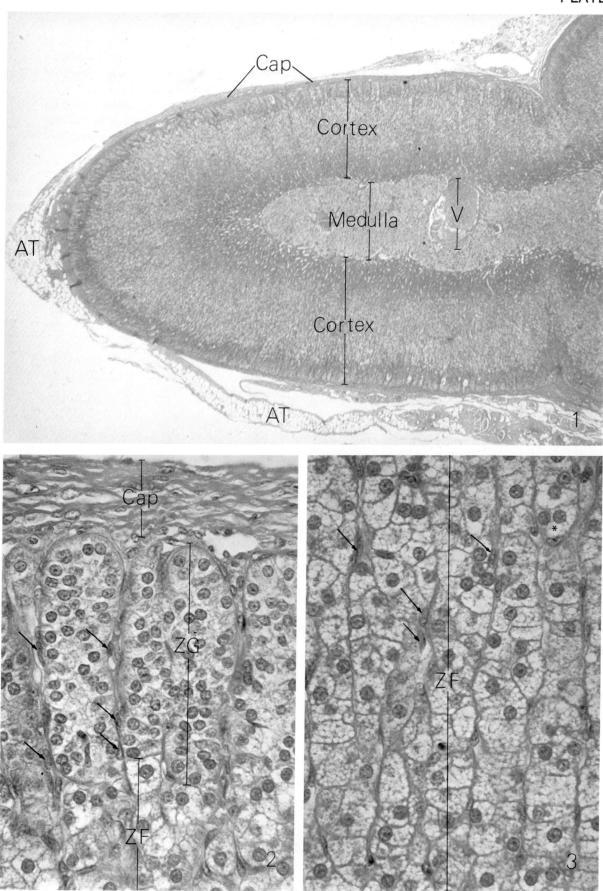

PLATE 105. Adrenal Gland II

The cells of the adrenal medulla develop from the same source as the postganglionic cells of the sympathetic nervous system. They are directly innervated by preganglionic cells of the sympathetic system and may be regarded as modified postganglionic cells that are specialized to secrete. These cells produce epinephrine and norepinephrine.

The adrenal medulla receives its blood supply via two routes: by arterioles that pass through the cortex and by capillaries that continue from the cortex, a type of portal circulation. Thus, some of the blood reaching the medulla contains cortical secretions.

FIGURE 1, adrenal gland, monkey, H&E ×400. The junction between the outer and inner parts of the zona fasciculata and the junction between the inner portion of the zona fasciculata and the zona reticularis are shown here. The outer part of the zona fasciculata, as described in the previous plate, consists of cells whose cytoplasm has a spongy appearance [ZF(S)]. It constitutes the bulk of the fascicular zone. The inner part of the zona fasciculata consists of slightly smaller cells [ZF(C)]. The cytoplasm of these cells appears more compact than that of the cells in the outer part, due to the considerably reduced number of lipid droplets. Throughout the entire zona fasciculata the cells appear as cords, and between the cords, one can see the elongated nuclei *(arrows)* that belong either to cells of the delicate connective tissue stroma or to endothelial cells.

The zona reticularis *(ZR)* is shown in the lower portion of this figure. This is the deepest part of the cortex, immediately adjacent to the medulla. It consists of interconnecting irregular cords and sheets of relatively small cells. The cords and sheets are narrower than those of the other parts of the cortex; in many places they are only one cell wide. Between the cords of cells are the capillaries that in this zone frequently appear dilated, compared with the collapsed appearance of the capillaries of the zona glomerulosa and outer fasciculata. As in the other parts of the gland, the elongated nuclei *(arrows)* belong to endothelial cells or to cells of the connective tissue stroma.

FIGURE 2, adrenal gland, monkey, H&E ×400. In mammals, the adrenal medulla is in the center of the gland, surrounded by the cortex. It consists of large cells that are organized in ovoid groups and short interconnecting cords. The cytoplasm of neighboring cells may stain with different intensity. These cells color when treated with chromate reagents, and for this reason, they are referred to as chromaffin cells. Elongated nuclei *(arrows)* of vascular or connective tissue cells can be seen in the delicate stroma that separates the groups of parenchymal cells. Ganglion cells *(GC)* are occasionally seen in sections of the adrenal medulla.

KEY

GC, ganglion cells	**ZF(S),** zona fasciculata, spongy cells	**arrows,** nuclei of endothelial cells or of connective tissue cells
ZF(C), zona fasciculata, compact cells	**ZR,** zona reticularis	**asterisk,** binucleate cell

PLATE 105

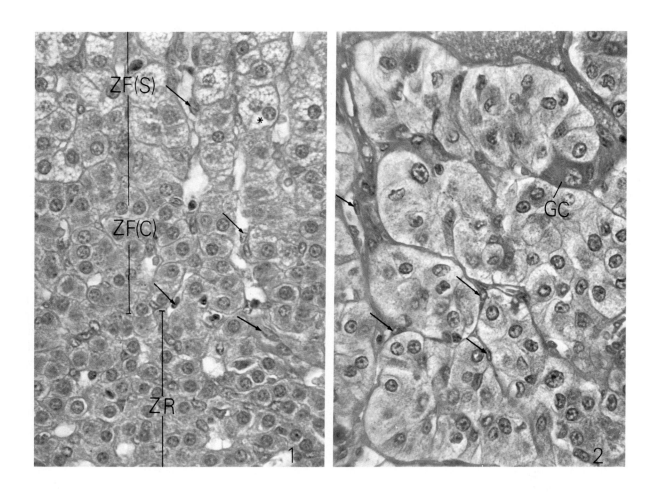

Male Reproductive System

21

The male reproductive system consists of the testes, epididymides and genital ducts, accessory reproductive glands, and penis (Fig. 21.1). The accessory glands include the seminal vesicles, prostate, and bulbourethral glands. The primary function of the testis is the production of sperm, the male gamete. The events of cell division that occur during production of these gametes, as well as those of the female, the ova, involve both normal division, *mitosis,* and reduction division, *meiosis.*

A brief description of mitosis and meiosis is included in Chapter 2, page 50. A basic understanding of these processes is essential in understanding the production of the gametes in both the male and the female.

TESTIS

The Testes Produce Sperm and Androgens

Androgens, especially *testosterone,* are steroid hormones secreted by the interstitial cells in the testes. They influence embryonic development, sexual maturation, and reproductive function:

- In the *embryo,* secretion of androgens is essential for the normal development of a male fetus.
- At *puberty,* secretion of testosterone is responsible for the initiation of sperm production, secretion in the accessory sex glands, and the development of the secondary sex characteristics.
- In the *adult,* secretion of testosterone is essential for the maintenance of sperm production (*spermatogenesis)* and for the maintenance of secondary sex characteristics, the genital ducts, and the accessory glands.

Spermatogenesis Requires That the Testes Be Maintained Below Normal Body Temperature

Shortly before birth the testes descend from the abdominal cavity through the inguinal canal into the scrotum. They carry with them an extension of the peritoneum, called the *tunica vaginalis,* that covers their anterolateral surface.

Within the scrotum the temperature of the testes is 2–3°C below body temperature. This lower temperature is essential for sperm production. If the testes are maintained at higher temperatures or if they fail to descend into the scrotum (cryptorchidism), sperm are not produced.

Each testis receives blood through a *testicular artery.* It is highly convoluted near the testis, where it is surrounded by the *venous pampiniform plexus.* This arrangement allows for heat exchange between the blood vessels. The cooler venous blood returning from the testis and scrotum cools the arterial blood before it enters the testis.

The Testes Have an Unusually Thick Connective Tissue Capsule, the Tunica Albuginea

A thick fibrous connective tissue capsule, the *tunica albuginea,* covers each testis (Fig. 21.2). The inner part of this capsule is the *tunica vasculosa,* a loose connective tissue layer that contains blood vessels. Each testis is divided into approximately 250 lobules by incomplete connective tissue septa that project from the capsule.

Along the posterior surface of the testis, the tunica albuginea thickens and projects inward as the *mediastinum testis.* Blood vessels, lymphatic vessels, and the genital ducts pass through the mediastinum as they enter or leave the testis.

Each Lobule Contains Several Highly Convoluted Seminiferous Tubules

Each lobule contains 1–4 *seminiferous tubules,* which produce the sperm, and a connective tissue stroma in which the *interstitial* or *Leydig cells* are contained (Fig. 21.3). Each tubule within the lobule forms a loop and, because of its considerable length, is highly convoluted, actually folding on itself within the lobule. The ends of the loop in the vicinity of the mediastinum assume a short straight course. This part of the seminiferous tubule is called the *tubuli recti* or straight tubule and is continuous with the *rete testis,* an anastomosing channel system within the mediastinum.

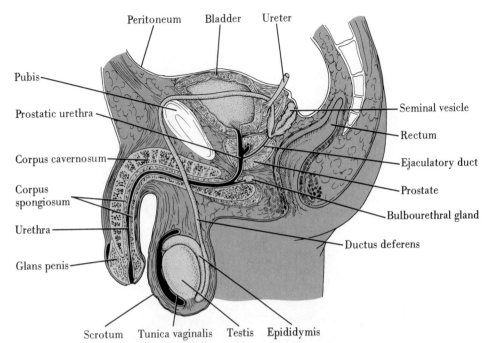

Figure 21.1. Schematic diagram demonstrating the components of the male reproductive system. Midline structures are depicted in sagittal section; bilateral structures including the testis, epididymis, vas deferens, and seminal vesicle are shown intact. (After Turner CD: In: Bloom W, Fawcett DW: *A Textbook of Histology,* 10th ed. Philadelphia, WB Saunders, 1975, p 805.)

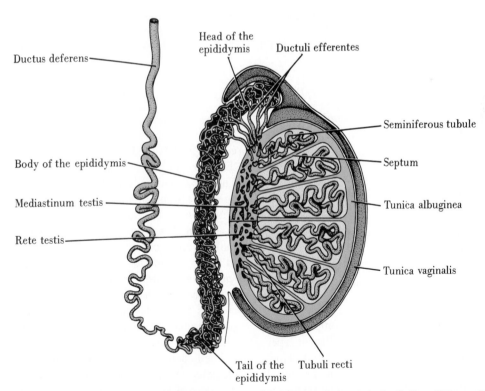

Figure 21.2. Schematic diagram of a longitudinal section through the human testis. The genital duct system, which includes the tubuli recti, rete testis, ductuli efferentes, ductus epididymis, and ductus deferens, is also shown. (Modified from Dym M: In: Weiss L (ed): *Cell and Tissue Biology, A Textbook of Histology,* 6th ed. Baltimore, Urban & Schwarzenberg, 1988, p 932.)

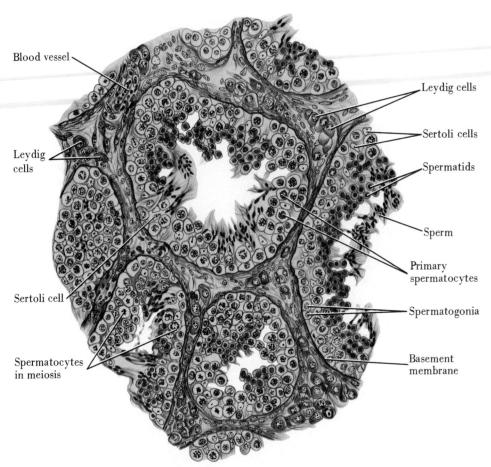

Figure 21.3. Drawing of a section of human testis. Several seminiferous tubules containing Sertoli and spermatogenic cells are shown. Leydig cells are seen in the interstitial tissue filling the interstices between the adjacent seminiferous tubules. (After Maximow AA: In: Bloom W, Fawcett DW: *A Textbook of Histology*, 10th ed. Philadelphia, WB Saunders, 1975, p 809.)

The Seminiferous Tubules Consist of a *Seminiferous Epithelium* Surrounded by a *Tunica Propria*

Each seminiferous tubule is approximately 50 cm (range 30–80 cm) in length and 150–250 μm in diameter. The *seminiferous epithelium* is a complex stratified epithelium composed of two basic populations of cells:

- *Spermatogenic cells,* which regularly replicate and differentiate into mature sperm
- *Sertoli cells,* also known as supporting or sustentacular cells, which do not undergo replication once puberty is reached

The Sertoli cells are columnar cells with complex apical and lateral processes that surround the adjacent spermatogenic cells and fill the spaces between them. However, the complex, elaborate configuration of the Sertoli cells cannot be seen distinctly in routine hematoxylin and eosin (H&E) preparation. The Sertoli cells give structural organization to the tubules as they extend through the full thickness of the seminiferous epithelium.

The spermatogenic cells are organized in poorly defined layers of progressive development between adjacent Sertoli cells (Fig. 21.4). The most immature spermatogenic cells, the *spermatogonia* or stem cells, rest on the basal lamina. The most mature cells, the *spermatids,* are attached to the apical portions of the Sertoli cell, where they border the lumen of the tubule.

The *tunica propria,* also called the lamina propria, is a multilayered connective tissue that lacks typical fibroblasts. In man, it consists of three to five layers of *myoid cells (peritubular contractile cells)* and collagen fibrils external to the basal lamina of the seminiferous epithelium. In rodents, animals frequently used to study spermatogenesis, the tunica propria consists of a single layer of myoid cells in an epithelioid arrangement. At the ultrastructural level, the myoid cells demonstrate features associated with smooth muscle cells, including the presence of a basal lamina and large numbers of actin filaments. They also exhibit a significant amount of rough endoplasmic reticulum (rER), a feature indicative of their role in collagen synthesis in the absence of typical fibroblasts. Rhythmic contractions of the myoid

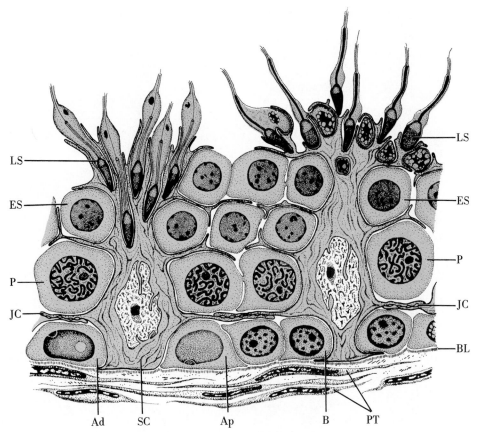

Figure 21.4. Schematic drawing of human seminiferous epithelium. The relationship of the Sertoli cells *(SC)* to the spermatogenic cells is indicated. The seminiferous epithelium rests on a basal lamina *(BL),* and a layer of peritubular cells *(PT)* surrounds the seminiferous tubule. The spermatogonia, type A pale *(Ap)*, type A dark *(Ad)*, and type B *(B)*, are located in the basal compartment of the seminiferous epithelium below the junctional complex *(JC)* between adjacent Sertoli cells. Pachytene primary spermatocytes *(P)*, early spermatids *(ES),* and late spermatids *(LS),* with partitioning residual cytoplasm that becomes the residual body, are seen in the adluminal compartment above the junctional complex. (Redrawn from Clermont Y: *American Journal of Anatomy* 112:35, 1963.)

HORMONAL REGULATION OF SPERMATOGENESIS

The endocrine function of the testis resides primarily in the Leydig cell population that synthesizes and secretes the principal circulating androgen, **testosterone.** Nearly all of the testosterone is produced by the testis; less than 5% is produced by the adrenal glands. It has been estimated in humans that the total Leydig cell population produces about 7 mg of testosterone per day. As the testosterone leaves the Leydig cells, it may pass into blood or lymphatic capillaries or through the peritubular tissue and enter the seminiferous tubules.

High local levels of testosterone within the testis (estimated to be as much as 200 times the circulating levels) are necessary for the proliferation and differentiation of the spermatogenic cells within the seminiferous epithelium. The lower peripheral level of testosterone influences

- Differentiation of the central nervous system and the genital apparatus and duct system
- Growth and maintenance of secondary sexual characteristics (such as growth of the beard, male distribution of pubic hair, and low-pitched voice)

- Growth and maintenance of the accessory sex glands (seminal vesicles, prostate, and bulbourethral), genital duct system, and the external genitalia
- Anabolic and general metabolic processes, including skeletal growth, skeletal muscle growth, distribution of subcutaneous fat, and kidney function
- Behavior, including libido

The steroidogenic and spermatogenic activities of the testis are regulated by hormonal interaction among the hypothalamus, adenohypophysis, and cells of the gonad, i.e., the Sertoli, spermatogenic, and Leydig cells. The adenohypophysis produces three hormones involved in this process: luteinizing hormone (LH), which in the male is sometimes referred to as interstitial cell-stimulating hormone (ICSH); follicle-stimulating hormone (FSH); and prolactin. In response to LH release by the pituitary, the Leydig cells produce increasing amounts of testosterone. Prolactin acts in combination with LH to increase the steroidogenic activity of the Leydig cells.

FSH and testosterone stimulate the process of sperm production within the seminiferous epithelium. The Sertoli cells are the primary target for FSH and androgens. Therefore, the Sertoli cells are the primary regulators of spermatogenesis.

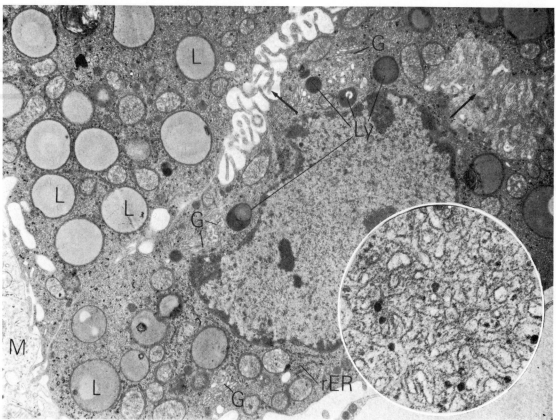

Figure 21.5. Electron micrograph of portions of several Leydig cells. The moderate electron density of the Leydig cell cytoplasm (compared with the lesser density of the small amount of cytoplasm of a microphage *(M)* included in the micrograph) is due to the abundant sER characteristic of Leydig cells. The **inset** shows, at higher magnification, the nature of the reticulum, particularly its close packing. The very dense particles represent glycogen. Other features characteristic of the Leydig cell seen in the lower-power micrograph are the numerous lipid droplets *(L)*, the segmented profiles of the Golgi complex *(G)*, and the presence of variable numbers of lysosomes *(Ly)*. Occasional profiles of rough endoplasmic reticulum *(rER)* are also seen. Note also the presence of microvilli along portions of the cell surface *(arrows)*. ×10,000; **inset,** ×60,000.

cells create peristaltic waves that help move spermatozoa and testicular fluid through the seminiferous tubules to the excurrent duct system. Blood and lymphatic vessels as well as the interstitial cells are present external to the myoid layer.

As a normal consequence of aging, the tunica propria increases in thickness. This is accompanied by a decrease in the rate of sperm production and an overall reduction in the size of the seminiferous tubules. Excessive thickening of the tunica propria earlier in life is also associated with infertility in the human male.

Leydig Cells

Leydig cells are large, polygonal, acidophilic cells that typically contain lipid droplets (Fig. 21.5). Lipochrome pigment is frequently seen in these cells. They also contain distinctive, rod-shaped cytoplasmic crystals, the ***crystals of***

Reinke (Fig. 21.6). In routine histologic preparations, the crystals are refractile and measure approximately 3 × 20 μm. Their function is unknown.

Like other steroid-secreting cells, Leydig cells have an elaborate smooth endoplasmic reticulum (sER). The enzymes necessary for the synthesis of testosterone from cholesterol are associated with the sER. Mitochondria with tubulovesicular cristae, another characteristic of steroid-secreting cells, are also present in Leydig cells.

Leydig cells differentiate and secrete testosterone during early fetal life. Secretion of testosterone is essential for the normal development of the male reproductive tract. The Leydig cells are active in the early differentiation of the male fetus and then undergo a period of inactivity beginning at about 5 months of fetal life. The inactive Leydig cells are difficult to distinguish from fibroblasts. When Leydig cells are exposed to gonadotropic stimulation at puberty, they again differentiate into androgen-secreting cells and remain active throughout life.

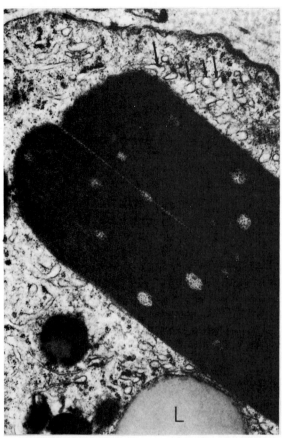

Figure 21.6. Electron micrograph of a Reinke crystal in the cytoplasm of a human Leydig cell. sER *(arrows)* and a lipid droplet *(L)* can be seen in the cytoplasm adjacent to the crystal. ×16,000. (Courtesy of Dr. D. F. Cameron.)

SPERMATOGENESIS

Spermatogenesis Is the Process by Which Spermatogonia Divide and Differentiate Into Spermatozoa (Sperm)

The process of spermatogenesis can be divided into three distinct phases:

- *Spermatogonial phase*
- *Spermatocyte phase (meiosis)*
- *Spermatid phase (spermiogenesis)*

Spermatogonial Phase

In the Spermatogonial Phase, Stem Cells Divide to Replace Themselves and to Provide a Population of Committed Spermatogonia

Human spermatogonia are classified into three types on the basis of the appearance of the nuclei in routine histologic preparations:

- *Type A dark (Ad) spermatogonia* have ovoid nuclei with intensely basophilic, finely granular chromatin.
- *Type A pale (Ap) spermatogonia* have ovoid nuclei with lightly staining, finely granular chromatin.
- *Type B spermatogonia* have generally spherical nuclei with chromatin that is condensed into large clumps along the nuclear envelope and around a central nucleolus (see Figs. 21.4 and 21.12).

Type Ad spermatogonia are thought to be the stem cells of the seminiferous epithelium. They divide at irregular intervals to give rise to either a pair of type Ad spermatogonia that remain as stem cells or to a pair of type Ap spermatogonia. The Ap spermatogonia are committed to the differentiation process that produces the sperm. They undergo several successive mitotic divisions, thereby increasing their number. An unusual feature of the division of an Ad spermatogonium into two type Ap spermatogonia is that the daughter cells remain connected by a thin cytoplasmic bridge. This same phenomenon occurs through each subsequent mitotic and meiotic division of the progeny of the original pair of Ap spermatogonia (Fig. 21.7). Thus, all of the progeny of an initial pair of Ap spermatogonia are connected, much like a strand of pearls. These cytoplasmic connections remain intact to the last stages of spermatid maturation. The connections are essential for the synchronous development of each clone from an original pair of Ap cells.

After several divisions, the type A spermatogonia differentiate into a type B spermatogonia. The appearance of type B spermatogonia represents the last event in the spermatogonial phase.

Spermatocyte Phase (Meiosis)

In the Spermatocyte Phase, Primary Spermatocytes Undergo Meiosis to Reduce Chromosome Number

The primary spermatocytes are produced by the mitotic division of the type B spermatogonia. They replicate their DNA shortly after they form, so that each primary spermatocyte contains the $4n$ amount of DNA before meiosis begins.

Meiosis is the process that results in reduction of both number of chromosomes and the amount of DNA to the haploid condition. Meiosis is described in detail in Chapter 2 (see page 51). A brief description of meiosis follows and is summarized in Figure 21.8.

The prophase of the first meiotic division, the stage during which the chromatin condenses into visible chromosomes, lasts up to 22 days in human primary spermatocytes. At the end of prophase, 44 autosomes and an X and a Y chromosome, each having two chromatin strands (chromatids), can be identified. Homologous chromosomes are paired as they line up on the metaphase plate.

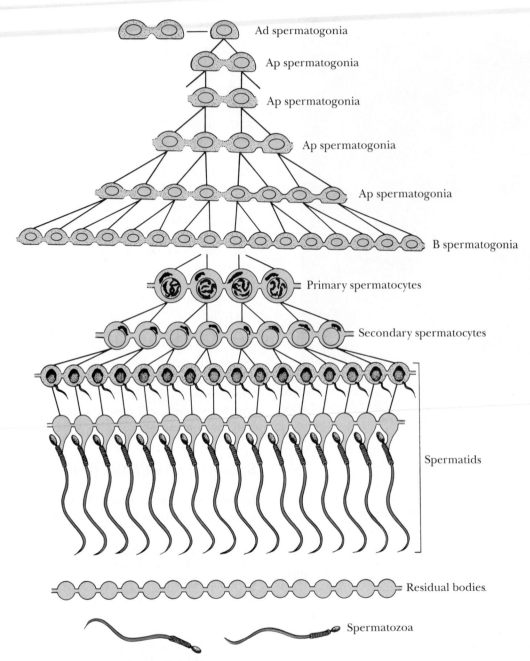

Ad spermatogonia

Ap spermatogonia

Ap spermatogonia

Ap spermatogonia

Ap spermatogonia

B spermatogonia

Primary spermatocytes

Secondary spermatocytes

Spermatids

Residual bodies

Spermatozoa

Figure 21.7. Schematic diagram illustrating the clonal nature of the various generations of spermatogenic cells. Cytoplasmic division is complete only in the primitive Ad spermatogonia that serve as stem cells. All other spermatogenic cells remain connected by intercellular bridges as they undergo mitotic and meiotic division and differentiation of the spermatids. The cells separate as individual spermatozoa as they are released from the seminiferous epithelium. The residual bodies left within the seminiferous epithelium remain interconnected. (From Dym M, Fawcett DW: *Biology of Reproduction* 4:195, 1971.)

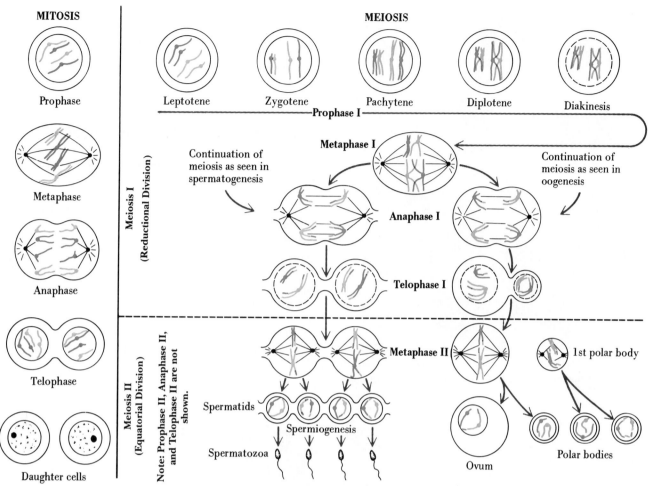

Figure 21.8. Comparison of mitosis and meiosis in a cell having two pairs of chromosomes (2*n*). The chromosomes of maternal and paternal origin are depicted in red and blue, respectively. The mitotic division produces daughter cells that are genetically identical with the parental cell (2*n*). The meiotic division, which has two components, a reductional division and an equatorial division, produces a cell that, unlike the parental cell, has only two chromosomes (*n*). In addition, during the chromosome pairing in prophase I of meiosis, there is exchange of chromosome segments, leading to further genetic diversity. Note that in the human the first polar body does not divide. Division of the first polar body does occur in some species.

The paired homologous chromosomes, called tetrads because they consist of four chromatids, exchange genetic material in a process called *crossing-over.* While the exchange is occurring, the four chromatids rearrange into a tripartite structure called a synaptonemal complex (Fig. 21.8, diplotene and diakinesis; and Fig. 21.9). This process ensures genetic diversity. Through genetic exchange, the four sperm produced from each primary spermatocyte are different from each other and from every other sperm. After crossing-over occurs, the homologous chromosomes separate and move to the opposite poles of the meiotic spindle (see Fig. 21.8). Thus, the tetrads, which have been modified by crossing-over, separate and become dyads again. The two chromatids of each original chromosome (although modified by crossing-over) remain together. This is just the opposite of what happens in mitotic division in which the

paired chromatids, representing template and newly synthesized DNA, respectively, separate.

The movement of a particular chromosome of a homologous pair to either pole of the spindle is random; i.e., maternally derived chromosomes and paternally derived chromosomes do not sort themselves out at the metaphase plate. This random sorting is another source of genetic diversity in the resulting sperm.

The cells derived from the first meiotic division are **secondary spermatocytes.** These cells immediately enter the prophase of the second meiotic division *without synthesizing new DNA* (i.e., without passing through an S phase; see page 51). Each secondary spermatocyte has 22 autosomes and an X or a Y chromosome. Each of these chromosomes consists of two sister chromatids. The secondary spermatocyte has the 2*n* (diploid) amount of DNA.

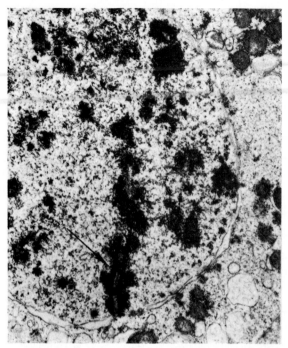

At metaphase of the second meiotic division, the chromosomes line up at the metaphase plate, and the sister chromatids separate and move to the opposite poles of the spindle. As the second meiotic division is completed and the nuclear membranes re-form, two spermatids are formed from each secondary spermatocyte (see Fig. 21.8).

Spermatid Phase (Spermiogenesis)

In the Spermatid Phase, Spermatids Differentiate Into Sperm

The cells that result from the second meiotic division are **spermatids**. Each spermatid is haploid in DNA content and in chromosome number (22 autosomes and an X or a Y chromosome). The haploid spermatids undergo a maturation process that produces the mature sperm. The normal diploid condition is restored when a sperm fertilizes an ovum.

Spermiogenesis consists of four phases:

- *Golgi phase*
- *Cap phase*
- *Acrosome phase*
- *Maturation phase*

Figure 21.9. Electron micrograph of synaptonemal complex *(arrow)* in the nucleus of a late pachytene primary spermatocyte. ×10,000.

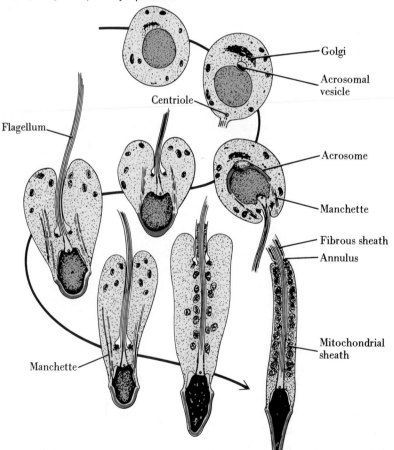

Figure 21.10. Schematic diagram of spermiogenesis in the human. The basic changes in the structure of the key organelles of the spermatid are illustrated (see text for detailed ex-planation). (Modified from Dym M: In: Weiss L (ed): *Cell and Tissue Biology, A Textbook of Histology,* 6th ed. Baltimore, Urban & Schwarzenberg, 1988, p 941.)

These phases in spermiogenesis occur while the spermatids are physically attached to the Sertoli cell plasma membrane by specialized junctions. The morphologic changes that occur during spermiogenesis are described now and are summarized in Figure 21.10.

During the *Golgi phase*, periodic acid-Schiff (PAS)-positive granules begin to accumulate in the Golgi complexes. These *proacrosomal granules*, rich in glycoproteins, coalesce into a membrane-bounded vesicle, the *acrosomal vesicle*, adjacent to the nuclear envelope. The vesicle enlarges, and its contents increase during this phase. The position of the acrosomal vesicle determines the anterior pole of the developing sperm.

Also during this phase, the centrioles migrate from the juxtanuclear region to the posterior pole of the spermatid, where the distal centriole aligns at right angles to the plasma membrane. The distal centriole initiates the synthesis of the nine peripheral microtubule doublets and two central microtubules that constitute the *axonemal complex* of the sperm tail (see Cilia and Flagella, page 74).

During the *cap phase*, the acrosomal vesicle spreads to cover the anterior half of the nucleus and becomes further condensed. This reshaped structure is called the *acrosomal cap*. The portion of the nuclear envelope beneath the acrosomal cap loses its pores and becomes thicker. The nuclear contents also become more condensed.

During the *acrosome phase*, the spermatid reorients itself so that the head becomes deeply embedded in the Sertoli cell and points toward the basal lamina. The developing flagellum extends into the lumen of the seminiferous tubule. The condensed nucleus of the spermatid flattens and elongates, the nucleus and its overlying acrosome move to a position immediately adjacent to the anterior plasma membrane, and the cytoplasm is displaced posteriorly. The cytoplasmic microtubules become organized into a cylindrical sheath, the *manchette,* that extends from the posterior rim of the acrosome toward the posterior pole of the spermatid.

The centrioles, which had earlier initiated the development of the flagellum, now move back to the posterior surface of the nucleus where the proximal centriole becomes attached to a shallow groove in the nucleus. They are then modified to form the *connecting piece* or *neck region* of the developing sperm. Nine coarse fibers develop from the centrioles attached to the nucleus and extend into the tail as the outer dense fibers peripheral to the microtubules of the axoneme. This unites the nucleus with the flagellum, hence the name, connecting piece.

As the plasma membrane moves posteriorly to cover the growing flagellum, the manchette disappears, and the mitochondria migrate from the rest of the cytoplasm to form a tight, helically wrapped sheath around the coarse fibers in the neck region and its immediate posterior extension (Fig. 21.11). This is the *middle piece* of the tail of the sperm. Distal to the middle piece, a *fibrous sheath* consisting of two longitudinal columns and numerous connecting ribs surrounds the nine longitudinal fibers of the *principal piece* and extends nearly to the end of the flagellum. This short segment of the tail distal to the fibrous sheath is the *end piece*.

During the last stage, the *maturation phase,* of spermatid differentiation, the excess cytoplasm is pinched off. This excess cytoplasm or *residual body* is then phagocytized by the Sertoli cells. The intercellular bridges that have characterized the developing gametes since the prespermatocyte stages remain with the residual bodies. This results in the release from the Sertoli cells of spermatids that are no longer attached to one another.

Structure of the Mature Sperm

The events of spermiogenesis, described above, produce a structurally unique cell. After further maturation of the sperm in the epididymis, it is capable of transporting its haploid content of DNA to the ovum. It carries with it an acrosome containing enzymes necessary for the penetration of the membranes covering the egg and only those other cellular components essential to provide the energy for its movement.

The mature human sperm is about 60 μm long. The sperm *head* is flattened and pointed and measures 4.5 μm long × 3 μm wide × 1 μm thick (Fig. 21.11). The acrosomal cap that covers the anterior two-thirds of the nucleus contains hyaluronidase, neuraminidase, acid phosphatase, and a trypsin-like protease called acrosin. These acrosomal enzymes are essential for the penetration of the zona pellucida of the ovum. The release of acrosomal enzymes as the sperm touches the egg is the first step in the *acrosome reaction.* This is a complex process that facilitates sperm penetration and subsequent fertilization and prevents the entry of additional sperm into the ovum.

The sperm *tail* is subdivided into the neck, the middle piece, the principal piece, and the end piece. The short neck contains the centrioles and the origin of the coarse fibers. The middle piece, about 7 μm long, contains the mitochondria, helically wrapped around the coarse fibers and the axonemal complex. These mitochondria provide the energy for movement of the tail and, thus, the motility of the sperm. The principal piece measures about 40 μm long and contains the fibrous sheath external to the coarse fibers and the axonemal complex. The end piece, approximately the last 5 μm of the flagellum in the mature sperm, contains only the axonemal complex.

Newly Released Sperm Are Nonmotile

The newly released sperm are carried from the seminiferous tubules in a fluid secreted by the Sertoli cells. The fluid and sperm flow through the seminiferous tubules, facilitated by contractions of the peritubular contractile cells, through the *straight tubules,* and enter the rete testis in the

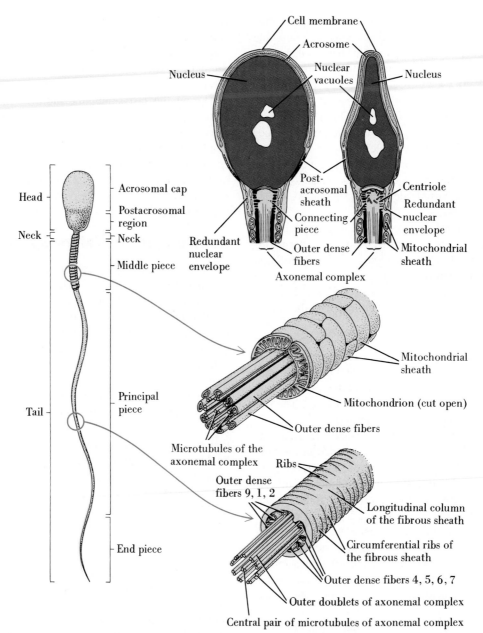

Figure 21.11. Diagram of a human spermatozoon. Regions of the spermatozoon are indicated on the left. Key ultrastructural features of the head (viewed in its major and minor dimensions) and the middle piece and principal piece of the spermatozoon are illustrated on the right. (After Pederson and Fawcett: In: Hafez ESE (ed): *Human Semen and Fertility Regulation in the Male.* St Louis, CV Mosby, 1976, figs. 7.1, 7.4, and 7.13.)

mediastinum. From the rete testis, they move through the extratesticular portion of the **efferent ductules,** the first part of the excurrent duct system, into the proximal portion of the **ductus epididymis.** As the sperm move through the 4–5 m of the highly coiled ductus epididymis, they acquire motility.

Contractions of the smooth muscle that surrounds the progressively distal and larger ducts continues to move the sperm by peristaltic action until they reach the distal portion of the *ductus epididymis* where they are stored before ejaculation.

Sperm can *live* for several weeks in the male excurrent duct system, but they will *survive* only 2–3 days in the female reproductive tract. They acquire the ability to fertilize the egg only after some time in the female tract. This process, which involves removal and replacement of glycocalyx components on the sperm membrane, is called **capacitation.**

SEMINIFEROUS TUBULES

Cycle of the Seminiferous Epithelium

Differentiating spermatogenic cells are not arranged at random in the seminiferous epithelium. There are specific associations of differentiating cell types. These associations occur because intercellular bridges are present between the progeny of each pair of type Ap spermatogonia and because

FACTORS AFFECTING SPERMATOGENESIS

Spermatogenic cells are very sensitive to noxious agents. Degenerative changes, such as premature sloughing of the cells or formation of multinucleated giant cells, are readily apparent following exposure to such agents. Factors that affect spermatogenesis include

- Dietary deficiencies
- General or local infections
- Elevated testicular temperature
- Steroid hormones and related medications
- Toxic agents such as mutagens, drugs, antimetabolites, and pesticides (particularly the short-chain halogenated hydrocarbons)
- Radiation

Proliferating cells are particularly sensitive to mutagenic agents and the absence of essential metabolites. Therefore, the nondividing Sertoli cells, the Leydig cells, and the reserve stem cells, which demonstrate low mitotic activity, are much less vulnerable than the actively dividing, differentiating spermatogenic cells.

Waves of the Seminiferous Epithelium

The *cycle* of the seminiferous epithelium describes changes that occur with time at any given site in the tubule; the *wave* of the seminiferous epithelium describes the distribution of patterns of cellular association (stages) along the length of the tubule. In rodents and other mammals that have been studied, including subhuman primates, each stage occupies a significant length of the seminiferous tubule, and the stages appear to occur sequentially along the length of the tubule. In the rat, there are approximately 12 waves in each tubule. A transverse section through the tubule will usually show only one pattern of cell associations (see Fig. 21.14*A*).

There are no waves in the human seminiferous epithelium. Each pattern of cellular associations (stage of the cycle) has a patch-like distribution in the human seminiferous tubule (see Fig. 21.14*B*). Patches do not extend around the circumference of the tubule, nor are they in sequence. Therefore, a transverse section through a human seminiferous tubule may show as many as 6 different stages of the cycle arranged in a pie-wedge fashion around the circumference of the tubule.

the synchronized cells spend specific times in each stage of maturation. All phases of differentiation occur sequentially at any given site in a seminiferous tubule as the progeny of stem cells remain connected by cytoplasmic bridges and undergo synchronous mitotic and meiotic divisions and differentiation (see Fig. 21.8).

Each recognizable grouping or *cell association* is considered a *stage* in a cyclic process. The series of stages that appears between two successive occurrences of the same cell association pattern at any given site in the seminiferous tubule constitutes the *cycle of the seminiferous epithelium.* In man, 6 stages or cell associations are defined in the cycle of the seminiferous epithelium (Fig. 21.12).

Using a pulse of tritiated thymidine, a specific generation of cells can be followed by sequential biopsies of the seminiferous tubules. In this way, the time needed for the labeled cells to go through the various stages can be determined. There may be several generations of developing cells in the thickness of the seminiferous epithelium at any given site and any given time. This produces the characteristic cell associations. The cycle of the seminiferous epithelium in man lasts about 16 days; 4.6 cycles are required for a spermatogonium to reach the time of release from the seminiferous epithelium as a sperm. Therefore, the total time required for the differentiation of a spermatogonium into a sperm is 74 days in man. The length of the cycle and the time required for spermatogenesis are constant and specific in each species.

The cycle of the seminiferous epithelium has been most thoroughly studied in rats, where 14 successive stages occur in linear sequence along the tubule (Figs. 21.13 and 21.14*A*). The 6 stages in man are not as clearly delineated as in rodents because in man the cellular associations occur in irregular patches that form a mosaic pattern (Fig. 21.14*B*).

Sertoli Cells

Sertoli Cells Constitute the True Epithelium of the Seminiferous Epithelium

Sertoli cells are tall, columnar, nonreplicating epithelial cells that rest on the thick, multilayered basal lamina (Fig. 21.16). They are the supporting cells for the developing sperm that become attached to their surface after meiosis. Sertoli cells contain an extensive sER, a well-developed rER, and stacks of annulate lamellae. They have numerous spherical and elongated mitochondria, a well-developed Golgi complex, and varying numbers of microtubules, lysosomes, lipid droplets, vesicles, glycogen granules, and filaments (Fig. 21.17). A sheath of 7–9-nm filaments surrounds the nucleus and separates it from other cytoplasmic organelles.

The euchromatic Sertoli cell nucleus, a reflection of this very active cell, is generally ovoid or triangular in shape and may have one or more deep infoldings. Its shape and location vary. It may be flattened, lying in the basal portion of the cell near and parallel to the base of the cell, or it may be triangular or ovoid, lying near or some distance from the base of the cell. In some species, the Sertoli cell nucleus contains a unique tripartite structure that consists of an RNA-containing nucleolus flanked by a pair of DNA-containing bodies called *karyosomes* (Fig. 21.17).

In man, characteristic inclusion bodies (of Charcot-Böttcher) are found in the basal cytoplasm. These are slender fusiform crystalloids that measure 10–25 μm long × 1 μm wide and are visible in routine histologic preparations.

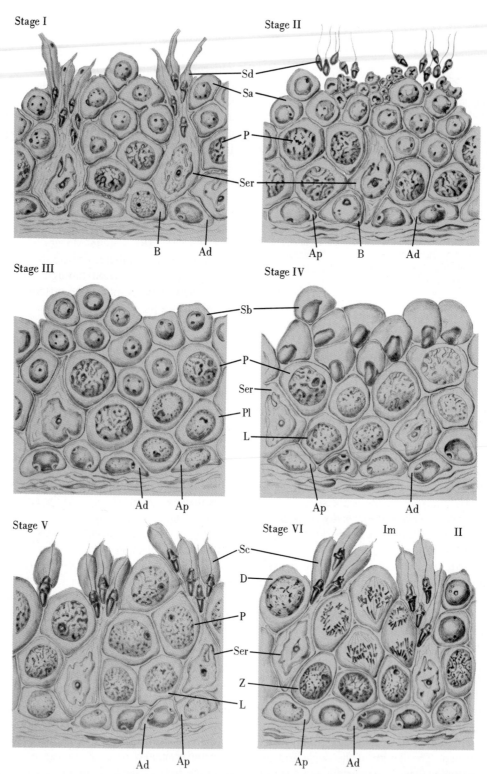

Figure 21.12. Schematic drawing of the six recognizable cell associations or stages of the cycle of the human seminiferous epithelium. *Ser,* Sertoli cells; *Ad,* type A dark spermatogonia; *Ap,* type A pale spermatogonia; *B,* type B spermatogonia; *Pl,* preleptotene spermatocytes; *L,* leptotene spermatocytes; *P,* pachytene spermatocytes; *D,* diplotene spermatocytes; *Im,* primary spermatocytes in division; *II,* secondary spermatocytes; and *Sa, Sb, Sc,* and *Sd,* spermatids in various steps of differentiation. (Based on Clermont Y: *American Journal of Anatomy* 112:50, 1963.)

SPERMATOGENESIS IN THE RAT

Numerous biochemical, physiologic, and morphologic studies utilizing the rat as an animal model system have contributed to our understanding of the events and control of spermatogenesis. Although a few aspects of spermatogenesis are unique in the human, the process in the rat is similar in many respects to that observed in other mammalian species, including primates. In the spermatogenic cycle of the rat shown in Figure 21.15, one can follow the successive changes an individual spermatogenic cell will undergo by starting with the A_1 cell located in the lower left-hand corner of the chart and following the path of differentiation indicated by the *arrows*. The most differentiated cell *(top row, column VIII)* is a spermatozoon that is being released from the seminiferous epithelium.

In the rat, six successive generations of spermatogonia (produced by mitotic divisions) with subtle morphologic differences have been described as types A_1, A_2, A_3, A_4, In, and B. Type A_1 spermatogonia are produced by the mitotic

division of the stem cells. (The superscript *m* in the diagram indicates the time of a mitotic division.) The mitotic divisions give rise to the cells of the next generation. Type B spermatogonia divide to produce preleptotene primary spermatocytes *(Pl)*. As the spermatogenic cells proceed through prophase of the first meiotic division, they pass through a series of morphologically distinct phases: preleptotene *(Pl)*, leptotene *(L)*, zygotene *(Z)*, pachytene *(P)*, diplotene *(D)*, and diakinesis. The secondary spermatocytes *(II)* produced by the first meiotic or reduction division immediately enter the second meiotic or equatorial division and give rise to the haploid spermatid.

During spermiogenesis, the maturation of the cells has been divided into a series of morphologically distinguishable *steps* indicated by Arabic numerals in Figure 21.15. The primary criteria used to identify the steps are alterations of the nucleus and acrosome. The drawings of the cells, indicated in the chart, are based on observations of PAS-hematoxylin-stained preparations. The PAS procedure stains the developing acrosome; hematoxylin stains the nucleus.

CYCLE OF THE SEMINIFEROUS EPITHELIUM IN THE RAT

The various generations of spermatogenic cells are not randomly distributed in the seminiferous epithelium but are organized into well-defined cellular associations. This can be explained by examining Figure 21.15. Identify the spermatid at step 6 enclosed in the vertical column outlined in red. The vertical column indicates a cellular association. Spermatids at step 6 of spermiogenesis are always associated with types A_1 and B spermatogonia, pachytene spermatocytes, and step 18 spermatids. As the step 6 spermatids pass to the next step in their differentiation, step 7, all the cells associated with them simultaneously pass to the next stage in their differentiation, i.e., the cellular association enclosed in the vertical column outlined in blue. The *vertical dashed lines* in Figure 21.15 enclose 14 such distinct cellular associations identified in the rat. The cellular associations, indicated by Roman numerals, are called *stages*. If the cellular association present in one portion of a rat seminiferous tubule were continually observed, one would see the cells passing successively through all 14 *stages*, and then a repeat of the initial association would be observed. This series of changes between the appearances of the same cellular association is defined as the *cycle of the seminiferous epithelium*. The number of stages in the cycle of the seminiferous epithelium is constant for a given species. In the human, 6 stages have been defined (see Fig. 21.12); in the mouse and monkey, 12.

In all species, with the exception of the human, a particular cellular association occupies a relatively long segment along a seminiferous tubule. Therefore, a cross section

through a tubule typically includes only one type of cellular association (see Fig. 21.14A). The spermatogenic cells in a cross section of a rat seminiferous tubule would consist of cells in 1 of the 14 cellular associations shown in Figure 21.15. This is *not* true of the human seminiferous tubule, where cellular associations occur in irregularly shaped areas along the tubule (see Fig. 21.14B). Therefore, a cross section through a tubule would reveal two or more distinct cellular associations.

Again except for the human, the segments of seminiferous tubules containing the various cellular associations are organized in an orderly sequence along the seminiferous tubule (see Fig. 21.13). The cellular associations in adjacent segments of a seminiferous tubule are always at the next higher or next lower stage of the cycle of the seminiferous epithelium. Thus, if one examines the cellular associations in the segments along the length of a seminiferous tubule, there is an orderly progression from one stage of the cycle to the next.

Autoradiographic studies utilizing tritiated thymidine, which is incorporated into meiotically and mitotically dividing cells during the period of DNA synthesis (S phase of the cell cycle), have revealed that the cycle of the seminiferous epithelium is of a constant duration, lasting about 16 days in humans. In humans it would require about 4.6 cycles (each of 16 days duration), or approximately 74 days, for a spermatogonium produced by a stem cell to complete the process of spermatogenesis. It would then require about 12 days for the spermatozoa to pass through the epididymis. Therefore, if a drug is given that inhibits the initial phases of spermatogenesis, it would require approximately 86 days to recognize the effect of that compound.

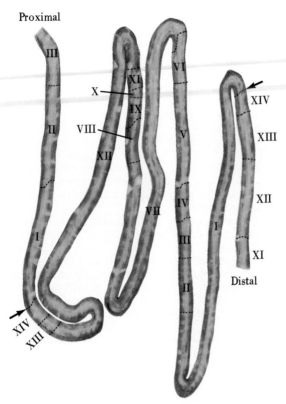

Proximal

Distal

Figure 21.13. Drawing of a portion of an isolated seminiferous tubule from rat testis. The 14 cellular associations identified in the rat (see Fig. 21.15) are arranged in a linear array of segments along the length of the tubule. *Roman numerals* on the segments indicate stages. *Arrows* indicate the beginning and end of a series of segments, including all stages of the cycle of the seminiferous epithelium in the rat. Proximal and distal ends of the isolated tubule are indicated. (After Perey B, Clermont Y, Leblond CP: *American Journal of Anatomy* 108:58, 1961.)

With transmission electron microscopy, they are resolved as bundles of poorly ordered, parallel or converging, straight, dense 15-nm-diameter filaments (see Fig. 21.16). Their chemical composition and function are as yet undetermined.

The Sertoli-Sertoli Junctional Complex Consists of a Structurally Unique Combination of Membrane and Cytoplasmic Specializations

Sertoli cells are bound to one another by an unusual junctional complex (Fig. 21.18). It is characterized, in part, by an exceedingly tight junction that includes more than 50 parallel fusion lines in the adjacent membranes. In addition, there are two cytoplasmic components that are part of this unique junctional complex:

- A *flattened cisterna of sER* parallels the plasma membrane in the region of the junction in each cell.
- *Actin filament bundles,* hexagonally packed, are interposed between the sER cisternae and the plasma membranes.

A similar-appearing junction is seen where the spermatids are attached to the Sertoli cells. There is no tight junction, however, and the spermatid lacks the flattened cisternae of the sER and the actin bundles (Figs. 21.17 and 21.18). Other junctional specializations of the Sertoli cells include gap junctions between Sertoli cells, desmosome-like junctions between Sertoli cells and early stage spermatogenic cells, and hemidesmosomes at the Sertoli cell-basal lamina interface.

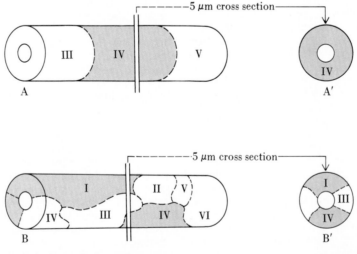

Figure 21.14. Schematic diagrams illustrating the difference in the organization of the seminiferous epithelium between most subhuman species **(A)** and man **(B)**. In subhuman species, a particular cellular association occupies a relatively long segment along the tubule. Therefore, in a typical cross section only a single cellular association is observed **(A')**. In man, cellular associations occur in irregularly shaped areas along the tubule, and therefore, a cross section typically shows two or more cellular associations **(B')**. (Modified from Dym M: In: Weiss L (ed): *Cell and Tissue Biology, A Textbook of Histology,* 6th ed. Baltimore, Urban & Schwarzenberg, 1988, p 949.)

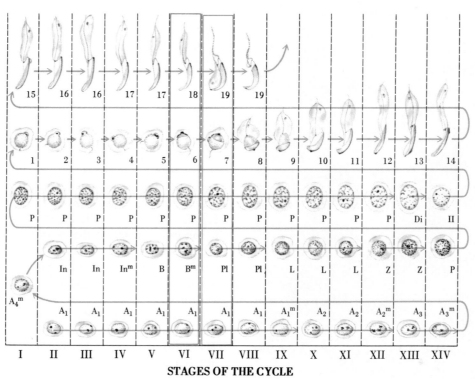

STAGES OF THE CYCLE

Figure 21.15. Schematic diagram depicting the spermatogenic cell associations of the 14 stages of the cycle of the seminiferous epithelium in the rat. Each numbered column *(Roman numerals)* shows the spermatogenic cell types present in the cellular associations found in cross sections of seminiferous tubules. See the text for an explanation of the progression of the cells through the stages of the cycle. *Arabic numerals 1–19* are used to indicate steps in the development of the spermatids, defined by changes in the appearance of the nucleus and acrosome. *Letters* are used to identify spermatogonia and spermatocytes: A_1, A_2, A_3, and A_4, four generations of type A spermatogonia; *In,* intermediate spermatogonia; *B,* type B spermatogonia; *Pl,* preleptotene spermatocytes; *L,* leptotene spermatocytes; *Z,* zygotene spermatocytes; *P,* pachytene spermatocytes; *Di,* diplotene spermatocytes; and *II,* secondary spermatocytes. The superscript *m* indicates mitotic division of the spermatogonia. (Modified from Dym M, Clermont Y: *American Journal of Anatomy* 128:269, 1970.)

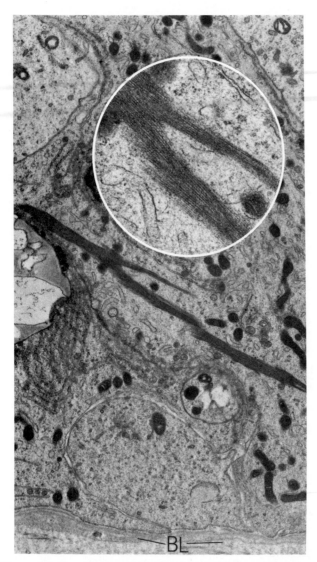

Figure 21.16. Electron micrograph of a human Sertoli cell. Characteristic crystalloid inclusion bodies of Charcot-Böttcher are present in the basal cytoplasm of the cell. The basal lamina *(BL)* is indicated for orientation. The filaments of the crystalloid can be seen in the **inset.** ×9,000; **inset,** ×27,000. (Courtesy of D. F. Cameron.)

The Sertoli-Sertoli Junctional Complex Divides the Seminiferous Epithelium Into Basal and Luminal Compartments

The Sertoli-Sertoli junctions establish a basal epithelial compartment and a luminal compartment (see Fig. 21.17). Spermatogonia and early primary spermatocytes are restricted to the basal compartment, i.e., between the Sertoli-Sertoli junctions and the basal lamina. More mature spermatocytes and spermatids are restricted to the luminal side of the Sertoli-Sertoli junctions. The early spermatocytes produced by mitotic division of the type B spermatogonia must pass through the junctional complex to get from the basal compartment to the luminal compartment. This occurs through the formation of a new junctional complex between Sertoli cell processes that extend beneath the newly formed spermatocytes and then the breakdown of the junction above them. Thus, in the differentiation of the spermatogenic cells, the processes of meiosis and spermiogenesis occur in the luminal compartment.

In both compartments, spermatogenic cells are surrounded by complex processes of the Sertoli cells. Because of the unusually close relationships between Sertoli cells and differentiating spermatogenic cells, it has been suggested that Sertoli cells serve as "nurse" or supporting cells. That is they function in the exchange of metabolic substrates and wastes between the developing spermatogenic cells and the circulatory system.

In addition, Sertoli cells phagocytize and breakdown the residual bodies formed in the last stage of spermiogenesis. They also phagocytize any spermatogenic cells that fail to differentiate completely.

The Sertoli-Sertoli Junctional Complex Is the Site of the Blood-Testis Barrier

In addition to the physical compartmentalization described above, the Sertoli-Sertoli junctional com-

---

SPERM-SPECIFIC ANTIGENS AND THE IMMUNE RESPONSE

In terms of the immunologic importance of the blood-testis barrier, two basic facts are well-established:

- Spermatozoa and spermatogenic cells possess molecules that are unique to this cell type and are recognized as "foreign" (not self) by the immune system.
- Spermatozoa are first produced at puberty long after the individual has become immunocompetent, i.e., capable of recognizing foreign molecules and producing antibodies against them.

Therefore, the blood-testis barrier serves an essential role in isolating the spermatogenic cells from the immune system.

Failure of the spermatogenic cells and spermatozoa to remain isolated results in the production of sperm-specific antibodies. Such an immune response is seen after vasectomy and in some cases of infertility. After vasectomy, sperm-specific antibodies are produced as the cells of the immune system are exposed to the spermatozoa that leak from the severed vas deferens. Thus, sperm no longer remain isolated from the immune system within the reproductive tract. In some cases of infertility, it has been shown that sperm-specific antibodies are present in the semen. These antibodies cause the sperm to agglutinate. This interferes with their movement and interaction with the ovum.

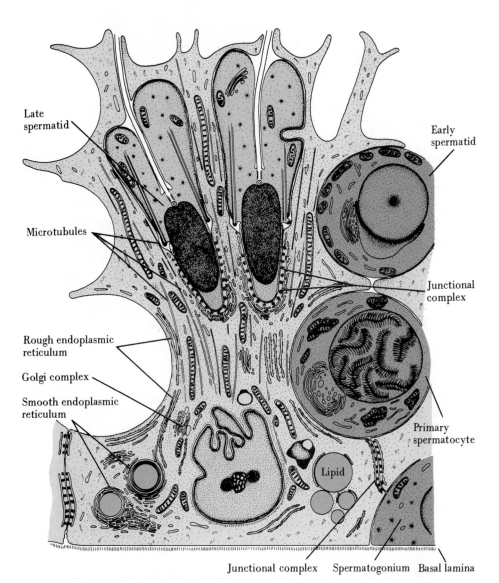

Figure 21.17. Schematic drawing of a Sertoli cell and adjacent spermatogenic cells showing their ultrastructural features. Junctional complexes between adjacent Sertoli cells and between the Sertoli cell and the late spermatids are illustrated. The late spermatids reside in recesses within the apical cytoplasm of the Sertoli cells. Lateral processes of the Sertoli cells extend over the surface of the spermatocytes and spermatids. (A karyosome is illustrated in the Sertoli cell nucleus.) (From Bloom W, Fawcett DW: *A Textbook of Histology,* 10th ed. Philadelphia, WB Saunders, 1975, p 813.)

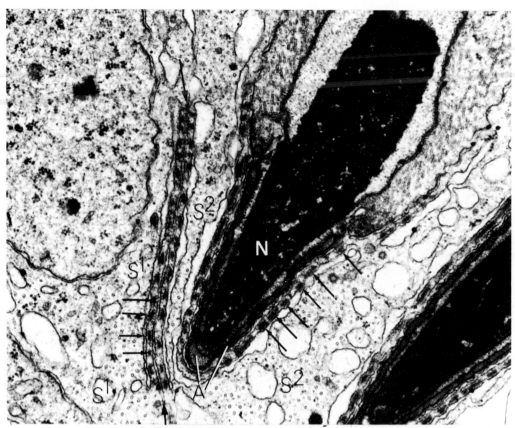

Figure 21.18. Electron micrograph demonstrating a Sertoli-Sertoli junctional complex and, in close proximity, a Sertoli-spermatid junctional specialization. Condensation and shaping of the spermatid nucleus *(N)* are well advanced. The acrosome *(A)* of the spermatid appears as a V-shaped profile, and in close association with it is the Sertoli cell junctional specialization characterized by bundles of microfilaments *(small arrows)* and the associated profile of endoplasmic reticulum, which resides immediately adjacent to the microfilament bundles. The Sertoli-Sertoli junction lies just to the left, joining one Sertoli cell *(S¹)* to the adjacent Sertoli cell *(S²)*. The *large arrows* indicate the limits of the junction. Note that the junction here reveals the same elements, the microfilament bundles *(small arrows)* and a profile of endoplasmic reticulum, as are seen in the Sertoli-spermatid junction. Not evident at this magnification is the tight junction associated with the Sertoli-Sertoli junctional complex. ×30,000.

plex also creates a physiologic compartmentalization of the seminiferous epithelium. The ionic, amino acid, carbohydrate, and protein composition of the fluid in the seminiferous tubules and excurrent ducts differs considerably from the composition of the blood plasma and the testicular lymph.

Plasma proteins *and circulating antibodies* are excluded from the lumen of the seminiferous tubules. The exocrine secretary products of the Sertoli cells, particularly ***androgen-binding protein (ABP),*** can become highly concentrated in the lumen. Most importantly, the barrier isolates the genetically and, therefore, antigenically different haploid germ cells (secondary spermatocytes, spermatids, and sperm) from the immune system of the adult male. Antigens produced by or specific to the sperm are prevented from reaching the systemic circulation. Conversely, γ-globulins, even specific sperm antibodies found in some individuals, are prevented from

reaching the developing spermatogenic cells in the seminiferous tubule.

Sertoli Cells Have Both Exocrine and Endocrine Secretory Functions

In addition to secreting fluid that facilitates passage of the maturing sperm into the intratesticular ducts, the Sertoli cells secrete ABP. ABP is necessary to concentrate testosterone in the lumen of the seminiferous tubule, where high concentrations of testosterone are essential for the normal maturation of the developing sperm.

Sertoli cells also secrete ***inhibin,*** a compound involved in the feedback loop that regulates FSH in the anterior pituitary gland. Sertoli cells, themselves, are stimulated by both FSH and testosterone; FSH is believed to be essential for the secretion of ABP (Fig. 21.19).

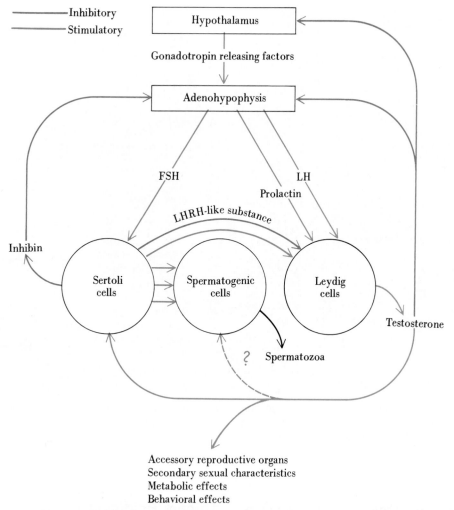

Inhibitory
Stimulatory

Hypothalamus

Gonadotropin releasing factors

Adenohypophysis

FSH

LH

Prolactin

LHRH-like substance

Inhibin

Sertoli cells

Spermatogenic cells

Leydig cells

Testosterone

? Spermatozoa

Accessory reproductive organs
Secondary sexual characteristics
Metabolic effects
Behavioral effects

Figure 21.19. Diagram depicting the hormonal regulation of male reproductive function. *Blue arrows* indicate stimulatory action on the system; *red arrows* indicate inhibitory feedback. See text for explanation. *LHRH,* luteinizing hormone-releasing hormone. (Modified from Dym M: In: Weiss L (ed): *Cell and Tissue Biology, A Textbook of Histology,* 6th ed. Baltimore, Urban & Schwarzenberg, 1988, p 959.)

INTRATESTICULAR DUCTS

Straight Tubules, the *Tubuli Recti,* Join the Seminiferous Tubules With the *Rete Testis* of the Mediastinum

At the end of each seminiferous tubule there is an abrupt transition to the *tubuli recti* or straight tubules. This short terminal section of the seminiferous tubule is lined only by Sertoli cells. Near their termination, the *tubuli recti* narrow, and their lining changes to a simple cuboidal epithelium.

The straight tubules empty into the *rete testis,* a complex series of interconnecting channels within the highly vascular connective tissue of the mediastinum (Fig. 21.20). A simple cuboidal or low columnar epithelium lines the channels

of the rete testis. These cell have a single apical cilium and few apical microvilli.

EXCURRENT DUCT SYSTEM

Efferent Ductules

The *Efferent Ductules* Connect the Rete Testis to the Epididymis

In man, approximately 20 *efferent ductules* (ductuli efferentes) connect the channels of the *rete testis* at the superior end of the mediastinum to the proximal portion of the *ductus epididymis.* As the *efferent ductules* exit the testis, they become highly coiled and form 6–10 conical

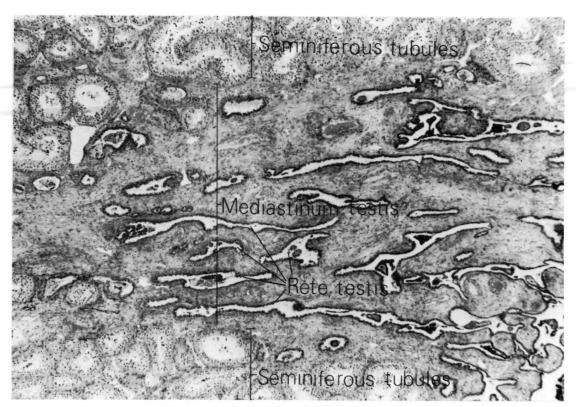

Figure 21.20. Photomicrograph of human testis. The section passes through the mediastinum of the testis. In this region the anastomosing channels of the rete testis are found. Semi-niferous tubules can be seen in the region adjacent to the mediastinum. ×40.

masses, the *coni vasculosi,* whose bases form part of the head of the epididymis. The coni vasculosi, each about 10 mm in length, contain highly convoluted ducts that measure 15–20 cm. At the base of the cones, the efferent ducts open into a single channel, the *ductus epididymis* (see Fig. 21.2).

The efferent ductules are lined with a pseudostratified columnar epithelium that contains clumps of tall and short cells, giving the luminal surface a sawtooth appearance (Fig. 21.21). Interspersed among the columnar cells are a few basal cells and intraepithelial lymphocytes. The tall columnar cells are generally ciliated. The short nonciliated cells have numerous microvilli and canalicular invaginations of the apical surface as well as numerous pinocytotic vesicles, membrane-bounded dense bodies, lysosomes, and other cytoplasmic structures associated with endocytic activity. *Most of the fluid secreted in the seminiferous tubules is reabsorbed in the efferent ductules.*

A muscular coat first appears at the beginning of the efferent ductules. The smooth muscle forms a layer several cells thick in which the cells are arrayed as a circular sheath in the wall of the ductule. Interspersed among the muscle cells are elastic fibers. Transport of the sperm in the efferent ductules is effected largely by both ciliary action and contraction of this fibromuscular layer.

Ductus Epididymis

The *Ductus Epididymis* Is a Highly Coiled Tube in Which Sperm Undergo Further Maturation

The *epididymis* lies along the posterior surface of the testis. It measures about 7.5 cm in length and consists of the *ductus epididymis* and its associated vascularized connective tissue, smooth muscle, and a fibrous connective tissue tunic (Fig. 21.22). The ductus epididymis is a highly coiled tube measuring 4–6 m in length. It is divided into a head (caput), a body (corpus), and a tail (cauda) (see Fig. 21.2). Sperm mature during their passage through the epididymis, acquiring motility and the ability to fertilize an egg. This maturation, like their earlier differentiation, is androgen dependent. During this process, changes occur in the sperm plasma membrane, including the addition to the glycocalyx of glycoproteins secreted by the epididymal epithelial cells.

The Principal Cells in the Pseudostratified Epithelium of the Epididymis Are Characterized by Stereocilia

Like most of the excurrent duct system, the ductus epididymis is also lined with a pseudostratified columnar ep-

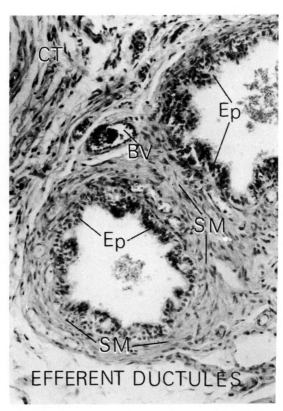

Figure 21.21. Photomicrograph of efferent ductules. The efferent ductules are lined with pseudostratified columnar epithelium *(Ep)*. The luminal surface has an uneven or wavy appearance due to the presence of alternating groups of tall columnar and cuboidal cells. Cilia are present on some cells. The ductules surrounded by circularly arranged smooth muscle *(SM)* are embedded in the connective tissue *(CT)*. BV, blood vessel. ×160.

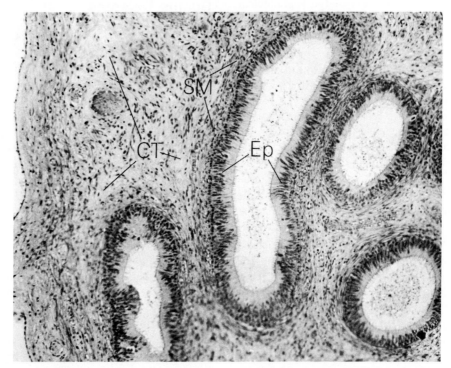

Figure 21.22. Photomicrograph of human epididymis. The section passes through the highly coiled ductus epididymis in several places. The epithelium *(Ep)* that lines the epididymis is pseudostratified columnar. The duct, which is surrounded by smooth muscle *(SM)*, is embedded in connective tissue *(CT)*. ×80.

ithelium. It contains **principal cells** (tall) and **basal cells** (short) (Fig. 21.23). The principal cells vary from about 80 μm in height in the head of the epididymis to about 40 μm in height in the tail. Numerous, long, modified microvilli called **stereocilia** extend from the luminal surface of the principal cells. The stereocilia vary in height from 25 μm in the head to about 10 μm in the tail. The small round basal cells rest on the basal lamina. They are the stem cells of the duct epithelium. In addition, intraepithelial lymphocytes called **halo cells** are found in the epithelium. Under normal conditions, this is the most proximal level of the excurrent duct system in which lymphocytes are present.

Epididymal Cells Function in Both Absorption and Secretion

Most of the fluid that is not absorbed by the efferent ductules is reabsorbed in the proximal portion of the epididymis. The epithelial cells also phagocytize any residual bodies not removed by the Sertoli cells as well as sperm that degenerate in the duct. The apical cytoplasm of the principal cells contains numerous invaginations at the bases of the stereocilia, along with coated vesicles, multivesicular bodies, and lysosomes (Fig. 21.24).

The principal cells secrete glycerophosphocholine, sialic acid, and glycoproteins, which add to the glycocalyx, and possibly steroids, which aid in the maturation of the sperm. They have numerous cisternae of rER surrounding the basally located nucleus and a remarkably large supranuclear Golgi complex. There are also profiles of sER and rER in the apical cytoplasm.

The Smooth Muscle Coat of the Ductus Epididymis Gradually Increases in Thickness to Become Three Layered in the Tail

In the head of the epididymis and most of the body, the smooth muscle coat consists of a thin layer of circular smooth muscle resembling that of the efferent ductules. In the tail, inner and outer longitudinal layers are added. These three layers are then continuous with the three smooth muscle layers of the **ductus deferens** (vas deferens), the next component of the excurrent duct system.

Differences in smooth muscle function parallel these morphologic differences. In the head and body of the epididymis, spontaneous, rhythmic peristaltic contractions serve to move the sperm along the duct. Few peristaltic contractions are seen in the tail of the epididymis, which serves as the principal reservoir for mature sperm. These sperm are forced into the vas deferens by intense contractions of the three smooth muscle layers after appropriate neural stimulation associated with ejaculation.

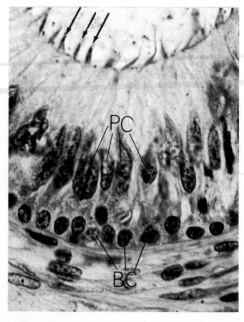

Figure 21.23. Photomicrograph of a portion of the tubular wall portion of the human ductus epididymis. Two epithelial cell types can be identified: principal cells *(PC)* and basal cells *(BC)*. Stereocilia *(arrows)* extend from the apical surface of the tall columnar principal cells. Nuclei of the basal cells are located adjacent to the basement membrane. ×640.

Ductus Deferens

The *Ductus Deferens (Vas Deferens),* the Terminal Portion of the Excurrent System, Ends in the Prostatic Urethra

The **ductus deferens** is a direct continuation of the tail of the epididymis (see Fig. 21.1). It ascends along the posterior border of the testis, close to the testicular vessels and nerves. It enters the abdomen as a component of the spermatic cord, as it passes through the inguinal canal. The vas deferens then descends to the pelvis, to the level of the bladder, where it connects to the prostatic urethra. The distal end of the ductus deferens enlarges to form the **ampulla**. It is joined there by the **duct of the seminal vesicle** and continues through the prostate gland to the urethra as the **ejaculatory duct**.

The ductus deferens is lined with a pseudostratified columnar epithelium that closely resembles that of the epididymis. The tall columnar cells also have long microvilli that extend into the lumen. The rounded basal cells rest on the basal lamina. Unlike the epididymis, however, the lumen of the duct does not appear smooth. In histologic preparations (Fig. 21.25), it appears to be thrown into deep longitudinal folds throughout most of its length, probably due

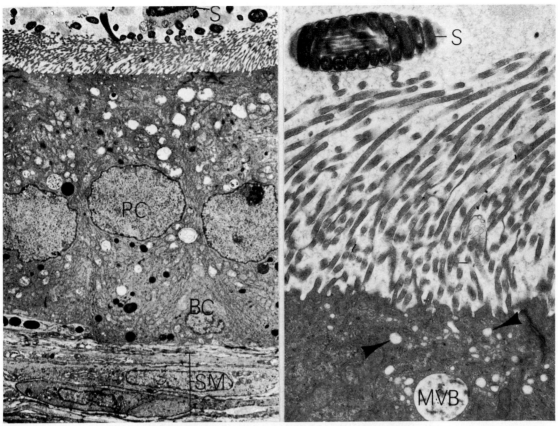

Figure 21.24. **a.** Electron micrograph of epididymal epithelium, showing principal cells *(PC)* extending to the lumen and a basal cell *(BC)* limited to the base of the epithelium. Smooth muscle *(SM)* is in the connective tissue below the epithelium. A portion of a sperm *(S)* is seen in the lumen. ×3,000. **b.** Apical surface of the epithelial cell with its numerous microvilli. Again, a portion of a sperm *(S)* is evident in the lumen. The large, light circular object is a multivesicular body *(MVB)*. The small, light circular profiles *(arrowheads)* are pinocytotic vesicles. ×13,000.

to contraction of the thick (1–1.5-mm) muscular coat of the duct during fixation.

The ***ampulla*** has taller, branched mucosal folds that often show glandular diverticula. The muscle coat surrounding the ampulla is thinner than that of the rest of the vas deferens, and the longitudinal layers disappear near the origin of the ejaculatory duct. The epithelium of the ampulla and of the ejaculatory duct appear to have a secretory function. The cells contain large numbers of yellow pigment granules. There is no muscularis layer in the wall of the ejaculatory duct; the fibromuscular tissue of the prostate substitutes for it.

ACCESSORY SEX GLANDS

Seminal Vesicles

The Paired *Seminal Vesicles* Secrete a Fluid That Is Rich in Fructose

The ***seminal vesicles*** are paired, elongate, highly folded tubular glands that have a muscular and fibrous coat (Fig. 21.26). They originate as evaginations of the vas deferens distal to the ampulla and, for that reason, resemble the ampulla. The mucosa is thrown into numerous primary, secondary, and tertiary folds that increase the secretory surface. All of the irregular chambers thus formed, however, communicate with the lumen.

The pseudostratified columnar epithelium contains tall, nonciliated columnar cells and short round cells that rest on the basal lamina. The short cells appear identical with those of the rest of the excurrent duct system. They also are assumed to be stem cells from which the columnar cells derive. The columnar cells have the morphology of protein-secreting cells, with a well-developed rER and large secretory vacuoles in the apical cytoplasm.

The secretion of the seminal vesicles is a whitish-yellow, viscous material. It contains fructose, which is the principal metabolic substrate for sperm, along with other simple sugars, amino acids, ascorbic acid, and prostaglandins. Although

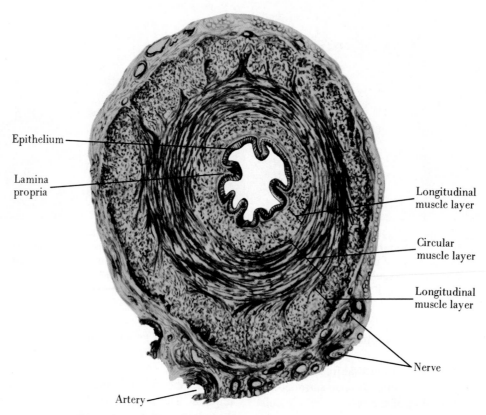

Epithelium

Lamina
propria

Longitudinal
muscle layer

Circular
muscle layer

Longitudinal
muscle layer

Nerve

Artery

Figure 21.25.   Drawing of a cross section through a human vas deferens. The thick muscularis is organized in three distinct smooth muscle layers: an inner longitudinal, middle circular, and outer longitudinal. Numerous elastic fibers are present in the lamina propria underlying the epithelium. ×30. (After Schaffer: In: Bloom W, Fawcett DW: *A Textbook of Histology,* 10th ed. Philadelphia, WB Saunders, 1975, p 848.)

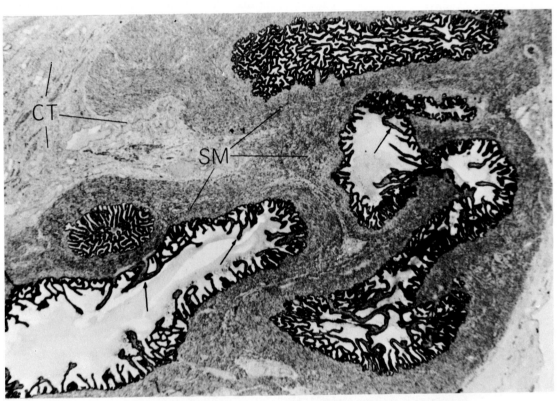

Figure 21.26. Photomicrograph of human seminal vesicle. The mucosa of the seminal vesicle is characterized by extensive folding *(arrows).* The mucosa rests on a thick smooth muscle *(SM)* investment that is organized in two layers: an inner circular layer and an outer longitudinal layer. ×16.

prostaglandins were first isolated from the prostate gland (hence the name), they are actually synthesized in large amounts in the seminal vesicles. Contraction of the smooth muscle coat of the seminal vesicles during ejaculation discharges their secretion into the ejaculatory ducts and helps to flush sperm out of the urethra. The secretory function and the morphology of the seminal vesicles are under the control of testosterone.

Prostate Gland

The Prostate, the Largest Accessory Sex Gland, Secretes Acid Phosphatase, Fibrinolysin, and Citric Acid

The prostate consists of a collection of 30–50 tubuloalveolar glands that surround the proximal urethra. The glands are arranged in three concentric layers: a mucosal layer, a submucosal layer, and the most peripheral layer containing the main prostatic glands (Fig. 21.27). The mucosal glands secrete directly into the urethra; the other two layers have ducts that open into the prostatic sinuses located on either side of the crest of the posterior wall of the urethra.

The epithelium is generally columnar but may have patches that are cuboidal, squamous, or pseudostratified (Fig. 21.28). It secretes protein enzymes, particularly acid phosphatase and fibrinolysin, along with citric acid. Acid phosphatase is also found in large amounts in lysosomes in the epithelial cells, and some acid phosphatase enters the circulation. In patients with prostatic cancer, blood levels of acid phosphatase are used to check for metastasis. The secretions are pumped into the urethra at the time of ejaculation by contraction of the fibromuscular tissue of the prostate. The fibrinolysin in the secretion serves to liquefy the semen. The epithelium of the prostate is also dependent on testosterone for normal morphology and function.

The prostatic alveoli, especially in older men, often contain *prostatic concretions (corpora amylacea)* of varied shape and size, often up to 2 mm in diameter (Fig. 21.28). They appear in sections as concentric lamellated bodies and are believed to be formed by precipitation of secretory material

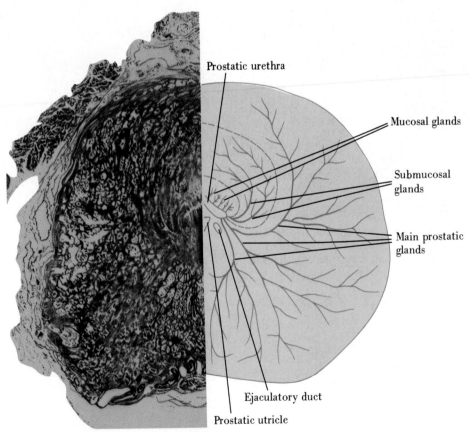

Prostatic urethra

Mucosal glands

Submucosal glands

Main prostatic glands

Ejaculatory duct

Prostatic utricle

Figure 21.27.   Human prostate gland. The survey micrograph on the left illustrates the basic morphology of the gland (see Fig. 21.28). The schematic diagram on the right illustrates the distribution of the glandular components within the prostate. The regions of the prostate containing mucosal, submucosal, and main prostate glands are indicated by the *dashed red lines*. (From Franks LM: *Annals of the Royal College of Surgeons of England* 14:92, 1954.)

BENIGN PROSTATIC HYPERTROPHY AND PROSTATIC CANCER

Benign prostatic hypertrophy (nodular hyperplasia) occurs in the mucosal and submucosal glands and can lead to partial or total obstruction of the urethra. This is believed to occur to some extent in all men by age 80 years. It is now routinely treated by transurethral removal of prostatic parenchyma. This procedure is called transurethral prostatectomy or TURP. Recently, several drugs have been introduced that "shrink" hypertrophic prostatic tissue in some men. They may actually act by relaxing the prostatic smooth muscle.

Cancer of the prostate is one of the most common cancers in the male, affecting approximately 1 in 20. Tumors usually develop peripherally, in the main glands. It is often not detected early because the abnormal growth may not impinge on the urethra and produce symptoms that demand prompt attention. Therefore, prostatic cancer is often inoperable by the time it is discovered.

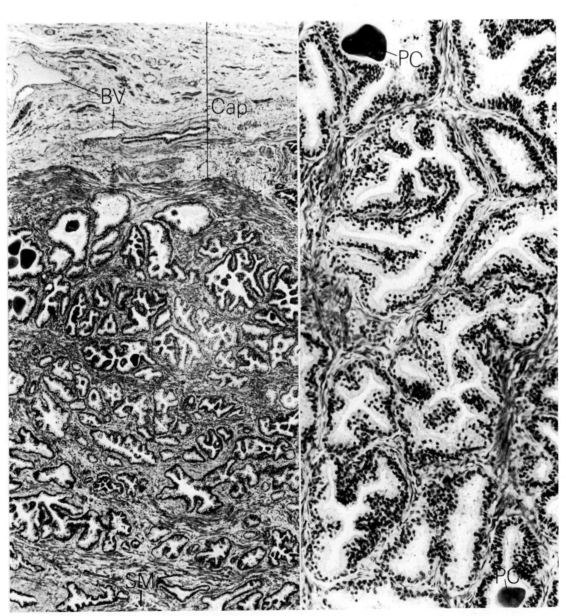

Figure 21.28. Photomicrograph of human prostate gland. **a.** The gland has a thick capsule *(Cap)* that contains numerous large blood vessels *(BV)*. Fibromuscular stroma composed of smooth muscle fibers *(SM)* and dense connective tissue surrounds the glandular component of the prostate. ×40. **b.** Prostatic concretions *(PC)* are commonly seen in the lumen of tubuloalveolar glands. ×145.

around cell fragments. They may become partially calcified.

Bulbourethral Glands (Cowper's Glands)

The Bulbourethral Glands Secrete Preseminal Fluid

The paired bulbourethral glands are pea-sized structures located in the urogenital diaphragm (see Fig. 21.1). The duct of each gland passes through the inferior fascia of the urogenital diaphragm and joins the initial portion of the penile urethra. The glands are compound tubuloalveolar glands that structurally resemble mucus secretory glands (Fig. 21.29). The simple columnar epithelium, which varies considerably in height depending on the functional state of the gland, is under the control of testosterone.

The clear, mucus-like glandular secretion contains considerable amounts of galactose and galactosamine, galacturonic acid, sialic acid, and methylpentose. Erotic stimulation causes release of the secretion, which constitutes the major portion of the preseminal fluid and probably serves as a lubricant of the penile urethra.

SEMEN

Semen Is the Combined Product of All of the Glandular Elements of the Male Reproductive System

Semen contains fluids and sperm from the testis and secretory products from the epididymis, vas deferens, prostate, seminal vesicles, and bulbourethral glands. It is alkaline and may help to neutralize the acid environment of the urethra and the vagina. Semen also contains prostaglandins that may influence sperm transit in both the male and female reproductive ducts and that may have a role in implantation of a fertilized ovum.

The volume of the average ejaculate of semen is about 3 mL. This normally contains up to 100 million sperm per mL, of which it is estimated that 20% are morphologically abnormal and nearly 25% are immotile.

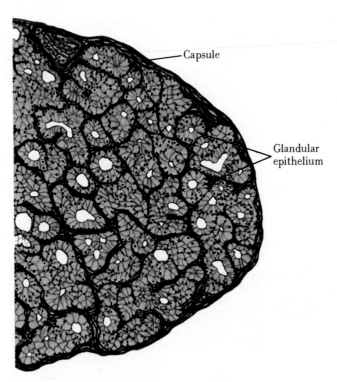

Capsule

Glandular epithelium

Figure 21.29.   Drawing of a portion of a bulbourethral gland lobule. The variation in the height of the epithelial cells of this compound tubuloalveolar gland reflects differences in their functional state.   ×120 (After Stieve H: Männliche Genitalorgane. In: von Möllendorf W (ed): *Handbuch der Mikroscopische Anatomie des Menschen*. Berlin, Springer, part 2, 1930, p 7.)

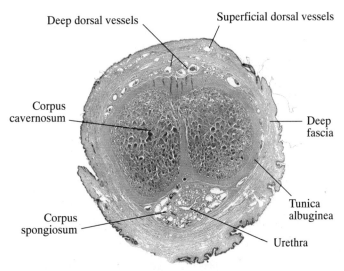

Figure 21.30. Photomicrograph of a histologic section of the penis.

PENIS

The penis is the termination of both the urinary system and the reproductive excurrent duct system in the male. The urethra, which originates at the bladder and extends through the penis, carries both semen and urine to the exterior.

Erection of the Penis Involves the Filling of the Vascular Sinuses of the Corpora Cavernosa and Spongiosum

The penis consists principally of two dorsal masses of erectile tissue, the ***corpora cavernosa,*** and a ventral mass of erectile tissue, the ***corpus spongiosum*** (corpus cavernosum urethrae), in which the urethra is embedded. A dense fibroelastic layer, the ***tunica albuginea,*** binds the three together and forms a capsule around each one (Fig. 21.30). The corpora cavernosa are lined with vascular endothelium. They increase in size and rigidity by filling with blood, principally derived from the ***helicine arteries.*** These arteries dilate under sexual stimulation to increase the blood flow to the penis. As the erectile tissue fills, the peripheral veins that normally drain it are increasingly compressed, and this may amplify the erectile response. The presence of an arteriovenous (AV) anastomosis between the deep artery of the penis and the peripheral venous system has recently been confirmed. Autonomic activity triggered by erotic stimulation regulates the flow of blood either into the corpora cavernosa or into the AV shunt.

The skin of the penis is thin and loosely attached to the underlying loose connective tissue except at the ***glans,*** where it is very thin and tightly attached. The skin of the glans is so thin that blood within its large, muscular anastomosing veins that drain the corpus spongiosum may give it a bluish color. There is no adipose tissue in the subcutaneous tissue. There is, however, a thin layer of smooth muscle that is continuous with the dartos layer of the scrotum. In uncircumcised males, the glans is covered with a fold of skin, the ***prepuce,*** that resembles a mucous membrane on its inner aspect. Numerous sebaceous glands are present in the skin of the penis just proximal to the glans.

The penis is innervated by spinal, sympathetic, and parasympathetic nerves. Many sensory nerve endings are distributed throughout the tissue of the penis, and sympathetic and parasympathetic visceral motor fibers innervate the smooth muscle of the trabeculae of the tunica albuginea and the blood vessels. Both sensory and visceral motor fibers play essential roles in the erectile and ejaculatory responses.

PLATE 106. Testis I

FIGURE 1, testis, monkey, hematoxylin and eosin (H&E) ×65. This section of the testis shows the seminiferous tubules, the tunica albuginea *(TA),* and the capsule of the organ. Extending from the very thick capsule are connective tissue septa *(S)* that divide the organ into compartments. Each compartment contains several seminiferous tubules and represents a lobule *(L).* Blood vessels *(BV)* are present within the inner portion of the capsule, the part referred to as the tunica vasculosa, and in the connective tissue septa.

The seminiferous tubules are convoluted; thus, the profiles they present in a section are variable in appearance. Not infrequently, the wall of a tubule is sectioned tangentially, thus obscuring the lumen and revealing what appears to be a solid mass of cells *(X).*

FIGURE 2, testis, monkey, H&E ×400. Examination at higher magnification, as in this figure, reveals a population of interstitial cells that occur in small clusters and lie in the space between adjoining tubules. They consist mostly of Leydig cells *(LC),* the chief source of testosterone in the male. They are readily identified by virtue of their location and by their small round nucleus and eosinophilic cytoplasm. Macrophages are also found in close association with the Leydig cells, but in lesser number. They are, however, difficult to identify in H&E sections.

A layer of closely apposed squamous cells forms a sheath-like investment around the tubule epithelium of each seminiferous tubule. In man, several layers of cells invest the tubule epithelium. The cells of this peritubular investment exhibit myoid features and account for the slow peristaltic activity of the tubules. Peripheral to the myoid layer is a broad lymphatic channel that occupies an extensive space between the tubules. In routine histologic sections, however, the lymphatic channels are usually collapsed and, thus, unrecognizable. The cellular elements that surround the tubule epithelium are generally referred to as a lamina propria *(LP)* or as a boundary tissue. As a lamina propria, it is atypical. It is not a loose connective tissue. Indeed, under normal circumstances, lymphocytes and other cell types related to the immune system are conspicuously absent.

Examination of the tubule epithelium reveals two kinds of cells: a proliferating population of spermatogenic cells and a nonproliferating population, the sustentacular, or Sertoli cells. The Sertoli cells are considerably fewer in number and can be recognized by their elongate, pale-staining nuclei *(Sn)* and conspicuous nucleolus. The Sertoli cell cytoplasm extends from the periphery of the tubule to the lumen.

The spermatogenic cells consist of successive generations arranged in concentric layers. Thus, the spermatogonia *(Sg)* are found at the periphery. The spermatocytes *(Sc),* most of which have large round nuclei with a distinctive chromatin pattern (due to their chromatin material being reorganized), come to lie above the spermatogonia. The spermatid population *(Sp)* consists of one or two generations and occupies the site closest to the lumen. The tubules in this figure have been identified according to their stage of development. The tubule at the upper right can be identified as stage VI. At this stage, the mature population of spermatids (identified by their dark-blue heads and eosinophilic thread-like flagella protruding into the lumen) are in the process of being released (spermiogenesis). The younger generation of spermatids is composed of round cells and exhibits round nuclei. Moving clockwise, the tubule indicated as stage VII is slightly more advanced. The mature spermatids are now gone. Progressing to stage VIII, the tubule at the bottom of the micrograph reveals that the spermatid population is undergoing a change in nuclear shape. Note the tapered nuclei *(arrows).* Further maturation of the spermatids is reflected in the tubule at the top of the micrograph, stage XI. Finally, the tubule marked as stage II, on the left, reveals slightly greater maturation of the luminal spermatids, and with the start of the new cycle (stage I), a newly formed spermatid population is now present. By examining the spermatid population and assessing the number of generations present, i.e., one or two, and the degree of maturation, it is possible with the aid of a chart to approximate the stage of a tubule.

KEY

BV, blood vessels
L, lobule
LC, Leydig cells
LP, lamina propria
S, connective tissue septa

Sc, spermatocytes
Sg, spermatogonia
Sn, Sertoli nuclei
Sp, spermatids

TA, tunica albuginea
X, tangential section of tubule with lumen obscured
arrows, spermatid nuclei displaying early shape change

PLATE 106

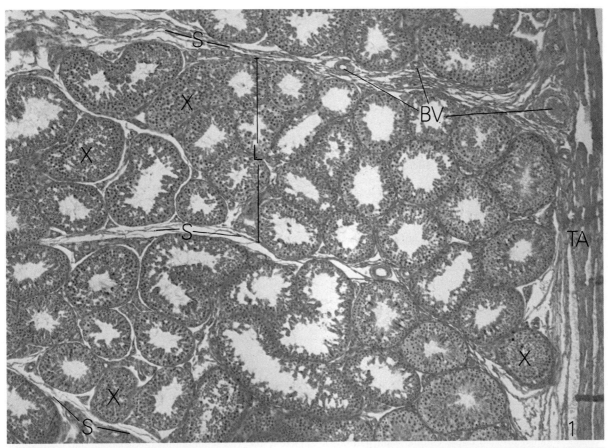

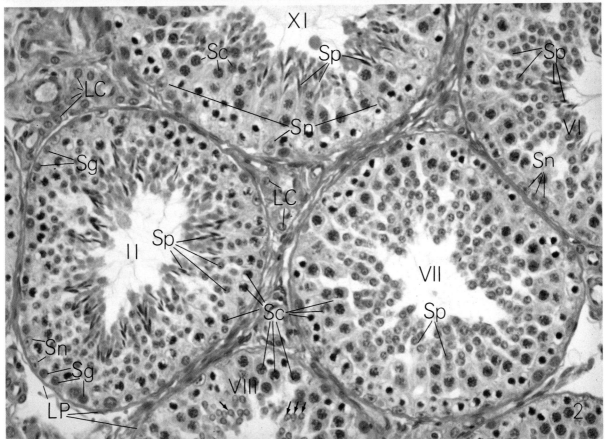

PLATE 107. Testis II

FIGURE 1, testis, newborn human, H&E ×180; inset ×360. *Prepubertal testis.* The various germ cell types representative of spermatogenesis in the mature seminiferous tubules are not present in the testis before puberty or in the postpubertal undescended testis. Instead, the "tubules" are represented by cords of cells in which a lumen is lacking. The seminiferous cords display the same tortuosity as in the adult; the tunica albuginea *(TA)* of the testis, though thinner, is of the same relative thickness.

The seminiferous cords are of considerably smaller diameter than the tubules of the adult and are composed of two cell types: the gonocyte or first-generation spermatogonium, derived from the primordial germ cell that migrates from the yolk sac to the developing gonad in the embryo; and a cell that resembles the Sertoli cell of the adult. The latter cell type predominates and comprises the bulk of the cord. The cells are columnar, and their nuclei are close to the basement membrane. The gonocytes *(G)* are the precursors of the definitive germ cells or spermatogonia. They are round cells that have a centrally placed, spherical nucleus. The cytoplasm takes little stain and usually appears as a light ring around the nucleus. This gives the gonocyte a distinctive appearance in histologic sections **(inset).** Generally, the gonocytes are found at the periphery of the cord, but many are also found more centrally placed. The gonocytes give rise to spermatogonia that begin to proliferate in males between the ages of 10 and 13 years. The seminiferous epithelium then becomes populated with cells at various stages of spermatogenesis, as seen in the adult.

The epithelial cords are surrounded by one or two layers of cells with long processes and flat nuclei. They resemble fibroblasts at the ultrastructural level and give rise to the myoid peritubular cells of the adult.

The interstitial cells of Leydig are conspicuous in the newborn, a reflection of the residual effects of maternal hormones. Leydig cells, however, regress and do not become conspicuous again until puberty. In this preparation, the Leydig cells *(LC)* can be seen between the cords **(inset).** They are ovoid or polygonal and are closely grouped, so that adjacent cells are in contact with each other. Overall, they have the same appearance as the Leydig cells of the adult.

FIGURE 2, testis, H&E ×65. *Straight tubules and rete testes.* In the posterior portion of the testis, the connective tissue of the tunica albuginea extends more deeply into the organ. This inward extension of connective tissue is called the mediastinum testis. It contains a network of anastomosing channels called the rete testis. Only a small portion of the mediastinum testis *(MT)* is evident in the figure. The area includes, however, a few seminiferous tubules *(ST)* in the upper portion of the micrograph and, fortuitously, the site where one of the seminiferous tubules terminates and joins the rete testis *(RT)*. This can be recognized in the area delineated by the *rectangle,* which is shown at higher magnification in Figure 3. As noted earlier, the seminiferous tubules are arranged in the form of a loop, with each end joining the rete testis. The seminiferous tubules open into the rete testis by way of a straight tubule or tubulus rectus. The tubuli recti are very short and are lined by Sertoli-like cells; no germ cell component is present.

FIGURE 3, testis, monkey, H&E ×400. The tubulus rectus *(TR)* in this figure appears to end on one side before it ends on the other. This is simply a reflection of the angle of section. When the straight tubule ends, however, the epithelial lining suddenly becomes cuboidal. This represents the rete testis, which constitutes an anastomosing system of channels that lead to the efferent ductules. The epithelial lining cells of the rete are sometimes more squamous than cuboidal or, occasionally, may be low columnar in appearance. Typically, they possess a single cilium; however, this is difficult to see in routine H&E preparations.

The connective tissue of the mediastinum is very dense but exhibits no other special features, nor is smooth muscle present. Adipose cells *(AC)* and blood vessels *(BV)*, particularly veins of varying size, are present within the connective tissue.

KEY

AC, adipose cells	**LC,** Leydig cells	**ST,** seminiferous tubules
BV, blood vessels	**MT,** mediastinum testis	**TA,** tunica albuginea
G, gonocytes	**RT,** rete testis	**TR,** tubulus rectus

PLATE 107

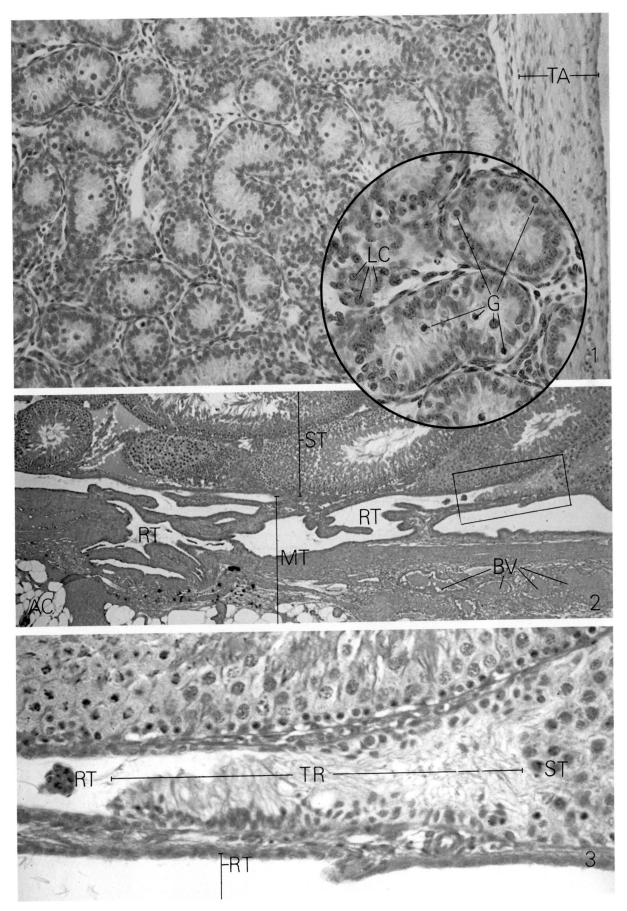

PLATE 108. Ductuli Efferentes and Epididymis

FIGURE 1, ductuli efferentes, monkey, H&E ×60; inset ×360. About 12–20 efferent ductules leave the testis and serve as channels from the rete testis to the ductus epididymis. Each of the efferent ductules undergoes numerous spiral windings and convolutions to form a group of conical structures; together they constitute the initial part of the head of the epididymis. When examined in a tissue section, the ductules exhibit a variety of irregular profiles due to their twisting and turning. This is evident in this figure on the right side of the micrograph.

The epithelium that lines the efferent ductules is distinctive in that groups of tall columnar cells alternate with groups of cuboidal cells, giving the luminal surface an unevenly contoured appearance. Thus, small cup-like depressions are created where the epithelium contains groups of cuboidal or low columnar cells. Typically, these shorter cells exhibit a brush border-like apical surface due to the microvilli that they possess (*arrowhead,* **inset**). The basal surface of the ductule, in contrast, has a smooth contour (see Fig. 2 and **inset**). Some of the cells, generally the tall columnar cells, possess cilia *(C)* **(inset).** Whereas the ciliated cells aid in moving the contents of the tubule toward the epididymis, the cells with the microvilli are largely responsible for absorbing fluid from the lumen. In addition to the columnar and cuboidal cells, basal cells are also present; thus, the epithelium is designated pseudostratified columnar. The basal cells possess little cytoplasm and presumably serve as a stem cell.

The efferent ductules possess a thin layer of circularly arranged smooth muscle cells *(SM,* **inset**). The muscle is close to the basal surface of the epithelial cells, being separated from it by only a small amount of connective tissue *(CT,* **inset**). Because of this close association, the smooth muscle may be overlooked or misidentified as connective tissue. Smooth muscle facilitates movement of luminal contents of the ductule to the ductus epididymis.

FIGURE 2, epididymis, monkey, H&E ×180. The epididymis, by virtue of its shape, is divided into a head, body, and tail. The initial part of the head contains the ductus epididymis, a single convoluted duct into which the efferent ductules open. The duct is, at first, highly convoluted but becomes less tortuous in the body and tail. A section through the head of the epididymis, as shown in Figure 1, cuts the ductus epididymis in numerous places, and as in the efferent ductules, different-shaped profiles are observed.

The epithelium contains two distinguishable cell types: tall columnar cells and basal cells similar to those of the efferent ductules. The epithelium is, thus, also pseudostratified columnar. The columnar cells are tallest in the head of the epididymis and diminish in height as the tail is reached. The free surface of the cell possesses stereocilia *(SC).* These are extremely long, branching microvilli. They evidently adhere to each other during the preparation of the tissue to form the fine tapering structures that are characteristically seen with the light microscope. The nuclei of the columnar cells are elongated and are located a moderate distance from the base of the cell. They are readily distinguished from the spherical nuclei of the basal cells that lie close to the basement membrane. Other conspicuous features of the columnar cells include a very large supranuclear Golgi apparatus (not seen at the magnification offered here), pigment accumulations *(P),* and, demonstrable with appropriate techniques, numerous lysosomes.

Because of the unusual height of the columnar cells and, again, the tortuosity of the duct, an uneven lumen appears in some sites; indeed, even "islands" of epithelium can be encountered in the lumen (see *arrows,* Fig. 1). Such profiles are accounted for by sharp turns in the duct where the epithelial wall on one side of the duct is partially cut. For example, a cut in the plane of the *double-headed arrow* indicated in this figure would create such an isolated epithelial island.

A thin layer of smooth muscle circumscribes the duct and appears similar to that associated with the efferent ductules. In the terminal portion of the epididymis, however, the smooth muscle acquires a greater thickness, and longitudinal fibers are also present. Beyond the smooth muscle coat there is a small amount of connective tissue *(CT)* that binds the loops of the duct together and carries the blood vessels *(BV)* and nerves.

KEY

AT, adipose tissue
BV, blood vessel
C, cilia
CT, connective tissue
P, pigment
SC, stereocilia
SM, smooth muscle
arrowhead (inset), brush border
arrows, "islands" of epithelium in the lumen

PLATE 108

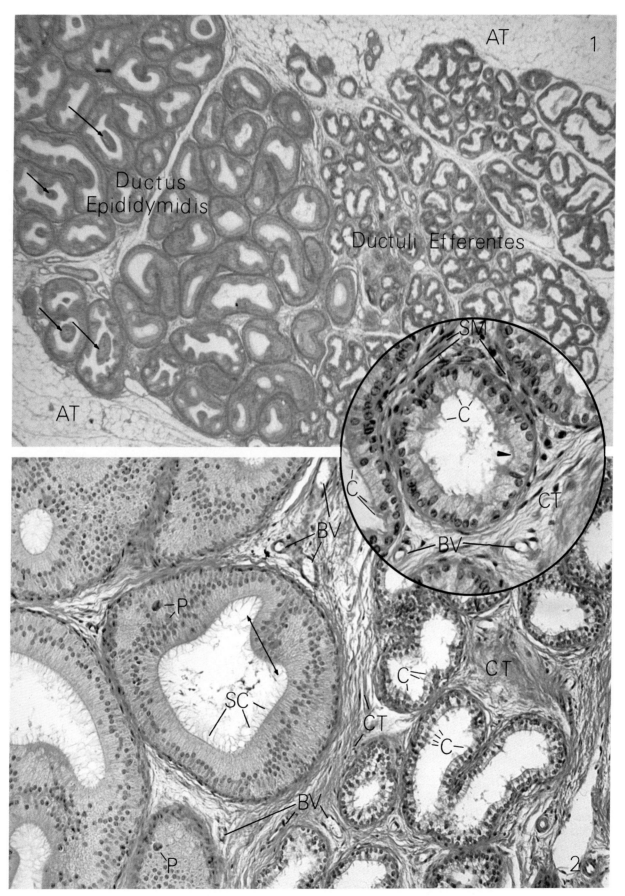

PLATE 109. Spermatic Cord and Ductus Deferens

The ductus (vas) deferens continues from the duct of the epididymis as a thick-walled muscular tube that leaves the scrotum and passes through the inguinal canal as a component of the spermatic cord. At the deep inguinal ring, it continues into the pelvis and, behind the urinary bladder, joins with the seminal vesicle to form the ejaculatory duct. The ejaculatory duct then pierces the prostate gland and opens into the urethra.

FIGURE 1, spermatic cord, human, H&E ×80. A cross section through the ductus deferens and some of the vessels and nerves that accompany the duct in the spermatic cord are shown in this figure. The wall of the ductus deferens is extremely thick, mostly due to the presence of a large amount of smooth muscle. The muscle contracts when the tissue is removed, causing the mucosa to form longitudinal folds. For this reason, in histologic sections, the lumen *(L)* usually appears irregular in cross section.

The smooth muscle of the ductus deferens is arranged as a thick outer longitudinal layer [*(L)*], a thick middle circular layer [*(C)*], and a thinner inner longitudinal layer [*(L)*]. Between the epithelium and the inner longitudinal smooth muscle layer there is a moderately thick cellular layer of loose connective tissue, the lamina propria *(LP)*. The connective tissue immediately surrounding the ductus deferens contains nerves and some of the smaller blood vessels that supply the duct. In fact, some of these vessels can be seen penetrating the outer longitudinal smooth muscle layer *(asterisks)*.

FIGURE 2, ductus deferens, human, H&E ×320; inset ×250. The epithelial lining of the ductus deferens consists of pseudostratified columnar epithelium with stereocilia *(arrowheads)*. It resembles the epithelium of the epididymis, but the cells are not as tall. The elongated nuclei of the columnar cells are readily distinguished from the spherical nuclei of the basal cells *(arrows)*. The epithelium rests on a loose connective tissue that extends to the smooth muscle; no submucosa is described.

A unique feature of the spermatic cord is the presence of a plexus of atypical veins (pampiniform plexus) that arise from the spermatic veins. These vessels receive the blood from the testis. (The pampiniform plexus also receives tributaries from the epididymis.) The plexus is an anastomosing vascular network that comprises the bulk of the spermatic cord. Portions of several of these veins *(BV)* are evident in the upper right of Figure 1 along with a number of nerves *(N)*. The unusual feature of the veins is their thick muscular wall that, at a glance, gives the appearance of an artery rather than a vein. Careful examination of these vessels **(inset)** shows that the bulk of the vessel wall is composed of two layers of smooth muscle—an outer circular layer *SM(C)* and an inner longitudinal layer *SM(L)*.

KEY

BV, blood vessels
CT, connective tissue
L, lumen of ductus deferens
LP, lamina propria
Lu, lumen of blood vessel

N, nerve
SM(C), circular layer of smooth muscle
SM(L), longitudinal layer of smooth muscle

arrowheads, stereocilia
arrows (Fig. 2), basal cell nucleus
asterisks (Fig. 1), small arteries supplying ductus deferens

PLATE 109

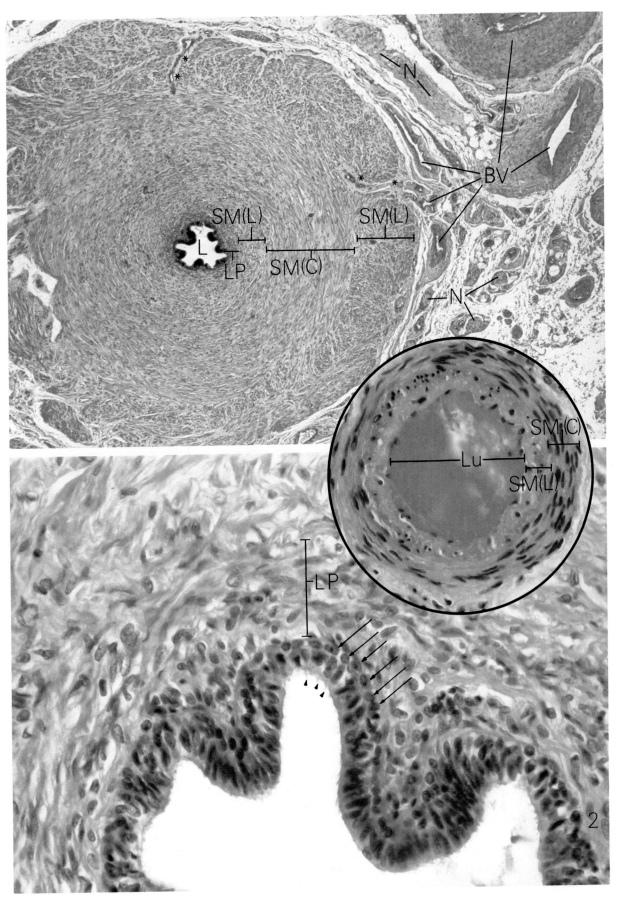

PLATE 110. Prostate Gland

The prostate gland surrounds the first part of the urethra. It consists of about 30–50 tubuloalveolar glands that are contained in a fibroelastic stroma. The stroma is characterized by the presence of numerous small bundles of smooth muscle, so that it can also be described as a fibromuscular stroma. Surrounding the gland is a fibroelastic capsule that also contains small bundles of smooth muscle. Ducts from the gland empty into the urethra.

FIGURE 1, prostate, human, H&E ×60. A section of the prostate gland is shown in this figure. The capsule *(Cap)* is in the upper part of the figure; the glandular components are in the lower part. The tubuloalveoli of the prostate gland vary greatly in form, as shown in this figure. They may appear as tubes, as alveoli, as alveoli with branches, or as tubes with branches. They may appear distended or may be collapsed. Frequently, in older individuals, precipitates [prostatic concretions *(PC)*] are present in the lumina. These stain with eosin and may have a concentric lamellar appearance. With time, they may become impregnated with calcium salts.

FIGURE 2, prostate, human, H&E ×145. The area enclosed within the *large rectangle* of Figure 1 is seen here at higher magnification and shows some characteristic features of the tubuloalveoli. In many places the epithelium bulges into the lumen; sometimes, the top of an epithelial fold is cut to give the impression of an island of cells in a lumen *(arrows)*. Large numbers of closely packed nuclei are seen when a fold is cut obliquely or crosswise *(arrowheads)*. This is one of the characteristic features of the prostate gland epithelium.

FIGURE 3, prostate, human, H&E ×64. This figure shows the epithelial cells at higher magnification. The epithelium consists mainly of columnar cells, although basal cells are also present. For this reason, the epithelium is classified as pseudostratified columnar. The columnar cells are described as containing secretion granules and lipid droplets, but these are not always evident. Many cells possess apical cytoplasmic protrusions *(arrows)* that seemingly break off into the lumen.

The various tubuloalveoli are surrounded by a fibroelastic stroma containing smooth muscle (fibromuscular stroma). The smooth muscle is not organized in a way that suggests that it belongs to any single tube or alveolus, as in the epididymis, but, rather, appears to be randomly dispersed in the stroma. In Figure 1, the staining of the muscle differs from the staining of the connective tissue. The muscle appears as the elongated dark fibers or as dark oval bodies *(SM)*, in either case surrounded by a more extensive continuous phase of the lighter-staining connective tissue. Some bundles of smooth muscle are also to be seen in the capsule.

FIGURE 4, prostate, human, H&E ×160. The *upper rectangle* in Figure 1, examined here at higher magnification, shows the smooth muscle cut in longitudinal [*(L)*] and cross section [*(X)*] and also reveals the presence of a nerve bundle *(N)*. The nerve stains very much like the connective tissue but can be recognized by virtue of its organization and the presence of a perineurial sheath. These features would be more evident at higher magnification.

KEY

BV, blood vessels
Cap, capsule
N, nerve bundle
PC, prostatic concretion
SM, smooth muscle
SM(L), smooth muscle, longitudinal section
SM(X), smooth muscle, cross section
arrowheads, nuclear clusters
arrows: Fig. 2, epithelial "islands;" Fig. 3, apical cytoplasmic protrusions

PLATE 110

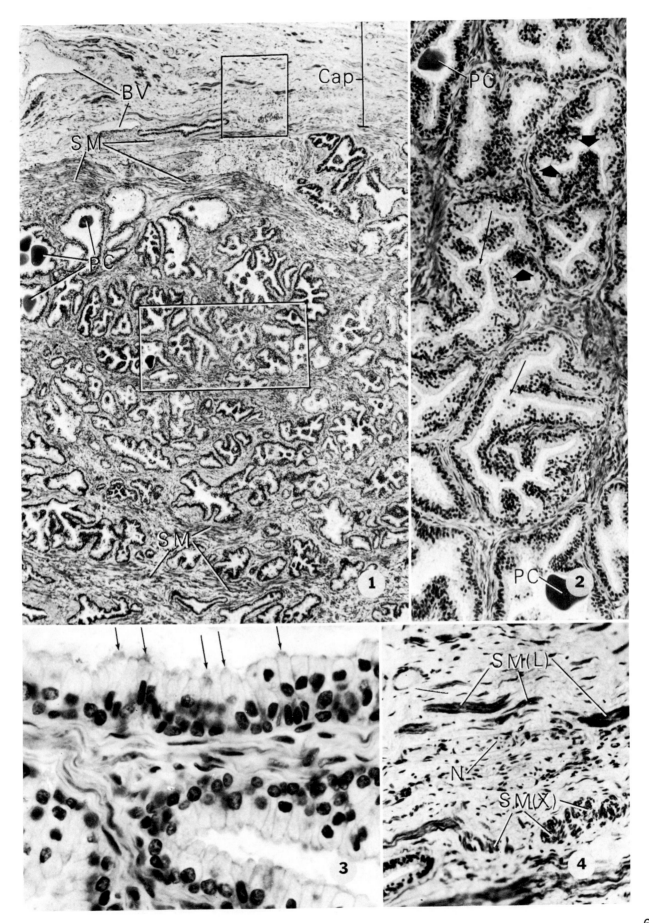

PLATE 111. Seminal Vesicle

The mucosa of the seminal vesicle rests on a thick layer of smooth muscle. The smooth muscle consists of an indistinct inner circular layer and an outer longitudinal layer, but these are difficult to distinguish. Beyond the smooth muscle is the connective tissue of the adventitia.

FIGURE 1, seminal vesicle, human, H&E ×30. This figure shows a cross section of a seminal vesicle. Due to the coiled nature of the vesicle, two almost distinct lumina, lying side by side, appear to be present. They are, however, connected so that, in effect, all of the internal spaces are continuous and what is seen here is actually a two-dimensional configuration reflecting a coiling of the tube.

The mucosa of the seminal vesicles is characterized by being extensively folded or ridged. The ridges vary in size and typically branch and interconnect with one another. The larger ridges may form recesses that contain smaller ridges, and when these are cut obliquely, they appear as mucosal arches that enclose the smaller folds *(arrows)*. When the plane of section is normal to the surface, the mucosal ridges appear as "villi." In some areas, particularly the peripheral region of the lumen, the interconnecting folds of the mucosa appear as alveoli. Each of these chambers is, however, simply a pocket-like structure that is open and continuous with the lumen.

The seminal vesicles are paired elongated sacs. Each vesicle consists of a single tube folded and coiled on itself with occasional diverticula in its wall. The upper extremity ends as a cul-de-sac; the lower extremity is constricted into a narrow straight duct that joins and empties into its corresponding ductus deferens.

FIGURE 2, seminal vesicle, human, H&E ×220. This higher magnification of the mucosal folds reveals the epithelium *(Ep)* and the underlying loose connective tissue *(CT)* or lamina propria *(LP)*. The epithelium is described as pseudostratified. It is composed of low columnar or cuboidal cells and small round basal cells. The latter are randomly interspersed between the larger principal cells, but they are relatively sparse in number. For this reason, the epithelium may not be readily recognized as pseudostratified. In some areas, the epithelium appears thick *(arrowhead)* and, based on the disposition of the nuclei, would seem to be multilayered. This is due to a tangential section of the epithelium and is not a true stratification. The lamina propria of the mucosa is composed of a very cellular connective tissue containing some smooth muscle cells *(SM)* and is rich in elastic fibers.

KEY

CT, connective tissue
Ep, epithelium
LP, lamina propria
SM, smooth muscle
arrowhead, oblique section of epithelium
arrows, mucosal arches

PLATE 111

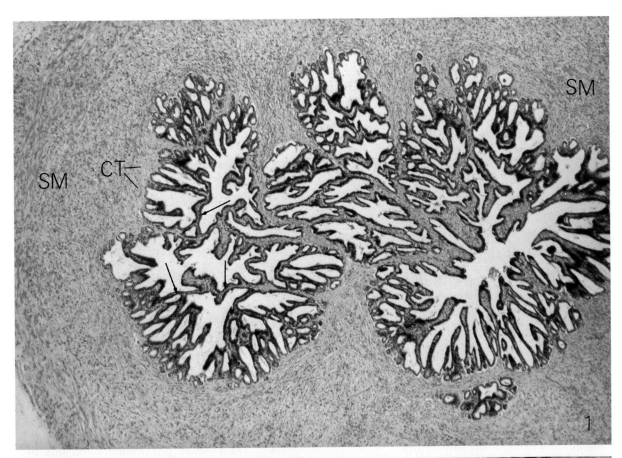

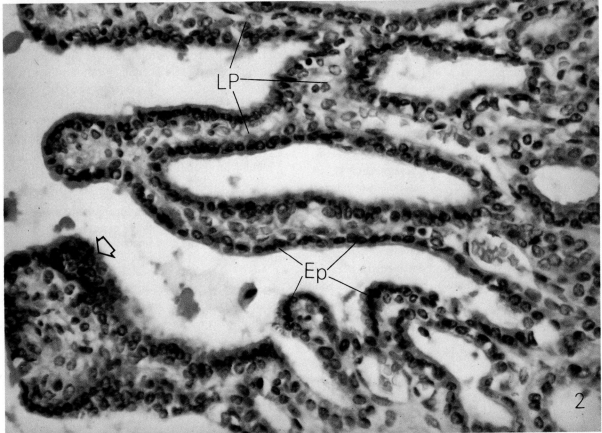

Female Reproductive System

22

The Female Reproductive System Consists of Internal Sex Organs and External Genital Structures

The internal female reproductive organs are located in the pelvis, and the external genital structures (external genitalia) are situated in the anterior part of the perineum known as the *vulva.*

- The internal organs are the *ovaries, oviducts, uterus,* and *vagina* (Fig. 22.1).
- The external genitalia include the *mons pubis, labia majora* and *minora, clitoris, vestibule* and *opening of the vagina,* and *external urethral orifice.*

The mammary glands are included in this chapter because their development and functional state are directly related to the hormonal activity of the female reproductive system. Similarly, the placenta is included because of its functional and physical relationship with the uterus in pregnancy.

The ovaries, oviducts, and uterus of the sexually mature female undergo marked structural and functional changes related to neural activity and changes in hormonal levels during each menstrual cycle and during pregnancy. These mechanisms also regulate the early development of the female reproductive system. The initiation of the menstrual cycle, referred to as the *menarche,* occurs in females between ages 9 and 14 years (average 13.5 years) and marks the end of puberty and the beginning of the reproductive life span. During this phase of life, the *menstrual cycle* averages about 28–30 days in length. Between ages 45 and 55 years, the menstrual cycles become increasingly infrequent and then cease. This change in reproductive function is referred to as the *menopause* or climacterium (commonly called the ''change of life''). The ovaries cease their reproductive function of producing ova and their endocrine function of producing hormones that regulate reproductive activity. Other organs, e.g., vagina and mammary glands, show other varying degrees of reduced function, particularly secretory activity.

OVARY

Production of Gametes and Production of Steroid Hormones Are the Two Major Functions of the Ovary

The ovaries have two interrelated functions: the production of gametes *(gametogenesis)* and the production of steroids *(steroidogenesis).* In the female, the production of gametes is called *oogenesis.* Developing gametes are called *oocytes;* mature gametes are called *ova.*

Two major groups of steroid hormones are secreted by the ovaries. They are the estrogens and the progestogens.

- *Estrogens* promote growth and maturation of internal and external sex organs and are responsible for the typical female characteristics that develop at the time of puberty. Estrogens also act on mammary glands to promote breast development by stimulating ductal and stromal growth and accumulation of adipose tissue.
- *Progestogens* prepare the internal sex organs, mainly the uterus, for pregnancy by promoting secretory changes in the endometrium (this is discussed in the section on cyclic changes in the endometrium). Progestogens also prepare the mammary gland for lactation by promoting lobular proliferation.

Both hormones play an important role in the menstrual cycle by preparing the uterus for implantation of a fertilized ovum. If implantation does not occur, the uterus undergoes degeneration of the endometrium followed by menstruation.

Ovarian Structure

In nulliparas (woman who have not borne children), the ovaries are paired, almond-shaped, pinkish-white structures measuring about 3 cm in length, 1.5 cm in width, and 1 cm in thickness.

Each ovary is attached to the posterior surface of the broad ligament by a peritoneal fold, the mesovarium (Fig. 22.1). The *superior (or tubal) pole* of the ovary is attached to the pelvic wall by the *suspensory ligament* of the ovary, which carries the ovarian vessels and nerves. The *inferior (or uterine) pole* is attached to the uterus by the *ovarian ligament.* This ligament is a remnant of the *gubernaculum,* the ligament that attaches the developing gonad to the floor of the pelvis. Before puberty, the surface of the ovary is smooth, but during reproductive life it becomes progressively scarred and irregular due to repeated ovulations. In postmenopausal women, the ovaries are about one-fourth the size observed during the reproductive period.

The Ovary Is Composed of a Cortex and a Medulla

A section through the ovary reveals two distinct regions:

- *Medulla* or *medullary region* located in the central portion of the ovary contains loose connective tissue, a mass of relatively large contorted blood vessels, lymphatic vessels, and nerves (Fig. 22.2).
- *Cortex* or *cortical region* found in the peripheral portion of the ovary surrounding the medulla contains the *ovarian follicles* embedded in a richly cellular connective tissue. Scattered smooth muscle fibers are present in the stroma around the follicles. The boundary between the medulla and cortex is indistinct. At the hilum, the cortex is interrupted, and the mesovarium is continuous with the medulla. Small, irregular blind ducts, the *rete ovarii,* which are remnants of the fetal indifferent gonad, may be found in this region.

"Germinal Epithelium" Instead of Mesothelium Covers the Ovary

The surface of the ovary is covered by a single layer of cuboidal, in some parts almost squamous cells. This cellular layer, known as the *germinal epithelium,* is continuous with the mesothelium that covers the mesovarium. The term *germinal epithelium* is a carryover from earlier days when it was incorrectly thought to be the site of germ cell formation in development. It is now known that the *primordial germ cells* (of both the male and female) are of extragonadal origin and that they migrate from the embryonic yolk sac into the cortex of the embryonic gonad where they differentiate and induce differentiation of the ovary. A dense connective tissue layer, the *tunica albuginea,* lies between the germinal epithelium and the underlying cortex.

Ovarian Follicles Provide the Microenvironment for the Developing Oocyte

Ovarian follicles of various sizes, each containing a single oocyte, are distributed in the stroma of the cortex. The size of a follicle is indicative of the developmental state of the oocyte. Early stages of oogenesis occur during fetal life when mitotic divisions massively increase the number of oogonia (see section on oogenesis). The oocytes present at birth remain arrested in their development at the first meiotic division (see page 51). As a young female passes through puberty, the ovaries begin a phase of reproductive activity

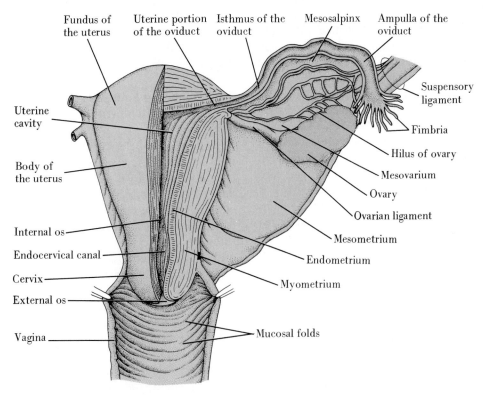

Figure 22.1. Schematic drawing of the components of the female reproductive system. (Based on Warwick R, Williams PL (eds): *Gray's Anatomy,* 35 ed. Edinburgh, Churchill Livingstone, 1973, p 1351.)

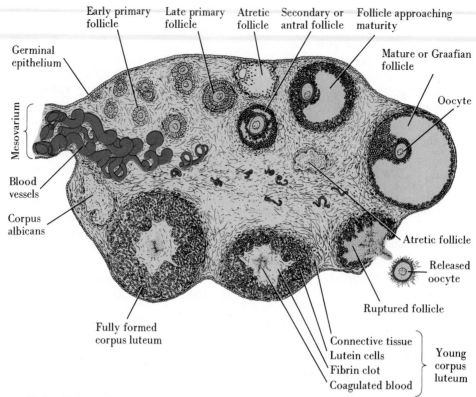

Figure 22.2. Schematic drawing of a section through the ovary. Highly coiled blood vessels are present in the hilum and medullary regions. (After C. E. Corliss.)

characterized by the cyclic growth and maturation of small groups of follicles. The first ovulation generally does not take place for a year or more following menarche. A cyclic pattern of follicular maturation and ovulation then continues in parallel with the menstrual cycle. Normally, only one oocyte reaches full maturity and is released from the ovary during each menstrual cycle. Obviously, the maturation and release of more than one egg at ovulation may lead to multiple zygotes. During the reproductive life span, a woman produces only about 400 mature ova. Most of the estimated 600,000–800,000 primary oocytes present at birth fail to complete maturation and are gradually lost through *atresia.* Atresia describes the spontaneous death and subsequent resorption of immature oocytes. This process begins as early as the fifth month of fetal life and reduces the number of primary oocytes from as many as 5 million in the fetus to less than 20% of that number at birth. The few oocytes that remain at menopause degenerate within a few years.

Follicle Development

Histologically, three basic types of ovarian follicles can be identified, based on developmental state:

• *Primordial follicles*
• *Growing follicles*
• *Mature* or *Graafian follicles* (Fig. 22.3)

The growing follicles are further subcategorized as *primary* and *secondary (or antral) follicles.* Some histologists identify additional stages in the continuum of follicular development. In the cycling ovary, follicles are found at all stages of development. The primordial follicles predominate.

The Primordial Follicle Is the Earliest Stage of Follicular Development

Primordial follicles first appear in the ovaries during the third month of fetal development. Early growth of the primordial follicles is independent of gonadotropin stimulation. In the developed, mature ovary, the primordial follicles are found in the stroma of the cortex just beneath the tunica albuginea. A single layer of squamous *follicular cells* surrounds the oocyte (Figs. 22.3 and 22.4). The outer surface of the follicular cells is bounded by a basal lamina. At this stage, the oocyte and the surrounding follicular cells are closely apposed to one another. The oocyte in the follicle measures about 30 μm in diameter and has a large eccentric nucleus that contains finely dispersed chromatin and one or more large nucleoli. The cytoplasm of the oocyte, referred to as ooplasm, exhibits a *Balbiani body.* At the ultrastructural level, this is identified as a localized accumulation of Golgi apparatus, endoplasmic reticulum, numerous mitochondria, and lysosomes. In addition, a human oocyte is seen to contain *annulate lamellae,* and numerous small vesicles are scattered throughout the cytoplasm along with small spherical mitochondria. Annulate lamellae resemble a stack of nuclear envelope profiles. Each layer of the stack includes pore structures morphologically identical with nuclear pores.

The Primary Follicle Is the First Stage of the Growing Follicle

As a primordial follicle makes the transition into a growing follicle, changes occur in the oocyte in the follicular cells and in the adjacent stroma. Initially, the oocyte enlarges and the surrounding flattened follicular cells proliferate and become cuboidal. At this stage, i.e., with the follicular cells becoming cuboidal, the follicle is identified as a *primary follicle.* As the oocyte grows, a homogeneous, deeply staining, acidophilic refractile layer called the *zona pellucida* appears between the oocyte and the adjacent follicular cells (Figs. 22.3 and 22.5). The zona pellucida is first apparent with the light microscope when the oocyte, surrounded by a single layer of cuboidal or columnar follicle cells, has grown to a diameter of 50–80 μm. The growing oocyte secretes this gel-like, periodic acid-Schiff (PAS)-positive layer that is rich in glycosaminoglycans and glycoproteins.

Follicular Cells Undergo Stratification to Form the Granulosa Layer of the Primary Follicle

Through rapid mitotic proliferation, the single layer of follicular cells gives rise to a stratified epithelium, the membrana granulosa, surrounding the oocyte. The follicular cells are then identified as the *granulosa cells.* The basal lamina retains its position between the outermost layer of the follicular cells, which become columnar, and the connective tissue stroma.

During follicular growth, extensive gap junctions develop between granulosa cells. Unlike Sertoli cells in the testis, however, the basal layer of the granulosa cells does not possess elaborate tight junctions (zonulae occludentes), an indication that there is not a blood-follicular barrier. Rather, movement of nutrients and small information macromolecules from the blood into the follicular fluid is essential for normal development of the ovum and the follicle.

Connective Tissue Cells Form the Theca Layers of the Primary Follicle

As the granulosa cells proliferate, stromal cells immediately surrounding the follicle form a sheath of connective tissue cells, known as the *theca folliculi,* just external to the basal lamina (Figs. 22.3 and 22.6). The theca folliculi further differentiates into two layers:

- The *theca interna* is the inner, highly vascularized layer of cuboidal secretory cells. The fully differentiated cells

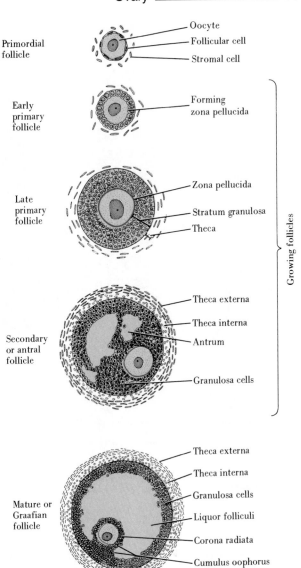

Figure 22.3. Schematic drawing of the stages in the development of ovarian follicles, beginning with the primordial follicle and ending with the mature or Graafian follicle. The secondary and the mature follicle are drawn at reduced size, thus, the smaller-appearing oocytes. The oocyte in a primordial follicle is arrested in the first meiotic prophase. As the follicle continues through its development, the oocyte progresses through the first meiotic division, which is completed just before the release of the oocyte from the mature follicle. The oocyte at this stage is referred to as a secondary oocyte (see text section on oogenesis and maturation of the ovum and fertilization). (Based on Junqueira LC, Carneiro J, Kelley RO: *Basic Histology,* 7th ed. Norwalk, CT, Appleton & Lange, 1992, p 443.)

of the theca interna possess ultrastructural features characteristic of steroid-producing cells. Cells of the theca interna possess a large number of luteinizing hormone (LH) receptors. In response to LH stimulation, they synthesize and secrete the androgens that are the precursors of estrogen. In addition to the secretory cells, the theca interna contains fibroblasts, collagen bundles, and a rich network of small vessels.

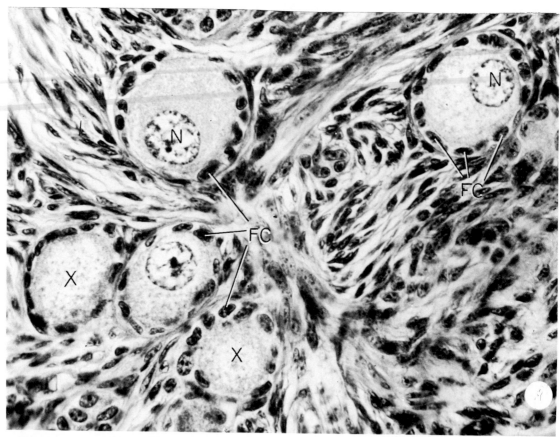

Figure 22.4. Photomicrograph of primordial follicles (monkey). The large oocyte in each follicle is surrounded by a single layer of flattened follicle cells *(FC)*. Usually, the nucleus *(N)* of the oocyte is in an eccentric position. Two oocytes in which the nucleus is not included in the plane of section are indicated *(X)*. ×640.

- The ***theca externa*** is the outer layer of connective tissue cells. It mainly contains smooth muscle cells and bundles of collagen fibers.

Boundaries between the thecal layers and between the theca externa and surrounding stroma are not distinct. However, the basal lamina between the granulosa layer and the theca interna establishes a distinct boundary separating these layers. It separates the rich capillary bed of the theca interna from the granulosa layer, which is avascular during the period of follicular growth.

Maturation of the Oocyte Occurs in the Primary Follicle

The distribution of organelles changes as the oocyte matures. Multiple, dispersed Golgi complexes derived from the single Balbiani body of the primordial oocyte become scattered in the cytoplasm. There is an increase in the number of free ribosomes, mitochondria, small vesicles, and multivesicular bodies and in the amount of rough endoplasmic reticulum (rER). Occasional lipid droplets and masses of lipochrome pigment can also be seen. The oo-

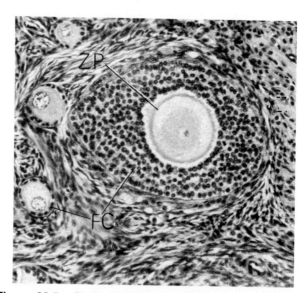

Figure 22.5. Photomicrograph of late primary follicle (monkey). In the late primary follicle, multiple layers of follicle cells *(FC)* surround the primary oocyte. At this stage, a homogeneous-appearing layer called the zona pellucida *(ZP)* is present between the oocyte and follicle cells. In the much smaller, adjacent primordial follicles, a single layer of flattened follicle cells can be seen. ×160.

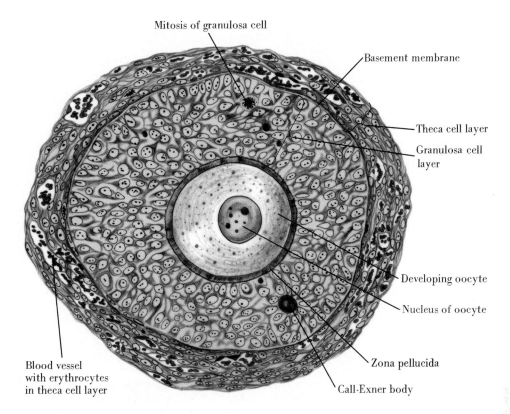

Figure 22.6. Drawing of growing follicle. A basement membrane separates the granulosa cell layer from the theca cell layer. The zona pellucida immediately surrounds the developing oocyte. ×375. (After Maximow AA: In: Bloom W, Fawcett DW: *A Textbook of Histology,* 10th ed. Philadelphia, WB Saunders, 1975, p 865.)

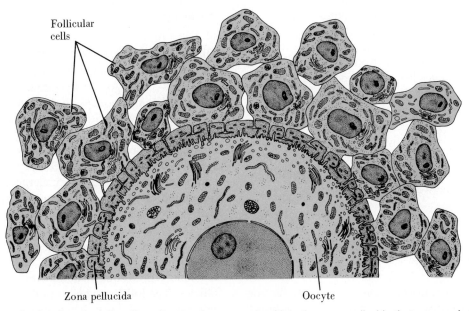

Figure 22.7. Schematic drawing depicting the ultrastructure of an oocyte and adjacent follicular cells. Numerous microvilli from the oocyte and slender processes from the follicular cells extend into the zona pellucida that surrounds the oocyte. (Based on Junqueira LC, Carneiro J, Kelley RO: *Basic Histology,* 7th ed. Norwalk, CT, Appleton & Lange, 1992, p 444.)

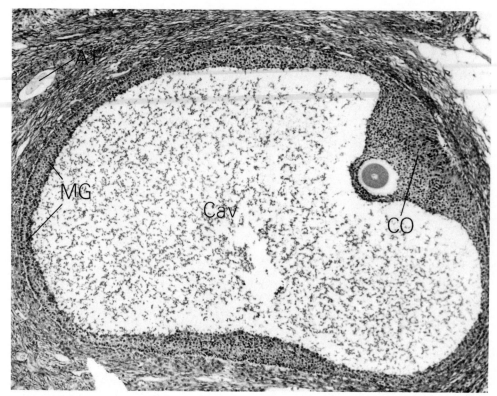

Figure 22.8. Photomicrograph of secondary follicle (monkey). The follicle is characterized by the presence of a large fluid-filled antrum or follicular cavity *(Cav)*. The oocyte is located in a mound of granulosa cells called the cumulus oophorus *(CO)*. The remaining follicle cells that surround the lumen are called the membrana granulosa *(MG)* or granulosa cells. An atretic follicle *(AF)* (upper left) can be seen near the secondary follicle. ×65.

cytes of many species, including those of mammals, exhibit specialized secretory vesicles known as **cortical granules.** They are located just beneath the plasma membrane **(oolemma).** The granules contained proteases that are released by exocytosis when the egg is activated by the sperm (discussed in the section on fertilization).

Numerous irregular microvilli from the oocyte project into the **perivitelline space** between the oocyte and the surrounding granulosa cells as the zona pellucida is deposited (Fig. 22.7). Slender processes from the granulosa cells develop at the same time and project toward the oocyte, intermingling with oocyte microvilli and, occasionally, invaginating into the oocyte plasma membrane. The processes may contact the plasma membrane but do not establish cytoplasmic continuity between the cells.

The Secondary Follicle Is Characterized by a Fluid-Containing Antrum

The primary follicle initially moves deeper into the cortical stroma as it increases in size, mostly through proliferation of the granulosa cells. Several factors are required for oocyte and follicular growth. They include

- *Follicle-stimulating hormone (FSH)*
- *Epidermal growth factor (EGF)*
- *Insulin-like growth factor I (IGF-I)*
- *Calcium ions (Ca^{2+})*

When the stratum granulosum reaches a thickness of 6–12 cell layers, fluid-filled cavities appear among the granulosa cells (Fig. 22.3). As the hyaluronic acid-rich fluid called *liquor folliculi* continues to accumulate among the granulosa cells, the cavities begin to coalesce, eventually forming a single crescent-shaped cavity called the **antrum.** The follicle is now identified as a **secondary** or **antral follicle.** The eccentrically positioned oocyte, which has attained a diameter of about 125 µm, undergoes no further growth. The inhibition of growth is achieved by the presence of a small 1–2-kD peptide known as **oocyte maturation inhibitor (OMI)** secreted by the granulosa cells into the antral fluid. A direct correlation is observed between the size of the secondary follicle and OMI concentration. The concentration is highest in small follicles and is lowest in mature follicles. The follicle, which was 0.2 mm in diameter as an early secondary follicle, when the fluid first appeared, continues to grow and reaches a size of 10 mm or more in diameter.

Cells of the Cumulus Oophorus Form a Corona Radiata Around the Secretory Follicle Oocyte

As the secondary follicle increases in size, the antrum, lined by several layers of granulosa cells, also enlarges (Fig. 22.8). The stratum granulosum has a relatively uniform thickness except for the region associated with the oocyte. Here, the granulosa cells form a thickened mound, the *cumulus oophorus,* that projects into the antrum. The cells of the cumulus oophorus that immediately surround the oocyte and remain with it at ovulation are referred to as the *corona radiata.* The corona radiata is made up of cumulus cells that send penetrating microvilli throughout the zona pellucida to communicate via gap junctions with microvilli of the oocyte (see Fig. 12.7). During follicular maturation, an increase in the number of surface microvilli of granulosa cells is observed and is correlated with an increased number of LH receptors on the free antral surface. Extracellular, densely staining, PAS-positive material called *Call-Exner bodies* may be seen between the granulosa cells. These bodies are secreted by the granulosa cells and contain hyaluronic acid and proteoglycans.

The Graafian Follicle Contains the Mature Secondary Oocyte

The mature follicle, also known as a *Graafian follicle,* has a diameter of 10 mm or more. Because of its very large size, it extends through the full thickness of the ovarian cortex and causes a bulge on the surface of the ovary. As the follicle nears its maximum size, there is a decrease in the mitotic activity of the granulosa cells. The stratum granulosum appears to become thinner as the antrum increases in size. As the spaces between the granulosa cells continue to enlarge, the oocyte and cumulus cells are gradually loosened from the rest of the granulosa cells in preparation for ovulation. The cumulus cells immediately surrounding the oocyte now form a single layer of cells of the corona radiata. These cells and loosely attached cumulus cells remain with the oocyte at the time of ovulation.

During this period of follicle maturation, the thecal layers become more prominent. Lipid droplets appear in the cytoplasm of the theca interna cells, and the cells demonstrate ultrastructural features associated with steroid-producing cells. In the human, LH stimulates the cells of the theca interna to secrete androgens, which serve as precursors for estrogens. Some of the androgens are transported to the smooth endoplasmic reticulum (sER) in the granulosa cells. In response to FSH, the granulosa cells catalyze the conversion of androgens to estrogens, which, in turn, stimulate the granulosa cells to proliferate and, thereby, increase the size of the follicle. Increased estrogen levels from both follicular and systemic sources are correlated with increased sensitization of gonadotropes to gonadotropin-releasing hormone. A surge in the release of FSH and/or LH is induced in the adenohypophysis approximately 24 hours before ovulation. In response to the LH surge, the LH receptors on granulosa cells are downregulated (desensitized), and granulosa cells no longer produce estrogens in response to LH. Triggered by this surge, the first meiotic division of the primary oocyte resumes. This occurs between 12 and 24 hours after the LH surge and before ovulation, resulting in the formation of the secondary oocyte and the first polar body. The granulosa and thecal cells then undergo luteinization and produce progesterone (see the section on corpus luteum).

Ovulation

Ovulation Is a Hormone-Mediated Process Resulting in the Release of the Secondary Oocyte

Ovulation is the process by which an oocyte is released from the Graafian follicle. The follicle destined to ovulate in any menstrual cycle is recruited from a cohort of several primary follicles in the first few days of the cycle. During ovulation, the oocyte must traverse the entire follicular wall including the germinal epithelium.

A combination of hormonal changes and enzymatic effects is responsible for the actual release of the secondary oocyte at the middle of the menstrual cycle, i.e., on the 14th day of a 28-day cycle. The factors include

- Increase in the volume and pressure of the follicular fluid
- Enzymatic proteolysis of the follicular wall by activated plasminogen
- Hormonally directed deposition of glycosaminoglycans between the oocyte-cumulus complex and the stratum granulosum
- Contraction of the smooth muscle fibers in the theca externa layer, triggered by prostaglandins

Just before ovulation, blood flow stops in a small area of the ovarian surface overlying the bulging follicle. This area of the germinal epithelium, known as the *macula pellucida* or the *stigma,* becomes elevated and then ruptures. The oocyte, surrounded by the corona radiata and cells of the cumulus oophorus, is forcefully expelled from the ruptured follicle (Fig. 22.9).

The oocyte is then transported into the abdominal ostium of the oviduct. At the time of ovulation, the fimbriae of the oviduct become closely apposed to the surface of the ovary, normally directing the oocyte into the oviduct and not allowing it to pass into the peritoneal cavity. After ovulation, the secondary oocyte remains viable for a period of approximately 24 hours. If fertilization fails to occur during this period, the secondary oocyte degenerates as it passes through the oviduct.

Ova that fail to enter the oviduct usually degenerate in the peritoneal cavity. Occasionally, however, one of these may become fertilized and implant on the surface of the ovary or the intestine or inside the rectouterine (Douglas) pouch. Such *ectopic implantations* usually do not develop beyond early fetal stages but may have to be removed surgically for the health of the mother.

Normally, only one follicle completes maturation in each cycle and ruptures to release its secondary oocyte. Rarely, oocytes are released from other follicles that have reached full maturity during the same cycle, leading to the possibility of multiple zygotes. Drugs, such as clomiphene citrate (Serophene), or human menopausal gonadotropins, given to stimulate ovarian activity, greatly increase the possibility of multiple births by causing the simultaneous maturation of several follicles.

POLYCYSTIC OVARIAN DISEASE (STEIN-LEVENTHAL SYNDROME)

The Stein-Leventhal syndrome is characterized by bilaterally enlarged polycystic ovaries. The individual is infertile due to lack of ovulation. Morphologically, the ovaries resemble a small white balloon filled with tightly packed marbles. The ovaries have a smooth pearl-white surface but do not show surface scarring, as no ovulations have occurred. The ovaries are often called oyster ovaries. The condition is due to the large number of fluid-filled follicular cysts and atrophic secondary follicles that lie beneath an unusually thick tunica albuginea. The pathogenesis is not clear but seems to be related to abnormal levels of different steroid hormones. The selection process of the follicles that undergo maturation seems to be disturbed. The individual has an anovulatory cycle characterized only by estrogenic stimulation of the endometrium (production of progesterone is inhibited by interruption in transformation of the Graafian follicle into a progesterone-producing corpus luteum). The treatment of choice is hormonal, to stabilize and reconstruct the estrogen/progesterone ratio, but in some cases, surgical intervention is necessary. A wedge-shaped cut is made into the ovary to expose the cortex, thus allowing the ova, following hormonal treatment, to leave the ovary without physical restrictions created by the preexisting thickened tunica albuginea.

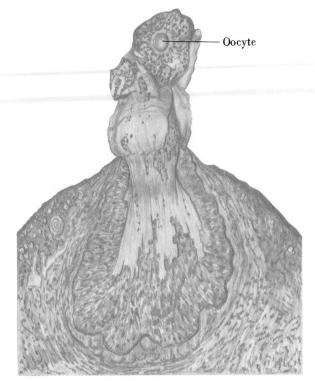

— Oocyte

Figure 22.9. Drawing of ovulation as observed in the rabbit. The oocyte, surrounded by the cumulus oophorus, is in the process of being expelled from the ruptured ovarian follicle. (Based on Weiss L, Greep RO: *Histology,* 4th ed. New York, McGraw-Hill, 1977, p 896.)

The Primary Oocyte Is Arrested for 12–50 Years in the Diplotene Stage of Prophase of the First Meiotic Division

The primary oocytes within the primordial follicles begin the first meiotic division in the embryo, but the process is arrested at the diplotene stage of meiotic prophase (see section on meiosis in Chapter 2). The completion of the first meiotic prophase does not occur until just before ovulation. Therefore, primary oocytes remain arrested in the first meiotic prophase for 12–50 years. This long period of meiotic arrest makes the primary oocyte more sensitive to adverse environmental influences and probably contributes to errors in meiotic division such as nondisjunction. This results in chromosomal anomalies such as trisomy of chromosome 21 (Down's syndrome).

As the first meiotic division (reduction division) is completed in the mature follicle (Fig. 22.10), each daughter cell of the **primary oocyte** receives an equal share of the chromatin, but one daughter cell receives the majority of the cytoplasm and becomes the **secondary oocyte.** It measures 150 μm in diameter. The other daughter cell receives a minimal amount of the cytoplasm and becomes the **first polar body.**

The Secondary Oocyte Is Arrested at Metaphase in the Second Meiotic Division Just Before Ovulation

As soon as the first meiotic division is completed, the secondary oocyte begins the second meiotic division. As the secondary oocyte surrounded by the cells of the corona radiata leaves the follicle at ovulation, the second meiotic division (equatorial division) is in progress. This division is arrested at metaphase and is completed only if the secondary oocyte is penetrated by a spermatozoon. If fertilization occurs, the secondary oocyte completes the second meiotic division and forms a mature **ovum** with the **maternal pronucleus** containing a set of 23 chromosomes. The other cell produced at this division is a **second polar body.** In the human, the first polar body does not divide; therefore, the fertilized egg can be recognized by the appearance nearby of the second polar body. The polar bodies, which are not capable of further development, degenerate.

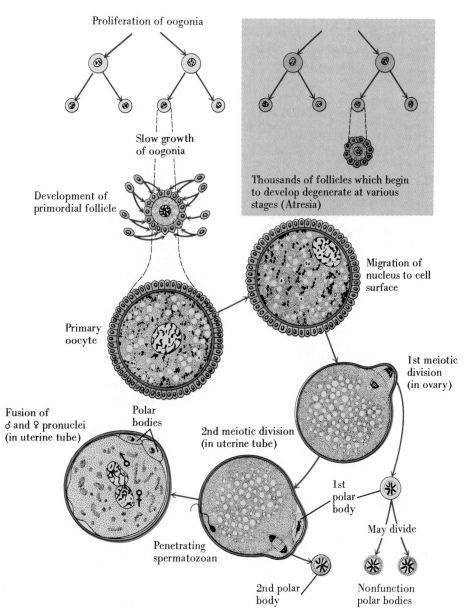

Proliferation of oogonia

Slow growth
of oogonia

Thousands of follicles which begin
to develop degenerate at various
stages (Atresia)

Development of
primordial follicle

Migration of
nucleus to cell
surface

Primary
oocyte

1st meiotic
division
(in ovary)

Fusion of
♂ and ♀ pronuclei
(in uterine tube)

Polar
bodies

2nd meiotic division
(in uterine tube)

1st
polar
body

May divide

Penetrating
spermatozoan

2nd polar
body

Nonfunction
polar bodies

Figure 22.10. Schematic diagrams illustrating changes that occur during the growth, maturation, and fertilization of the oocyte. In the initial development of the primordial follicle shown here, stromal cells migrate to the oogonium and form a surrounding layer. The oogonium then enlarges to form the primary oocyte. Note that the primary oocyte remains arrested in prophase I of meiosis. The first meiotic or reductional division is completed only if the oocyte progresses to ovulation. The second meiotic or equatorial division is not completed unless the secondary oocyte is penetrated by a spermatozoon. (After C. E. Corliss.)

FERTILIZATION

Fertilization Normally Occurs in the Ampulla of the Oviduct

To fertilize an egg, a spermatozoon must arrive at the site of fertilization. Usually, only a few hundred of the millions of spermatozoa in an ejaculate reach the site of fertilization, typically in the ampulla of the oviduct. On arrival, the spermatozoon penetrates the corona radiata, where the final steps of *capacitation* occur. Capacitation involves the release of the epididymal fluid glycoconjugate from the surface of the head of the spermatozoon. These surface glycosides added during sperm maturation in the epididymis inhibit binding to the zona pellucida receptor (see page 658). After capacitation, the spermatozoon is able to bind successfully to the zona pellucida receptors. Binding to the sperm receptor on the zona pellucida triggers the *acrosome reaction* in which enzymes that are released from the acrosome enable the spermatozoon to penetrate the zona pellucida. The penetration is accomplished by limited proteolysis of the zona pellucida in front of the advancing spermatozoon.

The nucleus of the sperm head that enters the secondary

oocyte forms a *male pronucleus* containing 23 paternal chromosomes. After the fusion of the two pronuclei, the resulting *zygote* with its diploid (2*n*) complement of 46 chromosomes undergoes a mitotic division or first cleavage. This two-cell stage marks the beginning of the embryo.

Several Spermatozoa May Penetrate the Zona Pellucida, But Only One Spermatozoon Completes the Fertilization Process

As the fertilizing spermatozoon penetrates the ooplasm, at least three types of postfusion reactions occur to prevent other spermatozoa from entering the egg (polyspermy). These events include

- *Fast block to polyspermy:* This is achieved by a large and long-lasting (up to 1 minute) depolarization of the oolemma. The depolarization creates a transient electrical block to polyspermy.
- *Cortical reaction:* Changes in the polarity of the oolemma then trigger release of Ca^{2+} from the ooplasmic stores. The Ca^{2+} propagates a cortical reaction wave. In this event the cortical granules move to the surface and fuse with the oolemma, leading to a transient increase in egg surface area and reorganization of the membrane. The contents of the cortical granules are released into the perivitelline space.
- *Zona reaction:* The released enzymes (proteases) of the cortical granules not only degrade the glycoprotein oocyte plasma membrane receptors for sperm binding but also form the *perivitelline barrier,* by cross-linking proteins on the surface of the zona pellucida. This creates the final and permanent block to polyspermy.

Corpus Luteum

The Collapsed Follicle Undergoes Reorganization into the Corpus Luteum After Ovulation

At ovulation, the follicular wall, composed of the remaining granulosa and thecal cells, is thrown into deep folds as the follicle collapses and is transformed into the *corpus luteum* (yellow body) or *luteal gland* (Fig. 22.11). At first, bleeding from the capillaries in the theca interna into the follicular lumen leads to the formation of the *corpus hemorrhagicum* with a central clot. Connective tissue from the stroma then invades the former follicular cavity. The cells of the granulosa and theca interna layers then undergo dramatic morphologic changes. These luteal cells increase in size and become filled with lipid droplets. A lipid-soluble pigment, lipochrome, in the cytoplasm of the cells gives them a yellow appearance in fresh preparations. At the ultrastructural level, the cells demonstrate features associated with steroid-secreting cells, namely, abundant sER and mitochondria with tubular cristae (Fig. 22.12).

Two types of luteal cells are identified:

- *Granulosa lutein cells,* very large (about 30 μm in diameter), centrally located cells derived from the granulosa cells
- *Theca lutein cells,* smaller (about 15 μm), more deeply staining, peripherally located cells derived from the cells of the theca interna layer

As the corpus luteum begins its formation, blood and lymphatic vessels from the theca interna rapidly grow into the granulosa layer. A rich vascular network is established within the corpus luteum. This highly vascularized structure located in the cortex of the ovary secretes progesterone and estrogens. These hormones stimulate the growth and

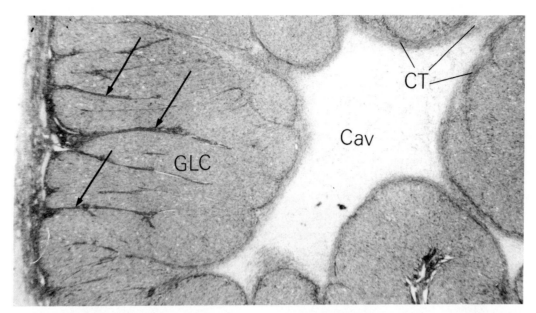

Figure 22.11. Photomicrograph of human corpus luteum. Granulosa lutein cells *(GLC)* derived from follicle cells form a thick, folded layer around the former follicular cavity *(Cav).* Connective tissue *(CT),* which has invaded the follicular cavity, and infoldings of the theca interna *(arrows)* can be seen in the corpus luteum. ×16.

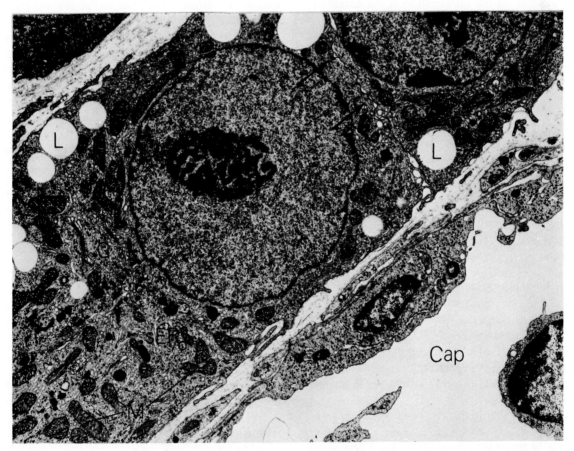

Figure 22.12. Electron micrograph of theca lutein cells from a corpus luteum of a monkey at an early implantation stage (day 10.5 of gestation). Membrane-bounded dense bodies are clustered near the Golgi region *(G);* most of the cytoplasm is packed with tubules of smooth endoplasmic reticulum *(sER),* lipid droplets *(L),* and mitochondria *(M).* Note the capillary *(Cap)* in the lower right and the closely apposed cell membranes of adjoining cells *(arrows).* ×10,000. (Courtesy of Dr. C. Booher.)

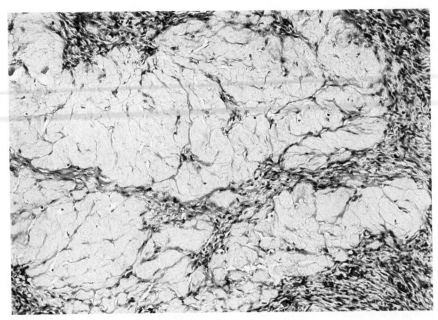

Figure 22.13. Photomicrograph of corpus albicans of a human ovary. Large amounts of intercellular hyaline material can be seen among the degenerating cells of the former corpus luteum. The corpus albicans is surrounded by ovarian stroma. ×125.

secretory activity of the lining of the uterus, the **endometrium,** to prepare it for the implantation of the developing zygote in the event that fertilization occurs.

The Corpus Luteum of Pregnancy Is Formed After Fertilization and Implantation

If fertilization and implantation *do occur*, the corpus luteum increases in size to form the ***corpus luteum of pregnancy.*** The corpus luteum is dependent for its existence and function on a combination of paracrine secretions, collectively described as ***luteotropins.***

Paracrine luteotropins are locally produced by the ovary. They include

- ***Estrogens***
- ***Insulin-like growth factors I and II (IGF-I and IGF-II)***

Endocrine luteotropins are produced at a distance from their target organ, the corpus luteum. They include

- ***Human chorionic gonadotropin (hCG),*** secreted by the trophoblast of the chorion, which stimulates the corpus luteum and prevents its degeneration
- ***Luteinizing hormone (LH)*** and ***prolactin,*** both secreted by the pituitary gland
- ***Insulin,*** produced by the pancreas

High levels of progesterone, produced from cholesterol by the corpus luteum, block the cyclic development of the ovarian follicles. In early pregnancy, the corpus luteum reaches a size of 2–3 cm, thereby filling most of the ovary. Its function begins gradually to decline after 8 weeks of pregnancy, although it persists throughout pregnancy. Although the corpus luteum remains active, the placenta produces sufficient amounts of estrogens and progestogens from maternal and fetal precursors to take over the function of the corpus luteum after 6 weeks of pregnancy. hCG can be detected in the serum as early as 6 days after conception and in the urine as early as 10–14 days of pregnancy. Detection of hCG in the urine forms the basis of most pregnancy tests.

The Corpus Luteum of Menstruation Is Formed in the Absence of Fertilization

If fertilization and implantation *do not occur*, the corpus luteum remains active only for 14 days; in this case it is called the ***corpus luteum of menstruation.*** In the absence of hCG and other luteotropins, the rate of secretion of progestogens and estrogens declines, and the corpus luteum begins to degenerate about 10–12 days after ovulation.

The corpus luteum degenerates and undergoes a slow involution after pregnancy or menstruation. The cells become loaded with lipid, decrease in size, and undergo autolysis. A white scar, the ***corpus albicans,*** is formed as intercellular hyaline material accumulates among the degenerating cells of the former corpus luteum (Fig. 22.13). The corpus albicans sinks deeper into the ovarian cortex as it slowly disappears over a period of several months.

Atresia

Most Ovarian Follicles Are Lost by Atresia

As previously stated, very few of the ovarian follicles that begin their differentiation in the embryonic ovary are destined to complete their maturation. Most of the follicles degenerate and disappear through a process called *follicular atresia*. Large numbers of follicles undergo atresia during fetal development, early postnatal life, and puberty. After puberty, groups of follicles begin to mature each menstrual cycle; normally, only one follicle completes its maturation. Atresia is now thought to be a mechanism whereby a few follicles are stimulated to maintain their development through the programmed death of the other follicles. Thus, a follicle in any stage of its maturation may undergo atresia. The process becomes more complex as the follicle progresses toward maturation.

In atresia of primordial and small, growing follicles, the oocyte becomes smaller and degenerates; similar changes occur in the follicular cells. As the cells are reabsorbed and disappear, the surrounding stromal cells migrate into the space previously occupied by the follicle, leaving no trace of its existence.

In atresia of large, growing follicles, the degeneration of the oocyte appears to occur secondarily to degenerative changes in the follicular wall, which include the following sequential events:

- Cessation of mitosis and expression of endonucleases and hydrolytic enzymes within the granulosa cells
- Invasion of the granulosa layer by neutrophils and macrophages
- Invasion of the granulosa layer by strands of vascularized connective tissue
- Sloughing of the granulosa cells into the antrum of the follicle
- Hypertrophy of the theca interna cells
- Collapse of the follicle as degeneration continues
- Invasion of connective tissue into the cavity of the follicle

The oocyte undergoes typical changes associated with degeneration and autolysis, and the remnants are phagocytized by invading macrophages. The zona pellucida, which is resistant to the autolytic changes occurring in the cells associated with it, becomes folded and collapses as it is slowly broken down within the cavity of the follicle. Macrophages in the connective tissue are involved in the phagocytosis of the zona pellucida and the remnants of the degenerating cells. The basement membrane between the follicular cells from the theca interna may separate from the follicular cells and increase in thickness, forming a wavy hyaline layer called the *glassy membrane*. This structure is characteristic of follicles in late stages of atresia.

Enlargement of the cells of the theca interna occurs in some atretic follicles. These cells, which are similar to theca lutein cells, become organized into radially arranged strands separated by connective tissue. A rich capillary network develops in the connective tissue. These atretic follicles, which resemble an old corpus luteum, are called *corpora lutea atretica*.

The Interstitial Gland Arises From the Theca Interna of the Atretic Follicle

As atretic follicles continue to degenerate, a scar with hyaline streaks develops in the center of the cell mass, giving it the appearance of a small corpus albicans. This structure eventually disappears as the ovarian stroma invades the degenerating follicle. In the ovaries of a number of mammals the strands of luteal cells do not degenerate immediately but become broken up and scattered in the stroma. These cords of cells contribute to the *interstitial gland* of the ovary and produce steroid hormones. The development of the interstitial gland is most extensive in animal species that have large litters.

In the human ovary, there are relatively few interstitial cells. They occur in the largest numbers in the first year of life and during the early phases of puberty, corresponding to times of increased follicular atresia. At menarche, there is involution of the interstitial cells; therefore, few are present during the reproductive life span and menopause. It has been suggested that in the human the interstitial cells are an important source of the estrogens that influence the growth and development of the secondary sex organs during the early phases of puberty. In other species, the interstitial cells have been shown to produce progesterone.

In the human, cells called *ovarian hilar cells* are found in the hilum of the ovary in association with vascular spaces and nonmyelinated nerve fibers. These cells, which structurally appear to be related to the interstitial cells of the testis, contain *Reinke crystalloids*. The hilar cells appear to respond to hormonal changes during pregnancy and at the onset of menopause. It has been suggested that the hilar cells secrete androgens, in that hyperplasia or tumors associated with these cells usually lead to masculinization.

Blood Supply and Lymphatics

Blood Supply to the Ovaries Comes From Two Different Sources: Ovarian and Uterine Arteries

The *ovarian arteries,* which are the branches of the abdominal aorta that pass to the ovaries through the suspensory ligaments, provide the principal arterial supply to the ovaries and oviducts. These arteries anastomose with the second blood source to the ovary, namely, the *ovarian branches of the uterine arteries,* which arise from the internal iliac arteries. Relatively large vessels arising from this region of anastomosis pass through the mesovarium and enter the hilum of the ovary. These large arteries are called *helicine arteries* because they branch and become highly coiled as they pass into the ovarian medulla (see Fig. 22.2).

Veins accompany the arteries and form a plexus, named

the *pampiniform plexus,* as they emerge from the hilum. The ovarian vein is formed from the plexus.

In the cortical region of the ovary, networks of lymphatic vessels in the thecal layers surround the large developing and atretic follicles and corpora lutea. The lymphatic vessels follow the course of the ovarian arteries as they ascend to para-aortic lymph nodes in the lumbar region.

Innervation

Ovaries Are Innervated by the Autonomic Ovarian Plexus

Sensory and autonomic nerve fibers that supply the ovary are conveyed mainly by the ovarian plexus. Although it is clear that the ovary receives both sympathetic and parasympathetic fibers, little is known of the actual distribution. Groups of parasympathetic ganglion cells are scattered in the medulla. Nerve fibers follow the arteries, supplying the smooth muscle in the walls of these vessels, as they pass into medulla and cortex of the ovary. Nerve fibers associated with the follicles do not penetrate the basal lamina. Sensory nerve endings are scattered in the stroma. The sensory fibers convey impulses via the ovarian plexus, to reach the dorsal root ganglia of the first lumbar spinal nerves. Therefore, ovarian pain is referred over the cutaneous distribution of these spinal nerves.

At ovulation, about 45% of women experience midcycle pain (''mittelschmerz''). This is usually a sharp lower abdominal pain lasting from a few minutes up to 24 hours and is frequently accompanied by a small amount of bleeding from the uterus. It is believed that this pain is related to smooth muscle cell contraction in the ovary as well as in its ligaments. The contraction is in response to an increased level of prostaglandin $F_{2\alpha}$ mediated by the surge of the LH.

OVIDUCT

The *oviducts* are paired tubes that extend bilaterally from the uterus toward the ovaries (see Fig. 22.1). The oviducts, also commonly referred to as the *uterine* or *Fallopian tubes,* transmit the ova from the ovary to the uterus and provide the necessary environment for fertilization and for initial development of the conceptus to the morula stage. One end of the tube is adjacent to the ovary and opens into the peritoneal cavity; the other end communicates with the uterine cavity.

The tube, which is approximately 10–12 cm long, can be divided into four segments by gross inspection:

- The *infundibulum* is the funnel-shaped segment of the tube adjacent to the ovary. At the distal end, it opens into the peritoneal cavity. The proximal end communicates with the ampulla. Fringed extensions, the *fimbriae,* extend from the mouth of the infundibulum toward the ovary.
- The *ampulla* is the longest segment of the tube, constituting about two-thirds the total length, and is the site of fertilization.
- The *isthmus* is the narrow, medial segment of the oviduct adjacent to the uterus.

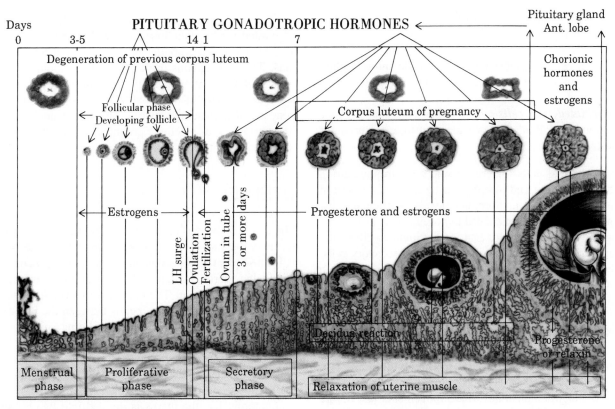

PITUITARY GONADOTROPIC HORMONES

Figure 22.14. Schematic diagram illustrating the morphologic changes in the endometrium and ovary during the menstrual cycle. The hormonal activities controlling these changes are indicated. For the purpose of this diagram, fertilization of the ovum is illustrated. Therefore, the decidua reaction is shown after the secretory phase of the endometrium. If fertilization had not occurred, the menstrual cycle would have repeated itself. (Modified from Pritchard JA, et al: *Williams' Obstetrics*, 17th ed. Norwalk, CT, Appleton-Century-Crofts, 1985, p 74.)

- The *uterine* or *intramural* part, measuring about 1 cm in length, lies within the uterine wall and opens into the cavity of the uterus.

The Wall of the Oviduct Is Composed of Three Layers

The oviduct wall resembles the wall of other hollow viscera, consisting of an external serosal layer, an intermediate muscular layer, and an internal mucosal layer. There is, however, no submucosa.

- The *serosa* or peritoneum consists of mesothelium and a thin layer of connective tissue.
- The *muscularis,* throughout most of its length, is organized into an inner, relatively thick circular layer and an outer, thinner longitudinal layer. The boundary between these layers is often indistinct.
- The *mucosa* exhibits relatively thin longitudinal folds that project into the lumen of the oviduct throughout its length. The folds, which are most numerous and complex in the ampulla (Fig. 22.15), become smaller in the isthmus.

The mucosal lining is simple columnar epithelium composed of two kinds of cells, ciliated and nonciliated

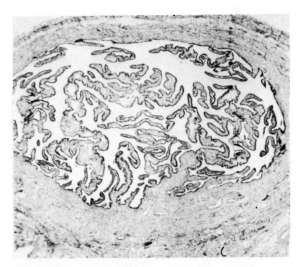

Figure 22.15. Photomicrograph of human uterine tube. The cross section is through the ampulla region of the uterine tube. The mucosa is thrown into extensive folds that project into the lumen of the tube. The muscularis is composed of a thick inner layer of circular fibers and an outer layer of longitudinal fibers. ×16.

(Fig. 22.16). They represent different functional states of a single cell type.

- *Ciliated cells* are most numerous in the infundibulum and ampulla. The wave of the cilia is directed toward the uterus.
- *Nonciliated, peg cells* are secretory cells that produce the oviductal fluid that provides nutritive material for the ovum.

The epithelial cells undergo cyclic hypertrophy during the follicular phase and atrophy during the luteal phase in response to changes in hormonal levels, particularly estrogens. Also, the ratio of ciliated to nonciliated cells changes during the hormonal cycle. Estrogen stimulates ciliogenesis, and progesterone increases the number of secretory cells. At about the time of ovulation, the epithelium reaches a height of about 30 μm and then reduces to about one-half of that height just before the onset of menstruation.

Oviduct Transport

Bidirectional Transport Occurs in the Oviduct

The oviduct demonstrates active movements just before ovulation as the fimbriae become closely apposed to the ovary and localize over the region of the ovarian surface where rupture will occur. As the egg is released, the ciliated cells in the infundibulum sweep it toward the opening of the oviduct and, thus, prevent it from passing into the peritoneal cavity. The egg is transported along the oviduct by peristaltic contractions. The mechanisms by which spermatozoa and the egg are transported from opposite ends of the oviduct are not fully understood. Evidence suggests that both ciliary movements and peristaltic muscular activity are involved in the movements of the egg. The move-

ment of the spermatozoa is much too rapid, however, to be accounted for by their intrinsic motility. Fertilization usually occurs in the ampulla, near its junction with the isthmus. The egg remains in the oviduct for about 3 days before it enters the uterine cavity. Several conditions that may alter the integrity of the tubal transport system (inflammation, use of intrauterine devices, surgical manipulation, tubal ligation) may cause ectopic pregnancies and, thus, are clinically important.

UTERUS

The uterus is the part of the female reproductive system that receives the rapidly developing morula from the oviduct. All subsequent embryonic and fetal development occurs within the uterus, which undergoes dramatic increases in size and development. The human uterus is a hollow, pear-shaped organ located in the pelvis between the bladder and rectum. In a woman who has never borne children (nulliparous), it weighs 30–40 g and measures 7.5 cm in length, 5 cm in width at its superior aspect, and 2.5 cm in thickness. Its lumen, which is also flattened, is continuous with the oviducts and the vagina.

Anatomically, the uterus is divided into two regions:

- The *body* is the large upper portion of the uterus. The anterior surface is almost flat; the posterior surface is convex. The upper, rounded part of the body that expands above the attachment of the uterine tubes is termed the *fundus.*
- The *cervix* is the lower, barrel-shaped part of the uterus separated from the body by the *isthmus* (see Fig. 22.1). The lumen of the cervix, the *cervical canal,* has a constricted opening or *os* at each end. The *internal os* communicates with the cavity of the uterus; the *external os,* with the vagina.

The uterine wall is composed of three layers. From the lumen outward they are

- *Endometrium,* the mucosa of the uterus.
- *Myometrium,* the thick muscular layer. It is continuous with the muscle layer of the oviduct and vagina. The smooth muscle fibers also extend into the ligaments connected to the uterus.
- *Perimetrium,* the external serous layer or visceral peritoneal covering of the uterus. The perimetrium is continuous with the pelvic and abdominal peritoneum and consists of a mesothelium and a thin layer of loose connective tissue. Underneath the mesothelium, a layer of elastic tissue is usually very prominent. The perimetrium covers the entire posterior surface of the uterus but only part of the anterior surface. The remaining part of the anterior surface consists of connective tissue or adventitia.

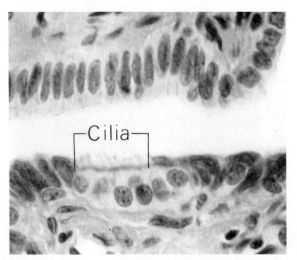

Figure 22.16. Photomicrograph of human uterine tube. The lumen of the tube is lined by simple columnar epithelium composed of ciliated and nonciliated cells. ×640.

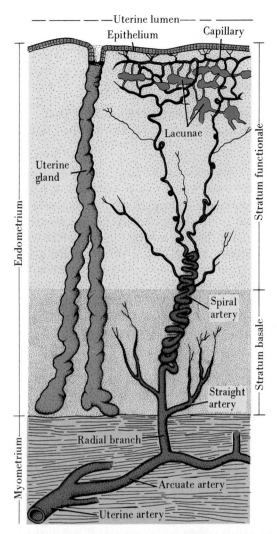

- Uterine lumen -
- Epithelium
- Capillary
- Lacunae
- Uterine gland
- Spiral artery
- Straight artery
- Radial branch
- Arcuate artery
- Uterine artery
- Endometrium
- Myometrium
- Stratum functionale
- Stratum basale

Figure 22.17. Schematic diagram illustrating the blood supply to the two layers—the stratum basale and stratum functionale—of the endometrium. (Based on Weiss L (ed): *Cell and Tissue Biology, A Textbook of Histology*, 6th ed. Baltimore, Urban & Schwarzenberg, 1988, p 869.)

The myometrium and the endometrium both undergo cyclic changes each month to prepare the uterus for implantation of an embryo. These changes constitute the *menstrual cycle*. If an embryo implants, the cycle stops, and both layers undergo considerable growth and differentiation during pregnancy (described below).

The Myometrium Forms a Structural and Functional Syncytium

The myometrium is the thickest layer of the uterine wall. It is composed of three indistinctly defined layers of smooth muscle:

- The *middle muscle layer* contains numerous large blood vessels (venous plexuses) and lymphatics and is called the *stratum vasculare*. It is the thickest layer and has

smooth muscle bundles described as oriented in a circular or spiral pattern interlaced with each other.
- The smooth muscle bundles in the *inner and outer layers* are described as predominantly oriented parallel to the long axis of the uterus.

As in most bulb-shaped hollow organs, such as the gallbladder and urinary bladder, however, distinctive muscular orientation is not seen. The muscle bundles seen in routine histologic sections appear to be randomly arrayed. This is consistent with their function of expelling the contents of the lumen through a narrow orifice.

In the nonpregnant uterus, the smooth muscle cells are about 50 μm in length. During pregnancy, the uterus undergoes enormous enlargement. The growth is primarily due to the hypertrophy of existing smooth muscle cells, which may reach more than 500 μm in length, and secondarily due to the development of new fibers through the division of existing muscle cells and the differentiation of undifferentiated mesenchymal cells. There is also an increase in the amount of connective tissue. As pregnancy proceeds, the uterine wall becomes progressively thinner as it stretches due to the growth of the fetus. After parturition, the uterus returns to near its original size. Some muscle fibers degenerate, but most return to their original size. The collagen produced during pregnancy to strengthen the myometrium is then enzymatically degraded by the cells that secreted it. The uterine cavity remains larger and the muscular wall remains thicker than before pregnancy.

Compared with the body of the uterus, the cervix has more connective tissue and less smooth muscle. Elastic fibers are abundant in the cervix but are found in appreciable quantities only in the outer layer of the myometrium of the body of the uterus.

The Endometrium Proliferates and Then Degenerates During a Menstrual Cycle

Throughout the reproductive life span, the endometrium undergoes cyclic changes each month that prepare it for the implantation of the embryo and the subsequent events of embryonic and fetal development. Changes in the secretory activity of the endometrium during the cycle are correlated with the maturation of the ovarian follicles (see Fig. 22.14). The end of each cycle is characterized by the partial destruction and sloughing of the endometrium, accompanied by bleeding from the mucosal vessels. The discharge of tissue and blood from the vagina, which usually continues for a period of 3–5 days, is referred to as *menstruation* or *menstrual flow*. The *menstrual cycle* is defined as beginning on the day when menstrual flow begins.

During reproductive life, the endometrium consists of two layers or zones that differ in structure and function (Fig. 22.17):

- ***Stratum functionale*** or ***functional layer:*** This layer is

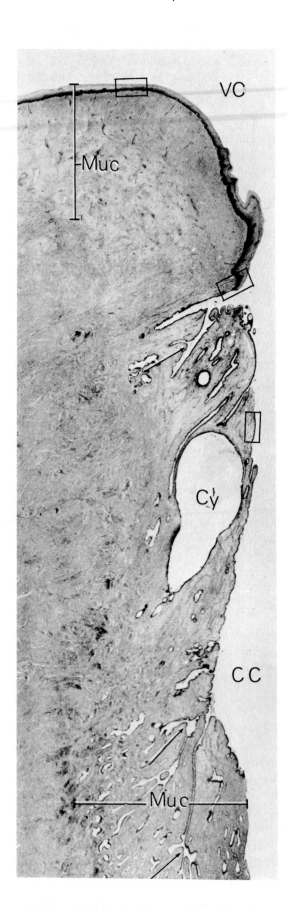

the thick part of the endometrium, which is sloughed off at menstruation.

- **Stratum basale** or **basal layer:** This layer is retained during menstruation and serves as the source for the regeneration of the stratum functionale.

The Stratum Functionale Is the Layer That Proliferates and Degenerates During the Menstrual Cycle

During the phases of the menstrual cycle, the endometrium varies from 1 to 6 mm in thickness. It is lined with a simple columnar epithelium with a mixture of secretory and ciliated cells. The surface epithelium invaginates into the underlying lamina propria, the **endometrial stroma,** forming **uterine glands.** These simple tubular glands, containing fewer ciliated cells, occasionally branch in the deeper aspect of the endometrium. The endometrial stroma, which resembles mesenchyme, is highly cellular and contains abundant intercellular ground substance. As in the oviduct, no submucosa separates the endometrium from the myometrium.

The Vasculature of the Endometrium Also Proliferates and Degenerates in Each Menstrual Cycle

The endometrium contains a unique system of blood vessels (Fig. 22.17). The uterine artery gives off 6–10 arcuate arteries that anastomose with one another in the myometrium. Branches from these arteries, the **radial arteries,** enter the basal layer of the endometrium where they give off **small straight arteries** that supply this region of the endometrium. The main branch of the radial artery continues upward and becomes highly coiled. It is called the **spiral artery.** Spiral arteries give off numerous arterioles that often anastomose with one another as they supply a rich capillary bed. The capillary bed includes thin-walled dilated segments called **lacunae.** Lacunae may also occur in the venous system that drains the endometrium. The straight arteries and the proximal part of the spiral arteries do not change during the menstrual cycle. The distal portion of the spiral arteries, under the influence of estrogens and progesterone, undergoes degeneration and regeneration with each menstrual cycle.

Figure 22.18. Photomicrograph of human cervix. The plane of section passes through the long axis of the cervix. The vaginal canal *(VC)* is present at the top of the photomicrograph; the cervical canal *(CC)* is on the right. The portion of the cervix that projects into the vagina, called the portio vaginalis, is covered with stratified squamous epithelium (see Fig. 22.19). The portion of the cervical mucosa *(Muc)* that faces the cervical canal is covered with simple columnar epithelium. An abrupt change in the surface epithelium occurs at the external os (see Fig. 22.20*a*). Cervical glands, which extend from the surface of the cervical canal into the underlying connective tissue, commonly develop into cysts *(Cy)* because of obstruction in their ducts. ×10.

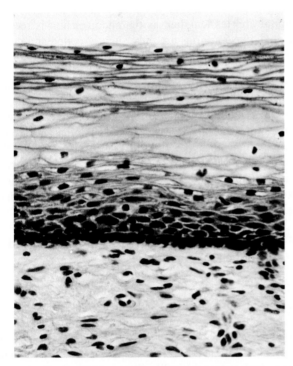

Figure 22.19. Photomicrograph of the portion of the human cervix that faces the vaginal canal. (The *upper rectangle* in Fig. 22.18 indicates the area shown in this figure.) This surface of the cervix is covered with stratified squamous epithelium. The larger cells of the middle and superficial layers of the epithelium have an empty appearance in this hematoxylin and eosin (H&E) preparation because their large content of glycogen was lost during fixation. ×3000.

Cervix

The Endometrium of the Cervix Differs From the Rest of the Uterus

The cervical mucosa, which measures about 2–3 mm in thickness, differs dramatically from the rest of the uterine endometrium, in that it contains large, branched glands (Fig. 22.18). Also, it lacks the spiral arteries. The cervical mucosa undergoes little change in thickness during the menstrual cycle and is not sloughed during the period of menstruation. During each menstrual cycle, however, the cervical glands undergo important functional changes that are related to the transport of spermatozoa within the cervical canal. The amount and properties of the mucus secreted by the gland cells vary during the menstrual cycle under the influence of the ovarian hormones. At midcycle, there is a 10-fold increase in the amount of mucus produced. This mucus is less viscous and appears to provide a more favorable environment for sperm migration. The cervical mucus at other times in the cycle restricts the passage of sperm into the uterus. Thus, hormonal mechanisms ensure that ovulation and changes in the cervical mucus are coordinated, thereby increasing the possibility that fertilization will occur if freshly ejaculated spermatozoa and the egg arrive simultaneously at the site of fertilization in the oviduct.

Blockage of the openings of the mucosal glands results in the retention of their secretions. This leads to formation of dilated cysts within the cervix, called *Nabothian cysts.* Nabothian cysts develop frequently but are clinically important only if numerous cysts produce marked enlargement of the cervix.

The Cervical External Os Is the Site of Transition Between Vaginal Stratified Squamous Epithelium and Cervical Simple Columnar Epithelium

The portion of the cervix that projects into the vagina, the *portio vaginalis,* is covered with a stratified squamous epithelium (Fig. 22.19). There is an abrupt transition just outside the external os between this squamous epithelium and the mucus-secreting columnar epithelium of the cervical canal (Fig. 22.20, *a* and *b*). Metaplastic changes in this transition zone constitute precancerous lesions of the cervix. The cervical epithelial cells are constantly exfoliated into the vagina. Stained preparations of the cervical cells (Papanicolaou cervical smear) are used routinely for screening and diagnosis of precancerous and cancerous lesions of the cervix.

Proliferative, Secretory, and *Menstrual Phases* Are the Defined Cyclic Changes of the Endometrium

The *menstrual cycle* is a continuum of developmental stages in the functional layer of the endometrium. It is controlled, ultimately, by gonadotropins secreted by the pars distalis of the pituitary gland that regulate the steroid secretions of the ovary. The cycle normally repeats every 28 days, during which the endometrium passes through a sequence of morphologic and functional changes. It is convenient to describe the cycle as having three successive phases:

- *Proliferative phase,* occurring concurrently with follicular maturation and influenced by ovarian estrogen secretion
- *Secretory phase,* coinciding with the functional activity of the corpus luteum and primarily influenced by progesterone secretion
- *Menstrual phase,* commencing as hormone production by the ovary declines with the degeneration of the corpus luteum (see Fig. 22.14)

It must be emphasized that the phases are part of a continuous process and that there is no abrupt change from one to the next.

The Proliferative Phase of the Menstrual Cycle Is Regulated by Estrogens

At the end of the menstrual phase, the endometrium consists of a thin band of connective tissue, about 1 mm thick, containing the basal portions of the uterine glands and the

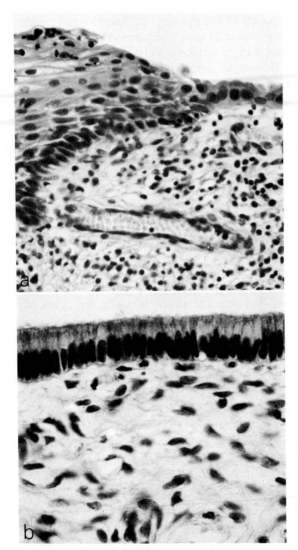

- Spiral arteries lengthen as the endometrium is reestablished; these arteries are only slightly coiled and do not extend into the upper third of the endometrium.

The proliferative phase continues for 1 day after ovulation, which occurs at about day 14 of a 28-day cycle. At the end of this phase, the endometrium has reached a thickness of about 3 mm. The glands have narrow lumina and are relatively straight but have a slightly wavy appearance (Fig. 22.22). Accumulations of glycogen are present in the basal portions of the epithelial cells. In routine histologic preparations, extraction of the glycogen gives an empty appearance to the basal cytoplasm.

The Secretory Phase of the Menstrual Cycle Is Under the Control of Progesterone

Under the influence of progesterone, dramatic changes occur in the stratum functionale, beginning a day or two after ovulation. The endometrium becomes edematous and may eventually reach a thickness of 5–6 mm. The glands enlarge and become corkscrew shaped, and their lumina become sacculated as they fill with secretory products (Fig. 22.23). The mucoid fluid being produced by the gland epithelium is rich in nutrients, particularly glycogen, required to support development if implantation occurs. Mitoses are now rare. The growth seen at this stage results from hy-

Figure 22.20. **a.** Photomicrograph of the surface epithelium of the cervix at the ostium of the cervix. The *middle rectangle* in Figure 22.18 indicates the area shown in this figure. The abrupt transition from stratified squamous epithelium to simple columnar epithelium can be seen. This transitional site is where cervical cancer most frequently develops. ×300. **b.** The simple columnar epithelium shown here came from the *lower rectangle* in Figure 22.18.

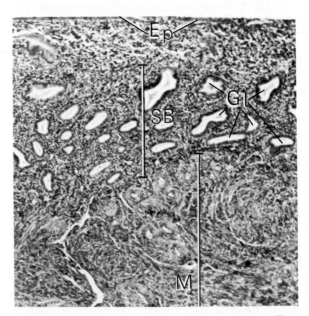

Figure 22.21. Photomicrograph of human uterus. The endometrium consists of a simple columnar epithelium and an extremely cellular connective tissue. A portion of the endometrium, the stratum functionale, undergoes dramatic change and is eventually sloughed during each menstrual cycle. The tissue shown here is at an early phase following sloughing. The resurfacing of the epithelium *(Ep)* is almost complete. The underlying stratum basale *(SB)*, which does not slough, contains glands *(Gl)* that give rise to new epithelium. Large numbers of blood vessels can be seen in the myometrium *(M)*, the muscle layer underlying the endometrium. ×40.

lower portions of the spiral arteries (Fig. 22.21). This layer is the **stratum basale;** the layer that was sloughed off was the **stratum functionale.** Under the influence of estrogens, the proliferative phase is initiated. Stromal, endothelial, and epithelial cells in the stratum basale proliferate rapidly, and the following changes can be seen:

- Epithelial cells in the basal portion of the glands reconstitute the glands and migrate to cover the denuded endometrial surface.
- Stromal cells proliferate and secrete collagen and ground substance.

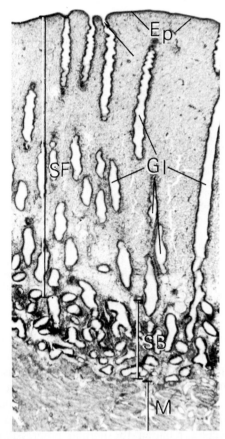

Figure 22.22. Photograph of monkey uterus. The endometrium is at the proliferative phase of the cycle. During this phase the stratum functionale (SF) greatly thickens. Long, slightly wavy glands (Gl) extend from the stratum basale (SB) to the surface epithelium (Ep). The junction between a gland and the surface epithelium is indicated by an *arrow. M,* myometrium. ×16.

pertrophy of the epithelial cells, an increase in vascularity, and edema of the endometrium. The spiral arteries, however, lengthen and become more coiled. They extend nearly to the surface of the endometrium.

The sequential influence of estrogens and progesterone on the *stromal cells* makes them capable of undergoing transformation into **decidual cells.** The stimulus for the transformation is the implantation of the blastocyst. Large pale cells rich in glycogen result from this transformation. Although the precise function of these cells is not known, it is clear that they provide a favorable environment for the nourishment of the embryo and that they create a specialized layer that facilitates the separation of the placenta from the uterine wall at the termination of pregnancy.

The Menstrual Phase Results From a Decline in the Ovarian Secretion of Progesterone and Estrogen

The corpus luteum remains active in hormone production for only about 10 days if fertilization does not occur. As the hormone levels rapidly decline, changes occur in the blood supply to the stratum functionale. Initially, periodic

contractions of the walls of the spiral arteries, lasting for several hours, cause the stratum functionale to become ischemic, the glands stop secreting, and the endometrium shrinks in height as the stroma becomes less edematous. After about 2 days, extended periods of arterial contraction, with only brief periods of blood flow, cause disruption of the surface epithelium and rupture of the blood vessels. It is important to realize that when the spiral arteries close off, blood flows into the stratum basale but not into the stratum functionale. Blood, uterine fluid, and sloughing stromal and epithelial cells from the stratum functionale constitute the vaginal discharge. As patches of tissue separate from the endometrium, the torn ends of veins, arteries, and glands are exposed. The desquamation continues until only the stratum basale remains. Clotting of blood is inhibited during this period of menstrual flow. Arterial blood flow is restricted except for the brief periods of relaxation of the walls of the spiral arteries. Blood continually seeps from the open ends of the veins. The period of menstrual flow normally lasts about 5 days. The average blood loss in the menstrual phase is 35–50 mL. Blood flow through the straight arteries maintains the stratum basale.

As noted, this is a cyclic process. Figure 22.14 shows a single cycle of the endometrium and then demonstrates a gravid state as it is established at the end of a secretory

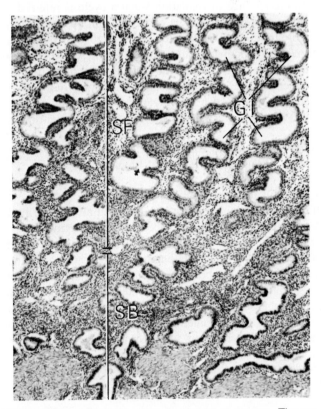

Figure 22.23. Photomicrograph of human uterus. The endometrium is at the secretory phase of the cycle. Glands (Gl) within the stratum functionale (SF) assume a corkscrew shape as the endometrium further increases in thickness. The stratum basale (SB) demonstrates less dramatic changes in its morphology. ×65.

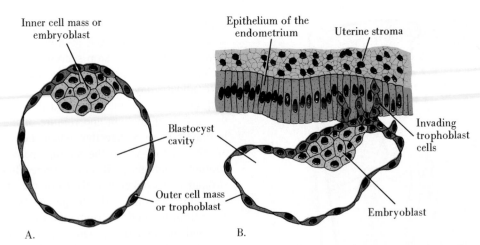

Figure 22.24. Schematic diagrams of sections through a human blastocyst at about 4½ days of development (A) and through a monkey blastocyst at about 9 days of development (B). The human blastocyst was recovered from the uterine lumen. At 9 days, the trophoblastic cells of the monkey blastocyst have begun to invade the epithelial cells of the endometrium. In the human, the blastocyst begins to invade the endometrium at about the fifth or sixth day of development. (After Sadler TW: *Langman's Medical Embryology*, 6th ed. Baltimore, Williams & Wilkins, 1990, p 32.)

phase. In the absence of fertilization, a cessation of bleeding would accompany the growth and maturation of new ovarian follicles. The epithelial cells would rapidly proliferate and migrate to restore the surface epithelium as the proliferative phase of the next cycle begins.

In the absence of ovulation (such a cycle is referred to as an *anovulatory cycle*), a corpus luteum does not form, and progesterone is not produced. In the absence of progesterone, the endometrium does not enter the secretory phase and continues in the proliferative phase until menstruation. In cases of infertility, biopsies of the endometrium can be used to diagnose such anovulatory cycles as well as other diseases of the ovary and disorders of the endometrium.

If Fertilization and Implantation Occur, a Gravid Phase Replaces the Menstrual Phase of the Cycle

If fertilization and subsequent implantation occur, decline of the endometrium is delayed until after parturition. As the blastocyst becomes embedded in the uterine mucosa in the early part of the second week, cells in the chorion of the developing placenta begin to secrete hCG and other luteotropins. These hormones maintain the corpus luteum and stimulate it to continue the production of progesterone and estrogens. Thus, the decline of the endometrium is prevented, and the endometrium undergoes further development during the first few weeks of pregnancy.

Implantation Is the Process in Which the Blastocyst Settles Into the Endometrium

The fertilized human ovum undergoes a series of changes as it passes through the oviduct and into the uterine cavity in preparation for becoming embedded in the uterine mucosa. The zygote undergoes cleavage, followed by a series of mitotic divisions without cell growth, resulting in a rapid increase in the number of cells in the embryo. Initially, the embryo is under the control of maternal informational macromolecules that have accumulated in the cytoplasm of the ovum during oogenesis. Later development is dependent on activation of the embryonic genome, which encodes various growth factors, cell junction components, and other macromolecules required for normal progression to the blastocyst stage.

The cell mass resulting from the series of mitotic divisions is known as a *morula* (fr. L. *morum*, mulberry), and the individual cells are known as *blastomeres.* Normally, during the third day after fertilization, the morula, which has reached a 12–16-cell stage and is still surrounded by the zona pellucida, enters the uterine cavity. The morula remains free in the uterus for about a day while continued cell division and development occur. The early embryo gives rise to a blastocyst, a hollow sphere of cells with a centrally located clump of cells. This *inner cell mass* will give rise to the tissues of the embryo proper; the surrounding layer of cells, the *outer cell mass,* will form the trophoblast and then the *placenta* (Fig. 22.24).

Fluid passes inward through the zona pellucida during this process, forming a fluid-filled cavity, the *blastocyst cavity.* This event defines the beginning of the *blastocyst.* As the blastocyst remains free in the uterine lumen for 1 or 2 days, undergoing further mitotic divisions, the zona pellucida disappears. The outer cell mass is now called the *trophoblast,* and the inner cell mass is referred to as the *embryoblast.*

Implantation Occurs During the *Implantation Window*

The attachment of the blastocyst to the endometrial epithelium occurs during the *implantation window,* the period that the uterus is receptive for implantation of the blastocyst. This short period results from the programmed se-

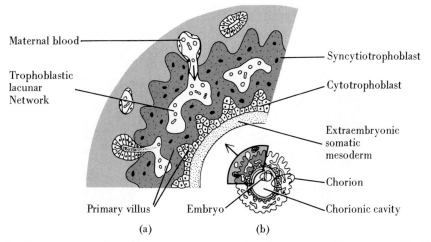

Maternal blood

Trophoblastic lacunar Network

Syncytiotrophoblast

Cytotrophoblast

Extraembryonic somatic mesoderm

Chorion

Chorionic cavity

Primary villus   Embryo

(a)   (b)

Figure 22.25. Schematic diagrams of sections through a human conceptus at 14 days of development. The relationship of the embryo to the chorionic sac is illustrated in **b.** A more detailed diagram of a section through the wall of the chorionic sac is shown in **a.** (After Moore KL, Persaud TVN: *The Developing Human,* 5th ed. Philadelphia, WB Saunders, 1993, p 46.)

quence of the action of progesterone and estrogens on the endometrium. Antiprogesterone drugs, such as RU 486 and its derivatives, compete for the receptors in the endometrial epithelium, thus blocking hormone binding. The failure of progesterone to gain access to its receptors prevents implantation, thus effectively closing the window. In the human, the implantation window begins on day 6 after the LH surge and is completed by day 10.

As contact is made with the uterine wall by the trophoblastic cells over the embryoblast pole, the trophoblast rapidly proliferates and begins to invade the endometrium. The invading trophoblast differentiates into the *syncytiotrophoblast* and the *cytotrophoblast.*

- The *cytotrophoblast* is a mitotically active inner cell layer producing cells that fuse with the syncytiotrophoblast, the outer erosive layer.
- The *syncytiotrophoblast* is not mitotically active and consists of a multinucleate cytoplasmic mass; it actively invades the epithelium and underlying stroma of the endometrium.

Through the activity of the trophoblast, the blastocyst is entirely embedded within the endometrium about the 11th day of development (further development of the syncytiotrophoblast and cytotrophoblast is described in the section on the placenta).

The syncytiotrophoblast has well-developed Golgi complexes, abundant sER and rER, numerous mitochondria, and relatively large numbers of lipid droplets. These features are consistent with the secretion of progesterone, estrogens, hCG, and lactogens by this layer. Recent evidence indicates that cytotrophoblasts may also be a source of steroid hormones and hCG.

After Implantation, the Endometrium Undergoes Decidualization

During pregnancy, the portion of the endometrium that undergoes morphologic changes is called the *decidua* or *decidua graviditas.* As its name implies, this layer will be shed with the placenta at parturition. The decidua includes all but the deepest layer of the endometrium. The stromal cells differentiate into large, rounded decidual cells (see page 698). The uterine glands enlarge and become more coiled during the early part of pregnancy and then become thin and flattened as the growing fetus fills the uterine lumen.

Three different regions of the decidua are identified by their relationship to the site of implantation (see Fig. 22.26):

- The *decidua basalis* is the portion of the endometrium that underlies the implantation site.
- The *decidua capsularis* is a thin portion of endometrium that lies between the implantation site and the uterine lumen.
- The *decidua parietalis* includes the remaining endometrium of the uterus.

By the end of the third month, the fetus grows to the point that the overlying decidua capsularis fuses with the decidua parietalis of the opposite wall, thereby obliterating the uterine cavity.

By the 13th day of development, an extraembryonic space, the *chorionic cavity,* has been established (Fig. 22.25). The cell layers that form the outer boundary of this cavity, i.e., the syncytiotrophoblast, the cytotrophoblast, and the extraembryonic somatic mesoderm, are collectively referred to as the *chorion.* The innermost membranes enveloping the embryo are called the *amnion* (Fig. 22.26).

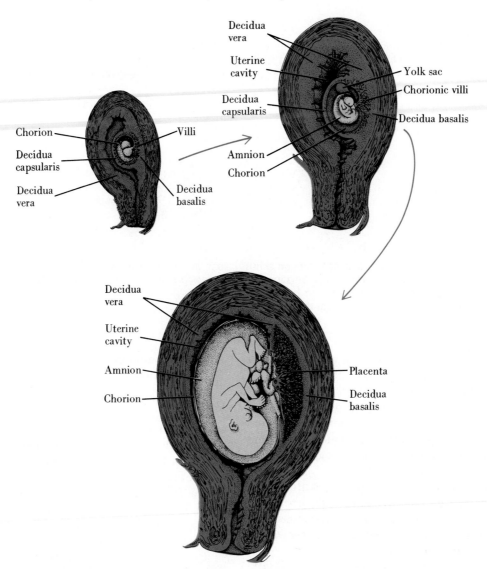

Figure 22.26. Schematic drawing of stages of human pregnancy that depicts the development of the placenta. Note that there is a gradual obliteration of the uterine lumen and disappearance of the decidua capsularis as the definitive discoid placenta is established. In this classic diagram the decidua parietalis is labeled decidua vera, an older term. (Modified from Williams J: *American Journal of Obstetrics and Gynecology* 13:1, 1927.)

PLACENTA

The Developing Fetus Is Maintained by the Placenta, Which Develops From Fetal and Maternal Tissues

The placenta consists of a fetal portion, formed by the *chorion,* and a maternal portion, formed by the *decidua basalis.* The two parts are involved in physiologic exchange of substances between the maternal and fetal circulation.

The *uteroplacental circulatory system* begins to develop around day 9, with development of vascular spaces called *trophoblastic lacunae* within the syncytiotrophoblast. Maternal sinusoids, which develop from capillaries of the maternal side, anastomose with the trophoblastic lacunae (see Fig. 22.25). The differential pressure between the arterial and venous channels that communicate with the la-

cunae establishes directional flow from the arteries into the veins, thereby establishing a primitive uteroplacental circulation. Numerous pinocytotic vessels present in the syncytiotrophoblast are indicative of the transfer of nutrients from the maternal vessels to the embryo.

Proliferation of the cytotrophoblast, growth of chorionic mesoderm, and blood vessel development successively give rise to

- *Primary chorionic villi*
- *Secondary villi*
- *Tertiary villi*

Beginning between days 11 and 13, the cytotrophoblast proliferates rapidly, sending cords or masses of cells, the *primary chorionic villi,* into the blood-filled trophoblastic lacunae in the syncytiotrophoblast (see Fig. 22.25).

Shortly after, about day 16, these villi begin to branch as chorionic mesoderm invades their bases, forming a central core of loose connective tissue. These *secondary villi,* composed of a core of mesenchyme surrounded by an inner layer of cytotrophoblast and an outer layer of syncytiotrophoblast, cover the entire surface of the chorionic sac (Fig. 22.27).

By the end of the third week, the secondary villi become *tertiary villi* after blood vessels have developed in the cores.

As the tertiary villi are forming, cytotrophoblastic cells in the villi continue to grow out through the syncytiotrophoblast. When they meet the maternal endometrium, they grow laterally and meet similar processes growing from neighboring villi. Thus, a thin layer of cytotrophoblastic cells, called the *trophoblastic shell,* is formed around the syncytiotrophoblast. The trophoblastic shell is interrupted only at sites where maternal vessels communicate with the intervillous spaces. Future growth of the placenta is accomplished by interstitial growth of the trophoblastic shell.

Two types of cells are recognized in the stroma of the villi: fibroblasts and *Hofbauer cells* (Fig. 22.28). The role of the Hofbauer cells, which are more common in the early placenta, is not known, but they have the morphologic characteristics of macrophages. The vacuoles in these cells contain lipids, glycosaminoglycans, and glycoproteins.

Early in Development, the Blood Vessels of the Villi Become Connected With Vessels From the Embryo

Blood begins to circulate through the primitive cardiovascular system and the villi at about 21 days. The intervillous spaces provide the site of exchange of nutrients, metabolic products and intermediates, and wastes between the maternal and fetal circulatory systems.

Through the first 8 weeks, villi cover the entire chorionic surface, but as the growth continues, villi on the decidua capsularis begin to degenerate, producing a smooth, relatively avascular surface called the *chorion laeve.* The villi adjacent to the decidua basalis rapidly increase in size and number and become highly branched. This region of the chorion, which is the fetal component of the placenta, is called the *chorion frondosum* or *villous chorion.* The layer of the placenta from which the villi project is called the *chorionic plate.*

During the period of rapid growth of the chorion frondosum, at about the fourth to fifth month, the fetal part of the placenta is divided by the *placental (decidual) septa* into 15–25 areas, called *cotyledons.* Wedge-like placental septa form the boundaries of the cotyledons, and because they do not fuse with the chorionic plate, maternal blood can circulate easily between them. Cotyledons are visible as the bulging areas on the maternal side of the basal plate.

The decidua basalis forms a compact layer, known as the *basal plate,* that is the maternal component of the placenta. Vessels within this part of the endometrium supply blood to the intervillous spaces. Except for relatively rare

rupturing of capillary walls, which is more common at delivery, fetal and maternal blood do not mix. This separation of the fetal and maternal blood, referred to as the *placental barrier,* is maintained primarily by the layers of fetal tissue. Starting at the fourth month, these layers become very thin in order to facilitate the exchange of products across the placental barrier. The thinning of the wall of the villus is, in part, due to the degeneration of the inner cytotrophoblast layer.

At its thinnest, the placental barrier consists of the

* Syncytiotrophoblast
* Discontinuous inner cytotrophoblast layer
* Basal lamina of the trophoblast
* Connective tissue of the villus
* Basal lamina of the endothelium
* Endothelium of the fetal placental capillary in the tertiary villus

This barrier bears a strong resemblance to the air-blood barrier of the lung, with which it has an important parallel function, viz., the exchange of oxygen and carbon dioxide, in this case between the maternal blood and the fetal blood. It also resembles the air-blood barrier by the presence in its connective tissue of a particular type of macrophage, in this instance, the Hofbauer cell.

The Placenta Is the Site of Exchange Between Maternal and Fetal Circulation

Fetal blood enters the placenta through a pair of *umbilical arteries* (Fig. 22.29). As they pass into the placenta, these arteries branch into several radially disposed vessels that give numerous branches in the chorionic plate. Branches from these vessels pass into the villi, forming extensive capillary networks in close association with the intervillous spaces. Exchange of gases and metabolic products occurs across the thin fetal layers that separate the two bloodstreams at this level. Antibodies can also cross this layer and enter fetal circulation to provide passive immunity against a variety of infectious agents, i.e., those of diphtheria, smallpox, and measles. Fetal blood returns through a system of veins that parallel the arteries except that they converge on a single *umbilical vein.*

Maternal blood is supplied to the placenta through 80–100 spiral endometrial arteries that penetrate the basal plate. Blood from these spiral arteries flows into the base of the intervillous spaces, which contain about 150 mL of maternal blood that is exchanged 3 or 4 times/min. The blood pressure in the spiral arteries is much higher than that in the intervillous spaces. As blood is injected into these spaces at each pulse, it is directed deep into the spaces. As the pressure decreases, the blood flows back over the surfaces of the villi and eventually enters endometrial veins also located in the base of the spaces.

Exchange of gases and metabolic products occurs as the blood passes over the villi. Normally, water, carbon diox-

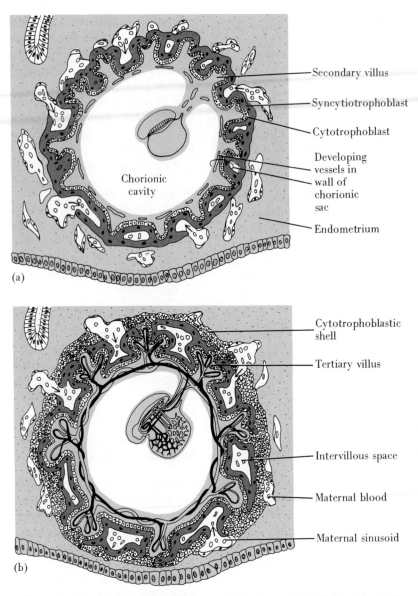

Secondary villus

Syncytiotrophoblast

Cytotrophoblast

Developing vessels in wall of chorionic sac

Endometrium

Chorionic cavity

(a)

Cytotrophoblastic shell

Tertiary villus

Intervillous space

Maternal blood

Maternal sinusoid

(b)

Figure 22.27. Schematic diagrams of section through a human embryo, chorionic sac, and placenta at 16 **(a)** and 21 **(b)** days of development. The diagrams illustrate the separation of the fetal and maternal blood vessels by the placental membrane composed of the endothelium of the capillaries, mesenchyme, cytotrophoblast, and syncytiotrophoblast. (After Moore KL, Persaud TVN: *The Developing Human*, 5th ed. Philadelphia, WB Saunders, 1993, p 66.)

ide, metabolic waste products, and hormones are transferred from the fetal blood to the maternal blood, and water, oxygen, metabolites, electrolytes, vitamins, hormones, and some antibodies pass in the opposite direction. The placental barrier does not exclude many potentially dangerous agents, such as alcohol, nicotine, viruses, drugs, exogenous hormones, and heavy metals. Therefore, during pregnancy, there is need to avoid exposure to or ingestion of such agents to reduce the risk of injury to the embryo or fetus.

Before the establishment of blood flow through the placenta, the growth of the embryo is supported, in part, by metabolic products that are synthesized by or transported through the trophoblast. The syncytiotrophoblast synthe-

sizes glycogen, cholesterol, and fatty acids, as well as other nutrients utilized by the embryo.

The Placenta Is a Major Endocrine Gland Producing Steroid and Protein Hormones

The placenta also functions as an endocrine organ, producing steroid and peptide hormones as well as prostaglandins that play an important role in the onset of labor. Immunocytochemical studies indicate that the syncytiotrophoblast is the site of synthesis of these hormones.

The steroid hormones, progesterone and estrogen, have essential roles in the maintenance of pregnancy. As pregnancy proceeds, the placenta takes over the major role in

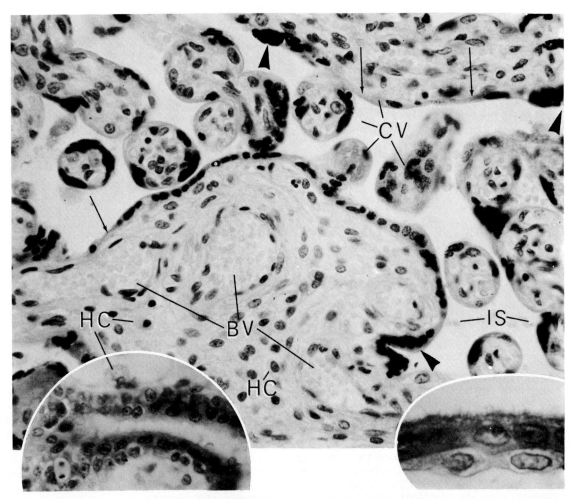

Figure 22.28. Photomicrograph of human placenta. The section is through the substance of a term placenta. Chorionic villi *(CV)* of various sizes and surrounding intervillous spaces *(IS)* can be seen. The connective tissue core of the villus contains branches and tributaries of the umbilical arteries and veins *(BV)*. Only capillaries are present in the smallest villi. The villi are covered by two cell layers **(insets).** The outer layer is the syncytiotrophoblast; immediately under this is the layer composed of cytotrophoblasts. Phagocytic cells, called Hofbauer cels *(HC)*, can be seen within the villi. *Arrowheads* indicate clusters of syncytiotrophoblast nuclei; *arrows* indicate attenuated syncytial cytoplasm. ×280; **insets,** ×1300.

the secretion of these steroids from the corpus luteum. The placenta produces enough progesterone by the end of the eighth week to maintain pregnancy if the corpus luteum is surgically removed or fails to function. In the production of placental estrogen, the *fetal adrenal cortex* plays an essential role, providing the precursors needed for estrogen synthesis. Because the placenta lacks the enzymes needed for the production of the estrogen precursors, a cooperative *fetoplacental (endocrine) unit* is established. Clinically, the monitoring of estrogen production during pregnancy can be used as an index of fetal development.

The following peptide hormones are secreted by the placenta:

- **Human chorionic gonadotropin (hCG),** the synthesis of which begins around day 6, even before syncytiotrophoblast formation, exhibits marked homology to pituitary TSH and stimulates the maternal thyroid gland to increase secretion of T_4. It also maintains the corpus luteum during the early pregnancy. Measurement of hCG is used to detect pregnancy and assess development during the early stages of the embryo.
- **Human chorionic somatomammotropin (hCS),** also known as human placental lactogen (hPL), is closely related to human growth hormone. Synthesized in the syncytiotrophoblast, it promotes general growth, regulates glucose metabolism, and stimulates mammary duct proliferation in the maternal breast. hCS effects on maternal metabolism are significant, but the role of this hormone in fetal development remains unknown.
- **Insulin-like growth factors I and II (IGF-I and IGF-II)** are produced by and stimulate proliferation and differentiation of the cytotrophoblast.
- **Endothelial growth factor (EGF)** exhibits an age-dependent dual action on the early placenta. In the 4–5-week-old placenta, EGF is synthesized by the cytotrophoblast and stimulates proliferation of the trophoblast. In the 6–12-week-old placenta, synthesis of

FETAL CIRCULATION

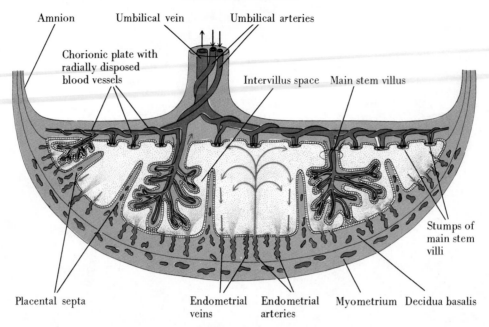

MATERNAL CIRCULATION

Figure 22.29. Schematic diagram of mature human placenta. The placenta is divided into subdivisions, called cotyledons, by placental septa that are formed by invaginations of the decidua basalis. Maternal blood enters the placenta through numerous endometrial spiral arteries that penetrate the basal plate. As the blood enters the cotyledon, it is directed deep into the intervillous space *(arrows)*. It then passes over the surface of the villi where the exchange of gases and metabolic products occurs. The maternal blood finally leaves the intervillous space through endometrial veins. The fetal blood enters the placenta through umbilical arteries that divide into several radially disposed arteries within the chorionic plate. Branches from the vessels pass into the main stem villi and there form extensive capillary networks. The veins within the villi then carry the blood back through a system of veins that parallels the fetal arteries. As noted above, exchange of gases and metabolic products occurs across the placental barrier as the maternal blood flows over the surface of the villi in close approximation to the fetal placental capillary beds within the villi. (After Moore KL, Persaud TVN: *The Developing Human,* 5th ed. Philadelphia, WB Saunders, 1993, p 177.)

EGF is shifted to the syncytiotrophoblast; it then stimulates and maintains the function of the differentiated trophoblast.

- ***Relaxin*** is synthesized by decidual cells and is involved in the "softening" of the cervix and the pelvic ligaments in preparation for parturition.
- ***Other growth factors*** stimulate cytotrophoblastic growth e.g., fibroblast growth factor, colony-stimulating factor (CSF-1), platelet-derived growth factor, and interleukins (IL-1 and IL-3) or inhibit trophoblast growth and proliferation (e.g., tumor necrosis factor).

VAGINA

The Vagina Is a Fibromuscular Tube Lined by Nonkeratinized *Stratified Squamous Epithelium*

The vagina is a fibromuscular sheath extending from the cervix to the vestibule, which is the area between the labia minora. In a virgin, the opening into the vagina may be surrounded by the hymen, folds of mucous membrane extending into the vaginal lumen. The hymen or its remnants are derived from the endodermal membrane that separated

---

FATE OF MATURE PLACENTA AT BIRTH

The mature placenta measures about 15–20 cm in diameter × 2–3 cm in thickness, covers 25–30% of the uterine surface, and weighs 500–600 g at term. The surface area of the villi in the human placenta is estimated to be about 10 m². The microvilli on the syncytiotrophoblast increase the effective area for metabolic exchange to more than 90 m². After birth, the uterus continues to contract, causing reduction of the luminal surface and placental separation from the uterine wall. The entire fetal portion of the placenta, fetal membranes, and the intervening projections of decidual tissue are released. During uncomplicated labor, the placenta is delivered approximately within half an hour after birth.

After delivery of the placenta, there is endometrial regeneration from the glands and stroma of the decidua basalis. Endometrial regeneration is completed by the end of the third week postpartum except at the placental site, where regeneration usually extends through the period of the next 3 weeks. In the first week after delivery, remnants of the decidua are shed and constitute the blood-tinged uterine discharge known as the ***lochia rubra.***

the developing vagina from the cavity of the definitive urogenital sinus in the embryo.

The vaginal wall consists of an

- Inner mucosal layer
- Intermediate muscular layer
- Outer adventitial layer (Fig. 22.30)

The *mucosa of the vagina* has numerous transverse folds or rugae (see Fig. 22.1) and is lined with stratified squamous epithelium (Fig. 22.31). Connective tissue papillae from the underlying lamina propria project into the epithelial layer. In humans and other primates, keratohyalin granules may be present in the epithelial cells, but under normal conditions, keratinization does not occur. Therefore, nuclei can be seen in epithelial cells throughout the thickness of the epithelium.

The Vaginal Mucosa Contains No Glands

The vaginal surface is lubricated by mucus produced by the cervical glands. The epithelium undergoes cyclic changes

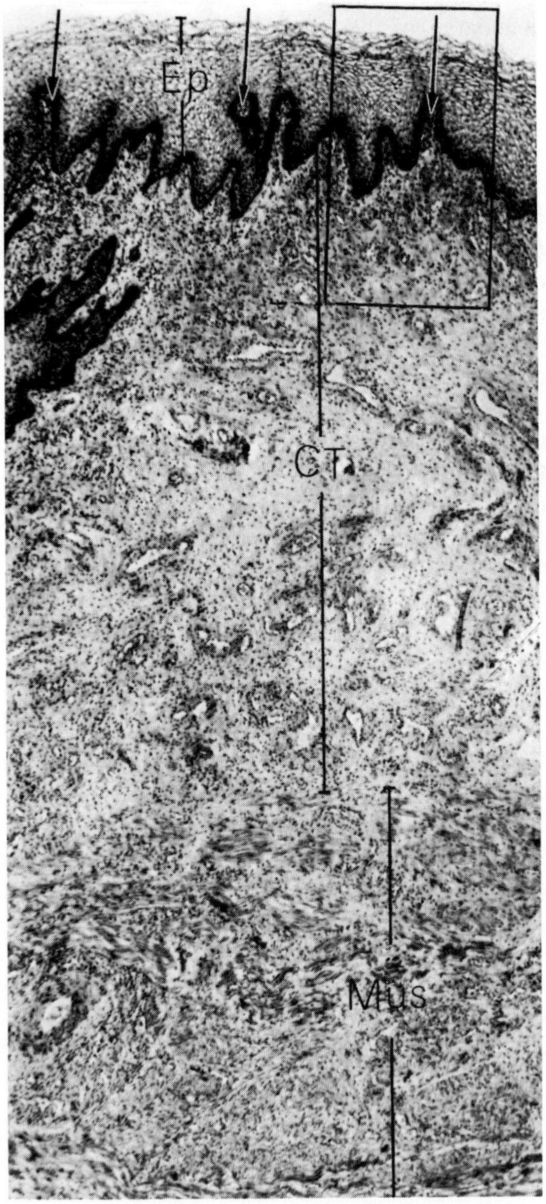

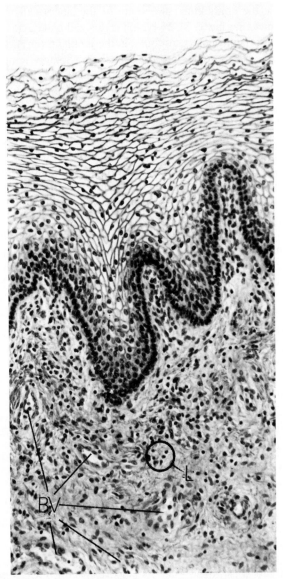

Figure 22.30. Photomicrograph of human vagina. The vaginal wall consists of three layers: a mucous membrane, a muscular layer *(Mus),* and an outer adventitia (not shown). The mucous membrane consists of a stratified squamous epithelium *(Ep)* and an underlying connective tissue layer *(CT).* Deep connective tissue papillae project into the undersurface of the epithelium *(arrows).* ×40.

Figure 22.31. Photomicrograph of human vaginal mucosa from the area of the *rectangle* in Figure 22.30. Projection of the connective tissue papillae into the epithelium gives the connective tissue-epithelial junction a very uneven appearance. Numerous blood vessels *(BV)* and leukocytes *(L)* are present in the connective tissue. The number of leukocytes varies with the ovarian cycle. The greatest number is found around the time of menstruation. ×180.

during the menstrual cycle. Under the influence of estrogens, during the follicular phase, the epithelial cells synthesize and accumulate glycogen as they migrate toward the surface. Cells are continuously desquamated, but near or during the menstrual phase the superficial layer of the vaginal epithelium may be shed.

The lamina propria exhibits two distinct regions. The outer region immediately below the epithelium is a highly cellular loose connective tissue. The deeper region, adjacent to the muscular layer, is more dense and may be considered a submucosa. The deeper region contains a large number of thin-walled veins that simulate erectile tissue during sexual arousal. Numerous elastic fibers are present immediately below the epithelium, and some of the fibers extend into the muscular layer. Many lymphocytes and leukocytes (particularly neutrophils) are found in the lamina propria. Many of these cells migrate into the epithelium. Solitary lymphatic nodules may also be present. The number of lymphocytes and leukocytes in the mucosa and vaginal lumen dramatically increases around the time of menstrual flow.

The **vaginal muscularis** is organized in two, sometimes indistinct, intermingling smooth muscle layers, an outer longitudinal layer and an inner circular layer. The outer layer, which is continuous with the corresponding layer in the uterus, is much thicker than the inner layer. Striated muscle fibers of the bulbospongiosus muscle are present at the vaginal opening.

The **vaginal adventitia** is organized into an inner dense connective tissue layer, adjacent to the muscularis, and an outer loose connective tissue layer that blends with the adventitia of the surrounding structures. The inner layer contains numerous elastic fibers that contribute to the elasticity and strength of the vaginal wall. The outer layer contains numerous blood and lymphatic vessels and nerves.

The vagina has few general sensory nerve endings. The sensory nerve endings that are more plentiful in the lower third of the vagina are probably associated primarily with pain and stretch sensations.

VAGINAL SMEARS

The examination of vaginal smears is a valuable diagnostic tool in evaluating estrogenic stimulation of the vaginal mucosa. The synthesis and the release of glycogen into the uterine lumen appear to be related directly to changes in the pH of the vaginal fluid. The pH of the vaginal fluid, which is normally low, around pH 4, becomes more acid near midcycle as *Lactobacillus acidophilus,* a lactic acid-forming bacterium in the vagina, metabolizes the glycogen. An alkaline environment is favorable for the growth of infectious agents such as staphylococci, *Corynebacterium vaginale, Trichomonas vaginalis,* and *Candida albicans,* causing an abnormal increase in vaginal secretions and inflammation of the vaginal mucosa and vulvar skin known as vulvovaginitis. Specific antimicrobial agents (antibiotics, sulfonamides) are used together with the nonspecific therapy (acidified 0.1% hexetidine gel) to restore the low pH in the vagina that retards the growth of the infectious agents.

EXTERNAL GENITALIA

The female external genitalia consist of the following parts that are collectively referred to as the **vulva** and have a stratified squamous epithelium:

- **Mons pubis:** The mons pubis is the rounded prominence over the pubic symphysis, formed by subcutaneous adipose tissue.
- **Labia majora:** The labia majora are two large longitudinal folds of skin, homologous to the skin of the scrotum, that extend from the mons pubis and form the lateral boundaries of the urogenital cleft. They contain a thin layer of smooth muscle, resembling the dartos muscle of the scrotum, and a large amount of subcutaneous adipose tissue. The outer surface, like that of the mons pubis, is covered with pubic hair. The inner surface is smooth and devoid of hair. Sebaceous and sweat glands are present on both surfaces.
- **Labia minora:** The labia minora are paired, hairless folds of skin that border the vestibule and are homologous to the skin of the penis. Abundant melanin pigment is present in the deep cells of the epithelium. The core of connective tissue within each fold is devoid of fat but does contain numerous blood vessels and fine elastic fibers. Large sebaceous glands are present in the stroma.
- **Clitoris:** The clitoris is an erectile structure that is homologous to the penis. Its body is composed of two small erectile bodies, the **corpora cavernosa;** the **glans clitoris** is a small, rounded tubercle of erectile tissue. The skin over the glans is very thin, forms the prepuce of the clitoris, and contains numerous sensory nerve endings.
- **Vestibule:** The vestibule is lined with stratified squamous epithelium. Numerous small mucous glands, the **lesser vestibular glands** (also called **Skene's glands**), are present primarily near the clitoris and around the external urethral orifice. The large, paired **greater vestibular glands** (also called **Bartholin's glands**) are homologous to the male bulbourethral glands. These glands, which are about 1 cm in diameter, are located in the lateral wall of the vestibule posterior to the bulb of the vestibule. The greater vestibular glands are tubuloalveolar glands that secrete a lubricating mucus (Fig. 22.32). The ducts of these glands open into the vestibule near the vaginal opening.

Numerous sensory nerve endings are present in the external genitalia:

- **Meissner's corpuscles** are particularly abundant in the skin over the mons pubis and labia majora.
- **Pacinian corpuscles** are distributed in the deeper layers of the connective tissue and are found in the labia majora and in association with the erectile tissue. The sensory impulses from these nerve endings play an important role in the physiologic response during sexual arousal.

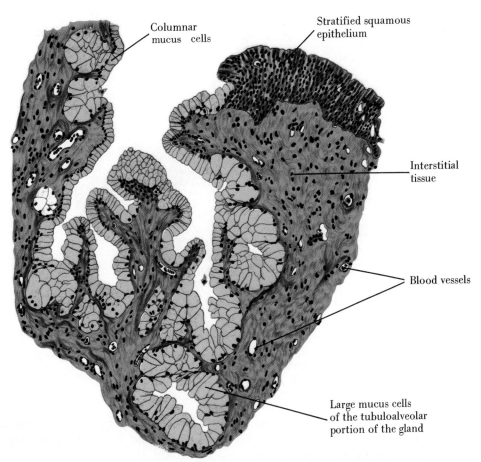

Columnar mucus cells

Stratified squamous epithelium

Interstitial tissue

Blood vessels

Large mucus cells of the tubuloalveolar portion of the gland

Figure 22.32. Drawing of a section of a greater vestibular or Bartholin's gland. Small ducts lined with columnar mucous cells extend from the tubuloalveolar terminal portions of the glands. Patches of stratified columnar epithelium are present in the larger ducts. ×185. (After Maximow AA: In: Bloom W, Fawcett DW: *A Textbook of Histology,* 10th ed. Philadelphia, WB Saunders, 1975, p 904.)

• *Free nerve endings* are present in great number and are equally distributed in the skin of the external genitalia.

MAMMARY GLANDS

The mammary glands or breasts are a distinguishing feature of mammals. During embryologic development, growth and development of the breast occur in both sexes. Multiple glands develop along paired epidermal thickenings, called the *mammary ridges (milk lines),* that extend from the developing axilla to the developing inguinal region. In the human, normally only one group of cells develops into a breast on each side. An extra breast (polymastia) or nipple (polythelia) may occur as an inheritable condition in about 1% of the female population. These relatively rare conditions may also occur in the male.

In the male, there is normally little additional development in postnatal life, and the glands remain rudimentary. In the female, the mammary glands undergo further development under hormonal influence. They are also influenced by changes in the ovarian hormone levels during each menstrual cycle. The actual initiation of milk secretion is induced by prolactin secreted by the adenohypophysis. The

ejection of the milk from the breast is stimulated by oxytocin released from the neurohypophysis. With the change in the hormonal environment at menopause, the glandular component of the breast regresses or involutes and is replaced by fat and connective tissue.

Mammary Glands Are Modified Apocrine Sweat Glands That Develop Under the Influence of Sex Hormones

The inactive adult mammary gland is composed of 15–20 irregular lobes of branched tubuloalveolar glands (Fig. 22.33). The lobes, separated by fibrous bands of connective tissue, radiate from the *mammary papilla* or *nipple* and are further subdivided into numerous lobules. Some of the fibrous bands, called *suspensory* or *Cooper's ligaments,* connect with the dermis. Abundant adipose tissue is present in the dense connective tissue of the interlobular spaces. The intralobular connective tissue is much less dense and contains little fat.

The epidermis of the adult nipple and areola is highly pigmented and somewhat wrinkled and has long dermal papillae invading into its deep surface (Fig. 22.34). It is covered by keratinized stratified squamous epithelium. The pig-

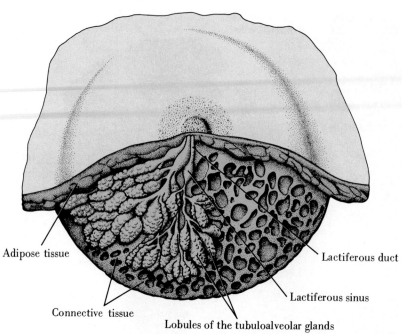

Adipose tissue

Lactiferous duct

Lactiferous sinus

Connective tissue

Lobules of the tubuloalveolar glands

Figure 22.33. Schematic drawing of the human breast as seen during lactation. The breast is composed of branched tubuloalveolar glands. (Based on Warwick R, Williams PL (eds): *Gray's Anatomy,* 35th ed. Edinburgh, Churchill Livingstone, 1973, p 1365.)

mentation of the nipple increases at puberty, and the nipple becomes more prominent. During pregnancy, the areola becomes larger, and the degree of pigmentation increases further. Deep to the areola and nipple, bundles of smooth muscle fibers are arranged radially and circumferentially in the dense connective tissue and longitudinally along the lactiferous ducts. These muscle fibers allow the nipple to become erect in response to various stimuli.

The areola contains sebaceous glands, sweat glands, and modified mammary glands (glands of Montgomery). These glands, which are described as having a structure intermediate between sweat glands and true mammary glands, produce small elevations on the surface of the areola. Numerous sensory nerve endings are present in the nipple. The areola contains fewer sensory nerve endings.

The tubuloalveolar glands, derived from modified sweat glands in the epidermis, lie in the subcutaneous tissue. Each gland ends in a *lactiferous duct* that opens through a constricted orifice onto the nipple. Beneath the *areola,* the pigmented area surrounding the nipple, each duct has a dilated portion, the *lactiferous sinus.* Near their openings, the lactiferous ducts are lined with stratified squamous epithelium. The epithelial lining of the duct shows a gradual transition to two layers of cuboidal cells in the lactiferous sinus and then becomes a single layer of columnar or cuboidal cells through the remainder of the duct system. Myoepithelial cells of ectodermal origin lie within the epithelium between the surface epithelial cells and the basal lamina. These cells, arranged in a basket-like network, are present in the secretory portion of the gland but are more apparent in the larger ducts.

The Morphology of the Secretory Portion of the Mammary Gland Varies With the Menstrual Cycle

In the *inactive gland,* the glandular component is sparse and consists chiefly of duct elements (Fig. 22.35). During the menstrual cycle, the inactive breast undergoes slight cyclic changes. Early in the cycle, the ducts appear as cords with little or no lumen. Under estrogen stimulation, at about the time of ovulation, the secretory cells increase in height, lumina appear in the ducts as small amounts of secretions accumulate, and fluid accumulates in the connective tissue.

Mammary Glands Undergo Dramatic Proliferation and Development During Pregnancy

The mammary glands exhibit a number of changes in preparation for lactation. The changes in the glandular tissue are accompanied by decreases in the amount of connective tissue and adipose tissue. Plasma cells, lymphocytes, and eosinophils infiltrate the fibrous component of the connective tissue as the breast develops. The development of the glandular tissue is not uniform, and variation in the degree of development is seen even within a single lobule. The cells vary in shape from flattened to low columnar. As the cells proliferate by mitotic division, the ducts branch and alveoli begin to develop. In the later stages of pregnancy, alveolar development becomes more prominent (Fig. 22.36). The actual proliferation of the stromal cells declines, and subsequent enlargement of the breast occurs through hypertrophy of the secretory cells and accumulation of secretory product in the alveoli.

Both Merocrine and Apocrine Secretion Are Involved in Production of Milk

The secreting cells contain abundant granular endoplasmic reticulum, a moderate number of large mitochondria, a supranuclear Golgi complex, and a number of dense lysosomes (Fig. 22.37). Depending on the secretory state, large lipid droplets and secretory granules may be present in the apical cytoplasm. The secretory cells produce two distinct products that are released by different mechanisms:

- *Merocrine secretion:* The protein component of the milk is synthesized in the rER, packaged into membrane-limited secretory granules for transport in the Golgi apparatus, and released from the cell by fusion of the granule's limiting membrane with the plasma membrane.
- *Apocrine secretion:* The fatty or lipid component of the milk arises as lipid droplets free in the cytoplasm. The lipid coalesces to form large droplets that pass to the apical region of the cell and project into the lumen of the acinus. The droplets are invested with an envelope of plasma membrane as they are released. A thin layer of cytoplasm is trapped between the plasma membrane and lipid droplet and is released with the lipid, but the *cytoplasmic loss in this process is minimal.*

The secretion released in the first few days after childbirth is known as **colostrum.** This premilk is an alkaline, yellowish secretion with a higher protein, vitamin A, sodium, and chloride content and a lower lipid, carbohydrate, and potassium content than milk. It contains considerable amounts of antibodies that provide the newborn with some degree

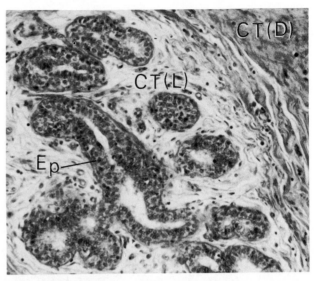

Figure 22.35. Photomicrograph of inactive or resting mammary gland. The epithelial (*Ep*) or glandular elements are embedded in loose connective tissue [*CT (L)*]. The epithelial cells within the lobule are primarily duct elements. The lobule is surrounded by dense connective tissue [*CT(D)*]. ×160.

of passive immunity. The antibodies in the colostrum are believed to be produced by the lymphocytes and plasma cells infiltrated into the stroma of the breast during its proliferation and development and secreted across the glandular cells as in salivary glands and intestine. As these wandering cells decrease in number after parturition, the production of colostrum stops, and lipid-rich milk is produced.

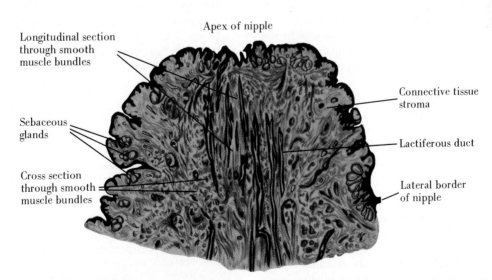

Figure 22.34. Drawing of perpendicular section through the nipple of a female breast. Keratinized stratified squamous epithelium covers the somewhat wrinkled surface of the nipple and areola. Bundles of smooth muscle fibers are embedded in the dense connective tissue that surrounds the lactiferous ducts located deep in the areola and nipple ×6. (After Schaffer: In: Bloom W, Fawcett DW: *A Textbook of Histology,* 10th ed. Philadelphia, WB Saunders, 1975, p 909.)

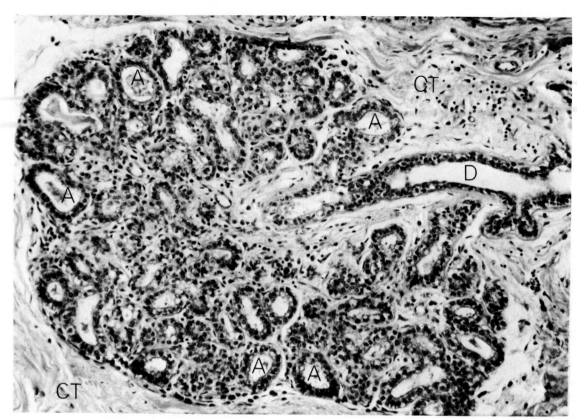

Figure 22.36. Photomicrograph of proliferative human mammary gland. During the early proliferative period, the development of the alveolar elements of the gland becomes conspicuous (compare with Fig. 22.35). Distinct alveoli (*A*) are present. Within a lobule, all these alveoli are joined to a duct. Loose, highly cellular connective tissue surrounds the alveoli. Dense connective tissue septa (*CT*) separate the individual lobules. ×160.

Hormonal Regulation of the Mammary Gland

The initial growth and development of the mammary gland at puberty occur under the influence of estrogens and progesterone being produced by the maturing ovary. Subsequent to this initial development, slight changes in the morphology of the glandular tissue occur during each ovarian cycle. During pregnancy, the corpus luteum and placenta continuously produce estrogens and progesterone. Estrogen present in the circulation stimulates proliferation of the lactiferous duct components, and progesterone stimulates growth of alveoli. It is now believed that the growth of the mammary glands is also dependent on the presence of prolactin, produced by the adenohypophysis; hCS, produced by the placenta; and adrenal glucocorticoids.

Lactation Is Under the Neurohormonal Control of the Adenohypophysis and Hypothalamus

Although estrogen and progesterone are essential for the physical development of the breast during pregnancy, both of these hormones also have an overriding suppressive effect on prolactin and hCS, the levels of which increase as pregnancy progresses. Immediately after birth, however, the sudden loss of estrogen and progesterone secretion from the placenta and corpus luteum allows the lactogenic effect of prolactin to assume its natural role. Production of milk also requires adequate secretion of growth hormone, adrenal glucocorticoids, and parathyroid hormones.

The act of suckling during breast-feeding initiates sensory impulses from receptors in the nipple to the hypothalamus. The impulses inhibit the release of prolactin-inhibiting factor, and prolactin is then released from the adenohypophysis. The sensory impulses also cause the release of oxytocin in the neurohypophysis. The oxytocin stimulates the myoepithelial cells that surround the base of the alveolar secretory cells and the base of the cells in the larger ducts, causing them to contract and eject the milk from the alveoli and the ducts. In the absence of suckling, secretion of milk ceases, and the mammary glands begin to regress. The glandular tissue then returns to an inactive condition.

LACTATION AND INFERTILITY

Almost 50% of fully breast-feeding women exhibit lactational amenorrhea (lack of menstruation during lactation) and infertility. This is due to high levels of serum prolactin, which suppress secretion of LH. Resumption of ovulation usually occurs after 6 months or earlier with decrease in suckling frequency. In cultures in which breast-feeding may continue for 2–3 years, lactational amenorrhea is the principal means of birth control.

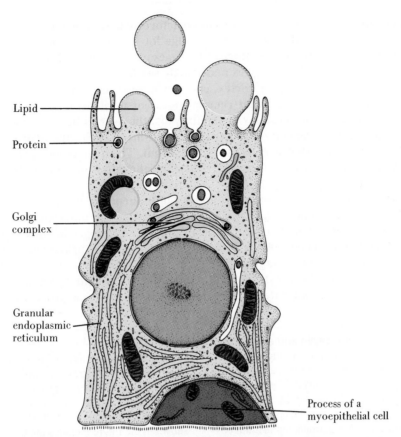

Lipid

Protein

Golgi complex

Granular endoplasmic reticulum

Process of a myoepithelial cell

Figure 22.37. Schematic diagram of a secretory epithelial cell from a lactating mammary gland. Large lipid droplets of the milk (shown in yellow) and a thin layer of adjacent cytoplasm are enclosed within an envelope of plasma membrane as the droplets are released (apocrine secretion). The protein component of the milk (shown in blue), which is synthesized in the granular endoplasmic reticulum and packaged in the Golgi complex, is released from the cell by fusion of the granule's limiting membrane with the plasma membrane (merocrine secretion). (Redrawn after Bloom W, Fawcett DW: *A Textbook of Histology,* 10th ed. Philadelphia, WB Saunders, 1975, p 914.)

Involution of the Mammary Gland

The mammary gland atrophies or involutes after menopause. In the absence of ovarian hormone stimulation, the secretory cells of the alveoli degenerate and disappear, but some ducts may remain. The connective tissue also demonstrates degenerative changes, marked by a decrease in the number of fibroblasts and collagen fibers, and loss of elastic fibers.

Blood Supply and Lymphatics

The arteries that supply the breast are derived from the thoracic branches of the axillary artery, the internal thoracic (internal mammary) artery, and anterior intercostal arteries.

Branches of the vessels pass primarily along the path of the alveolar ducts as they reach capillary beds surrounding the alveoli. Veins basically follow the path of the arteries as they return to the axillary and internal thoracic veins.

Lymphatic capillaries are located in the connective tissue surrounding the alveoli. The larger lymphatic vessels drain into axillary, supraclavicular, or parasternal lymph nodes.

Innervation

The nerves that supply the breast are anterior and lateral cutaneous branches from the second to sixth intercostal nerves. The nerves convey afferent and sympathetic fibers to and from the breast. The secretory function is primarily under hormonal control, but afferent impulses associated with suckling are involved in the reflex secretion of prolactin and oxytocin.

PLATE 112. Ovary I

The ovaries are small, paired, ovoid solid structures whose dimensions are roughly 3.0 × 1.5 × 1 cm. They possess a hilum on one edge for the transit of neurovascular structures. On this same edge they are attached to a mesovarium that joins them to the broad ligament. The ovaries produce oocytes and female sex hormones.

The outer part of the ovary, the cortex, contains numerous primordial follicles that are present at the time of birth and that remain quiescent until sexual maturation. At that time, under the influence of pituitary gonadotropins, the ovaries begin to undergo cyclical changes designated the ovarian cycle. During each ovarian cycle, the ovaries produce an oocyte (usually only one) that is ready for fertilization. The ovaries also produce estrogen and progesterone, the steroid hormones that bring about the uterine cycles and, in the human, menstruation.

At the beginning of the ovarian cycle, under the influence of a pituitary follicle-stimulating hormone (FSH), some of the primordial follicles begin to undergo changes that lead to the development of a mature (Graafian) follicle. These changes include a proliferation of cells and total enlargement of the follicle. Although several primordial follicles begin this series of developmental changes, usually only one reaches maturity and yields an oocyte. The discharge of the oocyte and its adherent cells is called ovulation. The other follicles that began to proliferate at the same time degenerate, a process referred to as atresia.

FIGURE 1, ovary, monkey, hematoxylin and eosin (H&E) ×120. The cortex of an ovary from a sexually mature individual is shown here. On the surface, there is a single layer of epithelial cells designated the germinal epithelium *(GEp)*. This epithelium is continuous with the serosa (peritoneum) of the mesovarium. Contrary to its name, the epithelium does not give rise to the germ cells. The germinal epithelium covers a dense fibrous connective tissue layer, the tunica albu-

ginea *(TA);* under the tunica albuginea are the primordial follicles *(PF)*. It is not unusual to see follicles at various stages of development or atresia in the ovary. In this figure, along with the large number of primordial follicles, there are four growing follicles *(SF)*, an atretic follicle *(AF)*, and part of a large follicle on the right. The region of the large follicle shown in the figure includes the theca interna *(TI)*, granulosa cells *(GC)*, and part of the antrum *(A)*.

FIGURE 2, ovary, monkey, H&E ×450. This figure shows several primordial follicles at higher magnification. Each follicle consists of an oocyte surrounded by a single layer of squamous follicular cells *(F)*. The nucleus *(N)* of the oocyte is typically large, but the oocyte itself is so large that the nucleus is often not included in the plane of section, as in the oocyte marked *X*. The group of epithelioid-appearing cells *(arrowhead)* are follicular cells of a primordial follicle that has been sectioned in a plane that just grazes the follicular surface. In this case, the follicular cells are seen en face.

FIGURE 3, ovary, monkey, H&E ×450. When a *primordial* follicle begins the changes leading to the formation of a mature follicle, the layer of squamous follicular cells becomes cuboidal, as in this figure. In addition, the follicular cells proliferate and become multilayered. A follicle undergoing these early changes is called a *primary* follicle. Thus, an early primary follicle may still be unilaminar, but it is surrounded by cuboidal cells, and this distinguishes it from the more numerous unilaminar primordial follicles that are surrounded by squamous cells.

FIGURE 4, ovary, monkey, H&E ×450. The primary follicle in this figure shows a multilayered mass of follicular cells *(FC)* surrounding the oocyte. The innermost layer of follicular cells is adjacent to a thick eosinophilic layer of extracellular homogeneous material called the zona pellucida *(ZP)*. At this stage of development, the oocyte has also enlarged slightly. The entire structure surrounded by the zona pellucida is actually the oocyte.

Surrounding the follicles are elongate cells of the highly cellular connective tissue, referred to as stromal cells. The stromal cells surrounding a secondary follicle become disposed into two layers designated the theca interna and the theca externa. As seen in Figure 1, stromal cells become epithelioid in the cell-rich theca interna *(TI)*.

KEY

A, antrum	**GEp,** germinal epithelium	**TI,** theca interna
AF, atretic follicle	**N,** nucleus of oocyte	**X,** oocyte showing only cytoplasm
F, follicle cells, primordial	**PF,** primordial follicles	**ZP,** zona pellucida
FC, follicle cells	**SF,** growing follicles	**arrowhead,** follicle cells in face
GC, granulosa cells	**TA,** tunica albuginea	view

PLATE 112

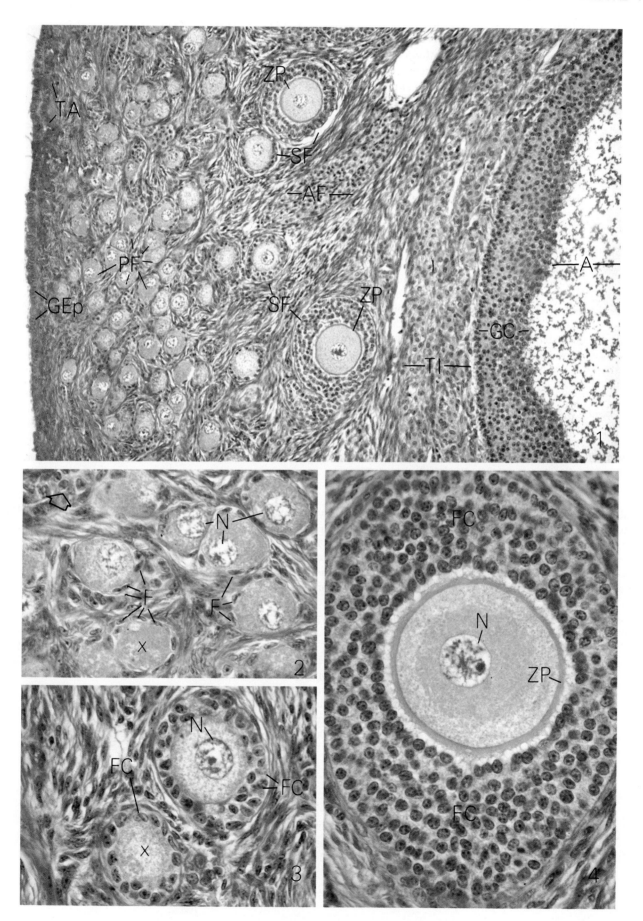

PLATE 113. Ovary II

Atresia of follicles is a regular event in the ovary, beginning in embryonic life. In any section through the ovary, follicles of various stages can be seen undergoing atresia. In all cases, the follicular cells show pyknosis of the nucleus and dissolution of the cytoplasm; the follicle is invaded by macrophages and other connective tissue cells. The oocyte degenerates, leaving behind the prominent zona pellucida. This may be folded inwardly or collapsed, but it usually retains its thickness and staining characteristics. Thus, when included in the plane of section, a partially disrupted zona pellucida serves as a reliable diagnostic feature of an atretic follicle.

In some ovaries, including the human ovary, clusters of epithelioid cells observed in the ovarian cortex are referred to collectively as interstitial glands. They are remnants of the theca interna of large degenerating follicles.

FIGURES 1 and 2, ovary, monkey, H&E ×120. Two follicles growing under the influence of FSH are shown in Figure 1. The more advanced follicle is a secondary follicle. The oocyte in this follicle is surrounded by several layers of follicular cells *(FC)* that, at this stage, are identified as granulosa cells. At a slightly earlier time, small lakes of fluid formed between the follicular cells, and these lakes have now fused into a well-defined larger cavity called the follicular antrum *(FA)* that is evident in the figure. The antrum is also filled with fluid and stains with the PAS reaction, although only lightly. The substance that stains with the PAS reaction has been retained as an eosinophilic precipitate in the antra of the secondary follicles shown here and in Figure 2. Immediately above the obvious secondary follicle is a slightly smaller follicle. Because no antral spaces are evident between the follicular cells, it is appropriate to classify it as a primary follicle. In both follicles, but particularly in the larger follicle with the antrum, the surrounding stromal cells have become altered to form two distinctive layers designated theca interna *(TI)* and theca externa *(TE)*. The theca interna is a more cellular layer, and the cells are epithelioid. When seen with the electron microscope, they display the characteristics of endocrine cells, particularly steroid-secreting cells. In contrast, the theca externa is a connective tissue layer. Its cells are more or less spindle-shaped.

In Figure 2, a later stage in the growth of the secondary follicle is shown. The antrum *(FA)* is larger, and the oocyte is off to one side, surrounded by a mound of follicular cells called the cumulus oophorus. The remaining follicular cells that surround the antral cavity are referred to as the membrana granulosa *(MG)* or simply as granulosa cells.

FIGURE 3, ovary, monkey, H&E ×65. Atretic follicles *(AF)* are shown here and at higher magnification in Figure 4. The two smaller atretic follicles can be identified by virtue of the retained zona pellucida *(ZP)* (see Fig. 4). The two larger, more advanced follicles do not display the remains of a zona pellucida, but they do display other features of follicular atresia.

FIGURE 4, ovary, monkey, H&E ×120. In atresia of a more advanced follicle, the follicular cells tend to degenerate more rapidly than the cells of the theca interna, and the basement membrane separating the two becomes thickened to form a hyalinized membrane, the glassy membrane *(arrows)* separates an outer layer of remaining theca interna cells *(TI)* from the degenerating inner follicular cells. The remaining theca interna cells may show cytologic integrity *(MG);* these intact theca cells remain temporarily functional in steroid secretion.

FIGURE 5, ovary, monkey, H&E ×120. Additional atretic follicles *(AF)* are shown here. Again, some show remnants of a zona pellucida *(ZP)*, and two show a glassy membrane *(arrows)*. Note that even though the atresia in these follicles is well advanced, some of the cells external to one of the glassy membranes still retain their epithelioid character *(open arrowhead)*. These are persisting theca interna cells.

KEY

AF, atretic follicle	**MG:** Fig. 2, membrana granulosa;	**arrows,** glassy membrane
FA, antrum of follicle	Fig. 4, persisting theca interna	**open arrowhead,** persisting theca
FC, follicle cells	cells	interna cells
	TE, theca externa	
	TI, theca interna	
	ZP, zona pellucida	

PLATE 113

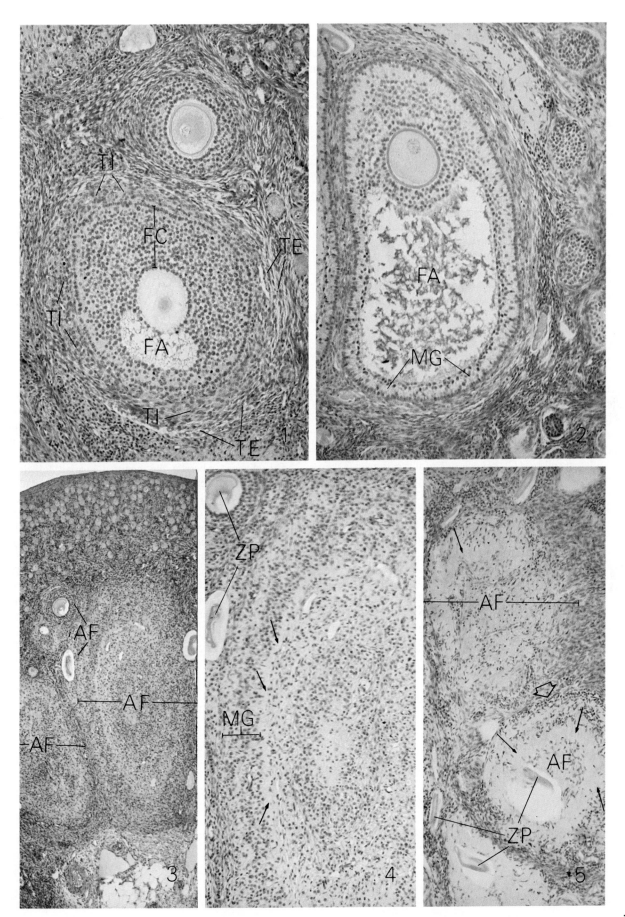

PLATE 114. Corpus Luteum

After the oocyte and surrounding cumulus cells are discharged from the mature ovarian follicle (ovulation), the remaining follicle cells (membrana granulosa) and the adjacent theca interna cells undergo changes that result in the formation of a new functional unit, the corpus luteum.

FIGURE 1, corpus luteum, human, H&E ×20. This figure shows ovarian cortex shortly after ovulation. The *arrowhead* points toward the surface of the ovary at the site of ovulation. The cavity *(FC)* of the former follicle has been invaded by connective tissue *(CT)*. The membrana granulosa has become plicated, and the granulosa cells, now transformed into cells of the corpus luteum, are called granulosa lutein cells. The plication of the membrana granulosa begins just before ovulation and continues as the corpus luteum develops. As the corpus luteum becomes more plicated, the former follicular cavity becomes reduced in size. At the same time, blood vessels *(BV)* from the theca of the follicle invade the former cavity and the transforming membrana granulosa cells *(TC)*. Cells of the theca interna follow the blood vessels into the outermost depressions of the plicated structure. These theca interna cells become transformed into cells of the corpus luteum called theca lutein cells.

FIGURE 2, corpus luteum, human, H&E ×20. A portion of a fully formed corpus luteum is shown here. Most endocrine cells are the granulosa lutein cells *(GLC)*. These form a folded cell mass that surrounds the remains of the former follicular cavity *(FC)*. External to the corpus luteum is the connective tissue of the ovary *(CT)*. Keep in mind that the theca interna was derived from the connective tissue stroma of the ovary. The location of theca lutein cells reflects this origin, and these cells *(TLC)* can be found in the deep outer recesses of the glandular mass, adjacent to the surrounding connective tissue.

FIGURES 3 and 4, corpus luteum, human, H&E ×65 (Fig. 3) and ×240 (Fig. 4). A segment of the plicated corpus luteum is shown in this figure at higher magnification. As already noted, the main cell mass is composed of granulosa lutein cells *(GLC)*. On one side of this cell mass is the connective tissue *(CT)* within the former follicular cavity; on the other side are the theca lutein cells. The granulosa lutein cells *(GLC)* contain a large spherical nucleus (see, also, *GLC,* Fig. 4) and a large amount of cytoplasm. The cytoplasm contains yellow pigment (usually not evident in routine H&E sections), hence the name, corpus luteum. Theca lutein cells also contain a spherical nucleus *(TLC)*, but the cells are smaller than the granulosa lutein cells. Thus, when identifying the two cell types, aside from location, note that the nuclei of adjacent theca lutein cells generally appear to be closer to each other than nuclei of adjacent granulosa lutein cells. The

connective tissue *(CT)* and small blood vessels that invaded the mass of granulosa lutein cells can be identified as the flattened and elongated components between the granulosa lutein cells.

The changes whereby the ruptured ovarian follicle is transformed into a corpus luteum occur under the influence of pituitary luteinizing hormone (LH). In turn, the corpus luteum itself secretes progesterone, which has a profound effect on the estrogen-primed uterus. If pregnancy occurs, the corpus luteum remains functional; if pregnancy does not occur, the corpus luteum regresses after having reached a point of peak development, roughly 2 weeks after ovulation. The regressing cellular components of the corpus luteum are replaced by fibrous connective tissue, and the structure is then called a corpus albicans.

KEY

BV, blood vessels
CT, connective tissue
FC, former follicular cavity
GLC, granulosa lutein cells
TC, cell transforming into the corpus luteum
TLC, theca lutein cells

PLATE 114

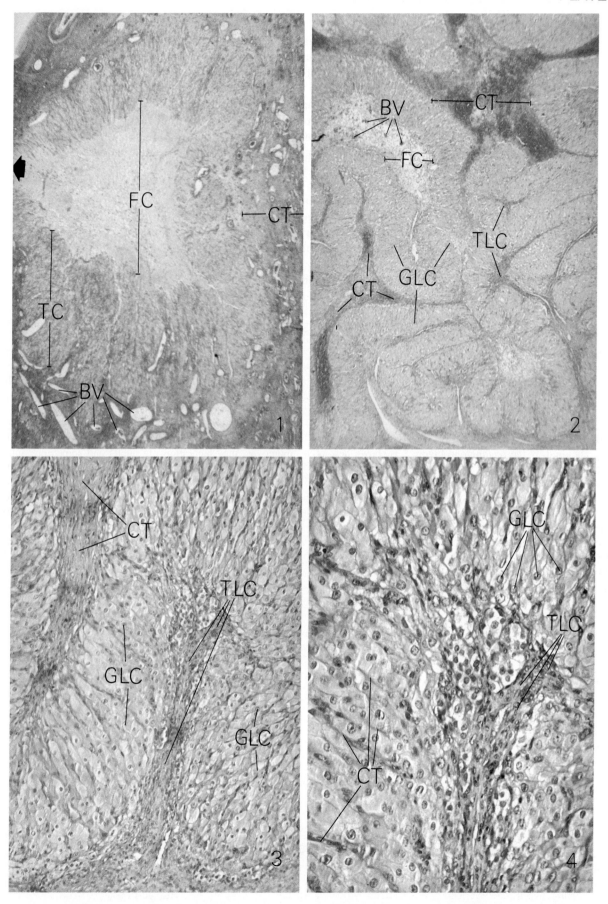

PLATE 115. Oviduct-Uterine Tube

The oviducts (uterine tubes, Fallopian tubes) are joined to the uterus and extend to the ovaries where they present an open flared end for entry of the ovum. The oviduct undergoes cyclical changes along with those of the uterus, but not nearly as pronounced. The epithelial cells increase in height during the middle of the cycle, just about the time the ovum will be passing through the tube, and become reduced during the premenstrual period. Some of the epithelial cells are ciliated. They depend on the ovaries for their viability. Not only do the number of ciliated cells increase during the follicular phase of the ovarian cycle, but removal of the ovaries in mature animals leads to atrophy of the epithelium and loss of ciliated cells.

The uterine tube varies in size and degree of mucosal folding along its length. The mucosal folds are more numerous near the open end (abdominal ostium) and less numerous near the uterus, where the tube is narrow and referred to as the isthmus. The next two-thirds of its length is an expanded form referred to as the ampulla. Near the opening, the tube flares outward and is called the infundibulum. It has fringed folded edges called fimbria.

Fertilization of the ovum usually occurs in the oviduct. For the first several days, the developing embryonic cells are contained in the tube as they travel to the uterus.

FIGURE 1, oviduct, human, H&E ×40. A cross section through the ampulla of the tube is shown here. Many mucosal folds project into the lumen *(L)*, and the complicated nature of the folds is evident by the variety of profiles that is seen. In addition to the mucosa, the remainder of the wall consists of a muscularis *(Mus)* and connective tissue.

The muscularis *(Mus)* consists of smooth muscle that forms a relatively thick layer of circular fibers and a thinner outer layer of longitudinal fibers. The layers are not clearly delineated, and no sharp boundary separates them.

FIGURE 2, oviduct, human, H&E ×160; inset ×320. The area enclosed by the *rectangle* in Figure 1 is shown here at higher magnification. The specimen shows a longitudinal section through a lymphatic vessel *(Lym)*. In other planes of section, the lymphatic vessels are difficult to identify. The fortuitously sectioned lymphatic vessel is seen in the core of the mucosal fold, along with a highly cellular connective tissue *(CT)* and the blood vessels *(BV)* within the connective tissue. The epithelium lining the mucosa is shown in the **inset.** The ciliated cells are readily identified by the presence of well-formed cilia *(C)*. Nonciliated cells, also called peg cells *(PC)*, are also readily identified by the absence of cilia; moreover, they have elongate nuclei and sometimes appear to be squeezed between the ciliated cells. The connective tissue *(CT)* contains cells whose nuclei are arranged in a typically random manner. They vary in shape, being elongated, oval, or round. Their cytoplasm cannot be distinguished from the intercellular material **(inset).** The character of the connective tissue is essentially the same from the epithelium to the muscularis, and for this reason, no submucosa is described.

KEY		
BV, blood vessels	**EP,** epithelium	**Muc,** mucosa
C, cilia	**L,** lumen	**Mus,** muscularis
CT, connective tissue	**Lym,** lymphatic vessel	**PC,** peg cells

PLATE 115

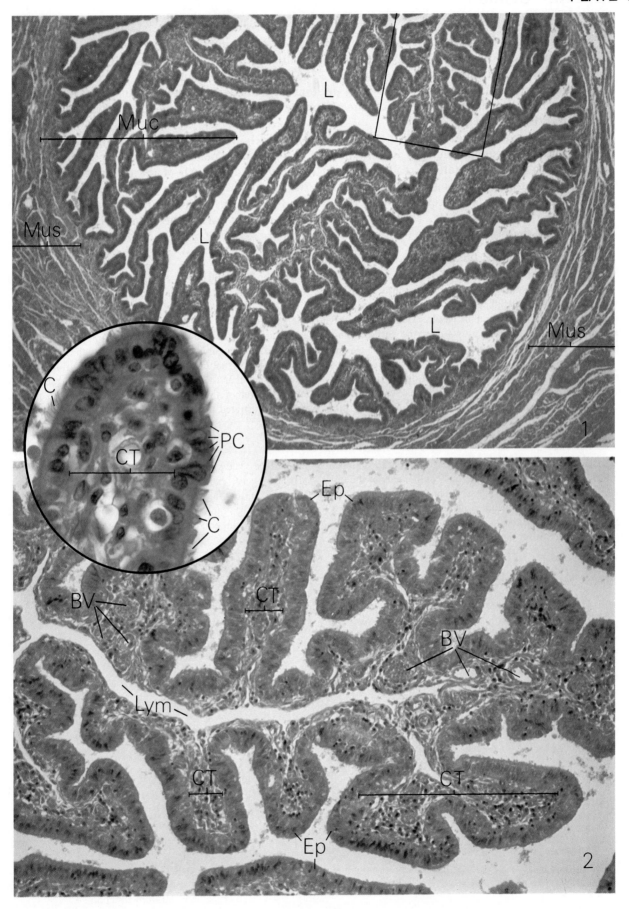

PLATE 116. Uterus I

The uterus is a hollow, pear-shaped organ with a thick muscular wall and, in the non-pregnant state, a narrow cavity. The uterine wall is composed of a mucosa, referred to as the endometrium; a muscularis, referred to as the myometrium; and, externally, a serosal cover, the perimetrium (visceral peritoneum). The serosa presents no special features. The myometrium consists of smooth muscle and connective tissue and contains the larger blood vessels.

The uterus undergoes cyclical changes that are largely manifested by the changes that occur in the endometrium. If implantation of an ovum does not occur after preparation for this event, the state of readiness is not maintained, and much of the endometrium degenerates and is sloughed off, constituting the menstrual flow. The part of the endometrium that is lost is referred to as the stratum functionale; the part that is retained is called the stratum basale. The stratum basale is the deepest part of the endometrium and adjoins the myometrium.

FIGURE 1, uterus, human, H&E ×25; inset ×120. After the stratum functionale is sloughed off, resurfacing of the raw tissue occurs. The epithelial resurfacing comes from the glands that remain in the stratum basale. The gland epithelium simply proliferates and grows over the surface. This figure shows the endometrium as it appears when resurfacing is complete. The area inscribed in the *upper small circle* is shown at higher magnification in the **inset** on the right. Note the simple columnar epithelium *(SEp)* that covers the endometrial surface and its similarity to the glandular epithelium *(Gl)*. The endometrium is relatively thin at this stage, and over half of it consists of the stratum basale *(SB)*. The area inscribed by the *lower small circle,* located in the region of the stratum basale, is shown at higher magnification in the **inset** on Figure 2. The glandular epithelium *(Gl)* of the deep portion of the glands is similar to that of the endometrial surface. Below the endometrium is the myometrium *(M),* in which a number of large blood vessels *(BV)* is present. A higher power of the interlacing bundles of smooth muscle cells is illustrated in Figure 4 of Plate 27, page 237.

FIGURE 2, uterus, human, H&E ×25; inset ×120. Under the influence of estrogen, the various components of the endometrium proliferate (proliferative stage), so that the total thickness of the endometrium is increased. As shown in this figure, the glands *(Gl)* become rather long and follow a fairly straight course within the stratum functionale *(SF)* to reach the surface. The stratum basale *(SB)* remains essentially unaffected by the estrogen and appears much the same as in Figure 1. In this figure, the stratum functionale *(SF),* on the other hand, has increased in thickness and constitutes about four-fifths of the endometrial thickness.

KEY		
BV, blood vessels	**M,** myometrium	**SEp (inset, Fig. 1),** surface epithelium
Gl, glands	**SB,** stratum basale	**SF,** stratum functionale

PLATE 116

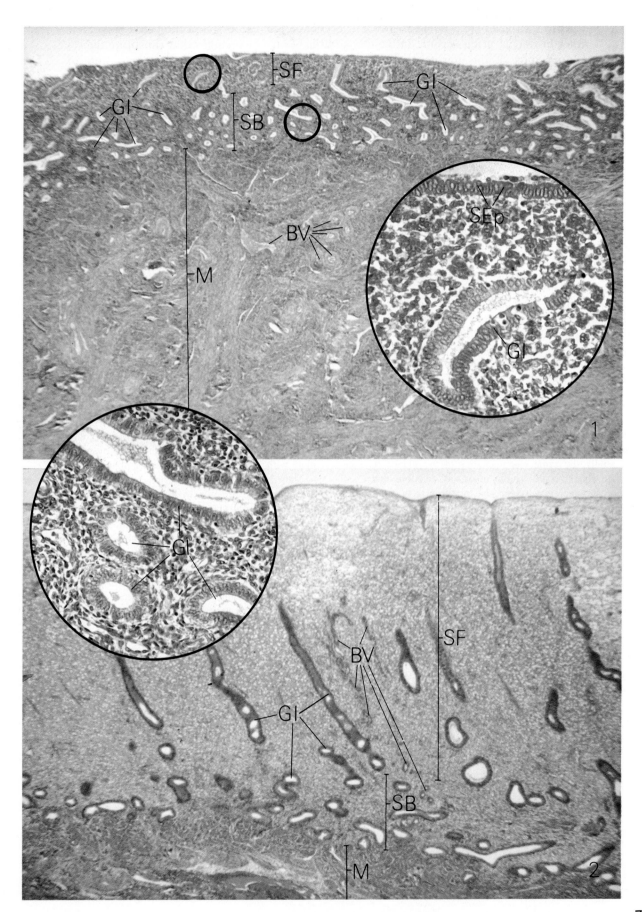

PLATE 117. Uterus II

After estrogen brings about the uterine events designated as the proliferative stage, another hormone, progesterone, influences additional uterine changes that constitute the secretory stage of the uterine cycle. This hormone brings the endometrium to a state of readiness for implantation, and as a consequence of its actions, the thickness of the endometrium increases further. There are conspicuous changes in the glands; these changes are primarily in the stratum functionale. The glands in the stratum functionale take on a more pronounced corkscrew shape and secrete mucus that accumulates in sacculations along their length.

As mentioned previously, if fertilization of the ovum and implantation of the embryonic cells do not occur, the stratum functionale is sloughed off, but the stratum basale remains behind. Associated with this partial loss of endometrium are vascular changes that occur in the stratum functionale but not in the stratum basale. The specialized, nonreacting arterial branches that supply the stratum basale are called straight arteries.

FIGURE 1, uterus, human, H&E ×25. This view of the endometrium in the secretory stage shows the stratum functionale *(SF),* the stratum basale *(SB),* and, in the lower left of the photomicrograph, a small amount of the myometrium *(M).* The uterine glands have been cut in a plane that is close to their long axes, and one gland *(arrow)* is seen opening at the uterine surface. Except for a few glands near the center of the diagram that resemble those of the proliferative stage, most of the glands *(Gl)* in this figure, including those that are labeled, show numerous shallow sacculations that give the profile of the glandular epithelium a serrated appearance. This is one of the distinctive features of the secretory stage. It is seen most advantageously in areas where the plane of section is close to the long axis of the gland. In contrast to the characteristic sinuous course of the glands in the stratum functionale, glands of the stratum basale more closely resemble those in the proliferative stage. They are not oriented in any noticeable relationship to the uterine surface, and many of their long profiles are even parallel to the plane of the surface.

FIGURE 2, uterus, human, H&E ×30; inset ×120. This slightly higher magnification of the stratum functionale shows essentially the same characteristics of the glands *(Gl)* described above; it also shows other modifications that occur during the secretory stage. One of these is that the endometrium becomes edematous. The increase in endometrial thickness due to edema is reflected by the presence of empty spaces between cells and other formed elements. Thus, many areas of this figure, especially the area within and near the *circle,* show histologic signs of edema.

In addition, in this stage, the glandular epithelial cells begin to secrete a mucoid fluid that is rich in glycogen. This product is secreted into the lumen of the glands, causing them to dilate. Typically, the glands of the secretory endometrium are more dilated than those of the proliferative endometrium, and this point can be readily discerned by comparing this plate with Figure 2 of the preceding plate.

The *circle* in this figure inscribes two glands that are shown at higher magnification in the **inset.** Each of these glands contains some substance within the lumen. The mucoid character of the substance within one of the glands can be surmised from its blue staining. Although not evident in routine H&E paraffin sections, the epithelial cells also contain glycogen during the secretory stage, and as already mentioned, this becomes part of the secretion. The *arrowheads* indicate stromal cells; some of these cells undergo enlargement late in the secretory stage. These modified stromal cells, called decidual cells, play a role in implantation.

KEY		
Gl, glands	**SB,** stratum basale	**arrowheads,** stromal cells
M, myometrium	**SF,** stratum functionale	

PLATE 117

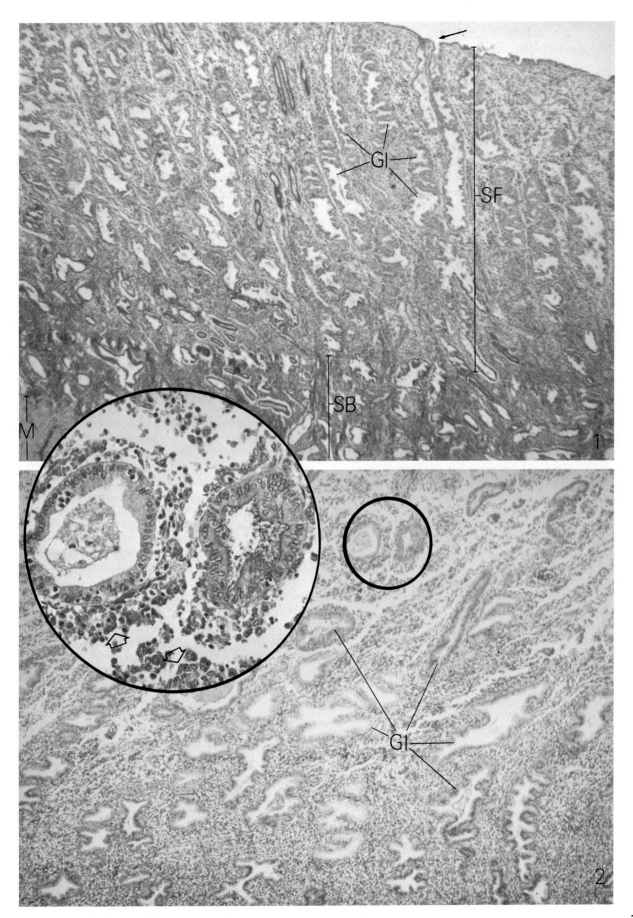

PLATE 118. Cervix

The cervix is the narrow or constricted inferior portion of the uterus, part of which projects into the vagina. A cavity referred to as the cervical canal traverses the cervix and provides a channel connecting the vagina and the uterine cavity. In its general features, the structure of the cervix resembles the remainder of the uterus in that it consists of a mucosa (endometrium) and a myometrium. There are, however, some differences in the mucosa.

The endometrium of the cervix does not undergo the cyclical loss of tissue that is characteristic of the body and fundus of the uterus. The amount and the character of its mucous secretion, however, vary at different times of the uterine cycle. The myometrium forms the major thickness of the cervix. It consists of interweaving bundles of smooth muscle cells situated in a more extensive, continuous network of fibrous connective tissue.

FIGURES 1 and 2, cervix, human, H&E ×15. The portion of the cervix that projects into the vagina, the portio vaginalis, is represented by the upper two-thirds of Figure 1. The lower third of the micrograph reveals the supravaginal portion of the cervix (portio supravaginalis). Figure 2 shows the supravaginal cervix at a slightly higher level, compared with Figure 1. The plane of section in both figures passes through the long axis of the cervical canal. The cervical canal *(CC)* is narrowed and cone shaped at its two ends. The upper end, the *internal os,* communicates with the uterine cavity, and the lower end, the *external os (OS),* communicates with the vagina. (For purposes of orientation, realize that only one side of the longitudinal section of the cervix is shown in these figures and that the actual specimen, as seen in a section, would present a similar image on the other side of the cervical canal.)

The mucosa *(Muc)* of the cervix differs according to the cavity it faces. The *two circles* in Figure 1 delineate representative areas of the mucosa that are shown at higher magnification in Figures 3 and 4, respectively.

Figure 2 emphasizes the nature of the cervical glands *(Gl).* The glands differ from those of the uterus in that they branch extensively. They secrete a mucous substance into the cervical canal that serves to lubricate the vagina.

FIGURE 3, cervix, human, H&E ×240. The surface of the portio vaginalis is stratified squamous epithelium *(SSEp).* The epithelium-connective tissue junction presents a relatively even contour in contrast to the irregular profile seen in the vagina. In other respects, the epithelium has the same general features as the vaginal epithelium. Another similarity is that the epithelial surface of the portio vaginalis undergoes cyclical changes similar to those of the vagina in response to ovarian hormones. The mucosa of the portio vaginalis, like that of the vagina, is devoid of glands.

FIGURE 4, cervix, human, H&E ×240. The mucosa of the cervical canal is covered with columnar epithelium. An abrupt change from stratified squamous epithelium *(SSEp)* to simple columnar epithelium *(CEp)* occurs at the opening of the cervical canal (external os). The *lower circle* in Figure 1 marks this site, known as the transition zone, and is shown at higher magnification here. Note the abrupt change in the epithelium at the point indicated by the *diamond-shaped marker,* as well as the large number of lymphocytes present in this region (compare with Fig. 3).

FIGURE 5, cervix, human, H&E ×500. Figure 5 shows, at high magnification, portions of the gland identified in the *circle* in Figure 2. Note the tall epithelial cells and the lightly staining supranuclear cytoplasm, a reflection of the mucin dissolved out of the cell during tissue preparation. The crowding and the change in shape of the nuclei *(asterisk)* seen at the bottom of one of the glands in this figure are due to a tangential cut through the wall of the gland as it passed out of the plane of section. (It is not uncommon for cervical glands to develop into cysts as a result of obstruction in the duct. Such cysts are referred to as Nabothian cysts.)

KEY

BV, blood vessels
CC, cervical canal
CEp, columnar epithelium
Gl, cervical glands
Muc, mucosa
Os, ostium of the uterus
SSEp, stratified squamous epithelium
asterisk (Fig. 5), tangential cut of the epithelial surface

PLATE 118

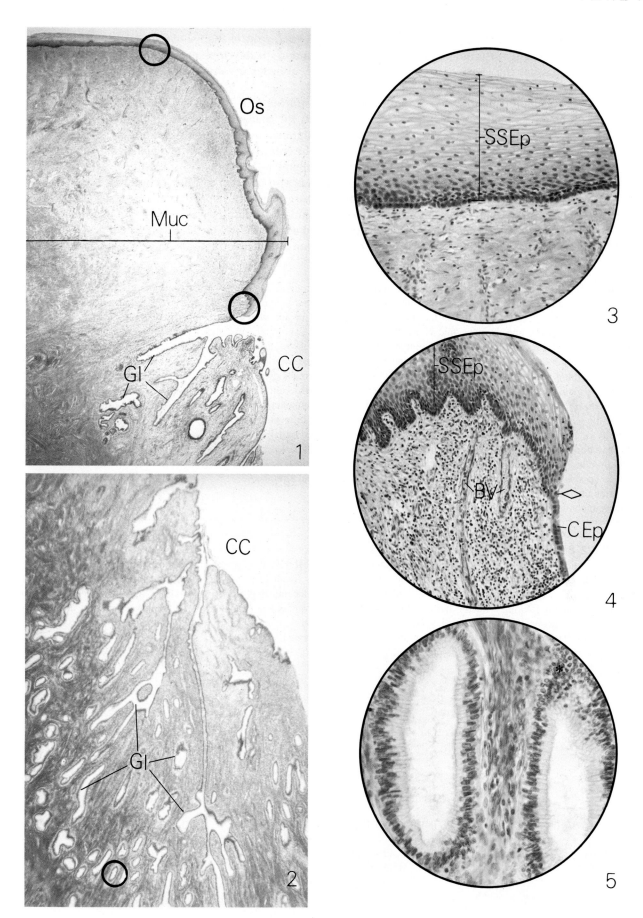

PLATE 119. Placenta I

The placenta is a discoid-shaped organ that serves for the exchange of materials between the fetal and maternal circulations during pregnancy. It develops primarily from embryonic tissue, the chorion frondosum; however, it also has a component derived from the uterus, namely, the basal plate.

One side of the placenta is embedded in the uterine wall; the other side faces the amniotic cavity that contains the fetus. After birth, the placenta separates from the wall of the uterus and is discharged along with the contiguous membranes of the amniotic cavity.

The umbilical cord connects the fetus to the placenta. It contains two arteries that carry blood to the placenta and a vein that returns blood to the fetus. The umbilical arteries have thick muscular walls. These are arranged as two layers: an inner longitudinal layer and an outer circular layer. Elastic membranes are poorly developed in these vessels and, indeed, may be absent. The umbilical vein is similar to the arteries, also having a thick muscular wall arranged as inner longitudinal and outer circular layers. Near its connection to the fetus, the umbilical cord may contain remnants of the allantois and yolk sac.

FIGURE 1, placenta, human, H&E ×16. A section extending from the amniotic surface into the substance of the placenta is shown here. This includes the amnion *(A)*, the chorionic plate *(CP)*, and the chorionic villi *(CV)*. The amnion consists of a layer of simple cuboidal epithelium and an underlying layer of connective tissue. The connective tissue of the amnion is continuous with the connective tissue of the chorionic plate as a result of their fusion at an earlier time. The plane of fusion, however, is not evident in H&E sections; the separation *(asterisks)* in parts of this figure in the vicinity of the fusion is an artefact.

The chorionic plate is a thick connective tissue mass that contains the ramifications of the umbilical arteries and vein. These vessels *(BVp)* do not have the distinct organizational features characteristic of arteries and veins; rather, they resemble the vessels of the umbilical cord. Although their iden-

tification as blood vessels is relatively simple, it is difficult to distinguish which vessels are branches of an umbilical artery and which are tributaries of the vein.

The main substance of the placenta consists of chorionic villi of different sizes (see Plate 120). These emerge from the chorionic plate as large stem villi that branch into increasingly smaller villi. Branches of the umbilical arteries and vein *(BVv)* enter the stem villi and ramify through the branching villous network. Some villi extend from the chorionic plate to the material side of the placenta and make contact with the maternal tissue; these are called ***anchoring villi***. Other villi, the ***free villi***, simply arborize within the substance of the placenta without anchoring onto the maternal side.

FIGURE 2, placenta, human, H&E ×70; inset ×370. The maternal side of the placenta is shown in this figure. The basal plate *(stratum basale, SB)* is on the right side of the illustration. This is the part of the uterus to which the chorionic villi anchor. Along with the usual connective tissue elements, the basal plate contains specialized cells called ***decidual cells*** *(DC)*. The same cells are shown at higher magnification in the **inset.** Decidual cells are usually found in

clusters and have an epithelial appearance. Because of these features, they are easily identified.

Septa from the basal plate extend into the portion of the placenta that contains the chorionic villi. The septa do not contain the branches of the umbilical vessels and, on this basis, can frequently be distinguished from stem villi or their branches.

KEY

A, amnion
BVp, blood vessel in chorionic plate
BVv, blood vessel in chorionic villi
CP, chorionic plate
CV, chorionic villi
DC, decidual cells
SB, stratum basale
asterisk, separation that is actually an artefact

PLATE 119

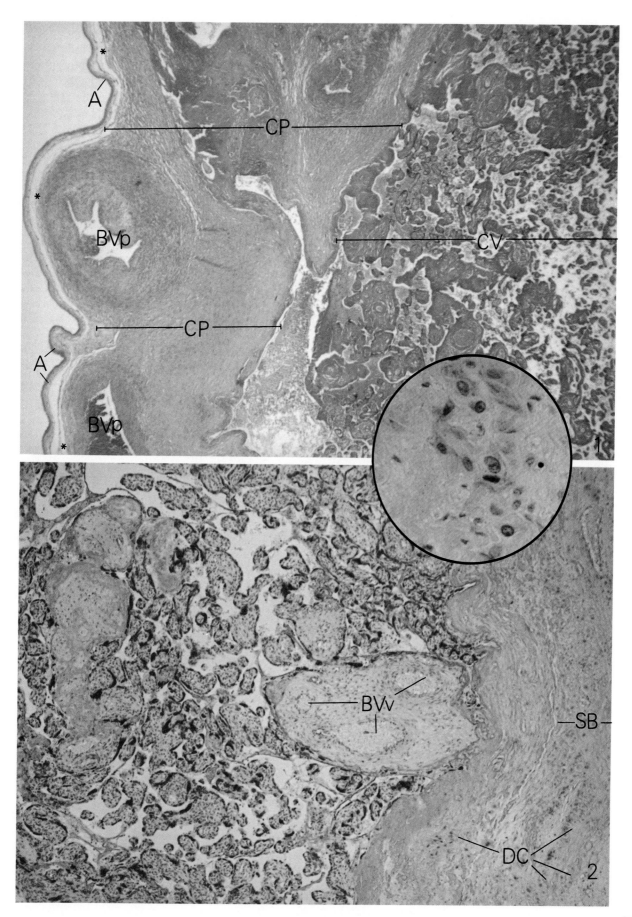

PLATE 120.   Placenta II

Chorionic villi consist of a connective tissue core and a two-layered cellular covering. The outermost cellular layer is the syncytiotrophoblast; immediately under this is another layer of cells referred to as cytotrophoblasts. The latter are numerous in the early placenta, but there are relatively few present in the placenta of late pregnancy.

The syncytiotrophoblast not only covers the surface of the chorionic villi but also extends from the anchoring villi onto the surface of the basal plate and onto the placental septa. As a consequence, the entire compartment in which maternal blood is contained is walled by syncytiotrophoblast.

Placenta, human, H&E ×280.   A section through the substance of a full-term placenta shows chorionic villi *(CV)* of different sizes and the surrounding intervillous space *(IS)*. The connective tissue of the villi contains branches and tributaries of the umbilical arteries and vein *(BV)*. The smallest villi contain only capillaries; larger villi contain correspondingly larger blood vessels. The intervillous space contains maternal blood. Maternal blood was drained from the specimen before its preparation, and therefore, few maternal blood cells are seen in the section.

The nuclei of the syncytiotrophoblast may be more or less evenly distributed, giving this layer an appearance (in H&E sections) similar to that of cuboidal epithelium. There are, however, sites where the nuclei are gathered in clusters *(arrowheads)*, as well as regions of syncytium relatively free of nuclei *(arrows)*. These stretches of syncytium may be so attenuated as to give the impression that the villous surface is devoid of a covering. It is thought that the nuclear clusters and the adjacent cytoplasm may separate from the villus and enter the maternal blood pool.

The syncytiotrophoblast contains microvilli that project into the intervillous space. These may appear as a striated border in paraffin sections, but they are not always adequately preserved and may not be evident.

In earlier placentas, the cytotrophoblasts form an almost complete layer of cells immediately deep to the syncytiotrophoblast. Cytotrophoblasts are the source of syncytiotrophoblasts. Cell division occurs in the cytotrophoblast layer, and the newly formed cells become incorporated into the syncytial layer. In this full-term placenta, only occasional cytotrophoblasts *(Cy)* can be discerned.

Most of the cells within the core of the villus are typical connective tissue fibroblasts. The nuclei of these cells stain well with hematoxylin, but the cytoplasm cannot be distinguished from the delicate intercellular fibrous material. Other cells have a recognizable amount of cytoplasm surrounding the nucleus. These are considered to be phagocytic and are named Hofbauer cells. The Hofbauer cells *(HC)* shown in the figure do not contain any distinctive cytoplasmic inclusions.

KEY		
BV, blood vessels	**HC,** Hofbauer cells	**arrows,** attenuated syncytial cytoplasm
CV, chorionic villi	**IS,** intervillous space	
Cy, cytotrophoblasts	**arrowheads,** clusters of syncytial trophoblast nuclei	**asterisk,** tangentially sectioned villus

PLATE 120

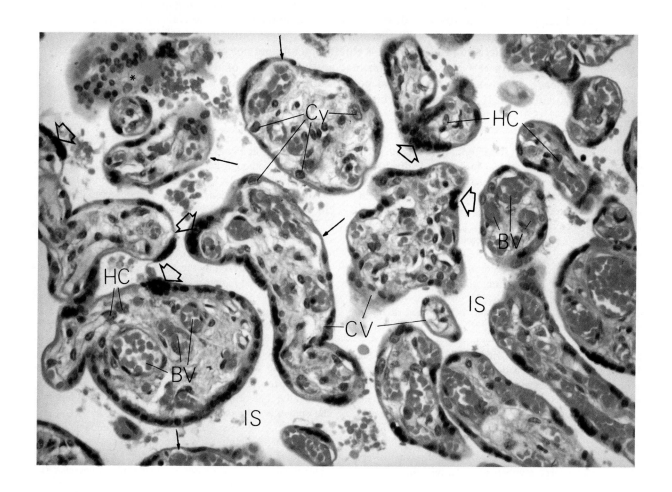

PLATE 121.   Vagina

The vagina is a fibromuscular tube that forms the opening of the female reproductive tract to the exterior. The wall of the vagina consists of three layers: a mucous membrane, a muscular layer, and an outer adventitia. At the lower end of the vagina, the opening is surrounded by the erectile tissue of the bulb of the vestibule. A relatively thin layer of striated muscle fibers, the bulbospongiosus muscle, lies just external to the bulb of the vestibule. Vaginal epithelium is influenced by ovarian hormones and undergoes cyclical changes that correspond to the ovarian cycle. In rodents, these changes are manifested by marked alterations in the cells. In humans, the epithelial changes are less pronounced but are, nevertheless, evident. The amount of glycogen stored in the epithelial cells increases under the influence of *estrogen*, whereas the rate of desquamation increases under the influence of *progesterone*.

Histologic study of the vagina should take into account the following points: (1) the epithelium does not keratinize and, except for the deepest layers, the cells appear to be empty in routine H&E sections; (2) the mucous membrane contains neither glands nor a muscularis mucosae; and (3) the muscle is chiefly smooth and not well ordered. This should be contrasted with the oral cavity, pharynx, and upper part of the esophagus in which the muscle is striated. The more distal portion of the esophagus, which contains smooth muscle, can be easily distinguished from the vagina because it has a muscularis mucosae.

FIGURE 1, vagina, human, H&E ×40; inset ×250. The mucous membrane of the vagina consists of stratified squamous epithelium *(Ep)* and an underlying connective tissue *(CT)*. The boundary between the two is readily identified, owing to the intense staining of the deep portion of the epithelium. Connective tissue papillae project into the undersurface of the epithelium, giving the epithelial-connective tissue junction an uneven appearance. The papillae *(arrows)* may be cut obliquely or in cross section and may, thus, appear as connective tissue islands within the epithelium.

The *rectangle* in this figure marks an area of vaginal epithelium and connective tissue that is examined at higher magnification in Figure 2. The epithelium is characteristically thick. Although keratohyalin granules may be present in the superficial cells, keratinization (in the human) does not occur. In this connection, nuclei can be observed throughout the entire thickness of the vaginal epithelium.

The muscular layer *(Mus)* of the vaginal wall is made up of smooth muscle. The smooth muscle is arranged in two ill-defined layers, with the outer one being somewhat longitudinal. The area marked by the *circle* in the upper left of this figure is shown at higher magnification in the **inset** to illustrate the smooth muscle cells. They are organized as small interlacing bundles surrounded by connective tissue.

FIGURE 2, vagina, human, H&E ×180. One of the features of vaginal epithelium that aids in its identification is that, except for the deepest layers, the cells have an empty appearance. This is due, in part, to the fact that the cells accumulate glycogen as they migrate toward the surface and, in the preparation of routine H&E sections, the glycogen is lost.

The connective tissue immediately under the vaginal epithelium contains large numbers of cells, most of which are lymphocytes *(L)*. The lymphocytes are characterized by their deep-staining, round nuclei. The number of lymphocytes varies during the ovarian cycle. Lymphocytes invade the epithelium around the time of menstruation, and they appear along with the epithelial cells in vaginal smears.

The connective tissue also contains large amounts of elastic material in addition to collagen fibers; however, this is not evident in H&E sections. The connective tissue also characteristically contains a large number of blood vessels *(BV)*.

KEY		
BV, bloods vessels	**Ep**, epithelium	**Mus**, muscular layer
CT, connective tissue	**L**, lymphocytes	**arrows**, connective tissue papillae

PLATE 121

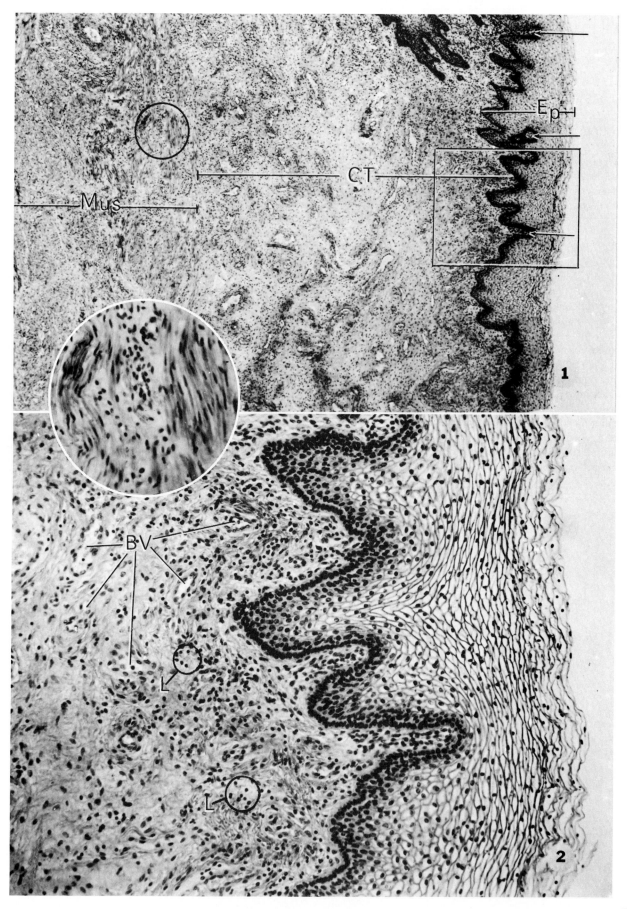

Ep

CT

Mus

1

BV

L

L

2

PLATE 122. Mammary Glands

The mammary glands are branched tubuloalveolar glands that develop from the epidermis and come to lie in the subcutaneous tissue (superficial fascia). They begin to develop at puberty in the female but do not reach a fully functional state until after pregnancy. The glands also develop in the male at puberty; the development is limited, however, and the glands usually remain in a stabilized state.

FIGURE 1, mammary gland, human, H&E ×80. This figure is a section through an inactive gland. The parenchyma is sparse and consists mainly of duct elements. Several ducts *(D)* are shown in the center of the field. A small lumen can be seen in each. The ducts are surrounded by a loose connective tissue [see *CT(L)*, Fig. 2], and together, the ducts and surrounding connective tissue constitute a lobule. Two lobules *(L)* are bracketed in this figure. Beyond the lobule, the connective tissue is more dense [*CT(D)*]. The two types of connective tissues can be distinguished at the low magnification of this figure.

FIGURE 2, mammary gland, human, H&E ×200; inset ×400. Additional details are evident at higher magnification. In distinguishing between the loose and dense connective tissue, recall that both extracellular and cellular features show differences that are evident in both the figure and the **inset.** Note the thicker collagenous fibers in the dense connective tissue in contrast to the much thinner fibers of the loose connective tissue. The loose connective tissue contains far more cells per unit area and a greater variety of cell types. This figure shows a cluster of lymphocytes *(L)* and, at still higher magnification **(inset)**, plasma cells *(P)* and individual lymphocytes *(L)*. Both plasma cells and lymphocytes are cells with a rounded shape, but plasma cells are larger and show more cytoplasm. In addition, regions of plasma cell cytoplasm display basophilia. Elongate nuclei in spindle-shaped cells belong to fibroblasts. In contrast, although the cell types in the dense connective tissue may also be diverse, a simple examination of equal areas of loose and dense connective tissue will, by far, show fewer cells in the dense connective tissue. Characteristically, the dense connective tissue contains numerous aggregates of adipocytes *(A)*.

The epithelial cells within the resting lobule are regarded as being chiefly duct elements. Usually, alveoli are not found; however, their precursors are represented as cellular thickenings of the duct wall. The epithelium of the resting lobule is cuboidal; in addition, myoepithelial cells are present. Reexamination of the **inset** shows a thickening of the epithelium in one location, presumably the precursor of an alveolus, and myoepithelial cells *(M)* at the base of the epithelium. As elsewhere, the myoepithelial cells are on the epithelial side of the basement membrane. During pregnancy, the glands begin to proliferate. This can be thought of as a dual process in which ducts proliferate and alveoli spring from the ducts.

KEY		
A, adipocytes	**D,** ducts	**M,** myoepithelial cells
CT(D), dense connective tissue	**L:** Fig. 1, lobules; Fig. 2 and inset, lymphocytes	**P,** plasma cells
CT(L), loose connective tissue		

PLATE 122

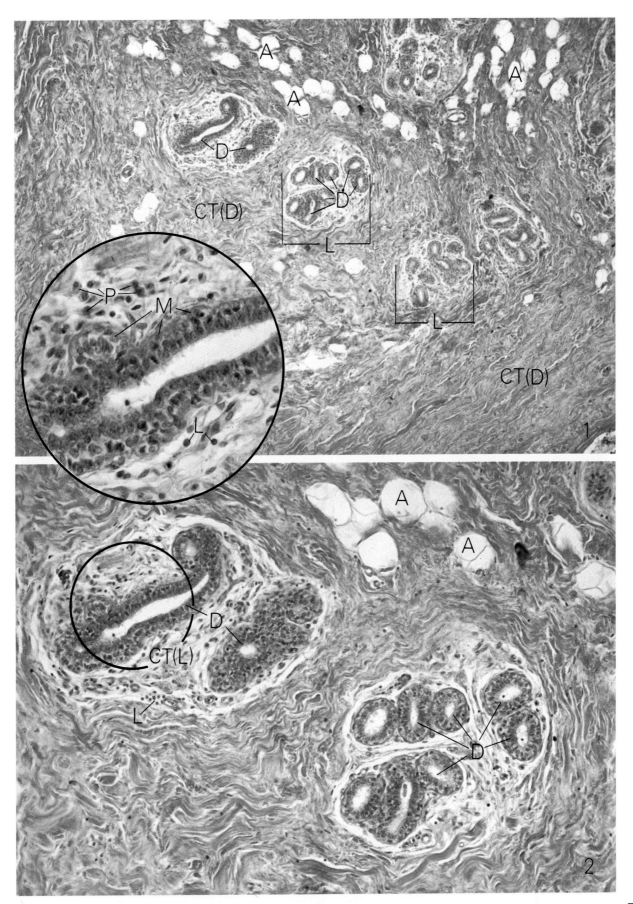

PLATE 123. Mammary Gland, Proliferative

FIGURE 1, mammary gland, human, H&E ×65; inset ×160. Whereas the development of the duct elements in the mammary gland is marked during the early proliferative period, the development of the alveolar elements becomes conspicuous at a later time. This figure shows several lobules *(L)* at a later stage of proliferation than is shown in the preceding plate. Distinct alveoli *(A)* can now be recognized. These are all joined to a duct *(D)*, although the connections are usually not seen in a two-dimensional section. Lobules are separated by dense connective tissue septa *(S)*, and some ducts can be recognized as being in an interlobular location. Although alveolar development is well under way, some regions of the gland are still in a relatively early stage of proliferation. For example, the **inset** shows where epithelial sprouting is occurring along the length of a duct *(arrowheads)*.

FIGURE 2, mammary gland, human, H&E ×160. A higher magnification of one of the proliferating lobules is shown here. Numerous alveoli *(A)* are evident. The alveoli consist of a single layer of cuboidal epithelium as well as myoepithelial cells. A small amount of precipitate is located in the lumen of some of the alveoli. This represents the early secretory product of the cells.

The duct *(D)* through which the alveoli will discharge their product is shown on the left, appearing as a stalk. It can be recognized because of its location and its elongated profile. Some of the flattened nuclei that are at the epithelium-connective tissue junction of the duct belong to myoepithelial cells.

The connective tissue *(CT)* surrounding the alveoli is loose and contains delicate collagenous fibers and large numbers of round cells *(arrows)*. The identity of these cells is difficult to establish at this magnification, although most are probably lymphocytes.

	KEY	
A, alveoli	**L**, lobule	**arrows**, round connective tissue
CT, connective tissue	**S**, septa	cells
D, duct	**arrowheads**, epithelial sprouts	

PLATE 123

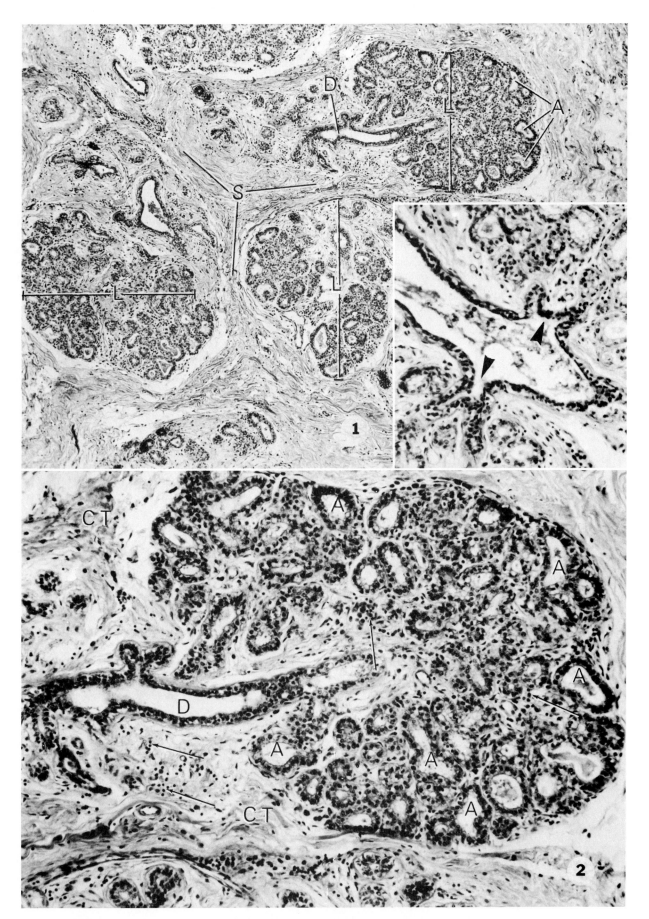

PLATE 124. Mammary Gland, Lactating

FIGURE 1, mammary gland, human, H&E ×160. The lactating mammary gland is characterized by the presence of large numbers of alveoli. Many of these appear as oval or spherical profiles, and in this respect, on cursory examination, the gland is easy to confuse with the thyroid gland. All of the alveoli in the mammary gland are joined to a duct, however, and the place where several alveoli open into a central channel can often be seen. These connections represent branchings of a terminal duct system. The presence of connected alveoli *(asterisks)* enables one to identify the lactating mammary gland and distinguish it from thyroid tissue even if the duct elements are not conspicuous. Sections of mammary glands usually include duct elements, but the small ducts are difficult to identify because they resemble the alveoli.

A large duct *(D)*, easily recognized by its size, is in the upper left of the figure. A number of connective tissue septa *(S)* separate the alveoli of neighboring lobules. Large blood vessels *(BV)* are within the connective tissue septa.

FIGURE 2, mammary gland, human, H&E ×640. This figure shows several alveoli at higher magnification. The alveoli of lactating mammary glands are made up of cuboidal epithelium and myoepithelial cells. Frequently, some precipitated product can be seen within the lumen of the alveolus. Only a small amount of connective tissue separates the neighboring alveoli. Capillaries *(Cap)* can be seen in this connective tissue.

FIGURE 3, mammary gland, human, Sudan black-B (or osmium tetroxide) ×640. This is a special preparation showing some of the lipid that is present in the mammary secretion. The lipid appears as the black spheres of various size within the alveolar lumen as well as within most of the cells. In its production, the lipid first appears as small droplets within the cells. These droplets become larger and, ultimately, are discharged into the alveolar lumen.

The lymphatic vessels of the mammary glands, which are important clinically, are usually not evident in histologic sections.

KEY

BV, blood vessels
Cap, capillaries
D, duct
S, septa
asterisks, branchings of terminal duct system

PLATE 124

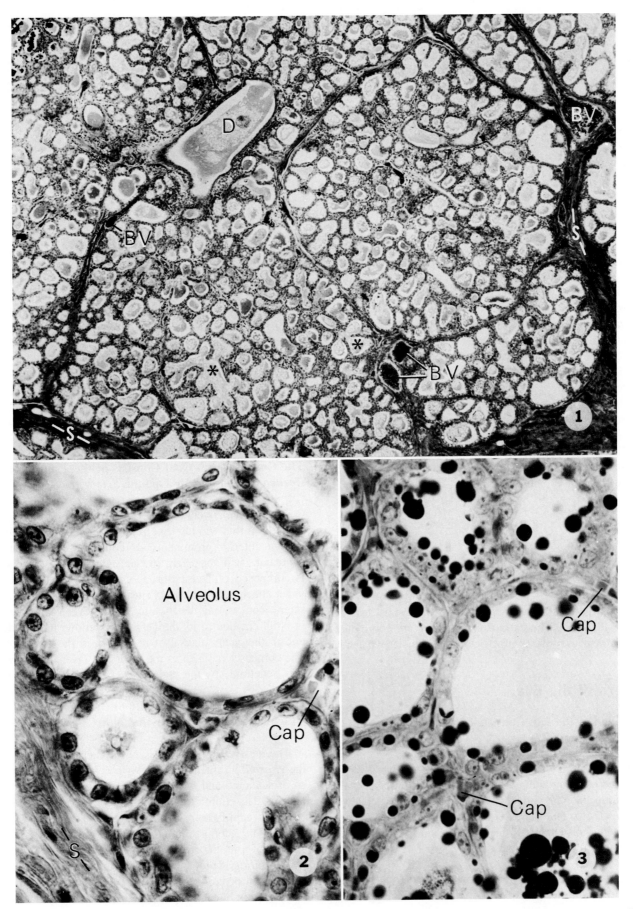

Eye

23

The eyes are complex sensory organs that provide us with the sense of sight. They are often compared to a simple camera with a lens to capture and focus the light and film to record the image. In the eye, the *cornea* and *lens* concentrate and focus light on the *retina*. Photoreceptors in the retina detect the intensity and color of the light striking them and encode the various parameters for transmission to the brain.

Because the eyes are paired, two somewhat different and overlapping images (visual fields) are sent to the brain. Therefore, complex neural mechanisms coordinate the movements of the eyes and perform the interpretation of the slightly different images. This is important because binocular vision enables us to perceive depth and distance to achieve a three-dimensional image.

GENERAL STRUCTURE OF THE EYE

The eye measures approximately 25 mm in diameter. It is suspended in the bony orbital socket by six extrinsic muscles that control its movement. A thick layer of adipose tissue partially surrounds and cushions the eye as it moves within the orbit. The extraocular muscles are coordinated so that the eyes move symmetrically about their own central axes.

Layers of the Eye

The Wall of the Eye Consists of Three Concentric Layers or Coats

The eyeball is organized in a manner such that it can be regarded as being composed of three structural layers. The layers are diagrammatically illustrated and color coded in Figure 23.1. The same color code is used in figures throughout this chapter to facilitate the study of each layer. The layers of the eye consist of the

- *Corneoscleral coat,* the outer or fibrous layer that includes the *sclera* and the *cornea*

- *Uvea,* the middle layer or vascular coat that includes the *choroid,* and the stroma of the *ciliary body* and *iris*
- *Retina,* the inner layer that includes an outer pigment epithelium, the inner neural retina, and the epithelium of the ciliary body and iris

On the anterior aspect of the eye, the layers are modified to admit and regulate the passage of light. The neural retina is continuous with the central nervous system through the **optic nerve.** The internal cavity of the eye is filled with a transparent gel, the *vitreous body,* that helps to maintain shape.

The Corneoscleral Coat Consists of the Transparent *Cornea* and the White Opaque *Sclera*

The *cornea* covers the anterior one-sixth of the eye (Fig. 23.1*a*). In this window-like region, the surface of the eye has an anterior prominence or convexity. The cornea is continuous with the *sclera* (fr. Gr. *skleros,* hard). The sclera is composed of dense fibrous connective tissue that provides attachment for the extrinsic muscles of the eye. The sclera, constituting the "white" of the eye, is slightly blue in children, due to its thinness, and yellow in the elderly, due to the accumulation of lipofuscin in its stromal cells. The corneosclera encloses the inner two layers except where it is penetrated by the optic nerve.

The *Uvea* Consists Principally of the *Choroid*, the Vascular Layer That Provides Nutrients to the Retina

The presence of blood vessels and melanin pigment gives the *choroid* an intense dark brown color. The pigment absorbs scattered and reflected light to minimize glare within the eye. The choroid, containing many venous plexuses and layers of capillaries, is firmly attached to the retina (Fig. 23.1*b*). The anterior rim of the uveal layer continues forward, where it forms the stroma of the *ciliary body* and *iris*.

The *ciliary body* is a ring-like thickening that extends inward just posterior to the level of the corneoscleral junction. Within the ciliary body is the ciliary (intraocular) muscle, a smooth muscle that is responsible for lens accommodation. Changes in the shape of the lens result from contraction of the ciliary muscle. This enables the lens to bring light rays from different distances to focus on the retina.

The *iris* is a contractile diaphragm that extends over the anterior surface of the lens. It also contains smooth muscle and melanin-containing pigment cells scattered in the connective tissue. The *pupil* is the central circular aperture of the iris. It appears black because one looks through the lens toward the heavily pigmented back of the eye. The pupil varies in size to control the amount of light that passes through the lens to reach the retina.

The Retina Consists of Two Components, the *Neural Retina* and *Pigment Epithelium*

The *retina* is a thin, delicate layer (Fig. 23.1c) that has two components:

- *Neural retina,* an inner layer that contains light-sensitive receptors and complex neuronal networks
- *Retinal pigment epithelium (RPE),* an outer layer that consists of simple cuboidal melanin-containing cells

Externally, the retina rests on the choroid; internally, it is associated with the vitreous body. The neural retina consists largely of *photoreceptor cells,* called retinal *rods* and *cones,* and interneurons. Visual information, encoded by the rods and cones, is sent to the brain via impulses conveyed through the optic nerve.

Chambers of the Eye

The Layers of the Eye and the Lens Serve as Boundaries for Three Chambers Within the Eye

The chambers of the eye are

- *Anterior chamber,* occupying the space between the cornea and the iris
- *Posterior chamber,* occupying the space between the posterior surface of the iris and the anterior surface of the lens
- *Vitreous space,* occupying the space between the posterior surface of the lens and the neural retina (Fig. 23.2)

The *vitreous body* is composed of a transparent gel substance that fills the vitreous space. It contains hyaluronic acid, widely dispersed collagen fibrils, and other proteins and glycoproteins.

The *Refractile Media* Components of the Eye Alter the Light Path to Focus It on the Retina

As light rays pass through the components of the eye, they are refracted. This focuses the light rays on the photoreceptors of the retina. Four transparent components of the eye, called the *refractile (or dioptric) media,* alter the path of the light rays. They are

- *Cornea,* the anterior window of the eye
- *Aqueous humor,* the watery fluid located in the anterior and posterior chambers
- *Lens,* a transparent crystalline biconcave structure suspended from the inner surface of the ciliary body by a ring of radially oriented fibers, the *zonule of Zinn*
- *Vitreous body* (or *humor*)

The cornea is the chief refractive element of the eye. It has a refractive index of 1.376 (air has a refractive index of 1.0). The lens is second in importance to the cornea in the refraction of light rays. Due to its elasticity, the lens can undergo slight shape change in response to the degree of tension of the ciliary muscle. The shape change is important in *accommodation* for proper focusing on near objects. The aqueous humor and the vitreous humor have

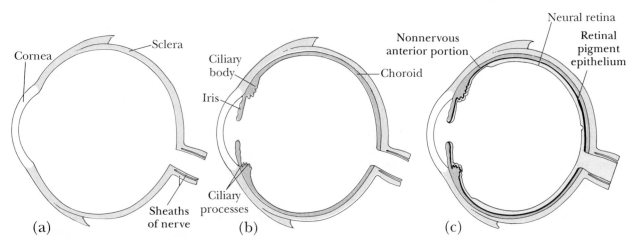

Figure 23.1. Schematic diagram of the layers of the eye. The layers are organized in three separate concentric layers: an outer supporting layer, the **corneoscleral coat (a)**; a middle vascular coat, the **uvea (b)**; and an inner photosensitive layer, the **retina (c)**.

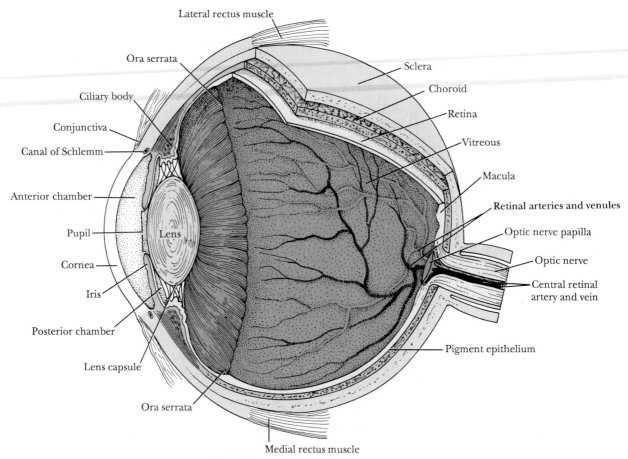

Lateral rectus muscle

Ora serrata

Ciliary body

Conjunctiva

Canal of Schlemm

Anterior chamber

Pupil

Cornea

Iris

Posterior chamber

Lens capsule

Ora serrata

Medial rectus muscle

Sclera

Choroid

Retina

Vitreous

Macula

Retinal arteries and venules

Optic nerve papilla

Optic nerve

Central retinal artery and vein

Pigment epithelium

Lens

Figure 23.2. Schematic diagram illustrating the internal structures of the human eye. (Modified from *The Anatomy of the Eye*, from an original drawing by Paul Peck. Copyright, Lederle Laboratories Division of American Cyanamid Company. All rights reserved. Reprinted with permission.)

only minor roles in the refraction of light rays. However, the aqueous humor plays an important role in providing nutrients to two avascular structures, the lens and cornea.

Blood Supply of the Eye

Two Systems of Blood Vessels Supply the Eye

Two independent arterial systems arise from the ophthalmic artery:

- The central retinal artery and its branches supply the optic nerve and the inner surface of the retina (these vessels are visualized with an ophthalmoscope in an eye examination).
- A second system supplies the outer coverings of the eye and the vascular layer.

The outer portions of the retina, including the photoreceptor cells and the outer pigment layer, receive blood from the choriocapillary layer of the vascular layer.

Development of the Eye

To understand the unusual structural and functional relationships in the eye, it is necessary to understand how it forms in the embryo.

The Tissues of the Eye Are Derived from Neuroectoderm, Surface Ectoderm, and Mesoderm

At the 22nd day of development, the eyes are evident as shallow grooves, the *optic sulci* or *grooves,* in the neural folds at the cranial end of the human embryo. As the neural tube closes, the paired grooves form outpocketings called *optic vesicles* (Fig. 23.3*A*). As each optic vesicle grows laterally, the connection to the forebrain becomes constricted into an optic stalk, and the overlying surface ectoderm thickens and forms a lens placode. This is followed by concomitant invagination of the optic vesicles and the lens placodes. The invagination of the optic vesicle results in the formation of a double-layered *optic cup* (Fig. 23.3*B*). The inner layer becomes the neural retina. The outer layer becomes the RPE.

Invagination of the central region of each lens placode

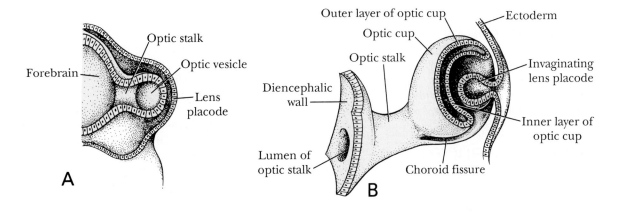

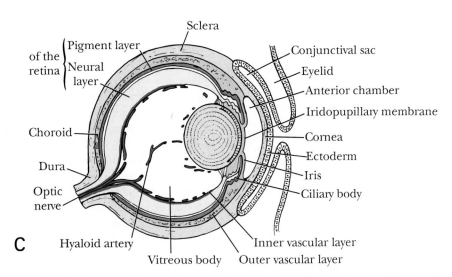

Figure 23.3. Schematic drawing illustrating the development of the eye. In **A,** the forebrain and developing optic vesicles are shown as they are seen in a 4-mm embryo. In **B,** the bilayered optic cup and invaginating lens vesicle are shown as they would be seen in a 7.5-mm embryo. The optic stalk connects the developing eye to the brain. In **C,** the eye is shown as it would appear in a 15-week fetus. All the layers of the eye are established, and the hyaloid artery can be seen traversing the vitreous body from the optic disc to the posterior surface of the lens. (Modified from Mann IC: *The Development of the Human Eye*, 3rd ed. (British Medical Association). New York, Grune & Stratton, 1974.)

results in the formation of the *lens vesicles.* By the fifth week of development, the lens vesicle loses its contact with the surface ectoderm and comes to lie in the mouth of the optic cup. After the lens vesicle detaches from the surface ectoderm, this same site again thickens to form the corneal epithelium. Mesenchymal cells from the periphery then give rise to the corneal endothelium and the corneal stroma.

Grooves in which blood vessels derived from mesenchyme form develop along the inferior surface of each optic cup and stalk. The grooves, called the *choroid fissures,* enable the hyaloid artery to reach the inner chamber of the eye. This artery and its branches supply the inner chamber of the optic cup, the lens vesicle, and the mesenchyme within the optic cup. The hyaloid vein returns blood from these structures. The distal portions of the hyaloid vessels degenerate, but the proximal portions remain as the *central artery* and *vein.* By the end of the seventh week, the edges of the choroid fissure fuse, and a round opening, the future pupil, is formed over the lens vesicle.

The outer layer of the optic cup forms a single layer of pigmented cells. Pigmentation begins at the end of the fifth week. The inner layer undergoes complicated differentiation into the nine layers of the neural retina. The photoreceptor (rod and cone) cells, as well as the bipolar, amacrine, and ganglion cells and nerve fibers are present by the seventh month. The macular depression begins to develop during the eighth month and is not complete until about 6 months after birth.

During the third month, growth of the optic cup gives rise to the ciliary body and the future iris, which forms a double row of epithelium in front of the lens. The mesoderm located external to this region becomes the stroma of the ciliary body and iris. Both epithelial layers of the iris become pigmented. In the ciliary body, however, only the outer layer is pigmented. At birth, the iris is light blue in fair-skinned people because pigment is usually not present. The dilator and sphincter pupillary muscles develop during the sixth month as derivatives of the neuroectoderm of the outer layer of the optic cup.

The embryonic origins of the individual eye structures are summarized in Table 23.1.

MICROSCOPIC STRUCTURE OF THE EYE

The External Layer—Corneosclera

The Cornea Consists of Five Layers: Three Cellular Layers and Two Lamellae

The transparent cornea (see Figs. 23.1 and 23.2, and Plate 125, page 761) is only 0.5 mm thick at its center and about 1 mm thick peripherally. It consists of three cellular layers that are distinct in both appearance and origin. These layers are separated from one another by two important lamellae that appear structureless when viewed with the light microscope. The five layers of the cornea that are seen in a transverse section are

- *Corneal epithelium*
- *Bowman's membrane*

_____

TABLE 23.1. Embryonic Origins of the Individual Structures of the Eye

SOURCE	DERIVATIVE
Surface ectoderm	Lens; epithelium of the cornea, conjunctiva, and lacrimal gland and its drainage system
Neural ectoderm	Vitreous body (derived partly from neural ectoderm of the optic cup and partly from mesenchyme); epithelium of the retina, iris, and ciliary body; muscle of pupillary sphincter and dilator; optic nerve
Mesoderm	Sclera; stroma of the cornea, conjunctiva, cilary body, iris, and choroid; extraocular muscles, eyelids (except epithelium and conjunctiva), hyaloid system (most of which degenerates before birth), and coverings of the optic nerve; connective tissue and blood vessels of the eye, bony orbit, and vitreous

- *Corneal stroma*
- *Descemet's membrane*
- *Corneal endothelium* (see Plate 128, page 767)

The Corneal Epithelium Is Nonkeratinized Stratified Squamous Epithelium

The corneal epithelium (see Plate 128, Fig. 1, page 767) measures about 50 μm in average thickness and is continuous with the conjunctival epithelium that overlies the adjacent sclera. The corneal cells adhere to neighboring cells via desmosomes that are present on short interdigitating processes. The cornea has remarkable regenerative capacity with a turnover time of approximately 7 days. As is typical of other stratified epithelium, such as that in the skin or conjunctiva, the cells proliferate from a basal layer and become squamous at the surface. These surface cells consist of one or two layers of nonkeratinized cells that have retained their nuclei. As the cells migrate to the surface, the cytoplasmic organelles gradually disappear, indicating a progressive decline in metabolic activity.

Numerous free nerve endings in the corneal epithelium provide it with extreme sensitivity to touch. Stimulation of these nerves, e.g., by small foreign bodies, elicits blinking of the eyelids, flow of tears, and often severe pain. Microvilli present on the surface epithelial cells help retain the tear film over the entire corneal surface. Drying of the corneal surface may cause it to ulcerate. Minor injuries of the corneal surface heal rapidly by the migration of cells to fill the defect.

Bowman's Membrane Is a Homogeneous Lamina on Which the Corneal Epithelium Rests

Bowman's membrane is a homogeneous, faintly fibrillar lamina that is approximately 8 μm thick. The collagen fibrils have a diameter of 18 nm and are randomly oriented. Bowman's membrane ends abruptly at the *limbus,* the junction of the cornea and sclera. Bowman's membrane provides strength to the cornea and is a barrier to the spread of infections. However, it does not regenerate. Therefore, if it is damaged, an opaque scar forms that may impair vision.

The *Corneal Stroma* Constitutes 90% of the Corneal Thickness

The stroma of the cornea, also called substantia propria, is composed of about 60 thin lamellae. Each lamella consists of parallel bundles of collagen fibrils. Between lamellae are nearly complete sheets of slender flattened fibroblasts. The fibrils measure approximately 23 nm in diameter and up to 1 cm in length. The collagen fibrils in each lamella are arranged at approximate right angles to those in the adjacent lamellae (Fig. 23.4). The ground substance contains **corneal proteoglycans,** sulfated glycos-

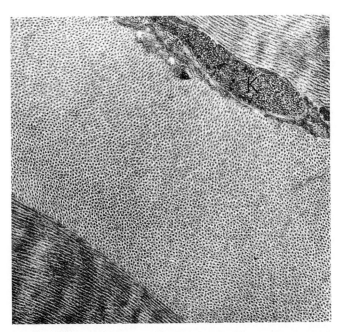

Figure 23.4. Electron micrograph of the corneal stroma showing parts of three lamellae and a portion of a corneal fibroblast [keratocyte (*K*)]. Note that the collagen fibrils in adjacent lamellae are oriented at right angles to one another. ×16,700.

aminoglycans (chiefly, keratan sulfate and chondroitin sulfate) covalently bound to protein.

It is believed that the uniform spacing of the collagen fibrils and the lamellae, as well as the *orthogonal array* of the lamellae (alternating layers at right angles), is responsible for the transparency to the cornea. The proteoglycans, along with collagen type V, regulate the precise diameter and spacing of the collagen fibrils. Swelling of the cornea following injury to the epithelium or endothelium disrupts this precise array and leads to translucency or opacity of the cornea.

The normal cornea contains no blood vessels or pigments. During an inflammatory response involving the cornea, large numbers of neutrophilic leukocytes and lymphocytes migrate from blood vessels of the limbus and penetrate between the lamellae of the stroma.

Descemet's Membrane Is an Unusually Thick Basal Lamina

Descemet's membrane is the basal lamina of the corneal endothelial cells. It is intensely periodic acid-Schiff positive and can be as much as 10 μm thick. It separates the corneal endothelium from the adjacent corneal stroma. Unlike Bowman's membrane, Descemet's membrane readily regenerates after injury. It also slowly increases in thickness with age. Descemet's membrane extends peripherally beneath the sclera as a meshwork called the *pectinate ligament.* Strands from the pectinate ligament insert into the ciliary muscle and the sclera and may help to maintain the normal curvature of the cornea by exerting tension on Descemet's membrane.

The *Corneal Endothelium* Provides Metabolic Exchange Between Cornea and Aqueous Humor

The corneal endothelium is a single layer of flattened cells covering the surface of the cornea that faces the anterior chamber. The cells are joined to each other by well-developed zonulae adherentes, by relatively leaky zonulae occludentes, and by desmosomes. Virtually all of the metabolic exchanges of the cornea occur across the endothelium. The endothelial cells contain many mitochondria and vesicles and an extensive rough endoplasmic reticulum (rER) and Golgi apparatus. They demonstrate endocytic activity and are engaged in active transport. Na^+-K^+-activated ATPase is localized on the lateral plasma membrane.

Transparency of the cornea requires the water content of the stroma to be precisely regulated. Physical or metabolic damage to the endothelium leads to rapid corneal swelling and, if the damage is severe enough, corneal opacity. Restoration of endothelial integrity is usually followed by deturgescence, although corneas can swell beyond their ability for self-repair. This can result in permanent focal opacities resulting from aggregation of collagen fibrils in the swollen cornea due to extraction of essential sulfated glycosaminoglycans.

The Sclera Is an Opaque Layer Consisting of Dense Connective Tissue

Flat collagen bundles pass in various directions in planes parallel to the surface of the sclera. Both the collagen bundles and the fibrils that form them are irregular in diameter and in their arrangement. Interspersed between the collagen bundles are fine networks of elastic fibers and a moderate amount of ground substance. Fibroblasts are scattered among these fibers.

The opacity of the sclera, like that of other dense connective tissues, is due primarily to the irregularity of its structure. The sclera is pierced by blood vessels, nerves, and the optic nerve (see Fig. 23.2). It is 1 mm thick posteriorly, 0.3–0.4 mm thick at its equator, and 0.7 mm thick at the corneoscleral margin or "limbus."

The sclera is divided into three rather ill-defined layers:

- ***Episclera,*** the external layer, is loose connective tissue adjacent to the periorbital fat.
- ***Sclera proper*** (also called ***Tenon's capsule***), the investing fascia of the eye, is composed of a dense network of thick collagen fibers.
- ***Lamina fusca,*** the inner aspect of the sclera, is located adjacent to the choroid and contains thinner collagen fibers as well as pigment cells and elastic fibers.

Tenon's (or the episcleral) space is located between the episclera and Tenon's capsule. This space and the surrounding periorbital fat allow the eye to rotate freely within the orbit. The tendons of the extraocular muscles attach to Tenon's capsule.

GLAUCOMA

Glaucoma is a clinical condition resulting from an increase in intraocular pressure. It can be caused by excessive secretion of aqueous humor or impedance of the drainage of aqueous humor from the anterior chamber. Nourishment of the internal tissues of the eye, particularly of the retina, is dependent on the diffusion of oxygen and nutrients from the intraocular vessels. To have normal flow of blood through these vessels (including the capillaries and veins), the hydrostatic pressure within the vessels must exceed the intraocular pressure. If the drainage of the aqueous humor is impeded, the intraocular pressure becomes elevated because the coverings of the eye do not allow the wall to expand. This increased pressure interferes with normal retinal nourishment and function. Visual deficits associated with glaucoma include blurring of vision and impaired dark adaptation (symptoms that indicate loss of normal retinal function) and halos around lights (a symptom indicating corneal endothelial damage). If the condition is not treated, the retina will be permanently damaged, and blindness will occur. Treatments are directed at decreasing the rate of production of aqueous humor or at eliminating the cause of the obstruction of normal drainage.

Limbus

The Limbus Is the Transitional Zone Between Cornea and Sclera

At the junction of the cornea and sclera (Fig. 23.5), Bowman's membrane ends abruptly. The overlying epithelium thickens from the 5 cell layers of the cornea to the 10–12 cell layers of the conjunctiva. It is at this junction that the corneal lamellae become less regular as they merge with the circular and oblique bundles of collagen fibers of the sclera. There is also an abrupt transition from the avascular cornea to the well-vascularized sclera.

It is the limbus region that contains the apparatus for the outflow of aqueous humor (Fig. 23.5, *upper enlargement*). In the stromal layer, endothelium-lined channels called the *trabecular meshwork* (or *spaces of Fontana*) merge to form the *canal of Schlemm.* This canal encircles the eye (Fig. 23.5). The aqueous humor is produced by the ciliary processes that border the lens in the posterior chamber of the eye. The fluid passes from the posterior chamber into the anterior chamber through the valve-like potential opening between the iris and lens. The fluid then passes through the openings in the trabecular meshwork in the limbus region

as it continues its course to enter the canal of Schlemm. Collecting trunks in the sclera, called *aqueous veins* because they convey aqueous humor instead of blood, transport the aqueous humor to (blood) veins located in the sclera.

Iris

The Iris Forms a Contractile Diaphragm Anterior to the Lens Surface

The iris arises from the anterior border of the ciliary body (see Plate 127, page 765). It is attached to the sclera about 2 mm posterior to the corneoscleral junction. The pupil is the central aperture of this thin disc. The iris is pushed slightly forward as it changes in size in response to light intensity.

The Iris Consists of Five Layers of Cells

The layers of the iris, from anterior to posterior, consist of

- Fibroblasts and melanocytes in a discontinuous layer, marked with ridges and grooves
- A thin avascular layer of stroma, the *anterior stromal sheet* or *lamella*
- A loose connective tissue layer that contains many small blood vessels and constitutes the main mass of the iris
- A discontinuous layer of smooth muscle that is derived from the anterior epithelial cells and is called the *posterior membrane*
- A double layer of pigmented epithelial cells (see Plate 128, page 767)

Two muscles, the *sphincter pupillae* and the *dilator pupillae,* form the posterior membrane. The cells of the dilator pupillae, located immediately adjacent to the anterior layer of the pigment epithelium, are derived from this layer and are called *(pigmented) myoepithelial cells.*

The size of the pupil is controlled by the contraction of the pupillary sphincter and dilator muscles. By increasing and decreasing the size of the opening, only the appropriate amount of light enters the eye. The *sphincter pupillae* is a circular band of smooth muscle located at the pupillary margin. It is innervated by parasympathetic nerves carried in the oculomotor nerve (cranial nerve III) and is responsible for reducing pupillary size in response to bright light.

Failure of the pupil to respond when light is shined into the eye—"pupil fixed and dilated"—is a sign of the lack of nerve or brain function. The *dilator pupillae* is a thin sheet of smooth muscle radially oriented near the posterior border of the iris. It is innervated by sympathetic nerves from the superior cervical ganglion and is responsible for increasing pupillary size in response to dim light.

The function of the pigment-containing cells in the iris is to absorb light rays. They are responsible for the color

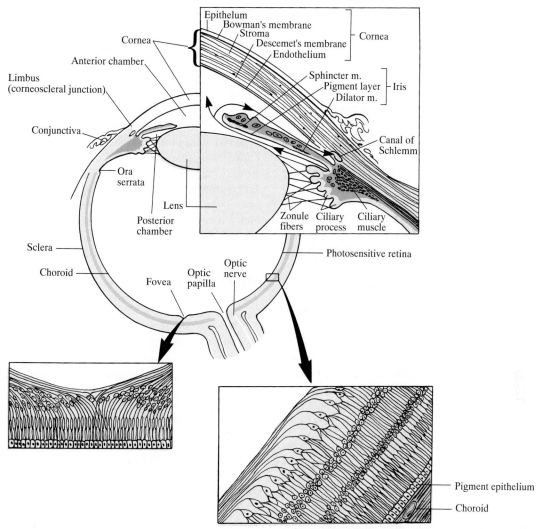

Figure 23.5. Schematic diagram of the structure of the eye. The *upper enlargement* depicts the anterior and posterior chambers in more detail and illustrates the direction of the flow of aqueous humor. The *lower enlargements* illustrate the organization of the cells of the retina in the retina proper *(right)* and the fovea *(left)*.

of the iris (i.e., eye color). The number of melanocytes in the stroma is responsible for variation in eye color. If there are few melanocytes in the stroma, eye color is derived from light reflected from the pigment present in the cells of the posterior surface of the iris, giving it a blue appearance. As the amount of pigment present in the stroma increases, the color changes from blue to shades of greenish-blue, gray, and, finally, brown.

The *Ciliary Body* Is a Thickened Anterior Portion of the Tunica Vasculosa, Located Between Iris and Choroid

The *ciliary body* extends for about 6 mm from the root of the iris, posterolaterally, to the *ora serrata* (see Fig. 23.2 and Plate 127, page 765). As seen from behind, the lateral edge of the ora serrata bears 17–34 grooves or crenelations. These grooves mark the anterior limit of both the retina and the choroid. The anterior third of the ciliary body has about 75 radial ridges or *ciliary processes*. The fibers of the zonule arise from the grooves between the ciliary processes.

The layers of the ciliary body are similar to those of the iris, consisting of a stroma and an epithelium. The stroma is divided into two layers:

- An outer layer of smooth muscle, the *ciliary muscle,* that makes up the bulk of the ciliary body
- An inner vascular region that extends into the ciliary processes

The epithelial layer covering the internal surface of the ciliary body is a direct continuation of the two layers of the retinal epithelium (see Fig. 23.1).

The Smooth Muscle of the Ciliary Body Is Organized in Three Functional Groups of Fibers

The smooth muscle of the ciliary body can be classified into three functional groups of fibers based on location:

- *Tensor portion,* consisting of meridional muscle fiber bundles bordering the scleral surface that are oriented longitudinally and function chiefly in stretching the choroid
- *Radial portion,* made up of muscle fibers bundles radiating in a fan-like fashion from their attachment to the scleral spur that insert into the circular portion of the ciliary muscle
- *Circular portion,* consisting of muscle fiber bundles occupying the inner and anterior part of the ciliary body that are oriented in a circular pattern forming a sphincter

The pull of the circular and radial fibers combine to reduce the tension on the zonule, so the lens becomes more spherical in shape. Forces generated by the longitudinal fibers on the scleral spur also open the angle of Schlemm and facilitate drainage of the aqueous humor.

Ciliary Processes Are Ridge-Like Extensions of the Ciliary Body From Which Zonule Fibers Emerge and Extend to the Lens

Ciliary processes, which measure approximately 2 mm in length, 1 mm in width, and 0.5 mm in height, are thickenings of the inner vascular region of the stroma. They are continuous with the vascular layers of the choroid. Scattered chromatophores and elastic fibers are present in the ciliary processes.

The Ciliary Epithelium Covers the Ciliary Body and Secretes Aqueous Humor

The ciliary epithelium is a double layer of columnar epithelial cells derived from the two layers of the optic cup. It has three principal functions:

- Secretion of aqueous humor
- Serving as the major component of the *blood-aqueous barrier* (part of the *blood-ocular barrier,* see below)
- Secretion and anchoring of the *zonular fibers* that form the *suspensory ligament of the lens*

The layer of the epithelium that has its basal lamina facing the posterior chamber is *nonpigmented.* The layer that has its basal lamina facing the connective tissue stroma of the ciliary body is *pigmented* and is directly continuous with the pigmented epithelial layer of the retina. The zonular fibers extend from the basal lamina of the nonpigmented epithelial cells of ciliary processes and insert into the lens capsule (the thickened basal lamina of the lens).

The cells of the nonpigmented inner layer have all the characteristics of a fluid transporting epithelium, including a complex junctional zone with a well-developed zonula occludens, complex lateral and basal plications, and localization of Na^+-K^+-ATPase in the lateral plasma membrane. In addition, they have an elaborate rER and Golgi complex, consistent with their role in secreting the zonular fibers. The cells of the pigmented layer have a less well-developed junctional zone and often exhibit large, irregular, lateral intercellular spaces. The apical surfaces of the two cell layers are held together by both desmosomes and gap junctions, creating discontinuous "luminal" spaces called *ciliary channels.*

The *aqueous humor* is similar in ionic composition to plasma but contains less than 0.1% protein (compared with 7% protein in plasma). The aqueous humor passes from the ciliary body toward the lens, then between the iris and lens, before it reaches the anterior chamber of the eye (Fig. 23.5). In the anterior chamber of the eye, the aqueous humor passes laterally to the angle formed between the cornea and iris. Here, it penetrates the tissues of the limbus as it enters the labyrinthine spaces and finally reaches the canal of Schlemm that communicates with the veins of the sclera.

The *Choroid* Is the Portion of the Vascular Layer That Lies Deep to the Retina

The *choroid* is a dark brown vascular sheet only 0.25 mm thick posteriorly and 0.1 mm thick anteriorly. It lies between the sclera and the retina (see Fig. 23.1).

Two layers can be identified in the choroid:

- *Choriocapillary layer,* an inner, vascular layer
- *Bruch's membrane,* a thin, amorphous, hyaline membrane

The choroid is attached firmly to the sclera at the margin of the optic nerve. A potential space, the *perichoroidal space* (between the sclera and retina), is traversed by thin lamellae or strands that pass from the sclera to the choroid. These lamellae form a layer called the *suprachoroid lamina.* The lamellae consist of large flat melanocytes scattered between connective tissue elements including collagen and elastic fibers, fibroblasts, macrophages, lymphocytes, plasma cells, and mast cells. The lamellae of the suprachoroid pass inward to surround the vessels in the remainder of the choroid layer. Free smooth muscle cells, not associated with blood vessels, are present in this tissue. Lymphatic channels called *epichoroid lymph spaces,* the long and short posterior ciliary vessels, and nerves on their way to the front of the eye are also present in the suprachoroid lamina.

Most of the blood vessels decrease in size as they approach the retina. The largest vessels continue forward beyond the ora serrata into the ciliary body. These vessels can be seen with an ophthalmoscope. The large vessels are mostly veins that course about in whorls before passing obliquely through the sclera as vortex veins. The inner layer of vessels, arranged in a single plane, is called the *choriocapillary layer.* The vessels of this layer provide nutrients to the cells of the retina. The fenestrated capillaries have lumina that are large and irregular in shape. In the region of the fovea, the choriocapillary layer is thicker, and the capillary network is more dense. This layer ends at the ora serrata.

Bruch's membrane measures 1–4 μm in thickness and

lies between the choriocapillary layer and the pigment epithelium of the retina. It is a thin, amorphous refractile layer, also called the *lamina vitrea.* In the transmission electron microscope (TEM), five different layers are identified in Bruch's membrane:

- The basal lamina of the endothelial cells of the choriocapillary layer
- A layer of collagen fibers approximately 0.5 μm thick
- A layer of elastic fibers approximately 2 μm thick
- A second layer of collagen fibers (thus, forming a sandwich around the intervening elastic tissue layer)
- The basal lamina of the retinal epithelial cells

RETINAL DETACHMENT

A potential space exists in the retina as a vestige of the space between the apical surfaces of the two epithelial layers of the optic cup. If this space expands, the neural retina separates from the pigment epithelium. This condition is called *retinal detachment.* If this condition is left uncorrected, blindness results. More commonly, as the vitreous body ages (in the sixth and seventh decades of life), it tends to shrink and pull away from the neural retina. This causes single or multiple tears in the neural retina that must be repaired by cryosurgery or laser surgery to prevent visual loss.

Retina

The retina, derived from the inner and outer layers of the optic cup, is the most internal of the three concentric layers of the eye (see Fig. 23.1c). It consists of two basic layers:

- *Neural retina* or *retina proper,* an inner layer that contains the photoreceptors
- *Retinal pigment epithelium,* an outer layer that rests on and is firmly attached to the choriocapillary layer of the choroid

A potential space exists between the two layers of the retina. The two layers may be separated mechanically from each other in the preparation of histologic specimens. Separation of the layers, ''retinal detachment,'' also occurs in the living state as a result of eye disease or trauma to the eye.

In the neural retina, two regions or portions that differ in function are recognized:

- The *nonphotosensitive region,* located anterior to the ora serrata, that lines the inner aspect of the ciliary body and the posterior surface of the iris (this portion of the retina has been described in the sections on the iris and ciliary body)
- The *photosensitive region* that lines the inner surface of

the eye posterior to the ora serrata except where it is pierced by the optic nerve

The site where the optic nerve joins the retina is called the *optic papilla* or *disc.* Because the optic papilla is devoid of photoreceptors, it is a blind spot in the visual field (see Plate 126, page 763). The *fovea centralis* is a shallow depression that is located about 2.5 mm lateral to the optic disc. It is the area of greatest visual acuity. The visual axis of the eye passes through the fovea. A yellow pigmented zone called the *macula lutea* surrounds the fovea. In relative terms, the fovea is the region of the retina that contains the highest concentration and most precisely ordered arrangement of the visual elements.

Ten Layers of Cells and Their Processes Constitute the Neural Retina

Before identifying the ten layers of the retina, it is important to identify the types of cells found there. This will aid in understanding the functional relationships of the cells. Studies of the retina in primates have identified at least 15 types of neurons that form at least 38 different types of synapses. For convenience, neurons and supporting cells can be classified into four groups of cells:

- *Photoreceptors*—the retinal *rods* and *cones*
- *Conducting neurons*—*bipolar* and *ganglion cells*
- *Association* and other *neurons*—*horizontal, centrifugal,* and *amacrine*
- *Supporting cells*—*Müller's cells* and *neuroglial cells*

The specific arrangement and associations of the nuclei and processes of these cells result in the retina being organized in eight to ten layers that are seen with the light microscope. Ten layers of the retina, from outside inward, are defined here (Fig. 23.6 and Plate 126, page 763):

1. *Pigment epithelium*—the outer layer of the retina not part of the neural retina but intimately associated with it
2. *Layer of rods and cones*—contains the outer and inner segments of photoreceptor cells
3. *External (or outer) limiting membrane*—the apical boundary of Müller's cells
4. *Outer nuclear layer*—contains the cell bodies (nuclei) of retinal rods and cones
5. *Outer plexiform layer*—contains the processes of retinal rods and cones and processes of the horizontal, amacrine, and bipolar cells that connect to them
6. *Inner nuclear layer*—contains the cell bodies (nuclei) of horizontal, amacrine, bipolar, and Müller's cells
7. *Inner plexiform layer*—contains the processes of horizontal, amacrine, and bipolar cells and processes of ganglion cells that connect to each other

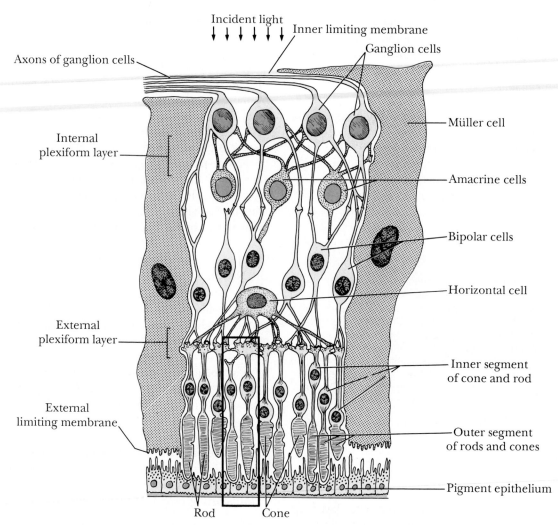

Figure 23.6. Schematic drawing of the layers of the retina. The interrelationship of the neurons is indicated. Light would enter the retina and pass through the internal layers of the retina before reaching the photoreceptors of the rods and cones that are closely associated with the pigment epithelium. The area in the *rectangle* is shown at higher magnification in Figure 23.7. (Modified from Dowling JE, Boycott BB: Organization of the primate retina: electron microscopy.)

8. *Ganglion cell layer*—contains the cell bodies (nuclei) of ganglion cells
9. *Layer of optic nerve fibers*—contains processes of ganglion cells that lead from the retina to the brain
10. *Internal (or inner) limiting membrane*—composed of the basal lamina of Müller's cells

Each of the layers is more fully described in the following sections (see corresponding numbers).

1. The Cells of the Retinal Pigment Epithelium Have Extensions that Surround the Processes of the Rods and Cones

The *retinal pigment epithelium (RPE)* is a single layer of cuboidal cells about 14 μm wide and 10–14 μm tall. The cells rest on Bruch's membrane of the choroid layer. The pigment cells are tallest in the fovea and adjacent regions. This accounts for the darker color of this region.

Adjacent RPE cells are connected by a junctional complex consisting of gap junctions and elaborate zonulae occludentes and adherentes. This junctional complex is the site of the *"blood-retinal barrier."*

The pigment cells have cylindrical sheaths on their apical surface that are associated with but do not directly contact the tip of the photoreceptor processes of the adjacent rod and cone cells. Complex cytoplasmic processes project for a short distance between the photoreceptors of the rods and cones. Numerous elongated melanin granules, unlike those found elsewhere in the eye, are present in many of these processes. They aggregate on the side of the cell nearest the rods and cones and are the most prominent feature of the cells. The nucleus, with its many convoluted infoldings, is located near the basal plasma membrane adjacent to Bruch's membrane. The cells also contain material, phagocytized from the processes of the photoreceptors, in the form of lamellar debris contained in residual bodies or phagosomes. A supranuclear Golgi apparatus and an extensive network of smooth endoplasmic reticulum surround the melanin granules and residual bodies that are present in the cytoplasm.

The RPE serves several important functions including

- *Absorption of light* passing through the neural retina to prevent reflection and the resultant glare.
- *Isolation of the retinal cells* from blood-borne substances. It serves as a major component of the **blood-retina barrier** via tight junctions between RPE cells.
- Participation in *restoration of photosensitivity* to visual pigments that were dissociated in response to light. The metabolic apparatus for visual pigment resynthesis is present in the RPE cells.
- *Phagocytosis and disposal* of membranous discs from the rods and cones of the retinal photoreceptor cells.

2. The Rods and Cones of the Photoreceptor Cells Extend From the Outer Layer of the Neural Retina to the Pigment Epithelium

The **rods and cones** are the outer segments of photoreceptor cells whose nuclei form the outer nuclear layer of the retina (Fig. 23.7). *It is important to recognize that the light that reaches the photoreceptors must first pass through all of the other, more internal layers of the neural retina.* The rods and cones are arranged in a palisade manner; therefore, with the light microscope, they appear as vertical striations.

The retina contains approximately 120 million rods and 7 million cones. The rods are about 2 μm in thickness and 50 μm long (ranging from about 60 μm at the fovea to 40 μm peripherally). The cones vary in length from 85 μm long at the fovea to 25 μm long at the periphery of the retina.

Functionally, the rods are more sensitive to light and are the receptors used during periods of low light intensity (e.g., at dusk or during the night). The visual image provided is one composed of gray tones (''a black and white picture''). In contrast, the cones exist in three forms that cannot be distinguished morphologically. They are less sensitive to low light and have maximal sensitivity to the red, green, or blue region of the visual spectrum. They provide a visual image composed of color and one that is believed to permit better visual acuity. The specificity of the cones provides a functional basis to explain color blindness that is believed to result from the lack of red-, green-, or (much less commonly) blue-sensitive cones.

Each rod and cone photoreceptor consists of three parts:

- **Outer segment**
- **Connecting stalk**
- **Inner segment**

The **outer segment** of the photoreceptor is roughly cylindrical or conical in shape (hence, the descriptive name rod or cone). This portion of the photoreceptor is intimately related to microvilli projecting from the adjacent pigment epithelial cells.

The **connecting stalk** contains a cilium composed of nine peripheral microtubule doublets extending from a basal body. The connecting stalk is seen as the constricted region of the cell that joins the inner to the outer segment. In this region, a thin, tapering process called the **calyceal process** extends from the distal end of the inner segment to surround the proximal portion of the outer segment (Fig. 23.7).

The **inner segment** is divided into an outer **ellipsoid** and an inner **myoid** portion. This segment contains a typical complement of organelles associated with a cell actively synthesizing proteins. A prominent Golgi apparatus, rER, and free polysomes are concentrated in the myoid region. Mitochondria are most numerous in the ellipsoid region. Microtubules are distributed throughout the inner segment. In the outer ellipsoid portion, cross-striated fibrous rootlets may extend from the basal body among the mitochondria.

The outer segment is the site of photosensitivity, and the inner segment contains the metabolic machinery to support the activity of the photoreceptors. The outer segment is considered to be a highly modified cilium because it is joined to the inner segment by the short connecting stalk.

In the TEM, 600–1000 regularly spaced horizontal discs are seen in the outer segment (Fig. 23.8). In rods, these discs are membrane-bounded structures measuring about 2 μm in diameter. They are enclosed within the plasma membrane of the outer segment (Fig. 23.8a). The parallel membranes of the discs are about 6 nm in thickness and are continuous at their ends. The central enclosed space is about 8 nm across. In both rods and cones, the plasma membrane in the region of the outer segment near the cilium has undergone repetitive transverse infolding to form the membranous discs. Autoradiographic studies have demonstrated that rods form new discs by infolding of the plasma membrane throughout their life span. Discs are formed in cones in a similar manner but are not replaced on a regular basis.

Rod discs lose their continuity with the plasma membrane from which they were derived soon after they are formed. They then pass like a stack of plates, proximally to distally, along the length of the cylindrical portion of the outer segment until they are eventually shed and phagocytosed by the pigment epithelial cells. Thus, each rod disc is a membrane-enclosed compartment within the cytoplasm. Discs within the cones retain their continuity with the plasma membrane (Fig. 23.8b).

The Interior of the Discs of Cones Is Continuous With the Extracellular Space

The basic difference in the structure of the rod and cone discs, i.e., the continuity with the plasma membrane, is correlated with the slightly different means by which the visual pigments are renewed in rods and cones. Newly synthesized rhodopsin is incorporated into the membrane of the rod disc as the disc is being formed at the base of the outer

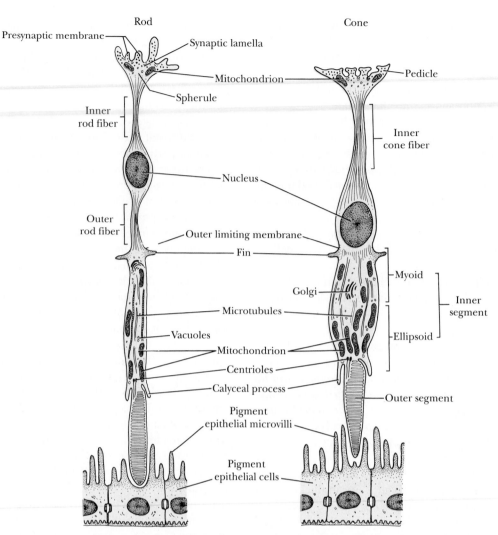

Figure 23.7. Schematic diagram of the ultrastructure of rod and cone cells. The outer segments of the rods and cones are closely associated with the adjacent pigment epithelium. (Modified from Dowling JE, Boycott BB: Organization of the primate retina: electron microscopy.) *Proceedings of the Royal Society of London* [*Biology*] 166:80, 1966.)

segment. It then takes several days for the disc to reach the tip of the outer segment. In contrast, although visual proteins are constantly being produced in retinal cones, the proteins are incorporated into cone discs located anywhere in the outer segment.

In Rod Cells, the Discs Contain the Pigment *Rhodopsin (Visual Purple)*

Rhodopsin initiates the visual stimulus as it is bleached by light. Rhodopsin is present in globular form on the outer surface of the lipid bilayer (on the cytoplasmic side) of the membranous discs. In the cone cells, the only visual pigment that has been isolated from the membranous discs is the photopigment *iodopsin.* However, it is known that the cones are specialized to respond maximally to one of the three colors (red, green, or blue). The visual pigments,

rhodopsin and iodopsin, are molecules that have a membrane-bound subunit called an *opsin* and a second component called a *chromophore.* The opsin of rods is *scotopsin;* the opsins of cones are *photopsins.* The chromophore of the rods is a vitamin A-derived carotenoid called *retinal.* Thus, an adequate intake of vitamin A is essential for normal vision. A prolonged dietary deficiency of vitamin A leads to the inability to see in dim light (''night blindness'').

Vision Is a Process by Which Light Striking the Retina Is Converted Into Electrical Impulses That Are Transmitted to the Brain

The impulses produced by light reaching the photoreceptors are conveyed by an elaborate network of nerves to the brain, where a visual image is produced. The conversion of the incident light into nerve impulses is called *transduction* and involves two basic steps:

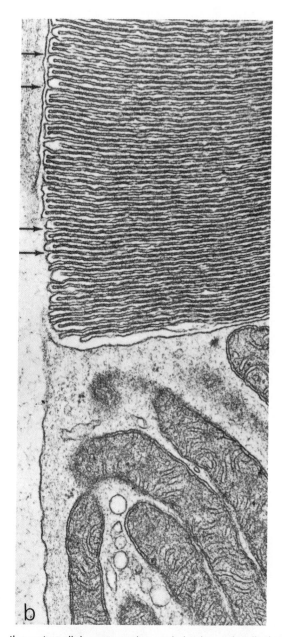

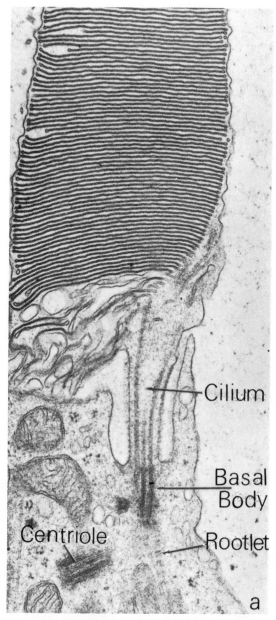

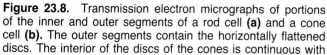

Figure 23.8. Transmission electron micrographs of portions of the inner and outer segments of a rod cell **(a)** and a cone cell **(b).** The outer segments contain the horizontally flattened discs. The interior of the discs of the cones is continuous with the extracellular space *(arrows).* In the rod cell, the plane of section passes through the connecting stalk and cilium. A centriole, cilium, basal body, and ciliary rootlet are identified. (Courtesy of T. Kuwabara.)

- Step 1 is a photochemical reaction that occurs in the outer segment of the rod and cone receptors as absorbed light energy causes *conformational changes in the chromophores.*
- Step 2 consists of *changes in concentration of internal transmitters* within the cytoplasm of the inner segment of the photoreceptors. These changes influence the ionic permeability of the plasma membrane and cause the photoreceptor to *become hyperpolarized,* thus initiating impulses that are conveyed to the brain.

In Rods, Absorbed Light Energy Causes Conformational Changes in *Retinal*, Converting It to *Retinol*

The conversion of retinal to retinol results in its being released from scotopsin (a reaction called "bleaching"). The cell becomes hyperpolarized as calcium diffuses from the receptor cell and reduces its permeability to sodium. The visual pigment is then reassembled, and calcium is transported back into the cell. The energy for this process is provided by the mitochondria located in the inner segment. Müller's cells and pigment epithelial cells also participate in the interconversion of *retinal and retinol* and the reactions necessary for the resynthesis of rhodopsin.

During the normal functioning of the photoreceptors, the membranous discs of the outer segment are shed and phagocytized by the pigment epithelial cells (Fig. 23.9). It is estimated that each of these cells is capable of phagocytizing and disposing of about 7500 shed discs/day. The discs are constantly turning over, and the production of new discs must be equal to the rate of disc shedding.

Discs Are Shed From Both Rods and Cones

In rods, there is a burst of disc shedding each morning, when, after a period of sleep, light first enters the eye. The time of disc shedding in cones is more variable. The shedding of discs in cones also enables the receptors to eliminate superfluous membrane. Although not fully understood, the shedding process in cones must also alter the size of the discs, so that the conical form is maintained as discs are released from the distal end of the cone.

3. The External (or Outer) Limiting Membrane Is Formed by a Row of Zonulae Adherentes Between Müller's Cells

The outer limiting membrane is not a true membrane. It is a row of zonulae adherentes between the apical ends of Müller's cells, i.e., the end that faces the pigment epithelium, with each other and with the rods and cones. Because Müller's cells end at the base of the inner segments of the receptors, they mark the location of this layer. Thus, the supporting processes of Müller's cells on which the rods and cones rest are pierced by the inner and outer segments of the photoreceptors.

4. The Outer Nuclear Layer Contains the Nuclei of the Retinal Rods and Cones

The region of the cytoplasm of the rods containing the nucleus is separated from the inner segment by a tapering process of the cytoplasm. In cones, the nuclei are located close to the outer segments, and similar tapering is not seen. The cone nuclei stain lightly and are larger and more oval than rod nuclei. Rod nuclei are surrounded by only a thin rim of cytoplasm. In contrast, a relatively thick investment of cytoplasm surrounds the cone nuclei.

5. The Outer Plexiform Layer Is Formed by the Processes of the Photoreceptor Cells and Neurons

The outer plexiform layer is formed by the processes of retinal rods and cones and the processes of horizontal, amacrine, and bipolar cells. The processes allow the photoreceptor cells to be coupled electrically to these specialized interneurons via synapses. A thin process extends from the region of the nucleus of each rod or cone to an

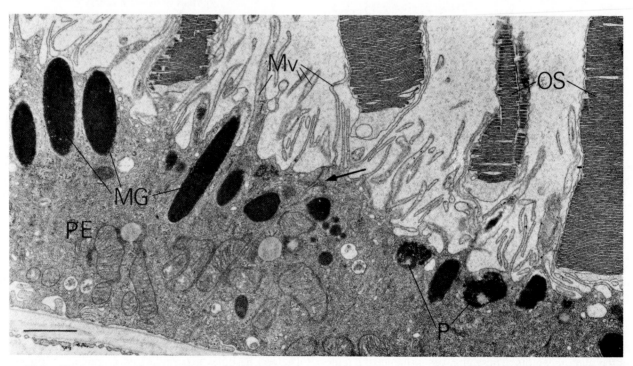

Figure 23.9. Transmission electron micrograph of the outer segments of rods and cones in association with the pigment epithelium. The pigment epithelial cells *(PE)* contain numerous elongated melanin granules *(MG)* that are aggregated against the side of the cell where the microvilli *(Mv)* extend from the surface toward the outer segments *(OS)* of rod and cone cells. The pigment epithelial cells contain numerous mitochondria and phagosomes *(P)*. The *arrow* indicates the location of the junctional complex between adjacent pigment epithelial cells. (Courtesy of T. Kuwabara.)

inner expanded portion with several lateral processes. The expanded portion is called a *spherule* in a rod or a *pedicle* in a cone. Normally, many photoreceptors converge onto one bipolar cell and form interconnecting neural networks. Cones located in the fovea, however, synapse with a single bipolar cell. The fovea is also unique in that the compactness of the inner neural layers of the retina causes the photoreceptors to be oriented obliquely. Horizontal cell dendritic processes synapse with photoreceptors throughout the retina and further contribute to the elaborate neuronal connections in this layer.

6. The Inner Nuclear Layer Consists of the Nuclei of Horizontal, Amacrine, Bipolar, and Müller's Cells

Müller's cells form the scaffolding for the whole retina. Their processes invest the other cells of the retina so completely that they fill most of the extracellular space. The basal and apical ends of Müller's cells form the internal and external limiting membranes, respectively. Microvilli extending from their apical border lie between the photoreceptors of the rods and cones. Capillaries from the retinal vessels extend only to this layer. The rods and cones carry on their metabolic exchanges with extracellular fluids transported across the blood-retinal barrier of the RPE.

The three types of conducting cells—*bipolar, horizontal,* and *amacrine*—found in this layer have distinct orientations (see Fig. 23.6). The processes of *bipolar cells* extend to both the inner and the outer plexiform layer. Through these connections, the bipolar cells establish synaptic connections with multiple cells in each layer except in the fovea, where the number of interconnected cells is reduced to provide greater visual acuity. The processes of *horizontal cells* extend to the external plexiform layer where they intermingle with processes of bipolar cells. The cells have synaptic connections with rod spherules, cone pedicles, and bipolar cells. This electrical coupling of cells is thought to affect the functional threshold between rods and cones and bipolar cells. The processes of *amacrine cells* branch extensively to provide sites of synaptic connections with axonal endings of bipolar cells and dendrites of ganglion cells.

In the peripheral regions of the retina, the axons of bipolar cells pass to the inner plexiform layer where they synapse with several ganglion cells. In the fovea, they may synapse with a single ganglion cell, again reflecting the greater visual acuity in this region. Amacrine cell processes pass inward, contributing to a complex interconnection of cells. They synapse in the inner plexiform layer with bipolar, ganglion, and other amacrine cells (see Fig. 23.6).

7. The Inner Plexiform Layer Consists of a Complex Array of Intermingled Neuronal Cell Processes

The inner plexiform layer consists of a complex intermingling of the processes of the amacrine, bipolar, and ganglion cells. The processes have a course that parallels the inner limiting membrane, thus giving the appearance of horizontal striations to this layer.

8. The Ganglion Cell Layer Consists of the Cell Bodies of Large Multipolar Neurons

The cell bodies of large multipolar nerve cells up to 30 μm in diameter constitute the ganglion cell layer. They have lightly staining round nuclei with prominent nucleoli and have Nissl bodies in their cytoplasm. An axonal process emerges from the rounded cell body, passes into the nerve fiber layer, and then into the optic nerve. The dendrites extend from the opposite end of the cell to ramify in the inner plexiform layer. In the peripheral regions of the retina, a single ganglion cell may synapse with a hundred bipolar cells. In marked contrast, in the macular region, surrounding the fovea, the bipolar cells are smaller (some authors refer to them as "midget" bipolar cells), and there tends to be a single connection between a midget bipolar cell and a ganglion cell. Over most of the retina, the ganglion cells are only a single layer of cells. At the macula, however, they are piled up to eight deep, although they are absent over the fovea itself. Scattered among the ganglion cells are small neuroglial cells with densely staining nuclei.

9. The Layer of Optic Nerve Fibers Contains Axons of the Ganglion Cells

The axonal processes of the ganglion cells form a flattened layer running parallel to the retinal surface. This layer increases in depth as the axons converge at the optic disc. The axons are thin, nonmyelinated processes measuring up to 5 μm in diameter.

10. The Internal (or Inner) Limiting Membrane Consists of a Basal Lamina Separating the Retina From the Vitreous Body

The internal limiting membrane is the basal lamina of Müller's cells.

Specialized Regions of the Retina. The *fovea* appears as a shallow depression located at the posterior pole of the optical axis of the eye. Its central region, known as the *fovea centralis,* is about 200 μm in diameter. Most of the layers of the retina except the layer of the photoreceptors are markedly reduced or are absent in this region (see Fig. 23.5). Here, that layer is composed entirely of cones that are longer and are more slender and rod-like than they are elsewhere. The adjacent pigment epithelial cells and choriocapillaris are also thickened in this region.

The *macula lutea* is the area surrounding the fovea. It is yellowish due to the presence of yellow pigment (xanthophyll). Retinal vessels are absent in this region. Here, the retinal cells and their processes, especially the ganglion cells, are heaped up on the sides of the fovea so that light may pass unimpeded to this most sensitive area of the retina.

Vessels of the Retina. The *central retinal artery* and *vein,* the vessels that can be seen and assessed with an ophthalmoscope, pass through the center of the optic nerve to enter the bulb of the eye at the optic disc (see Fig. 23.2 and the section on the developing eye). The artery branches immediately into upper and lower branches, each of which divides again. Veins undergo a similar pattern of branching. The vessels initially lie between the vitreous body and inner limiting membrane. As the vessels pass laterally, they pass deeper within the inner retinal layers. Branches from these vessels form a capillary plexus that does not extend beyond the inner nuclear layer. The branches of the central retinal artery do not anastomose with each other and, therefore, are classified as anatomical end arteries. Evaluation of the retinal vessels and optic disc during the physical examination of a patient not only provides important information on the state of the eye but also provides early clinical signs of a number of conditions including elevated intracranial pressure, hypertension, glaucoma, and diabetes.

Crystalline Lens

The lens is a transparent, avascular, biconvex structure. It is suspended between the edges of the ciliary body by the *zonule* or *suspensory ligament.* The pull of the zonular fibers keeps the lens in a flattened condition. Release of that tension causes the lens to fatten or *accommodate* to bend light rays originating close to the eye so that they focus on the retina.

The lens has three principal components (see Plate 128, Fig. 3, page 767):

- *Lens capsule,* a thick basal lamina measuring approximately 10–20 μm, produced by the anterior lens cells
- *Subcapsular epithelium,* a cuboidal layer of cells present only on the anterior surface of the lens
- *Lens fibers,* structures derived from subcapsular epithelial cells

The *lens capsule,* composed primarily of type IV collagen and proteoglycans, is elastic. It is thickest at the equator where the fibers of the zonule attach to it.

The cuboidal cells of the *subcapsular epithelium* are connected by gap junctions. They have few cytoplasmic organelles and stain faintly. The apical region of the cell is directed toward the internal aspect of the lens and the lens fibers with which they form junctional complexes. The lens increases in size during normal growth and then continues, at an ever-decreasing rate, the production of new lens fibers throughout life. The new lens fibers develop from the subcapsular epithelial cells located near the equator. Cells in this region increase in height and then differentiate into lens fibers.

As the *lens fibers* develop, they become highly elongated and appear as thin, flattened structures. They lose their nu-

clei and other organelles as they become filled with proteins called *crystallins.* Mature lens fiber attain a length of 7–10 mm, a width of 8–10 μm, and a thickness of 2 μm. Near the center of the lens, in the *nucleus,* the fibers are compressed and condensed to such a degree that it is impossible to recognize individual fibers. Despite this density and the protein content, the lens is normally transparent.

Changes in the Lens Are Associated With Aging

With increasing age, the lens gradually loses its elasticity and ability to accommodate. This condition, called *presbyopia,* usually occurs in the fourth decade of life. This is easily corrected by wearing reading glasses or using a magnifying lens.

Loss of transparency of the lens or its capsule is also a relatively common condition associated with aging. This condition, called *cataract,* may be due to conformational changes or cross-linking of proteins. The development of a cataract may also be related to disease processes, metabolic or hereditary conditions, trauma, or exposure to a deleterious agent (such as ultraviolet radiation). Cataracts that significantly impair vision can usually be corrected surgically by removing the lens and replacing it with a plastic lens implanted in the posterior chamber.

Vitreous Humor

Vitreous Humor Is the Transparent Jelly-Like Substance That Fills the Posterior Segment (Vitreous Space) of the Eye

The vitreous humor is loosely attached to the surrounding structures, including the limiting membrane of the retina. The main body of the vitreous is a homogeneous gel containing about 99% water, collagen, and glycosaminoglycans (principally hyaluronic acid). The hyaloid canal (or Cloquet's canal), which is not always visible, runs through the center of the vitreous from the optic disc to the posterior lens capsule. It is the remnant of the pathway of the hyaloid artery of the developing eye.

Accessory Structures of the Eye

The Conjunctiva Lines the Space Between the Inner Surface of the Eyelids and the Anterior Surface of the Eye Lateral to the Cornea

The conjunctiva is a thin, transparent mucous membrane that extends from the lateral margin of the cornea, across the sclera, and covers the internal surface of the eyelids. It consists of a stratified columnar epithelium containing numerous goblet cells and rests on a lamina propria composed of loose connective tissue.

The Primary Function of the Eyelids Is to Protect the Eye

The skin of the lids is loose and elastic to accommodate their movement. Within each eyelid is a flexible support, the *tarsal plate,* consisting of dense fibrous and elastic tissue. The undersurface of the tarsal plate is covered by conjunctiva (Fig. 23.10).

The eyelid contains three types of glands:

- *Meibomian glands,* long sebaceous glands embedded in the tarsal plates that appear as vertical yellow streaks in the tissue deep to the conjunctiva
- *Glands of Zeis,* small modified sebaceous glands that are connected with and empty their secretion into the follicles of the eyelashes
- *Glands of Moll,* sweat glands with unbranched sinuous tubules that begin as a simple spiral

About 25 *Meibomian glands* are present in the upper eyelid, and 20 are present in the lower eyelid. The sebaceous secretion of the Meibomian glands produces an oily layer on the surface of the tear film that retards the evaporation of the normal tear layer.

The eyelashes emerge from the most anterior edge of the lid margin, in front of the openings of the Meibomian glands. The lashes are short, stiff, curved hairs and may occur in double or triple rows. The lashes on the same eyelid margin may have different lengths and diameters.

The Lacrimal Gland Produces Tears That Moisten the Cornea and Pass to the Nasolacrimal Duct

Tears are produced by *lacrimal* and *tarsal glands.* The *lacrimal gland* is located beneath the conjunctiva on the upper lateral side of the eye. The *tarsal glands* (also called

the *accessory tear glands*) are compound serous tubuloalveolar glands that have distended lumina. They are located on the inner surface of the upper and lower eyelids (Fig. 23.10).

The lacrimal gland consists of several separate lobules of tubuloacinar serous glands. The acini have large lumina lined with columnar cells. Myoepithelial cells, located below the epithelial cells within the basal lamina, aid in the release of tears. Approximately 12 ducts drain from the lacrimal gland into the conjunctival space beneath the upper eyelid.

Tears Are Sterile and Contain the Antibacterial Enzyme *Lysozyme*

Tears keep the conjunctiva and corneal epithelium moist, wash foreign material from the eye as they flow across the corneal surface toward the medial angle of the eye (Fig. 23.10), and protect the eye through their bacteriocidal properties. The *lacrimal puncta,* the small openings of the *lacrimal canaliculi* through which the tears drain from the eye, are located at the medial angle. The upper and lower canaliculi join to form the *common canaliculus* that opens into the *lacrimal sac.* The sac is continuous with the *nasolacrimal duct* that opens into the nasal cavity below the inferior turbinate. A pseudostratified ciliated epithelium lines the lacrimal sac and the nasolacrimal duct.

The Eye Is Moved Within the Orbit by the Extraocular Muscles

Six *extraocular muscles* (also called *extrinsic muscles*) attach to each eye. These are the medial, lateral, superior, and inferior rectus muscles and the superior and inferior oblique muscles. The superior oblique muscle is innervated by the *trochlear nerve (cranial nerve IV).* The lateral rectus muscle is innervated by the *abducens nerve (cranial*

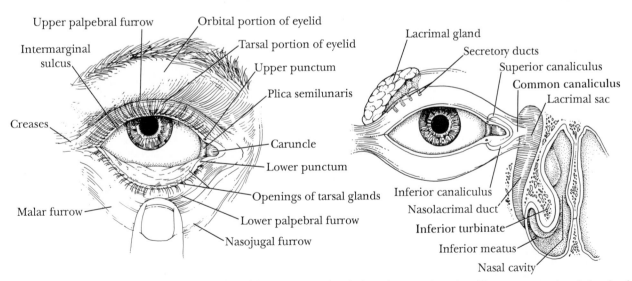

Figure 23.10. Schematic diagrams of the eye and its accessory structures. The *drawing* on the *right* shows a coronal section passing through the lacrimal bone and associated bones bordering the nasal cavity. The components of the lacrimal drainage system are shown.

nerve VI). All of the remaining extraocular muscles are innervated by the *oculomotor nerve (cranial nerve III).* The combined and precisely controlled action of these muscles allows vertical, lateral, and rotational movement of the eye. Normally, the actions of the muscles of both eyes are coordinated so that they eyes move in parallel *(conjugate gaze).*

ATLAS PLATES

125–128

PLATE 125. Eye I

This micrograph of a meridional section through the eyeball illustrates most of the structural features of the eye at low magnification and provides orientation for the plates that follow.

The wall of the eyeball consists of three layers: the retina, the uvea, and an outer fibrous layer, the corneoscleral coat.

Eye, human, hematoxylin and eosin (H&E) ×7. The innermost layer is the retina *(R)*, which consists of several layers of cells. Among these are receptor cells (rods and cones), neurons (e.g., bipolar and ganglion cells), supporting cells, and a pigment epithelium (see Plate 126). The receptor components of the retina are situated in the posterior three-fifths of the eyeball. At the anterior boundary of the receptor layer, the ora serrata *(OS)*, the retina becomes reduced in thickness, and nonreceptor components of the retina continue forward to cover the posterior or inner surface of the ciliary body *(CB)* and the iris *(I)*. This anterior nonreceptor extension of the inner layer is highly pigmented, and the pigment (melanin) is evident as the black inner border of these structures.

The uvea, the middle layer of the eyeball, consists of the choroid, the ciliary body, and the iris. The choroid is a vascular layer; it is relatively thin and difficult to distinguish in the accompanying figure except by location. On this basis, it is identified *(Ch)* as being just external to the pigmented layer of the retina. The choroid is also highly pigmented; the choroidal pigment is evident as a discrete layer in several parts of the section.

Anterior to the ora serrata, the uvea is thickened; here, it is called the ciliary body *(CB)*. This contains the ciliary muscle (see Plate 127, page 765), which brings about adjustments of the lens for the focusing of light. The ciliary body also contains processes to which the zonular fibers are attached. These fibers function as suspensory ligaments of the lens *(L)*. The iris *(I)* is the most anterior component of the uvea and contains a central opening, the pupil.

The outermost layer of the eyeball, the fibrous layer, consists of the sclera *(S)* and the cornea *(C)*. Both of these contain collagenous fibers as their main structural element; however, the cornea is transparent, and the sclera is opaque. The extrinsic muscles of the eye insert into the sclera and effect movements of the eyeball. These are not included in the preparation except for a small piece of a muscle insertion *(arrow)* in the upper left of the illustration. Posteriorly, the sclera is pierced by the emerging optic nerve *(ON)*.

The lens is considered in Plate 128, page 767. Just posterior to the lens is the large cavity of the eye, the vitreous cavity, which is filled with a thick jelly-like material, the vitreous humor or body. Anterior to the lens are two additional, fluid-filled chambers of the eye, the anterior *(AC)* and posterior chambers *(PC)*, separated by the iris.

KEY		
AC, anterior chamber	**I,** iris	**PC,** posterior chamber
C, cornea	**L,** lens	**R,** retina
CB, ciliary body	**ON,** optic nerve	**S,** sclera
Ch, choroid	**OS,** ora serrata	**arrow,** muscle insertion

PLATE 125

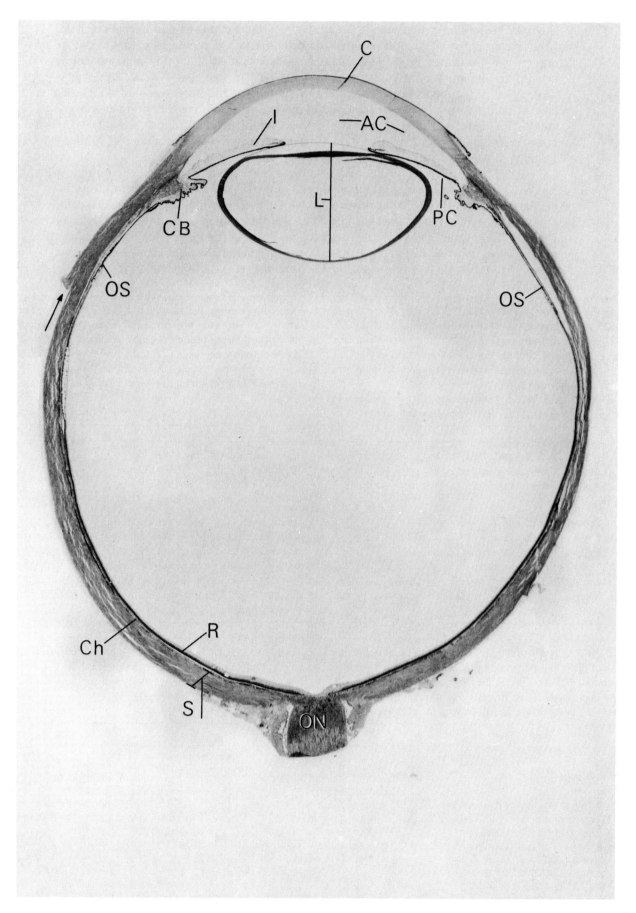

PLATE 126. Eye II

The optic nerve and retina are, in effect, a projection of the central nervous system, and the fibrous cover of the optic nerve is an extension of the meninges of the brain. As a consequence, pressure within the cranial cavity, transmitted along this channel, can be detected by examination of the optic disc.

Müller's cells are supporting cells comparable with neuroglia. Processes of Müller's cells ramify virtually through the entire thickness of the retina. The internal limiting membrane is the basal lamina of Müller's cells; the external limiting membrane is actually not a membrane; rather, it represents junctional complexes between the processes of Müller's cells and photoreceptor cells (rods and cones).

Aside from the pigment epithelium and Müller's cells, the other cells of the retina are neural elements arranged sequentially in three layers: (1) the rods and cones; (2) an intermediate neuronal layer (bipolar, horizontal, and amacrine cells); and (3) ganglion cells. Nerve impulses originating in the rods and cones are transmitted to the intermediate layer and then to the ganglion cells. Synaptic connections occur in the inner and outer plexiform layers, resulting in some degree of neuronal integration. Finally, the ganglion cells send their axons to the brain as components of the optic nerve.

FIGURE 1, eye, human, H&E ×65. The site where the optic nerve leaves the eyeball is called the optic disc *(OD)*. It is characteristically marked by a depression, evident here. Receptor cells are not present at the optic disc, and because it is not sensitive to light stimulation, it is sometimes referred to as the blind spot.

The fibers that give rise to the optic nerve originate in the retina, more specifically, in the ganglion cell layer (see be-

low). They traverse the sclera through a number of openings *(arrows)* to form the optic nerve. The region of the sclera that contains these openings is called the lamina cribrosa *(LC)*. The optic nerve contains a central artery and vein (not seen here) that also traverse the lamina cribrosa. Branches of these blood vessels *(BV)* supply the inner portion of the retina.

FIGURE 2, eye, human, H&E ×325. On the basis of structural features that are evident in histologic sections, the retina is divided into ten layers as listed below and labeled in this figure.

1. Pigment epithelium *(PEp)*
2. Layer of rods and cones *(R&C)*
3. External limiting membrane *(ELM)*
4. Outer nuclear layer (nuclei of rod and cone cells) *(ONL)*
5. Outer plexiform layer *(OPL)*
6. Inner nuclear layer (nuclei of bipolar, horizontal, amacrine, and Müller's cells) *(INL)*

7. Inner plexiform layer *(IPL)*
8. Layer of ganglion cells *(GC)*
9. Nerve fiber layer *(NFL)*
10. Internal limiting membrane *(ILM)*

This figure also shows the innermost layer of the choroid *(Ch)*. There is a cell-free membrane, the lamina vitrea *(LV)*, also called Bruch's membrane. Electron micrographs reveal that it corresponds to the basement membrane of the pigment epithelium. Immediately external to the lamina vitrea is the capillary layer of the choroid (lamina choriocapillaris). These vessels supply the outer part of the retina.

FIGURE 3, eye, human, H&E ×440. The posterior portion of the retina contains a small depression called the fovea centralis *(FC)*. This part of the retina contains only cone cells. The depression of the fovea is due to a spreading apart of the inner layers of the retina, leaving the cone elements rel-

atively uncovered. The fovea centralis is associated with acute vision. As one moves from the fovea toward the ora serrata, the number of cone cells decreases and the number of rod cells increases.

KEY

BV, blood vessels
Ch, choroid
ELM, external limiting membrane
FC, fovea centralis
GC, layer of ganglion cells
ILM, internal limiting membrane
INL, inner nuclear layer (nuclei of bipolar, horizontal, amacrine, and Müller's cells)

IPL, inner plexiform layer
LC, lamina cribrosa
LV, lamina vitrea
NFL, nerve fiber layer
OD, optic disc
ONL, outer nuclear layer (nuclei of rod and cone cells)

OPL, outer plexiform layer
PEp, pigment epithelium
R&C, layer of rods and cones
arrows, openings in sclera (lamina cribrosa)

PLATE 126

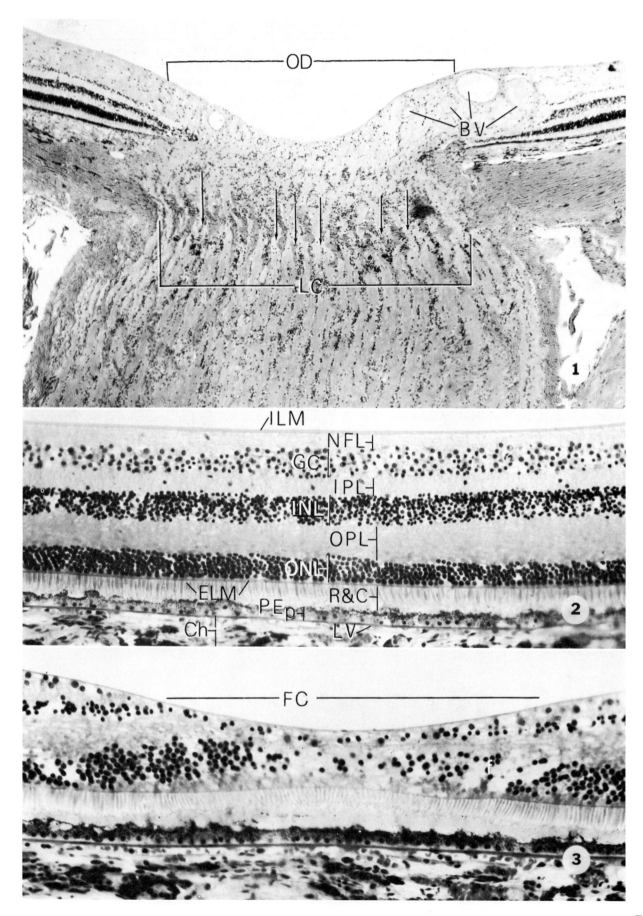

PLATE 127. Eye III

FIGURE 1, eye, human, H&E ×30; inset ×300. A portion of the anterior segment of the eye, shown in this figure, includes parts of the cornea *(C)*, sclera *(S)*, iris *(I)*, ciliary body *(CB)*, anterior chamber *(AC)*, posterior chamber *(PC)*, lens *(L)*, and zonular fibers *(ZF)*. The zonular fibers function as the suspensory ligament of the lens.

The cornea is considered in detail in Plate 128. However, the relationship of the cornea to the sclera is illustrated to advantage here. The junction between the two *(arrows)* is marked by a change in staining, with the substance of the cornea appearing lighter than that of the sclera. The corneal epithelium *(CEp)* is continuous with the conjunctival epithelium *(CjEp)* that covers the sclera. (The junction between these is marked by the *small circle* and shown at higher magnification in the **inset**.) The conjunctival epithelium is separated from the dense fibrous component of the sclera by a loose vascular connective tissue. Together, this connective tissue and the epithelium constitute the conjunctiva *(Cj)*. The epithelial-connective tissue junction of the conjunctiva is irregular; in contrast, the undersurface of the corneal epithelium presents an even profile.

Just lateral to the junction of the cornea and sclera is a canal, seen in cross section, the canal of Schlemm (see *CS*, Fig. 2). This canal takes a circular route about the perimeter of the cornea. It communicates with the anterior chamber through a loose trabecular meshwork of tissue called the spaces of Fontana. These spaces can only be seen adequately in ideal preparations and are not evident in this plate. The canal of Schlemm also communicates with episcleral veins. By means of its communications, the canal of Schlemm provides a route for the fluid in the anterior and posterior chambers to reach the bloodstream. The canal may form more than one channel as it encircles the cornea.

The iris and lens are considered in Plate 128. The *rectangles* mark those areas of the lens that are shown in Plate 128 (Fig. 3 and its **inset**).

FIGURE 2, eye, human, H&E ×65; inset ×570. Immediately internal to the anterior margin of the sclera *(S)* is the ciliary body *(CB)*. The inner surface of this forms radially arranged, ridge-shaped elevations, the ciliary processes *(CP)*, to which the zonular fibers *(ZF)* are anchored. From the outside in, the components of the ciliary body are the ciliary muscle *(CM)*, the connective tissue (vascular) layer *(VL)*, the lamina vitrea *(LV*, **inset**), and the ciliary epithelium *(CiEp*, **inset**). The ciliary epithelium consists of two layers **(inset)**, the pigmented *(P)* and the nonpigmented layer *(nP)*. The ciliary epithelium plays a role in the formation of the aqueous humor. The lamina vitrea is a continuation of the same layer of the choroid: It is the basement membrane of the pigmented ciliary epithelial cells.

The ciliary muscle is arranged in three patterns. The outer layer is immediately deep to the sclera. These are the meridionally arranged fibers of Brücke. The outermost of these continues more posteriorly into the choroid and is referred to as the tensor muscle of the choroid. The middle layer is the radial group. It radiates from the region of the sclerocorneal junction into the ciliary body. The innermost layer of muscle cells is circularly arranged. These are seen in cross section. The circular artery and vein *(CAV)* for the iris, also cut in cross section, are just anterior to the circular group of muscle cells.

KEY

AC, anterior chamber
C, cornea
CAV, circular artery and vein
CB, ciliary body
CEp, corneal epithelium
CiEp, ciliary epithelium
Cj, conjunctiva
CjEp, conjunctival epithelium
CM, ciliary muscle
CP, ciliary processes
CS, canal of Schlemm
I, iris
L, lens
LV, lamina vitrea
nP, nonpigmented layer of the ciliary epithelium
P, pigmented layer of the ciliary epithelium
PC, posterior chamber
S, sclera
VL, vascular layer (of ciliary body)
ZF, zonular fibers
arrows, junction between cornea and sclera

PLATE 127

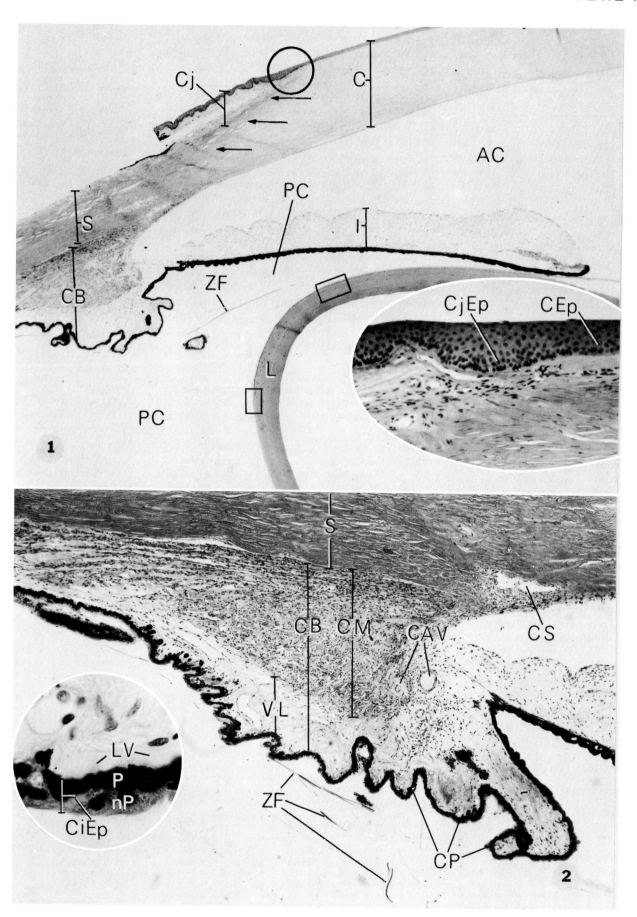

PLATE 128. Eye IV

The cornea is the transparent portion of the eye, anterior to the iris. It consists of five layers, three of which are cellular: the epithelium; Bowman's membrane, which is acellular; the substantia propria (corneal stroma); Descemet's membrane, also acellular; and the endothelium.

FIGURE 1, cornea, human, H&E ×135; insets ×600. The full thickness of the cornea is illustrated here; the two surfaces are shown at higher magnification in the **insets.** The epithelium *(Ep)* is stratified squamous, about five or six cells in thickness. The basal cells exhibit a columnar or polyhedral shape; cells become progressively flattened as they migrate toward the surface. They do not keratinize, and accordingly, each cell contains a nucleus. The cells are joined by desmosomes that appear as "intercellular bridges" *(arrow)* in light micrographs **(inset).**

The undersurface of the corneal epithelium presents a smooth profile. It rests on a homogeneous-appearing substance called Bowman's membrane *(BwM)*. The substantia propria *(SP, corneal stroma)* forms most of the thickness of the cornea; it is avascular. It consists of regularly arranged sheets or lamellae of collagen fibrils and fibroblasts. The collagen fibrils within each lamella are parallel to each other but at right angles to the fibrils of adjacent lamellae. This orientation contributes to the transparency of the cornea. Indeed, opacity due to scarring of the cornea (e.g., after a wound) is accompanied by a failure to reestablish the normal orientation. The substantia propria is separated from the corneal endothelium by Descemet's membrane *(DM)*. Like Bowman's membrane, this appears homogeneous with the light microscope. It is the thick basal lamina of the corneal endothelium. The endothelium *(En)* consists of a single layer of low cuboidal cells whose lateral cell margins are sometimes evident.

Although the stroma is avascular, after injury, white blood cells migrate into the cornea from the vessels in the sclera. Even in noninflammatory states, a few lymphocytes may be seen in the cornea. The corneal epithelium is richly supplied with nerve endings; however, these are not evident in H&E sections.

FIGURE 2, iris, human, H&E ×250. The pupillary margin of the iris is shown here at higher magnification than in Plate 127. The major portion of the iris consists of connective tissue *(CT)* that contains pigment cells *(PC)* to a varying degree (only in the albino are these absent). The posterior surface of the iris consists of two layers of pigmented epithelial cells *(PE)*. The cells of the anterior of these two layers contain myofilaments and are called pigmented myoepithelial cells *(PMyE)*; they are derived from the epithelial cells of the embryonic anterior layer. These cells make up the radial or dilator muscle fibers of the iris. The myoid character of these cells is largely obscured by the pigment. In addition, the iris contains smooth muscle cells arranged circularly around the pupil. These are seen in cross section in this figure *[SM(C)]*. These circularly arranged muscle cells make up the pupillary constrictor of the iris.

FIGURE 3, lens, human, H&E ×800; inset ×250. The lens consists entirely of epithelial cells surrounded by a homogeneous capsule *(LCap)* to which the zonular fibers *(ZF)* are joined. The lens capsule is also a thick basal lamina, that of the lens epithelial cells. On the anterior surface of the lens, the cells have a cuboidal shape. At the lateral margin, however, the cells are extremely elongated **(inset),** and their cytoplasm extends toward the center of the lens. These elongated columns of epithelial cytoplasm are also referred to as lens fibers *(LF)*. New cells are produced at the margin of the lens and displace the older cells toward the center. As the cells differentiate, the older cells (called lens fibers) lose their nucleus.

KEY

BwM, Bowman's membrane	**LF,** lens "fibers"	**SM(C),** circular smooth muscle
CT, connective tissue	**PC,** pigment cells	**SP,** substantia propria
DM, Descemet's membrane	**PE,** pigment epithelium	**ZF,** zonular fibers
En, corneal endothelium	**PMyE,** pigmented myoepithelial	**arrow,** intercellular bridges
Ep, corneal epithelium	cells	
LCap, lens capsule		

PLATE 128

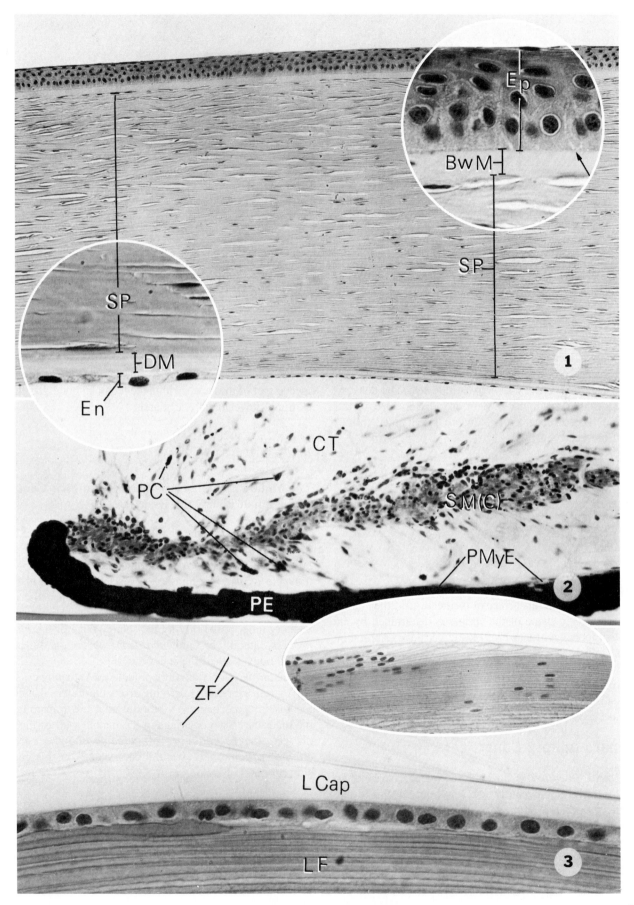

Ear

24

The ear is a three-chambered sensory structure that in the *auditory system* functions in the perception of sound and in the *vestibular system* functions in the maintenance of balance (Fig. 24.1). Each of the three divisions of the ear, the *external ear,* the *middle ear,* and the *internal ear,* is an essential part of the auditory system. The external and middle ear collect and conduct sound energy to the inner ear, where auditory sensory receptors transduce that energy into the electrical energy of nerve impulses. The sensory receptors of the vestibular system are also located in the inner ear. These receptors respond to gravity and movement of the head.

EXTERNAL EAR

The External Ear Is Composed of an *Auricle* and an *External Auditory Meatus*

Auricle

The *auricle (pinna)* is the oval-shaped appendage that projects from the lateral surface of the head, i.e., the "ear." The characteristic shape of the auricle is determined by an internal supporting structure of elastic cartilage. Thin skin with hair follicles, sweat glands, and sebaceous glands covers the auricle. The auricle is considered to be a nearly vestigial structure in humans, compared with its development and role in other animals. However, it is an essential component in sound localization and amplification.

External Auditory Canal

The canal *(meatus)* is an air-filled tubular space that follows a slightly S-shaped course for about 25 mm to the *tympanic membrane (eardrum).* The wall of the canal is continuous externally with the auricle. The wall of the lateral one-third of the canal is cartilaginous and is continuous with the elastic cartilage of the auricle. The medial two-thirds of the canal is contained within the temporal bone.

The lateral part of the canal is lined by skin that contains

hair follicles, sebaceous glands, and *ceruminous glands.* The coiled tubular apocrine ceruminous glands are modified sweat glands. Their secretion mixes with that of the sebaceous glands and with desquamated cells to form *cerumen* or *earwax.* The cerumen lubricates the skin and coats the meatal hairs to impede the entry of foreign particles into the ear. Excessive accumulation of cerumen can plug the meatus, however, resulting in conductive hearing loss. The medial part of the canal, within the temporal bone, has thinner skin and fewer hairs and glands.

MIDDLE EAR

The Middle Ear Is an Air-Filled Space That Contains Three Small Bones, the Ossicles

The middle ear is an air-filled space in the temporal bone, the *tympanic cavity* (Fig. 24.2). It is spanned by three small bones, the *auditory ossicles,* that are connected by two movable joints. The middle ear also contains the *auditory tube (Eustachian tube)* as well as the muscles that move the ossicles. The middle ear is bounded anteriorly by the auditory tube, posteriorly by the spongy bone of the *mastoid process,* laterally by the *tympanic membrane,* and medially by the bony wall of the inner ear.

The primary function of the middle ear is to convert sound waves (air vibrations) arriving from the external auditory meatus into mechanical vibrations that are transmitted to the inner ear. Two openings in the medial wall of the middle ear, the *vestibular (oval) window* and the *cochlear (round) window,* are essential components in this conversion process.

The Tympanic Membrane (Eardrum) Separates the External Auditory Canal From the Middle Ear

The eardrum is the medial boundary of the external auditory canal and the lateral wall of the middle ear. The layers of the tympanic membrane from outside to inside are

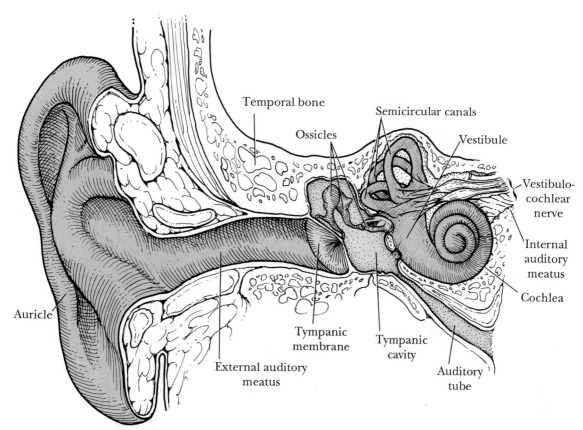

Figure 24.1. Schematic illustration of the three divisions of the ear: external ear (auricle and external auditory meatus), middle ear (tympanic cavity, ossicles, tympanic membrane, and auditory tube), and inner ear (semicircular canals and cochlea).

- The skin of the external auditory canal
- A core of radially and circularly arranged collagen fibers (Fig. 24.3)
- The epithelial lining (mucous membrane) of the middle ear (See Fig. 24.5)

One of the auditory ossicles, the *malleus,* is attached to the tympanic membrane. Sound in the form of airwaves causes the tympanic membrane to vibrate, and these vibrations are transmitted to the attached auditory ossicles that link the external ear to the inner ear. Perforation of the tympanic membrane may cause transient or permanent hearing impairment.

The Auditory Ossicles Connect the Tympanic Membrane to the Oval Window

The three small bones, the *malleus,* the *incus,* and the *stapes,* cross the space of the middle ear in series (Fig. 24.4) and connect the tympanic membrane to the oval window. These bones help to convert sound waves, i.e., vibrations in air, to mechanical (hydraulic) vibrations in tissues and fluid-filled chambers. Movable joints connect the bones, which are named according to their approximate shape:

- *Malleus (hammer),* attached to the tympanic membrane
- *Stapes (stirrup),* whose footplate fits into the oval window
- *Incus (anvil),* linking the malleus to the stapes

Muscles Attach to the Ossicles and Affect Their Movement

The *tensor tympani muscle* lies in a bony canal above the auditory tube; its tendon inserts on the malleus. Contraction of this muscle increases tension on the tympanic membrane. The *stapedius muscle* lies in a bony eminence on the posterior wall of the middle ear; its tendon inserts on the stapes. Contraction of the stapedius tends to dampen the movement of the stapes at the oval window. The stapedius, only a few millimeters in length, is the smallest of all the skeletal muscles.

The two muscles of the middle ear are responsible for a protective reflex called the *attenuation reflex.* Contraction of the muscles makes the chain of ossicles more rigid, thus reducing the transmission of vibrations to the inner ear. This protects the inner ear from the damaging effects of very loud sound.

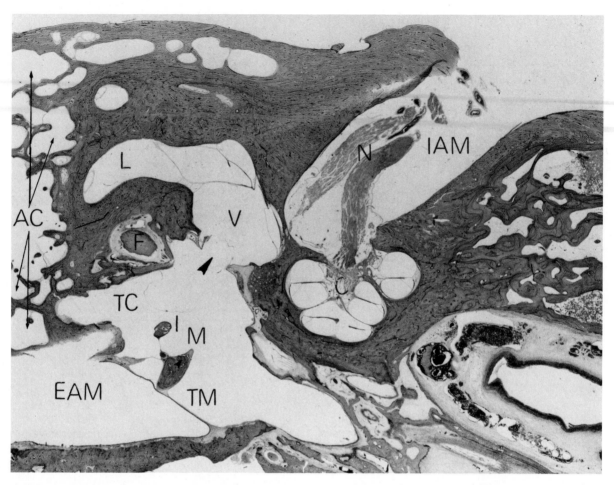

Figure 24.2. Horizontal section of a human temporal bone. The relationships of the three divisions of the ear within the temporal bone can be observed. The tympanic membrane *(TM)* separates the external auditory meatus *(EAM)* from the middle ear space or tympanic cavity *(TC)*. Within the tympanic cavity, cross sections of the malleus *(M)* and incus *(I)* can be seen. The posterior wall of the tympanic cavity is associated with the mastoid air cells *(AC)*. The lateral wall of the cavity is formed principally by the tympanic membrane. The opening to the inner ear or oval window *(arrowhead)* is seen in the medial wall of the cavity (the stapes has been removed). The facial *(F)* nerve can be observed near the oval window. The cochlea *(C)*, the vestibule *(V)*, and a portion of the lateral semicircular canal *(L)* of the inner ear are identified. The cochlear and vestibular divisions of cranial nerve VIII *(N)* can also be observed within the internal auditory meatus *(IAM)*. ×6.5.

The Auditory (Eustachian) Tube Connects the Middle Ear to the Nasopharynx

The auditory tube, a narrow flattened channel lined with ciliated pseudostratified columnar epithelium, is approximately 3.5 cm long (Fig. 24.6). It vents the middle ear, allowing pressure in the middle ear to equilibrate with atmospheric pressure. The walls of the tube are normally pressed together but separate during yawning and swallowing. It is common for infections to spread from the pharynx to the middle ear via the auditory tube (causing *otitis media*). A small mass of lymphatic tissue, the tubal tonsil, is often found at the pharyngeal orifice of the auditory tube.

The *Mastoid Air Cells* Extend From the Middle Ear Into the Temporal Bone

A system of air cells projects into the mastoid portion of the temporal bone from the middle ear. The epithelial lining of these air cells is continuous with that of the tympanic cavity and rests on periosteum. This continuity allows infections in the middle ear to spread into these air cells, resulting in a condition called *mastoiditis.* Before the development of antibiotics, repeated episodes of otitis media and mastoiditis usually led to deafness.

INNER EAR

The Inner Ear Consists of Two Labyrinthine Compartments, One Contained Within the Other

The *bony (osseous) labyrinth* is a complex system of interconnected cavities and canals in the petrous portion of the temporal bone. The *membranous labyrinth* lies within the bony labyrinth and consists of a complex system of small sacs and tubules that also form a continuous space enclosed within a wall of epithelium and connective tissue.

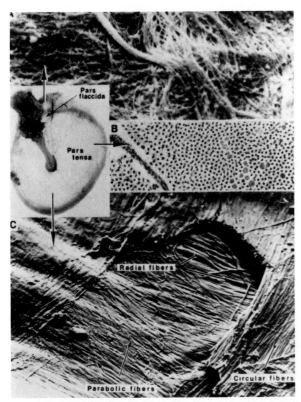

Figure 24.3. Electron micrographs of the tympanic membrane. **A.** Scanning electron micrograph that demonstrates the irregular arrangement of collagen and elastic fibers in the upper one-fifth of the membrane (pars flaccida). **B.** Cross section of fibers of the lower four-fifths of the tympanic membrane (pars tensa). The majority of profiles seen in this region are round collagen fibrils. **C.** Scanning electron micrograph of a partially dissected human tympanic membrane. Observe the arrangement of fibers in the pars tensa. (From Lim DJ: Scanning electron microscope morphology of the ear. In: Paparella MM, Shumrick DA (eds): *Otolaryngology*. Philadelphia, WB Saunders, chap 18, 1980.)

There are three fluid-filled spaces in the inner ear:

- *Endolymphatic spaces,* contained within the membranous labyrinth
- *Perilymphatic space,* lying between the wall of the bony labyrinth and the wall of the membranous labyrinth
- *Cortilymphatic space,* lying within the organ of Corti

The *endolymph* of the membranous labyrinth is a fluid similar to *intra*cellular fluid because it has a high potassium concentration and a low sodium concentration. The *perilymph* is a fluid similar in ionic content to *extra*cellular fluid. The third space, the *cortilymphatic space,* lies within the organ of Corti (see below) and is a true intercellular space. The cells surrounding the space loosely resemble an absorptive epithelium. The cortilymphatic space is filled with *cortilymph,* a fluid also having a composition similar to that of extracellular fluid.

The Bony Labyrinth Consists of Three Connected Spaces Within the Temporal Bone

The three spaces of the bony labyrinth, as illustrated in Figure 24.7, are

- *Semicircular canals*
- *Vestibule*
- *Cochlea*

The Vestibule Is the Central Space That Contains the *Utricle* and *Saccule* of the Membranous Labyrinth

The vestibule is the central space of the bony labyrinth. The *utricle* and *saccule* of the membranous labyrinth lie in an elliptical and spherical recess, respectively. The *semicircular canals* extend from the vestibule posteriorly, and the *cochlea* extends from the vestibule anteriorly. The vestibular (oval) window into which the footplate of the stapes inserts lies in the lateral wall of the vestibule.

The Semicircular Canals Are Bony Walled Tubes That Lie at Right Angles to Each Other

These three narrow bony-walled tubes, each forming about three-quarters of a circle, extend from the wall of the

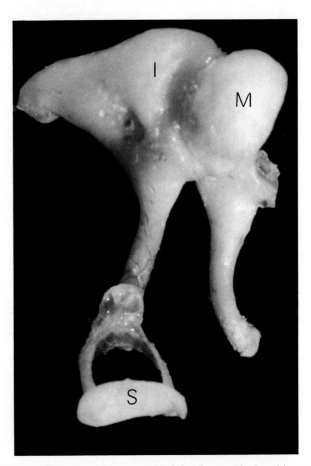

Figure 24.4. Photomicrograph of the three articulated human middle ear ossicles: the malleus *(M)*, the incus *(I)*, and the stapes *(S)*. ×10.

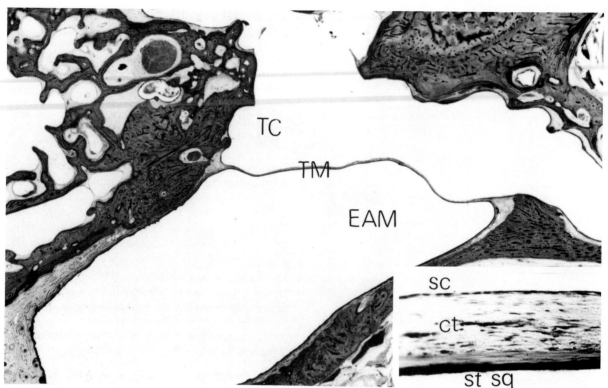

Figure 24.5. Cross section through a human tympanic membrane. The tympanic membrane (TM), external auditory meatus (EAM), and tympanic cavity (TC) can be seen. ×9. **Inset.** Higher magnification of the tympanic membrane. The outer epithelial layer of the membrane consists of stratified squamous epithelium (st sq), and the inner epithelial layer of the membrane consists of low simple cuboidal epithelium (sc). A middle layer of connective tissue (ct) lies between the two epithelial layers. ×190.

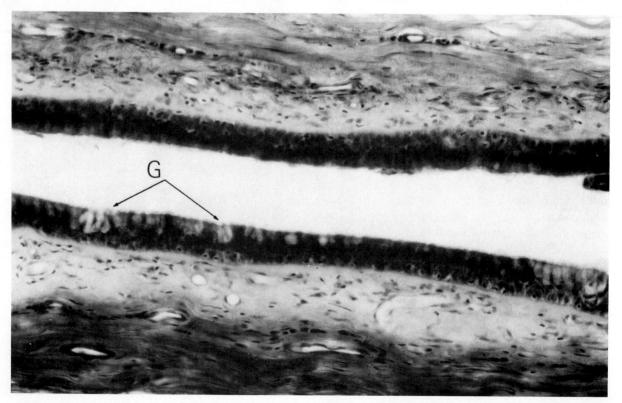

Figure 24.6. Photomicrograph of a human auditory tube near the nasopharynx. In this region, the auditory tube is lined by ciliated, pseudostratified columnar epithelium. Goblet cells (G) are seen interspersed among the epithelial cells. ×180.

vestibule. The semicircular canals lie at approximately right angles to each other in superior, posterior, and horizontal planes. At the lateral end of each semicircular canal, close to the vestibule, is a dilation called an *ampulla* (Fig. 24.7*b*). Each inner ear has three ampullae. The three canals open into the vestibule through five orifices, with the superior and posterior semicircular canals sharing a *common crus* medially.

The Cochlea Is a Conically Shaped Helix Connected to the Vestibule

The lumen of the cochlea, like that of the semicircular canals, is continuous with that of the vestibule. It connects to the vestibule on the side opposite the semicircular canals. Between its base and the apex, the cochlea makes about $2^3/_4$ turns around a central bony core called the *modiolus*. A sensory ganglion, the *spiral ganglion,* lies in the modiolus. One opening of the canal, the cochlear (round) window on its inferior surface near the base, is covered by a thin membrane *(the secondary tympanic membrane).*

Membranous Labyrinth, Like Bony Labyrinth, Is Divided Into Three Subcompartments

The subcompartments of the membranous labyrinth are

- *Membranous semicircular ducts*
- *Utricle* and *saccule*
- *Membranous cochlea,* also called the *cochlear duct* (Fig. 24.7, *c* and *d*)

The membranous semicircular ducts lie within the bony semicircular canals and are continuous with the utricle. The utricle and saccule are contained in recesses in the vestibule and are connected by the membranous *utriculosaccular duct.* The membranous cochlear duct is contained within the bony cochlea and is continuous with the saccule (Fig. 24.7*c*).

The membranous semicircular ducts, utricle, and saccule are components of the *vestibular system.* The membranous cochlea is part of the *auditory system.* They are innervated by the vestibular and cochlear divisions, respectively, of the *auditory nerve (vestibulocochlear nerve, cranial nerve VIII).*

Specialized Sensory Cells Are Located in Six Regions in the Membranous Labyrinth

Six regions of sensory receptors project from the wall of the membranous labyrinth into the endolymphatic space in each inner ear (Fig. 24.7*d*):

- Three *cristae ampullaris* located in the ampullae of the semicircular ducts
- Two *maculae,* one in the utricle *(macula utriculi)* and the other in the saccule *(macula sacculi)*
- The *organ of Corti* that projects into the endolymph of the cochlear duct

The three *cristae ampullaris* are sensitive to angular acceleration of the head (i.e., turning of the head). The *maculae* of utricle and saccule sense the position of the head and linear movement. The *organ of Corti* functions as the sound receptor. Despite having different specific functions, all six receptors share similar structural specializations and characteristics.

The Hair Cell, a Nonneuronal Mechanoreceptor, Is the Common Receptor Cell of the Vestibulocochlear System

The several different functions of the receptors of the inner ear are performed by cells that are remarkably similar in structure. They also have a common basis of function in the initiation of nerve impulses.

Several important characteristics are common to hair cells:

- All are *epithelial cells.*
- Each possesses numerous *stereocilia,* modified microvilli, called *sensory "hairs"* (Fig. 24.8).
- In the vestibular system, each hair cell possesses a single true cilium called a *kinocilium* (Fig. 24.8).
- In the auditory system, hair cells lose their cilium during development but do have a *residual basal body.*
- All hair cells are associated with both *afferent* and *efferent nerve endings.*
- All hair cells are *transducers;* i.e., they convert mechanical energy to electrical energy that can be transmitted via the vestibulocochlear nerve to the brain.

VERTIGO

The sense of rotation without equilibrium (dizziness, vertigo) is the major clinical sign of dysfunction of the vestibular system. Causes of vertigo range from the administration of specific drugs to a tumor (acoustic neuroma). These tumors develop in or near the internal auditory meatus and exert pressure on the vestibular division of cranial nerve VIII or branches of the labyrinthine artery. Vertigo can be produced normally in individuals by excessive stimulation of the semicircular ducts. Similarly, excessive stimulation of the utricle can produce motion sickness (seasickness, carsickness, or airsickness) in some individuals.

Some diseases of the inner ear affect both hearing and equilibrium. For example, patients who are diagnosed as having Ménière's disease initially complain of episodes of dizziness and tinnitus (ringing) and later develop a low-frequency hearing loss. Although the etiologic agent of Ménière's disease has not been determined, it is known that the membranous labyrinth becomes distended (endolymphatic hydrops). This distension is thought to be a result of malabsorption of endolymph within the endolymphatic sac.

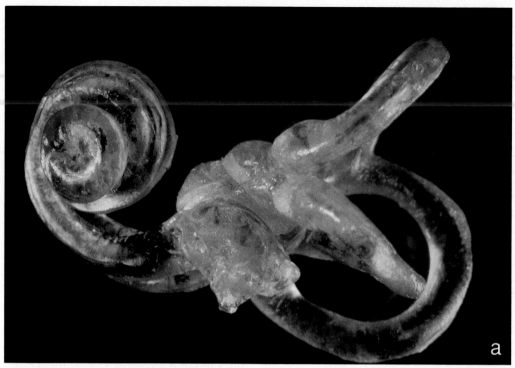

Figure 24.7. Photograph **(a)** and diagrams **(b–d)** of the human inner ear. **a.** Cast of human inner ear bony labyrinth. The cochlear portion of the labyrinth appears blue-green, and the region of the vestibular bony labyrinth appears orange. (Courtesy of Dr. Merle Lawrence.) **b.** Components of the bony labyrinth. Divisions of the bony inner ear labyrinth are the vestibule, cochlea, and three semicircular canals. The openings of the oval window and the round window can be observed. Lateral view of left bony labyrinth. **c.** Diagram of membranous inner ear labyrinth lying within the bony labyrinth. The cochlear duct can be seen spiraling within the bony cochlea. The saccule and utricle are positioned within the vestibule, and the three semicircular ducts are lying within their respective canals. This is a medial view of the right membranous labyrinth, allowing the endolymphatic duct and sac to be observed from this perspective. **d.** Diagram of the sensory regions of the inner ear for equilibrium and hearing. These regions are the macula of the saccule, the cristae ampullaris of the three semicircular ducts, and the organ of Corti of the cochlear duct. Medial view of right membranous labyrinth.

The number of stereocilia varies. There are 50–100 stereocilia/cell in the vestibular system and on the ***inner hair cells*** of the organ of Corti. The ***outer hair cells*** of the organ of Corti have 100–300 stereocilia.

In the vestibular system, there are two types of hair cells and associated nerve endings (Fig. 24.9). ***Type I hair cells*** are piriform in shape with a rounded base and a thin neck and are surrounded by an afferent nerve chalice and a few efferent nerve fibers. ***Type II hair cells*** are cylindrical in shape and have afferent and efferent bouton nerve endings synapsing basally.

All Receptor (Hair) Cells Have a Common Basis of Receptor Cell Function

All receptor (hair) cells of the inner ear appear to function by the bending or flexing of their stereocilia (sensory hairs). The means by which the stereocilia are bent varies from receptor to receptor and is discussed in the section on each specific receptor area. Stretching of the plasma membrane caused by the bending of the stereocilia generates transmembrane potential changes in the receptor cell that are conveyed to the afferent nerve ending(s) associated with each hair cell. When a kinocilium is present, its location relative to the bending of the stereocilia is important. Stereocilia that are bent away from the kinocilium cause hyperpolarization of the receptor cell; stereocilia that are bent toward the kinocilium cause depolarization of the receptor cell and consequent generation of an action potential (Figs. 24.10 and 24.11).

Cristae Ampullaris: Sensors of Angular Movement

Each of the three cristae ampullaris is the sensory region of one of the semicircular ducts in the semicircular canals (Fig. 24.12) and lies in the ampulla of the semicircular canal (see Fig. 24.7d). Each crista is a thickened epithelial ridge that is oriented perpendicular to the long axis of the sem-

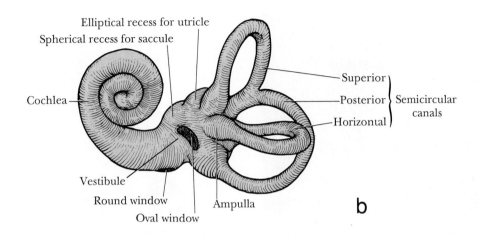

Elliptical recess for utricle
Spherical recess for saccule
Cochlea
Superior
Posterior } Semicircular canals
Horizontal
Vestibule
Round window
Oval window
Ampulla

b

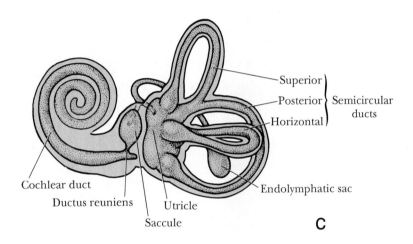

Superior
Posterior } Semicircular ducts
Horizontal
Cochlear duct
Ductus reuniens
Utricle
Saccule
Endolymphatic sac

c

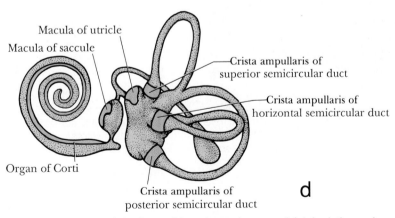

Macula of utricle
Macula of saccule
Crista ampullaris of superior semicircular duct
Crista ampullaris of horizontal semicircular duct
Organ of Corti
Crista ampullaris of posterior semicircular duct

d

Figure 24.7. **b–d.** Diagrams of the bony (**b**) and membranous (**c**) labyrinths and sensory region (**d**) of the human inner ear.

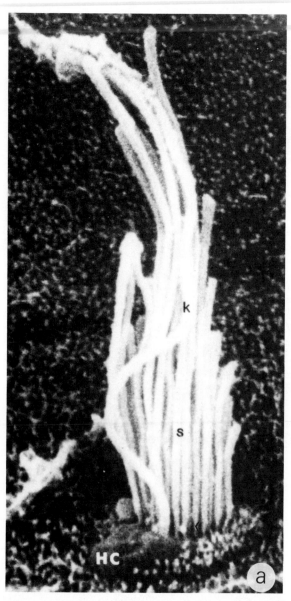

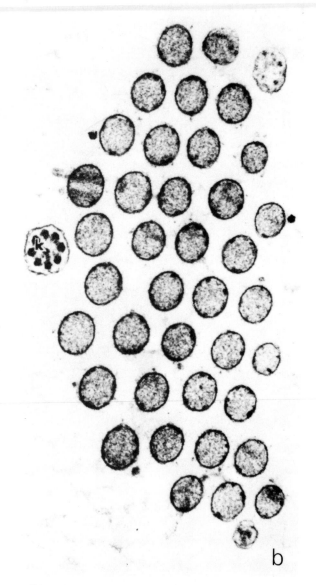

Figure 24.8.   Electron micrographs of the kinocilium and stereocilia of a vestibular sensory hair cell. **a.** Scanning electron micrograph of the apical surface of a sensory hair cell *(HC)* from the macula of the utricle. Note the relationship of the kinocilium *(k)* to the stereocilia *(s)*. **b.** Transmission electron micrograph of the kinocilium and stereocilia of a vestibular hair cell in cross section. The kinocilium *(k)* has a greater diameter than the stereocilia. ×47,500. (From Hunter-Duvar IM, Hinojosa R: Vestibule: sensory epithelia. In: Friedmann I, Ballantyne J (eds): *Ultrastructural Atlas of the Inner Ear.* London, Butterworths, 1984, figs. 9.11 and 9.12.)

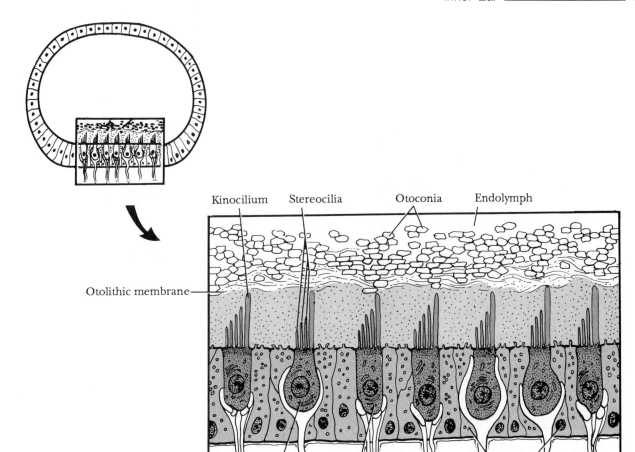

Kinocilium   Stereocilia   Otoconia   Endolymph

Otolithic membrane

Type I hair cell   Type II hair cell   Supporting cells

Figure 24.9. Diagram of a cross section of the utricle. A more detailed diagram of the cellular organization of the macula of the utricle is shown in the *enlarged rectangle*. Supporting cells can be seen lying between the two principal types of sensory hair cells (types I and II). The stereocilia and kinocilium of each sensory hair cell are embedded in the otolithic membrane on which otoconia are lying.

icircular canal and consists of hair cells with stereocilia and supporting epithelial cells.

A *cupula* is a gelatinous structure that is attached to the hair cells of each crista. The cupula projects into the lumen and is surrounded by endolymph. During rotational movement of the head, the walls of the semicircular canal and the membranous semicircular ducts move, but the endolymph contained within the ducts tends to lag behind because of inertia. The cupula, projecting into the endolymph, is swayed by the movement differential between the crista fixed to the wall of the duct and the endolymph. Bending of the stereocilia in the narrow space between the hair calls and the cupula leads to the generation of nerve impulses in the associated nerve endings.

Macula Sacculi and Macula Utriculi: Sensors of Gravity and Linear Movement

The maculae are innervated sensory thickenings of the epithelium facing the endolymph in the saccule and utricle of the vestibule (see Fig. 24.7d). As in the cristae, each macula consists of hair cells of both types, supporting cells, and nerve endings associated with the hair cells. The maculae of the utricle and saccule are oriented at right angles to one another. When a person is standing, the ***macula utriculi*** is in a horizontal plane, and the ***macula sacculi*** is in a vertical plane.

The gelatinous material that overlies the maculae is called the ***otolithic membrane.*** It contains 3–5 μm crystalline

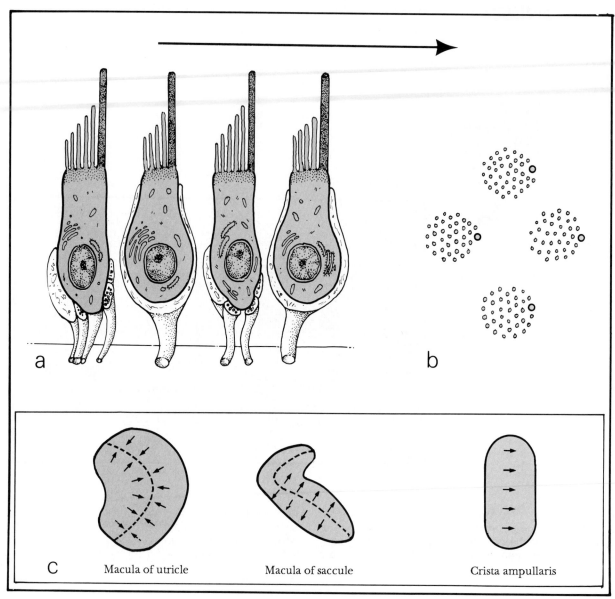

Figure 24.10. Diagram of the morphologic polarization of vestibular hair cells. (From Lindenman HH: Anatomy of the otolith organs. *Advances in Oto-Rhino-Laryngology* 20:405–433, 1973, S Karger AG, Basel.)

particles of calcium carbonate and protein, the *otoliths (otoconia)* on its outer surface (Fig. 24.13). This surface of the otolithic membrane lies opposite to the surface in which the stereocilia of the hair cells are embedded. The otolithic membrane moves on the macula in a manner analogous to that by which the cupula moves on the crista. Stereocilia of the hair cells are bent by gravity in the stationary individual when the otolithic membrane and its otolith pull on the stereocilia. They are also bent during linear movement when the individual is moving in a straight line and the otolithic membrane drags on the stereocilia because of inertia.

Organ of Corti: Sensor of Sound Vibrations

The cochlear duct divides the cochlear canal into three parallel compartments or *scalae:*

- *Scala media,* the middle compartment in the cochlear canal
- *Scala vestibuli*
- *Scala tympani* (Fig. 24.14)

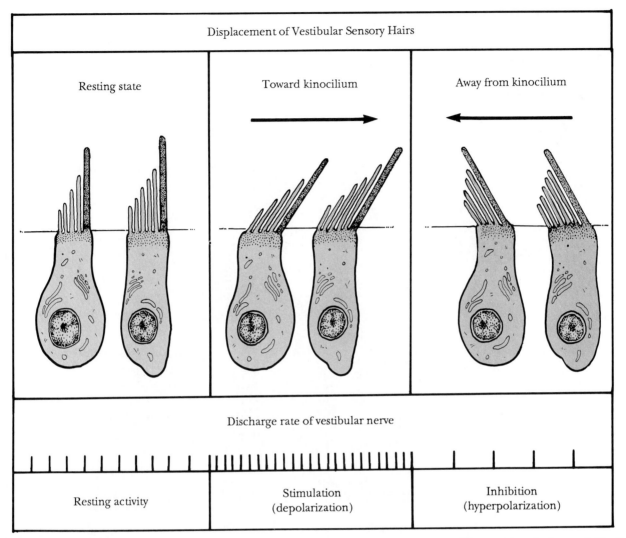

Displacement of Vestibular Sensory Hairs

Resting state | Toward kinocilium | Away from kinocilium

Discharge rate of vestibular nerve

Resting activity | Stimulation (depolarization) | Inhibition (hyperpolarization)

Figure 24.11. Diagram illustrating the functional aspects of the vestibular hair cells. (From Wersall J, Gleisner L, Lundquist P-G: Ultrastructure of the vestibular end organs. In: DeReuck AVS, Knight J (eds): *Myotatic, Kinesthetic, and Vestibular Mechanisms.* Boston, Little, Brown, 1967.)

The cochlear duct, itself, is the scala media. The scala vestibuli and scala tympani are the spaces above and below, respectively, the scala media. The scala media is an endolymph-containing space that is continuous with the lumen of the saccule and contains the organ of Corti, which rests on its lower wall.

The scala vestibuli and the scala tympani are perilymph-containing spaces and communicate with each other at the apex of the cochlea through a small channel called the *helicotrema*. The scala vestibuli is described as beginning at the oval window, and the scala tympani is described as ending at the round window.

The Scala Media Is a Triangular-Shaped Space With Its Acute Angle Attached to the Modiolus

In transverse section, the scala media appears as a triangular space with its most acute angle attached to a bony extension of the modiolus, the ***osseous spiral lamina*** (Fig. 24.14). The upper wall of the scala media, which separates it from the scala vestibuli, is the ***vestibular (Reissner's) membrane*** (Fig. 24.15). The lateral or outer wall of the scala media is the ***stria vascularis*** (Fig. 24.16). It is lined with a thick, pseudostratified epithelium that may be the

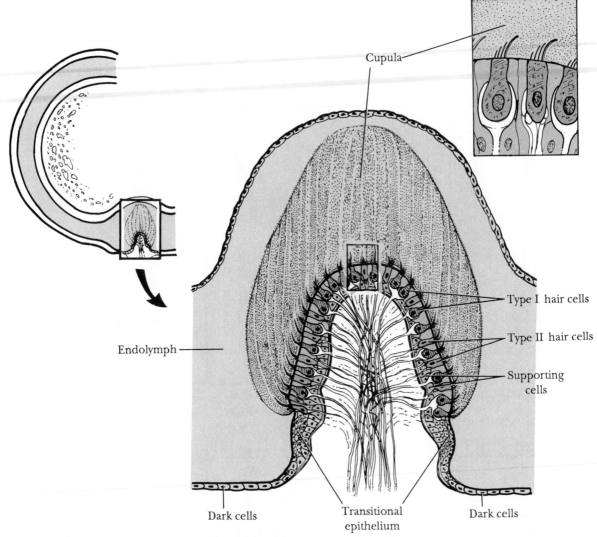

Figure 24.12. Diagram of a typical semicircular duct within its canal. The cellular organization of the sensory region, i.e., the crista ampullaris, of a semicircular duct is shown in the *large diagram* and the *enlarged rectangle* form it. The crista ampullaris is composed of both type I and type II sensory hair cells and supporting cells. The stereocilia and kinocilium of each hair are embedded in the cupula that projects toward the nonsensory wall of the ampulla.

site of synthesis of endolymph. The lower wall or floor of the scala media is the **basilar membrane.** The organ of Corti rests on the basilar membrane and is overlain by the **tectorial membrane.**

The Organ of Corti Is Composed of Hair Cells, Phalangeal Cells, and Pillar Cells

The organ of Corti is a complex epithelial layer on the floor of the scala media. It is formed by

- **Inner** (close to the spiral lamina) and **outer** (farther from the spiral lamina) **hair cells**
- **Inner** and **outer phalangeal (supporting) cells**
- **Pillar cells**

Several other named cell types of unknown function are also described in the organ of Corti. Those interested should consult monographs and specialized texts for more detailed descriptions.

The Hair Cells Are Arranged in an Inner and an Outer Row of Cells

The inner hair cells form a single row of cells throughout all $2^3/_4$ turns of the cochlear duct. The number of cells forming the width of the continuous row of outer hair cells is variable. Three ranks of hair cells are found in the basal part of the coil (Fig. 24.17). The width of the row gradually increases to five ranks of cells at the apex of the cochlea.

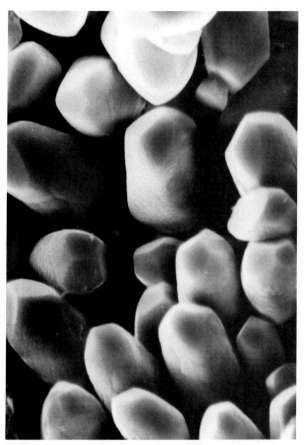

Figure 24.13. Scanning electron micrograph of human otoconia. Each otoconium has a long cylindrical body with a three-headed facet on each end of its body. ×5000.

The Phalangeal and Pillar Cells Provide Support for the Hair Cells

The phalangeal cells are supporting cells for both rows of hair cells. Each hair cell is intimately associated with a reticular cell that completely surrounds the basal portion of the sensory cell, preventing it from touching the basilar membrane. The phalangeal cells associated with the inner hair cells surround the cells completely (Fig. 24.18). The phalangeal cells associated with the outer hair cells surround only the basal portion of the hair cell completely and send apical processes toward the endolymphatic space (Fig. 24.19). These processes flatten near the apical ends of the hair cells and form a complete plate of phalangeal cell surface around the hair cells (Fig. 24.20).

The apical ends of the phalangeal cells are tightly bound to one another and to the hair cells by elaborate tight junctions. They form the *reticular lamina* that seals the endolymphatic compartment from the true intercellular spaces of the organ of Corti (Figs. 24.19 and 24.20). The extracellular fluid in this intercellular space is *cortilymph.* It has a composition similar to other extracellular fluids and to perilymph.

Pillar cells have broad apical and basal surfaces that form plates and a narrowed cytoplasm. The inner pillar cells rest on the tympanic lip of the spiral lamina; the outer pillar cells rest on the basilar membrane. Between them they form a triangular-shaped tunnel, the **tunnel of Corti.**

The Tectorial Membrane Extends From the Spiral Limbus Over the Cells of the Organ of Corti

The tectorial membrane is attached medially to the modiolus. Its lateral free edge projects over and attaches to the organ of Corti by the stereocilia of the hair cells. It is usually described as a keratin-like layer containing fibrils embedded in a dense amorphous ground substance.

Sound Perception

As described on page 769, sound waves striking the tympanic membrane are translated into simple mechanical vibrations. The ossicles of the middle ear convey these vibrations to the cochlea.

HEARING LOSS—VESTIBULAR DYSFUNCTION

There are several types of disorders that can affect the auditory and vestibular system, resulting in deafness, dizziness (vertigo), or both. Auditory disorders are classified as either conductive or sensorineural in nature. Conductive hearing loss results when sound waves are impeded mechanically from reaching the auditory sensory receptors within the inner ear. This type of hearing loss principally involves the external ear or structures of the middle ear. One example of a conductive hearing loss is the disease of otosclerosis, characterized by the growth of new spongy bone within the bony labyrinth near the oval window. This spongy bone growth can cause the fixation of the base of the stapes (ankylosis) in the oval window. This results in a decrease in the efficiency of sound conduction to the inner ear.

Sensorineural hearing impairment may also occur after injury to the auditory sensory hair cells within the inner ear or to cochlear division of cranial nerve VIII. Such hearing losses may be congenital or acquired. Causes of acquired sensorineural hearing loss include infections of the membranous labyrinth (e.g., meningitis, chronic otitis media), acoustic trauma (i.e., exposure to excessive noise for a long time), and administration of certain classes of antibiotics and diuretics.

A third example of sensorineural hearing loss is that which often occurs during the process of aging. A loss of the sensory hair cells or associated nerve fibers occurs beginning in the basal turn of the cochlea and progressing apically over time. The characteristic impairment is a high-frequency hearing loss. This type of hearing loss is termed presbycusis (see presbyopia, page 756).

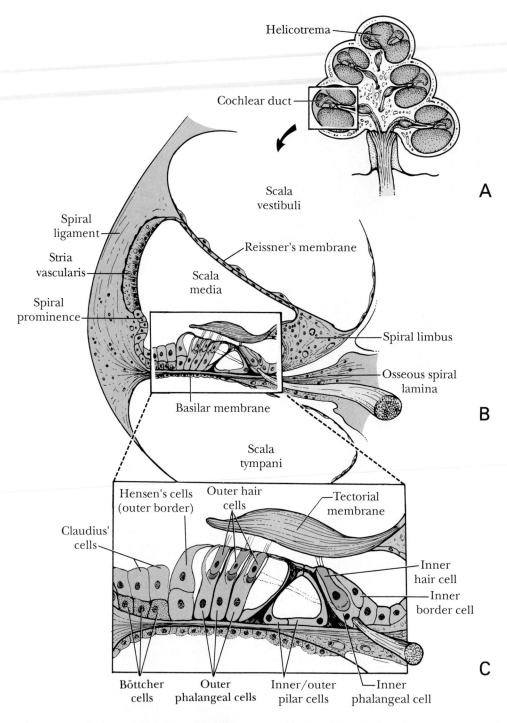

Figure 24.14.   A. Schematic diagram of a midmodiolar section of the cochlea that illustrates the position of the cochlear duct within the $2^3/_4$ turns of the bony cochlea. Observe that the scala vestibuli and scala tympani are continuous apically (helicotrema). **B.** Cross section of basal cochlear duct. The cochlear duct and the osseous spiral lamina divide the cochlea into the scala vestibuli and the scala tympani, which contain perilymph. The scala media, i.e., the space within the cochlear duct, is filled with endolymph. **C.** Diagram of the sensory and supporting cells of the organ of the Corti. The sensory cells are divided into an inner row of sensory hair cells and three rows of outer sensory hair cells. The supporting cells are inner and outer pillar cells, inner and outer (Deiters') phalangeal cells, border cells, Hensen's cells, Claudius' cells, and Böttcher's cells. (Modified from Goodhill V: *Ear, Diseases, Deafness, and Dizziness.* Hagerstown, MD, Harper & Row, 1979, figs 1.66, 1.68, and 1.70.)

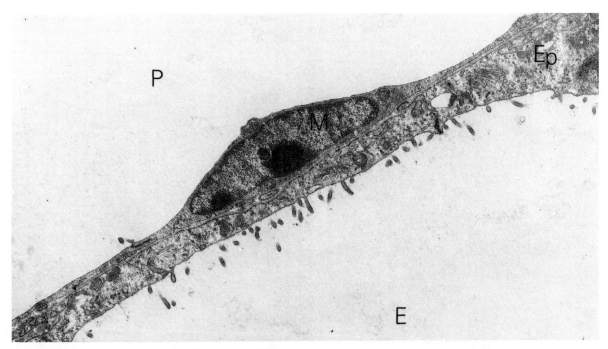

Figure 24.15. Transmission electron micrograph of vestibular (Reissner's) membrane. Two cell types can be observed: a mesothelial cell *(M)*, which faces the scala vestibuli and is bathed by perilymph *(P)*, and an epithelial cell *(Ep)*, which faces the scala media and is bathed by endolymph *(E)*. ×8400.

In the Inner Ear the Vibrations of the Ossicles Are Transformed Into Waves in the Perilymph

Movement of the stapes in the oval window of the vestibule sets up vibrations or traveling waves in the perilymph of the scala vestibuli. The vibrations are transmitted through the vestibular membrane to the scala media (cochlear duct), which contains endolymph, and are also propagated to the perilymph of the scala tympani. Pressure changes in this closed perilymphatic-endolymphatic system are reflected in movements of the membrane that covers the round window in the base of the cochlea.

As a result of sound vibrations entering the inner ear, a traveling wave is set up in the basilar membrane (Fig. 24.21). A sound of specified frequency causes displacement of a relatively long segment of the basilar membrane, but the region of maximal displacement is narrow. High-frequency sounds cause maximal vibration of the basilar membrane near the base of the cochlea; low-frequency sounds cause maximal displacement nearer the apex. The point of maximal displacement of the basilar membrane is specified for a given frequency of sound, and this is the morphologic basis of frequency discrimination. Amplitude discrimination, i.e., perception of sound intensity or loudness, depends on the degree of displacement of the basilar membrane at any given frequency range.

Movement of the Stereocilia of the Hair Cells in the Cochlea Initiates Neuronal Transduction

Hair cells are attached, through the phalangeal cells, to the basilar membrane, which vibrates during sound reception. The stereocilia of these hair cells are, in turn, attached to the tectorial membrane, which also vibrates. The tectorial membrane and the basilar membrane are, however, hinged at different points. Thus, a shearing effect occurs between the basilar membrane (and the cells attached to it) and the tectorial membrane when sound vibrations impinge on the inner ear.

The stereocilia of the hair cells, inserted into the tectorial membrane, are the only structures that connect the basilar membrane and its complex epithelial layer to the tectorial membrane. The shearing effect between the basilar membrane and the tectorial membrane distorts the stereocilia of the hair cells and, thus, the apical portion of the hair cells, and this distortion generates membrane potentials that are conveyed to the brain via the ***cochlear nerve (cochlear division of the vestibulocochlear nerve, cranial nerve VIII).***

Innervation of the Sensory Regions of the Inner Ear

The vestibulocochlear nerve or cranial nerve VIII innervates the sensory regions of the inner ear membranous

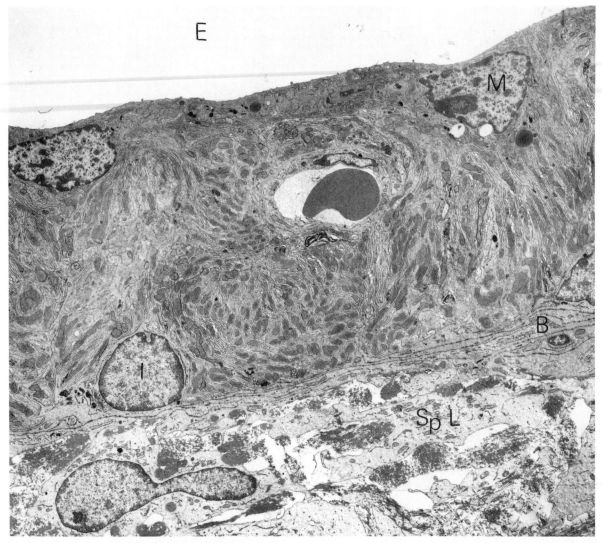

Figure 24.16. Transmission electron micrograph of stria vascularis. The apical surfaces of the marginal cells *(M)* of the stria are bathed by endolymph *(E)*. Intermediate cells *(I)* are positioned between the marginal cells and the basal cells *(B)*, which separate the other cells of the stria vascularis from the spiral ligament *(Sp L)*. ×4700.

labyrinth. Cranial nerve VIII is divided into a vestibular division, which innervates the sensory receptors associated with the vestibular system, and a cochlear division, which innervates the sensory receptors associated with the auditory system (Fig. 24.22).

The vestibular nerve is subdivided into a superior division and an inferior division. The superior division innervates the

- Macula of the utricle
- Part of the macula of the saccule
- Cristae ampullaris of the superior and lateral semicircular ducts

The inferior division innervates the

- Macula of the saccule
- Crista ampullaris of the posterior semicircular duct

Bipolar neurons of the vestibular division have their cell bodies (ganglion of the vestibular nerve, Scarpa's ganglion) located in the internal auditory meatus. Dendritic processes of the vestibular nerve fibers synapse at the base of the vestibular sensory hair cells, either as a chalice around a type I (inner) hair cell or as a bouton associated with a type II (outer) hair cell. The axons of the vestibular nerve fibers enter the brain stem and terminate in the vestibular nuclei.

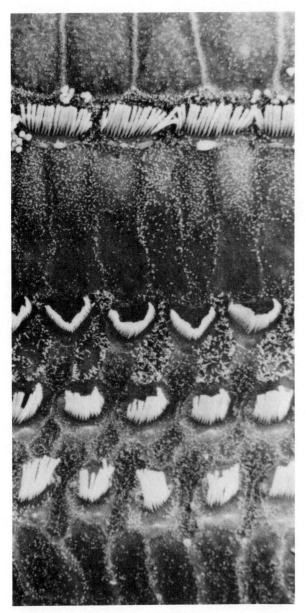

Figure 24.17. Scanning electron micrograph illustrating the configuration of stereocilia on the apical surfaces of the inner row and three outer rows of cochlear sensory hair cells. ×3250.

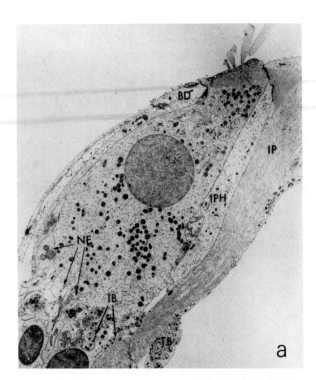

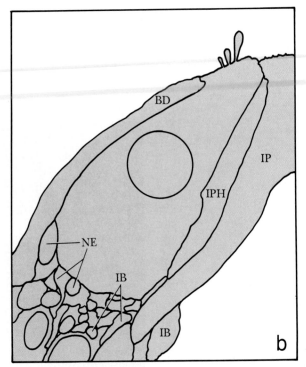

Figure 24.18. Electron micrograph **(a)** and accompanying diagram **(b)** of an inner sensory hair cell. Observe the rounded base and constricted neck of the inner hair cell. Nerve endings *(NE)* from afferent nerve fibers *(IB)* to inner hair cells are seen basally. Afferent nerve fibers *(IB)* to outer hair cells are seen in a tunnel lateral to an inner pillar cell *(IP)*. *IPH,* inner phalangeal cell; and *BD,* border cell. ×6300. (From Kimura RS: Sensory and accessory epithelia of the cochlea. In: Friedmann I, Ballantyne J (eds): *Ultrastructural Atlas of the Inner Ear.* London, Butterworths, 1984, fig 5.3.)

Some secondary neuronal fibers travel to the cerebellum and to the nuclei of cranial nerves III, IV, and VI that innervate the muscles of the eye. Other secondary fibers descend into the cervical segments of the spinal cord as the vestibulospinal tracts.

Nerve fibers of the cochlear nerve division enter the bony cochlea through the modiolus from the internal auditory meatus. Neurons of the cochlear nerve fibers are also bipolar and have their cell bodies located in the spiral ganglion within the modiolus. Dendritic processes of the afferent cochlear nerve fibers exit the modiolus through foramina nervosa and enter the organ of Corti. The dendritic processes are divided into two branches. Fifteen to twenty dendritic processes of one branch will innervate only one inner-row sensory hair cell. Ninety-five percent of all afferent neurons will make up this branch. Dendritic processes of the other branch innervate the sensory hair cells of the outer rows. One dendritic nerve fiber of this branch will innervate 10 outer-row hair cells. The axons of the cochlear nerve fibers enter the brain stem and terminate in the cochlear nuclei of the medulla. Nerve fibers from these nuclei pass to the geniculate nucleus of the thalamus and then to the auditory cortex of the temporal lobe.

Efferent fibers conveying impulses from the brain pass parallel to the ascending afferent nerve fibers of the vestibulocochlear nerve (cochlear efferents of Rasmussen). Efferent nerve fibers from the brain stem pass through the vestibular nerve. They synapse either on afferent endings of the inner hair cell or on the basal aspect of an outer hair cell. Efferent fibers are thought to effect control of auditory and vestibular input to the central nervous system, presumably enhancing some afferent signals while suppressing other signals.

Blood Vessels of the Membranous Labyrinth

The blood supply to the external ear, middle ear, and the bony labyrinth of the inner ear is derived from vessels associated with the external carotid arteries. The arterial blood supply to tissues of the membranous labyrinth of the inner ear is derived intracranially from the labyrinthine artery, a common branch of the anterior inferior cerebellar or basilar artery. The labyrinthine artery is a terminal artery, in that it has no anastomoses with other surrounding arteries. Therefore, interruption of blood flow in this artery can have severe consequences for the inner ear function. Experimental disruption of blood flow for only 15 seconds can cause the loss of electrical potentials from excitable nerve

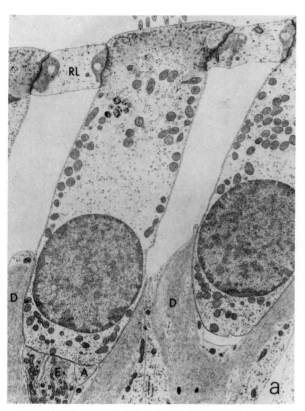

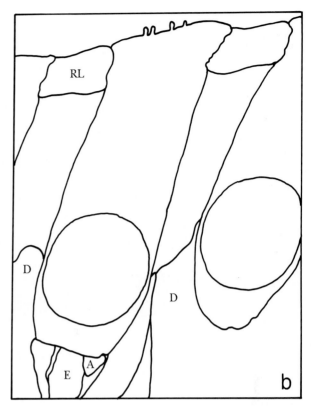

Figure 24.19. Electron micrograph **(a)** and accompanying diagram **(b)** of outer sensory hair cells. Afferent *(A)* and efferent *(E)* nerve endings are seen basally. Outer phalangeal cells (Deiters' cells) are seen surrounding the outer hair cells basally. Their apical projections form the reticular lamina *(RL)*.

Observe that the midexternal surfaces of the outer hair cells are not surrounded by supporting cells. ×6300. (From Kimura RS: Sensory and accessory epithelia of the cochlea. In: Friedmann I, Ballantyne J (eds): *Ultrastructural Atlas of the Inner Ear*. London, Butterworths, 1984, fig 5.11.)

fibers of the inner ear. Irreversible loss of fibers and cells can result from the prolonged occlusion of the arterial supply.

The labyrinthine artery lies in the internal auditory canal where it divides into the common cochlear artery and the anterior vestibular artery (Fig. 24.23). The common cochlear artery divides into the main cochlear artery and the vestibulocochlear artery. The vestibulocochlear artery branches into the posterior vestibular artery and the cochlear branch. The main cochlear artery distributes to three-fourths of the cochlea, and the cochlear branch supplies the basal one-fourth of the cochlea. The anterior vestibular artery supplies the

- Macula of the utricle
- Part of the macula of the saccule
- Cristae ampullaris of the superior and lateral semicircular ducts

The posterior vestibular artery supplies the

- Macula of the saccule
- Crista ampullaris of the posterior semicircular duct

This arterial arrangement exactly parallels the distribution of the superior and inferior divisions of the vestibular nerve.

Radiating arterioles arise from the main arterial divisions and distribute to various regions of the membranous labyrinth. In the cochlear tissues, arterioles are distributed to the spiral limbus, basilar membrane, and lateral cochlear wall. There are no arterioles distributed to the tissues of the organ of Corti. Oxygen and nutrients to the sensory hair cells diffuse through the surrounding tissues.

Venous drainage from the cochlea is via the posterior and anterior spiral modiolar veins (Fig. 24.24) that form the common modiolar vein. The common modiolar vein and the vestibulocochlear vein form the vein of the cochlear aqueduct. The latter empties into the inferior petrosal sinus.

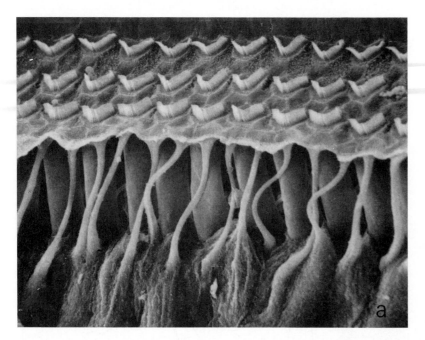

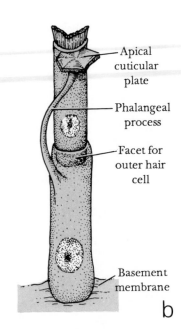

Figure 24.20. Scanning electron micrograph **(a)** and accompanying diagram **(b)** that illustrate the architecture of the outer phalangeal (Deiters') cells. Each Deiters' cell cups the basal surface of an outer sensory hair cell and extends its phalangeal process apically to form an apical plate that supports the outer sensory hair cells. ×2400.

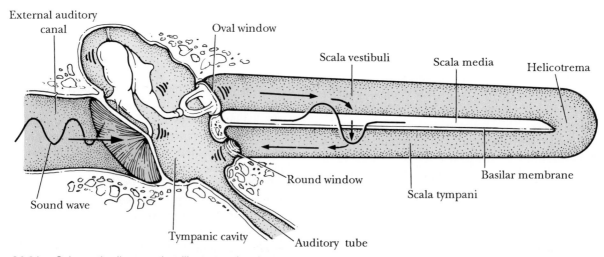

Figure 24.21. Schematic diagram that illustrates the dynamics of the three divisions of the ear. Sound waves are collected and transmitted from the external ear to the middle ear, where they are converted into mechanical vibrations. The mechanical vibrations are then converted at the oval window into fluid vibrations within the inner ear. Fluid vibrations cause displacement of the basilar membrane on which rest the auditory sensory hair cells. Such displacement leads to stimulation of the hair cells and a discharge of neural impulses from them. (Modified from Karmody CS: *Textbook of Otolaryngology*. Philadelphia, Lea & Febiger, 1983, p 40.)

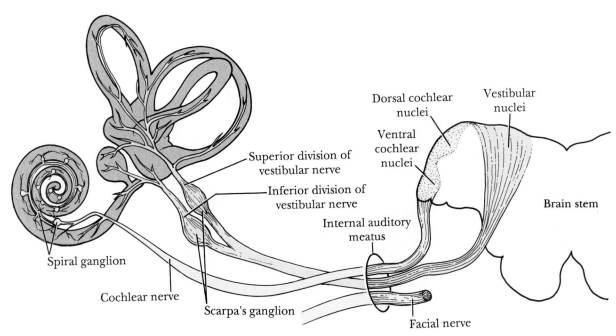

Figure 24.22. Diagram illustrating the innervation of sensory regions of the inner ear. (Modified from Hawke M, Keene M, Alberti PW: In: *Classical Otoscopy, A Text and Colour Atlas.* Edinburgh, Churchill Livingstone, 1984.)

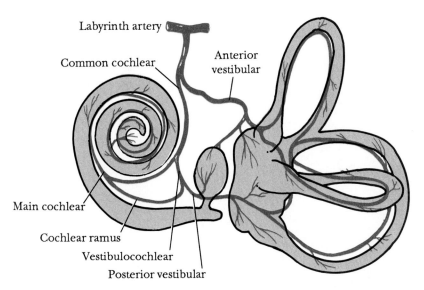

Figure 24.23. Diagram of the arterial supply of the membranous labyrinth of the inner ear. (Modified from Schuknecht HF: *Pathology of the Ear.* Reprinted by permission of Harvard University Press, Cambridge, MA, 1974.)

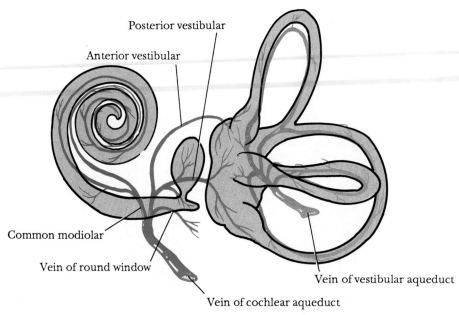

Figure 24.24.   Diagram of the venous drainage of the membranous labyrinth of the inner ear. (Modified from Schuknecht HF: *Pathology of the Ear*. Reprinted by permission of Harvard University Press, Cambridge, MA, 1974.)

The anterior vestibular vein drains blood from the utricle and superior and lateral semicircular ducts, whereas the posterior vestibular vein drains the saccule and posterior semicircular duct. The anterior and posterior vestibular veins join the vein of the round window to form the vestibulo-cochlear vein. The semicircular canals and the endolymphatic duct and sac are drained by the vein of the vestibular aqueduct, which drains into the sigmoid venous sinus.

ATLAS PLATES

129–130

PLATE 129. Ear

The inner ear consists of a system of chambers and canals in the temporal bone that contain a network of membranous channels. These are referred to, respectively, as the bony labyrinth and membranous labyrinth. In places, the membranous labyrinth forms the lining of the bony labyrinth; in other places, there is a separation of the two. Within the space lined by the membranous labyrinth is a watery fluid called endolymph. External to the membranous labyrinth, i.e., between the membranous and bony labyrinths, is additional fluid called perilymph.

The bony labyrinth is divided into three parts: the cochlea, the semicircular canals, and the vestibule. The cochlea and semicircular canals contain membranous counterparts of the same shape; however, the membranous components of the vestibule are more complex in their form, being composed of ducts and two chambers, the utricle and saccule. The cochlea contains the receptors for hearing, i.e., the organ of Corti; the semicircular canals contain the receptors for movement; and the saccule and utricle contain receptors for position.

FIGURE 1, ear, guinea pig, hematoxylin and eosin (H&E) ×20. In this section through the inner ear, bone surrounds the entire inner ear cavity. Because of its labyrinthine character, in sections the inner ear appears as a number of separate chambers and ducts. These, however, are all interconnected (except that the perilymphatic and endolymphatic spaces remain separate). The largest chamber is the vestibule *(V)*. The left side of this chamber *(black arrow)* leads into the cochlea *(C)*. Just below the *black arrow* and to the right is the oval ligament *(OL)* surrounding the base of the stapes *(S)*. Both structures have been cut obliquely and are not seen in their entirety. The facial nerve *(FN)* is in an osseous tunnel to the left of the oval ligament. The communication of the vestibule with one of the semicircular canals is marked by the *white arrow*. At the upper right are cross sections of the membranous labyrinth through components of the duct system *(DS)*.

The cochlea is a spiral structure having the general shape of a cone. The specimen illustrated here makes $3^1/_2$ turns (in humans, there are $2^3/_4$ turns). The section goes through the central axis of the cochlea. This consists of a bony stem called the modiolus *(M)*. It contains the beginning of the cochlear nerve *(CN)* and the spiral ganglion *(SG)*. Because of the plane of section and the spiral arrangement of the cochlear tunnel, the tunnel is cut crosswise in seven places (note $3^1/_2$ turns). A more detailed examination of the cochlea and the organ of Corti is provided in Plate 130.

FIGURE 2, ear, guinea pig, H&E ×225. A higher magnification of one of the semicircular canals and of the crista ampullaris *(CA)* within the canal seen in the lower right of Figure 1 is provided here. The receptor for movement, the crista ampullaris (note its relationships in Fig. 1), is present in each of the semicircular canals. The epithelial *(Ep)* surface of the crista consists of two cell types, sustentacular (supporting) cells and hair (receptor) cells. (Two types of hair cells are distinguished with the electron microscope.) It is difficult to identify these cells on the basis of specific characteristics; they can, however, be distinguished on the basis of location (see **inset**), as the hair cells *(HC)* are situated in a more superficial location than the sustentacular cells *(SC)*. A gelatinous mass, the cupula *(Cu)*, surmounts the epithelium of the crista ampullaris. Each receptor cell sends a hair-like projection deep into the substance of the cupula.

The epithelium rests on a loose, cellular connective tissue *(CT)* that also contains the nerve fibers associated with the receptor cells. The nerve fibers are difficult to identify because they are not organized as a discrete bundle.

KEY		
C, cochlea	**Ep,** epithelium	**SC,** sustentacular cell
CA, crista ampullaris	**FN,** facial nerve	**SG,** spiral ganglion
CN, cochlear nerve	**HC,** hair cell	**V,** vestibule
CT, connective tissue	**M,** modiolus	**black arrow,** entry to cochlea
Cu, cupula	**OL,** oval ligament	**white arrow,** entry to semicircular
Ds, duct system (of membranous labyrinth)	**S,** stapes	canal

PLATE 129

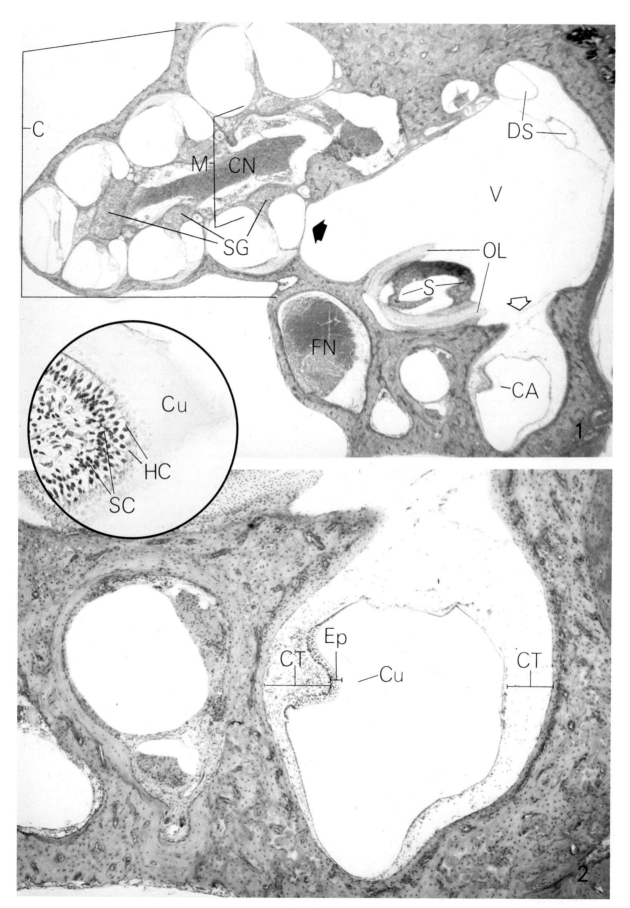

PLATE 130.   Organ of Corti

FIGURE 1, ear, guinea pig, H&E ×65; inset ×380. A section through one of the turns of the cochlea is shown here. The most important functional component of the cochlea is the organ of Corti, enclosed by the *rectangle* and shown at higher magnification in Figure 2. Other structures are included in this figure. The spiral ligament *(SL)* is a thickening of the periosteum on the outer part of the tunnel. Two membranes, the basilar membrane *(BM)* and the vestibular membrane *(VM)*, join with the spiral ligament and divide the cochlear tunnel into three parallel canals, namely, the scala vestibuli *(SV)*, the scala tympani *(ST)*, and the cochlear duct *(CD)*. Both the scala vestibuli and scala tympani are perilymphatic spaces; these communicate at the apex of the cochlea. The cochlear duct, on the other hand, is the space of the membranous labyrinth and is filled with endolymph.

It is thought that the endolymph is formed by the portion of the spiral ligament that faces the cochlear duct, the stria vascularis *(StV)*. This is highly vascularized and contains specialized "secretory" cells.

A shelf of bone, the osseous spiral lamina *(OSL)*, extends from the modiolus to the basilar membrane. Branches of the cochlear nerve *(CN)* travel along the spiral lamina to the modiolus, where the main trunk of the nerve is formed. The components of the cochlear nerve are bipolar neurons whose cell bodies constitute the spiral ganglion *(SG)*. These cell bodies are shown at higher magnification in the **inset** (upper right). The spiral lamina supports an elevation of cells, the limbus spiralis *(LS)*. The surface of the limbus is composed of columnar cells.

FIGURE 2, ear, guinea pig, H&E ×180; inset ×380. The components of the organ of Corti, beginning at the limbus spiralis *(LS)*, are as follows: inner border cells *(IBC)*; inner phalangeal and hair cells *(IP&HC)*; inner pillar cells *(IPC)*; (the sequence continues, repeating itself in reverse) outer pillar cells *(OPC)*; hair and outer phalangeal cells *(HC&OP)*; and outer border cells or cells of Hensen *(CH)*. Hair cells are receptor cells; the other cells are collectively referred to as supporting cells. The hair and outer phalangeal cells can be distinguished in this figure by their location (see **inset**) and because their nuclei are well aligned. Because the hair cells rest on the phalangeal cells, it can be concluded that the upper three nuclei belong to outer hair cells, whereas the lower three nuclei belong to outer phalangeal cells.

The supporting cells extend from the basilar membrane to the surface of the organ of Corti (this is not evident here but can be seen in the **inset**), where they form a reticular membrane *(RM)*. The free surface of the receptor cells fits into openings in the reticular membrane, and the "hairs" of these cells project toward and make contact with the tectorial membrane *(TM)*. The latter is a cuticular extension from the columnar cells of the limbus spiralis. In ideal preparations, nerve fibers can be traced from the hair cells to the cochlear nerve. In their course from the basilar membrane to the reticular membrane, groups of supporting cells are separated from other groups by spaces that form spiral tunnels. These tunnels are named the inner tunnel *(IT)*, the outer tunnel *(OT)*, and the internal spiral tunnel *(IST)*. Beyond the supporting cells are two additional groups of cells, the cells of Claudius *(CC)* and the cells of Böttcher *(CB)*.

KEY

BM, basilar membrane
CB, cells of Böttcher
CC, cells of Claudius
CD, cochlea duct
CH, cells of Hensen
CN, cochlear nerve
HC&OP, hair and outer phalangeal cells
IBC, inner border cells

IP&HC, inner phalangeal and hair cells
IPC, inner pillar cells
IST, internal spiral tunnel
IT, inner tunnel membrane
LS, limbus spiralis
OPC, outer pillar cells
OSL, osseous spiral lamina
OT, outer tunnel

RM, reticular membrane
SG, spiral ganglion
SL, spiral ligament
ST, scala tympani
StV, stria vascularis
SV, scala vestibuli
TM, tectorial membrane
VM, vestibular membrane

PLATE 130

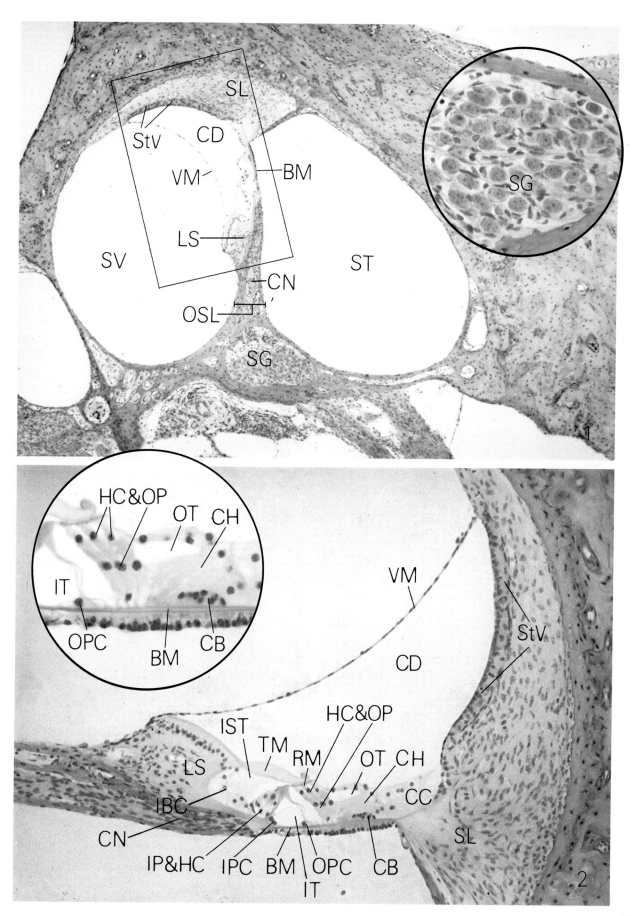

Index